NEUROIMMUNOMODULATION

PERSPECTIVES AT THE NEW MILLENNIUM

C. Cicum

ANNALS OF THE NEW YORK ACADEMY OF SCIENCES
Volume 917

NEUROIMMUNOMODULATION

PERSPECTIVES AT THE NEW MILLENNIUM

Edited by
Ario Conti, Georges J.M. Maestroni, Samuel M. McCann,
Esther M. Sternberg, James M. Lipton, and Craig C. Smith

The New York Academy of Sciences
New York, New York
2000

Library of Congress Cataloging-in-Publication Data

Neuroimmunomodulation : perspectives at the new millennium / editor by Ario Conti ... [et al.].
    p.; cm. — (Annals of the New York Academy of Sciences, ISSN 0077-8923 ; v. 917)
Includes bibliographical references.
ISBN 1-57331-287-8 (cloth : alk. paper) — ISBN 1-57331-288-6 (paper : alk. paper)
    1. Neuroimmunology—Congresses. I. Conti, Ario. II. International Congress ISNIM
(4th : 1999 : Lugano, Switzerland) III. Series.
[DNLM: 1. Neuroimmunomodulation—Congresses. 2. Autoimmune
Diseases–immunology–Congresses. 3. Cytokines–immunology–Congresses. 4.
Melatonin–immunology–Congresses. 5. Mental Disorders–immunology–Congresses.
6. Nervous System Diseases–immunology–Congresses. W1 AN626YL v.917 2000]
Q11 .N5 vol. 917
[QP356.47]
500 s—dc00
[616.8'0479 21; aa05 10-17]

                                                      00-045235
                                                           CIP

K-M Research/PCP
Printed in the United States of America
ISBN 1-57331-287-8 (cloth)
ISBN 1-57331-288-6 (paper)
ISSN 0077-8923

ANNALS OF THE NEW YORK ACADEMY OF SCIENCES

Volume 917

NEUROIMMUNOMODULATION

PERSPECTIVES AT THE NEW MILLENNIUM[a]

Editors
ARIO CONTI, GEORGES J.M. MAESTRONI, SAMUEL M. MCCANN,
ESTHER M. STERNBERG, JAMES M. LIPTON, AND CRAIG C. SMITH

Conference Organizers
G.J.M. MAESTRONI, A. CONTI, E. PEDRINIS,
P. LUSCIETI, G. FRIGO, AND S. LECCHINI

Advisory Board
N.G. ABRAHAM (USA), R. ADER (USA), A. ANGELI (ITALY),
E. ARTZ (ARGENTINA), T. BARTFAI (SWEDEN), H. BESEDOVSKY (GERMANY),
A. CATANIA (ITALY), M. DARDENNE (FRANCE), A. DEL REY (GERMANY),
E. FERRARI (ITALY), P. GAILLARD (SWITZERLAND), T. GIRALDI (ITALY),
V. GEENEN (BELGIUM), M. GUERRERO (SPAIN), A.B. GROSSMAN (UK),
F. HALBERG (USA), C. HEIJNEN (THE NETHERLANDS),
D. HELLHAMMER (GERMANY), T. HORI (JAPAN), E.A. KORNEVA (RUSSIA),
J.M. LIPTON (USA), W. MASLINSKI (POLAND), L. MATERA (ITALY),
G. NORBIATO (ITALY), U. OTTEN (SWITZERLAND), A. OVADIA (ISRAEL),
A. PANERAI (ITALY), N.J. ROTHWELL (UK), W. SAVINO (BRAZIL),
G. SOLOMAN (USA), M. SCHWARTZ (ISRAEL), M. SCHEDLOWSKI (POLAND),
J.F. SHERIDAN (USA), J. SZELENYI (HUNGARY), AND R.L. WILDER (USA)

CONTENTS

Part I. Plenary Lectures

[a]This volume contains the papers from a conference entitled **4th International Congress of the International Society for Neuroimmunomodulation**, which was held on September 29–October 2, 1999, in Lugano, Switzerland.

Part V. Neurodegenerative Diseases and Neural-Immune Communications in Normal and Injured Brain

Part VI. Melatonin, NIM, and Hematopoiesis

Part VII. Behavior, Emotional Disorders, and Immunity

Part VIII. Prolactin and GB in Neuroimmunomodulation

Part IX. Neuroimmunomodulation: Perspectives in Oncology

Part X. Cytokines and Neuroendocrine Functions

Part XI. HPA Axis, Sex Hormones, and NOS

Part XII. Neuroendocrine Control of Thymic Physiology

Part XIII. Opiates and the Immune System

Part XIV. Autoimmune Diseases

Part XV. Stress, Neuroendocrine Responses, and Allergy

Part XVI. Bacterial, Parasite, and Non-AIDS Viral Infections

Part XVII. Hormonal and Immune Disorders in HIV Infection

Financial assistance was received from:

Major Funders

- Department of Education, State of Canton Ticino, Switzerland
- Medical School, University Of Insubria, Italy
- Swiss Cancer League
- Lega Ticinese per la Lotta Contro il Cancro

Contributors

- Institut Biochimique, SA, Lugano, Switzerland
- Nuova Linnea, Riazzino, Switzerland
- Institut de Recherche Internationales Servier, Courbevoie, France
- Glaxo Wellcome AG, Shönbül, Switzerland
- Dako Diagnostic AG, Zug, Switzerland
- Canberra Packard AG, Zürich, Switzerland
- Leica Mikroskopie Systeme AG, Glattbrugg, Switzerland
- Merck AG, Basel, Switzerland
- Olympus Optical AG, Volketswil, Switzerland
- Municipality Of Lugano
- Morwell Diagnostic GmbH, Egg, Switzerland

NEUROIMMUNOMODULATION

PERSPECTIVES AT THE NEW MILLENNIUM

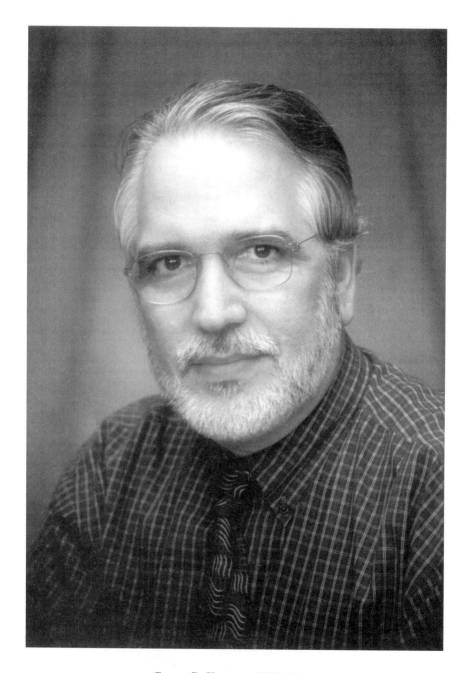

George P. Chrousos, M.D., Sc.D.

1999 Novera Herbert SpectorAward for Significant Contributions in Both Leadership and Research in Neuroimmunomodulation

Recipient: George P. Chrousos, M.D., Sc.D.

Dr. George P. Chrousos is Director of the Pediatric Endocrinology Program at the U.S. National Institute of Child Health and Human Development (NICHD), the National Institutes of Health (NIH), and professor of pediatrics and physiology at Georgetown University Medical School.

Recognized as an outstanding researcher in endocrinology and metabolism, his contributions include research on the regulation of the hypothalamic–pituitary–adrenal axis, and the pathophysiologic and molecular mechanisms of the syndromes of glucocorticoid hormone resistance and congenital isolated glucocorticoid deficiency. His research team introduced corticotropin-releasing hormone (CRH) as a diagnostic test for Cushing's syndrome and adrenal insufficiency. Their research also elucidated the pathophysiology of hypothalamic–pituitary–adrenal axis alterations in a number of developmental/psychiatric states, including major affective disorder, anorexia nervosa, chronic strenuous exercise, atypical depression, the chronic fatigue/fibromyalgia syndromes, and the adolescent and postpartum blues/depression syndromes. Dr. Chrousos and his colleagues determined the neuropeptide feedback and cytokine regulation of the hypothalamic CRH neuron. His research team isolated "tissue corticotropin-releasing factor," and demonstrated that it is a major determinant of peripheral inflammation. He cloned the regulatory region and studied the regulation of the human CRH gene. He and his colleagues elucidated neural and hormonal mechanisms through which the stress system influences the immune and inflammatory reaction and predisposes individuals to allergic, autoimmune, infectious and neoplastic disorders.

Dr. Chrousos is the recipient of, among others, the Endocrine Society's Richard Weitzman Award (1987) "for outstanding research achievements in Endocrinology and Metabolism"; the Superior Service Award of the U.S. Public Health Service (1992) "for pioneering studies on the hypothalamic-pituitary-adrenal axis function, leading to new insights into the pathophysiology of adrenal diseases"; the Endocrine Society's Clinical Investigator Award (1997) "for major achievements in clinical investigation"; the Hans Selye Award of the Hans Selye Foundation (1997) for "outstanding contributions to stress research"; and the Endocrine Society's Pharmacia International Award (1999) "for excellence in published clinical research."

Preface

This is the fourth in a series of proceedings of congresses of the International Society for NeuroImmunoModulation to be published as one of the *Annals of the New York Academy of Sciences*. The Fourth International Congress of the International Society for NeuroImmunoModulation, organized by Drs. Georges Maestroni and Ario Conti, took place in October 1999 in Lugano, Switzerland: 292 scientists from 33 countries attended the conference, and a significant proportion of these were not members of the Society, indicating one of the most important characteristics of this growing field. Not only has there been explosive growth of the field, but it is now expanding beyond the original group of scientists who were involved at its inception.

Scientists and physicians from overlapping areas in neuroscience, immunology, endocrinology, psychiatry and psychology are increasingly recognizing the importance of integrative research in this borderland area between disciplines. ISNIM is clearly filling a significant need of the world community in bringing together high-profile, internationally recognized experts in their specialties, to share and disseminate their latest findings. This volume reflects that level of excellence in the breadth and depth of research that is covered, from studies of molecular mechanisms, and neuroanatomical and neuroendocrine pathways, to clinical relevance of neural-immune interactions in health and disease.

Papers presented reflect advances in detailed immunological analyses of the impact of neural variables, including stress, on specific cellular and molecular events that take place over the full time course of autoimmune, inflammatory or allergic responses and infectious diseases. Although older dogmas held that glucocorticoids are uniformly immunosuppressive, more recent work presented in this volume indicates a clearly immunomodulatory role for these stress hormones on immune responses, in some cases even stimulating immune responses. Furthermore, although glucocorticoids were initially thought to exert their effects primarily as systemic blood-borne hormones, it is clear that the full synthetic machinery for glucocorticoids exists in the thymus and plays an important role in lymphocyte selection. More emphasis is also now being placed on the immune regulatory role of hormones and neurotransmitters in addition to the glucocorticoids, including gonadal hormones, leptin and neuropeptides such as MSH and sympathetic and parasympathetic mechanisms. Furthermore the molecular mechanisms of action of these mediators are being studied at increasingly detailed levels to gain an understanding of second messengers, such as nitric oxide, that play a role in the transduction of their effects.

Advances in the detailed understanding of the effects of cytokines on brain function, sickness behaviors and neural growth and development are elucidating the role that the afferent communication arm of immune-to-nervous system signaling plays in health and disease of the nervous system. The role of neural-immune pathways in physiological processes has gone beyond fever to include the role of cytokines in such processes as sleep, learning and aging.

Indeed, the range of diseases in which neural-immune mechanisms are being studied has also greatly expanded beyond the traditional autoimmune diseases such as multiple sclerosis and ocular immune diseases, to include nerve trauma, Alzheimer's disease, schizophrenia, depression, and autoimmune diseases such as Sjogren's and rheumatoid arthritis. Important advances in these illnesses include detailed elucidation of genetic as well as environmental factors in their pathogenesis.

For those of us present since the inception of the modern phase of this ancient discipline, the developments summarized by the papers at this conference, and presented in this volume, represent both a culmination and a new beginning for this important interdisciplinary and integrative field.

ESTHER STERNBERG, M.D.
Bethesda, MD, USA

Does Stress Make You Sick and Belief Make You Well?

The Science Connecting Body and Mind

ESTHER M. STERNBERG[a]

National Institute of Mental Health, CNE/National Institutes of Health,
Bethesda, Maryland 20892-1284, USA

The notion that stress makes you sick and belief makes you well has been part of the popular culture for thousands of years. These ideas are universal throughout all cultures. In Western culture this notion held sway from before the time of Hippocrates, when the Greeks built temples to Aesclepius, the god of healing, all the way through to modern times, when Norman Cousins and Norman Vincent Peale have espoused the idea that laughter and positive thinking heals. Perhaps because of their very popularity, most scientists have until very recently rejected the concept that emotions can affect disease and that disease can affect our emotional health. In part this may be because until recently, scientists have not had the technological tools to prove these connections. But, in the last decade we have finally developed the technology in immunology and neuroscience to prove that these connections between emotions and disease, between the brain and the immune system, the mind and the body, are real.

Thus, with molecular biology we can prove that immune molecules, the interleukins, signal the brain through many routes—through the bloodstream and through nerve pathways. And we can prove that when the brain receives such signals we experience a set of feelings and behaviors that, lumped together, are called "sickness behavior." We know that immune modulatory molecules can also stimulate the brain's hormonal stress response and start a cascade of hormones that finally result in the adrenal gland's release of antiinflammatory corticosteroid hormones. Thus, the brain's stress response keeps the immune system turned down when an immune response is no longer needed to fight off a foreign invader. This can be good or bad, for too many of these antiinflammatory stress hormones at the wrong time, such as during chronic stress, can predispose a stressed host to more infection. On the other hand, too little can predispose to autoimmune diseases such as arthritis, since the immune response is not shut off and can go on unchecked. Many studies have now proven that a blunted hormonal stress response in animals and humans, whether present on a genetic basis, because of drug therapy, or because of surgical intervention, can all lead to increased susceptibility to inflammatory disease. These diseases include arthritis, systemic lupus erythematosus, allergic asthma, and atopic dermatitis. Knowing this can help treat such diseases, or can lead to development of new treatments for such illnesses based on stimulating various parts of the hormonal stress response.

But immune molecules, the interleukins, do not simply act as hormones to stimulate brain function. They also act as growth factors when expressed in brain. These molecules are made by the scaffolding cells in the brain—those cells that are not nerve cells that provide an essential milieu to help nerve cells survive or kill them off. So through this science we know that interleukins play an important role in nerve cell death and survival and therefore in nerve regeneration and repair. Thus, interactions between the immune and nervous systems play a role in diseases such as Alzheimer's, stroke, neuroAIDS, and nerve trauma. Understanding exactly how such molecules and immune cells interact with nerve cells is helping us develop new treatments for these diseases. Interactions in the other direction are also true—that is, nerve chemicals play a role in keeping the immune system active. In this way, adrenalin-like molecules released from nerve endings in the spleen can help restore lost immune cell function that occurs during aging. Drugs that stimulate growth of such nerve endings can thus be used to enhance the diminished immune responses seen in aging. There are still more communications between these systems that occur at a local level, where nerve endings feed tissues, such as the lining of joints. Nerve chemicals released from such nerve endings during inflammation can increase inflammation, and thus drugs that block such nerve chemicals can be used to treat arthritis.

What does the future hold? All of these discoveries just touch the surface, and each leads to many more questions, which, when answered in depth, will lead to more specific ways to manage stress effects on immune function, local effects of nerve chemicals on inflammation, and effects of immune molecules on nerve growth and death. Studies showing the effects of interleukins on sickness behavior raise the question of whether these molecules play a role in illnesses such depression, in the absence of infection. We now have the tools to answer these questions by combining molecular biology and modern imaging technologies. With such technologies, we should also be able to take studies of the effects of stress on immune responses to the next level, by asking how learning and memory and early experience and development affect the stress response. With sophisticated new genetic and mathematical modeling techniques, we can determine what part of our stress responsiveness we are born with and how much is under environmental control. These sorts of studies will help us understand not only the reasons for individual differences in stress responsiveness that affect susceptibility to inflammatory disease, but will also point the way to using old and developing new behavioral strategies that can change the set point of different individuals' stress responses. So this science can help explain why meditation, crystals, or other alternative therapies do work to ameliorate disease. By studying the neurobiology of the placebo effect, we can not only understand such phenomena that have been around for thousands of years in all cultures, but also physicians can shed the bias that has stigmatized the lowly placebo effect: rather than trying to control for and exclude this effect, researchers can use this very powerful biological tool judiciously to help heal.

More than anything else this field of neuroimmunomodulation—the brain–immune connection, the science of the mind–body connections—embodies the marriage of the beliefs of the popular culture with technological advances across many disciplines, from the molecular through to the systems interaction level. That is the most important contribution of this field to modern science and medicine—it pushes and pulls science out of a narrow reductionist view rooted in the sixteenth century philosophy of Descartes, back into the holistic view of entwined body and soul embodied in Hippocrates' thought. But it does so with a modern technological twist that empowers us to apply this science to discover new treatments for a whole host of diseases.

So, this very old science, born before recorded history, has now, with modern scientific technology, been reborn. Not only can this science help physicians and scientists believe their patients when they say that stress makes them sick and belief makes them well, but it can help us develop new therapies to treat many diseases, from arthritis to Alzheimer's disease and stroke, from nerve trauma to the immunosuppression of aging.

The Mechanism of Action of Cytokines to Control the Release of Hypothalamic and Pituitary Hormones in Infection

S.M. McCANN,[a,b] M. KIMURA,[c] S. KARANTH,[b] W.H. YU,[b]
C.A. MASTRONARDI,[b] AND V. RETTORI[d]

[b]Pennington Biomedical Research Center (LSU), Baton Rouge,
Louisiana 70808-4124, USA

[c]Institute for Medical and Dental Engineering, Tokyo Medical and Dental University,
2-3-10 Kanda-Surugadai, Chiyoda-ku, Tokyo 101, Japan

[d]Centro de Estudios Farmacologicos y Botanicos, Consejo Nacional de Investigaciones
Cientificas y Tecnicas (CEFYBO-CONICET), Serrano 665, 1414 Buenos Aires, Argentina

ABSTRACT: During infection, bacterial and viral products, such as bacterial lipopolysaccharide (LPS), cause the release of cytokines from immune cells. These cytokines can reach the brain by several routes. Furthermore, cytokines, such as interleukin-1 (IL-1), are induced in neurons within the brain by systemic injection of LPS. These cytokines determine the pattern of hypothalamic–pituitary secretion that characterizes infection. IL-2, by stimulation of cholinergic neurons, activates neural nitric oxide synthase (nNOS). The nitric oxide (NO) released diffuses into corticotropin-releasing hormone (CRH)–secreting neurons and releases CRH. IL-2 also acts in the pituitary to stimulate adrenocorticotropic hormone (ACTH) secretion. On the other hand, IL-1α blocks the NO-induced release of luteinizing hormone-releasing hormone (LHRH) from LHRH neurons, thereby blocking pulsatile LH but not follicle-stimulating hormone (FSH) release and also inhibiting sex behavior that is induced by LHRH. IL-1α and granulocyte macrophage colony-stimulating factor (GMCSF) block the response of the LHRH terminals to NO. The mechanism of action of GMCSF to inhibit LHRH release is as follows. It acts on its receptors on γ-aminobutyric acid (GABA)ergic neurons to stimulate GABA release. GABA acts on GABAa receptors on the LHRH neuronal terminal to block NOergic stimulation of LHRH release. IL-1α inhibits growth hormone (GH) release by inhibiting GH-releasing hormone (GHRH) release, which is mediated by NO, and stimulating somatostatin release, also mediated by NO. IL-1α-induced stimulation of PRL release is also mediated by intra-hypothlamic action of NO, which inhibits release of the PRL-inhibiting hormone dopamine. The actions of NO are brought about by its combined activation of guanylate cyclase-liberating cyclic guanosine monophosphate (cGMP) and activation of cyclooxygenase (COX) and lipoxygenase (LOX) with liberation of prostaglandin E_2 and leukotrienes, respectively. Thus, NO plays a key role in inducing the changes in release of hypothalamic peptides induced in infection by cytokines. Cytokines, such as IL-1β, also act in the anterior pituitary

[a]Address for correspondence: S.M. McCann, Pennington Biomedical Research Center (LSU), 6400 Perkins Road, Baton Rouge, LA 70808-4124. Voice: 225-763-3042; fax: 225-763-3030.

mccannsm@mhs.pbrc.edu

4

gland, at least in part via induction of inducible NOS. The NO produced inhibits release of ACTH. The adipocyte hormone leptin, a member of the cytokine family, has largely opposite actions to those of the proinflammatory cytokines, stimulating the release of FSHRF and LHRH from the hypothalamus and FSH and LH from the pituitary directly by NO.

INTRODUCTION

Our knowledge of neuroimmunomodulation has undergone explosive growth since the discovery of the structure of many pro- and antiinflammatory cytokines and the revelation that certain other hormones are members of the cytokine family, which includes PRL, growth hormone (GH), and the newly discovered adipocyte hormone leptin. Nearly all of these cytokines have roles as autocrine, paracrine, and hormonal agents that play an important part not only in normal homeostasis of the body, but also in the response to infections.

The induction of fever following injection of bacterial lipopolysaccharide (LPS) was the first example of neuroimmunomodulation, because it was early shown that LPS not only apparently induced fever on its own, but also released an endogenous pyrogen that circulated to the brain and induced fever. In the early 1960s, it was discovered that injection of purified LPS into dogs induced fever after a delay and a concomitant increase in plasma cortisol. These findings suggested that endogenous pyrogen reached the brain and induced not only fever, but also release of corticotropin-releasing hormone (CRH) that activated adrenocorticotropic hormone (ACTH) followed by cortisol release.[1] Because of the high potency of cytokines, the amounts circulating in the blood after LPS were too small to isolate and determine structure of these compounds. In the 1980s and 1990s, however, the structure of many of them was revealed, and it is now apparent that endogenous pyrogen was at least in part interleukin-1 (IL-1).

Understanding of the mechanism of action of cytokines to alter hypothalamic–pituitary function was also made possible by discovery of the many classical transmitters and hypothalamic peptides that control the release of the various pituitary hormones from the anterior lobe of the pituitary gland. The release of the various pituitary hormones is controlled by neurohormones that are released into the hypophyseal portal vessels that transport them to the anterior pituitary gland where they stimulate or inhibit particular pituitary cell types.[2,3] There is a family of peptides that stimulates the release of the pituitary hormones, namely, corticotropin-releasing hormone (CRH), luteinizing hormone-releasing hormone (LHRH), follicle-stimulating hormone (FSH)-releasing factor (FSHRF), GH-releasing hormone (GHRH), GH release-inhibiting hormone (somatostatin), prolactin (PRL)-inhibiting and -stimulating factors, and thyrotropin (T)RH. Several other peptides, in particular vasopressin, oxytocin, and atrial natriuretic peptide, have modifying actions on the release of pituitary hormones by actions directly on the gland, whereas catecholamines can also influence the secretion of pituitary hormones by direct action on the gland, the principal effect being the inhibitory action of dopamine (DA), the most potent PRL-inhibiting hormone. The pattern of release of pituitary hormones in infection is brought about by cytokine-induced release of hypothalamic peptides, which alter the release of pituitary hormones. Furthermore, direct actions of these cytokines on the pituitary gland itself can alter pituitary hormone release and responsiveness of the gland to hypothalamic peptides.[4]

Introduction of bacteria into the body causes the liberation of toxic, soluble products of the bacterial cell wall, for example, LPS, which circulates in the blood and acts on immune cells, particularly monocytes and macrophages. LPS combines with its receptors on these cells and induces the synthesis and release of various cytokines, such as IL-1, tumor necrosis factor (TNF), IL-6, IL-2, γ-interferon, and others. The pattern of release probably depends on the infective agent and the severity of the infection.[4]

Because there is no arterial blood supply to the anterior pituitary gland, cytokines released into the circulation only reach the hypophyseal portal capillaries in the median eminence (ME) of the tuber cinereum via the anterior hypophyseal arteries.[5] Cytokines (molecular mass 15 kDa) diffuse into the ME, because there is little or no blood–brain barrier there. Therefore, the concentration of cytokines delivered to the anterior lobe sinusoids by the long hypophyseal portal veins will be lower than in arterial blood. The concentration of cytokines in blood reaching the anterior lobe via the short portal vessels draining the neural lobe of the pituitary is similarly reduced by diffusion into neural lobe tissue. One-third of the blood supply of the anterior lobe is provided by these vessels.[5]

Transport of cytokines to the hypothalamus presents a more difficult problem except in regions where the blood–brain barrier is defective in the ME and other circumventricular organs: the organum vasculosum lamina terminalis, the subfornical organ, the subcommissural organ, the area postrema, and the pineal gland.[6] Permeability is probably also enhanced in the choroid plexus. Banks and Kastin[7] have reported a transport system that carries IL-1 and other cytokines into the brain. Clearly, peripherally injected cytokines effectively reach the brain, because IL-1 injected intravenously (i.v.) can induce fever and increase ACTH secretion by hypothalamic action.[4]

Evidence is also mounting for the production of various cytokines by glial elements within the brain. This appears to be the case for IL-1, IL-2, and IL-6 and perhaps for others.[6] Bacterial LPS appears to be capable of increasing the production of cytokines such as IL-6 in the anterior pituitary.[8]

In addition, a neuronal system that produces IL-1β has been described in humans.[9] The cell bodies of these neurons are located in the paraventricular nucleus (PVN) with axons projecting to the ME, so that IL-1β released from these neurons could reach the anterior lobe and even the peripheral circulation after uptake by portal vessels.

The research to be reviewed here indicates that NO has a powerful influence on the secretion of not only the hypothalamic peptides, but also classical synaptic transmitters, such as catecholamines and γ-amino butyric acid (GABA). NO also has a powerful effect in suppressing or stimulating the release of pituitary hormones directly. NO is formed in the body by NOS, an enzyme that converts arginine in the presence of oxygen and several cofactors into equimolar quantities of citrulline and NO. In aqueous solutions, NO, a free radical, decomposes to nitrate, which, in the presence of superoxide, further decomposes into two free radicals, nitrite and hydroxyl ions. All of these free radicals are powerful oxidizing agents. The half-life of NO in aqueous solutions is 5 to 10 seconds. However, the half-life of the soluble gas in living systems is prolonged by combination with other substances to form nitroso compounds, which slowly release the gas.[10]

There are three isoforms of the enzyme. One, termed inducible NOS (iNOS), is formed principally by immune cells, such as macrophages, but also by other cells, such as vascular endothelial cells. Bacterial infection leads to release of products of their cell walls, such as bacterial LPS, which combines with receptors on the surface of macrophages and these other cells. The LPS–receptor combination acts in the nucleus to induce synthesis of iNOS mRNA, which then synthesizes iNOS. The induction of iNOS mRNA occurs within an hour or two, and NO synthesis begins within 2 hours. It reaches a peak at 18 hours, declining to nearly control levels by 24 hours following a single injection of LPS. LPS also induces mRNA for various cytokines, such as IL-1, -2, -6, and TNF-α, which are then synthesized. These also act on the cell surface receptors of the above-mentioned cells to produce iNOS mRNA and iNOS formation. The large quantities of NO produced then interact with the bacteria or viruses and cause cell death by inactivating metabolic enzymes. These amounts of NO are also toxic to neighboring cells, but not to the cells containing iNOS, and cause apoptosis and cell death in the region of production of NO.[10,11]

The endothelial NOS (eNOS) is formed in vascular endothelial cells following cholinergic stimulation. It is a constitutive enzyme that requires an increase in intracellular free calcium (CA^{2+}) stimulated by the activated muscarinic-type cholinergic receptors on the endothelial cells. The increased [CA^{2+}] interacts with calmodulin and activates the enzyme. The activated enzyme produces NO, which diffuses to overlying smooth muscle, and activates soluble guanylate cyclase (GC), which converts guanosine triphosphate (GTP) to cyclic guanosine monophosphate (cGMP). This relaxes the vascular smooth muscle. It probably plays an important role in control of vascular tone, and the large amounts of NO produced by iNOS during infection can cause vascular collapse in the toxic shock syndrome.[10]

Garthwaite *et al.*[12] found evidence for NO production in incubates of hippocampal slices that were stimulated to produce long-term potentiation. Palmer *et al.*[13] showed that this substance was indeed NO, leading Bredt and Snyder[14] to isolate neural NOS (nNOS). They studied the distribution of the enzyme by immunocytochemistry. Thus, NO is the first gaseous transmitter that, instead of acting on cell surface receptors, diffuses into the cell to activate or inhibit intracellular enzymes.

nNOS is found in the cerebellum and various regions of the cerebral cortex and also in various ganglion cells of the autonomic nervous system. Large numbers of nNOS-containing neurons were also found in the hypothalamus, particularly in the paraventricular and supraoptic nuclei with axons projecting to the ME and neural lobe, which also contained large amounts of nNOS. These findings indicated that the enzyme was synthesized at all levels of the neuron from perikaryon to axon terminals.[15]

Because of this distribution in the hypothalamus in regions that contain peptidergic neurons that control pituitary hormone secretion, we decided to determine the role of this soluble gas in hypothalamic–pituitary function. The approach was to incubate medial basal hypothalamic (MBH) explants with sodium nitroprusside (NP), which spontaneously liberates NO, and determine whether this altered the release of various hypothalamic transmitters. Hemoglobin, which scavenges NO by a reaction with the heme group on the molecule, and inhibitors of NOS (such as N^G-monomethyl-L-arginine (NMMA), a competitive inhibitor of NOS), was also used to determine the effects of decreased NO. Two types of studies were performed. In the first set of experiments, MBH explants were preincubated *in vitro* and then exposed to neurotransmitters that modify the release of the various hypothalamic peptides in the presence or absence of inhibitors of the release of NO. The response to NO itself, provided by sodium NP, was also evaluated. Anterior pituitaries were incubated similarly *in vitro*, and the effects of these compounds that increase or decrease the release of NO into the tissue were examined.

In order to determine whether the results *in vitro* also held *in vivo*, substances were injected into the third ventricle of the brain of conscious, freely moving animals to determine the effect on pituitary hormone release.

ROLE OF THE HYPOTHALAMIC–PITUITARY–ADRENAL SYSTEM IN INFECTION

The hypothalamic–pituitary response to infection can be mimicked by the injection of bacterial LPS i.v. or i.p. This induces an identical pattern of pituitary hormone secretion as that seen in infection. There is a very rapid increase in plasma ACTH and PRL within a few minutes following i.v. injection of LPS. The response is dose-related and is accompanied by a rapid inhibition of LH and TSH but not FSH secretion. GH secretion is stimulated in humans but suppressed in the rat.[16]

Recent work indicates that central nervous system infection is a powerful inducer of cytokine production in glia and neurons of the brain, which causes induction of iNOS and production of potentially toxic quantities of NO. Following i.v. injection of an intermediate dose of LPS, there was an induction of IL-1α immunoreactive neurons in the preoptic–hypothalamic region.[16] These cells were shown to be neurons by the fact that double staining revealed the presence of neuron-specific enolase. The neurons were found in saline-injected control animals, suggesting that they are normally present, but they increased in number by a factor of two within two hours after injection of LPS. They are located in a region that also contains the thermosensitive neurons. They may be the neurons that are stimulated to induce fever following injection of LPS. They have short axons that did not clearly project to the areas containing the various hypothalamic-releasing and -inhibiting hormones, but they could also be involved in the stimulation or inhibition of their release, which occurs following infection.

This study led to further research, which demonstrated that i.p. injection of a moderate dose of LPS induced IL-1β and iNOS mRNA in the brain, anterior pituitary, and pineal glands. The results were very exciting because an induction of IL-1β and iNOS mRNA occurred with the same timecourse as found in the periphery following injection of LPS, namely, clear induction of IL-1β followed by iNOS mRNA within two hours, reaching a peak in 4–6 hours, followed by a decline to near basal levels at the next measurement by 24 hours after the injection. The induction of both mRNAs occurred in the meninges; the choroid plexus; the circumventricular organs, such as the subfornical organ and ME; in the ependymal cells lining the ventricular system; and very suprisingly in parvocellular neurons of the PVN and arcuate nucleus (AN), areas of particular interest because they contain the hypothalamic-releasing and -inhibiting hormone-producing neurons and also other neurotransmitters controlled by NO.[17]

The greatest induction occurred in the anterior lobe of the pituitary, where the iNOS mRNA was increased at two hours by a factor of 45 and in the pineal where the activity was increased by a factor of 7 at six hours, whereas the increase in the PVN was fivefold. At six hours, the MBH was found to have an increased content of NOS measured *in vitro*, and the collected cerebrospinal fluid (CSF) had increased concentrations of the NO metabolite nitrate. These results indicate that the increase in iNOS mRNA was followed by de novo synthesis of iNOS that liberated NO into the tissue and also into the CSF. Presumably, LPS was bound to its receptors in the circumventricular organs and in the choroid plexus. These receptors, as in macrophages, activated DNA-directed IL-1β mRNA synthesis which, in turn, caused the synthesis of IL-1β. IL-1β then activated iNOS mRNA and synthesis.[17]

How can neurons in the AN and PVN be activated if they are inside the blood–brain barrier? In the case of the AN, the neurons may have axons that project to the ME. These neurons may have LPS receptors on their cell surfaces which then induce IL-β mRNA and IL-1β synthesis. IL-1β then induces iNOS mRNA followed by NO synthesis. Alternatively, LPS acting on its receptors may simultaneously induce IL-β mRNA and iNOS mRNA.

Active transport mechanisms for IL-1 and other cytokines,[7] and perhaps LPS, are present in the choroid plexus. On the basis of our results, the cells of the choroid plexus must have LPS receptors on them. LPS then stimulates IL-1β and iNOS mRNA, followed by synthesis of IL-1β and iNOS in the choroid plexus. LPS and IL-1β are then transported into the CSF. LPS is carried by CSF flow to the third ventricle, where it either crosses the ependyma or acts on terminals of PVN neurons in the ependyma to induce IL-1β and iNOS mRNA.

This massive delayed increased NO production should further increase the effects of NO to maintain the pattern of hypothalamic hormone secretion already induced by LPS. Unfortunately, the effect of inhibitors of NOS on these later stages in the response to LPS or infection have not yet been studied. Interestingly enough, in studies on LHRH release induced by NO, it has been shown that increasing concentrations of NO provided by release from sodium NP produce a bell-shaped dose–response curve in terms of LHRH release with values reaching a peak and then declining as the concentration of NO increases.[18] Therefore, the massive increase in NO produced by iNOS, several hours after injection of LPS, might actually reduce the effects of NO on releasing hormone discharge below the peaks achieved earlier.

In addition to inducing production of proinflammatory cytokines such as IL-1, IL-2, IL-6, and TNFα, LPS also induces production of antiinflammatory cytokines, such as IL-10 and IL-13 and IL-1 receptor antagonist in the brain, pituitary, and pineal gland.[42] In the periphery these inhibit the inflammatory response induced by the proinflammatory cytokines. Limited studies indicate that these antiinflammatory cytokines antagonize the actions of the proinflammatory cytokines in the brain as well as the hypothalamic–pituitary response to infection.[19]

The initial response to LPS is mediated by the constitutive nNOS present in the brain. There is no participation of the NO synthesized by iNOS in this initial response. Indeed, the initial response must be due to action on receptors for LPS on the endings of vagal afferents and also in areas where the blood–brain barrier is not present, such as the choroid plexus, ME, OVLT, area postrema, and other circumventricular organs. Input to the hypothalamus from LPS by vagal afferents occurs at least in part by activation of the locus ceruleus that sends noradrenergic axons to the hypothalamus to activate CRH release.[20] The noradrenergic axons apparently synapse on cholinergic interneurons in the region of the PVN.[21]

CRH release from hypothalami incubated *in vitro* is controlled by muscarinic cholinergic receptors because it can be blocked by atropine.[21,22] The acetylcholine-producing interneurons in the hypothalamus release acetylcholine, which stimulates a muscarinic-type receptor, which in turn stimulates CRH release from the CRH neurons. Nicotinic receptors also appear to play a stimulatory role.[22] nNOS has been located in neurons in the PVN of the hypothalamus. Stimulated CRH release can be blocked by NMMA, a competitive inhibitor of all forms of NOS. Consequently, CRH release from the neurons in the PVN is stimulated by cholinergic neurons that synapse on these NOergic neurons to activate NOS. NOS synthesizes NO, which diffuses into the CRH neurons and activates CRH release by activating cyclooxygenase I (COX I), leading to the generation of prostaglandin E_2 (PGE_2) from arachidonate (AA). PGE_2 activates CRH via activation of adenylyl cyclase (AC) and generation of cyclic adenosine monophosphate (cAMP). cAMP activates protein kinase A (PKA), which induces exocytosis of CRH secretory granules into the hypophyseal portal vessels which then activates ACTH release from the corticotrophs of the anterior pituitary gland. NO activates not only COX, but also lipoxygenase (LOX), which also plays a role in the activation of CRH release.[23] NO also activates GC, which converts guanosine triphosphate into cGMP. cGMP is postulated to increase the intracellular $[Ca^{2+}]$ required to activate phospholipase A_2 (PLA_2), which converts membrane phospholipids into AA, the substrate for COX and LOX, permitting generation of PGs and leukotrienes, respectively.[21,24]

Activation of CRH release can be blocked by the synthetic glucocorticoid dexamethasone[23,24] and also by blockers of the three pathways of AA metabolism, such as clotrimazol, which blocks epoxygenase which converts AA into epoxides; indomethacin, which inhibits COX; and by 5′8′11-eicisotrionoic acid, which blocks LOX. Thus, CRH release is activated by the AA cascade.[23] α-Melanotcyte-stimulating hormone (αMSH) also inhibits CRH release.[24] Cyclosporin inhibits CRH release as well,[25] probably by inhibiting calcineurin. Calcineurin dephosphorylates NOS, rendering it inactive.

Of the many proinflammatory cytokines, it has been shown that IL-1α or β, TNFα, IL-6, and IL-2 can stimulate ACTH release from the anterior pituitary *in vitro* and *in vivo*.[4] The principal action is probably, at least acutely, on the release of CRH and vasopressin from the hypothalamus, but there are also clear effects at the pituitary level. There have been few studies on the mechanism of this direct pituitary action of cytokines; however, several cytokines such as IL-6 have been found to be produced in pituitaries, and nNOS is also present in the gland as indicated earlier. There are indications that NO participates in inhibiting the response of ACTH to vasopressin.[26] Whether it plays a role in the stimulatory action of the various proinflammatory cytokines on ACTH secretion has not yet been studied.

In our studies LPS itself had no acute effect on ACTH release from hemianterior pituitaries *in vitro*.[16] However, LPS induces cytokine production in the pituitary. Cytokine production would be increased in a few hours and undoubtedly would modify the responses of the pituitary to the continued altered secretion of releasing and inhibiting hormones.

In addition to the proinflammatory cytokines that we have discussed extensively, it is now clear that there are a number of antiinflammatory cytokines, the first one to be discovered being IL-I receptor antagonist, but IL-10 and IL-13 also serve this role, as indicated above. These are also induced in the brain by LPS and may play roles at the hypothalamic and pituitary levels to diminish the response to the proinflammatory cytokines.

EFFECT OF CYTOKINES AND NO ON THE RELEASE OF LHRH

Our most extensive studies were carried out with regard to the release of LHRH, which controls the release of LH from the pituitary gland. LHRH release is not continuous, but instead is pulsatile, with the frequency of pulses determined by the species and gonadal hormone status, with considerable variation in individual animals of a given species.[2,3] LH then circulates to the gonads and causes the production of gonadal steroids. In the female, after secretion of FSH to develop the ovarian follicles, LH produces ovulation and formation of the corpus luteum. Not only does LHRH act after its secretion into the hypophyseal–portal vessels to stimulate LH and to a lesser extent FSH release, but it also induces mating behavior in rats.[27]

Our experiments showed that release of NO from NP promoted LHRH release in vitro and that the action was blocked by hemoglobin, a scavenger of NO.[28] NP also caused an increased release of PGE_2 from the tissue,[29] which previous experiments showed played an important role in the release of LHRH. Furthermore, it caused the biosynthesis and release of prostanoids from [^{14}C]AA. The effect was most pronounced for PGE_2, but there also was release of LOX products, which have been shown to play a role in LHRH release. Inhibitors of COX, the enzyme responsible for prostanoid synthesis, such as indomethacin and salicylic acid, blocked the release of LHRH induced by norepinephrine (NE), providing further evidence for the role of NO in the control of LHRH release via the activation of COX I.[30] Needleman's group[31] later showed that NO activates COX I and COX II in cultured fibroblasts. The action is probably mediated by a combination of NO with the heme group of COX altering its conformation. The action on LOX is similar; although it contains ferrous iron, the actual presence of heme in LOX has yet to be demonstrated.

The previously accepted pathway for the physiologic action of NO is by activation of soluble GC by interaction of NO with the heme group of this enzyme, thereby causing conversion of GTP into cGMP, which mediates the effects on smooth muscle by decreasing the intracellular $[Ca^{2+}]$ as described above. On the other hand, Muallem's group[32] has shown in incubated pancreatic acinar cells that cGMP has a biphasic effect on intracellular $[Ca^{2+}]$, elevating it at low concentrations and lowering it at higher concentrations. We postulate that the NO released from the NOergic neurons near the LHRH neuronal terminals diffuses into the terminals and activates GC. The cGMP synthesized increases the intracellular $[Ca^{2+}]$ required to activate PLA_2. PLA_2 causes the conversion of membrane phospholipids in the LHRH terminal to AA, which then can be converted to PGE_2 via the activated COX. The released PGE_2 activates AC, causing an increase in cAMP release, which activates PKA, leading to exocytosis of LHRH secretory granules into the hypophyseal–portal capillaries for transmission to the anterior pituitary gland.[30]

NE has previously been shown to be a powerful releasor of LHRH. In the present experiments, we show it acted by activation of the NOergic neurons, since the activation of these neurons and the release of LHRH could be blocked by phentolamine, an α-receptor blocker, and prazosine, an α_1-receptor blocker. Therefore, the action is by α_1-adrenergic receptors.[28,30]

We measured the effect of NE on the content of nNOS in the MBH explants at the end of the experiments by homogenizing the tissue and adding [^{14}C]arginine and measuring its conversion to citrulline on incubation of the homogenate, a modification of the method of Bredt and Snyder.[15,30] Because arginine is converted to equimolar quantities of NO and citrulline, measurement of citrulline production provides a convenient estimate of the activity of the enzyme. The NO disappears rapidly, making its measurement very difficult. NE caused an increase in citrulline formation, suggesting that NE had increased the content of nNOS during the 30-minute incubation of MBH explants. We confirmed that we had actually increased the content of enzyme by isolating the enzyme according to the method of Bredt and Snyder[15] and then measuring the conversion of labeled arginine to citrulline. The conversion was highly significantly increased by NE.[30]

Glutamic acid, at least in part by means of n-methyl-D-aspartate (NMDA) receptors, also plays a physiologically significant role in controlling the release of LHRH. Therefore, we evaluated where glutamic acid fit into the picture. It also acted via NO to stimulate LHRH release, but we showed that the effect of glutamic acid could be completely obliterated by the α-receptor blocker phentolamine. Consequently, we concluded that glutamic acid acts by stimulation of the noradrenergic terminals in the MBH to release NE, which then initiated NO release and stimulation of LHRH release.[33]

Oxytocin has actions within the brain to promote mating behavior in the female and penile erection in the male rat. Because LHRH mediates mating behavior, we hypothesized that oxytocin would stimulate LHRH release, which mediates LH release from the pituitary. Consequently, we incubated MBH explants and demonstrated that oxytocin induced concentration-dependent LHRH release (10^{-7}–10^{-10} M) via NE stimulation of nNOS. Therefore, oxytocin may be very important as a stimulator of LHRH release. Furthermore, the released NO acts as a negative feedback to inhibit oxytocin release.[34]

One of the few receptors to be identified on LHRH neurons is the GABAa receptor. Consequently, we evaluated the role of GABA on LHRH release and the participation of NO in this. The experiments showed that GABA blocked the response of the LHRH neurons to NP, which acts directly on the LHRH terminals. We concluded that GABA suppressed LHRH release by blocking their response to NE. Additional experiments showed that NO stimulated the release of GABA, providing thereby an inhibitory feed-forward pathway to inhibit the pulsatile release of LHRH initiated by NE. As NE stimulated the release of NO, this would stimulate the release of GABA, which would then block the response of the LHRH neuron to the NO released by NE.[35]

Other studies indicated that NO would suppress the release of DA and NE. We have already described the ability of NE to stimulate LHRH release. DA also acts as a stimulatory transmitter in the pathway. Therefore, there is an ultrashort-loop negative feedback mechanism to terminate the pulsatile release of LHRH, because the NO released by NE would diffuse to the noradrenergic terminals and inhibit the release of NE, thereby terminating the pulse of NE, LHRH, and finally LH.[36]

β-Endorphin blocks release of LHRH into the hypophyseal portal vessels by stimulating μ opiate receptors, thereby inhibiting secretion of LH. Our results indicate that β-endorphin stimulates μ opioid receptors on NOergic neurons to inhibit the activation and consequent synthesis of NOS in the MBH. β-Endorphin also blocks the action of NO on PGE_2 release, and consequently on LHRH release, by stimulating GABAergic inhibitory input to LHRH terminals that blocks NO-induced activation of COX and consequent PGE_2 secretion.[37]

We further examined the possibility that other products from this system might have inhibitory actions. Indeed, we found that as we added increasing amounts of NP, we obtained a bell-shaped dose–response curve of the release of LHRH, such that the release increased with increasing concentrations of NP up to a maximum at around 600 μM and then declined with higher concentrations. When the effect of NP on NOS content at the end of the experiment was measured, we found that high concentrations of NP lowered the NOS content. Furthermore, NP could directly decrease NOS content when incubated with MBH homogenates, results that indicate a direct inhibitory effect on NOS probably by interaction of NO with the heme group on the enzyme. Thus, when large quantities of NO are released, as could occur following induction of iNOS in the brain during infections, the release of NO would be decreased by an inhibitory action on the enzyme at these high concentrations. Furthermore, cGMP released by NO also acted in the explants or even the homogenates at high concentrations to suppress the activation of NOS. This pathway could also be active in the presence of high concentrations of NO, as in infection.[18] Thus, high concentrations of NO produced in the MBH by iNOS produced by arcuate neurons could inactive NOS, leading to decreased NO stimulation of LHRH and decreased LH released and loss of libido.

EFFECT OF CYTOKINES (IL-1 AND GMCSF) ON THE NOErgic CONTROL OF LHRH RELEASE

The cytokines so far tested, for example, interleukin-1 and granulocyte macrophage colony-stimulating factor (GMCSF), act within the hypothalamus to suppress the release of LHRH as revealed in both *in vivo* and *in vitro* studies. We have examined the mechanism of this effect and found that for IL-1, it occurs by inhibition of COX, as shown by the fact that there is a blockade of the conversion of labeled AA to prostanoids, particularly PGE_2, and the release of PGE_2 induced by NE is also blocked.[38] LOX was also inhibited by IL-1α, as indicated by decreased leukotriene formation. Leukotrienes also increase LHRH release.

A principal mechanism of action is by suppression of the LHRH release induced by NO donors such as NP.[38] We first believed that there were IL-1 and GMCSF receptors on the LHRH neuron that blocked the response of the neuron to NO. However, since we had also shown that GABA blocks the response to NP and earlier work had shown that GABA receptors are present on the LHRH neurons, we evaluated the possibility that the action of cytokines could be mediated by stimulation of GABAergic neurons in the MBH. Indeed, in the case of GMCSF, its inhibitory action on LHRH release can be reversed by GABAa receptor blocker, bicuculline, which also blocks the inhibitory action of GABA itself on the response of the LHRH terminals to NO. Therefore, we believe that the inhibitory action of cytokines on LHRH release is mediated, at least in part, by stimulation of GABA neurons.[39]

ROLE OF NO IN MATING BEHAVIOR

LHRH controls lordosis behavior in the female rat and is also involved in mediating male sex behavior. Studies in vivo have shown that NO stimulates the release of the LHRH involved in inducing sex behavior. This behavior can be blocked by inhibitors of NOS. Apparently, there are two LHRH neuronal systems: one with axons terminating on the hypophyseal portal vessels; and the other with axons terminating on neurons that mediate sex behavior.[27] NO is also involved in inducing penile erection by the release of NO from NOergic neurons innervating the corpora cavernosa penis. The role of NO in sex behavior in both sexes has led us to refer to NO as the "sexual gas".[40] The suppression of LHRH release by cytokines may be responsible for the decreased libido characteristic of infections.

EFFECT OF CYTOKINES AND NO ON THE RELEASE OF OTHER HYPOTHALAMIC PEPTIDES

Pulsatile GH release is controlled by GHRH release, and this can be blocked by intraventricular injection of NMMA, indicating that NO is also responsible for GHRH release.[41] Somatostatin release and mRNA synthesis are also stimulated by NO.[42] Injection of IL-1α into the third ventricle inhibits GH release by blocking the release of GHRH and stimulating the release of somatostatin.[37] NO induces the PRL release from injection of IL-1α by inhibiting release of the PRL-inhibiting hormone, DA.[43]

ACTION OF CYTOKINES AND NO TO CONTROL RELEASE OF ANTERIOR PITUITARY HORMONES

NOS is localized in LH gonadotropes and folliculostellate cells, which are modified glial cells that bear a resemblance to macrophages, as revealed by immunocytochemistry.[44] When pituitaries are incubated in vitro, most pituitary hormones are secreted only in small quantities. The exception to this rule is PRL, which is secreted in large amounts because of removal of inhibitory hypothalamic control by DA.[45] The other anterior pituitary hormones are secreted at low levels because of lost stimulatory hypothalamic input, and NO donors have little effect on this basal release in the case of GH. On the other hand, in the case of PRL, which is released in large amounts, NO donors suppress the release of the hormone; and inhibitors of NOS usually enhance the release, indicating that there is still some capability for the gland to increase release of PRL *in vitro*.

DA is the most important PRL-inhibiting hormone by action on D^2 receptors in the gland. The dramatic inhibitory action of DA can be prevented by D^2 receptor blockers and also is prevented by incubation in the presence of inhibitors of NOS. Therefore, we conclude that the primary inhibitory action of DA is mediated by its action to stimulate D^2 receptors on the NOS-containing cells in the pituitary gland with resultant release of NO, which diffuses to the lactotropes and activates GC, causing the release of cGMP which mediates the inhibition of PRL secretion. Consistent with this hypothesis is the fact that NO donors suppress PRL release and the addition of cGMP can also lower the release of the hormone from incubated pituitaries. NO probably also inhibits ACTH release.[45] By contrast NO mediates the stimulation of FSH and LH induced by FSHRF, LHRH, and leptin, presumably by activation of specific receptors on the gonadotropes. NO converts GTP to cGMP that induces release of FSH and LH secretory granules.

During infection, cytokines, secreted by folliculostellate cells, are also released within the pituitary gland, resulting in activation of iNOS leading to generation of NO.[17] Therefore, NO should mediate, at least in part, the actions of cytokines directly on the pituitary gland.

THE ADIPOCYTE HORMONE LEPTIN

Leptin is a member of the cytokine family of hormones and has actions that are quite different from those of the inflammatory cytokines, which in some ways resemble those of the antiinflammatory cytokines. Instead of inhibiting LHRH release, as is the case with the proinflammatory cytokines, leptin combines with its receptors in the arcuate region to activate LHRH release by stimulating the release of NO from NOergic neurons. Rather surprisingly, it also activates not only FSH, but also LH release from hemipituitaries incubated *in vitro* at concentrations similar to those of LHRH itself. Again, the action is mediated by NO[47] and is modified by estrogen.[47,49] Evidence is mounting that these actions of leptin to stimulate gonadotropin secretion are of physiological importance and may play an important role in induction of puberty and in the amenorhea that follows malnutrition, as in the case of anorexia nervosa.[50]

Like other cytokines, leptin release is stimulated by LPS. The mechanism of this has yet to be determined, but the increase in leptin can be blocked completely by the glucocorticoid dexamethasone. The action of leptin on the hypothalamic–pituitary axis in this situation has not yet been studied, but leptin also elevates body temperature and inhibits feeding. These are responses to LPS and it may be that leptin plays a role in the anorexia, decreased libido and fever induced by infection.[51]

REFERENCES

1. CHOWERS, I., H.T. HAMMEL, J. EISENMAN *et al.* 1966. A comparison of the effects of environmental and preoptic heating and pyrogen on plasma cortisol levels. Am. J. Physiol. **210:** 606–610.

2. McCann, S.M. & S.R. Ojeda. 1996. The anterior pituitary and hypothalamus. *In* Textbook of Endocrine Physiology. Third edit. J.E. Griffin & S.R. Ojeda, Eds.: 101–133. Oxford University Press. Oxford, England.

3. Reichlin, S. 1992. Neuroendocrinology. *In* Textbook of Endocrinology. D.W. Foster & J.D. Wilson, Eds.: 135–219. Saunders. Philadelphia, PA.

4. McCann, S.M., S. Karanth, A. Kamat *et al.* 1994. Induction by cytokines by the pattern of pituitary hormone secretion in infection. Neuroimmunomodulation **1:** 2–13.

5. Porter, J.C., J.F. Sisom, J. Arita & M.J. Reymond. 1983. The hypothalamic–hypophysial vasculature and its relationship to secretory cells of the hypothalamus and pituitary gland. Vitam. Horm. **40:** 145–174.

6. Koenig, J.I. 1991. Presence of cytokines in the hypothalamic–pituitary axis. Prog. Neuroendocrinimmunol. **4:** 143.

7. Banks, W.A., A.J. Kastin, W. Huang *et al.* 1996. Leptin enters the brain by a saturable system independent of insulin. Peptides **17:** 305–311.

8. Spangelo, B.L., R.M. MacLeod & P.C. Isakson. 1990. Production of interleukin-6 by anterior pituitary cells *in vitro.* Endocrinology **126:** 582–586.

9. Breder, C.D., C.A. Dinarello & C.B. Saper. 1988. Interleukin-1 immunoreactive innervation of the human hypothalamus. Science **240:** 321–324.

10. McDonald, L.J. & F. Murad. 1996. Nitric oxide and cyclic GMP signaling. Proc. Soc. Exp. Biol. Med. **211:** 1–6.

11. Dawson, V.L. & T.M. Dawson. 1996. Nitric oxide in neuronal degeneration. Proc. Soc. Expl. Biol. Med. **211:** 33–40.

12. Garthwaite, J., S.J. Charles & R. Chess-Williams. 1988. Endothelium-derived relaxing factor release on activation of NMDA receptors suggests role as intercellular messenger in the brain. Nature (London) **336:** 385–388.

13. Palmer, R.M.J., A.G. Ferrige & S. Moncada. 1987. Nitric oxide release accounts for the biological activity of endothelium-derived relaxing factor. Nature (London) **327:** 424–526.

14. Bredt, D.S. & S.H. Snyder. 1990. Isolation of nitric oxide synthetase, a calmodulin requiring enzyme. Proc. Natl. Acad. Sci. USA **87:** 682–685.

15. Bredt, D.S., P.M. Hwang & S.H. Snyder. 1990. Localization of nitric oxide synthase indicating a neural role for nitric oxide. Nature (London) **347:** 768–770.

16. Rettori, V., W.L. Dees, J.K. Hiney *et al.* 1994. An interleukin-1-α-like neuronal system in the preoptic–hypothalamic region and its induction by bacterial lipopolysaccharide in concentrations which alter pituitary hormone release. Neuroimmunomodulation **1:** 251–258.

17. Wong, M-L., V. Rettori, A. Al-Shekhlee *et al.* 1996. Inducible nitric oxide synthase gene expression in the brain during systemic inflammation. Nat. Med. **2:** 581–584.

18. Canteros, G., V. Rettori, A. Genaro *et al.* 1996. Nitric oxide synthase content of hypothalamic explants: increased by norepinephrine and inactivated by NO and cGMP. Proc. Natl. Acad. Sci. USA **93:** 4246–4250.

19. Wong, M-L., P.B. Bongiorno, V. Rettori *et al.* 1997. Interleukin (IL) 1β, IL-1 receptor antagonist, IL-10, and IL-13 gene expression in the central nervous system and anterior pituitary during systemic inflammation: pathophysiological implications. Proc. Natl. Acad. Sci. USA **94:** 227–232.

20. Franci, J., C. Franci, J. Antunes-Rodrigues & S.M. McCann. 1999. The effect of locus ceruleus lesions on stress-induced alterations in anterior pituitary hormone release in male rats. Brain Res. Submitted.

21. Karanth, S., K. Lyson & S.M. McCann. 1993. Role of nitric oxide in interleukin 2-induced corticotropin-releasing factor release from incubated hypothalami. Proc. Natl. Acad. Sci. USA **90:** 3383–3387.

22. Karanth, S., K. Lyson & S.M. McCann. 1999. Effects of cholinergic agonists and antagonists on interleukin-2-induced corticotropin-releasing hormone release from the mediobasal hypothalamus. Neuroimmunomodulation **6:** 168–174.

23. Lyson, K. & S.M. McCann. 1992. Involvement of arachidonic acid cascade pathways in interleukin-6-stimulated corticotropin-releasing factor release *in vitro*. Neuroendocrinology **55:** 708–713.

24. Karanth, S., K. Lyson, M.C. Aguila & S.M. McCann. 1995. Effects of luteinizing-hormone-releasing hormone, α-melanocyte-stimulating hormone, naloxone, dexamethasone and indomethacin on interleukin-2-induced corticotropin-releasing factor release. Neuroimmunomodulation **2:** 166–173.

25. Karanth, S., K. Lyson & S.M. McCann. 1994. Cyclosporin A inhibits interleukin-2-induced release of corticotropin releasing hormone. Neuroimmunomodulation **1:** 82–85.

26. Turnbull, A.V. & C.L. Rivier. 1999. Regulation of the hypothalmic–pituitary–adrenal axis by cytokines: actions and mechanisms of action. Physiol. Rev. **79:** 1–71.

27. Mani, S.K., J.M.C. Allen, V. Rettori *et al.* 1994. Nitric oxide mediates sexual behavior in female rats by stimulating LHRH release. Proc. Natl. Acad. Sci. USA **91:** 6468–6472.

28. Rettori, V., N. Belova, W.L. Dees *et al.* 1993. Role of nitric oxide in the control of luteinizing hormone-releasing hormone release *in vivo* and *in vitro*. Proc. Natl. Acad. Sci. USA **90:** 10130–10134.

29. Rettori, V., M. Gimeno, K. Lyson & S.M. McCann. 1992. Nitric oxide mediates norepinephrine-induced prostaglandin E_2 release from the hypothalamus. Proc. Natl. Acad. Sci. USA **89:** 11453–11546.

30. Canteros, G., V. Rettori, A. Franchi *et al.* 1995. Ethanol inhibits luteinizing hormone-releasing hormone (LHRH) secretion by blocking the response of LHRH neuronal terminals to nitric oxide. Proc. Natl. Acad. Sci. USA **92:** 3416–3420.

31. Salvemini, D., T.P. Misko, J.L. Masferrer *et al.* 1993. Nitric oxide activates cyclooxygenase enzymes. Proc. Natl. Acad. Sci. USA **90:** 7040–7044.

32. Xu, X., R.A. Star, G. Tortorici & S. Muallem. 1994. Depletion of intracellular Ca^{2+} stores activatess NOS to generate cGMP and regulate Ca^{2+} influx. J. Biol. Chem. **269:** 12645–12653.

33. Kamat, A., W.H. Yu, V. Rettori & S.M. McCann. 1995. Glutamic acid stimulated luteinizing-hormone releasing hormone release is mediated by alpha adrenergic stimulation of nitric oxide release. Brain. Res. Bull. **37:** 233–235.

34. Rettori, V., G. Canteros, A. Faletti *et al.* 1997. Oxytocin stimulates the release of luteinizing hormone-releasing hormone from medial basal hypothalamic explants by releasing nitric oxide. Proc. Natl. Acad. Sci. USA **94:** 2741–2744.

35. Seilicovich, A., B.H. Duvilanski, D. Pisera *et al.* 1995. Nitric oxide inhibits hypothalamic luteinizing hormone-releasing hormone release by releasing γ-aminobutyric acid. Proc. Natl. Acad. Sci. USA **92:** 3421–3424.

36. Seilicovich, A., M. Lasaga, M. Befumo *et al.* 1995. Nitric oxide inhibits the release of norepinephrine and dopamine from the medial basal hypothalamus of the rat. Proc. Natl. Acad. Sci. USA **92:** 11299–11302.

37. Faletti, A.G., C.A. Mastonardi, A. Lomniczi *et al.* 1999. β-Endorphin blocks luteinizing hormone-releasing hormone release by inhibiting the nitricoxidergic pathway controlling its release. Proc. Natl. Acad. Sci. USA **96:** 1722–1726.

38. Rettori, V., N. Belova, A. Kamat *et al.* 1994. Blockade by interleukin-1-α of the nitricoxidergic control of luteinizing hormone-releasing hormone release *in vivo* and *in vitro*. Neuroimmunomodulation **1:** 86–91.

39. Kimura, M., W.H. Yu, V. Rettori & S.M. McCann. 1997. Granulocyte-macrophage colony stimulating factor suppresses LHRH release by inhibition of nitric oxide synthase and stimulation of γ-aminobutyric acid release. Neuroimmunomodulation **4:** 237–243.

40. McCann, S.M. & V. Rettori. 1996. The role of nitric oxide in reproduction. Proc. Soc. Exp. Biol. Med. **211:** 7–15.

41. Rettori, V., N. Belova, W.H. Yu *et al.* 1994. Role of nitric oxide in control of growth hormone release in the rat. Neuroimmunomodulation **1:** 195–200.

42. Aguila, M.C. 1994. Growth hormone-releasing factor increases somatostatin release and mRNA levels in the rat periventricular nucleus via nitric oxide by activation of guanylate cyclase. Proc. Natl. Acad. Sci. USA **91:** 782–786.

43. RETTORI, V., N. BELOVA, M. GIMENO & S.M. MCCANN. 1994. Inhibition of nitric oxide synthase in the hypothalamus blocks the increase in plasma prolactin induced by intraventricular injection of interleukin-1α in the rat. Neuroimmunomodulation **1:** 116–120.

44. CECCATELLI, S., A.L. HULTING, X. ZHANG, L. GUSTAFSSON, M. VILLAR & T. HOK-FELT. 1993. Proc. Natl. Acad. Sci. USA **90:** 11292–11296.

45. DUVILANSKI, B.H., C. ZAMBRUNO, A. SEILICOVICH et al. 1995. Role of nitric oxide in control of prolactin release by the adenoypophysis. Proc. Natl. Acad. Sci. USA **92:** 170–174.

46. MCCANN, S.M., M. KIMURA, A. WALCZEWSKA et al. 1998. Hypothalamic control of gonadotropin secretion by LHRH, FSHRF, NO, cytokines and leptin. Domest. Anim. Endocrinol. **15:** 333–344.

47. YU, W.H., M. KIMURA, A. WALCZEWSKA et al. 1997. Role of leptin in hypthalamic–pituitary function. Proc. Natl. Acad. Sci. USA **94:** 1023–1028.

48. YU, W.H., A. WALCZEWSKA, S. KARANTH & S.M. MCCANN. 1997. Nitric oxide mediates leptin-induced luteinizing hormone-releasing hormone (LHRH) and LHRH and leptin-induced LH release from the pituitary gland. Endocrinology **138:** 5055–5058.

49. WALCZEWSKA, A., W.H. YU, S. KARANTH & S.M. MCCANN. 1999. Estrogen and leptin have differential effects on FSH and LH release in female rats. Proc. Soc. Exp. Biol. Med. **222:** 170–177.

50. LICINIO, J., A.B. NEGRAO, C. MANTZOROS et al. 1998. Synchronicity of frequently-sampled 24-hour concentrations of circulating leptin, luteinizing hormone, and estradiol in healthy women. Proc. Natl. Acad. Sci. USA **95:** 2541–2546.

51. MASTRONARDI, C., W.H. YU & S.M. MCCANN. 1999. Lipopolysaccharide (LPS)-induced leptin (L) release is not mediated by nitric oxide (NO), but is blocked by dexamethasone (DEX) [abstract]. Experimental Biology '99, Washington, DC, April 17–21: #594.9, p A750, part II.

Bidirectional Heterologous Desensitization of Opioid and Chemokine Receptors

T.J. ROGERS,[a,b] A.D. STEELE,[b] O.M.Z. HOWARD,[c] AND J.J. OPPENHEIM[c]

[b]Department of Microbiology and Immunology, Center for Substance Abuse Research, and the Fels Institute for Cancer Research and Molecular Biology, Temple University School of Medicine, Philadelphia, Pennsylvania 19140, USA

[c]Laboratory of Molecular Immunoregulation, Division of Basic Sciences, National Cancer Institute, Frederick Cancer Research and Development Center, Frederick, Maryland 21702-1201, USA

ABSTRACT: Opioids are known to suppress a number of elements of the immune response, including antimicrobial resistance, antibody production, and delayed-type hypersensitivity. Phagocytic cells may be particularly susceptible to opioid administration, since reduced production of the cytokines IL-1, IL-6 and TNF-α, monocyte-mediated phagocytosis, and both neutrophil and monocyte chemotaxis have all been well established. Earlier studies have shown that both μ- and δ-opioid agonists induce a chemotactic response in monocytes and neutrophils. In addition, μ- and δ-opioid administration inhibited the chemotactic response of these cell populations to a number of chemokines through a process of heterologous desensitization. We report here that μ-, δ-, and κ-opioid agonists also induce a chemotactic response in T lymphocytes. Using the human T-cell line Jurkat, we have confirmed previous observations that pre-incubation with met-enkephalin (MetEnk), an endogenous opioid agonist, prevents the subsequent chemotactic response to the chemokine RANTES. On the other hand, treatment with MetEnk does not alter the response to the chemokine SDF-1α. Moreover, we found that pretreatment with RANTES prevented a subsequent response of monocytes to the μ-opioid agonist DAMGO. These results suggest that activation of members of the opioid and chemokine receptor families leads to downregulation of each other's leukocyte migratory activities.

It is well established that intravenous opiate drug abusers have a greater incidence of infection than do nonabusers.[1,2] Moreover, the natural killer (NK) cell activity and antibody-dependent cellular cytotoxicity of peripheral blood mononuclear cells of heroin abusers is suppressed,[3,4] and there is also evidence that abusers have alterations in the numbers and proportion of CD2+, CD4+, and CD8+ cells.[3–7] On the other hand, heroin addicts are reported to have increased levels of serum IgA, IgM, and IgG.[3] Addicts are reported to have a much greater prevalence of viral hepatitis A, B, and C, bacterial pneumonias, tuberculosis, central nervous system infections, and endocarditis.[2,8,9]

[a]Address for correspondence: Department of Microbiology and Immunology, Temple University School of Medicine, 3400 N. Broad Street, Philadelphia, PA 19140. Voice: 215-707-3215; fax: 215-707-7788.

rogerst@astro.ocis.temple.edu

It is apparent from experimental analysis that both endogenous and exogenous opioid compounds exert a direct effect on the immune system. It is well established that opioid administration leads to altered antibody responses,[10–12] suppression of delayed-type hypersensitivity,[13–15] and reduced NK cell activity.[16–18] The mechanism of this immunomodulation is uncertain, but is likely to be due to an interaction of the opioid compound with multiple populations of immune cells. Both macrophage and T-cell functions can be altered following treatment with opioid compounds, and this includes a reduction in macrophage microbicidal and tumoricidal activity,[19–21] macrophage phagocytic activity,[22–25] and the production of the T-cell products IL-2, IL-4, and γ-IFN.[26–29]

In contrast to the inhibition of phagocytic activity following opioid administration, morphine and the endogenous opioids β-endorphin, met-enkephalin (MetEnk), and dynorphin induce chemotaxis of human monocytes and neutrophils.[30–33] On the other hand, pretreatment with opioids leads to the inhibition of chemotaxis of neutrophils and monocytes both to complement-derived chemotactic factors[34,35] and to the chemokines MIP-1α, RANTES, MCP-1 and IL-8.[33] In these studies the administration of morphine, heroin, MetEnk, the more selective μ-agonist [D-ala^2, N-MePhe^4, Gly-ol^5]enkephalin (DAMGO), or the selective δ-agonist [D-Pen^2, D-Pen^5]enkephalin (DPDPE) inhibited the subsequent chemotaxis of human peripheral blood neutrophils and monocytes. The results of Grimm et al.[33] suggest that the activation of the μ- and δ-opioid receptors leads to the desensitization of the chemokine receptors CCR1, CCR2, CXCR1, and CXCR2. This opioid-induced desensitization appears to be due to phosphorylation of the chemokine receptor.

Both the opioids and chemokines mediate their effects on leukocytes through the activation of G protein–coupled seven transmembrane receptors. There are three major types of opioid receptors (μ, κ, and δ), and four families of chemokine receptors, the classification of the latter being based on the amino acid sequence at the amino-terminal cysteine of the chemokine ligand (C, CC, CXC, and CX$_3$C). The generation of chemotactic activity by these ligands is due to the activation of a complex series of signaling events that must be tightly regulated in order to permit the appropriate directed migration of leukocytes from one anatomical site to another. A major aspect of this regulation involves inactivation of the receptor, a process in which the native ligand at high concentration (or following repeated administration) typically induces receptor phosphorylation and is known as "homologous" desensitization. On the other hand, activation of G protein–coupled receptors at a low ligand concentration may initiate signaling pathways that induce "heterologous" desensitization of other unrelated receptors.

The aim of this study was to examine the interactions of opioid and chemokine receptors expressed by T cells and monocytes. Earlier work established that opioid receptor activation in neutrophils and monocytes results in the heterologous desensitization of certain chemokine receptors.[33] We report results that demonstrate that opioid receptor activation in T cells leads to the selective desensitization of receptors for RANTES, but not of the receptor for SDF-1α. Conversely, we demonstrate that the activation of chemokine receptors by RANTES, but not by SDF-1α, leads to an inhibition of the function of the μ-opioid receptor.

μ-, δ- AND κ-OPIATES INDUCE T-CELL CHEMOTAXIS

In our initial studies, we examined the chemotactic activity of μ-, κ-, and δ-opioids to induce a chemotactic response in human T cells. Chemotactic analysis was carried out as previously described,[33,36] using standard 48-well microchemotaxis chambers with the Jurkat T-cell line. These T cells exhibited a significant chemotactic response to the endogenous opioid MetEnk at concentrations at or near 10 nM (see FIGURE 1). Previous work clearly established that human monocytes and neutrophils exhibit a chemotactic response to morphine[37]; however, in the present experiments Jurkat T cells failed to migrate in response to this exogenous opiate (data not shown).

On the basis of a number of studies with various cell types, it is believed that MetEnk is primarily an agonist for the δ-opioid receptor. In an effort to further examine the nature of the chemotactic response of T cells to opioids, we transfected Jurkat cells with the μ-, κ-, or δ-opioid receptor. Parental Jurkat cells were transfected by electroporation with opioid receptor plasmid constructs that permit the stable expression of protein in mammalian cells. The resulting transfected cells were cloned in the presence of antibiotic selection, and positive clones were identified following both RT-PCR analysis, and radiolabeled binding analysis. Using RT-PCR, we verified earlier published results[38] and have shown that the parental Jurkat cell line expresses low, but detectable levels of the δ-opioid receptor. The transfected clones that express the μ- (J-MOR5.1), δ- (J-DOR2.2) and κ- (J-KOR8) opioid receptors were compared with the nontransfected T cells for their response to a battery of selective opioid receptor agonists. The results show (see FIGURE 2) that the δ-opioid-selective opioid agonist DPDPE induces a chemotactic response in both J-DOR2.2 and in the parental cell line. This result is consistent with the MetEnk results shown above. On the other hand, the J-MOR5.1 cell line, but not parental cells, show a response to the selective μ-opioid agonist DAMGO. Finally, the J-KOR8 line, but not parental cells, gives a chemotactic response to the selective κ-opioid agonist trans-3,4-dichloro-N-methyl-*N*-[7-(1-pyrrolidinyl) cyclohexyl] benzene-acetamide methanesulfonate (U50,488H). The failure of the parental cells to respond to morphine is most likely due to the fact that these cells do not express the receptor for this moderately selective μ-opioid agonist.

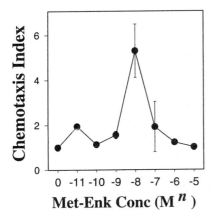

FIGURE 1. Chemotaxis of Jurkat T cells induced by MetEnk. Chemotaxis was assessed by using a standard 48-well microchemotaxis chamber with MetEnk dilutions in the lower chamber and T cells at 2×10^6/ml in the upper chamber, separated by a 5-μm-pore polycarbonate membrane. The chemotaxis index is a ratio of the cells/high-powered field (hpf) for the chemoattractant over the cells/hpf for medium. Data are expressed as the mean chemotaxis index ±SD for a representative experiment.

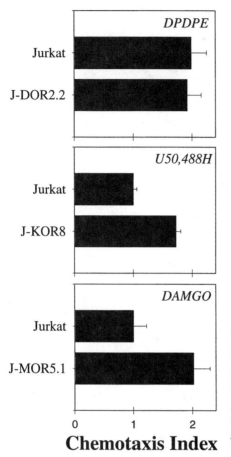

FIGURE 2. Chemotaxis of Jurkat T cells (Jurkat) and transfected Jurkat cell clones that express the δ-opioid receptor (J-DOR2.2), κ-opioid receptor (J-KOR8), or the μ-opioid receptor (J-MOR5.1). The parental Jurkat cells or transfected cells were tested for the chemotaxis to the δ-opioid agonist DPDPE (*top panel*), the κ-opioid agonist U50,488H (*middle panel*), or the μ-opioid agonist DAMGO (*bottom panel*).

INHIBITION OF T-CELL CHEMOTAXIS BY OPIATES

   T cells were preincubated with MetEnk to assess the effect on chemokine-induced chemotaxis. Incubation of cells with a concentration of 10 nM for 60 min at 37°C was utilized, based on the finding that this was the optimal chemotactic concentration for these cells (FIG. 1). The results (see FIGURE 3) show that Jurkat T cells respond to the chemokine RANTES with maximal chemotaxis at a concentration of 50 ng/ml. However, MetEnk pretreated cells failed to manifest a significant chemotactic response to RANTES (an 81% inhibition of specific migration). Jurkat T cells also exhibit a chemotactic response to the chemokine SDF-1α (see FIGURE 4), and, importantly, pretreatment with MetEnk does not alter the response to this CXCR4 ligand. These results suggest that selective signaling mechanisms are responsible for opioid-induced heterologous desensitization.

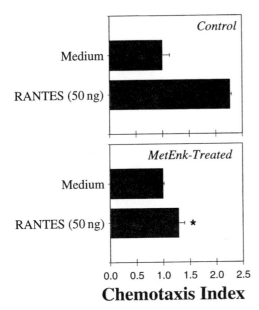

FIGURE 3. Inhibition of RANTES-induced chemotaxis of Jurkat cells by pretreatment with MetEnk. The parental Jurkat cells were treated for 1 hour with 10 nM MetEnk, washed thoroughly, and subjected to analysis of RANTES-induced chemotaxis. Results are presented for the optimal chemotactic concentration (50 ng/ml) of RANTES. Comparison of the response to RANTES by control and MetEnk-treated cells: $p < 0.02$.

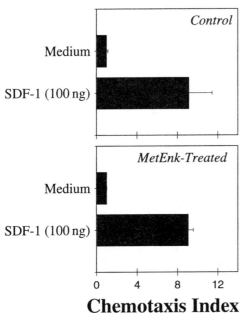

FIGURE 4. Inhibition of SDF 1α-induced chemotaxis of Jurkat cells by pretreatment with MetEnk. Jurkat cells were treated for 1 hour with 10 nM MetEnk, washed, and subjected to analysis of SDF-1-induced chemotaxis. Results are presented for the optimal chemotactic concentration (100 ng/ml) of SDF-1α.

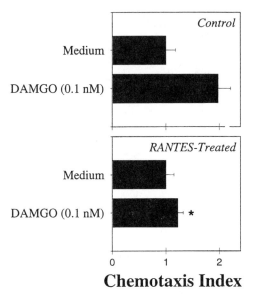

FIGURE 5. Inhibition of DAMGO-induced chemotaxis of monocytes by pretreatment with RANTES. Monocytes were treated for 1 hour with RANTES (50 ng/ml), washed, and subjected to analysis of DAMGO-induced chemotaxis. Results are presented for the optimal chemotactic concentration (0.1 nM) of DAMGO.

INHIBITION OF OPIOID-INDUCED T-CELL CHEMOTAXIS BY CHEMOKINES

In order to further examine the nature of the cross-desensitization between opioid and chemokine receptors, we carried out experiments with primary human peripheral blood monocytes and both Jurkat T cells and the human HaCaT keratinocyte cell line. Freshly isolated monocytes were incubated with the chemokine RANTES, or medium as a control, for 60 min at 37°C at a concentration of 50 ng/ml. The results (see FIGURE 5) show that the control monocytes respond to the μ-opioid agonist DAMGO with a maximal response at 0.1 nM. Monocytes pretreated with RANTES failed to exhibit a chemotactic response to DAMGO (FIG. 5) or the δ-opioid agonist DPDPE (data not shown). Additional experiments show that pretreatment of Jurkat T cells or HaCaT keratinocytes with RANTES inhibits the subsequent response to MetEnk or DAMGO, respectively (data not shown).

RANTES STIMULATION RESULTS IN PHOSPHORYLATION OF THE μ-OPIOID RECEPTOR

The process of homologous desensitization of most G protein–coupled seven transmembrane receptors involves the activation of a protein kinase and receptor phosphorylation. Previous results have shown that pretreatment of U937 promonocyte cells with MetEnk results in the phosphorylation of CXCR2[33] suggesting that heterologous desensitization of at least some chemokine receptors is also dependent on receptor phosphorylation. We investigated whether the desensitization of opioid receptors following chemokine administration involves opioid receptor phosphorylation. In order to carry out these experiments, the HaCaT keratinocyte cell line was treated with RANTES for 30 min at 37°C, followed by whole-cell lysis and immunoprecipitation with a combination of anti-phosphoserine and anti-threonine antibodies. The immunoprecipitates were subjected to Western blot analysis using an anti-μ-opioid receptor antibody as a probe. The results show that treatment of HaCaT cells with RANTES leads to phosphorylation of the μ-opioid receptor. Control experiments carried out with RANTES treatment of μ-opioid receptor-transfected CHO cells, in the absence of receptors for RANTES, does not result in μ-opioid receptor phosphorylation.

DISCUSSION

We have extended earlier studies,[33,37] which showed that opioid treatment selectively inhibits the chemotactic response of monocytes and neutrophils to the chemoattractants IL-8, MIP-1α, RANTES, and MCP-1, but not NAP-1, MIP-1β or fMLP. We report results here that show that T cells also possess the cellular signaling capacity that is responsible for opioid-induced chemokine desensitization. Pretreatment of T cells with MetEnk leads to the inhibition of the response to RANTES, but not SDF-1α. These results reveal an additional element of selectivity in the opioid-induced cross-desensitization, since RANTES receptors (primarily CCR1 and CCR5), but not CXCR4, are affected. On the basis of our work, the selectivity of the cross-desensitization induced by opioid receptor activation is apparent in several cell types we have analyzed, including human monocytes, neutrophils, T cells, keratinocytes, and murine thymocytes.

The phenomenon of heterologous desensitization is common to many members of the G protein–coupled receptor superfamily. It is clear that there is a degree of selectivity in the signaling processes that are responsible for the cross-desensitization of unrelated receptors. Studies with a number of chemoattractant receptors have shown, for example, that fMLP receptor activation leads to desensitization of the receptors for C5a, IL-8, PAF, and LTB$_4$.[39–41] However, CXCR1 activation does not fully desensitize receptors for fMLP, PAF, or LTB$_4$. The process of homologous desensitization appears to involve the function of one or more members of the G protein–coupled receptor kinase (GRK) family, and these GRKs specifically phosphorylate activated receptors and recruit arrestin proteins.[42,43] The binding of arrestin is believed to result in a stabilized receptor–GRK–arrestin complex that interrupts the receptor–G protein interactions and assists in internalization of the receptor from the membrane.[44] The selectivity of the cross-desensitization process may be determined in part by the specific members of the GRK and arrestin family members that are recruited to the receptor. For example, CCR5 is a substrate primarily for both GRK2 and GRK3; however, studies with transfected HEK-293 cells suggest that CCR5 phosphorylation requires overexpression of both the GRKs and either β-arrestin 1 or 2 in this cell line.[45] These results suggest that the susceptibility of a particular G protein–coupled receptor to desensitization may be dictated by the particular target cell population and the endogenous level of GRKs and arrestins. The regulation of either GRK or arrestin expression and function are not fully understood. Recent studies suggest that GRK4, 5, and 6 function is regulated in part by negatively charged phospholipids such as PIP_2.[46] The activity of GRK2 is stimulated following phosphorylation by protein kinase C, whereas the function of GRK5 is inhibited either by phosphorylation or by interaction with calmodulin.[47–51]

This report provides the first direct evidence that chemokines are capable of selectively regulating the function of the opioid receptor family. These G protein–coupled receptors are critical for the maintenance of analgesia by the endogenous opioid peptides and are the targets for common alkaloid analgesic drugs such as morphine. Our results suggest that the production of chemokines in the brain may have an impact on the function of opioid receptors in the central nervous system and have the potential to alter both central and peripheral neurological function. In the periphery, chemokines, by reducing analgesic effects of opioids, may increase the perception of pain at inflammatory sites.

ACKNOWLEDGMENTS

This work was supported in part by National Institutes of Health Grants DA-06650 and DA-11130.

REFERENCES

1. HUSSEY, H.H. & S. KATZ. 1950. Infections resulting from narcotic addiction. Am. J. Med. **9:** 186–193.
2. LOURIA, D.B., T. HENSLE & J. ROSE. 1967. The major medical complications of heroin addiction. Ann. Int. Med. **67:** 1–22.
3. NOVICK, D.M., M. OCHSHORN, V. GHALI et al. 1989. Natural killer cell activity and lymphocyte subsets in parenteral heroin abusers and long-term methadone maintenance patients. J. Pharmacol. Exp. Ther. **250:** 606–610.
4. KREEK, M.J., E. KHURI, N. FLOMENBERG et al. 1990. Immune status of unselected methadone maintained former heroin addicts. Prog. Clin. Biol. Res. **328:** 445–448.
5. DONAHOE, R.M., C. BUESO-RAMOS, F. DONAHOE et al. 1987. Mechanistic implications of the findings that opiates and other drugs of abuse moderate T-cell surface receptors and antigenic markers. In Neuroimmune Interactions: Proceedings of the Second International Workshop on Neuroimmunomodulation. B.D. Jankovic´, B.M. Markovic´ & N.H. Spector, Eds. Ann. N.Y. Acad. Sci. **496:** 711–721.
6. MCDONOUGH, R., J. MADDEN, A. FALEK et al. 1980. Alteration of T and null lymphocyte frequencies in the peripheral blood of hyman opiate addicts: In vivo evidence for opiate receptor sites on T lymphocytes. J. Immunol. **125:** 2539–2543.
7. DONAHOE, R.M., J.K.A. NICHOLSON, J.J. MADDEN et al. 1986. Coordinate and independent effects of heroin, cocaine, and alcohol abuse on T-cell E-rosette formation and antigenic marker expression. Clin. Immunol. Immunopathol. **41:** 254–264.
8. REICHMAN, L.B., C.P. FELTON & J.R. EDSALL. 1979. Drug dependence, a possible new risk factor for tuberculosis disease. Arch. Intern. Med. **139:** 337–339.
9. HAVERKOS, H.W. & R.W. LANGE. 1990. Serious infections other than human immunodeficiency virus among intravenous drug users. J. Infect. Dis. **161:** 894–902.
10. JOHNSON, H.M., E.M. SMITH, B.A. TORRES & J.E. BLALOCK. 1982. Regulation of the in vitro antibody response by neuroendocrine hormones. Proc. Natl. Acad. Sci. USA **79:** 4171–4174.
11. TAUB, D.D., T.K., EISENSTEIN, E.B. GELLER et al. 1991. Immunomodulatory activity of μ- and κ-selective opioid agonists. Proc. Natl. Acad. Sci. USA **88:** 360–364.

12. BUSSIERE, J.L., M.W. ADLER, T.J. ROGERS & T.K. EISENSTEIN. 1992. Differential effects of morphine and naltrexone on the antibody response in various mouse strains. Immunopharmacol. Immunotoxicol. **14:** 657–673.

13. PELLIS, N.R., C. HARPER & N. DAFNY. 1986. Suppression of the induction of delayed hypersensitivity in rats by repetitive morphine treatments. Exp. Neurol. **93:** 92–97.

14. BRYANT, H.U. & R.E. ROUDEBUSH. 1990. Suppressive effects of morphine pellet implants on *in vivo* parameters of immune function. J. Pharmacol. Exp. Ther. **255:** 410–414.

15. MOLITOR, T.W., A. MORILLA, J.M. RISDAHL *et al.* 1992. Chronic morphine administration impairs cell-mediated immune responses in swine. J. Pharmacol. Exp. Ther. **260:** 581–586,

16. WEBER, R.J. & A. PERT. 1989. The periaqueductal gray matter mediates opiate-induced immunosuppression. Science **245:** 188–190.

17. SHAVIT, Y., R. YIRMIYA & B. BEILIN. 1990. Stress neuropeptides, immunity and neoplasia. *In* The Neuroendocrine-Immune Network. S. Freier, Ed.: 163–175. CRC Press. Boca Raton, FL.

18. BAYER, B.M., S. DAUSSIN, M. HERNANDEZ & L. IRVIN. 1990. Morphine inhibition of lymphocyte activity is mediated by an opioid dependent mechanism. Neuropharmacology **29:** 369–374.

19. TUBARO, E., G. BORELLI, C. CROCE *et al.* 1983. Effect of morphine on resistance to infection. J. Infect. Dis. **148:** 656–666.

20. TUBARO, E., C. SANTIANGELI, L. BELOGI *et al.* 1987. Methadone vs. morphine: comparison of their effect on phagocytic functions. Int. J. Immunopharmacol. **9:** 79–88.

21. HAGI, K., K. UNO, K. INABA & S. MURAMATSU. 1994. Augmenting effect of opioid peptides on murine macrophage activation. J. Neuroimmunol. **50:** 71–76.

22. FORIS, G., A. MEDGYESI, E. GYIMESI & M. HAUCK. 1984. Met-enkephalin induced alterations of macrophage functions. Mol. Immunol. **21:** 747–750.

23. FORIS, G., G.A. MEDGYESI & M. HAUK. 1986. Bidirectional effect of met-enkephalin on macrophage effector functions. Mol. Cell. Biochem. **69:** 127–137.

24. ROJAVIN, M., I. SZABO, J.L. BUSSIERE *et al.* 1993. Morphine treatment in vitro or in vivo decreases phagocytic functions of murine macrophages. Life Sci. **53:** 997–1006.

25. SZABO, I., M. ROJAVIN, J.L. BUSSIERE *et al.* 1993. Suppression of peritoneal macrophage phagocytosis of *Candida albicans* by opioids. J. Pharmacol. Exp. Ther. **267:** 703–706.

26. BROWN, S.L. & D.E. VAN EPPS. 1986. Opioid peptides modulate production of interferon-gamma by human mononuclear cells. Cell. Immunol. **103:** 19–26.

27. PETERSON, P.K., B. SHARP, G. GEKKER *et al.* 1987. Opioid-mediated suppression of interferon-γ production by cultured peripheral blood mononuclear cells. J. Clin. Invest. **80:** 824–831.

28. BESSLER, H., M.B. SZTEIN & S.A. SERRATE. 1990. β-Endorphin modulation of IL-1-induced IL-2 production. Immunopharmacology **19:** 5–14.

29. VAN DEN BERGH, P., R. DOBBER, S. RAMLAL *et al.* 1994. Role of opioid peptides in the regulation of cytokine production by murine CD4$^+$ T cells. Cell. Immunol. **154:** 109–122.

30. VAN EPPS, D.E. & L. SALAND. 1984. β-Endorphin and met-enkephalin stimulate human peripheral blood mononuclear cell chemotaxis. J. Immunol. **132:** 3046–3053.

31. RUFF, M.R., S.M. WAHL, S. MERGENHAGEN & C.B. PERT. 1985. Opiate receptor-mediated chemotaxis of human monocytes. Neuropeptides **5:** 363–366.

32. MAKMAN, M.H., T.V. BILFINGER & G.B. STEFANO. 1995. Human granulocytes contain an opiate alkaloid-selective receptor mediating inhibition of cytokine-induced activation and chemotaxis. J. Immunol. **154:** 1323–1330.

33. GRIMM, M., A. BEN-BARUCH, D.D. TAUB *et al.* 1998. Opiates transdeactivate chemokine receptors: delta and mu opiate-receptor mediated heterologous desensitization. J. Exp. Med. **188:** 317–325.

34. PEREZ-CASTRILLON, J.P., J. PEREZ-ARELLANO, J. GARCIA-PALOMO *et al.* 1992. Opioids depress in vitro human monocyte chemotaxis. Immunopharmacology **23:** 57–61.

35. LIU, Y., D.J. BLACKBOURN, L.F. CHUANG *et al.* 1992. Effects of in vivo and in vitro administration of morphine sulfate upon *Rhesus macaque* polymorphonuclear cell phagocytosis and chemotaxis. J. Pharmacol. Exp. Ther. **265:** 533–539.
36. WANG, J.M., D.W. MCVICAR, J.J. OPPENHEIM & D.J. KELVIN. 1993. Identification of RANTES receptors on human monocytic cells: competition for binding and desensitization by homologous desensitization by homologous chemotactic cytokines. J. Exp. Med. **177:** 699–705.
37. GRIMM, M.C., A. BEN-BARUCH, D.D. TAUB *et al.* 1998. Opiate inhibition of chemokine-induced chemotaxis. Ann. N.Y. Acad. Sci. **840:** 9–20.
38. CHUANG, L.F., T.K. CHUANG, K.F. KILLAM, JR. *et al.* 1994. Delta opioid receptor gene expression in lymphocytes. Biochem. Biophys. Res. Commun. **202:** 1291–1299.
39. TOMHAVE, E.D., R.M. RICHARDSON, J.R. DIDSBURY *et al.* 1994. Cross-desensitization of receptors for peptide chemoattractants. Characterization of a new form of leukocyte regulation. J. Immunol. **153:** 3267–3275.
40. FOXMAN, E.F., J.J. CAMPBELL & E.C. BUTCHER. 1997. Multistep navigation and the combinatorial control of leukocyte chemotaxis. J. Cell Biol. **139:** 1349–1360.
41. CAMPBELL, J.J., E.F. FOXMAN & E.C. BUTCHER. 1997. Chemoattractant receptor cross talk as a regulatory mechanism in leukocyte adhesion and migration. Eur. J. Immunol. **27:** 2571–2578.
42. CARMAN, C.V. & J.L. BENOVIC. 1998. G-protein-coupled receptors: turn-ons and turn-offs. Curr. Opin. Neurobiol. **8:** 335–344.
43. ARAGAY, A.M., A. RUIZ-GOMEZ, P. PENELA *et al.* 1998. G protein–coupled receptor kinase 2 (GRK2): mechanisms of regulation and physiological function. FEBS Lett. **430:** 37–40.
44. GUREVICH, V.V., R. PALS-RYLAARSDAM, J.L. BENOVIC *et al.* 1997. Agonist-receptor-arrestin, an alternative ternary complex with high agonist affinity. J. Biol. Chem. **272:** 27497–27500.
45. ARAMORI, I., J. ZHANG, S.S. FERGUSON *et al.* 1997. Molecular mechanisms of desensitization of the chemokine receptor CCR-5: receptor signaling and internalization are dissociable from its role as an HIV-1 co-receptor. EMBO J. **16:** 4606–4616.
46. PITCHER, J.A., Z.L. FREDERICKS, W.C. STONE *et al.* 1996. Phosphatidylinositol 4,5-bisphosphate (PIP$_2$)-enhanced G protein–coupled receptor kinase (GRK) activity: Location, structure, and regulation of the PIP$_2$ binding site distinguishes the GRK subfamilies. J. Biol. Chem. **271:** 24907–24913.
47. WISTEL, R., S. FREUND, C. KRASEL *et al.* 1995. Protein kinase cross-talk: membrane targeting of the β-adrenergic receptor kinase by protein kinase C. J. Biol. Chem. **270:** 2105–2109.
48. CHUANG, T.T., H. LEVINE, 3RD & A. DE BLASI. 1995. Phosphorylation and activation of β-adrenergic receptor kinase by protein kinase C. J. Biol. Chem. **270:** 18660–18665.
49. CHUANG, T.T., L. PAOLUCCI & A. DE BLASI. 1996. Inhibition of G protein–coupled receptor kinase subtypes by Ca^{2+}/calmodulin. J. Biol. Chem. **271:** 28691–28696.
50. PRONIN, A.N. & J.L. BENOVIC. 1997. Regulation of the G protein–coupled receptor kinase GRK5 by protein kinase C. J. Biol. Chem. **272:** 3806–3812.
51. PRONIN, A.N., D.K. SATPAEV, V.Z. SLEPAK & J.L. BENOVIC. 1997. Regulation of G protein–coupled receptor kinases by calmodulin and localization of the calmodulin binding domain. J. Biol. Chem. **272:** 18273–18280.

Neurohormones and Catecholamines as Functional Components of the Bone Marrow Microenvironment

GEORGES J.M. MAESTRONI[a]

Center for Experimental Pathology, Istituto Cantonale di Patologia, Locarno, Switzerland

ABSTRACT: A variety of cytokines and growth factors exert a finely tuned control on the complex series of proliferative and differentiative events called hematopoiesis. Recent studies have shown that neuroendocrine and neural factors may also regulate hematopoiesis. In particular, besides its important immunoenhancing properties, the pineal neurohormone melatonin can also rescue hematopoiesis from the toxic effect of anti-cancer drugs via the action of T-helper cell novel opioid cytokines. In turn, these substances bind κ-opioid receptors expressed in GM-CSF-activated macrophage-like stromal cells and seem to stimulate IL-1. Adrenergic agents can also affect hematopoiesis. We demonstrated that pre-B cells express α_{1B}-adrenoceptors (α_{1B}-AR) and that their activation by catecholamines results in suppressed myelopoiesis *in vitro* or protection *in vivo* against supralethal doses of carboplatin. Most recently, we found that α_{1B}-AR gene knockout mice show a deranged hematopoietic recovery after sublethal irradiation. Regeneration of pre-B cells (the cell type expressing α_{1B}-AR) and of erythrocytes was much faster in knockout than in wild-type mice. Most interesting, bone marrow cells can synthesize both melatonin and catecholamines. As far as melatonin is concerned, human and murine bone marrow cells contain and synthesize melatonin at a concentration that is three orders of magnitude higher than that normally found in serum. Catecholamines are also present in substantial amounts and originate both from nerve endings and bone marrow cells. These findings open interesting new perspectives and include hematology among the disciplines that would benefit from the integrative NIM approach.

INTRODUCTION

The hematopoietic microenvironment that supports blood and immunocompetent cell generation is mainly constituted of bone marrow stromal cells and their products.[1] A variety of soluble factors and cytokines released by stromal cells exert both positive and negative effects on cell growth and differentiation.[2–4] Neuropeptides and/or neurotransmitters, which also seem to be produced by stromal cells, are gradually recognized to take part in this complex regulation of hematopoiesis.[5–8] Consistently, hormonal and neurotransmitter receptors have been described in a variety of immunohematopoietic cells.[6,9–11] In the past several years, our contribution in this field has been focused on the hematopoietic role of the pineal hormone melatonin and of catecholamines. Accordingly, FIGURE 1 shows a scheme of the hematopoietic microenvironment with catecholamines and melatonin highlighted.

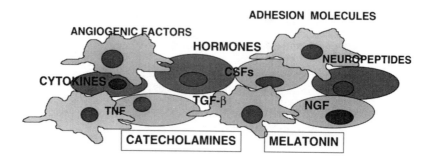

FIGURE 1. The bone marrow microenvironment. Stromal cells and their products are schematized. Among growth factors, transforming growth factor-β (TGF-β) and nerve growth factor (NGF) seem to play an important role. Relatively new entries include catecholamines and the pineal neurohormone melatonin.

CATECHOLAMINES

We have shown that chemical sympathectomy by 6-hydroxydopamine or administration of the α_1-adrenergic antagonist prazosin enhances myelopoiesis and exerts an inhibitory effect on lymphopoiesis.[12–14] These results suggest that the function of the blood-forming system is under sympathetic nervous regulation. Such regulation might be exerted directly on bone marrow cells or indirectly via other mechanisms. To verify this, we investigated whether adrenergic agonists could influence hematopoietic functions *in vitro*. As a matter of fact, we found that when added directly into bone marrow cultures, adrenergic agonists proved to inhibit the number of granulocyte/macrophage colony-forming units (GM-CFU).[14] Also the α_1-selective adrenergic agonist methoxamine and, to a much lesser extent, the α_2-agonist clonidine proved to exert an inhibitory action when added to the GM-CFU assay.[14] The relative potency of these adrenergic agonists in inhibiting the number of GM-CFUs and α-adrenergic antagonists in counteracting this effect were consistent with the presence of α_1-adrenergic receptors (α_1-ARs) on bone marrow cells.[14] As a matter of fact, binding studies revealed the presence of two saturable and specific binding sites (K_d high: 0.98 ± 0.32 nM; K_d low: 55.9 ± 8.2 nM). Competition experiments performed with a variety of α-adrenergic agonists and antagonists gave IC_{50} and K_d values that were compatible with the presence of a high-affinity α_{1B}-AR on bone marrow cells.[14] The remaining site was characterized less clearly, and the results obtained were compatible with a low-affinity α_1-AR. Further studies showed that the high-affinity α_1-AR is present on loosely adherent Mac1⁻B220⁺sIgM⁻ (pre-B) cells. Conversely, the low-affinity α_1-AR seems to be present on Mac1⁺B220⁻ cells.[15] We also showed that norepinephrine administration in mice rescued hematopoiesis from a lethal dose of the non-cell-cycle–specific chemotherapeutic agent carboplatin. At its most effective dose (3 mg/kg s.c.), norepinephrine protected 77% of the mice injected i.v. with 200 mg/kg of carboplatin (LD 100:170 mg/kg)]. The simultaneous administration of the α_1-AR antagonist prazosin brought the proportion of surviving mice down to 30%, indicating that α_1-ARs mediated most of the norepinephrine-induced hematopoietic rescue.[16] More recently, we demonstrated that murine bone marrow contains a substantial amount of catecholamines. Norepinephrine and dopamine showed a circadian rhythm with peak values during the night. The rhythm was disrupted by chemical sympathectomy, whereas epinephrine did not show any rhythmicity or sensitivity to 6-hydroxydopamine (see FIGURE 2).[16] Moreover, norepinephrine and dopamine were found in both short-term and long-term bone marrow cultures. These findings indicate that endogenous catecholamines in the bone marrow have both neural and cellular origin.[17] On the other hand, in a different experimental model, a recent report shows that surgical denervation decreased femoral cellularity as well as hematopoietic progenitor cell concentration.[18]

The cell types that produce catecholamines are unknown. It has been recently reported that catecholamines and their metabolites are present in single lymphocytes and extracts of T- and B-cell clones and that they downregulate lymphocyte function via an autocrine loop.[19] Therefore, bone marrow catecholamines might derive, in part, from bone marrow lymphocytes or from their precursors. Both for lymphocyte function and hematopoiesis, the role of catecholamines seems to be inhibitory.[12–14,19] To mention just one recent finding, in the case of hematopoiesis, this inhibition might be exploited in modulating the bone marrow sensitivity to myelotoxic anti-cancer drugs.[16]

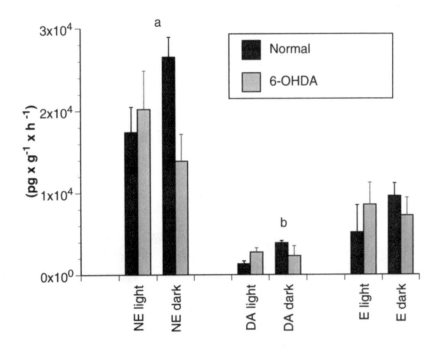

FIGURE 2. Bone marrow catecholamines in the light and dark phase of the photoperiod. Eleven mice were sacrificed per group at different times of a 12-hour light–12-hour dark photoperiod. The area under the curve was obtained by plotting the concentration of catecholamines against time and was calculated using the trapezoidal rule and taken as an index of catecholamine input into the bone marrow over a given time interval. The values represent the mean picograms per gram of tissue per hour. **(a)** $p < 0.02$; **(b)** $p < 0.001$.

HEMATOPOIESIS IN α_{1B}-AR GENE KNOCKOUT MICE

Most recently we had the opportunity to study hematopoiesis in mice with the α_{1B}-AR gene knocked out (KO). First of all, we found that bone marrow cells of WT mice express α_{1A}-AR and α_{1B}-AR mRNA, whereas bone marrow cells of KO mice express only the α_{1A}-AR mRNA (FIG. 3). FIGURE 3 also shows that the α_{1B}-AR is apparently expressed in the murine pre-B cell line 70Z3, confirming our previous pharmacological studies.[15] No difference in blood parameters between KO and WT

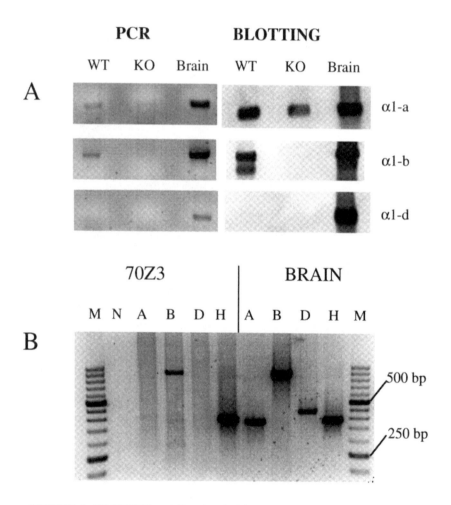

FIGURE 3. (A) RT-PCR and digoxigenin-labeled hybridization of Southern blotting of α_1-AR genes in bone marrow cells. **(B)** RT-PCR of α_1-AR genes in the murine pre-B cell line 70Z3. M: molecular weight markers; N: negative control (no RNA); A: α_{1A}-AR, 375 bp; B: α_{1B}-AR, 687 bp; D: α_{1D}-AR, 428 bp; H: hypoxanthine-phosphoribosyl-transferase, 390 bp. Brain RNA was used as a positive control.

mice under normal physiological conditions was found. Also, the concentration of bone marrow hematopoietic precursors as well as the number of thymocytes and myeloid cells and B and T lymphocytes in the spleen did not show significant differences (data not shown). On the contrary, after sublethal irradiation, that is, during bone marrow regeneration, KO mice showed higher bone marrow cellularity and a concentration of pre-B cells that was at least threefold higher (see FIGURE 4).

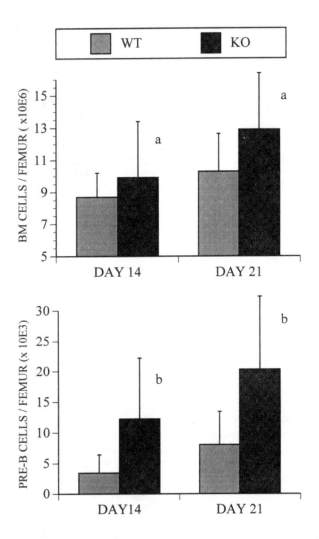

FIGURE 4. Bone marrow cellularity and pre-B cell concentration after sublethal irradiation. Mice were exposed to a total body irradiation of 5 Gy. The values represent the mean ± the standard deviation from 18 mice per group at 14 days and 22 and 24 mice at 21 days after irradiation for WT and KO mice, respectively. **(a)** $p < 0.05$; **(b)** $p < 0.001$.

Due to its vital importance, the hematopoietic function is controlled by a complex network of regulatory mechanisms. It is, therefore, not surprising that, in a steady-state, physiological situation, KO mice did not show significant hematopoietic differences from WT mice. However, this was not the case after sublethal total body irradiation, for example, during bone marrow regeneration. Regeneration of pre-B cells was apparently much faster in KO mice than in WT mice. A more active lymphopoiesis was reflected by higher blood lymphocyte counts (Togni and Maestroni, this volume) and possibly by the higher bone marrow cellularity shown by KO mice. These results, together with the fact that the α_{1B}-AR is expressed in pre-B cells,[15] suggest that the α_{1B}-AR is involved in directly controlling B-cell development. B lymphocytes are produced throughout life, and this process is characterized by large-scale apoptotic cell death constituting an important control mechanism for eliminating potentially harmful cells and regulating the number of mature B cells entering the immune system.[20,21] Many cells at the level of pro-B cells fail to make productive IgH gene rearrangement or sustain errors of DNA recombination and become apoptotic.[21] Surviving cells develop in pre-B cells that then synthesize L chains to form B lymphocytes expressing IgM at the cell surface. A second checkpoint at this stage deletes many cells expressing potentially self-reactive IgM.[21] The α_{1B}-AR might therefore be involved at the level of this second checkpoint as the receptors seem to be expressed only in pre-B cells and not in pro-B or B cells (Maestroni and Togni, unpublished results). The role of the pre-B cells α_{1B}-AR might be relevant in emergency situations such as infections, in which large numbers of B cells have to be recruited and newly formed. Future studies will investigate the humoral immunity of α_{1B}-AR gene KO mice as well as their proneness to develop autoimmune diseases. Taken together, these findings are indicative of a physiological role of catecholamines in hematopoiesis.

MELATONIN

Activation of melatonin receptors enhances the release of Th1 cytokines, such as interferon-γ and IL-2, as well as of novel opioid cytokines.[22–24] Melatonin has also been reported to enhance the production of IL-1, IL-6, and tumor necrosis factor from human monocytes.[24,25] Through these mediators, melatonin may counteract secondary immunodeficiencies, protect mice against lethal viral and bacterial diseases, synergize with IL-2 in cancer patients, and influence hematopoiesis.[26] We have reported that melatonin could rescue hematopoiesis from the toxic effect of cancer chemotherapeutic compounds in Lewis lung carcinoma–bearing mice. Interestingly, a most recent reports confirms the protective effect of melatonin in rats treated with myelotoxic drugs.[27] In contrast, a recent double-blind clinical study in advanced lung cancer patients did not show any myeloprotective effect of melatonin.[22,28] A reason for this failure might be a very deranged immune status due to the advanced stage of the disease. A state of immune activation seems to facilitate the melatonin action. In fact, melatonin may influence the blood-forming system in mice via the induction or stimulation of T-helper-cell–derived cytokines that are recognized by anti-common opioid sequence (Tyr-Gly-Gly-Phe), anti-IL-4 and anti-dynorphin mAbs.[29,30] The mechanism of these melatonin-induced opioids (MIO), which have

TABLE 1. Melatonin in mouse bone marrow and long-term bone marrow culture (LTBMC)

	No. of Mice	pg/mg BM
C57BL/6	5	225.69 ± 89.20
C3H/He	3	195.60 ± 105.70
SJL/J	3	413.82 ± 81.52
LTBMC		74.2 PG/10^6 cells

NOTE: Data represent the mean ± SD. BM, bone marrow.

an apparent molecular weight of 15 and 67 kDa, is dependent on the binding to κ-opioid receptors present in bone marrow macrophages and involves the release of IL-1.[22]

These results suggest a hematopoietic role for melatonin. Recently, we investigated whether bone marrow cells synthesize melatonin directly. We found that both human and murine bone marrow contain high concentrations of melatonin and the enzymatic machinery needed for its synthesis.[31] TABLE 1 shows the melatonin concentration in bone marrow cells from three different strains of mice and from a long-term bone marrow culture. It is noteworthy that melatonin was present in the adherent stromal cells of the culture[31]; that is, melatonin seems to be a component of the bone marrow microenvironment.

CONCLUSION AND PERSPECTIVES

The results reviewed briefly here show that, in analogy with the immune system, the hematopoietic system is also regulated by neural and neuroendocrine agents. The basic finding is perhaps that hematopoietic precursors and/or bone marrow stromal cells may directly synthesize these factors as components of the hematopoietic microenvironment. This does not exclude the possible participation of classical neural or neuroendocrine mechanisms but rather underlines the importance of the hematopoietic role played by these agents. In particular, the role of catecholamines and melatonin is intriguing because it seems to reveal an unsuspected environmental influence on hematopoiesis. The catecholaminergic tone is, in fact, well known to be associated with the rest–activity rhythm, while melatonin is the transducer of basic circadian cues such as the photoperiod. This subtle environmental influence of the blood-forming system might be even more fundamental than that exerted by the cytokine network. Our findings indicate that the endogenous release of multiple hematopoietic regulators may be controlled by neural or neuroendocrine factors. It seems that one has sighted the tip of an iceberg representing a mechanism of hematopoietic regulation capable of transducing environmental information to the blood-forming system. This new, fascinating research avenue calls for further studies. A central question is whether the neural regulation of hematopoiesis plays any role in aplastic anemia, leukemia, and immune-based diseases or during emergencies such as acute infections and/or stress events. Any positive answer to this question might provide a conceptual framework in which new pharmacological strategies to prevent or correct pathological situations could be devised.

REFERENCES

1. DORSCHKIND, K. 1990. Regulation of hemopoiesis by bone marrow stromal cell and their products. Annu. Rev. Immunol. **8:** 11–137.

2. KITTLER, E.L., H. MCGRATH, D. TEMELES et al. 1992. Biologic significance of constitutive and subliminal growth factor production by bone marrow stroma. Blood **79:** 3168–3178.

3. CLARK, B.R. & A. KEATING. 1995. Biology of bone marrow stroma. Ann. N.Y. Acad. Sci. **770:** 70–78.

4. LEMISCHKA, I.R. 1997. Microenvironmental regulation of hematopoietic stem cells. Stem Cells **15:** 63–68.

5. RAMESHWAR, P., D. GANEA & P. GASCON. 1994. Induction of IL-3 and granulocyte-macrophage colony-stimulating factor by substance P in bone marrow cells is partially mediated through the release of IL-1 and IL-6. J. Immunol. **152:** 4044–4054.

6. ADER, R., N. COHEN & D. FELTEN. 1995. Psychoneuroimmunology: interactions between the nervous system and the immune system. Lancet **345**(8942): 99–103.

7. RAMESHWAR, P. & P. GASCON. 1996. Induction of negative hematopoietic regulators by neurokinin-A in bone marrow stroma. Blood **88:** 98–106.

8. AUFFRAY, I., S. CHEVALIER, J. FROGER et al. 1996. Nerve growth factor is involved in the supportive effect by bone marrow derived stomal cells of the factor-dependent human cell line UT-7. Blood **88:** 1608–1618.

9. FELDMAN, R.D., G.W. HUNNINGHAKE & W.L. MACARDLE. 1987. β-Adrenergic-receptor-mediated suppression of interleukin-2 receptors in human lymphocytes. J. Immunol. **139:** 3355–3359.

10. MALEC, P. & Z. NOWAK. 1988. Propranolol enhances in vitro interleukin-2 receptor expression on human lymphocytes. Immunol. Lett. **17:** 319–321.

11. SPENGLER, R.N., R.M. ALLEN, D.G. REMICK et al. 1990. Stimulation of α-adrenergic receptors augments the product of macrophage-derived tumor necrosis factor. J. Immunol. **145:** 1430–1434.

12. MAESTRONI, G.J.M., A. CONTI & E. PEDRINIS. 1992. Effect of adrenergic agents on hematopoiesis after syngeneic bone marrow transplantation in mice. Blood **5:** 1178–1182.

13. MAESTRONI, G.J.M. & A. CONTI. 1994. Noradrenergic modulation of lymhohematopoiesis. Int. J. Immunopharmacol. **16:** 117–122.

14. MAESTRONI, G.J.M. & A. CONTI. 1994. Modulation of hematopoiesis via α_1-adrenergic receptors on bone marrow cells. Exp. Hematol. **22:** 314–321.

15. TOGNI, M. & G.J.M. MAESTRONI. 1996. Hematopoietic rescue via α_1-adrenoceptors on bone marrow B cell precursors and endogenous transforming growth factor-β. In Molecular Biology of Hematopoiesis. Vol. 5. N.G. Abraham, S. Asano, G. Brittinger et al., Eds.: 609–617. Plenum. New York.

16. MAESTRONI, G.J.M., M. TOGNI & V. COVACCI. 1997. Norepinephrine protects mice from acute lethal doses of carboplatin. Exp. Hematol. **25:** 491–494.

17. MAESTRONI, G.J.M., M. COSENTINO, F. MARINO et al. 1998. Neural and endogenous catecholamines in the bone marrow. Circadian association of norepinephrine with hematopoiesis? Exp. Hematol. **26:** 1172–1177.

18. AFAN, A.M., C.S. BROOME, S.E. NICHOLLS et al. 1997. Bone marrow innervation regulates cellular retention in the murine haemopoietic system. Br. J. Haematol. **98:** 569–577.

19. BERGQUIST, J., A. TARKOWSKI, R. EKMAN & A. EWING. 1994. Discovery of endogenous catecholamines in lymphocytes and evidence for catecholamine regulation of lymphocyte function via an autocrine loop. Proc. Natl. Acad. Sci. USA **91:** 12912–12916.

20. LU, L. & D.G. OSMOND. 1997. Apoptosis during B lymphopoiesis in mouse bone marrow. J. Immunol. **158:** 5136–5145.

21. MELCHERS, F., A. ROLINK, U. GRAWUNDER et al. 1995. Positive and negative selection events during B lymphopoiesis. Curr. Opin. Immunol. **7:** 214–227.

22. MAESTRONI, G., F. ZAMMARETTI & E. PEDRINIS. 1999. Hematopoietic effect of melato-
    nin. Involvement of type 1 κ-opioid receptor on bone marrow macrophages and
    interleukin-1. J. Pineal Res. **27:** 145–153.
23. GARCIA-MAURIÑO, S., M.G. GONZALES-HABA, J.R. CALVO et al. 1997. Melatonin
    enhances IL-2, Il-6, and IFN-γ production by human circulating CD4+ cells. J.
    Immunol. **159:** 574–581.
24. GARCIA-PERGANEDA, A., D. POZO, J.M. GUERRERO & J.R. CALVO. 1997. Signal trans-
    duction for melatonin in human lymphocytes. Involvement of a pertussis toxin-sensi-
    tive G protein. J. Immunol. **159:** 3774–3781.
25. BARJAVEL, M.J., Z. MAMDOUH, N. RAGHBATE & O. BAKOUCHE. 1998. Differential
    expression of the melatonin receptor in human monocytes. J. Immunol. **160:** 1191–
    1197.
26. MAESTRONI, G.J.M. 1998. The photoperiod transducer melatonin and the immune
    hematopoietic system. J. Photochem. Photobiol. B: Biology **43:** 186–192.
27. ANWAR, M.M., H.A. MAHFOUZ & A.S. SAYED. 1998. Potential protective effects of
    melatonin on bone marrow of rats exposed to cytotoxic drugs. Comp. Biochem.
    Physiol. **119:** 493–591.
28. GHIELMINI, M., O. PAGANI, Y. DE YONG et al. 1998. Double blind randomized study
    on the myeloprotective effect of melatonin given in combination with carboplatin
    and etoposide in advanced lung cancer. Br. J. Cancer **80:** 1058–1061.
29. MAESTRONI, G.J.M., A. CONTI & P. LISSONI. 1994. Colony-stimulating activity and
    hematopoietic rescue from cancer chemothereapy compounds are induced by mela-
    tonin via endogenous interleukin 4. Cancer Res. **54:** 4740–4743.
30. MAESTRONI, G.J.M. & A. CONTI. 1996. Melatonin and the immune–hematopoietic sys-
    tem. Therapeutic and adverse pharmacological correlates. Neuroimmunomodulation
    3: 325–332.
31. CONTI, A., S. CONCONI, E. HERTENS et al. 2000. Evidence for melatonin synthesis in
    mouse and human bone marrow cells. J. Pineal Res. **28:** 193–202.

The Stress Response and Immune Function: Clinical Implications

The 1999 Novera H. Spector Lecture

GEORGE P. CHROUSOS[a]

Pediatric Endocrinology Section, Pediatric and Reproductive Endocrinology Branch, National Institute of Child Health and Human Development, National Institutes of Health, Bethesda, Maryland 20892, USA

> *The soul sympathizes with the diseased and traumatized body and the body suffers when the soul is ailing.*
> —ARISTOTLE, 4TH CENTURY B.C.E.

INTRODUCTION

The neuroendocrine and immune systems play major roles in the adaptation and, hence, survival of the organism.[1,2] Any "stressor" or threat to the stability or "homeostasis" of the internal milieu is counteracted by adaptive forces of the organism, collectively called "the adaptive response." The central nervous system (CNS) effector of this response is the "stress system" with its main components, the corticotropin-releasing hormone (CRH)/arginine-vasopressin (AVP) and locus ceruleus–noradrenaline (LC-NA)/autonomic (sympathetic) neurons of the hypothalamus and brain stem. These, respectively, regulate the peripheral activities of the hypothalamic–pituitary–adrenal (HPA) axis and the systemic/adrenomedullary sympathetic nervous systems (SNS). Activation of the HPA axis and LC-NA/autonomic system result in systemic elevations of glucocorticoids and catecholamines (CAs), respectively, which act in concert to maintain homeostasis. It is primarily through the stress system that stress influences the innate and specific immune response.

Since Selye's time in the late 1930s, the adrenal glands have been known to shrink the thymus and lymph nodes.[2] Subsequently, the glucocorticoids were found to inhibit lymphocyte proliferation, migration, and cytotoxicity and to suppress the secretion of certain cytokines, such as interleukin-2 (IL-2) and interferon-γ (IFN-γ). These observations and the broad use of glucocorticoids as potent antiinflammatory/immunosuppressant agents over the last 50 years led to the initial conclusion that stress was, in general, immunosuppressive. Recently, however, there has been convincing evidence that corticotropin-releasing hormone (CRH), glucocorticoids, and CAs—as well as other products of the stress system—influence the immune response both at their baseline levels and/or at elevated levels observed during stress.

[a]Address for correspondence: George P. Chrousos, M.D., NICHD, NIH, Bldg. 10/9D42, Bethesda, MD 20892-1583. Voice: 301-496-5800; fax 301-402-0884.
Chrousog@mail.nih.gov

This new understanding helps explain some well-known, but often contradictory, effects of stress on the immune system and on the onset and course of certain infectious, autoimmune/inflammatory, allergic, and neoplastic diseases. In this overview, the current understanding of interactions of the stress and immune systems is presented, and the physiologic and pathophysiologic implications of these interactions are discussed. To avoid extensive citation, several review articles containing many of the original references are included.

HISTORIC MILESTONES

Inflammation was known in antiquity, and almost 2,000 years ago Celsus defined in writing four of the five cardinal signs of inflammation; Eustachius described the adrenal glands in 1563.[1-3] How the brain communicates with the immune system remained an unanswered question until recently. Yet evidence that lymphoid organs are innervated dates back to the end of last century, when nerves were found to enter lymph nodes.

In 1898, von Fürth described a bioactive principle in extracts from animal adrenal glands, which he called "suprarenin." Three years later, Takamine and Aldrich independently isolated suprarenin in crystalline form and named it adrenaline, now also known as epinephrine. Noradrenaline or norepinephrine was formally isolated and identified from tissues a little over 40 years later.

At the turn of this century, Metchnicoff and Ehrlich, respectively, developed the concepts of cellular and humoral immunity, whereas Loeper and Crouzon were the first to describe a pronounced leukocytosis after subcutaneous injection of epinephrine in humans in 1904. In the 1920s Metal'nikov and Chorine showed that immune reactions could be conditioned by classic Pavlovian means, and in the 1930s, Selye described involution of the thymus in animals exposed to stressors. At the same time, he expanded upon the concept of the stress response initially introduced by Cannon. Indeed, Cannon had called this response the "fight or flight" reaction and linked it to stress and to CA secretion.

In the 1940s, von Euler isolated noradrenaline from a lymphoid organ, the spleen, and later provided evidence that NE was the major neurotransmitter released from sympathetic nerves. Cortisone, the ketone metabolite of the active principle of the adrenal glands, was isolated by Kendal and Reichstein in the late 1940s and shown to suppress immune functions. These scientists, along with Hench, received the Nobel Prize in Medicine or Physiology after Hench showed that cortisone produced a spectacular amelioration of rheumatoid arthritis. Interestingly, in the 1950s Dougherty and Frank noticed a 400% increase of what they called "stress lymphocytes" within 10 min after subcutaneous injection of epinephrine. These cells had the morphology of large granular lymphocytes or natural killer (NK) cells, whose function and characteristics were described in the late 1970s.

In the 1970s and 1980s, Besedovsky and coworkers demonstrated that classic hormones and the newly described cytokines were involved in a functionally relevant *crosstalk* between the brain and the immune system. They showed that an immune response induced an increase of plasma glucocorticoid concentrations, altered the activity of hypothalamic noradrenergic neurons and decreased the content of NE in the spleen.

At about the same time, the first comprehensive morphologic studies provided evidence that both primary and secondary lymphoid organs were innervated by sympathetic nerve fibers. Furthermore, it was shown conclusively that classic behavioral conditioning of stressful stimuli or lesions in specific regions of the brain reproducibly altered immune function. Finally, we and others obtained evidence that in experimental animals the susceptibility to autoimmune/inflammatory diseases was determined to a great extent by the activity of the stress system and that stress mediators exerted both pro- and antiinflammatory effects.[1-4]

ORGANIZATION OF THE STRESS SYSTEM

The HPA axis and the SNS are peripheral limbs of the stress system, whose main function is to maintain basal and stress-related homeostasis.[1,2] The central components of this system are located in the hypothalamus and the brainstem (see FIGURE 1). They include the parvocellular neurons of the paraventricular nuclei of the hypothalamus that release CRH and AVP, the CRH neurons of the paragigantocellular and parabrachial nuclei of the medulla, and the A1, A2, A3, and A6 (locus ceruleus, LC) mostly noradrenergic (NA) cell groups of the medulla and pons (the LC–NA system).

Each of the paraventricular nuclei has three parvocellular divisions: a medial group, producing mostly CRH and projecting and secreting into the hypophysial portal system; an intermediate group, producing mostly AVP and also projecting and secreting into the hypophysial portal system; and a lateral group, producing primarily CRH and projecting to and innervating noradrenergic and other neurons of the stress system in the brainstem (see FIGURE 2). Some parvocellular neurons contain and secrete both CRH and AVP, and this neural population increases with stress. Other paraventricular CRH neurons project to and innervate proopiomelanocortin (POMC)-containing neurons of the central stress system in the arcuate nucleus of the hypothalamus, as well as neurons of pain control areas of the hind brain and spinal cord (FIGS. 1 and 2). Activation of the stress system leads to CRH-induced secretion of POMC-derived and other opioid peptides, which enhance analgesia. These peptides also simultaneously inhibit the activity of the stress system by suppressing CRH and NE secretion.

CRH stimulates the secretion of ACTH by the corticotrophs of the anterior pituitary. Its effect on the pituitary is also permissive, because when CRH is absent, very little ACTH secretion takes place. AVP alone has very little ACTH secretagogue activity but is a potent synergistic factor with CRH. CRH and AVP may act synergistically on other target tissues with CRH and AVP receptors in the CNS and perhaps the periphery.

Every hour, the parvocellular neurons secrete two or three mostly synchronous pulses of CRH and AVP into the hypophysial portal system. In early morning, the amplitudes of these pulses are highest, increasing the amplitude and apparent frequency of ACTH and cortisol secretory episodes. The frequency appears to increase because previously undetectable pulses of ACTH and cortisol become measurable by standard assays. During acute stress, the amplitude of CRH and AVP pulses also increases, resulting in increases in the amplitude and apparent frequency of ACTH and cortisol pulses; in this case, the stress system recruits additional secretagogues of CRH, AVP, or ACTH, such as magnocellular AVP and angiotensin II.

Circulating ACTH of pituitary origin is the key regulator of glucocorticoid secretion by the adrenal gland's *zona fasciculata*. Other hormones, including CAs, neuropeptide Y (NPY) and CRH coming from the adrenal medulla, and additional autonomic neural input to the adrenal cortex, also influence glucocorticoid secretion.

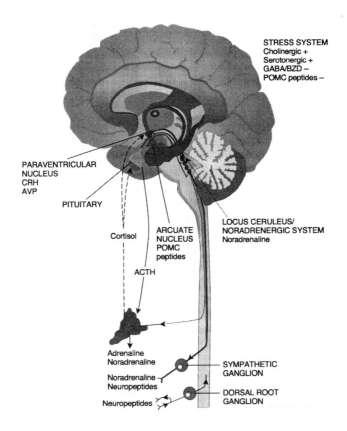

FIGURE 1. Major components of the central and peripheral stress system. The paraventricular nucleus and the locus ceruleus/noradrenergic system are shown along with their peripheral limbs, the pituitary–adrenal axis, and the adrenomedullary and systemic sympathetic systems. The hypothalamic corticotropin-releasing hormone (CRH) and central noradrenergic neurons mutually innervate and activate each other, while they exert presynaptic autoinhibition through collateral fibers. Arginine vasopressin (AVP) from the paraventricular nucleus synergizes with CRH on stimulating corticotropin (ACTH) secretion. The cholinergic and serotonergic neurotransmitter systems stimulate both components of the central stress system, while the γ-aminobutyric acid/benzodiazepine (GABA/BZD) and arcuate nucleus proopiomelanocortin (POMC) peptide systems inhibit it. The latter is directly activated by the stress system and is important in the enhancement of analgesia that takes place during stress. (Reprinted from G.P. Chrousos[2] by permission.)

The sympathetic system, which originates in nuclei within the brainstem, gives rise to preganglionic efferent fibers that leave the CNS through the thoracic and lumbar spinal nerves ("thoracolumbar system"). Most of the sympathetic preganglionic fibers terminate in ganglia located in the paravertebral chains that lie on either side of the spinal column; the remaining preganglionic sympathetic neurons terminate in prevertebral ganglia, which lie in front of the vertebrae. From these ganglia, postganglionic sympathetic fibers run to the tissues innervated. Most postganglionic sympathetic fibers release NE; there are subpopulations of neurons, though, that secrete other active substances as well, including NPY and CRH. Adrenal medulla contains chromaffin cells, embryologically and anatomically homologous to the sympathetic

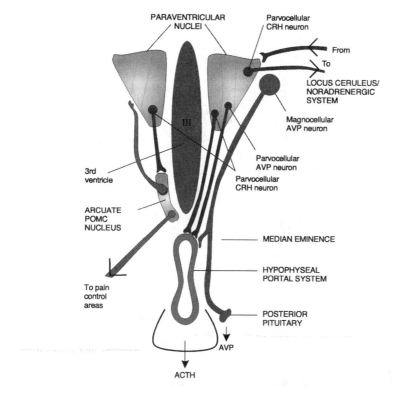

FIGURE 2. A close-up view of the paraventricular nuclei of the hypothalamus. Parvocellular CRH- and arginine vasopressin (AVP)-secreting neurons project to and secrete into the hypophysial portal system. Parvocellular CRH neurons also project to the brain stem to innervate neurons of the locus ceruleus/noradrenergic system. Magnocellular AVP-secreting neurons terminate at the posterior pituitary and secrete into the systemic circulation; they also have collateral terminals in the portal system, however. CRH is permissive for and stimulates pituitary corticotropin (ACTH) secretion, while AVP has a major synergistic role with CRH in the secretion of ACTH. The arcuate proopiomelanocortin (POMC) nucleus is shown, along with the mutual innervation between CRH and POMC peptide–secreting neurons. (Reprinted from G.P. Chrousos[2] by permission.)

ganglia also derived from the neural crest. The adrenal medulla, unlike the postganglionic sympathetic nerve terminals, releases mainly epinephrine, and to a lesser extent NE in an approximate ratio of 4:1; typical preganglionic sympathetic nerve terminals, whose main neurotransmitter is acetylcholine, innervate the chromaffin cells of the adrenal medulla.

Role of Stress System in Maintaining Basal and Stress-Related Homeostasis

The stress system has a baseline, circadian activity, but also responds on demand to physical and emotional stressors.[1,2] Both at rest and during stress and primarily through CRH, glucocorticoids, and CAs, the stress system maintains basal and stress-related *homeostasis*. These substances are major regulators of behavior, fuel metabolism, cardiovascular function, and thermogenesis and adjust these functions according to need. This system integrates and responds to a great diversity of distinct circadian, neurosensory, blood-borne, and limbic signals. This includes humoral and neural signals from the immune and inflammatory reaction. Indeed, any immune challenge that threatens the stability of the internal milieu can be regarded as a stressor, that is, a stimulus to the organism that activates the stress system to help re-attain homeostasis.

Functionally, the CRH and LC-NA systems seem to participate in a positive, reverberatory feedback loop so that activation of one system tends to activate the other as well.[1,2] This includes projections of CRH-secreting neurons from the lateral PVN to the central sympathetic systems in the brainstem, and conversely, projections of catecholaminergic fibers from the LC-NA system, via the ascending noradrenergic bundle, to the PVN in the hypothalamus. Thus, CRH stimulates noradrenaline secretion through its specific receptors, while noradrenaline stimulates CRH secretion primarily through α_1-noradrenergic receptors. Autoregulatory, ultrashort negative feedback loops are also present in these neurons, with CRH and norepinephrine collateral fibers acting in an inhibitory fashion on presynaptic CRH and α_2-noradrenergic receptors, respectively. The CRH, AVP, and noradrenergic neurons receive stimulatory input from the serotonergic, cholinergic, and histaminergic systems and inhibitory input from the γ-aminobutyric acid (GABA)/benzodiazepine and opioid peptide neuronal systems of the brain. Centrally secreted substance P has inhibitory actions on the hypothalamic CRH, but not AVP, neurons and stimulatory effects on the central noradrenergic system.

Activation of the stress system leads to adaptive behavioral and physical changes. Centrally, the behavioral changes include enhanced arousal and accelerated motor reflexes, better attention span and cognitive function, decreased feeding and sexual behavior, and increased ability to withstand pain. Peripherally, the activation of the stress system results in increased sympathetic output, that is, increase of the release of NE from the sympathetic nerve terminals and epinephrine/NE from the adrenal medulla and in increased secretion of glucocorticoids by the adrenal cortex. These changes are related to the physical adaptation that includes changes in cardiovascular function, intermediary metabolism, and modulation of the immune and inflammatory reaction.

Innervation of Lymphoid Organs

Sympathetic/noradrenergic and sympathetic/NPY postganglionic nerve fibers innervate both the smooth muscle of the vasculature and the parenchyma of specific compartments of primary and secondary lymphoid organs.[3] These nerve fibers and their varicosities do travel in plexuses that run adjacent to and along the blood vessels in these organs; it is hence possible that both NA and NPY, released from these fibers, play a role in controlling blood flow to these organs and the traffic of leukocytes within their vessels. However, some noradrenergic fibers, which are not associated with blood vessels, are present in the parenchyma of lymphoid tissues. NE released from their nerve fibers may exert immunomodulatory roles by altering the activity of local leukocytes. Noradrenergic innervation of lymphoid tissues appears to be regional and specific; generally, zones of T cells, macrophages, and plasma cells are richly innervated, while nodular and follicular zones of developing or maturing B cells are poorly innervated.

The main target cells of the noradrenergic innervation of lymphoid organs appear to be immature and mature thymocytes, thymic epithelial cells (TEC), T lymphocytes, macrophages, mast cells, plasma cells, and enterochromaffin cells. Noradrenergic nerve fibers in the thymus are closely associated with mast cells within both the perivascular and parenchymal zones, suggesting a possible humoral role for NE and histamine in the maturation of T cells. Noradrenergic innervation is present early in development, and the arrival of the fibers generally precedes the development of the cellular compartment of the immune system, suggesting a role for NE and/or other products of the SNS in the development of this system.

In addition to the autonomic/sympathetic innervation, all lymphoid organs also receive sensory peptidergic innervation that is confined mostly to the parenchyma. The most abundantly present neuropeptides are the tachykinins, substance P and neurokinin A, calcitonin gene-related peptide (CGRP), and vasoactive intestinal polypeptide/peptide histidine isoleucine (VIP/PHI). Double immunofluorescence reveals coexistence of tachykinins with CGRP and of TH with NPY. This coexistence pattern conforms to the general scheme described for the peripheral innervation of nonimmune organs.

A close spatial relationship between peptidergic nerve fibers and mast cells, T cells, or macrophages is observed in immune organs. Peptidergic nerves, however, are sparse in pure B-cell regions. Neuro-mast cell contacts are present in lymphoid organs, except the spleen. Mast cells bear receptors for and respond to substance P (SP) and CRH; the latter trigger the release of granules containing histamine, cytokines, and lipid mediators of inflammation, including leukotrienes. NA, on the other hand, through the stimulation of α_2- or β_2-adrenoreceptors, stimulates or inhibits the release of granules containing histamine and other proinflammatory substances from mast cells. Thus, apart from their direct immunomodulatory effects, SP antidromically released from sensory nerves, or NA released from postganglionic noradrenergic nerve terminals, may exert indirect immunomodulatory effects via changes in mast cell degranulation within the parenchyma of lymphoid organs.

Neuro-mast cell connections and neuro-macrophage connections, as well as neuro–T-cell contacts, are not restricted to the preformed lymphoid organs and tissues, but are also regularly encountered in most nonimmune tissue. Mast cells, T cells, and macrophages are regularly seen contacted by the terminals of peripheral nerves from the sympathetic and sensory ganglia. In the skin postcapillary venules, macrophages, mast cells, and peptidergic nerves stained for tachykinins/CGRP form a typical quadrad, while in the outer wall of larger blood vessels, the quadrad is joined by TH/NPY fibers. Further, close interrelations but no coincidence of TH/NPY and SP/CGRP immunoreactive fibers are frequently observed in perivascular regions.

THE IMMUNE RESPONSE AND THE INFLAMMATORY REACTION

Any immune response involves, first, recognition of a pathogen, and second, mounting of a reaction against it. Broadly speaking, the different types of immune response fall into two categories: the *innate* (or nonspecific) and the *adaptive* (or specific) immune response.

Phagocytic cells, such as monocytes, macrophages, and polymorphonuclear neutrophils bind to microorganisms, internalize them and kill them. Because they use primitive "nonspecific" recognition systems, which allow them to bind to a variety of injurious agents, they mediate innate immune responses, acting as a first line of defense. However, a subgroup of lymphocytes known as large granular lymphocytes (LGLs) also have the capacity to recognize surface changes that occur on a variety of tumor or virally infected cells and to destroy these cells also using "nonspecific" recognition systems; this action is often called "natural killer" (NK) cell activity. Both monocytes/macrophages and LGLs may also recognize and destroy target cells (or pathogens) coated with specific antibody.

The phagocytic cells that initiate the innate immune response produce a set of proinflammatory cytokines, namely, TNF-α, interleukin (IL)-1, and IL-6 in the form of a cascade, which amplify the inflammatory response locally, influence the adaptive immune response, and serve as signals of an inflammatory response to the CNS (see below).

Lymphocytes, such as T lymphocytes (or T cells) and B lymphocytes (or B cells) are central components of the adaptive immune response, since they specifically recognize individual pathogens, whether they are inside host cells or outside in the tissue fluids or blood. B cells combat extracellular pathogens and their products by releasing antibodies, which specifically recognize and bind target molecules, the antigens. Antigens may be molecules on the surface of pathogens or soluble toxins, produced by them. One group of lymphocytes, the T-helper (Th) cells, exert regulatory function, that is, they interact with B cells and help them divide, differentiate, and make antibody; this group also interacts with mononuclear lymphocytes and helps them destroy intracellular pathogens. Another group of T cells, the T-cytotoxic (Tc) cells, are responsible for the destruction of host cells that have become infected by viruses or other intracellular pathogens. T cells use a specific receptor, the T-cell antigen receptor (TCR), to recognize antigens, but only in association with familiar markers on host cells. This receptor is related, both in structure and function, to the surface antibody, which B cells use as their antigen receptors. T cells generate their effects either by releasing cytokines or by direct cell–cell interactions.

The cells of the immune system are widely distributed throughout the body, but if an infection occurs, it is necessary to mobilize a large number of them at the site of infection. The process by which this occurs manifests itself as inflammation and includes (1) increased blood supply to the infected area by local vasodilatation and (2) increased capillary permeability to permit diapedesis of leukocytes and exudation of plasma containing soluble mediators of immunity. The migration of leukocytes is assisted by a process of chemical attraction known as chemotaxis exerted by cytokines called chemokines (see FIGURE 3).

The cells that participate in the inflammatory reaction are monocytes, polymorphonuclear leukocytes, including neutrophils, basophils and eosinophils, and lymphocytes, all attracted from the blood to the inflammatory site, and local immune accessory cells, such as endothelial cells, mast cells, tissue fibroblasts, and resident macrophages. In the earliest stages of inflammation, neutrophils are particularly

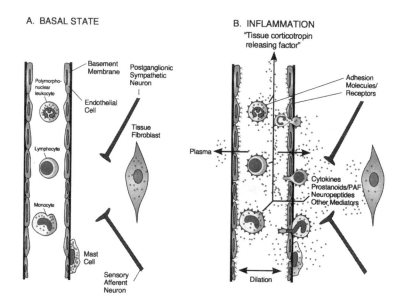

FIGURE 3. Major components and events of inflammation. Quiescent circulating leukocytes, local immune accessory cells, and the terminals of peripheral postganglionic sympathetic and sensory afferent neurons are shown (*left panel*). In inflamed tissue (*right panel*), there is vasodilation, increased permeability of the vessel, and exudation of plasma. Activated leukocytes and endothelial cells express adhesion molecules and adhesion-molecule receptors. Cells attach to the vessel wall, and diapedesis takes place, with chemotaxis towards a chemokine gradient at the focus of inflammation. Activated circulating cells, migrant cells, local immune accessory cells, and peripheral nerves secrete cytokines, prostanoids, platelet-activating factor, neuropeptides, and other mediators of inflammation. Some of these substances, such as interleukin-6, leukotrienes, complement component 5α, corticotropin-releasing hormone, and transforming growth factor-β have chemokinetic activity. Some substances, such as the inflammatory cytokines, tumor necrosis factor α, interleukin-1, and interleukin-6, escape in the systemic circulation, causing systemic symptoms and activating the hypothalamic–pituitary–adrenal axis. Because of such effects, these substances were historically referred to as "tissue corticotropin-releasing factor (CRF)" (Reprinted from G.P. Chrousos[2] by permission.)

prevalent, but in the later stages monocytes and lymphocytes take on a primary role. Local generation of secretory products, including cytokines, lipid mediators of inflammation, and neuropeptides, is crucial for further chemoattraction of cells and for the coordinated activation of the effector cells. Most of the time, these events are clinically undetectable. Occasionally, however, clinical inflammation occurs, generating high concentrations of local and circulating levels of cytokines and other mediators of inflammation associated with systemic illness manifestations and activation of the stress system.

The postganglionic sympathetic neurons and the sensory afferent fibers and of the peripheral nervous system also influence inflammation (FIG. 3). The neuropeptide CRH and the neurotransmitter NA that are released from the postganglionic sympathetic nerve fibers, respectively, exert mostly proinflammatory and antiinflammatory effects locally (see text below). The sensory fibers sense the local threat and not only send signals to the central nervous system, but also secrete proinflammatory or antiinflammatory substances, such as, respectively, the neuropeptides substance P or somatostatin, in the site of inflammation.

Role of Th1 and Th2 Cells and Type 1 and Type 2 Cytokines in the Regulation of Cellular and Humoral Immunity

Immune responses are regulated by antigen-presenting cells (APC), such as monocytes/macrophages, dendritic cells, and other phagocytic cells that are components of *innate immunity,* and by the recently described lymphocyte subclasses Th1 and Th2, which are components of *adaptive immunity.* Th1 cells primarily secrete IFN-γ, IL-2, and TNF-β, which promote cellular immunity, whereas Th2 cells secrete a different set of cytokines, primarily IL-4, IL-10, and IL-13, which promote humoral immunity (see FIGURE 4).

Naive CD4$^+$ (antigen-inexperienced) Th0 cells are clearly bipotential and serve as precursors of Th1 and Th2 cells. Among the factors currently known to influence the differentiation of these cells towards Th1 or Th2, cytokines produced by cells of the innate immune system are the most important. Thus, IL-12, produced by activated monocytes/macrophages or other APCs, is a major inducer of Th1 differentiation and hence cellular immunity; this cytokine acts in concert with NK-derived IFN-γ to further promote Th1 responses. APC-derived IL-12 and TNF-α, in concert with NK cell- and Th1 cell-derived IFN-γ, stimulate the functional activity of T cytotoxic (Tc) cells, NK cells, and activated macrophages, that is, the major components of cellular immunity. All three cytokines, IL-12, TNF-α, and IFN-γ, also stimulate the synthesis of nitric oxide (NO) and other inflammatory mediators that drive chronic delayed type inflammatory responses. Because of these crucial and synergistic roles in inflammation, IL-12, TNF-α, and IFN-γ are considered major proinflammatory cytokines.

Th1 and Th2 responses are mutually inhibitory. Thus, IL-12 and IFN-γ inhibit Th2, and, *vice versa,* IL-4 and IL-10 inhibit Th1 responses. IL-4 and IL-10 promote humoral immunity by stimulating the growth and activation of mast cells and eosinophils, the differentiation of B cells into antibody-secreting B cells, and B cell immunoglobulin switching to IgE. Importantly, these cytokines inhibit macrophage activation, T-cell proliferation, and the production of proinflammatory cytokines. Thus, IL-4 and IL-10 are major antiinflammatory cytokines (FIG. 4).

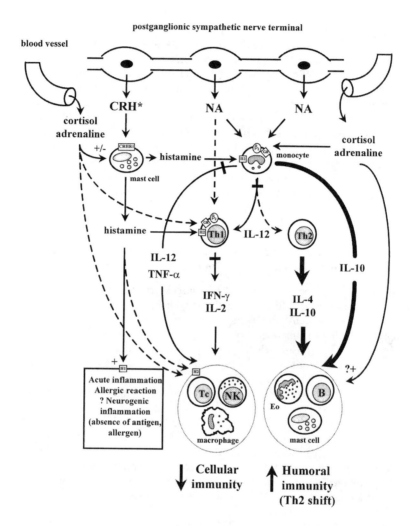

FIGURE 4. Effect of corticotropin-releasing hormone–mast cell–histamine axis, glu-cocorticoid, and catecholamines on Th1/Th2 balance and, hence, cellular and humoral immunity. Stress and CRH influence immune/inflammatory and allergic responses by stim-ulating glucocorticoid, catecholamines, and peripheral (immune) CRH secretion and by altering the production of key regulatory cytokines and histamine (see text). *CRH is also released from sensory nerves upon their activation. *Solid lines* represent stimulation, and *dashed lines* represent inhibition. Abbreviations: CRH, peripheral (immune) corticotropin-releasing hormone; NA, noradrenaline, NK, natural killer cell; GR, glucocorticoid receptor; T, T cell; B, B cell; Th, T-helper cell; Tc, T-cytotoxic cell; Eo, eosinophil; IL, interleukin, TNF, tumor necrosis factor; IFN, interferon. (Reprinted from I.J. Elenkov & G.P. Chrousos[4] by permission.)

EFFECTS OF THE HPA AXIS AND THE SNS ON THE IMMUNE AND INFLAMMATORY REACTION

Adrenocortical Hormones

The antiinflammatory and immunosuppressive properties of glucocorticoids, exerted via their ubiquitous intracellular receptors, make them invaluable therapeutic agents in numerous diseases.[2,5,6] The glucocorticoid receptor is a 777–amino acid cytoplasmic protein with three major functional domains and several subdomains. The carboxy-terminal region binds glucocorticoid, and the middle portion domain binds to specific sequences of DNA in the regulatory regions of glucocorticoid-responsive genes (glucocorticoid-responsive elements).

Glucocorticoids influence the traffic of circulating leukocytes and inhibit many functions of leukocytes and immune accessory cells. They suppress the immune activation of these cells, inhibit the production of cytokines and other mediators of inflammation, and cause cytokine resistance. Subgroups of T lymphocytes are particularly affected by glucocorticoids. Thus, these hormones suppress Th1 function and stimulate apoptosis of eosinophils and certain groups of T lymphocytes. Glucocorticoids also inhibit the expression of adhesion and adhesion receptor molecules on the surface of immune and other cells and potentiate the acute-phase reaction. All of these effects depend on altering the transcription rates of glucocorticoid-responsive genes or changing the stability of messenger RNAs of several proteins involved in inflammation. For instance, glucocorticoids suppress production of IL-6 and IL-1 by decreasing both the transcription rate of the genes for these interleukins and the stability of their messenger RNA.

Among the many proteins regulated by glucocorticoids are the phospholipase A2, cyclooxygenase 2, and inducible nitric oxide synthetase 2 genes. Suppression of these proteins decreases production of prostanoids, platelet-activating factor, and nitric oxide, three key molecules in the inflammatory response. The activated glucocorticoid receptor also inhibits the proinflammatory activity of many growth factors and cytokines by directly interacting with and blocking the third-messenger systems for these hormones. These include the transcription factors c-jun, NF-κB, and CREB. In a mutual fashion, elevated intracellular concentrations of these factors prevent the activated glucocorticoid receptor from exerting its effects on the genome.

Several circadian immune functions cause disease-associated diurnal changes that correspond to plasma glucocorticoid levels.[2] For example, the delayed hypersensitivity reaction, which is particularly sensitive to glucocorticoids, is greatest in the evening, when glucocorticoids are low, and least in the morning, when they are high. The same is true for the cytokine IL-6, whose levels in plasma have a circadian rhythm with peaks in the evening and the early morning hours.

The secretion of adrenal androgens, which, like cortisol, follow the circadian pattern of ACTH, is associated with a distinct developmental pattern with highest levels *in utero,* puberty, and early adulthood.[7] Adrenal androgens with the Δ^5 configuration in the A ring have been suggested as modulators of immune function. An orphan receptor of the steroid-thyroid receptor superfamily specific for Δ^5-adrenal androgens has been detected in T lymphocytes and presumably mediates the potentiation of Th1 cells by these androgens, enhancing cellular immunity.

Catecholamines

Lymphocyte traffic and circulation are under the influence of SNS and CAs.[2,3] In the short term, acutely (less than 30 min), CAs mobilize NK cells from depots; whereas in the long term, chronically, CAs decrease the number of lymphocytes, and particularly of NK cells in the peripheral blood. CAs or β-adrenoreceptor (AR) agonists inhibit the T-cell proliferation induced by mitogens. This is usually accompanied by an increase of cAMP in lymphocytes, and the amount of cAMP produced by T cells stimulated with isoproterenol, a β-AR agonist, is proportional to the degree of inhibition of the proliferation. β-AR agonists exert a similar inhibitory effect on the proliferative response of human highly purified T cells stimulated with immobilized anti-CD3 monoclonal antibody through the CD3/TCR complex.

In vitro and *in vivo* studies reveal that CAs mediate, both acutely and chronically, an inhibition of NK cell activity. Central administration of CRH, which is known to increase the sympathetic autonomic outflow, is accompanied by decreased NK activity in the periphery, an effect that is independent of adrenocortical activation. This effect of central CRH is also rapid: within 20 min of the infusion, lytic values of splenic NK cells decline by nearly 50%, whereas the cytotoxicity of peripheral NK cells is reduced within one hour.

Moreover, several lines of evidence suggest that stress, which is accompanied by increased levels of peripheral CAs, inhibits several components of cellular immunity and particularly NK cell activity, an effect that is mediated mainly by the CRH-SNS axis. Thus, in animals, the central application of anti-CRH antibodies completely blocks the inhibitory effect of footshock stress on NK activity. It appears that NK cells are the most "sensitive" cells to the suppressive effect of stress, and, not surprisingly, NK cell activity has become a *bona fide* index of stress-induced suppression of cellular immunity, employed in many studies. Apart from a direct and acute effect, chronically, during subacute or chronic stress, CAs may suppress NK activity indirectly, though their potent inhibition of the production of IL-12 and IFN-γ, cytokines that are essential for NK activity (see text below).

CAs appear to mediate both inhibitory and stimulatory effects on macrophage activity. This process is influenced by several factors, such as availability of type 1/ proinflammatory cytokines; presence or absence of antigen; presence in the microenvironment of proinflammatory mediators such as SP; peripheral (immune) CRH and histamine, released from the sensory and postganglionic–sympathetic neurons or mast cells, respectively; and the state of activation or differentiation of macrophages, which may determine β-AR responsiveness and the expression of α-ARs. CAs also exert enhancing effects on the initiation of Tc responses, in contrast to inhibition of effector Tc cell function. CAs inhibit both neutrophil phagocytosis and the release of lysosomal enzymes from neutrophils. Furthermore, the superoxide generation and formation of oxygen radicals that play an important microbicidal role are suppressed at nanomolar concentrations of epinephrine, an effect mediated by β_2-ARs.

When B cells and Th cells are exposed to Th cell-dependent antigen, NE, through stimulation of β_2 receptors exerts an enhancing effect on B-cell antibody (Ab) production. One mechanism for this enhancement may involve a β_2-AR-induced increase in the frequency of B cells differentiating into Ab-secreting cells. Moreover, Th cells not only activate B cells via cell-to-cell interaction, but also they (Th2 cells) provide the cytokines necessary for B-cell growth. Here again CAs may play an important modulatory role through their differential effect on type 1 and type 2 cytokine production (see text below). Thus, the β-AR agonists salbutamol and fenoterol potentiate IL-4-induced IgE production by human PBMC, whereas they inhibit IFN-γ production by the same cells. Furthermore, salbutamol induces an increase of the *ex vivo* release of IL-4, IL-6, and IL-10 by human PBMC.

Stress Hormones Suppress Cellular and Potentiate Humoral Immunity

Effects of Glucocorticoids

Glucocorticoids suppress the production of TNF-α, IFN-γ, and IL-2 *in vitro* and *in vivo* in animals and humans.[2,3] As recently shown, glucocorticoids also act through their classic cytoplasmic/nuclear receptors on APCs to suppress the production of the main inducer of Th1 responses IL-12 *in vitro* and *ex vivo*. Because IL-12 is extremely potent in enhancing IFN-γ and inhibiting IL-4 synthesis by T cells, the inhibition of IL-12 production may represent a major mechanism through which glucocorticoids affect the Th1/Th2 balance. Thus, glucocorticoid-treated monocytes/macrophages produce significantly less IL-12, leading to a decreased capacity of these cells to induce IFN-γ production by antigen-primed CD4[+] T cells; the same treatment of monocytes/macrophages is also associated with an increased production of IL-4 by T cells, probably resulting from disinhibition from the suppressive effects of IL-12 on Th2 activity (FIG. 4).

Furthermore, glucocorticoids potently downregulate the expression of IL-12 receptors on T and NK cells. This explains why human peripheral blood mononuclear cells stimulated with immobilized anti-CD3 lose their ability to produce IFN-γ in the presence of glucocorticoids. Thus, although glucocorticoids may have a direct suppressive effect on Th1 cells, the overall inhibition of IFN-γ production by these cells appears to result mainly from the inhibition of IL-12 production by APCs and from the loss of IL-12 responsiveness of NK and Th1 cells.

It is particularly noteworthy that glucocorticoids have no effect on the production of the potent anti-inflammatory cytokine IL-10 by monocytes; yet lymphocyte-derived IL-10 production is upregulated by glucocorticoids. Thus, rat CD4[+] T cells pretreated with dexamethasone exhibit increased levels of mRNA for IL-10. Similarly, during experimental endotoxemia or cardiopulmonary bypass, or in multiple sclerosis patients having an acute relapse, the treatment with glucocorticoids is associated with increased plasma IL-10 secretion. This might have resulted from a direct stimulatory effect of glucocorticoids on T-cell IL-10 production and/or from the disinhibition of the restraining inputs of IL-12 and IFN-γ on monocyte/lymphocyte IL-10 production.

Effects of Catecholamines

CAs drive a Th2 shift at the level of both APCs and Th1 cells (FIG. 4). We recently demonstrated that NA and adrenaline potently inhibited or enhanced the production of IL-12 and IL-10, respectively, in human whole-blood cultures stimulated with LPS *ex vivo*.[8] These effects are mediated by stimulation of β-ARs, because they are completely prevented by propranolol, a β-AR antagonist. Our findings were subsequently extended by other laboratories showing that nonselective β- and selective

β_2-AR agonists inhibited the production of IL-12 *in vitro* and *in vivo*. In conjunction with their ability to suppress IL-12 production, β_2-AR agonists inhibited the development of Th1-type cells while promoting Th2 cell differentiation.

β_2-ARs are expressed on Th1 cells, but not on Th2 cells. This may provide an additional mechanistic basis for a differential effect of CAs on Th1/Th2 functions. In fact, in both murine and human systems, β_2-AR agonists inhibit IFN-γ production by Th1 cells, but do not affect IL-4 production by Th2 cells. Importantly, the differential effect of CAs on Th1/Th2 cytokine production also operates in *in vivo* conditions. Thus, increasing sympathetic outflow in mice by selective α_2-AR antagonists or application of β-AR agonists results in inhibition of LPS-induced TNF-α and IL-12 production; in humans, the administration of the β_2-AR agonist salbutamol results in inhibition of IL-12 production *ex vivo* and acute brain trauma that is followed by massive release of CAs triggers secretion of substantial amounts of systemic IL-10.

CAs exert inhibition on the production of proinflammatory cytokines *in vivo*. Application of propranolol, a β-AR antagonist that blocks their inhibitory effect on cytokine-producing cells, results in substantial increases of LPS-induced secretion of TNF-α and IL-12 in mice. Thus, systemically, both glucocorticoids and CAs, respectively, through inhibition and stimulation of Th1 and Th2 cytokine secretion, cause selective suppression of cellular immunity and a shift towards Th2-mediated humoral immunity. This is further substantiated by studies showing that stress hormones inhibit effector function of cellular immunity components, that is, the activity of NK, Tc, and activated macrophages.

The above general conclusion on the effects of stress hormones on Th1/Th2 balance may not pertain to certain conditions or local responses, at specific compartments of the body. Thus, the synthesis of TGF-β, another type 2 cytokine with potent antiinflammatory activities, is differentially regulated by glucocorticoids: it is enhanced in human T cells but suppressed in glial cells. In addition, NA, via stimulation of α_2-ARs, can augment LPS-stimulated production of TNF-α from mouse peritoneal macrophages, whereas hemorrhage, a condition associated with elevations of systemic CA concentrations, increases through stimulation of α-AR, the expression of TNF-α and IL-1 by lung mononuclear cells.

Because the response to β-AR agonist stimulation wanes during maturation of the human monocyte to macrophage, it is possible that at certain compartments of the body, the α-AR-mediated effect of CAs becomes transiently dominant. Through this mechanism, CAs may actually boost local cellular immune responses in a transitory fashion. This is further substantiated by the finding that CAs potentiate the production of IL-8 from PBMC and epithelial cells of the lung, thus probably promoting recruitment of polymorphonuclear leukocytes to this organ. The "paradoxic" stress-induced potentiation of inflammation in the lung may explain why the "adult respiratory distress" syndrome develops frequently in patients with major infections associated with profound activation of the stress system. Thus, in summary, while stress hormones suppress Th1 responses and proinflammatory cytokine secretion and boost Th2 responses systemically, they may affect certain local responses differently. Further studies are needed to address this question.

The CRH–Mast Cell–Histamine Axis

Central hypothalamic CRH influences the immune system indirectly, through activation of the end-products of the peripheral stress response, that is, glucocorticoids and CAs. CRH, however, is also secreted peripherally at inflammatory sites (*peripheral* or *immune* CRH) and influences the immune system directly through local modulatory actions.[2] We first localized immunoreactive CRH in inflamed tissues of animals with experimental carrageenin-induced subcutaneous aseptic inflammation and streptococcal-cell-wall- and adjuvant-induced arthritis and retinol-binding-protein (RBP)-induced uveitis, and in human tissues from patients with various autoimmune/inflammatory diseases, including rheumatoid arthritis, autoimmune thyroid disease, and ulcerative colitis. The demonstration of CRH-like immunoreactivity in the dorsal horn of the spinal cord, dorsal root ganglia, and sympathetic ganglia support the hypothesis that the majority of immune CRH in early inflammation is of peripheral nerve rather than of immune cell origin.

Peripheral CRH has proinflammatory and vascular permeability-enhancing and vasodilatory actions. Thus, systemic administration of specific CRH antiserum blocks the inflammatory exudate volume and cell number in carrageenin-induced inflammation and RBP-induced uveitis, and inhibits stress-induced intracranial mast cell degranulation. In addition, CRH administration to humans or nonhuman primates causes major peripheral vasodilation manifested as flushing and increased blood flow and hypotension; an intradermal CRH injection induces a marked increase of vascular permeability and mast cell degranulation.[9] Importantly, this effect is blocked by a CRH type 1 receptor antagonist and is stronger than the effect of an equimolar concentration of C48/80, a potent mast cell secretagogue.

Thus, it appears that the mast cell is a major target of immune CRH. This has an anatomic prerequisite: in blood vessels, periarterial sympathetic plexuses are closely associated with mast cells lining the perivascular regions, and plexuses of nerve fibers (noradrenergic and peptidergic) within lymphoid parenchyma are also closely associated with clusters of mast cells. Histamine, a major product of mast cell degranulation, is a well-recognized mediator of acute inflammation and allergic reactions. These actions are mainly mediated by activation of H1 histamine receptors and include vasodilation, increased permeability of the vessel wall, edema, and in the lungs bronchoconstriction. Thus, it is conceivable that CRH activates mast cells via a CRH receptor type 1–dependent mechanism, leading to release of histamine and other contents of the mast cell granules that subsequently cause vasodilatation, increased vascular permeability, and other manifestations of inflammation (FIG. 4).

The last 10–15 years have provided strong evidence that histamine may have important immunoregulatory functions via H2 receptors expressed on immune cells. We have recently found that histamine, via stimulation of H2 receptors on peripheral monocytes and subsequent elevation of cAMP, inhibits the secretion of human IL-12 and stimulates the production of IL-10.[9] Our data are consistent with previous studies showing that histamine, via H2 receptors, also inhibits TNF-α production from monocytes and IFN-γ production by Th1-like cells, but has no effect on IL-4 production from Th2 clones. Thus, histamine, similarly to CAs, appears to drive a Th2 shift both at the level of APCs and Th1 cells. Thus, the activation of CRH–mast cell–histamine axis through stimulation of H1 receptors may induce acute inflammation and allergic reactions, whereas through activation of H2 receptors it may induce suppression of Th1 responses and a Th2 shift (FIG. 4).

Some Generalizations on the Effects of Stress on the
Immune and Inflammatory Responses

The evidence presented above, accumulated over the last decade, strongly suggests that stress hormones differentially regulate Th1/Th2 patterns and type 1/type 2 cytokine secretion. Although interest in the Th2 response was initially directed at its protective role in helminthic infections and its pathogenic role in allergy, this response may have important regulatory functions in countering the tissue-damaging effects of macrophages and Th1 cells. Thus, an excessive immune response, through activation of the stress system and hence through glucocorticoids and CAs, suppresses the Th1 response and causes a Th2 shift. This may protect the organism from "overshooting" by type 1/proinflammatory cytokines and other products of activated macrophages with tissue-damaging potential.

Locally, stress may exert pro- or antiinflammatory effects. This may be influenced by several factors, such as the organ involved, the nature of the response, the presence or absence of antigen, the nature of antigen, and/or the presence and relative expression of particular receptor subtypes on the surface of immune cells (e.g., β_2- versus α_2-adrenergic or H1- versus H2-histaminergic receptors). Despite some stereotypy, stress is not a uniform, nonspecific reaction; and this includes its effects on the immune and inflammatory reaction. Indeed, different types of stressors with their own central neurochemical and peripheral neuroendocrine "signatures" might have different effects on the immune response.

EFFECTS OF THE IMMUNE AND INFLAMMATORY REACTIONS ON THE HPA AXIS AND THE SNS

The last two to three decades have provided evidence that during an immune response, certain cytokines can signal the CNS, which through a complex CRH-dependent pathway triggers activation of both the HPA axis and the SNS.[2] Most of the HPA axis–stimulating activity in plasma comes from three cytokines, TNF-α, IL-1, and IL-6, which are produced at inflammatory sites and elsewhere in response to inflammation. In most situations, TNF-α appears first, followed by tandem secretion of IL-1 and IL-6. All three cytokines stimulate their own secretion from the cells that produce them. In addition, TNF-α and IL-1 stimulate secretion of IL-6, whereas IL-6 inhibits secretion of TNF-α and IL-1. IL-6 acts synergistically with glucocorticoids in stimulating production of acute-phase reactants. Secretion of systemic IL-6 is also increased during stress of noninflammatory etiology, presumably stimulated by stress-induced CAs through a β_2-adrenergic receptor mechanism.

All three inflammatory cytokines independently activate the HPA axis; in combination, their effects are synergistic. Activation can be blocked with CRH-neutralizing antibodies, glucocorticoids, and prostanoid synthesis inhibitors. All three cytokines also directly stimulate CRH secretion in rat hypothalamic explants, and this effect can also be blocked by glucocorticoids and prostanoid synthesis inhibitors *in vitro*. The three inflammatory cytokines also mediate the stimulatory effect of bacterial lipopolysaccharide on the HPA axis. Antibodies to IL-6 almost completely inhibit this effect, suggesting a central role for IL-6 in axis stimulation.

The elevations of ACTH and cortisol attained by IL-6 in human beings are well above those observed with maximal stimulating doses of CRH, suggesting that IL-6 in addition to CRH stimulates parvocellular AVP and other ACTH secretagogues.[11] ACTH levels are already maximal at doses of IL-6 that do not increase peripheral AVP levels. At higher doses, however, IL-6 causes peripheral elevations of AVP, indicating that this cytokine can also activate magnocellular AVP-secreting neurons. This suggests that elevations of IL-6 may be a common etiologic factor in the syndrome of inappropriate secretion of antidiuretic hormone observed in diverse states, such as infectious or inflammatory diseases or trauma.

The HPA axis and the SNS are involved in a long feedback loop between the immune system and the CNS. The afferent limb of this loop seems to operate by blood-borne cytokines, which via circulation or through the afferents of the vagus nerve activate the central components of the stress system. How inflammatory cytokines reach the hypothalamic CRH and AVP neurons is unclear, given that the blood–brain barrier protects the cellular bodies of both kinds of neurons. The cytokines may cause the endothelial and glial cells to secrete prostanoids and IL-6 and other mediators of inflammation, which reach the CRH and AVP neurons in a cascade-like fashion. Alternatively, a special transport system may be present for one or more of the inflammatory cytokines. Also, the inflammatory cytokines may directly activate the terminals of the CRH and AVP neurons in the median eminence, which is outside the blood–brain barrier. Because NA released in this region might exert tonic inhibitory control on CRH release through stimulation of α_2-ARs, it was suggested that TNF-α, by inhibiting NA release, that is, by disinhibition of this control, might trigger an increase of CRH release and subsequently an increase of ACTH from the anterior pituitary.

Inflammation may also activate the HPA axis indirectly, by stimulation of the central noradrenergic stress system through cytokines and other mediators, which act first on stress system neurons of the area postrema that lie outside the blood–brain barrier or on neuron bodies inside the barrier through the endothelial–glial–neuronal cascade mentioned above. In addition, nociceptive, visceral, and somatosensory afferent neurons of the peripheral nervous system from inflammatory sites acutely stimulate the noradrenergic and CRH stress systems through an ascending neural spinal or cerebral nerve route. In fact, several lines of evidence indicate that certain cytokines, such as IL-1 and INF-α, stimulate both the central and peripheral components of the SNS. Thus, administration of IL-1 in the periphery increases the turnover of NA in the hypothalamus and increases peripheral NA and epinephrine plasma levels. Intracerebroventricular and peripheral injection of interferon (IFN)-α or IL-1β produces a long-lasting increase of the sympathetic activity of the splenic nerve and an increased turnover of NA in the spleen.

In addition to their acute effects on the hypothalamus, the inflammatory cytokines can apparently directly stimulate pituitary ACTH and adrenal cortisol secretion at high concentrations or given adequate time for interaction with these tissues.[2,11] Normally, the anterior pituitary and adrenal glands produce IL-6, TGF-β, and other cytokines, which may influence local hormone production. These cytokines may not always stimulate the pituitary gland or the adrenal cortex, however. IL-6, TNF-α, and interferon-γ inhibit the stimulatory effect of CRH on anterior pituitary cell cultures, whereas TNF-α and TGF-β are potent inhibitors of ACTH-induced cortisol production by cultured adrenocortical cells.

Other inflammatory mediators and cytokines, including INF-α, IL-2, epidermal growth factor, TGF-β, prostanoids, and platelet-activating factor (PAF), may also participate in the modulation of the HPA axis activity by inflammation (TABLE 1). The interferons IL-2 and IL-12 may do so indirectly, by causing secretion of inflammatory cytokines. Prostanoids and platelet-activating factor, however, are autacoid amplifiers of hypothalamic CRH and AVP secretion. Receptors for these substances are present in the PVN, and CRH and AVP neurons respond to them.

Certain cytokines or combinations of cytokines have been shown to cause their target tissues to become resistant to glucocorticoids.[2,6] IL-2 and IL-4 together cause glucocorticoid resistance in T cells by markedly decreasing the affinity of the glucocorticoid receptor for its ligand by an as-yet unclear mechanism. In addition, changes in the intracellular metabolism of cortisol into less active or inactive metabolites in cells of the immune system alter the sensitivity of these cells to glucocorticoids.

Inflammatory Stress: A Compound Syndrome

The last 15 years have provided evidence that certain cytokines, and particularly the proinflammatory ones, including tumor necrosis factor (TNF)-α, IL-1, and IL-6, activate both the HPA axis and the LC-NE/SNS system.[2,11] Moreover, these cytokines induce anorexia/nausea, fatigue and/or depressive affect, hyperalgesia with or

TABLE 1. Cytokines and other mediators of inflammation that influence the hypothalamic–pituitary–adrenal axis

Inflammatory Chemokines
Tumor necrosis factor-α
Interleukin-1α and interleukin-1β
Interleukin-6
Interleukin-8
Other Cytokines
Interferon-α
Interferon-γ
Interleukin-2
Interleukin-12
Growth Factors
Epidermal growth factor
Transforming growth factor-β
Lipid Mediators
Prostanoids
Platelet-activating factor

TABLE 2. Inflammatory stress syndrome as a compound of two major biological programs of adaptation

Sickness Syndrome	Classic Stress Syndrome
Anorexia/nausea	Anorexia/stimulation of appetite[a]
Fatigue and/or depressed affect	Motivation/stimulated affect
Somnolence	Arousal
Hyperalgesia ± Headache	Analgesia
Elevated temperature/fever	Antipyrectic
Increased metabolic rate	Increased metabolic rate/return to normal[b]
Acute-phase reaction	Acute-phase reaction
Molecular Effectors	
Inflammatory cytokines, mediators of inflammation	CRH, AVP, glucocorticoids, catecholamines, immune CRH

[a]Initially stimulation of anorexia via CRH; then stimulation of appetite by glucocorticoids.
[b]Initially stimulation of metabolic rate by CRH and CA; then return to normal by glucocorticoids.

without headache, somnolence, sleep disturbances, temperature elevation or fever, and increases of the basal metabolic rate, changes collectively referred to as "sickness syndrome"; these cytokines also activate the hepatic and other tissue synthesis of acute-phase proteins, such as C-reactive protein, cell adhesion molecules, fibrinogen, and plasminogen activator inhibitor 1, a phenomenon referred to as the "acute-phase reaction." Stress that is associated with an immune challenge has been called immune or inflammatory stress, which in fact is a combination of the sickness and classic stress syndromes, along with their effects on the pain/afferent neural systems and the acute-phase reaction (TABLE 2).

AMPHIDROMOUS INTERACTIONS BETWEEN THE STRESS AND IMMUNE SYSTEMS

Short- and Long-Term Adaptations

Chronic activation of either the HPA axis and the SNS or the immune and inflammatory reaction results in reciprocally protective adaptations.[2] Thus, the immune suppression of patients with chronic endogenous Cushing syndrome is quite mild, suggesting that these patients become somewhat tolerant to glucocorticoids. Indeed, even though neutrophilia and eosinopenia persist, the lymphocyte phenotypes and function in these patients are similar to those of age- and gender-matched controls. Animals with chronic inflammatory disease, on the other hand, have mild rather than severe hypercortisolism, which is surprisingly associated with low CRH and high AVP messenger RNA expression and peptide secretion in the hypothalamus.

Peripheral inflammation-induced hypothalamic elevation of substance P, an inhibitor of CRH secretion, has been considered the mechanism by which CRH neuron suppression occurs in certain painful inflammatory states. In addition, elevated levels of certain cytokines, such as TNF-α and TGF-β, may participate in the restraint of the HPA axis by blocking the stimulatory effects of CRH and ACTH on the pituitary gland and adrenal cortex, respectively. Human examples of this are certain patients with septic shock or AIDS and most patients with African trypanosomiasis, who have impaired adrenal responses to stress or exogenous stimuli like CRH and corticotropin.

Chronic activation of the HPA axis is also associated with another adrenocortical adaptation, which leads to a relative decrease in the production of Δ^5-adrenal androgens. This in turn may alter the T-helper phenotype of chronically affected patients towards predominance of Th2.

Influences of Reproductive Hormones

In general, autoimmune diseases affect females more than males.[2] In animal models, androgens usually suppress, whereas estrogens stimulate, certain components of the immune response. The mechanisms of these effects are insufficiently characterized, although estrogens are known to stimulate adhesion molecules and adhesion molecule receptors in immune and immune accessory cells and to activate NO synthase in the vasculature, while the CRH gene and hence immune CRH expression are responsive to estrogen.[12] Prolactin also potentiates the immune and inflammatory reaction *in vitro* and in animals. Inhibition of pituitary prolactin secretion in humans with autoimmune disease has not been effective therapeutically, perhaps because local, autacoid prolactin production may not respond to dopaminergic inhibition.

DISTURBANCES IN THE INTERACTION BETWEEN THE STRESS AND IMMUNE SYSTEMS

Defects of the HPA Axis and/or SNS

Disturbances of the feedback relationship between the HPA axis and the immune and inflammatory reaction have been observed in animals and human states[2] (TABLE 3). An excessive HPA response to inflammation can mimic the stress or hypercortisolemic state, increase susceptibility to certain infectious agents and tumors, and cause resistance to autoimmune or inflammatory disease. Conversely, a defective HPA axis response can mimic the glucocorticoid-deficient state and thus cause resistance to infections and neoplasms, but increased susceptibility to autoimmune and inflammatory disease. Indeed, such properties were identified in Fischer and Lewis rats, two highly inbred strains selected for their resistance (Fischer) or susceptibility (Lewis) to inflammatory disease. In the Lewis rat, the responsiveness of the HPA axis to inflammatory stimuli is decreased, whereas in the Fischer rat HPA axis responsiveness to the same stimuli is increased.

Lewis rats are susceptible to a host of inflammatory diseases such as a rheumatoid arthritis-like syndrome in response to streptococcal cell-wall peptidoglycan, uveitis in response to immunization with retinol-binding protein, and encephalomyelitis in response to myelin basic protein. Fischer rats, by contrast, resist these experimentally

TABLE 3. States potentially associated with suppression or activation of the immune and inflammatory reaction through defects in the hypothalamic–pituitary–adrenal (HPA) axis or its target tissues[a]

Suppression of immune and inflammatory reaction	Activation of immune and inflammatory reaction and sickness syndrome
Increased HPA axis activity	*Decreased HPA axis activity*
Cushing's syndrome	Adrenal insufficiency
Melancholic depression	Rheumatoid arthritis
Chronic active alcoholism	Atypical/seasonal depression
Chronic stress	Chronic fatigue/fibromyalgia
Chronic excessive excercise	Hypothyroidism
Pregnancy (last trimester)	Posttraumatic stress disorder
	Nicotine withdrawal
	Post-Cushing's syndrome cure
	Post glucocorticoid therapy
	Postpartum period
	Late luteal phase
	Climactery
	Post chronic stress
	(Lewis rat)
	(Obese chicken, autoimmune thyroidits)
Hypersensitivity to glucocorticoids	*Resistance to glucocorticoids*
HIV-1 infection (Vpr)	Rheumatoid arthritis
	Steroid-resistant asthma
	AIDS and glucocorticoid resistance
	Degenerative osteoarthritis
	Crohn's disease
	Systemic lupus erythematosus[b]

[a]Taken from G.P. Chrousos.[2]
[b]Secondary to increased catabolism of cortisol in target tissues.

induced diseases. The defect in the Lewis rat was localized to the hypothalamic CRH neuron, which was globally defective in its response to all stimulatory neurotransmitters. The overall HPA axis response to stress was decreased in the Lewis rat; in addition, these animals exhibited chronic elevations of vasopressin as well as behaviors reminiscent of atypical depression in humans, a state characteristized by low hypothalamic CRH secretion.

Do the abnormalities in Lewis rats have parallels in humans? A subgroup of patients with active rheumatoid arthritis might qualify.[2] These patients have low or normal circadian concentrations of ACTH and cortisol despite elevated plasma concentrations of IL-1β and IL-6.[13] Such patients have a poor response to the stress associated with of major surgery, such as large joint replacement, despite dramatic postoperative elevations of IL-1β and IL-6. Like Lewis rats, these patients also have consistently elevated levels of circulating AVP. Similarly to Lewis rats with streptococcal cell wall peptidoglycan-induced arthritis, the inflamed joints of these patients have markedly elevated concentrations of immunoreactive CRH. None of these abnormalities of the HPA axis were present in "control" patients with osteomyelitis (inflammatory disease) or degenerative osteoarthritis.

A key question about human rheumatoid arthritis is whether the hyporesponsiveness of the HPA axis is genetic, constitutional or secondary to a particular type of chronic inflammation or both. To date, the data point to a genetic disturbance that defines increased susceptibility. Prospective studies of families with autoimmune inflammatory disease should test this hypothesis, using a quantifiable benign inflammatory stimulus such as recombinant IL-6.[11]

Other examples suggest that a defective HPA axis increases susceptibility to autoimmune disease or increased immune reactivity (TABLE 3). Given the many behavioral effects of the inflammatory cytokines and CRH, it is not surprising that fatigue, dysthymia, irritability, or even frank depression are frequent in many of these low-CRH states in which one would expect amplification of some sickness syndrome manifestations.

Defects of the Glucocorticoid Target-Tissues

Glucocorticoid hypersensitivity of the immune system can mimic the immunosuppression of hypercortisolism, while glucocorticoid resistance of the immune system may result in excessive immune and inflammatory activity[2,6] (TABLE 3). Six diseases illustrate this mechanism. In rheumatoid arthritis, the concentration of glucocorticoid receptors in circulating leukocytes is reduced by approximately 50%. This phenomenon cannot be attributed to hypercortisolism. Leukocyte resistance to glucocorticoids also occurs in steroid-resistant asthma. Most patients with this disorder have marked but reversible decreases of affinity of glucocorticoid receptors in T-lymphocytes, suggesting an acquired problem, probably associated with elevations of transcription factors such as cjun, NF-κB, and CREB that interact with and neutralize activated glucocorticoid receptors; however, in a small subgroup of patients, glucocorticoid receptor concentrations are irreversibly decreased in all leukocyte subtypes, suggesting a congenital syndrome. In some patients with AIDS, leukocytes also have a marked decrease in the affinity of glucocorticoid receptors for cortisol. In these patients, the glucocorticoid resistance may be generalized, since there are signs of glucocorticoid deficiency, including postural hypotension and hyponatremia, despite elevated levels of corticotropin and cortisol. A fourth disease in which the reduced expression of glucocorticoid receptors and glucocorticoid resistance may have a role is degenerative osteoarthritis. Osteoarthritic chondrocytes contain approximately half of the glucocorticoid receptors of normal chondrocytes and resist dexamethasone-induced suppression of metalloprotease synthesis. Metalloprotease participates in the limited inflammatory destruction of the cartilage in the joints of patients with osteoarthritis. Finally, glucocorticoid resistance has also been observed in patients with Crohn's disease and in patients with systemic lupus erythematosus.

Stress-Induced Th2 Shift: Clinical Implications

A major factor governing the outcome of infectious diseases is the selection of Th1- versus Th2-predominant adaptive responses during and after the initial invasion of the host.[4] Thus, stress and, hence, a stress-induced Th2 shift, may have a profound effect on the susceptibility of the organism to an infection and/or may influence its course, the defense against which is primarily through cellular immunity mechanisms. As an example, cellular immunity, and particularly IL-12 and IL-12-dependent IFN-γ secretion in humans, seems essential in the control of mycobacterial infections and may be of importance in the control of *Helicobacter pylori* infections.

Also, HIV[+] patients have IL-12 deficiency, and their disease progression has been correlated with a Th2 shift.[4] The sympathetic/noradrenergic innervation of lymphoid tissue may be particularly relevant to HIV infection, since lymphoid organs represent the primary site of HIV pathogenesis. NA, the major sympathetic neurotransmitter released locally in lymphoid organs, directly accelerates HIV-1 replication in acutely infected human PBMCs. The effect of NA on viral replication is transduced via the β-AR-adenylyl cyclase–cAMP–PKA signaling cascade. The HIV-1 itself may contribute to the induction of intracellular cAMP through an immunosuppressive, retroviral envelope peptide that causes a shift in the cytokine balance toward suppression of cell-mediated immunity.

Progression of HIV infection is also characterized by increased cortisol secretion in both the early and late stages of the disease. Thus, progressive, albeit mildly increasing glucocorticoid production triggered by the chronic infection, was recently proposed to contribute to HIV progression. Kino *et al.* found that one of the HIV-1 accessory proteins, Vpr, acts as a potent coactivator of the host glucocorticoid receptor rendering lymphoid cells hyperresponsive to glucocorticoids.[14] Thus, on the one hand, stress hormones suppress cellular immunity and directly accelerate HIV replication, while, on the other hand, the virus itself suppresses cell-mediated immunity using the same pathways by which stress hormones, including CAs and glucocorticoids, alter the Th1/Th2 balance.

Major injury (serious traumatic injury and major burns) or major surgical procedures often lead to severe immunosuppression that contributes to delayed wound healing and infectious complications and, in some cases, to sepsis, the most common cause of late death after trauma.[4] A strong stimulation of the SNS and the HPA axis correlates with the severity of both cerebral and extracerebral injury and an unfavorable prognosis. The suppressed cellular immunity is associated with diminished production of IFN-γ and IL-12 and increased production of IL-10, that is, a Th2 shift.

In rheumatoid arthritis (RA), multiple sclerosis (MS), type 1 diabetes mellitus, autoimmune thyroid disease (ATD), and Crohn's disease (CD), the T-helper balance is skewed towards Th1 and an excess of IL-12 and TNF-α production, while Th2 activity and the production of IL-10 are deficient.[4] This appears to be a critical factor that determines the proliferation and differentiation of Th1-related autoreactive cellular immune responses in these disorders. On the other hand, systemic lupus erythematosus (SLE) is associated with a Th2 shift and an excessive production of IL-10, while IL-12 and TNF-α production appear to be deficient.

The effect of stress in the vulnerability to and the onset and progression of autoimmune disorders is extremely complex; often stress is related to both triggering/exacerbation and amelioration of disease activity.[2,4] Animal studies and certain clinical observations suggest that a hyperactive or hypoactive stress system may be associated with decreased or increased vulnerability to different types of autoimmune diseases. Thus, Fischer rats, which have a hyperactive stress system, are extremely resistant to experimental induction of Th1-mediated autoimmune states, including arthritis, uveitis, and experimental allergic encephalomyelitis (EAE). Similarly, women in the third trimester of pregnancy, who have increased levels of cortisol, experience remission of Th1-type-mediated autoimmune diseases, such as RA, MS, type 1 diabetes mellitus, and ATD, possibly via suppression of proinflammatory (IL-12 and TNF-α) and potentiation of antiinflammatory (IL-4 and IL-10) cytokine production. Through a reciprocal mechanism, Th2-type-mediated autoimmune disorders mainly driven by IL-10, such as SLE, may flare up in high cortisol and CA output states, that is, during stress or pregnancy.

Conversely, Lewis rats, which possess a hypoactive HPA axis, are extremely prone to develop experimentally induced Th1-mediated states, such as arthritis, uveitis, or EAE. Similarly, clinical situations associated with decreased stress system activity are associated with increased expression or susceptibility to Th1-type-mediated autoimmune diseases such as RA, MS, and ATD (TABLE 3). These are the postpartum period and the period that follows cure of endogenous Cushing's syndrome or discontinuation of glucocorticoid therapy.[2,12] This might also include the period that follows cessation of chronic stress or a rebound effect upon relief from stressors.

Epidemiologic studies suggest that severe stress, as reported by many patients, often precedes the development of certain Th1-mediated autoimmune states.[4] Viral induction of autoimmunity is thought to occur by either bystander T-cell activation or molecular mimicry. Recent studies suggest that tissue-tropic Coxsackie B4 virus is associated by bystander damage with the development of type 1 diabetes mellitus, while human parvoviruses may be causative agents for rheumatoid arthritis. If future studies confirm these hypotheses, severe stress and, hence, severe suppression of cellular immunity may turn to be a critical factor that facilitates the establishment of pathogenic and tissue-tropic viral infection followed by "autoimmune" tissue damage. At a later stage, severe stress, by skewing the balance towards Th2, may ameliorate disease activity, while acute stress and peripheral release of immune CRH, through its proinflammatory effects, may in some cases exacerbate disease activity.

Allergic reactions, such as asthma, eczema, hay fever, urticaria, and food allergy, are characterized by dominant Th2 responses, overproduction of histamine, and a shift to IgE production.[4] As in the case of autoimmunity, the effects of stress on atopic reactions are complex, act at multiple levels, and can act in either direction. Stress hormones acting at the level of APCs and lymphocytes may induce a Th2 shift, and thus facilitate or sustain atopic reactions; however, this can be antagonized by their effects on the mast cell. Glucocorticoids and CAs (through β_2-ARs) suppress the release of histamine by mast cells, thus abolishing its proinflammatory, allergic, and bronchoconstrictor effects. Thus, reduced levels of epinephrine and cortisol and increased levels of IL-6 in the very early morning could contribute to nocturnal wheezing and have been linked to high circulating histamine levels in asthmatics.

Several lines of evidence suggest that stress can increase the susceptibility to tumors, tumor growth, and metastases.[4] The amount of IL-12 available at the tumor site appears to be critical for tumor regression. Thus, low levels of IL-12 have been associated with tumor growth, as opposed to tumor regression observed with administration of IL-12 delivered *in situ* or systemically. On the other hand, local overproduction of IL-10 and TGF-β, by inhibiting the production of IL-12 and TNF-α and the cytotoxicity of NK and Tc cells, seems to play an inappropriate immunosuppressive role, allowing increased malignant tumor growth. In humans, the augmentation of the rate of tumor progression and cancer-related death has been associated with stress, whereas treatment with cimetidine, an H2 histamine antagonist, correlated with increased survival in patients with gastric and colorectal cancer. These data suggest that stress hormone/histamine-induced suppression of cellular immunity may contribute to increased growth of certain tumors.

SYSTEMIC INFLAMMATION AND WELL-BEING

Like the stress response, the inflammatory reaction of an individual is crucial for survival of the self and species.[1,2] Also like the stress response, inflammation is meant to be tailored to the stimulus and time-limited. A fully fledged systemic inflammatory reaction consists of activation of immune and immune accessory cells and resultant stimulation of two major programs: (1) the sickness syndrome and (2) the classic stress syndrome. As a result, the acute-phase reaction and the pain program, mediated by the afferent sensory and autonomic systems, are also activated (TABLE 2).

Be it an inflammatory focus with spillover of inflammatory effector molecules into the systemic circulation or a truly generalized, systemic inflammatory reaction, the programs that are activated during inflammation have both synergistic and antagonistic actions. For instance, the inflammatory cytokines stimulate coreactive protein production by the liver, and this effect is potentiated by glucocorticoids, which, however, also inhibit the secretion of inflammatory cytokines, bringing inflammation to a close.[2] Most of the manifestations of sickness syndrome, including anorexia/nausea, fatigue, and/or depressed affect, somnolence, hyperalgesia with or without headache, fever, and an increased metabolic rate, are all suppressed by glucocorticoids. Yet, peripheral neuronal CRH activated by stress or the inflammatory reaction, and substance P activated by the inflammatory reaction potentiate inflammation.[1,2]

Chronic systemic inflammation, depending on its degree, varies from asymptomatic to mildly symptomatic, to severely symptomatic. Regardless of the presence of overt sickness syndrome manifestations, chronic elevations of circulating inflammatory cytokines and/or activation of the stress system result in a combination of immune and metabolic disturbances, including endothelial inflammation and/or a Th1 to Th2 switch, osteoporosis, hypercoagulability of the blood, dyslipidemia, insulin resistance, carbohydrate intolerance and/or diabetes type 2, and hypertension.[15,16] Many of these manifestations constitute the visceral fat syndrome, which deteriorates with time in patients with chronic inflammation and/or stress; this represents an exacerbation of a phenomenon that commonly occurs with advancing age in both men and women.[11] These chronic immune and metabolic changes increase all-cause mortality, primarily cardiovascular due to atherosclerosis, but also cancer- and infection-related mortality; they also cause significant morbidity, potentially including clinically significant osteoporosis.

Chronic or intermittent but frequent inflammation due to the presence of inflammatory foci, such as those of allergic rhinitis, bronchial asthma, periodontitis, *Helicobacter pylori* infection, or multiple sclerosis, may be responsible for varying degrees and patterns of sickness syndrome manifestations in these patients and may be associated with the chronic immune, metabolic, and cardiovascular complications of chronic inflammation and stress mentioned above.

Hypercytokinemia is not limited to conditions characterized by classic inflammatory stress, such as trauma and burns, infectious illnesses, autoimmune inflammatory diseases, and allergic inflammatory states (TABLE 4). Inflammatory phenomena in the CNS as seen, for example, Alzheimer's disease or schizophrenia, as well as noninflammatory stress are associated with elevations of IL-6. Interestingly, obesity, especially the visceral type, is associated with chronic elevations of IL-6 in the circulation (see below).

The Chronic Pain and Fatigue Syndromes

Several chronic pain and fatigue syndromes, such as fibromyalgia and the chronic fatigue syndrome, have been associated with chronic sickness syndrome manifestations, such as fatigue and hyperalgesia, and with hypoactivity of the stress system[17] (TABLE 3). Interestingly, these clinical manifestations and the hypocortisolism of these patients are quite reminiscent of mild glucocorticoid deficiency (Addison's disease). Patients with glucocorticoid deficiency have elevated levels of proinflammatory cytokines such as IL-6, which may explain their typical sickness syndrome manifestations.[11,18] When we administered human recombinant IL-6 to such patients, we induced an explosive sickness syndrome which was markedly more severe than that observed in healthy controls; in contrast, patients with endogenous hypercortisolism showed very little or no response to IL-6 (unpublished data). It is tempting to speculate that patients with chronic pain and fatigue syndrome suffer from an imbalance between the immune and inflammatory response and the stress response, which results in excessive sickness syndrome manifestations of the former versus the antithetical effects of the latter (TABLE 2).

TABLE 4. **States associated with hypercytokinemia**

Trauma/burns
Infectious illness
Autoimmune inflammatory disease
Allergic inflammation
CNS inflammation
Noninflammatory stress
Obesity/visceral obesity
Aging

Obesity as a Chronic Inflammatory State

Adipose tissue secretes large amounts of TNF-α and IL-6 in a neurally, hormonally, and metabolically regulated fashion.[19] The plasma levels of these cytokines are proportional to the body mass index (BMI) and are further elevated in patients with visceral obesity.[20,21] The secretion of inflammatory cytokines has a circadian pattern, with elevations in the evening and in the early morning hours.[22] This pattern is maintained in patients with inflammatory diseases and in obese subjects, albeit at a higher level, is affected by the quality and quantity of sleep, and correlates with manifestations of the sickness syndrome. In obesity, the hypercytokinemia is associated frequently with some manifestations of the sickness syndrome, such as fatigue and somnolence, and with the other programs that may be activated during the inflammatory reaction, especially the acute-phase reaction. Thus, obesity, especially the visceral type, can be considered as a chronic inflammatory state, with many of the behavioral, immune, metabolic, and cardiovascular sequelae of such a state.

THERAPEUTIC PERSPECTIVES

Glucocorticoids and agents that potentiate their actions are options for treatment of autoimmune inflammatory diseases. "Designer" anti-inflammatory glucocorticoids with little metabolic activity have reached the preclinical level. By potentiating the secretion or the effects of hypothalamic CRH with CRH secretagogues, CRH agonists, or CRH-binding protein antagonists that cross the blood–brain barrier, it may be possible to prevent the development of inflammatory disease in susceptible persons with a hypofunctional HPA axis and at the same time correct central nervous system symptoms of CRH deficiency. Such an action could be envisioned for nonpeptidic substance P antagonists, which would be expected to reverse the CRH suppression that occurs in chronic inflammatory states and at the same time act as a local antiinflammatory agent.

Antagonists of proinflammatory peptides such as substance P and CRH may control inflammatory diseases or processes in which these peptides have a primary pathogenic role. Depending on their ability to cross the blood–brain barrier and the location of the therapeutic target, these antagonists could be used systemically or in a compartmentalized fashion. We recently employed a nonpeptidic CRH receptor type 1 antagonist, antalarmin, in the treatment of rodent inflammation.[23,24] Antalarmin suppressed acute neurogenic and chronic autoimmune inflammation in animals.

Once the mechanisms of acquired glucocorticoid resistance in rheumatoid arthritis, steroid-resistant asthma, SLE, and other inflammatory diseases are elucidated, therapy with the appropriate intracellular agents that will sensitize the cascade of glucocorticoid action in immune cells, treatment with cytokines or their antagonists, or pharmacological agents that influence their secretion and action may become available for the management of these disorders.

The potential immunopotentiating effects of Δ⁵-adrenal androgens on Th1 cells may be useful in the treatment of diseases such as systemic lupus erythematosus and the final stages of AIDS. A prospective, placebo-controlled study of dehydroepiandrosterone administration to patients with lupus was associated with marked clinical improvement and minimal adverse effects. A similar therapy might be beneficial in other such diseases.

Moreover, blocking the effect of stress by means of β_2-AR and/or H2 antagonists may result in boosting Th1 responses that may be useful in the management of certain infections or tumors, whereas the combined administration of β_2-AR agonists and glucocorticoids may help in the management of certain Th1-mediated autoimmune diseases. Finally, CRH antagonists such as antalarmin may help prevent stress-induced Th1 suppression and triggering of stress-induced allergic or vasokinetic phenomena.[22,23]

REFERENCES

1. CHROUSOS, G.P. & P.W. GOLD. 1992. The concepts of stress and stress system disorders: overview of physical and behavioral homeostasis. JAMA **267:** 1244–1252.
2. CHROUSOS, G.P. 1995. The hypothalamic–pituitary–adrenal axis and immune-mediated inflammation. N. Engl. J. Med. **332:** 1351–1362.
3. CHROUSOS, G.P. & I. ELENKOV. 2000. Interactions of the endocrine and immune systems. *In* Endocrinology. 4th edit. L. DeGroot & L. Jameson, Eds. W.B. Saunders Co. Philadelphia. In press.
4. ELENKOV, I.J. & G.P. CHROUSOS. 1999. Stress hormones, Th1/Th2-patterns, pro/anti-inflammatory cytokines and susceptibility to disease. Trends Endocrinol. Metab. **10:** 359–368.
5. MAGIAKOU, M.A. & G.P. CHROUSOS. 1997. Corticosteroid therapy, nonendocrine disease, and corticosteroid withdrawal. Curr. Ther. Endocrinol. Metab. Sixth edit. C.W. Bardin, Ed.: 138–142. Mosby. St. Louis, MO.
6. BAMBERGER, C.M., H.M. SCHULTE & G.P. CHROUSOS. 1996. Molecular determinants of glucocorticoid receptor function and tissue sensitivity. Endocrine Rev. **17:** 221–244.
7. MASTORAKOS, G. & G.P. CHROUSOS. 1995. Adrenal hyperandrogenism. Chapter 79. *In* Reproductive Endocrinology, Surgery, and Technology. E. Adashi, J. Rock & Z. Rosenwak, Eds.: 1539–1553. Raven Press. New York.
8. ELENKOV, I.J., D.A. PAPANICOLAOU, R.L. WILDER & G.P. CHROUSOS. 1996. Modulatory effects of glucocorticoids and catecholamines on human interleukin-12 and interleukin-10 production: clinical implications. Proc. Assoc. Am. Physiol. **108:** 374–381.
9. THEOHARIDES, T.C., L.K. SINGH, W. BOUCHER *et al.* 1998. Corticotropin-releasing hormone induces skin mast cell degranulation and increased vascular permeability, a possible explanation for its proinflammatory effects. Endocrinology **139:** 403–413.
10. LINK, A.A., T. KINO, J.A. WORTH *et al.* 2000. Ligand activation of the adenosine A2α receptors inhibits IL-12 production by human monocytes, J. Immunol. **164:** 436–442.
11. PAPANICOLAOU, D.A., R.L. WILDER, S.C. MANOLAGAS & G.P. CHROUSOS. 1998. The pathophysiologic roles of interleukin-6 in humans. Ann. Intern. Med. **128:** 127–137.
12. CHROUSOS, G.P., D. TORPY & P.W. GOLD. 1998. Interactions between the hypothalamic–pituitary–adrenal axis and the female reproductive system: clinical implications. Ann. Intern. Med. **129:** 229–240.
13. CROFFORD, L.J., K.T. KALOGERAS, G. MASTORAKOS *et al.* 1997. Circadian relationships between interleukin (IL)-6 and hypothalamic–pituitary–adrenal axis hormones: failure of il-6 to cause sustained hypercortisolism in patients with early untreated rheumatoid arthritis. J. Clin. Endocrinol. Metab. **82:** 1279–1283.
14. KINO, T., A. GRAGEROV, J.B. KOPP *et al.* 1999. The HIV-1 virion-associated protein Vpr is a coactivator of the human glucocorticoid receptor. J. Exp. Med. **89:** 51–61.
15. CHROUSOS, G.P. & P.W. GOLD. 1998. A healthy body in a healthy mind- and *vice versa*: the damaging power of "uncontrollable" stress. (Editorial) J. Clin. Endocrinol. Metab. **83:** 1842–1845.

16. GOLD, P.W. & G.P. CHROUSOS. 1999. The endocrinology of melancholic and atypical depression: relation to neurocircuitry and somatic consequences. Proc. Assoc. Am. Physicians **111:** 22–34.
17. CLAUW, D.J. & G.P. CHROUSOS. 1997. Chronic pain and fatigue syndromes: overlapping clinical and neuroendocrine features and potential pathogenic mechanisms. NeuroImmunoModulation **4:** 134–153.
18. PAPANICOLAOU, D.A., C. TSIGOS, E.H. OLDFIELD & G.P. CHROUSOS. 1996. Acute glucocorticoid deficiency is associated with plasma elevation of interleukin-6: does the latter participate in the symptomatology of the steroid withdrawal syndrome and adrenal insufficiency? J. Clin. Endocrinol. Metab. **81:** 2303–2306.
19. ORBAN, Z., A.T. REMALEY, M. SAMPSON *et al.* 1999. The differential effect of food intake and adrenergic stimulation of adipose-derived hormones and cytokines in man. J. Clin. Endocrinol. Metab. **84:** 2126–2133.
20. VGONTZAS, A.N., D.A. PAPANICOLAOU, E.O. BIXLER *et al.* 1997. Elevation of plasma cytokines in disorders of excessive daytime sleepiness: role of sleep disturbance and obesity. J. Clin. Endocrinol. Metab. **82:** 1313–1316.
21. VGONTZAS, A.N., D.A. PAPANICOLAOU, E.O. BIXLER *et al.* 2000. Sleep apnea and daytime sleepiness and fatigue: relations with visceral obesity, insulin resistance, and hypercytokinemia. J. Clin. Endocrinol. Metab. **85:** 1151–1158.
22. VGONTZAS, A.N., D.A. PAPANICOLAOU, E.O. BIXLER *et al.* 1999. Circadian interleukin-6 secretion and quality and depth of sleep. J. Clin. Endocrinol. Metab. **84:** 2603–2607.
23. WEBSTER, E.L., D.B. LEWIS, D.J. TORPY *et al.* 1996. In vivo and in vitro characterization of antalarmin, a nonpeptide corticotropin-releasing hormone (CRH) receptor antagonist: suppression of pituitary acth release and peripheral inflammation. Endocrinology **137:** 5747–5750.
24. BORNSTEIN, S.R., E.L. WEBSTER, D.J. TORPY *et al.* 1998. Chronic effects of a nonpeptide corticotropin-releasing hormone type 1 receptor antagonist on pituitary–adrenal function, and body weight and metabolic regulation. Endocrinology **139:** 1546–1555.

Oncology in Neuroimmunomodulation

What Progress Has Been Made?

ARIO CONTI[a]

*Istituto Cantonale di Patologia, Centre for Experimental Pathology,
Casella postale, 6601 Locarno 1, Switzerland*

ABSTRACT: In 1987 in Dubrovnik, Yugoslavia, N.H. Spector named a new discipline: Neuroimmunomodulation. R. Ader called this new discipline psychoneuroimmunomodulation when the major emphasis was on its behavioral aspects. Neuroimmunomodulation (NIM) is devoted to the study of the interactions at different morphologic and functional levels among the immune, nervous, and endocrine systems. In fact, this science is the modern manifestation of an old science: in the words of B.D. Jankovic (1987), "Neuroimmunomodulation is a modern reflection in neurosciences and immunosciences of the ideas and experience of philosophers and ingenious observers of ancient Egypt, Greece, China, India, and other civilizations that the mind is involved in the defense against diseases." Twelve years ago NIM was regarded by many conventional scientists almost as a form of witchcraft. Today it may be the fastest growing area of biomedical science research in the world. Important clinical applications will not be far behind. NIM research has also progressed in the field of oncology research. Topics such as treatment of hormone-dependent cancer with analogues of hypothalamic hormones, the role of opioids and T cells in cancer, stress–cancer–immune connections, the anticancer role of melatonin and cytokines, immunotherapy of cancer, and the role of psychotherapy in cancer patients represent some lines of research that have been or are being investigated by scientists. Some areas remain to be thoroughly investigated such as the influence of physical exercise (sports), music (classical or modern), and/or relaxation techniques (e.g. yoga) on the development of human cancer. This paper reviews the role of NIM in oncology and provides some perspectives for further research and development of clinical applications.

INTRODUCTION

Science and art need not be in conflict: both require the use of imagination, cognitive insight, discipline, and creative application. During the last two decades of the millenium, conceptual shifts in neuroimmunoscience have provided new evidence to support intuitive beliefs regarding the connection between the mind–body unit, external and/or internal stimuli such as viruses and bacteria, and primordial environmental stimuli such as the light:dark cycle, moon cycle, tides, magnetic forces, and humidity. Moreover, many new factors such as climate changes, air pollution, the

[a]Address for correspondence: Dr. Ario Conti, Ph.D., Istituto Cantonale di Patologia, Centre for Experimental Pathology, via in Selva 24, 6601 Locarno 1, Switzerland. Voice: ++41 91 756 26 72; fax: ++41 91 796 20 43.
ario@bluewin.ch

rise in world population, particularly in developing countries, the rise of poverty in developed countries, and their social and environmental effects are becoming increasingly sophisticated. Consequently, the role of human management of the ecosystem has begun to be reconsidered by each and every one of us, scientists, politicians, and the lay public.

In light of this new knowledge, the interdisciplinary research of neuroimmuno-modulation (NIM)[1,2] (and psychoneuroimmunomodulation[3]), spanning immunology, neurobiology, neuroendocrinology, and behavioral sciences, is growing. The international society for NIM has active members in 50 countries. This revolution in the basic science will undoubtedly lead in the next century to a corresponding revolution in clinical practice and, most importantly, in the area of preventive medicine.

The interactions among the nervous, endocrine, and immune systems have been investigated from the subcellular to the behavioral levels, using the modern tools of receptor and membrane physiology, biochemistry, pharmacology, immunology, chronobiology, and genetics. Moreover, scientists working in basic research have also become interested in establishing NIM connections with cancer and tumors. Nevertheless, the interest in NIM does not seem to involve the majority of clinicians: until now, oncologists remain skeptical about NIM and integrative studies as applied to cancer.

In fact, a critical analysis reveals that the literature on the relationships between cancer, tumor, oncology, and NIM and their influence on immunocompetence did not involve oncologists except in rare cases and furthermore is so heterogeneous that it seriously challenges the observer's capacity to find any order at all among these studies. For these reasons, I will not attempt here to summarize all papers related to NIM, cancer, and oncology that have been published in the last decades. Instead, I offer only a short and selected review that will address the question posed in the title: What progress has been made in NIM in oncology? I also hope to stimulate basic scientists to involve clinicians (i.e. oncologists) as partners in this beautiful and promising field of research.

CITATIONS FROM 1986 TO AUGUST 1999

Medline, which provides access to nine million citations and other related databases, reports 872 citations from 1982 until August 1999 for the keyword "neuroimmunomodulation (NIM)." Among these, further searching the keywords "NIM-cancer," "NIM-tumor," and "NIM-oncology" yields 63, 125, and 11 citations (1986–August 1999), respectively. Proceedings of four different ISNIM congresses constitute a four-volume, state-of-the-art collection representing most of the areas of research in the field of neuroimmunomodulation.[1,4–6] The tables of contents of these basic books of NIM research suggest the depth and breadth of the subject matter. Nevertheless, despite several years of experimental observations, the clinical application of neuroimmunomodulation, that is, oncology, is still at the beginning stages.

OPIOIDS, OPIATES, MET-ENKEPHALINS, LEUCINE ENKEPHALIN, β-ENDORPHIN, AND PROOPIOMELANOCORTIN AND CANCER

In recent years it has become certain that neuroimmune mechanisms play a role in the defense against cancer. However, these interactions are highly complex, and many variations are possible according to the nature of the neoplasm involved. Recently, a complete review has been published on the connection between neuroimmunomodulation and cancer.[7]

Since 1979, opioids that exert potent modulatory effects on a large variety of reactions[1,8] have been shown to be involved in modulation of tumor growth,[9–11] and therefore they have been studied in many immune functions in cancer patients. Effects of endogenous opioids have been studied on NK activity, α-interferon, interleukin-2, chemotaxis, release of histamine from mast cells, and other actions.[9–12] In particular, methionine enkephalin and leucine enkephalin effects on natural killer cell (NK) activity in isolated peripheral blood lymphocytes from cancer patients indicated a difference in the dose–response effects of both enkephalins between lymphocytes from cancer patients and normal volunteers.[13] Correlations between neuroendocrine (opioid, such as β-endorphin and melatonin secretion) and immune functions (T4/T8 ratio) have been studied in 40 cancer patients with early or advanced neoplastic disease, suggesting that melatonin and β-endorphin secretion have no role in determining immune dysfunctions in cancer.[14] Proopiomelanocortin (POMC), which is the precursor of the multiple-function molecules ACTH, α-MSH, and β-endorphin, has also been reported to be involved in the disease progression of cancer.[15]

INTERLEUKINS

Since their discovery, cytokines (also known as immunocompetent products) appear to exert an important hormonal effect on the endocrine system.[16] The most studied interleukin in cancer diseases and the one most considered as a potential immunotherapeutic agent is interleukin-2 (IL-2). One of the first studies on the immunomodulatory role of IL-2 reported that human glial cells secrete a factor (GSF) that suppresses the mitogen responsiveness of normal human peripheral blood lymphocytes (PBL), expressed as IL-2 production, in a dose-dependent manner. Cellular defects induced by GSF closely parallel the observed defects noted in T cells obtained from patients with gliomas, indicating that the factor elicited from glial tumors may be responsible for the immunological deficits observed in patients with primary malignant intracranial tumors.[17] An advance in the understanding of psychoneuroimmune interactions involved in the control of tumor growth by manipulating host anticancer defenses through a neuroimmunotherapeutic strategy has been achieved by Lissoni. Lissoni's work (1986–1994) has been largely reviewed[18]: his strategy to cope with cancer is based on a neuroimmunotherapeutic approach that proposes a concomitant administration of the pineal neurohormone melatonin with IL-2. Melatonin has been largely confirmed to amplify the antitumor efficacy of IL-2 in humans in different types of tumors.[19–35]

Moreover, two most important immunosuppressive events occurring during IL-2 therapy, that is, macrophage-related suppressive events and release of IL-10, may be abrogated by a concomitant administration of melatonin and IL-12, respectively. Therefore, the association of IL-12 could further amplify IL-2 efficacy with respect to IL-2 alone or IL-2 plus melatonin.[29] Moreover, low-dose recombinant IL-2 (rIL-2) is not only less toxic than high-dose rIL-2 therapy, but is also considered the most physiologic immunotherapeutic strategy to activate the anticancer immune response *in vivo.*[31]

Effects of IL-3 have been also been investigated in non–small cell lung cancer patients in whom serum growth hormone (GH) increased significantly in response to IL-3, whereas prolactin showed a progressive but not statistically significant decrease. Other hormones such as FSH, LH, TSH, melatonin, cortisol, and β-endorphin did not show any variation upon IL-3 injection.[23]

IL-6[36,37] and IL-7[38] have also been reviewed, as have other interleukins. IL-6, mainly produced by monocytes and macrophages, is known to influence the secretions of anterior pituitary hormones and is considered to play an important role in the interaction between the immune and the endocrine systems. IL-6 is considered not only a lymphocyte hormone but also an endocrine messenger because of its secretion by folliculo-stellate (FS) cells (which have been identified as intrapituitary sources of IL-6), whereas in pituitary adenomas the cytokine is produced by tumor cell themselves. According to Renner's work IL-6 may be involved in function and growth of normal and adenomatous endocrine pituitary cells.[37]

HORMONES AND PEPTIDES

Various hormones and peptides have been studied in connection with neuroimmunomodulation and different forms of tumors. Vasointestinal peptide (VIP) stimulated cytotoxicity against human colon cancer cells (CaCo-2),[39,40] but secretin was found to be more effective against erythroleukemia cells (K-562),[41] demonstrating the concept that gastrointestinal peptides can play a role in the regulation of cellular toxicity against tumor cells.[41] The neuropeptide substance P (SP) appears to be involved in the B-cell differentiation process. In fact, SP receptors have been found on a large variety of leukocytes,[42] and receptor-positive cells respond to *in vitro* stimulation with SP in a variety of ways. For example, SP has been shown to enhance IgA and IgM responses by Payer's patch and splenic B cells and can directly interact with clonal B-lymphoma cells and highly purified splenic B cells, suggesting that SP is implicated as a late-acting B-cell differentiation factor that requires an additional triggering mechanism to initiate the B-cell differentiation process.[43] Little is known about the regulation of expression of SP or its receptor in leukocytes. However, early evidence suggests that genes used by neuronal cells and macrophages to encode SP and its receptor are similar if not identical.[43] SP has also been involved in neurohematopoietic communications via a neurokinin-1 receptor (NK-1R) and growth factors. Molecular studies demonstrated in particular that this neuropeptide mediates and induces the production of IL-1 and stem cell factor (SCF) in stroma bone marrow cells, and these cytokines have the potential to autoregulate NK-1 receptors.[44]

Growth hormone (GH) is produced not only by the endocrine system but also by immunocompetent cells. A question arises about the structure of the GH produced by immunocompotent cells. In fact, two human lymphocyte cell lines, a T-cell line and a B-cell line (H9) and (IM9), were shown to produce and secrete an immunoreactive growth hormone (irGH) to Nb2 lymphoma cells whose molecular size is similar to that of pituitary GH as well as irGH secreted by peripheral blood lymphocytes; however, the two molecules are not exactly identical.[42]

Besides VIP and GH, prolactin (PRL) is involved in a wide range of physiological effects and has been cloned in several species. Its immunoregulatory role in different experimental models has already been well documented.[45,46] PRL has been studied in connection with the immune system and tumors[47]: PLR receptors have been detected in human, mouse, and rat lymphoid tissues; and the action of PRL on mitogenesis has been studied on the Nb2 rat lymphoma cell line.[47] Moreover, PRL induces a number of genes after the stimulation of quiescent Nb2 T cells, including c-fos, c-myc, ornithine decarboxylase, interferon regulatory factor-1, and many others.[48] Growth hormone (GH), prolactin (PRL), and insulin-like growth factors have been largely reviewed by Kelley.[49,50]

Luteinizing-hormone-releasing hormone (LHRH), LHRH receptor, and gene expression of LHRH have been implicated in neuroimmunomodulation since the observation that prolactin induced stimulation in the rat Nb2 T- cell line. In fact, LHRH functions in a cytokine-like manner, and results have been clearly demonstrated on rat immature lymphoma T-cell line Nb2, in which the LHRH gene is regulated by PRL at various times during the cell cycle.[48]

New peptides have been purified from tumor cells; for example, a survival-promoting peptide has been purified from medium conditioned by Y79 human retinoblastoma cells and the HN33.1 mouse hippocampal cell line. This peptide maintains cells and their processes *in vitro* for the HN33.1 cell line treated with H_2O_2 and *in vivo* for cortical lesions of the cerebral cortex. It has been demonstrated that such peptides operate by diffusion to regulate and modulate the immune response and thereby rescue neurons that would usually degenerate after cortical lesions.[51] Recently, on the basis of their work on hematopoiesis and bone marrow, which are known to produce positive and negative growth regulators, Maestroni *et al.* reported that adherent bone marrow cells, when mixed with tumor cells, release a bone marrow stromal factor(s) that inhibits the primary growth and metastases formation in mice transplanted with Lewis lung carcinoma or B16 melanoma.[52]

STRESS, CANCER, AND NEUROIMMUNOMDULATION

Neuroimmunomodulation has been associated with the concept of stress, psychosocial and physical stress and life events. The belief that cancer might be related to temperament or distress has been emphasized throughout the history of medicine. The field of psychneuroimmunology, as defined by Ader,[3] has its origins in psychosomatic medicine and has evolved to the investigation of complex interactions between psyche and the nervous, immune, and endocrine systems.[18,53–57] A critical bibliographic search of the literature about psychosocial, primary stress-related variables and their influence on immunocompetence is so heterogeneous and based so much on anecdotal evidence that it is difficult to find anything useful. Immunologic alterations have been noted in a variety of human conditions as, for example, early childhood losses and bereavement, separation, caretaking of seriously ill family members, marital discord, examinations, unemployment, and even commonplace stressors. Experiments using more psychophysiologic stressors, like parachute jumping and space flight, have also revealed immunologic alterations. Most immunologic changes are transient in nature, and their relevance for pathologic conditions is widely unclear. Diverse measures of a range of psychosocial stressors for different populations are related to any of a number of indicators of immune functioning. A given psychosocial stressor may be associated with some markers of immunocompetence but not with others. In humans, some studies provide a clear-cut definition and quantification of stress, but they give little attention to the question of how a particular stressor is perceived and handled by the individual.

Thus, conflicting results have been obtained in a number of psychoneuroimmunologic investigations, especially when the effect of chronic stressors is measured. In human subjects, as opposed to animal models, the immunologic response to a stressor appears to be dependent not only on the nature, duration, and severity of the stressor, but also on its interplay with host factors such as genetic factors, early and other previous experience, age, cognitive functions, ego strength, and psychophysiologic vulnerability. Moreover, not only psychic states, but also personality traits and coping ability appear to be of importance.

Stress acts as an influence that changes the psychophysiologically nonadapted organism's biologic responses and thus influences its reactivity. Depending on the nature, quantity, quality, and duration of the stressor, but also on host variability, the consequences could be on the one hand immune-enhancing and thus salutogenic, and on the other hand, immunosuppressive and interacting with other factors that could be detrimental and pathogenic. In human studies, the evaluation of the individual's coping style has been neglected, as low-anxious, high-anxious, repressive, and defensive coping modes may result in different immune reactions, particularly in subjects dealing with severe and long-lasting adverse life events such as cancer.

At the present, both biobehavioral and psychoneuroimmunology have not developed integrative concepts that unify the different approaches. Bridging this apparent gap in research cannot be left to psychoneuroimmunologists and neuroscientists alone: it requires close and integrative cooperation between those studying the neurological reactions and and those studying the behavioral/social events.[53,54,58,59] In more recent studies in humans, physicians working with cancer patients frequently reported that severe emotional losses and grief occurred in some cases before cancer was diagnosed. In some cases, however, stress apparently does not create cancer, but it might contribute by activating of a latent neoplasia and/or by impairing immunosurveillance during a critical life phase.[60]

Awareness of the interactive relation between psychosocial stressors, neuroendocrine and immunological processes, and tumor progression in patients with cancer appears to be important for clinicians. However, it is not established yet how the available knowledge can be applied therapeutically. For example, in the case of breast cancer hormonal factors play a part in the carcinogenesis of breast cancer where the growth is influenced by several endocrine hormones. Therapeutically, antiestrogen therapy is effective in the treatment of breast cancer. However, several components of the immune system are related to the course of disease in these patients. Psychosocial stressors influence neuroendocrine, that is, corticotropin-releasing hormone (CRH), cortisol, and estrogen, and immunological functions. Clinicians have to consider that psychosocial stressors may be linked to recurrence or survival and that certain coping mechanisms, even those of a negative nature, and the social network of the patient may have therapeutic value. Because recurrence of the disease is still possible many years after curative surgery, multifactorial effects on the course of disease are likely.[56]

In contrast to human studies, a great number of studies using many different animal models with a considerable amount of data on the effects of psychosocial factors on tumor incidence and progression is available in the animal research literature.[61] Generally, these studies have shown that immune functions and/or development of cancer can be altered by early environmental stressors, for example, handling,[62] separation,[63,64] uncontrollable situations,[62] changes in the social environment, and changes in bonding.

Different models of stress (e.g., spatial disorientation, rotational stress, restraint stress, social stress, swim stress, and abdominal surgery)[65–70] and tumors (e.g., Lewis lung carcinoma, TXL5 lymphoma, hepatocellular carcinoma, F344 tumor, CRNK-16 leukemia, A-Rad leukemia, MADB106 mammary carcinoma, and CO47 colon cancer)[68,70–73] and size of inoculum and/or combination with chemotherapeutic agents (e.g. cyclophosphamide)[65–67,69,70,74] have been developed. Psychological and experimental stressors can modulate, presumably via neuroendocrine mechanisms, the host's antitumor responses, which can control metastases and primary tumors independently of each other.

Moreover, a high heterogeneity appears both for the animal tumor system used and for the characteristics of the stressor employed.[67,69,70] Results support the view that mechanisms underlying the tumor-enhancing action of stressors involve the psychoneuroendocrine network and indicate the relevance of chronobiology in experimental cancer research, that is, oncology and neuroimmunomodulation.[70,75]

Overexpression of the gene encoding human transforming growth factor alpha (TGFα),[68] adrenergic modulation of immune resistance factors in controlling metastasis development,[76] and adrenergic[77] and melatonin[71,78–81] modulation of hematopoiesis indicate a possible role in monitoring the use and effects of such drugs in cancer patients.

MELATONIN, NIM, CANCER, AND ONCOLOGY

Interactions of pineal gland and melatonin with other organs, that is, the immune system, as well as with hypothalamic hormones, represent one important approach to the investigation of the etiology and pathogenesis of and therapeutic approach to neoplastic diseases. Between 1966 and 1999, 514 scientific papers were published in the field including the keywords "melatonin and cancer and/or tumor," but only few papers consider the keyword "neuroimmunomodulation." The majority of papers are devoted to basic studies and fewer to clinical investigations.

Altered secretion of neurohormones such as melatonin and β-endorphin in the immunocompetence of 40 patients affected by early or advanced neoplastic disease was first investigated in 1988–1981,[82] and a major clinical study on the effect of melatonin combined with the different interleukins has been reviewed. (See the INTERLEUKINS section.)

In the past several years, interest in the immunophysiological role of the pineal gland and melatonin has grown to the extent that now their immunoregulatory role is widely recognized.[83] Melatonin has immunoenhancing properties, and it is able to counteract the immunodepression induced by acute stress, drug treatment (i.e. anticancer drugs), and viral infections.[83–89] The clinical and therapeutic importance of melatonin in oncology has been reviewed.[18] This review summarizes a series of reports from 1986 through 1994 in which patients affected by metastatic solid tumors, metastatic non–small cell lung cancer, advanced solid neoplasms, myelodysplastic syn-drome, hepatocellular carcinoma, and advanced endocrine tumors were studied. The general conclusion is that melatonin protects against IL-2 and synergizes with the IL-2 anticancer action. This combined strategy represents a well-tolerated intervention to control tumor growth. In most cases performance status and quality of life seem improved.[18] Other pineal hormones, however, have immuno-modulatory activity, in particular 5-methoxytryptophol (5-MTT), which is mainly produced during the light phase of the day. A study was carried out to evaluate the efficacy of low-dose IL-2 in association with both MLT and 5-MTT. The study included 14 untreatable advanced solid-tumor patients (lung cancer: 4; gastric cancer: 3; mesothelioma: 2; hepatocarcinoma: 2; pancreatic cancer: 1; melanoma: 1; colon cancer: 1). The clinical results, as evaluated by WHO criteria after each cycle, consisted of partial response (PR) in 4/14 (29%) (lung cancer: 2; hepatocarcinoma: 1; mesothelioma: 1), stable disease (SD) in 6, and progressive disease in the last 4 patients. The treatment was extremely well tolerated in all patients, and no fever greater than 38°C occurred. These preliminary results show that the neuroimmunotherapy with low-dose IL-2 plus two pineal hormones, MLT and 5-MTT, is a well-tolerated and potentially effective cancer therapy of patients with untreatable advanced solid tumor, with results apparently superior compared to those previously described with IL-2 plus MLT alone.[32]

SPORTS, CANCER, AND NIM

Mens sana in corpore sano. This famous adage postulates that physical exercise is good for health and might prevent the development of diseases such as psychiatric diseases and cancer (or tumors). Scientifc data that confirm such sayings are very few and in some cases controversial.

A first epidemiological study aimed at verifying the relationship between physical exercise (high, moderate, or low) and breast cancer development in women did not seem to confirm the postulate. In fact, the authors concluded that awareness of breast cancer, beliefs about breast self-examination, or engaging in regular physical exercise as a preventive health behavior do not affect the practice of self examination.[90]

On the other hand the prevalence (lifetime occurrence) rate of cancer of the female reproductive system (uterus, ovary, cervix, and vagina) and breast cancer in long-term athletic training may indicate a lower risk of breast cancer and cancers of the reproductive system[91] and a lower prevalence of benign diseases of the breast and benign tumors of the reproductive system among former college athletes compared to nonathletes.[92] The relationship between various indicators of physical activity and endometrial cancer risk was analyzed using data of a case-control study conducted in 1988 to 1991 in Switzerland and Italy on 274 histologically confirmed cases and 572 controls admitted to hospital for acute, nonneoplastic, nonhormone-related diseases. A case-control study was performed in western New York state among 232 women with newly diagnosed endometrial cancer. These studies suggest that a moderate or high physical activity is an indicator of reduced endometrial cancer risk, although these observations still require epidemiologic confirmation and clearer definition from a pathogenic point of view.[93,94] The study of the relationship between physical activity and endometrial cancer (405 endometrial cancer cases and 297 population controls) suggests that physically inactive women may be at increased risk of endometrial cancer because they are more likely to be overweight or obese. Future studies should attempt to obtain more detailed assessments of physical activity, including the intensity with which an individual is engaged in an activity and the actual time involved in exertion.[95]

The most frequently diagnosed cancer in men is prostate cancer. Exercise has been studied as an alterable risk factor that may reduce the incidence, morbidity, and mortality due to this cancer. Unlike other forms of cancer, the bulk of the evidence at this time does not seem to support an overwhelmingly beneficial effect for exercise on prostate cancer risk.[96]

Sport activity and personality and behavior are reported to be important elements in preventing cancer and coronary heart disease.[97] Evidence that physical activity may protect against various forms of cancer has been evaluated in relation to occupational demands, leisure activities, and participation in sports. Some studies suggest that a physically active occupation offers some protection against colon cancer, and an application of Bradford Hill's criteria generally supports the causal nature of the relationship between physical inactivity and an increased risk of intestinal neoplasia. In women active leisure seems to be associated with a reduced prevalence of breast and reproductive system cancer. Physical activity potentially encourages a healthy lifestyle, and it could have more direct effects on certain forms of carcinogenesis.[98] A preventive anticancer strategy associated with physical activity should be considered together with appropriate dietary habits. Among a limited range of foods and beverages, the consumption of rice, green tea, and instant coffee tended to be associated with a decreased risk of adenomatous polyps of the sigmoid colon. Although the associations observed with dietary habits still need to be substantiated, the findings on physical activity lend further evidence to the hypothesis that physical activity may be protective against the development of colon cancer, colorectal cancer, and colorectal adenomas.[99,100]

Important aspects in the aftercare of patients with cancer of head and neck can be realized by physical training in a sports group where this practice can improve subjective quality of life: this concept of rehabilitation should not be missing in the aftercare of patients with malignant cancer[101] or during radiation therapy treatment for breast cancer.[102] The effects of an aerobic exercise program (walking on a treadmill 1 month after bone marrow transplantation) designed to improve the physical performance of patients undergoing bone marrow transplantation have been published.

These results contrast with literature reports indicating that spontaneous recovery of physical functioning after BMT can take many months and that about 30% of patients experience long-lasting impairment of physical performance. The study concludes that fatigue and loss of physical performance in patients undergoing BMT can be corrected with adequate rehabilitative measures.[103] Moreover, a self-paced, home-based walking exercise program can help manage symptoms and improve physical functioning during radiation therapy.[102]

Do physical exercise and sports prevent the development of cancer? It seems that, generally, physical activity may protect against various form of cancer. Nevertheless, existing reports that have been rewiewed are by no means conclusive. Therefore a need remains for well-designed epidemiological studies of this issue. It should be taken into consideration that there are also potential negative effects from some types of exercise, particularly excessive exposure to ultraviolet light in certain water sports. Because moderate exercise seems to elevate mood and help conserve lean tissue, it may be a helpful component of treatment after a neoplasm has been diagnosed. Future work on this topic should (1) attempt to obtain more detailed assessements of physical activity, including the intensity with which an individual engages in an activity and the actual time involved in exertion; (2) investigate in detail the frequency, intensity, and duration pf physical activity as well as the type of activity and period during a person's lifetime exercise might be beneficial; (3) focus on topics such as identifying the role of neuroendocrine factors (hormones, cytokines, peptides, etc.) regulating the immune response to exercise and vice versa, understanding the effect and the appropriate type of physical exercise in patients with diseases that involve the immune system (cancer, autoimmune diseases, viral and infectious diseases, etc.); and (4) individuate the possible long-term role of regular physical activity and/or exercise in preventing such diseases and/or the decline in immune functions that normally occur during the aging process.

MUSICOTHERAPY, TUMORS, AND NEUROIMMUNOMODULATION

The last 20 years have brought oncology and critical care patients great progress but also unique and complex problems. With the explosion of technology and advances in medicine, many intensive care units are seeing an increase in oncology patients. Intensive care units are stressful and frightening. In the hands of a trained music therapist, the use of music therapy in pain and symptom management of patients with long-term and life-threatening illnesses, such as advanced malignant disease, has proven to be a potent nonpharmacologic tool for reducing pain and suffering and improving quality of life. The diversity of its potential applications is particularly suited to the diversity of the challenges—physical, psycho-social and spiritual—that these patients present.[104–108] By altering affective, cognitive, and sensory processes, music may decrease pain perception[109] by distraction, increased control, use of prior skills, and relaxation. Data on the mechanisms and effects of music therapy on mood are controversial and include nonrelevant effects[109] or positive effects.[110] On the other hand, music therapy can decrease a patient's anxiety and side effects when receiving chemotherapy.[111]

CONCLUSIONS AND PERSPECTIVES

I will conclude this paper as I began: science and art need not be in conflict because both require the use of imagination, cognitive insight, discipline, and creative application. Over the last few decades, basic scientific research eliciting connections between cancer, tumors, and NIM has expanded to the point that prospective clinical studies can now be based on a solid rationale.

Additionally, the arts are now viewed as an integral component of holistic care for patients and families. By offering opportunities to engage in the arts and creative expression, persons with cancer can be enabled to mourn, grieve, celebrate life, be empowered to endure their situation, and find healing and meaning. Comprehensive supportive care for cancer patients requires the efforts of an interdisciplinary team (scientists, physicians, pharmacologists, artists, parents of the patients, etc.), and the interdisciplinary and integrative science of neuroimmunomodulation must focus on new strategies to facilitate communication and balance between the mind and body of the patient.

REFERENCES

1. JANKOVÌC, B.D., B.M. MARKOVIC & N.H. SPECTOR, Eds. 1987. Neuroimmune Interactions: Proceedings of the Second International Workshop on Neuroimmunomodulation. Ann. N.Y. Acad. Sci. **496.**
2. SPECTOR, N.H. 1987. Epilogue. *In* Neuroimmune Interactions: Proceedings of the Second International Workshop on Neuroimmunomodulation. B.D. Jankovìc, B.M. Markovic & N.H. Spector, Eds. Ann. N.Y. Acad. Sci. **496:** 750–751.
3. ADER, R. 1981. Psychoneuroimmunology. Academic Press. New York.
4. SPECTOR, N.H., K. BULLOCH, B.H. FOX *et al.* 1985. Neuroimmunomodulation: Proceedings of the First International Workshop on Neuroimmunomodulation. Papers from the workshop held by the International Group on Neuroimmunomodulation (IWGN) at the National Library of Medicine (of the National Institutes of Health) on November 27–December 3, 1984, Bethesda, MD. Gordon and Breach. London.
5. FABRIS, N., B.D. JANKOVIC, N.H. MARKOVIC & N.H. SPECTOR, Eds. 1992. Ontogenetic and Phylogenetic Mechanisms of Neuroimmunomodulation: From Molecular Biology to Psychosocial Sciences. Ann. N.Y. Acad. Sci. **650.**
6. MCCANN, A.M., E.M. STERNBERG, J.M. LIPTON *et al*, Eds. 1998. Neuroimmunomodulation: Molecular Aspects, Integrative Systems, and Clinical Advances. Ann. N.Y. Acad. Sci. **840.**
7. BERCZI, I., D.A. CHOW, E. BARAL & E. NAGY. 1998. Neuroimmunoregulation and cancer (review). Int. J. Oncol. **13:** 1049–1060.
8. PLOTNIKOFF, N.P., R.E. FAITH, A.J. MUNGO & R.A. GOOD. 1986. Enkephalins and Endorphins: Stress and the Immune System. Plenum Press. New York.
9. ZAGON, I.S. & P.J. MCLAUGHLIN. 1983. Opioid antagonists inhibit the growth of metastatic murine neuroblastoma. Cancer Lett. **21:** 89–94.
10. MORLEY, J.E., N. KAY, J. ALLEN *et al.* 1985. Endorphins, immune function and cancer. Psychopharmacol. Bull. **21:** 485–488.
11. AYLESWORTH, C.F., C.A. HODSON & J. MEITES. 1979. Opiate antagonists inhibit mammary tumor growth in rats. Proc. Soc. Exp. Biol. Med. **161:** 18–20.
12. WYBRAN, J.T., T. APPELBOOM, J.P. FARALY & A. GOVAERTS. 1979. Suggestive evidence for morphine and methionine-enkephaline-like receptors on normal blood T lymphocytes. J. Immunol. **123:** 1068–1070.
13. FAITH, R.E., H.J. LIANG, N.P. PLOTNIKOFF *et al.* 1987. Neuroimmunomodulation with enkephalins: in vitro enhancement of natural killer cell activity in peripheral blood lymphocytes from cancer patients. Nat. Immun. Cell. Growth Regulat. **6:** 88–98.

14. BARNI, S., P. LISSONI, M. CAZZANIGA *et al.* 1992. Neuroimmunotherapy with subcutaneous low-dose interleukin-2 and the pineal hormone melatonin as a second-line treatment in metastatic colorectal carcinoma. Tumori **78:** 383–387.
15. SLOMINSKI, A., R. PAUS & J. WORTSMAN. 1993. On the potential role of proopiomelanocortin in skin physiology and pathology. Mol. Cell. Endocrinol. **93:** C1–6.
16. KNIGHT, R., N. SARLIS & A. STEPHANOU. 1992. Interleukins and neurohormones: a common language. Postgrad. Med. J. **68:** 603–605.
17. ELLIOTT, L.H., W.H. BROOKS & T.L. ROSZMAN. 1992. Suppression of high affinity IL-2 receptors on mitogen activated lymphocytes by glioma-derived suppressor factor. J. Neurooncol. **14:** 1–7.
18. CONTI, A. & G.J.M. MAESTRONI. 1995. The clinical neuroimmuno-therapeutic role of melatonin in oncology. J. Pineal Res. **19:** 103–110.
19. LISSONI, P., F. BRIVIO, S. BARNI *et al.* 1990. Neuroimmunotherapy of human cancer with interleukin-2 and the neurohormone melatonin: its efficacy in preventing hypotension. Anticancer Res. **10:** 1759–1761.
20. LISSONI, P., S. BARNI, C. ARCHILLI *et al.* 1990. Endocrine effects of a 24-hour intravenous infusion of interleukin-2 in the immunotherapy of cancer. Anticancer Res. **10:** 753–757.
21. LISSONI, P., S. BARNI, F. ROVELLI *et al.* 1990. The biological significance of soluble interleukin-2 receptors in solid tumors. Eur. J. Cancer **26:** 33–36.
22. LISSONI, P., E. TISI, F. BRIVIO *et al.* 1991. Modulation of interleukin-2-induced macrophage activation in cancer patients by the pineal hormone melatonin. J. Biol. Regul. Homeost. Agents **5:** 154–156.
23. LISSONI, P., F. ROVELLI, E. TISI *et al.* 1992. Endocrine effects of human recombinant interleukin-3 in cancer patients. Int. J. Biol. Markers **7:** 230–233.
24. LISSONI, P., S. BARNI, A. ARDIZZOIA *et al.* 1992. Immunological effects of a single evening subcutaneous injection of low-dose interleukin-2 in association with the pineal hormone melatonin in advanced cancer patients. J. Biol. Regul. Homeost. Agents. **6:** 132–136.
25. LISSONI, P., S. BARNI, G. TANCINI *et al.* 1993. A study of the mechanisms involved in the immunostimulatory action of the pineal hormone in cancer patients. Oncology **50:** 399–402.
26. LISSONI, P., S. BARNI, F. ROVELLI *et al.* 1993. Neuroimmunotherapy of advanced solid neoplasms with single evening subcutaneous injection of low-dose interleukin-2 and melatonin: preliminary results. Eur. J. Cancer **2:** 185–189.
27. LISSONI, P., A. ARDIZZOIA, E. TISI *et al.* 1993. Amplification of eosinophilia by melatonin during the immunotherapy of cancer with interleukin-2. J. Biol. Regul. Homeost. Agents **7:** 34–36.
28. LISSONI, P., S. BARNI, A. ARDIZZOIA *et al.* 1994. A randomized study with the pineal hormone melatonin versus supportive care alone in patients with brain metastases due to solid neoplasms. Cancer **73:** 699–701.
29. LISSONI, P., S. PITTALIS, F. ROVELLI *et al.* 1995. Interleukin-2, melatonin and interleukin-12 as a possible neuroimmune combination in the biotherapy of cancer. J. Biol. Regul. Homeost. Agents **9:** 63–66.
30. LISSONI, P., S. BARNI, V. FOSSATI *et al.* 1995. A randomized study of neuroimmunotherapy with low-dose subcutaneous interleukin-2 plus melatonin compared to supportive care alone in patients with untreatable metastatic solid tumor. Support Care Cancer **3:** 194–197.
31. LISSONI, P. 1996. Effects of low-dose recombinant interleukin-2 in human malignancies. Cancer J. Sci. Am. **3:** S115–120.
32. LISSONI, P., L. FUMAGALLI, F. PAOLOROSSI *et al.* 1997. Anticancer neuroimmunomodulation by pineal hormones other than melatonin: preliminary phase II study of the pineal indole 5-methoxytryptophol in association with low-dose IL-2 and melatonin. J. Biol. Regul. Homeost. Agents **11:** 119–122.
33. LISSONI, P., F. PAOLOROSSI, A. ARDIZZOIA *et al.* 1997. A randomized study of chemotherapy with cisplatin plus etoposide versus chemoendocrine therapy with cisplatin, etoposide and the pineal hormone melatonin as a first-line treatment of advanced non-small cell lung cancer patients in a poor clinical state. J. Pineal Res. **23:** 15–19.

34. LISSONI, P., G. TANCINI, S. BARNI et al. 1997. Treatment of cancer chemotherapy-induced toxicity with the pineal hormone melatonin. Support Care Cancer 5: 126–129.

35. LISSONI, P., M. CAZZANIGA, G. TANCINI et al. 1997. Reversal of clinical resistance to LHRH analogue in metastatic prostate cancer by the pineal hormone melatonin: efficacy of LHRH analogue plus melatonin in patients progressing on LHRH analogue alone. Eur. Urol. 31: 178–181.

36. LOTZ, M. 1995. Interleukin-6: a comprehensive review. Cancer Treat. Res. 80: 209–233.

37. RENNER, U., J. GLODDEK, M.P. PEREDA et al. 1998, Regulation and role of intrapituitary IL-6 production by folliculostellate cells. Domest. Anim. Endocrinol. 15: 353–362.

38. APPASAMY, P.M. 1995. Interleukin-7 and lymphopoiesis: biological and clinical implications. Cancer Treat. Res. 80: 235–233.

39. MUTT, V. 1988. Vasoactive intestinal polypeptide and related peptides: isolation and chemistry. Ann. N.Y. Acad. Sci. 527: 1–19.

40. GOETZL, E.J., R.P. PANKHANIYA, G.O. GAUFO et al. 1998. Selectivity of effects of vasoactive intestinal petide on macrophages and lymphocytes in compartmental immune responses. In Neuroimmunomodulation: Molecular Aspects, Integrative Systems, and Clinical Advances. A.M. McCann, E.M. Sternberg, J.M. Lipton et al., Eds. Ann. N.Y. Acad. Sci. 840: 540–550.

41. VAN TOL, E.A., H.W. VERSPAGET, A.S. PENA et al. 1991. Modulatory effects of VIP and related peptides from the gastrointestinal tract on cell mediated cytotoxicity against tumor cells in vitro. Immunol. Invest. 20: 257–267.

42. BOST, K.L., S.A. BREEDING & D.W. PASCUAL. 1992. Modulation of the mRNAs encoding substance P and its receptor in rat macrophages by LPS. Reg. Immunol. 4: 105–112.

43. PASCUAL, D.W., K.L. BOST, J. XU-AMANO et al. 1992. The cytokine-like action of substance P upon B-cell differentiation. Reg. Immunol. 4: 100–104.

44. RAMESHWAR, P. & P. GASCON. 1995. Substance P (SP) mediates production of stem cell factor and interleukin-1 in bone marrow stroma: potential autoregulatory role for these cytokines in SP receptor expression and induction. Blood 86: 482–490.

45. GOFFIN, V., B. BOUCHARD, C.J. ORMANDY et al. 1998. Prolactin: a hormone at the crossroads of neuroimmunoendocrinology. In Neuroimmunomodulation: Molecular Aspects, Integrative Systems, and Clinical Advances. A.M. McCann, E.M. Sternberg, J.M. Lipton et al., Eds. Ann. N.Y. Acad. Sci. 840: 498–509.

46. WALKER, S.A., R.W. MCMURRAY, J.M. HOURI et al. 1998. Effects of prolactin in stimulating disease activity in systemic lupus erythematosus. In Neuroimmunomodulation: Molecular Aspects, Integrative Systems, and Clinical Advances. A.M. McCann, E.M. Sternberg, J.M. Lipton et al., Eds. Ann. N.Y. Acad. Sci. 840: 762–772.

47. FERRAG, F., J.J. LEBRUN, P. TOURAINE et al. 1994. Prolactin and the immune system. Immunomethods 5: 21–30.

48. WILSON, T.M., L.Y. YU-LEE & M.R. KELLEY. 1995. Coordinate gene expression of luteinizing hormone-releasing hormone (LHRH) and the LHRH receptor after prolactin stimulation in the rat Nb2 T-cell line: implications for a role in neuroimmunomodulation and cell cycle gene expression. Mol. Endocrinol. 9: 44–53.

49. KELLEY, K.W., S. ARKINS & Y.M. LI. 1992. Growth hormone, prolactin and insulin-like growth factors: new jobs for old players. Brain Behav. Immun. 6: 317–326.

50. KELLEY, K.K., W.A. MEIER, C. MINSHALL et al. 1998. Insulin growth factor-I inhibits apoptosis in haematopoietic progenitor cells. In Neuroimmunomodulation: Molecular Aspects, Integrative Systems and Clinical Advances. A.M. McCann, E.M. Sternberg, J.M. Lipton et al., Eds. Ann. N.Y. Acad. Sci. 840: 518–524.

51. CUNNINGHAM, T.J., L. HODGE, D. SPEICHER et al. 1998. Identification of a survival-promoting peptide in medium conditioned by oxidatively stressed cell lines of nervous system origin. J. Neurosci. 18: 7047–7060.

52. MAESTRONI, G.J.M., E. HERTENS & P. GALLI. 1999. Factor(s) from nonmacrophage bone marrow stromal cells inhibit Lewis lung carcinoma and B16 melanoma growth in mice. CMLS. Cell. Mol. Life. Sci. **55:** 663–667.

53. BALTRUSCH, H.J., E. GEHDE, I. TITZE & H.J. HEINZE. 1992. Early socialization and development of cancer in later life: biopsychosocial and psychoneuroimmunologic aspects. Ann. N.Y. Acad. Sci. **650:** 355–362.

54. BALTRUSCH, H.J. & W. STANGEL. 1991. Stress, cancer and immunity. New developments in biopsychosocial and psychoneuroimmunologic research. Acta Neurol. **13:** 315–327.

55. FIFE, A., P.J. BEASLEY & D.L. FERTIG. 1996. Psychoneuroimmunology and cancer: historical perspectives and current research. Adv. Neuroimmunol. **6:** 179–190.

56. BOERMEESTER, M.A. & R.M. BUTZELAAR. 1998. Interaction between breast cancer, psychosocial stress and the immune response. Ned. Tijdschr. Geneeskd. **143:** 83–842.

57. KIECOLT-GLASER, J.K. & R. GLASER. 1999. Psychoneuroimmunology and immunotoxicology: implications for carcinogenesis. Psychosom. Med. **61:** 271–272.

58. NELSON, E., P. SLOPER, A. CHARLTON & D. WHILE. 1994. Children who have a parent with cancer: a pilot study. J. Cancer Educ. **9:** 30–36.

59. GIRALDI, T., M.G. RODANI, G. CARTEI & L. GRASSI. 1997. Psychosocial factors and breast cancer: a 6-year Italian follow-up study. Psychother. Psychosom. **66:** 229–236.

60. BIONDI, M., A. COSTANTINI & A. PARISI. 1996. Can loss and grief activate latent neoplasia? A clinical case of possible interaction between genetic risk and stress in breast cancer. Psychother. Psychosom. **65:** 102–105.

61. JUSTICE, A. 1985. Review of the effects of stress on cancer in laboratory animals: importance of time of stress application and type of tumor. Psychol. Bull. **98:** 108–138.

62. DECHAMBRE, R.P. & R.C. LA BARBA. 1978. The effect of neonatal tactile stimulation on adult response to Ehrlich carcinoma in mice. IRCS Med. Sci. **6:** 472.

63. COE, C.L., L.T. ROSENBERG & S. LEVINE. 1988. Immunological consequences of maternal separation in infant primates. *In* Neuroimmunomodulation. N.H. Spector, Ed.: 213–216. Gordon & Breach. New York.

64. KLING, A., R. LLOYD, K. TACHIKI *et al.* 1990. Effect of social separation on immune function and brain neurotransmitters in Cebus monkey. Abstracts of the International Congress of the ISNIM, Florence. No. 244.

65. GIRALDI, T., L. PERISSIN, S. ZORZET, P. PICCINI & V. RAPOZZI. 1989. Effects of stress on tumor growth and metastasis in mice bearing Lewis lung carcinoma. Eur. J. Cancer Clin. Oncol. **25:** 1583–1588.

66. PERISSIN, L., S. ZORZET, P. PICCINI *et al.* 1991. Effects of rotational stress on the effectiveness of cyclophosphamide and razoxane in mice bearing Lewis lung carcinoma. Clin. Exp. Metastasis **9:** 541–549.

67. PERISSIN, L., S. ZORZET, V. RAPOZZI & T. GIRALDI. 1993. A noninvasive simple method for measurement of urinary excretion of melatonin in undisturbed mice. J. Pineal Res. **15:** 138–140.

68. HILAKIVI-CLARKE, L. & R.B. DICKSON. 1995. Stress influence on development of hepatocellular tumors in transgenic mice overexpressing TGF alpha. Acta Oncol. **34:** 907–912.

69. GIRALDI, T., L. PERISSIN, S. ZORZET *et al.* 1994. Metastasis and neuroendocrine system in stressed mice. Int. J. Neurosci. **74:** 265–278.

70. PERISSIN, L., S. ZORZET, V. RAPOZZI *et al.* 1998. Seasonal effects of rotational stress on Lewis lung carcinoma metastasis and T lymphocyte subsets in mice. Life Sci. **63:** 711–719.

71. CONTI, A., N. HARAN-GHERA & G.J. MAESTRONI. 1992. Role of pineal melatonin and melatonin-induced immuno-opioids in murine leukemogenesis. Med. Oncol. Tumor Pharmacother. **9:** 87–92.

72. PERISSIN, L., V. RAPOZZI, S. ZORZET & T. GIRALDI. 1997. Survival time in mice bearing TLX5 lymphoma subjected to rotational stress and chemotherapy with CCNU. Anticancer Res. **17:** 4355–4357.

73. BEN-ELIYAHU, S., G.G. PAGE, R. YIRMIYA & G. SHAKHAR. 1999. Evidence that stress and surgical interventions promote tumor development by suppressing natural killer cell activity. Int. J. Cancer **80:** 880–888.
74. ZORZET, S., L. PERISSIN, V. RAPOZZI & T. GIRALDI. 1998. Restraint stress reduces the antitumor efficacy of cyclophosphamide in tumor-bearing mice. Brain Behav. Immunol. **12:** 23–33.
75. PERISSIN, L., S. ZORZET, V. RAPOZZI et al. 1994. Seasonal dependency of the effects of experimental stressors on tumor metastasis in mice bearing Lewis lung carcinoma. Chronobiologia **21:** 99–103.
76. PERISSIN, L., V. RAPOZZI, S. ZORZET & T. GIRALDI. 1996. Blockers of adrenergic neurons and receptors, tumor progression and effects of rotational stress in mice. Anticancer Res. **16:** 3409–3413.
77. MAESTRONI, G.J.M. 1998. Is haematopoiesis under the influence of neural and neuroendocrine mechanisms? Histol. Histopathol. **13:** 271–274.
78. MAESTRONI, G.J.M. & A. CONTI. 1996. Melatonin and the immunehaematopietic system. Therapeutic and adverse pharmacological correlates. Neuroimmunomodulation **3:** 325–332.
79. CONTI, A. & G.J.M. MAESTRONI. 1998. Endogenous melatonin in serum, pineal gland and bone marrow of inbred and outbred mice. Thymus and pineal gland in neuroimmunoendocrinology. Swieradow Zdrog Abstract 22B.
80. CONTI, A., S. CONCONI, E. HERTENS et al. 1999. Evidence for melatonin synthesis in mouse and human bone marrow cells. J. Pineal Res. **28:** 193–202.
81. TAN, D., L.C. MANCHESTER, J.R. REITER et al. 2000. Identification of extremely high levels of melatonin in bone marrow: its origin and significance. Biochem. Biophys. In press.
82. BARNI, S., P. LISSONI, S. CRISPINO et al. 1988. Neuroimmunomodulation in cancer patients: correlations between melatonin and β-endorphin blood levels and T helper/suppressor ratio. Int. J. Biol. Markers **3:** 82–86.
83. MAESTRONI, G.J.M., A. CONTI & R.J. REITER, Eds. 1994. Advances in Pineal Research. Libbey. London.
84. MAESTRONI, G.J.M., A. CONTI & P. LISSONI. 1999. Colony-stimulating activity and haematopoietic rescue from cancer chemotherapy compounds are induced by melatonin via endogenous interleukin-4. Cancer Res. **54:** 4740–4743.
85. MAESTRONI, G.J.M., V. COVACCI & A. CONTI. 1999. Haematopoietic rescue via T-cell-dependent, endogenous GM-CSF by the pineal neurohormone melatonin in tumor bearing mice. Cancer Res. **54:** 2429–2432.
86. BEN-NATHAN, D., G.J.M. MAESTRONI & A. CONTI. 1995. Protective effect of melatonin in mice infected with encephalitis viruses. Arch. Virol. **140:** 223–230.
87. BARTSCH, C. & H. BARTSCH. 1993. Melatonin secretion in oncologic patients: current results and methodological considerations. In Advances in Pineal Research. G.J.M. Maestroni, A. Conti & R.J. Reiter, Eds.: 283–301. Libbey. London.
88. BLASK, D.E. 1993. Melatonin in oncology. In Melatonin: Biosynthesis, Physiological Effects, and Clinical Applications. H-S. Yu & R. Reiter, Eds.: 447–477. CRC Press. Boca Raton, FL.
89. MAESTRONI, G.J.M. & A. CONTI. 1996. Melatonin in human breast cancer tissue: association with nuclear grade and estrogen receptor status. Lab. Invest. **75:** 557–561.
90. SCHLUETER, L.A. 1982. Knowledge and beliefs about breast cancer and breast self-examination among athletic and nonathletic women. Nurs. Res. **31:** 348–353.
91. FRISCH, R.E., G. WYSHAK, N.L. ALBRIGHT et al. 1985. Lower prevalence of breast cancer and cancers of the reproductive system among former college athletes compared to nonathletes. Br. J. Cancer **52:** 885–891.
92. WYSHAK, G., R.E. FRISCH, N.L. ALBRIGHT et al. 1986. Lower prevalence of benign diseases of the breast and benign tumours of the reproductive system among former college athletes compared to nonathletes. Br. J. Cancer **54:** 841–845.
93. LEVI, F., C. LA VECCHIA, E. NEGRI & S. FRANCESCHI. 1993. Selected physical activities and the risk of endometrial cancer. Br. J. Cancer **67:** 846–851.
94. OLSON, S.H., J.E. VENA, J.P. DORN et al. 1997. Exercise, occupational activity, and risk of endometrial cancer. Ann. Epidemiol. **7:** 46–53.

95. STURGEON, S.R., L.A. BRINTON, M.L. BERMAN *et al.* 1993. Past and present physical activity and endometrial cancer risk. Br. J. Cancer **68:** 584–589.
96. OLIVERIA, S.A. & I.M. LEE. 1997. Is exercise beneficial in the prevention of prostate cancer? Sports Med. **23:** 271–278.
97. GROSSARTH-MATICEK, R., H.J. EYSENCK, G. UHLENBRUCK *et al.* 1990. Sport activity and personality as elements in preventing cancer and coronary heart disease. Percept. Motor Skills **71:** 199–209.
98. SHEPHARD, R.J. 1990. Physical activity and cancer. Int. J. Sports Med. **11:** 413–420.
99. KONO, S., K. SHINCHI, N. IKEDA *et al.* 1991. Physical activity, dietary habits and adenomatous polyps of the sigmoid colon: a study of self-defense officials in Japan. J. Clin. Epidemiol. **44:** 1255–1261.
100. SANDLER, R.S., M.L. PRITCHARD & S.I. BANGDIWALA. 1995. Physical activity and the risk of colorectal adenomas. Epidemiology **6:** 602–606.
101. SEIFERT, E., S. EWERT & J. WERLE. 1992. Exercise and sports therapy for patients with head and neck tumors. Rehabilitation (Stuttgart) **31:** 33–37.
102. MOCK, V., K.H. DOW, C.J. MEARES *et al.* 1997. Effects of exercise on fatigue, physical functioning, and emotional distress during radiation therapy for breast cancer. Oncol. Nurs. Forum **24:** 991–1000.
103. DIMEO, F., H. BERTZ, J. FINKE *et al.* 1996. An aerobic exercise program for patients with haematological malignancies after bone marrow transplantation. Bone Marrow Transpl. **18:** 1157–1160.
104. MUNRO, S. & B. MOUNT. 1978. Music therapy in palliative care. Can. Med. Assoc. J. **119:** 1029–1034.
105. SALMON, D. 1993. Music and emotion in palliative care. J. Palliat. Care **9:** 48–52.
106. JOHNSTON, K. & J. ROHALY-DAVIS. 1996. An introduction to music therapy: helping the oncology patients in the ICU. Crit. Care Nurs. Q. **18:** 54–60.
107. BREWER, J.F. 1998. Healing sounds. Compl. Ther. Nurs. Midwifery **4:** 7–12.
108. TOBIA, D.M., E.F. SHAMOS, D.M. HARPER *et al.* 1999. The benefits of group music at the 1996 music weekend for women with cancer. J. Cancer Educ. **14:** 115–119.
109. BECK, S.L. 1991. The therapeutic use of music for cancer-related pain. Oncol. Nurs. Forum **18:** 1327–1337.
110. MAGILL-LEVREAULT, L. 1993. Music therapy in pain and symptom management. J. Palliat. Care **9:** 42–48.
111. SABO, C.E. & S.R. MICHAEL. 1996. The influence of personal message with music on anxiety and side effects associated with chemotherapy. Cancer Nurs. **19:** 283–289.

The Role of Pro- and Antiinflammatory Cytokines in Neurodegeneration

STUART M. ALLAN[a]

School of Biological Sciences, 1.124 Stopford Building, University of Manchester, Oxford Road, Manchester, M13 9PT, United Kingdom

ABSTRACT: Experimental and clinical damage to the brain leads to rapid upregulation of an array of cytokines predominantly by glia. These cytokines may exert neurotoxic or neuroprotective actions. This paper will focus on the pro-inflammatory cytokine interleukin-1 (IL-1), which participates in diverse forms of brain damage including ischemia, brain trauma, and excitotoxic injury. Administration of low doses of IL-1 markedly exacerbates these forms of brain damage, whereas blocking IL-1 release or actions reduces neuronal death. IL-1 receptor antagonist (IL-1ra) is also upregulated by brain damage (mainly by neurons) and acts as an endogenous inhibitor of neurodegeneration, presumably by blocking IL-1 actions on its receptor. We have studied the actions of both IL-1 and IL-1ra in experimental models of ischemic and neurotoxic injury in rats, and have found site-specific effects within the striatum. On the basis of this and further work, we propose that IL-1 can exacerbate cell death in these conditions by modifying polysynaptic anterograde pathways leading from the striatum to the cortex. The precise nature of these pathways remains undetermined, as do the underlying mechanisms by which IL-1 can exert its effects, but appear to involve induction of IL-1 in specific brain regions and activation of cortical glutamatergic pathways.

INTRODUCTION

A number of pro- and antiinflammatory cytokines are induced in the brains of humans and experimental animals in response to various insults or injury leading to neurodegeneration.[1] In general proinflammatory cytokines such as interleukin-1 (IL-1) are neurotoxic, whereas the "classical" antiinflammatory cytokines such as IL-1ra, IL-4, and IL-10 are neuroprotective. However for the proinflammatory cytokines IL-6 and TNFα, both effects have been described.[2,3] It appears therefore that there are complex interactions between different cytokines to affect cell death, although the precise mechanisms of action and interaction of these cytokines is not yet fully understood.

IL-1 is one of the most widely studied cytokines in terms of its role in neurodegeneration and much of our work has focused on this. The IL-1 family comprises three known ligands (IL-1α, IL-1β, and IL-1ra), two membrane-bound receptors, receptor accessory proteins, soluble receptors, and other components.[1,4] IL-1α and β are agonists, whereas IL-1ra is a naturally occurring receptor antagonist.[5] The IL-1

[a]Address for correspondence: Voice: +44 161 275 5356; fax: +44 161 275 5948.
stuart.allan@man.ac.uk

proteins are all formed as precursors that are cleaved by different enzymes to the mature form. IL-1β differs from IL-1α in that the pro-form is inactive and therefore requires cleavage by IL-1β converting enzyme (ICE),[6] a member of the caspases, a family of cysteine proteases involved in apoptosis.[7] In the periphery IL-1α and IL-1β are thought to exert identical effects, whereas it is not clear if this is also the case in the CNS, where IL-1β is believed to be more important, particularly in neurodegeneration.[1,8]

Effects of the members of the IL-1 family are mediated through actions on the IL-1 receptor, IL-1RI (80 kDa), which exists in both membrane-bound and soluble forms.[9,10] Signal transduction requires binding of IL-1RI to the membrane-bound IL-1 receptor accessory protein (IL-1RAcP).[11] The 68-kDa type 2 receptor (IL-1RII) lacks an intracellular signaling domain and is believed to act as a "decoy" receptor in that it is shed from the membrane and binds IL-1, thereby preventing access of the ligand to the functional IL-1RI.[12]

The majority of the work on IL-1 receptors has been performed in the periphery, and much speculation surrounds the existence of novel or atypical receptors in the brain, especially because the known receptors are expressed at low levels, particularly in brain regions where IL-1 is thought to exert its effects.

IL-1 EXPRESSION AND ACTION IN THE CNS

Basal expression of IL-1 and its receptors is barely detectable, particularly in the rodent brain.[13] However, regional distribution of both IL-1β mRNA and protein has been described in the normal rat brain, in the cerebellum, frontal cortex, olfactory tubercle, and certain regions of the hippocampus and hypothalamus.[14,15] Although the basal levels are very low, rapid upregulation, particularly of IL-1β, in the brain is observed in response to both systemic and local insults.[16,17]

IL-1 has a number of diverse actions in the CNS to modify feeding behavior, fever, and neuroendocrine responses, mainly through actions in the hypothalamus.[2,9,18] IL-1 also affects many neurotransmitters, neuropeptides, and neurotrophic factors in different brain regions, while electrophysiological studies have shown it to inhibit long-term potentiation and affect synaptic transmission.[2,19,20] In addition, IL-1 has been implicated in many forms of neurodegeneration.[1,8]

IL-1 AND NEURODEGENERATION

IL-1 has been proposed to mediate acute neurodegeneration mainly on the basis of *in vivo* studies, where its release or action has been blocked. Administration or overexpression of IL-1ra and caspase inhibitors in experimental animals has been shown to significantly reduce the extent of cell death following a number of insults including ischemia, trauma, and excitotoxicity.[21–28]

In addition, IL-1β injected in the rat brain at the time of experimental ischemic or traumatic injury causes increased cell death and edema.[22,26,29] We have also observed that IL-1β, when co-injected with the selective excitotoxin S-AMPA in the striatum of the rat brain, can produce extensive distant cortical injury that is not seen with either S-AMPA or IL-1β injected alone (see FIGURE 1), although direct injection of IL-1β into different areas of the rat brain in the absence of any other insult does not cause any cell death.[24] The mechanism of this potent effect of IL-1β is not known, although in focal cerebral ischemia, exacerbating effects of IL-1β and neuroprotective actions of IL-1ra are mediated through actions in the striatum that influence cortical damage.[30]

Further support of a role for IL-1β in acute neurodegeneration comes from studies that have found increased expression of IL-1β and its receptors in the brain in response to ischemic, traumatic, or excitotoxic injury.[13,31–39] Increased expression of IL-1β is usually seen within the area of injury or in areas that subsequently undergo cell loss and has been observed as rapidly as 15 minutes after trauma, which is consistent with an active role for IL-1β in the subsequent cell death.[33] Immunohistochemical studies in our laboratory have demonstrated that the localization and cell source of IL-1β expression after excitotoxin administration[37] or fluid percussion

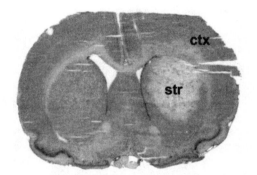

S-AMPA + Vehicle

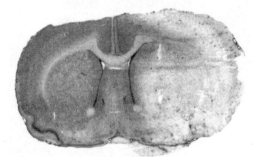

S-AMPA + hrIL-1ß

FIGURE 1. Representative coronal brain sections to demonstrate the effect of intrastriatal co-injection of vehicle or hrIL-1β (10 ng) with S-AMPA (7.5 nmol) on neuronal damage in the rat brain. The pale (white) region is nonviable neuronal tissue and the dark region represents viable tissue. Note the extensive region of the cortex, which is damaged after treatment with hrIL-1β. *ctx*, cortex; *str*, striatum.

injury (S. Toulmond, personal communication) in the rat is time-dependent. Early expression (less than 24 h) of immunoreactive IL-1β is confined to microglia, whereas later expression (24 h to 3 days) is seen predominantly in astrocytes. It is possible these two cell sources are involved with different actions of IL and that the delayed expression occurs after injury is complete.

SITES OF IL-1 ACTION IN NEURODEGENERATION

Our recent data have demonstrated that IL-1β appears to have site-specific effects in the rat CNS to affect neuronal damage.[30,40] In focal cerebral ischemia, IL-1β increases damage in both the striatum and the cortex when administered into the striatum, but has no effect when injected into the cortex.[30] Likewise, IL-1ra reduces the infarct volume resulting from MCAO when injected into the striatum, but has no effect when administered directly into the cortex.[41] Interestingly, injection of IL-1ra in the contralateral striatum also significantly inhibits neuronal damage following MCAO.

These results are supported by other studies on excitotoxic brain damage. Co-injection of IL-1ra with the AMPA receptor agonist S-AMPA or the NMDA receptor agonist methanoglutamate (MGlu) in the striatum results in a significant inhibition of the lesion volume produced by either excitotoxin alone. However, co-injection of IL-1ra with either of these agonists directly into the cerebral cortex fails to affect the outcome. In addition, striatal co-injection of IL-1β with S-AMPA results in a dramatic exacerbation of cell death throughout the ipsilateral cortex (FIG. 1). However, IL-1β when injected directly in the cortex together with S-AMPA or MGlu does not affect the resultant lesion volume.[24] We have also found that the lesion volume produced by direct S-AMPA or MGlu infusion in the cortex is significantly increased by administration of IL-1β into either the ipsilateral or contralateral striatum.[24] These data suggest that IL-1β acts in the rat striatum to affect neuronal cell death after either excitotoxin injection or MCAO. The underlying mechanisms of this effect are not clear, but we propose that IL-1β could cause distant injury via an action on polysynaptic anterograde pathway(s) leading from the striatum back to the cortex, possibly via the thalamus.

Specific areas of the striatum (ventral striatum and lateral shell of the nucleus accumbens) appear to be more responsive to IL-1β. Thus co-injection of IL-1β and S-AMPA fails to cause cortical death when injected into some striatal regions but are particularly effective in the shell of the nucleus accumbens and the ventrolateral striatum.[40] These areas of the striatum show quite distinct connections with other regions of the brain[42,43] and could be important in mediating the effects of IL-1β. Indeed, recent evidence suggests that hypothalamic IL-1 is involved in mediating the observed effects on striatal AMPA-mediated cell death.[44] This is particularly intriguing given the known actions of IL-1 in the hypothalamus to affect other systems, and the existence of both direct and indirect connections from the hypothalamus to the cortex.[43]

MECHANISMS OF IL-1 ACTION IN NEURODEGENERATION

How IL-1β acts to produce its effects after excitotoxin administration or cerebral ischemia is not clear, but there are a number of possibilities. Given that coadministration of IL-1ra can reduce the lesion volume resulting from striatal S-AMPA or MGlu infusion suggests that effects of IL-1β on cell death are mediated downstream of glutamate receptor activation.[24] This is supported by experiments in our laboratory where we have shown that IL-1β has no effect on the release of glutamate from isolated presynaptic nerve terminals (synaptosomes) prepared from the striatum.[45] However, this is in contrast to findings in other brain regions such as the hippocampus, where IL-1β has been shown to reduce glutamate release.[46]

There are no direct connections between the striatum and the cortex, but IL-1β may have retrograde actions on corticostriatal projections whereby it is internalized at the nerve terminal of the corticostriatal fiber and transported back to the cortex, where it can act directly, or via the release of some other factor(s) to increase the vulnerability of the cortical cells. Internalization of IL-1 and the retrograde transport of neuropeptides and growth factors have been described,[47] but since direct injection of IL-1β into the cortex does not affect local cell death produced by intracortical excitotoxin administration this mechanism is unlikely.[24] Nonetheless it is a possible mechanism of action, and it remains to be seen how cortical IL-1β administration affects damage produced by striatal S-AMPA. It could be that the activation of AMPA receptors and the resultant afferent pathways from the striatum are required for IL-1β to produce its effects.

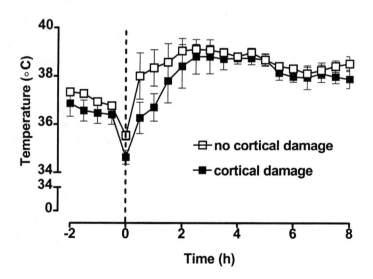

FIGURE 2. Correlation between body temperature and the production of cortical cell death after striatal co-infusion of S-AMPA (7.5 nmol) and hrIL-1β (10 ng) in the rat brain. Zero (*dotted line*) indicates the time of infusion. Body temperature was monitored by intraperitoneal radiotransmitter.

IL-1β is a known pyrogen,[48,49] and increases in body temperature have been shown to dramatically increase cell death, particularly in response to cerebral ischemia.[50–53] This is supported by evidence that IL-1β injections in the striatum can produce a marked rise in temperature.[54] However, we have found that intracerebroventricular injection of IL-1β produces a similar increase in core temperature but has no effect on the extent of cell death resulting from striatal S-AMPA infusion. Likewise, within the group of animals injected with S-AMPA and IL-1β in the striatum, some animals exhibit cortical damage and some show no cortical cell death (i.e., it appears to be an "all or nothing" event), whereas their temperature profiles are very similar (see FIGURE 2). It would be expected that animals with greater amounts of damage would display more of a temperature rise. It appears, therefore, that increases in body temperature per se are not responsible for the observed effects of IL-1β on AMPA-mediated cell death, although modifications in brain temperature cannot be ruled out.[54–56]

Finally, as discussed earlier there are a number of known anterograde pathways connecting the striatum to the cortex,[43,57,58] and we believe that IL-1β could be acting via these to affect cell viability in the cortex.

OTHER CYTOKINES

A number of other cytokines, both pro- and antiinflammatory, are expressed in response to clinical or experimental neurodegenerative insults.[3,16] Administration of the recombinant cytokines or blockade of their release or action has been demonstrated to influence the outcome after insults such as ischemia, brain injury, and excitotoxin administration. Thus, for example, IL-6 has been shown to inhibit neuronal damage caused by striatal N-methyl-D-aspartate (NMDA) infusion[59] or focal cerebral ischemia in the rat.[60] In contrast, transgenic mice overexpressing IL-6 in the brain show severe neurodegeneration.[61] Conflicting data exist over the effects and role of TNFα in neurodegeneration. A number of studies have proposed a role for TNF in mediating neuronal damage, in that blockade of its actions can reduce experimentally induced cell death.[62–64] In contrast, mice rendered genetically unresponsive to TNF through deletion of TNF receptors show enhanced ischemic damage compared to wild-type animals, thereby suggesting a neuroprotective role for TNF.[65] In support of the latter, we have found that administration of TNFα can reduce the lesion volume produced by striatal injection of S-AMPA (S.M. Allan and N.J. Rothwell, unpublished data).

CONCLUSION

We have demonstrated site-specific actions of IL-1 and IL-1ra in ischemic and excitotoxic brain damage in the rat, which can lead to distant cortical injury via activation of polysynaptic pathways. Understanding the underlying mechanisms and pathways involved in these effects may be beneficial to future therapeutic strategies for the treatment of a number of acute neurodegenerative conditions such as stroke and head trauma.

ACKNOWLEDGMENTS

Many thanks to Professor Nancy Rothwell and Dr. Giamal Luheshi for their assistance in the preparation of this manuscript.

REFERENCES

1. ROTHWELL, N.J. & S.J. HOPKINS. 1995. Cytokines and the nervous system II: Actions and mechanisms of action. Trends Neurosci. **18:** 130–136.
2. RELTON, J.K., T.J. NEUBERGER, A.M. BENDELE et al. 1997. Cytokines: neurotoxicity and neuroprotection. In Neuroprotection in CNS Diseases. P.R. Bär & M.F. Beal, Eds.: 225–241. Marcel Dekker. New York.
3. WATKINS, L.R., M.K. HANSEN, K.T. NGUYEN et al. 1999. Dynamic regulation of the proinflammatory cytokine, interleukin-1β: molecular biology for non-molecular biologists. Life Sci. **65:** 449–481.
4. DINARELLO, C.A. & R.C. THOMPSON. 1991. Blocking IL-1: interleukin-1 receptor antagonist in vivo and in vitro. Immunol. Today **12:** 404–410.
5. THORNBERRY, N.A., H.G. BULL, J.R. CALAYCAY et al. 1992. A novel heterodimeric cysteine protease is required for interleukin-1β processing in monocytes. Nature **356:** 768–774.
6. NICHOLSON, D.W. & N.A. THORNBERRY. 1997. Caspases: killer proteases. Trends Biochem. Sci. **22:** 299–306.
7. ROTHWELL, N., S. ALLAN & S. TOULMOND. 1997. The role of interleukin 1 in acute neurodegeneration and stroke: pathophysiological and therapeutic implications. J. Clin. Invest. **100:** 2648–2652.
8. DINARELLO, C.A. 1996. Biologic basis for interleukin-1 in disease. Blood **87:** 2095–2147.
9. SIMS, J.E. & S.K. DOWER. 1994. Interleukin-1 receptors. Eur. Cytokine Netw. **5:** 539–546.
10. GREENFEDER, S.A., P. NUNES, L. KWEE et al. 1995. Molecular cloning and characterization of a second subunit of the interleukin 1 receptor complex. J. Biol. Chem. **270:** 13757–13765.
11. SIMS, J.E., M.A. GAYLE, J.L. SLACK et al. 1993. Interleukin 1 signaling occurs exclusively via the type 1 receptor. Proc. Natl. Acad. Sci. USA **90:** 6155–6159.
12. GABELLEC, M.M., M. CRUMEYROLLE-ARIAS, F. LE SAUX et al. 1999. Expression of interleukin-1 genes and interleukin-1 receptors in the mouse brain after hippocampal injury. Neurosci. Res. **33:** 251–260.
13. BANDTLOW, C.E., M. MEYER, D. LINDHOLM et al. 1990. Regional and cellular codistribution of interleukin 1β and nerve growth factor mRNA in the adult rat brain: possible relationship to the regulation of nerve growth factor synthesis. J. Cell Biol. **111:** 1701–1711.
14. LECHAN, R.M., R. TONI, B.D. CLARK et al. 1990. Immunoreactive interleukin-1β localization in the rat forebrain. Brain Res. **514:** 135–140.
15. HOPKINS, S.J. & N.J. ROTHWELL. 1995. Cytokines and the nervous system. I: Expression and recognition. Trends Neurosci. **18:** 83–88.
16. BENVENISTE, E.N. 1997. Cytokines: influence on glial cell gene expression and function. In Neuroimmunoendocrinology. Vol. 69. J.E. Blalock, Ed.: 31–75. Karger. Basel.
17. ROTHWELL, N.J. & G. LUHESHI. 1994. Pharmacology of interleukin-1 actions in the brain. Adv. Pharmacol. **25:** 1–20.
18. VEZZANI, A., N. CONTI, A. DE LUIGI et al. 1999. Interleukin-1β immunoreactivity and microglia are enhanced in the rat hippocampus by focal kainate application: functional evidence for enhancement of electrographic seizures. J. Neurosci. **19:** 5054–5065.
19. O'CONNOR, J.J. & A.N. COOGAN. 1999. Actions of the pro-inflammatory cytokine IL-1β on central synaptic transmission. Exp. Physiol. **84:** 601–614.

20. RELTON, J.K. & N.J. ROTHWELL. 1992. Interleukin-1 receptor antagonist inhibits ischaemic and excitotoxic neuronal damage in the rat. Brain Res. Bull. **29:** 243–246.
21. LODDICK, S.A. & N.J. ROTHWELL. 1996. Neuroprotective effects of human recombinant interleukin-1 receptor antagonist in focal cerebral ischaemia in the rat. J. Cereb. Blood Flow Metab. **16:** 932–940.
22. TOULMOND, S. & N.J. ROTHWELL. 1995. Interleukin-1 receptor antagonist inhibits neuronal damage caused by fluid percussion injury in the rat. Brain Res. **671:** 261–266.
23. LAWRENCE, C.B., S.M. ALLAN & N.J. ROTHWELL. 1998. Interleukin-1 and the interleukin-1 receptor antagonist act in the striatum to modify excitotoxic brain damage in the rat. Eur. J. Neurosci. **10:** 1188–1195.
24. HAGAN, P., J.D.E. BARKS, M. YABUT et al. 1996. Adenovirus-mediated overexpression of interleukin-1 receptor antagonist reduces susceptibility to excitotoxic brain injury in perinatal rats. Neuroscience **75:** 1033–1045.
25. YAMASAKI, Y., N. MATSUURA, H. SHOZUHARA et al. 1995. Interleukin-1 as a pathogenetic mediator of ischemic brain damage in rats. Stroke **26:** 676–681.
26. YANG, G.-Y., Y.-J. ZHAO, B.L. DAVIDSON & A.L. BETZ. 1997. Overexpression of interleukin-1 receptor antagonist in the mouse brain reduces ischemic brain injury. Brain Res. **751:** 181–188.
27. LODDICK, S.A., A. MACKENZIE & N.J. ROTHWELL. 1996. An ICE inhibitor, z-VAD-DCB attenuates ischaemic brain damage in the rat. Neuroreport **7:** 1465–1468.
28. TOULMOND, S., J.K. RELTON, C. LAWRENCE et al. 1993. Neurotoxic effects of interleukin-1 (IL-1) in vivo. Soc. Neurosci. Abstr. **23:** 771.19.
29. STROEMER, R.P. & N.J. ROTHWELL. 1998. Exacerbation of ischemic brain damage by localized striatal injection of IL-1ß in the rat. J. Cereb. Blood Flow Metab. **18:** 833–839.
30. BUTTINI, M., A. SAUTER & H.W.G.M. BODDEKE. 1994. Induction of interleukin-1β mRNA after focal cerebral ischaemia in the rat. Mol. Brain Res. **23:** 126–134.
31. FAN, L., K.G. PERLMAN, P.C. MCDONNELL et al. 1993. Experimental traumatic brain injury induces expression of interleukin-1β mRNA in the rat brain. Soc. Neurosci. Abstr. **19:** 1880–1880.
32. MINAMI, M., Y. KURAISHI, K. YABUUCHI et al. 1992. Induction of interleukin-1β mRNA in rat brain after transient forebrain ischemia. J. Neurochem. **58:** 390–392.
33. YABUUCHI, K., M. MINAMI, S. KATSUMATA & M. SATOH. 1993. In situ hybridization study of interleukin-1β mRNA induced by kainic acid in the rat brain. Mol. Brain Res. **20:** 153–161.
34. HAGAN, P., S. POOLE, A.F. BRISTOW et al. 1996. Intracerebral NMDA injection stimulates production of interleukin-1β in perinatal rat brain. J. Neurochem. **67:** 2215–2218.
35. DAVIES, C.A., S.A. LODDICK, S. TOULMOND et al. 1999. The progression and topographic distribution of interleukin-1β expression after permanent middle cerebral artery occlusion in the rat. J. Cereb. Blood Flow Metab. **19:** 87–98.
36. PEARSON, V.L., N.J. ROTHWELL & S. TOULMOND. 1999. Excitotoxic brain damage in the rat induces interleukin-1β protein in microglia and astrocytes: correlation with the progression of cell death. Glia **25:** 311–323.
37. SAIRANEN, T.R., P.J. LINDSBERG, M. BRENNER & A.-L. SIREN. 1997. Global forebrain ischemia results in differential cellular expression of interleukin-1β (IL-1β) and its receptor at mRNA and protein level. J. Cereb. Blood Flow Metab. **17:** 1107–1120.
38. NISHIYORI, A., M. MINAMI, S. TAKAMI & M. SATOH. 1997. Type 2 interleukin-1 receptor mRNA is induced by kainic acid in the rat brain. Mol. Brain Res. **50:** 237–245.
39. GRUNDY, R.I., N.J. ROTHWELL & S.M. ALLAN. 1998. Site of action of IL-1 on AMPA receptor mediated excitotoxicity within the rat striatum. Soc. Neurosci. Abstr. **24:** 568.15.
40. STROEMER, R.P. & N.J. ROTHWELL. 1997. Cortical protection by localized striatal injection of IL-1ra following cerebral ischemia in the rat. J. Cereb. Blood Flow Metab. **17:** 597–604.
41. HEIMER, L., G.F. ALHEID, J.S. DE OLMOS et al. 1997. The accumbens: beyond the core-shell dichotomy. J. Neuropsychiatry Clin. Neurosci. **9:** 354–381.

42. RISOLD, P.Y., R.H. THOMPSON & L.W. SWANSON. 1997. The structural organization of connections between hypothalamus and cerebral cortex. Brain Res. Rev. **24:** 197–254.

43. ALLAN, S.M., C.B. LAWRENCE & N.J. ROTHWELL. 1998. Interleukin-1β and interleukin-1 receptor antagonist do not affect glutamate release or calcium entry in rat striatal synaptosomes. Mol. Psychiatry **3:** 178–182.

44. ALLAN, S.M., L.C. PARKER & B. COLLINS. 2000. Cortical cell death induced by interleukin-1 is mediated via actions in the hypothalamus of the rat. Proc. Natl. Acad. Sci. USA **97:** 5580–5585.

45. MURRAY, C.A., B. MCGAHON, S. MCBENNETT & M.A. LYNCH. 1997. Interleukin-1β inhibits glutamate release in hippocampus of young, but not aged, rats. Neurobiol. Aging **18:** 343–348.

46. LADURON, P.M. 1995. Functional consequences of retrograde axonal transport of receptor-bound neurotensin. Trends Pharmacol. Sci. **16:** 338–343.

47. KLUGER, M.J. 1991. Fever: role of pyrogens and cryogens. Physiol. Rev. **71:** 93–127.

48. KLUGER, M.J., W. KOZAK, L.R. LEON et al. 1995. Cytokines and fever. Neuroimmunomodulation **2:** 216–223.

49. MALBERG, J. & L. SEIDEN. 1998. Small changes in ambient temperature cause large changes in 3,4-methylenedioxymethamphetamine (MDMA)-induced serotonin neurotoxicity and core body temperature in the rat. J. Neurosci. **18:** 5086–5094.

50. BUSTO, R., W.D. DIETRICH, M.Y.T. GLOBUS et al. 1987. Small differences in intraischemic brain temperature critically determine the extent of ischemic neuronal injury. J. Cereb. Blood Flow Metab. **7:** 729–738.

51. MINAMISAWA, H., C.H. NORDSTRÖM, M.L. SMITH & B.K. SIESJÖ. 1990. The influence of mild body and brain hypothermia on ischemic brain damage. J. Cereb. Blood Flow Metab. **10:** 365–374.

52. GINSBERG, M.D. 1998. Temperature influence on ischemic brain injury. *In* Ischemic Stroke: From Basic Mechanisms to New Drug Development. Vol. 16. C.Y. Hsu, Ed.: 65–88. Karger. Basel.

53. GRUNDY, R.I., N.J. ROTHWELL & S.M. ALLAN. 1999. Dissociation between the effects of interleukin-1 (IL-1) on excitotoxic brain damage and body temperature in the rat. Brain Res. **830:** 32–37.

54. HARA, S., T. MUKAI, F. KURIIWA et al. 1997. Inhibition of NMDA-induced increase in brain temperature by *N*-ω-nitro-L-arginine and indomethacin in rats. Brain Res. **756:** 301–304.

55. MORIKAWA, E., M.D. GINSBERG, W.D. DIETRICH et al. 1992. The significance of brain temperature in focal cerebral ischemia: histopathological consequences of middle cerebral artery occlusion in the rat. J. Cereb. Blood Flow Metab. **12:** 380–389.

56. PARENT, A. & L.-N. HAZRATI. 1995. Functional anatomy of the basal ganglia. I. The cortico-basal ganglia-thalamo-cortical loop. Brain Res. Rev. **20:** 91–127.

57. GROENEWEGEN, H.J., C.I. WRIGHT & H.B. UYLINGS. 1997. The anatomical relationships of the prefrontal cortex with limbic structures and the basal ganglia. J. Psychopharmacol. **11:** 99–106.

58. TOULMOND, S., V.D. FAGE & J. BENAVIDES. 1992. Local infusion of interleukin-6 attenuates the neurotoxic effects of NMDA on rat striatal cholinergic neurons. Neurosci. Lett. **144:** 49–52.

59. LODDICK, S.A., A.V. TURNBULL & N.J. ROTHWELL. 1998. Cerebral interleukin-6 is neuroprotective during permanent focal cerebral ischemia in the rat. J. Cereb. Blood Flow Metab. **18:** 176–179.

60. CAMPBELL, I.L., C.R. ABRAHAM, E. MASLIAH et al. 1993. Neurologic disease induced in transgenic mice by cerebral overexpression of interleukin 6. Proc. Natl. Acad. Sci. USA **90:** 10061–10065.

61. DAWSON, D.A., D. MARTIN & J.M. HALLENBECK. 1996. Inhibition of tumor necrosis factor-α reduces focal cerebral ischemic injury in the spontaneously hypertensive rat. Neurosci. Lett. **218:** 41–44.

62. MEISTRELL, M.E.I., G.I. BOTCHKINA, H. WANG et al. 1997. Tumor necrosis factor is a brain damaging cytokine in cerebral ischemia. Shock **8:** 341–348.

63. LAVINE, S.D., F.M. HOFMAN & B.V. ZLOKOVIC. 1998. Circulating antibody against tumor necrosis factor-α protects rat brain from reperfusion injury. J. Cereb. Blood Flow Metab. **18:** 52–58.
64. BRUCE, A.J., W. BOLING, M.S. KINDY *et al.* 1996. Altered neuronal and microglial responses to excitotoxic and ischemic brain injury in mice lacking TNF receptors. Nature Med. **2:** 788–794.

Neuroendocrine Regulation of IL-12 and TNF-α/IL-10 Balance

Clinical Implications

ILIA J. ELENKOV,[a,b,c] GEORGE P. CHROUSOS,[c] AND RONALD L. WILDER[b]

[b]Inflammatory Joint Diseases Section, Arthritis and Rheumatism Branch,
National Institute of Arthritis and Musculoskeletal and Skin Diseases,
National Institutes of Health, Bethesda, Maryland 20892, USA

[c]Pediatric Endocrinology Section, Pediatric and Reproductive Endocrinology Branch,
National Institute of Child Health and Human Development,
National Institutes of Health, Bethesda, Maryland 20892, USA

ABSTRACT: Interleukin-12 and tumor necrosis factor (TNF)-α promote T-helper (Th) 1 responses and cellular immunity, whereas IL-10 suppresses Th1 activities and stimulates Th2 and humoral immune responses. Recent evidence indicates that glucocorticoids, norepinephrine, epinephrine, histamine, and adenosine inhibit the production of human IL-12 and TNF-α, whereas they do not affect or even stimulate the production of IL-10. Through this mechanism these neuroendocrine mediators may cause a selective suppression of Th1 responses and a Th2 shift rather than generalized Th suppression. The substantial Th2-driving force of endogenous stress mediators, as well as histamine and adenosine, can be amplified to a great extent during certain conditions and may play a role in increased susceptibility of the organism to various infections that are normally cleared by Th1 responses. In addition, conditions that contribute to a substantial increase or decrease of local or systemic concentrations of these mediators via modulation of IL-12, TNFα/IL-10 balance may also play a role in induction, expression, and progression of certain autoimmune diseases, allergic/atopic reactions, and tumor growth. These conditions include: acute or chronic stress; cessation of chronic stress or chronic hypoactivity of the stress system; severe exercise; serious surgical procedures or traumatic injuries; major burns; severe ischemia or hypoxia; pregnancy and the postpartum period. Thus, better understanding of the neuroendocrine regulation of IL-12, TNF-α/IL-10 balance might help the development of new therapeutic strategies for the treatment of Th1- and Th2-mediated human diseases.

INTRODUCTION

Interleukin (IL)-12, tumor necrosis factor (TNF)-α, and IL-10 are key regulators of T helper (Th) 1/Th2 balance, which is critically skewed, one way or the other, in several infections, autoimmunity, atopy, and tumors.[1,2] Importantly, neutralization

[a]Address for correspondence: Dr. Ilia J. Elenkov, Pediatric Endocrinology Section, PREB, NICHD, Building 10, Room 9D42, 10 Center Drive MSC 1583, NIH, Bethesda, MD 20892. Voice: 301-496-5800; fax: 301-402-0884.
elenkovi@mail.nih.gov

of IL-12 and TNF-α activities shows promise in ameliorating certain types of Th1-driven autoimmune diseases,[3] whereas exogenous application of IL-12 appears to be beneficial in experimentally induced tumors.[4] Thus, the regulation of the production of these three cytokines has recently attracted considerable interest.

Although genetic and immunologic factors undoubtedly play a role, recent evidence suggests that certain neuroendocrine mediators are also involved in regulation of IL-12 and TNFα/IL-10 balance. Thus, data accumulated over the last five years indicate that glucocorticoids, norepinephrine (NE), epinephrine, histamine, and adenosine induce a Th2 shift, a process mediated through their differential effect on type 1 and type 2 cytokine production. This new concept helps explain some well-known, but often contradictory, effects of these mediators on the immune system and on the onset and course of certain infectious, autoimmune, atopic, and neoplastic diseases.

ROLE OF IL-12, TNF-α, AND IL-10 IN IMMUNOREGULATION

Th1 cells secrete IFN-γ, IL-2, and TNF-β, which promote cellular immunity; whereas Th2 cells secrete IL-4, IL-10, and IL-13, which promote humoral immunity[1,2] (see FIGURE 1). IL-12, produced by activated monocytes/macrophages or other antigen-presenting cells (APCs), is a major inducer of Th1 differentiation and, hence, cellular immunity; this cytokine acts in concert with natural killer (NK) cell-derived IFN-γ to further promote Th1 responses.[5] APC-derived IL-12 and TNF-α, in concert with NK cell– and Th1 cell–derived IFN-γ, stimulate the functional activity of T cytotoxic (Tc) cells, NK cells, and activated macrophages, that is, the major components of cellular immunity. Type 1 cytokines, such as IL-12, TNF-α, and IFN-γ are also considered the major proinflammatory cytokines because they stimulate the synthesis of nitric oxide and other inflammatory mediators that drive chronic delayed-type inflammatory responses.[1,2,5]

Th1 and Th2 responses are mutually inhibitory. Thus, IL-12 and IFN-γ inhibit Th2, and, vice versa, IL-4 and IL-10 inhibit Th1 responses. Type 2 cytokines, such as IL-4 and IL-10, promote humoral immunity by stimulating the growth and activation of mast cells and eosinophils, the differentiation of B cells into antibody-secreting B cells, and B-cell immunoglobulin switching to IgE. Importantly, type 2 cytokines inhibit macrophage activation, T-cell proliferation, and the production of proinflammatory cytokines. Thus, IL-4 and IL-10 are considered the major antiinflammatory cytokines[1,2] (FIG. 1).

STRESS HORMONES MEDIATE A TH2 SHIFT

Effects of Glucocorticoids

Glucocorticoids act on APCs to suppress the production of the main inducer of Th1 responses IL-12 *in vitro* and *ex vivo*.[6,7] Because IL-12 is extremely potent in enhancing IFN-γ and inhibiting IL-4 synthesis by T cells, the inhibition of IL-12 production may represent a major mechanism by which glucocorticoids affect the Th1/Th2 balance. Indeed, glucocorticoid-treated monocytes/macrophages produce significantly

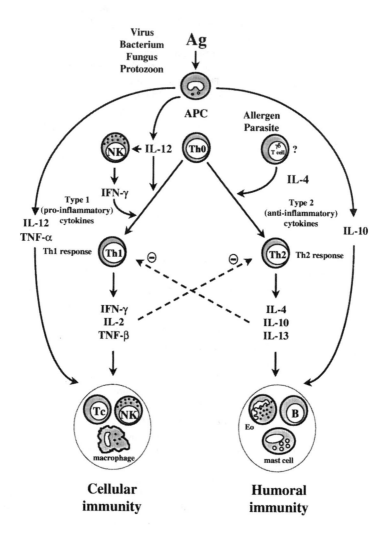

FIGURE 1. Role of Th1 and Th2 cells, and type 1 and type 2 cytokines in the regulation of cellular and humoral immunity. Cellular immunity provides protection against intracellular bacteria, protozoa, fungi, and several viruses; whereaas humoral immunity provides protection against multicellular parasites, extracellular bacteria, some viruses, soluble toxins, and allergens (see text). *Solid lines* represent stimulation, and *dashed lines* inhibition. ABBREVIATIONS: Ag, antigen; APC antigen-presenting cell; NK, natural killer cell; T, T cell; B, B cell; Th, T-helper cell; Tc, T-cytotoxic cell; Eo, eosinophil; IL, interleukin; TNF, tumor necrosis factor; IFN, interferon. (From Elenkov and Chrousos.[35] Reproduced by permission.)

less IL-12, leading to a decreased capacity of these cells to induce IFN-γ production by antigen-primed CD4[+] T cells; the same treatment of monocytes/macrophages is also associated with an increased production of IL-4 by T cells, probably resulting from disinhibition from the suppressive effects of IL-12 on Th2 activity.[8] Furthermore, glucocorticoids potently downregulate the expression of IL-12 receptors on T and NK cells. This may explain why human peripheral blood mononuclear cells stimulated with immobilized anti-CD3 lose their ability to produce IFN-γ in the presence of glucocorticoids.[9] Thus, although glucocorticoids may have a direct suppressive effect on Th1 cells, the overall inhibition of IFN-γ production by these cells appears to result mainly from the inhibition of IL-12 production by APCs and from the loss of IL-12 responsiveness of NK and Th1 cells.

It is particularly noteworthy that glucocorticoids have no effect on the production of the potent antiinflammatory cytokine IL-10 by monocytes,[6,10] yet lymphocyte-derived IL-10 production appears to be upregulated by glucocorticoids. Thus, rat CD4[+] T cells pretreated with dexamethasone exhibit increased levels of mRNA for IL-10.[11] Similarly, during experimental endotoxemia or cardiopulmonary bypass, or in multiple sclerosis patients having an acute relapse, the treatment with glucocorticoids is associated with increased plasma IL-10 secretion.[10,12,13] This might have resulted from a direct stimulatory effect of glucocorticoids on T-cell IL-10 production and/or from the disinhibition of the restraining inputs of IL-12 and IFN-γ on monocyte/lymphocyte IL-10 production.

Effects of Catecholamines

Catecholamines (CAs), that is, norepinephrine (NE) and epinephrine, drive a Th2 shift both at the level of APCs and Th1 cells. We recently demonstrated that NE and epinephrine potently inhibited or enhanced the production of IL-12 and IL-10, respectively, in human whole-blood cultures stimulated with bacterial lipopolysaccharide (LPS) *ex vivo*.[6] These effects are mediated by stimulation of β-adrenoreceptors (ARs) since they are completely prevented by propranolol, a β-AR antagonist. Our findings were subsequently extended by other laboratories showing that nonselective β- and selective β_2-AR agonists inhibited the production of IL-12 *in vitro* and *in vivo*.[14,15] β_2-ARs are expressed on Th1 cells, but not on Th2 cells.[16] This may provide an additional mechanistic basis for a differential effect of CAs on Th1/Th2 functions. In fact, in both murine and human cultures, β_2-AR agonists inhibit IFN-γ production by Th1 cells, but do not affect IL-4 production by Th2 cells.[16,17]

The differential effect of CAs on type 1/type 2 cytokine production also operates under *in vivo* conditions. Thus, increasing sympathetic outflow in mice by selective α_2-AR antagonists or application of β-AR agonists results in inhibition of LPS-induced TNF-α and IL-12 production[15,18,19]; in humans, the administration of the β_2-AR agonist salbutamol results in inhibition of IL-12 production *ex vivo*,[14] and acute brain trauma that is followed by massive release of CAs triggers secretion of substantial amounts of systemic IL-10.[20] Thus, systemically, both glucocorticoids and CAs, respectively, through their effects on type 1 and type 2 cytokine secretion cause selective suppression of cellular immunity and a shift towards Th2-mediated humoral immunity.

HISTAMINE SUPPRESSES IL-12 AND TNF-α AND STIMULATES IL-10 PRODUCTION VIA H2 RECEPTORS

Histamine is a well-recognized mediator of acute inflammation and allergic reactions. These actions are mainly mediated by activation of H1 histamine receptors and include vasodilation, increased permeability of the vessel wall, edema, and in the lungs bronchoconstriction. Recent evidence indicates, however, that histamine may also have important immunoregulatory functions via H2 receptors expressed on immune cells.[21,22] Thus, histamine inhibits TNF-α, but potentiates IL-6 production.[23,24] Because TNF-α is primarily a type 1 cytokine and IL-6 promotes B-cell differentiation, these data suggest that histamine may promote humoral immunity. We have recently found that histamine inhibits the secretion of human IL-12 and stimulates the production of IL-10 in whole blood and monocyte cultures stimulated with LPS.[25] Cimetidine, an H2 receptor antagonist, blocked the effects of histamine on IL-12 and IL-10 production, whereas dimaprit, an H2 receptor agonist, mimicked dose-dependently the effect of histamine. Monocytes are the main IL-12– and IL-10–producing cells in LPS-stimulated human peripheral blood, and human monocytes express H2 receptors.[25,26] Because Ro 20-1724, a phosphodiesterase inhibitor, potentiates the effect of histamine on both IL-12 and IL-10 secretion, it appears that H2 receptors on monocytes mediate the effects of histamine via an increase of intracellular cAMP. Our data are consistent with a recent study showing that histamine, via H2 receptors, inhibits IFN-γ production by Th1-like cells, but has no effect on IL-4 production from Th2 clones.[27] Thus, histamine, similar to CAs, appears to drive a Th2 shift at the level of both APCs and Th1 cells. Through this mechanism allergen/antigen-IgE-induced-release of histamine might participate in a positive-feedback loop that promotes and sustains a shift to IgE production.

ACTIVATION OF ADENOSINE A2A RECEPTORS INHIBITS IL-12 AND TNF-α, AND STIMULATES IL-10 PRODUCTION BY MONOCYTES

Inflammation, ischemia, and tissue injury represent pathologic states in which intracellular ATP metabolism is accelerated, resulting in enhanced release from metabolically active cells of the endogenous purine nucleoside adenosine. Adenosine exerts potent antiinflammatory and immunosuppressive effects mediated mainly by A2 receptors: diminished leukocyte accumulation, inhibition of C2 production, and reduction of the superoxide anion generation.[28–30]

We have recently demonstrated that the adenosine analogues NECA and CGS-21680 dose-dependently inhibit the production of IL-12 induced by LPS in whole-blood and isolated human monocyte cultures.[31] Because A2a receptors are characterized by their high-affinity binding of the agonist CGS-21680, this pharmacological profile of the response implies involvement of A2a receptors. Moreover, the inhibitory effect of CGS-21680 is potentiated by a phosphodiesterase inhibitor and prevented by an inhibitor of the type I and II PKA. Thus, ligand activation of A2a receptors through stimulation of the cAMP/PKA pathway appears to mediate the inhibition of IL-12 production by human monocytes.[31] This is consistent with previous studies showing that adenosine analogues inhibit, also via stimulation of

A2 receptors, the secretion of the proinflammatory cytokine TNF-α by human monocytes.[32]

Adenosine analogues potentiate, however, the production of IL-10 *in vitro* by human monocytes, in human whole blood *ex vivo* and *in vivo* in endotoxemic mice.[31,33,34] This indicates that adenosine expresses a Th1/Th2 modulatory profile similar to CAs and histamine. Thus, conditions related to increased local concentrations of adenosine, through inhibition of IL-12 and TNF-α, and potentiation of IL-10 production from monocytes, may simultaneously mediate an inhibition of Th1 responses and a shift towards Th2 dominance.

CLINICAL IMPLICATIONS

Infections

A major factor governing the outcome of infectious diseases is the selection of Th1- versus Th2-predominant adaptive responses during and after the initial invasion of the host. Thus, a Th2 shift, induced by stress hormones, histamine, or adenosine, may have a profound effect on the susceptibility of the organism to and/or may influence the course of an infection, the defense against which is primarily through cellular immunity mechanisms[6,35] (TABLE 1). For example, cellular immunity, and particularly IL-12- and IL-12-dependent IFN-γ secretion in humans, seems essential in the control of mycobacterial infections.[36] Individuals who have experienced stressful life events are more likely to develop tuberculosis and less likely to recover (cf. Ref. 37). Thus, stress hormone–induced inhibition of IL-12 and IFN-γ production and the consequent suppression of cellular immunity may explain, at least in part, the pathophysiologic mechanisms of these observations (TABLE 1).

Chronic gastritis, which in some cases progresses to peptic ulcer, is largely caused by an *Helicobacter pylori* infection against which Th1 responses appear to have a protective role.[38] The role of stress in promoting peptic ulcers has been recognized for many years. Thus, increased systemic stress hormone levels, in concert with an increased local concentration of histamine induced by inflammatory or stress-related mediators, may skew the local responses towards Th2 and, thus, may allow the onset or progression of a *Helicobacter pylori* infection.

Infectious Complications after Major Injury and Hypoxic/Ischemic Conditions

Major injury (serious traumatic injury and major burns) or major surgical procedures often lead to severe immunosuppression, which contributes to infectious complications and in some cases to sepsis, the most common cause of late death after trauma. Strong stimulation of the sympathetic/adrenomedullary system and the hypothalamic–pituitary–adrenal (HPA) axis correlates with the severity of both cerebral and extracerebral injury and an unfavorable prognosis (cf. Ref. 20). In patients with traumatic major injury and in animal models of burn injury, suppressed cellular immunity is associated with diminished production of IFN-γ and IL-12 and increased production of IL-10 (a Th2 shift).[39] A recent study indicated that systemic release of IL-10 triggered by sympathetic nervous system activation might be a key mechanism of immunosuppression observed after injury. Thus, high levels of

TABLE 1. Putative pathophysiologic roles of stress hormone–induced alterations of Th1/Th2 balance in certain infections, infectious complications after major injury, autoimmune/inflammatory, allergic, or neoplastic diseases

Condition	Host response	Pathogenic response	Role of stress
Infections Mycobacterium tuberculosis Helicobacter pylori HIV Common cold viruses	Th1 protects	Suppressed cellular immunity, deficit of IL-12 and IFN-γ, Th2 shift with progression of infection	Stress-induced Th2 shift may contribute to increased susceptibility to or progression of these infections
Major injury	Th2 protects?	Suppressed cellular immunity and IL-12, and IFN-γ production, overproduction of IL-10, Th2 shift	Increased levels of stress hormones may contribute to suppression of cellular immunity resulting in infectious complications
Autoimmunity RA, MS, ATD, type 1 diabetes mellitus	Excessive Th1 response	Th1 shift, overproduction of IL-12, TNF-α, IFN-γ; deficit of IL-10	A hypoactive stress system may facilitate/sustain the Th1 shift and flares of these autoimmune diseases[a]
SLE	Excessive Th2 response	Th2 shift, deficit of IL-12 and TNF-α, overproduction of IL-10	Stress (Th2 shift) may induce/facilitate flares of SLE
Allergy (Atopy)	Excessive Th2 responses	Th2 shift, deficit of IL-12, overproduction of IL-4, IL-10	Stress hormone- (and histamine)-induced Th2 shift may induce/facilitate/sustain allergic reactions[a]
Tumors	Th1 protects	Suppressed cellular immunity, deficit of IL-12, TNF-α, overproduction of IL-10	Stress hormone- (and histamine)-induced Th2 shift may contribute to increased susceptibility to or progression of certain tumors

[a]The role of stress in autoimmunity and atopy is more complex, see text for details.

ABBREVIATIONS: Th, T helper; IL, interleukin; TNF, tumor necrosis factor; IFN, interferon; RA, rheumatoid arthritis; MS, multiple sclerosis; ATD, autoimmune thyroid disease; SLE, systemic lupus erythematosus.

SOURCE: From Elenkov and Chrousos.[35]

systemic IL-10 documented in patients with "sympathetic storm", resulting from acute accidental or iatrogenic brain trauma, were associated with a high incidence of infection.[20]

During ischemia or hypoxia, local adenosine concentrations increase to the micromolar range.[40] Thus, a massive release of adenosine during major injury may mediate, through inhibition of IL-12 and TNF-α and potentiation of IL-10 production, part of the substantial immunosuppression that occurs in these patients. Therefore, stress hormones, histamine, and adenosine secretion triggered by major injury, may contribute via an induction of a Th2 shift to the severe immunosuppression observed in these conditions.

Autoimmunity

In rheumatoid arthritis (RA), multiple sclerosis (MS), type 1 diabetes mellitus, autoimmune thyroid disease (ATD), and Crohn's disease (CD), Th1/Th2 balance is skewed towards Th1 responses and an excess of IL-12 and TNF-α production, while Th2 activity and the production of IL-10 are deficient.[41–43] This appears to be a critical factor that determines the proliferation and differentiation of Th1-related autoreactive cellular immune responses in these disorders.[44] On the other hand, systemic lupus erythematosus (SLE) is associated with a Th2 shift and an excessive production of IL-10, while IL-12 and TNF-α production appear to be deficient[45–47] (TABLE 1).

The effect of stress on autoimmunity is extremely complex; often stress is related to both induction/exacerbation and amelioration of disease activity.[35,48,49] Hyperactive or hypoactive stress systems may be associated with decreased or increased vulnerability to different types of autoimmune diseases. Thus, F344 rats, which have a hyperactive stress system, are resistant to experimental induction of Th1-mediated autoimmune states, including arthritis, uveitis, and experimental allergic encephalomyelitis (EAE).[49] Similarly, women in the third trimester of pregnancy, who have increased levels of cortisol, frequently experience remission of Th1 type–mediated autoimmune diseases, such as RA and MS, possibly via suppression of proinflammatory (IL-12 and TNF–α) cytokine production.[49,50] Through a reciprocal mechanism, Th2 type-mediated autoimmune disorders mainly driven by IL-10, such as SLE, may flare up in high cortisol and CAs output states, that is, during stress or pregnancy.[49,50]

Conversely, LEW and DA rats, which possess a hypoactive HPA axis, are extremely prone to developing experimentally induced Th1-mediated states, such as arthritis, uveitis, or EAE.[49] Similarly, clinical situations associated with decreased stress system activity are associated with increased expression or susceptibility to Th1 type-mediated autoimmune diseases such as RA, MS, and ATD. These are the postpartum period and the period that follows cure of endogenous Cushing's syndrome or discontinuation of glucocorticoid therapy.[6,49,51] This might also include the period that follows cessation of chronic stress or a rebound effect on relief from stressors.[35]

Interestingly, recent studies indicate that methotrexate and sulfasalazine, the most effective second-line agents for the treatment of RA, enhance extracellular adenosine concentrations.[28,52] Excessive production of IL-12 and TNF-α appears to play a critical role in RA. Thus, our results suggest that methotrexate via release of adenosine and through A2a receptors inhibits IL-12 and TNF-α production, which may explain, at least in part, the beneficial effects of these drugs in RA patients.[31]

Allergy/Atopy

Dominant Th2 responses and a shift to IgE production characterize atopic reactions, such as asthma, eczema, hay fever, and urticaria. As in the case of autoimmunity, the effects of stress on atopic reactions are complex, occur at multiple levels, and can be exerted in either direction. Stress hormones acting at the level of APCs and Th1 cells may induce a Th2 shift and thus facilitate or sustain atopic reactions; however, this can be antagonized by their effects on mast cells (for details see Ref. 35).

In vivo and *in vitro* exposure to glucocorticoids and β_2-agonists result in a reduction of IL-12 production, which persists at least several days.[6,8,14] Thus, glucocorticoid and β_2-AR-agonist therapy in asthma is likely to reduce the capacity of APC to produce IL-12, to suppress type 2 cytokine synthesis in activated but not resting T cells, and to abolish eosinophilia.[8] If, however, resting (cytokine-uncommitted) T cells are subsequently activated by APCs preexposed to glucocorticoids and/or β_2-AR agonists, enhanced IL-4 production, but limited IFN-γ synthesis, could be induced.[8] This suggests that, while in the short term the effect of glucocorticoids and β_2-AR agonists may be beneficial in asthma, their long-term effects might be to sustain the increased vulnerability of the patient to this condition. This is further supported by the observations that both glucocorticoids and β_2-AR agonists potentiate the IgE production *in vitro* and *in vivo*.[53,54]

Tumor Growth

Low levels of IL-12 have been associated with tumor growth, as opposed to the tumor regression observed with administration of IL-12 delivered *in situ* or systemically.[4] On the other hand, local overproduction of IL-10 and TGF-β, by inhibiting the production of IL-12 and TNF-α and the cytotoxicity of NK and Tc cells, seems to play an inappropriate immunosuppressive role, as is seen in melanoma.[55]

Stress can increase the susceptibility to tumors, tumor growth, and metastases. In animals, β-AR stimulation suppresses NK cell activity and compromises resistance to tumor metastases[56]; stress decreases the potential of spleen cells to turn into anti-tumor Tc against syngeneic B16 melanoma, and it significantly suppresses the ability of tumor-specific CD4+ cells to produce IFN-γ and IL-2.[57] High concentrations of histamine have been measured within colorectal and breast cancer tissues, and treatment with cimetidine, an H2 histamine antagonist, correlates with increased survival in patients with colorectal cancer.[25,58] Our results suggest that by preventing the effect of histamine on IL-12 and IL-10 production, cimetidine may contribute to a restoration of Th1 and a local cellular immune responses.

The above-described adenosine-induced inhibition of IL-12 production may be relevant to the immunosuppression observed in solid tumors, where hypoxic conditions cause accumulation of high concentrations of extracellular adenosine that may contribute to inhibition of cellular immunity.[59] These data suggest that stress hormone-, histamine-, and/or adenosine-induced inhibition of IL-12 and potentiation of IL-10 production and subsequent suppression of cellular immunity may contribute to the increased growth of certain tumors.

REFERENCES

1. FEARON, D.T. & R.M. LOCKSLEY. 1996. The instructive role of innate immunity in the acquired immune response. Science **272:** 50–53.

2. MOSMANN, T.R. & S. SAD. 1996. The expanding universe of T-cell subsets: Th1, Th2 and more. Immunol. Today **17:** 138–146.

3. BUTLER, D.M., A.M. MALFAIT, R.N. MAINI *et al.* 1999. Anti-IL-12 and anti-TNF antibodies synergistically suppress the progression of murine collagen-induced arthritis. Eur. J. Immunol. **29:** 2205–2212.

4. COLOMBO, M.P., M. VAGLIANI, F. SPREAFICO *et al.* 1996. Amount of interleukin 12 available at the tumor site is critical for tumor regression. Cancer Res. **56:** 2531–2534.

5. TRINCHIERI, G. 1995. Interleukin-12: a proinflammatory cytokine with immunoregulatory functions that bridge innate resistance and antigen-specific adaptive immunity. Annu. Rev. Immunol. **13:** 251–276.

6. ELENKOV, I.J., D.A. PAPANICOLAOU, R.L. WILDER & G.P. CHROUSOS. 1996. Modulatory effects of glucocorticoids and catecholamines on human interleukin-12 and interleukin-10 production: clinical implications. Proc. Assoc. Am. Physicians **108:** 374–381.

7. BLOTTA, M.H., R.H. DEKRUYFF & D.T. UMETSU. 1997. Corticosteroids inhibit IL-12 production in human monocytes and enhance their capacity to induce IL-4 synthesis in CD4+ lymphocytes. J. Immunol. **158:** 5589–5595.

8. DEKRUYFF, R.H., Y. FANG & D.T. UMETSU. 1998. Corticosteroids enhance the capacity of macrophages to induce Th2 cytokine synthesis in CD4+ lymphocytes by inhibiting IL-12 production. J. Immunol. **160:** 2231–2237.

9. WU, C.Y., K. WANG, J.F. MCDYER & R.A. SEDER. 1998. Prostaglandin E_2 and dexamethasone inhibit IL-12 receptor expression and IL-12 responsiveness. J. Immunol. **161:** 2723–2730.

10. VAN DER POLL, T., A.E. BARBER, S.M. COYLE & S.F. LOWRY. 1996. Hypercortisolemia increases plasma interleukin-10 concentrations during human endotoxemia—a clinical research center study. J. Clin. Endocrinol. Metab. **81:** 3604–3606.

11. RAMIERZ, F., D.J. FOWELL, M. PUKLAVEC *et al.* 1996. Glucocorticoids promote a TH2 cytokine response by CD4+ T cells in vitro. J. Immunol. **156:** 2406–2412.

12. TABARDEL, Y., J. DUCHATEAU, D. SCHMARTZ *et al.* 1996. Corticosteroids increase blood interleukin-10 levels during cardiopulmonary bypass in men. Surgery **119:** 76–80.

13. GAYO, A., L. MOZO, A. SUAREZ *et al.* 1998. Glucocorticoids increase IL-10 expression in multiple sclerosis patients with acute relapse. J. Neuroimmunol. **85:** 122–130.

14. PANINA-BORDIGNON, P., D. MAZZEO, P.D. LUCIA *et al.* 1997. β2-Agonists prevent Th1 development by selective inhibition of interleukin 12. J. Clin. Invest. **100:** 151–1519.

15. HASKO, G., C. SZABO, Z.H. NEMETH *et al.* 1998. Stimulation of β-adrenoceptors inhibits endotoxin-induced IL-12 production in normal and IL-10 deficient mice. J. Neuroimmunol. **88:** 57–61.

16. SANDERS, V.M., R.A. BAKER, D.S. RAMER-QUINN *et al.* 1997. Differential expression of the β2-adrenergic receptor by Th1 and Th2 clones: implications for cytokine production and B-cell help. J. Immunol. **158:** 4200–4210.

17. BORGER, P., Y. HOEKSTRA, M.T. ESSELINK *et al.* 1998. β-Adrenoceptor-mediated inhibition of IFN-γ, IL-3, and GM-CSF mRNA accumulation in activated human T lymphocytes is solely mediated by the β2-adrenoceptor subtype. Am. J. Respir. Cell Mol. Biol. **19:** 400–407.

18. HASKO, G., I.J. ELENKOV, V. KVETAN & E.S. VIZI. 1995. Differential effect of selective block of α2-adrenoreceptors on plasma levels of tumour necrosis factor-α, interleukin-6 and corticosterone induced by bacterial lipopolysaccharide in mice. J. Endocrinol. **144:** 457–462.

19. ELENKOV, I.J., G. HASKO, K.J. KOVACS & E.S. VIZI. 1995. Modulation of lipopolysac-charide-induced tumor necrosis factor-α production by selective α- and β-adrenergic drugs in mice. J. Neuroimmunol. **61:** 123–131.

20. WOICIECHOWSKY, C., K. ASADULLAH, D. NESTLER *et al.* 1998. Sympathetic activation triggers systemic interleukin-10 release in immunodepression induced by brain injury. Nat. Med. **4:** 808–813.

21. ROCKLIN, R.E. 1990. Histamine and H2 antagonists in inflammation and immunodefi-ciency. Marcel Dekker. New York and Basel.

22. FALUS, A. & K. MERETEY. 1992. Histamine: an early messenger in inflammatory and immune reactions. Immunol. Today **13:** 154–156.

23. VANNIER, E., L.C. MILLER & C.A. DINARELLO. 1991. Histamine suppresses gene expression and synthesis of tumor necrosis factor alpha via histamine H2 receptors. J. Exp. Med. **174:** 281–284.

24. VANNIER, E. & C.A. DINARELLO. 1994. Histamine enhances interleukin (IL)-1-induced IL-6 gene expression and protein synthesis via H2 receptors in peripheral blood mononuclear cells. J. Biol. Chem. **269:** 9952–9956.

25. ELENKOV, I.J., E. WEBSTER, D.A. PAPANICOLAOU *et al.* 1998. Histamine potently sup-presses human IL-12 and stimulates IL-10 production via H2 receptors. J. Immunol. **161:** 2586–2593.

26. SMIT, M.J., R. LEURS, S.R. SHUKRULA *et al.* 1994. Rapid desensitization of the hista-mine H2 receptor on the human monocytic cell line U937. Eur. J. Pharmacol. **288:** 17–25.

27. LAGIER, B., B. LEBEL, J. BOUSQUET & J. PENE. 1997. Different modulation by hista-mine of IL-4 and interferon-γ (IFN-γ) release according to the phenotype of human Th0, Th1 and Th2 clones. Clin. Exp. Immunol. **108:** 545–551.

28. CRONSTEIN, B.N., D. NAIME & E. OSTAD. 1993. The antiinflammatory mechanism of methotrexate. Increased adenosine release at inflamed sites diminishes leukocyte accumulation in an in vivo model of inflammation. J. Clin. Invest. **92:** 2675–2682.

29. CRONSTEIN, B.N., E.D. ROSENSTEIN, S.B. KRAMER *et al.* 1985. Adenosine: a physio-logic modulator of superoxide anion generation by human neutrophils. Adenosine acts via an A2 receptor on human neutrophils. J. Immunol. **135:** 1366–1371.

30. LAPPIN, D. & K. WHALEY. 1984. Adenosine A2 receptors on human monocytes modu-late C2 production. Clin. Exp. Immunol. **57:** 454–460.

31. LINK, A.A., T. KINO, J.A. WORTH *et al.* 1999. Ligand activation of adenosine A2a receptors inhibits IL-12 production by human monocytes. J. Immunol. **164:** 436–442.

32. PRABHAKAR, U., D.P. BROOKS, D. LIPSHLITZ & K.M. ESSER. 1995. Inhibition of LPS-induced TNF-α production in human monocytes by adenosine (A2) receptor selec-tive agonists. Int. J. Immunopharmacol. **17:** 221–224.

33. LE MOINE, O. 1996. Adenosine enhances IL-10 secretion by human monocytes. J. Immunol. **156:** 4408–4414.

34. HASKO, G., C. SZABO, Z.H. NEMETH *et al.* 1996. Adenosine receptor agonists differen-tially regulate IL-10, TNF-α, and nitric oxide production in RAW 264.7 macroph-ages and in endotoxemic mice. J. Immunol. **157:** 4634–4640.

35. ELENKOV, I.J. & G.P. CHROUSOS. 1999. Stress hormones, Th1/Th2 patterns, pro/anti-inflammatory cytokines and susceptibility to disease. Trends Endocrinol. Metabol. **10:** 359–368.

36. ALTARE, F., A. DURANDY, D. LAMMAS *et al.* 1998. Impairment of mycobacterial immunity in human interleukin-12 receptor deficiency. Science **280:** 1432–1435.

37. LERNER, B.H. 1996. Can stress cause disease? Revisiting the tuberculosis research of Thomas Holmes, 1949–1961. Ann. Intern. Med. **124:** 673–680.

38. KARTTUNEN, R.A., T.J. KARTTUNEN, M.M. YOUSFI *et al.* 1997. Expression of mRNA for interferon-γ, interleukin-10, and interleukin-12 (p40) in normal gastric mucosa and in mucosa infected with *Helicobacter pylori*. Scand. J. Gastroenterol. **32:** 2–27.

39. O'SULLIVAN, S.T., J.A. LEDERER, A.F. HORGAN *et al.* 1995. Major injury leads to pre-dominance of the T helper-2 lymphocyte phenotype and diminished interleukin-12 production associated with decreased resistance to infection. Ann. Surg. **222:** 482–490.

40. VAN BELLE, H., F. GOOSSENS & J. WYNANTS. 1987. Formation and release of purine catabolites during hypoperfusion, anoxia, and ischemia. Am. J. Physiol. **252:** H886–H893.

41. FELDMANN, M., F.M. BRENNAN & R.N. MAINI. 1996. Role of cytokines in rheumatoid arthritis. Annu. Rev. Immunol. **14:** 397–440.

42. KOTAKE, S., H.R.J. SCHUMACHER, C.H. YARBORO *et al.* 1997. In vivo gene expression of type 1 and type 2 cytokines in synovial tissues from patients in early stages of rheumatoid, reactive, and undifferentiated arthritis. Proc. Assoc. Am. Physicians **109:** 286–301.

43. BRALEY-MULLEN, H., G.C. SHARP, H. TANG *et al.* 1998. Interleukin-12 promotes activation of effector cells that induce a severe destructive granulomatous form of murine experimental autoimmune thyroiditis. Am. J. Pathol. **152:** 1347–1358.

44. SEGAL, B.M., B.K. DWYER & E.M. SHEVACH. 1998. An interleukin (IL)-10/IL-12 immunoregulatory circuit controls susceptibility to autoimmune disease. J. Exp. Med. **187:** 537–546.

45. PARK, Y.B., S.K. LEE, D.S. KIM *et al.* 1998. Elevated interleukin-10 levels correlated with disease activity in systemic lupus erythematosus. Clin. Exp. Rheumatol. **16:** 283–288.

46. GRONDAL, G., H. KRISTJANSDOTTIR, B. GUNNLAUGSDOTTIR *et al.* 1999. Increased number of interleukin-10-producing cells in systemic lupus erythematosus patients and their first-degree relatives and spouses in Icelandic multicase families. Arthritis Rheum. **42:** 1649–1654.

47. HORWITZ, D.A., J.D. GRAY, S.C. BEHRENDSEN *et al.* 1998. Decreased production of interleukin-12 and other Th1-type cytokines in patients with recent-onset systemic lupus erythematosus. Arthritis Rheum. **41:** 838–844.

48. ROGERS, M.P. & M. FOZDAR. 1996. Psychoneuroimmunology of autoimmune disorders. Adv. Neuroimmunol. **6:** 169–177.

49. WILDER, R.L. 1995. Neuroendocrine–immune system interactions and autoimmunity. Annu. Rev. Immunol. **13:** 307–338.

50. ELENKOV, I.J., J. HOFFMAN & R.L. WILDER. 1997. Does differential neuroendocrine control of cytokine production govern the expression of autoimmune diseases in pregnancy and the postpartum period? Mol. Med. Today **3:** 379–383.

51. CHROUSOS, G.P. 1995. The hypothalamic–pituitary–adrenal axis and immune-mediated inflammation. N. Engl. J. Med. **332:** 1351–1362.

52. MORABITO, L., M.C. MONTESINOS, D.M. SCHREIBMAN *et al.* 1998. Methotrexate and sulfasalazine promote adenosine release by a mechanism that requires ecto-5′-nucleotidase-mediated conversion of adenine nucleotides. J. Clin. Invest. **101:** 295–300.

53. ZIEG, G., G. LACK, R.J. HARBECK *et al.* 1994. In vivo effects of glucocorticoids on IgE production. J. Allergy Clin. Immunol. **94:** 222–230.

54. COQUERET, O., B. DUGAS, J.M. MENCIA-HUERTA & P. BRAQUET. 1995. Regulation of IgE production from human mononuclear cells by β_2-adrenoceptor agonists. Clin. Exp. Allergy **25:** 304–311.

55. CHOUAIB, S., C. ASSELIN-PATUREL, F. MAMI-CHOUAIB *et al.* 1997. The host–tumor immune conflict: from immunosuppression to resistance and destruction. Immunol. Today **18:** 493–497.

56. SHAKHAR, G. & S. BEN-ELIYAHU. 1998. In vivo β-adrenergic stimulation suppresses natural killer activity and compromises resistance to tumor metastasis in rats. J. Immunol. **160:** 3251–3258.

57. LI, T., M. HARADA, K. TAMADA *et al.* 1997. Repeated restraint stress impairs the antitumor T cell response through its suppressive effect on Th1-type CD4[+] T cells. Anticancer Res. **17:** 4259–4268.

58. MATSUMOTO, S. 1995. Cimetidine and survival with colorectal cancer. Lancet **346:** 115.

59. HOSKIN, D.W., T. REYNOLDS & J. BLAY. 1994. Adenosine as a possible inhibitor of killer T-cell activation in the microenvironment of solid tumours. Int. J. Cancer **59:** 854–855.

Hypothalamic Mechanisms of Pain Modulatory Actions of Cytokines and Prostaglandin E$_2$

T. HORI,[a,b] T. OKA,[b,c] M. HOSOI,[b,c] M. ABE,[b,d] AND K. OKA[b]

[b]Department of Integrative Physiology, Kyushu University
Graduate School of Medical Sciences, Fukuoka 812-8582, Japan

[c]Departments of Psychosomatic Medicine, Kyushu University Graduate School of
Medical Sciences, Fukuoka 812-8582, Japan

[d]Departments of Anesthesiology, Kyushu University Graduate School of Medical
Sciences, Fukuoka 812-8582, Japan

ABSTRACT: A decrease and subsequent increase in nociceptive threshold in the whole body are clinical symptoms frequently observed during the course of acute systemic infection. These biphasic changes in nociceptive reactivity are brought about by central signal substances induced by peripheral inflammatory messages. Systemic administration of lipopolysaccharide (LPS) or interleukin-1β (IL-1β), an experimental model of acute infection, may mimic the biphasic changes in nociception, hyperalgesia at small doses of LPS, and IL-1β and analgesia at larger doses. Our behavioral and electrophysiological studies have revealed that IL-1β in the brain induces hyperalgesia through the actions of prostaglandin E$_2$ (PGE$_2$) on EP3 receptors in the preoptic area and its neighboring basal forebrain, whereas the IL-1β-induced analgesia is produced by the actions of PGE$_2$ on EP1 receptors in the ventromedial hypothalamus. An intravenous injection of LPS (10–100 μg/kg) produced hyperalgesia only during the period before fever develops and was abolished by microinjection of NS-398 (an inhibitor of cyclooxygenase 2) into the preoptic area, but not into the other areas in the hypothalamus. The hyperalgesia induced by the cytokines PGE$_2$ and LPS may explain the systemic hyperalgesia clinically observed in the early phase of infectious diseases, which probably warns the organisms of infection before the full development of sickness symptoms. The switching of nociception from hyperalgesia to analgesia accompanied by sickness symptoms may reflect changes in the host's strategy for fighting microbial invasion as the disease progresses.

Inflammation is primarily a local response to injurious and inflammatory stimuli, and it is subject to positive and negative controls by pro- and antiinflammatory substances released locally, such as kinins, peptides, eicosanoids, and cytokines. Proinflammatory substances, directly or indirectly, stimulate and/or sensitize nociceptors, thereby producing local hyperalgesia. However, if inflammation is severe enough or spreads systemically, global changes in nociceptive thresholds occur in association, more or less, with a variety of sickness symptoms such as fever.[1,2]

[a]Address for correspondence: Dr. Tetsuro Hori, Department of Integrative Physiology, Kyushu University, Graduate School of Medical Sciences, Fukuoka 812-8582, Japan. Voice: +81-92-642-6085; fax: +81-92-642-6093.

thori@physiol.med.kyushu-u.ac.jp

Experiments involving intraplantar injection of interleukin-1β (IL-1β), for instance, have shown that increased levels of IL-1β may produce hyperalgesia at distant peripheral sites.[3] Peripheral administration of lipopolysaccharide (LPS) may cause a biphasic change in systemic nociceptive reactivity, that is, hyperalgesia initially at low doses of LPS, which is followed by analgesia if the doses are higher.[4] Apparently, these changes in nociception are brought about by altered activities of central pain-modulating systems in response to various signal substances in the brain such as eicosanoids and cytokines.

BIPHASIC CHANGES IN NOCICEPTIVE REACTIVITY DURING ACUTE INFLAMMATION

Hyperalgesia such as myalgia and arthralgia is one of the early clinical signs of acute systemic infection. Hyperalgesia is observed in animal models of acute inflammation that are induced by peripheral administration of LPS. For instance, an intravenous (i.v.) or intraperitoneal (i.p.) injection of LPS or lithium chloride produces hyperalgesia as assessed by spinally mediated pain reflex (tail-flick test) and supraspinally mediated nociceptive behaviors (hot-plate test and formalin test) in rats.[4–8] Because the tail-flick response to an innocuous stimulus (touch) is not affected by lithium chloride, the hyperalgesic response appears to be modality-specific.[7] A biphasic change of nociceptive threshold has also been demonstrated in rats.[4] LPS (i.v.) at lower doses reduces the tail-flick latency during the rising phase of monophasic fever and the first (early) phase of the biphasic fever. On the other hand, LPS (i.v.) at higher doses prolonged the tail-flick latency during the second (late) phase of the biphasic fever and the subsequent period showing hypothermia.[4]

CYTOKINES AND HYPERALGESIA

The enhancement of the nociceptive tail-flick response caused by LPS and lithium chloride (i.p.) is blocked by subcutaneous (s.c.) injection of IL-1 receptor antagonist (IL-1ra), suggesting the mediation by IL-1.[5] Indeed, IL-1 (i.p.) reduces the tail-flick latency and the paw-withdrawal latency in the rat[5,9] (see FIGURE 1). This raises a question whether the source of such IL-1 and its site(s) of actions for eliciting hyperalgesia are the peripheral tissues or central nervous system or both. On the basis of the findings on effects of subdiaphragmatic vagotomy, spinal cord lesion, and decerebration on LPS- and lithium chloride (i.p.)–induced hyperalgesia, Watkins *et al.*[6] have concluded that the illness-inducing agents produce hyperalgesia by the following means: By activating vagal afferents, presumably through production of IL-1 in hepatic Kupffer and endothelial cells, rather than by generating a blood-borne mediator of the blood–brain barrier, the vagal neural signals eventually reach as yet unknown brain site(s) rostral to the mid-mesencephalon, centrifugally, a descending pathway arising from the nucleus raphe magnus through the dorsolateral funiculus of the spinal cord. We have revealed that hyperalgesia induced by i.p. injection of IL-1β is completely abolished by intracerebroventricular (i.c.v.) injection of dichlophenac, an inhibitor of cyclooxygenase (COX), and α-melanocyte-stimulating hormone (α-MSH), a potent

A Diclofenac   B α-MSH

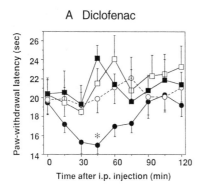 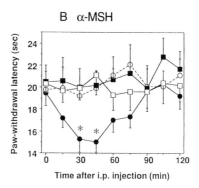

FIGURE 1. The inhibitory effects of i.c.v. injection of diclofenac (**A**) and α-MSH (**B**) on the rhIL-1β (i.p.)-induced hyperalgesia. In (**A**), rats were injected with diclofenac (1 ng, i.c.v.) + rhIL-1β (100 ng/kg, i.p.) (■), physiological saline (i.c.v.) + rhIL-1β (100 ng/kg, i.p.) (●), diclofenac (1 ng, i.c.v.) + vehicle (i.p.) (□), and physiological saline (i.c.v.) + vehicle(i.p.) (○). In (**B**), rats were injected with α-MSH (100 ng, i.c.v.) + rhIL-1β (100 ng/kg, i.p.) (■), physiological saline (i.c.v.) + rhIL-1β (100 ng/kg, i.p.) (●), α-MSH (100 ng, i.c.v.) + vehicle (i.p.) (□), and physiological saline (i.c.v.) + vehicle(i.p.) (○). I.c.v. injection of diclofenac, α-MSH or physiological saline was performed 10 min before the i.p. injection of either rhIL-1β or vehicle. Each point represents mean ±SEM. Symbols adjacent to points represent the level of significance when compared with saline (i.c.v.) + vehicle (i.p.) controls. *$p < 0.05$. (From Oka *et al.*[9] with permission from Elsevier Science, Oxford, U.K.)

antiinflammatory peptide, at doses that had no effect when peripherally given (FIG. 1).[9] These findings suggest that brain mechanisms involving the production of eicosanoids and an α-MSH-sensitive process is involved in hyperalgesia evoked by peripheral IL-1β.

HYPOTHALAMIC CYTOKINES AND BIPHASIC MODULATION OF NOCICEPTIVE REACTIVITY

It is well established that pro- and antiinflammatory cytokines are synthesized in the brain by microglia, astrocytes, vascular endothelial cells, meningeal macrophages, and probably also by neurons. The receptors and the binding sites of these cytokines have also been described in the brain. (See Wong *et al.*[10] for review.) The induction of proinflammatory cytokines (IL-1, IL-6, and tumor necrosis factor-α [TNF-α]) in the brain occurs during peripheral inflammation as well as during pathological processes in the brain such as central infection and ischemia.[10,11] An i.p. or i.v. administration of LPS is known to increase the levels of IL-1β, TNF-α, and IL-6 and their mRNA in the brain.[12–16] These brain-derived cytokines cause a variety of acute sickness symptoms, including biphasic modulation of pain, that are almost identical with those observed during peripheral infection. It has been reported that i.c.v. injection of IL-1β, IL-6, and TNF-α induce either hyperalgesia,[17–22] analgesia,[23–26] or no effect[27] (see TABLE 1). These contradictory findings may be explained by differences in the concentration of IL-1 administered,[28] the sites of its actions in the hypothalamus,[29,30] and the types of stimulated receptors for prostaglandin E$_2$ (PGE$_2$), which is a principal mediator of proinflammatory cytokines.[31] It is therefore possible to suggest that brain-derived cytokines are involved in the biphasic changes of nociceptive reactivity after i.p. injection of LPS. But the appearance of IL-1-like immunoreactivity is observed in the brain 90 min after peripheral administration of LPS.[12] Therefore, centrally induced cytokines are unlikely to contribute to, at least, the early phase of LPS-induced hyperalgesia that starts 5 min after LPS administration; rather they are responsible for the maintenance of LPS-induced hyperalgesia, which lasts at least 90 min.[6,8]

HYPOTHALAMIC PGE$_2$ AND BIPHASIC MODULATION OF NOCICEPTIVE REACTIVITY

As has already been described, thermal hyperalgesia induced by IL-1β (i.p.) administration at nonpyrogenic doses (10–100 ng/kg = ca. 3.25–32.5 ng) is mediated by central mechanisms involving the production of eicosanoids and an α-MSH-sensitive process.[9] Moreover, hyperalgesia produced by an i.v. injection of LPS (10–100 μg/kg) is abolished by microinjection of dichlophenac (a nonselective inhibitor of COX-1 and COX-2) or NS398 (a selective COX-2 inhibitor) into the medial preoptic area (MPO), but not into the other hypothalamic nuclei.[8]

The complete blocking of LPS (i.v.)-induced hyperalgesia by COX inhibitors at the MPO region suggests the obligatory role of local synthesis of eicosanoids for the manifestation of hyperalgesia. There is ample evidence that PGE$_2$ at the preoptic area (POA) and the neighboring basal forebrain is a principal, if not the sole, mediator of hyperalgesia. First, an injection of LPS (i.p.) or IL-1β (i.v.) produces an increase in the PGE$_2$ levels in the POA region of rats and guinea pigs that is detectable within 30 min.[32,34] Second, rat hypothalamic explants, when stimulated with IL-1β, release only PGE$_2$.[35] Third, the other eicosanoids, such as PGI$_2$ and PGD$_2$, induce analgesia in rats.[36–38] Fourth, there are dense PGE$_2$ binding sites[39,40] and PGE$_2$ receptor mRNA is expressed in the hypothalamus including the POA region.[41] Finally, a majority of neurons in the POA region decrease their discharge rates in response to direct application of PGE$_2$.[42]

BIPHASIC MODULATION OF NOCICEPTION BY CENTRAL INJECTION OF PGE$_2$ AND ITS AGONISTS

Dose-Dependent Modulation of Nociception by PGE$_2$

To verify the hypothesis that central PGE$_2$ modulates pain, we studied the effects of i.c.v. injection of PGE$_2$ and its agonists on the paw-withdrawal latency on the hot plate in rats.[31] An i.c.v. injection of PGE$_2$ produced a biphasic effect on the nociceptive behavior depending on the doses administered; that is, it produced long-lasting (5–60 min after injection) hyperalgesia by PGE$_2$ at low, nonpyrogenic doses (10 pg/kg–10 ng/kg = ca. 3.25 pg–3.25 ng = ca. 9 fmol–9 pmol) and a rapid, short-lasting (5 min) analgesia at a high (pyrogenic) dose (1 μg/kg = ca. 325 ng = ca.900 pmol) (see FIGURES 2A and 2B).[29] Consistent with the behavioral findings, an i.c.v. injection of

TABLE 1. Effects of central injection of cytokines and PGE$_2$ on nociception

Cytokines and PGE$_2$	Effect	Dose	Duration sites of action	Animal	Method	Possible involvement	Other effects	Reference
i.c.v. injection								
IL-1β	Hyperalgesia	10 pg/kg–1 ng/kg[a]	5–60 min	Rat	Hot-plate test	IL-1R, PGs	10 ng/kg–1 μg/kg[a]: no effect	17
	Hyperalgesia	10 pg/kg–1 ng/kg[a]	5–60 min	Rat	WDR neuron	IL-1R, PGs	10 ng/kg–1 μg/kg[a]: no effect	18
	Hyperalgesia	10 pg	15–30 min	Rat	Hot-plate test		100 ng: no effect	22
	Hyperalgesia	5–50 ng	15–55 min	Rat	Tail-flick test			19
	No effect	125–2000 IU (0.25–4 ng)		Rat	Cold-water tail-flick, hot-plate test		Fever	27
	Bimodal			Rat	Paw-pressure test			28
	Hyperalgesia	10–100 pg	60–180 min			IL-1R, PGs, CRF		
	Analgesia	1–10 ng	120–180 min			IL-1R, CRF	Fever	
IL-1α	No effect	250–1000 IU (2.5–10 ng)		Rat	Cold-water tail-flick, hot plate test		Fever	27
	Analgesia	48 ng/kg[b]	5–20 min	Mouse	Writhing test			23
	Analgesia	1 ng		Mouse	Writhing test	Peripheral CRF		25
	Analgesia	2.5–15 ng	3–5 min	Rat	Hot-plate test			24
	Analgesia	5 ng	3 min	Rat	Hot-plate test	Central CRF and NA		26
IL-6	Hyperalgesia	300 pg–300 ng	15–30 min	Rat	Hot-plate test	PGs		20
TNFα	Hyperalgesia	10 pg–1 ng	60 min	Rat	Plantar test	IL-1, PGs	10 ng: no effect	21
	Analgesia	1–3.5 ng	3–5 min	Rat	Hot-plate test	IL-1	Decreased locomotion	24

TABLE 1./continued

Cytokines and PGE₂	Effect	Dose	Duration sites of action	Animal	Method	Possible involvement	Other effects	Reference
PGE₂	Bimodal			Rat				
	Hyperalgesia	10 pg/kg–10 ng/kg[a]	5–60 min		Hot-plate test	EP3R		31
	Hyperalgesia	3.5 pg	15–30 min		WDR neuron	EP3R		43, 47
	Analgesia	1 μg/kg[a]	5 min		Hot-plate test	EP1R		31
	Analgesia	350 ng	5–15 min		WDR neuron	EP1R		43, 47
Microinjection								
IL-1β	Hyperalgesia	5 pg/kg–50 pg/kg[c]	MPO	Rat	Hot-plate test	IL-1R, PGs	0.2–2 ng/kg[c]: no effect	29
		20 pg/kg	MnPO, LPO, DBB	Rat	Hot-plate test			
		5 ng	PVH	Rat	Hot-plate test			30
	Analgesia	20 pg/kg–50 pg/kg[c]	VMH	Rat	Hot-plate test	IL-1R, PGs		29
		5 ng	CM, G	Rat	Hot-plate test			30
PGE₂	Hyperalgesia	5–50 fg	MPO	Rat	Hot-plate test	EP3R	50 ng: no effect but produced fever	48
			MnPO, LPO, DBB[d]	Rat	Hot-plate test			
	Analgesia	5 pg–50 ng	VMH	Rat	Hot-plate test	EP1R		49

ABBREVIATIONS: IL-1R, IL-1 receptor; PG, prostaglandin; WDR, wide dynamic range; CRF, corticotropin releasing factor; NA, noradrenaline; EP3R, EP3 receptor; EP1R, EP1 receptor; MPO, medial preoptic area; MnPO, median preoptic nucleus; LPO, lateral preoptic area; DBB, diagonal band of Broca; PVH, paraventricular nucleus of the hypothalamus; VMH, ventromedial hypothalamus; CM, centromedial thalamic nucleus; G, gelatinosus thalamic nucleus.
[a]Rats weighing 300–350 g.
[b]50% inhibition in 20-g mice.
[c]Rats weighing 320–350 g.
[d]These sites were determined by the injection of M&B28767, an EP3 receptor agonist.

PGE_2 at low doses (1–10 fmol) enhanced the firing rate responses of wide dynamic range (WDR) neurons in the trigeminal nucleus caudalis to noxious pinching of facial skin 15–25 min after injection, whereas that of PGE_2 at higher doses (100 pmol–1 nmol) inhibited them 5–15 min after injection (FIGS. 2C and 2D).[43] Low-threshold mechanoreceptive neurons in the same nucleus, which relay the innocuous, tactile signals, did not change their responsiveness to skin brushing after i.c.v. injection of PGE_2 at both 10 fmol and 1 nmol. This indicates that the modulatory effect of PGE_2 on the responsiveness of somatosensory neurons is modality-specific.

Biphasic Modulation of Nociception through Different Types of PGE_2 Receptors

Four subtypes of the PGE_2 receptors, EP1, EP2, EP3, and EP4, have been cloned from mouse,[44] human,[45] and rat.[46] They are known to couple to different signal transduction pathways, that is, mobilization of intracellular Ca^{2+} (EP1), activation (EP2 and EP4), or inhibition (EP3) of adenylate cyclase. We have demonstrated that

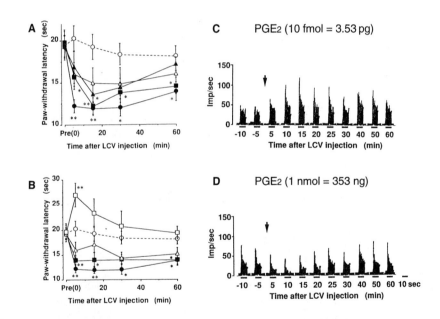

FIGURE 2. Effects of i.c.v. injection of PGE_2 on nociception as assessed by a hot-plate test (A and B) and by changes in the firing rate responses of WDR neurons in the trigeminal nucleus caudalis to noxious stimuli (C and D). In (**A**), rats were injected with PGE_2 at 1 pg/kg (△), 10 pg/kg (▲), 100 pg/kg (■), and 1 ng/kg (●), and physiological saline (○). In (**B**), rats were injected with PGE_2 at 1 ng/kg (●), 10 ng/kg (■), 100 ng/kg (△), and 1 μg/kg (□), and physiological saline (○). Data of rats injected with PGE_2 at 1 ng/kg and physiological saline shown in A are also illustrated in B for comparison. Each point represents mean ±SEM. Symbols adjacent to points represent the level of significance when compared with saline-injected controls. *$p < 0.05$; **$p < 0.01$. In (**C**) and (**D**), noxious pinching was applied during the underlined 10-sec periods. (From Oka *et al.*[31] and Oka *et al.*[43] with permission from Elsevier Science, Oxford, U.K.)

an i.c.v. injection of an EP3 receptor agonist (M&B28767) at 1 pg/kg–100 pg/kg (ca. 0.9–90 fmol) decreases the paw-withdrawal latency on a hot-plate 15–60 min after injection[31] and the injection of M&B28767 at 1–100 fmol augments the nociceptive responses of the trigeminal WDR neurons in a similar time course with that of the nociceptive behavioral response (see FIGURE 3).[47] In contrast, an i.c.v. administration of an EP1 receptor agonist (17-phenyl-ω-trinor PGE$_2$) at 50 μg/kg (ca. 42 nmol) and 1–10 nmol prolongs the paw-withdrawal latency[31] and inhibits the nociceptive responses of WDR neurons[47] 5–15 min after injection, respectively (FIG. 3). Moreover, an EP1 receptor antagonist (SC19220) at 300 nmol (i.c.v.) abolished the PGE$_2$ (1 nmol, i.c.v.)-induced analgesic effects on the nociceptive behavior[31] and the nociceptive responses of WDR neurons.[47] On the other hand, an i.c.v. injection of butaprost (an EP2 receptor agonist) at 100 fmol and 10 nmol had no effect on nociceptive threshold examined behaviorally[31] and electrophysiologically.[47] Thus, PGE$_2$

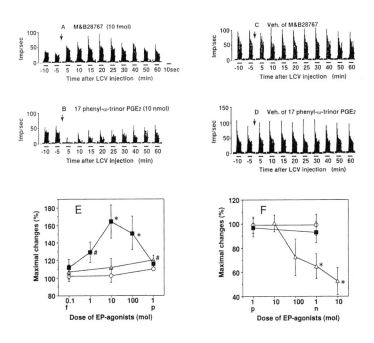

FIGURE 3. Effects of i.c.v. injection of EP-receptor agonists on the firing rate responses of the trigeminal WDR neurons to noxious pinching. M&B28767 at 10 fmol (**A**), 17-phenyl-ω-trinor PGE$_2$ at 10 nmol (**B**), vehicle of M&B28767 (**C**), and vehicle of 17-phenyl-ω-trinor PGE$_2$ (**D**) were injected into the lateral cerebroventricle at time zero. (**E, F**) Dose-related effects of EP receptor agonists on the responses of WDR neurons to noxious pinching. The maximal changes during the observation period (enhancement (**E**) and suppression (**F**)) in the nociceptive neuronal responses after injection of 17-phenyl-ω-trinor PGE$_2$ (△), butaprost (○), and M&B28767 (■) are plotted. Noxious pinching was applied during the underlined 10-sec periods. Each point represents mean ±SEM. Symbols adjacent to points represent the level of significance when compared with the nociceptive responses after treatment with corresponding vehicles. *$p < 0.05$, **$p < 0.01$. (From Oka *et al.*[47] with permission from Elsevier Science, Oxford, U.K.)

in the brain at lower levels produces hyperalgesia through its actions on EP3 receptors and at higher levels produces analgesia through its actions on EP1 receptors.

Biphasic Modulation of Nociception by Actions of PGE₂ on Different Sites in the Hypothalamus

We then investigated another, additional possibility that the biphasic modulation of nociception of PGE₂ is caused by its actions on different sites in the hypothalamus and neighboring basal forebrain where i.c.v.-administered PGE₂ is most likely to

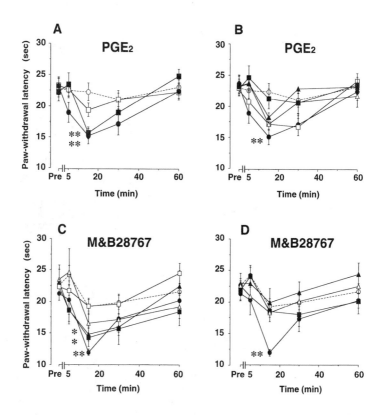

FIGURE 4. Effects of microinjection of PGE₂ **(A, B)** and M&B28767 **(C, D)** into the MPO on paw-withdrawal latency on a hot plate. In **(A)**, rats were microinjected with PGE₂ at 0.5 fg (□), 5 fg (■), and 50 fg (●), and saline (○). In **(B)**, rats were microinjected with PGE₂ at 50 fg (●), 500 fg (□), 5 pg (△), 50 pg (▲), and 500 pg (■), and saline (○). Data of rats microinjected with PGE₂ at 50 fg (●) and saline (○) shown in A are also illustrated in B for comparison. In **(C)**, rats were microinjected with M&B28767 at 0.005 fg (□), 0.05 fg (▲), 0.5 fg (●), 5 fg (■), and 50 fg (△), and vehicle (○). In **(D)**, rats were microinjected with M&B28767 at 0.5 fg (●), 500 fg (▲), 5 pg (■), and 50 pg (△), and vehicle (○). Data of rats microinjected with M&B28767 at 0.5 fg (●) and vehicle (○) shown in C are also illustrated in D for comparison. Symbols adjacent to points represent the level of significance. *$p < 0.05$, **$p < 0.01$. (From Hosoi et al.[48] with permission from the International Association for the Study of Pain, Seattle, Washington.)

reach. We found that the most sensitive sites to microinjected PGE$_2$ (5–50 fg, non-pyrogenic doses) and M&B28767 (0.05–5 fg) in producing hyperalgesic behavior are located in the POA region, that is, the medial and the lateral parts of POA, the median preoptic nucleus (MnPO), and the diagonal band of Broca (DBB) (see Figure 4).[48] These areas contain neurons that alter the firing rate in response to direct application of PGE$_2$[42] and express EP3 receptors mRNA at high levels.[41] Neither the microinjection of 17-phenyl-ω-trinor PGE$_2$ (an EP1 agonist) nor of butaprost (an EP2 agonist) affected nociception in the POA region.

On the other hand, the site most sensitive to injected PGE$_2$ (5 pg–50 ng) and 17-phenyl-ω-trinor PGE$_2$ (500 pg) for evoking analgesia was found to be the VMH.[49] Furthermore, the analgesia after intra-VMH administration of PGE$_2$ (500 pg) was abolished by co-injection of SC19220 (150 ng). In comparison with the high levels of EP3 receptor mRNA in the brain, the transcript of EP1 receptors is poorly expressed in the brain and is found only in the supraoptic nucleus and the paraventricular nucleus of the hypothalamus.[50] The cloned murine and rat EP3 receptors have a higher affinity to PGE$_2$ than EP1 receptors.[46,51] The differences in the densities of EP1 and EP3 receptor transcripts may explain the higher sensitivity to PGE$_2$ in inducing EP3 receptor-mediated hyperalgesia and the lower sensitivity in evoking the EP1 receptor-mediated analgesia. In line with the failure of butaprost (an EP2 agonist) to modulate nociception, the EP2 receptor mRNA is not detectable in the brain.[52] The disappearance of the hyperalgesic effects of PGE$_2$ and M&B28767 at the higher doses may be due to the desensitization of EP3 receptors that occurs during exposure to high levels of PGE$_2$.[53–55] Thus, PGE$_2$ at low levels produces hyperalgesia through its actions on EP3 receptors in the POA, MnPO, and DBB, whereas PGE$_2$ at high levels induces analgesia through its actions on EP1 receptors in the VMH. The switching from hyperalgesia to analgesia with an increase in PGE$_2$ levels is associated with the development of systemic acute-phase responses such as fever. It is interesting that fever and activation of the splenic sympathetic nerve are brought about by stimulation of EP1 receptors in the brain.[56–58]

CENTRAL NEURAL PATHWAYS FOR MODULATION OF PAIN BY PERIPHERAL LPS

Regarding the issue of how peripherally (i.p. or i.v.) administered LPS increases PGE$_2$ levels in the hypothalamus, the following mechanisms may be considered (see Figure 5A): (1) LPS or LPS-induced signal substances (e.g., cytokines and complements) stimulate peripheral sensory nerves, particularly the vagus in the case of i.p. injection.[66,59] (2) The neural signals reach the medullary adrenergic neurons (A1/A2) by way of the nucleus of tractus solitarius, and (3) then they are conveyed to the MPO region via the ventral noradrenergic bundle, where (4) locally released noradrenaline acts on as yet unknown cells to activate the arachidonate metabolism.[59] Another mechanism proposed is that PGE$_2$ is synthesized *de novo* from endothelial cells of cerebral microvessels, perivascular microglia, and/or meningeal macrophages. It has been demnstrated that systemic injection of LPS induces COX-2 and its mRNA in these nonneuronal cells associated with cerebral microvessels, leptomeninges, and choroid plexus.[60–62] It is suggested that COX-2 induces PGE$_2$ to alter

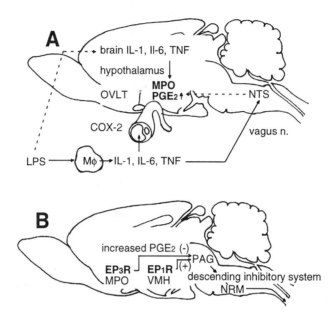

FIGURE 5. Summary and possible mechanisms of peripheral LPS- and cytokine-induced systemic hyperalgesia (**A**) and opposing effects of PGE_2 in the MPO and the VMH.

the activity of nearby brain regions that participate in different functions. Both mechanisms do not seem to be mutually exclusive, and they might work synergistically and/or contribute to different phases of LPS-induced changes in nociceptive reactivity.

It is not fully understood how the PGE_2-induced alteration of neuronal activities in the POA and VMH regions produce hyperalgesia and analgesia, respectively. One possible mechanism is that altered activities of hypothalamic neurons may influence the activity of neurons in the descending pain inhibitory system (DPIS) in the lower brainstem (FIG. 5B). (See Jones[63] for review.) Histological studies have revealed the direct neural connection from the POA and VMH regions to the periaqueductal grey matter (PAG) and the nucleus raphe magnus (NRM), principal nuclei in the DPIS.[64] Electrical stimulation of both the POA and VMH regions is known to produce behavioral analgesia[65] and an inhibition of nociceptive neuronal responses of the spinal dorsal horn in cats and rats[66–68] and the trigeminal nucleus caudalis in rats.[69] The analgesic effects of stimulation of the POA and VMH regions have been shown to be mediated by the activation of the DPIS69,[70] rather than their direct projection to the spinal cord and the trigeminal sensory nucleus. Electrophysiological studies have shown that PGE_2 and IL-1β predominantly reduce the discharge rate of neurons in the POA region[71–73] and IL-1β facilitates the firing rate of VMH neurons[74] in a prostaglandin-dependent way. Therefore, it is suggested that the reduced activity of POA neurons and increased activity of VMH neurons by PGE_2 and IL-1β suppresses and augments the activity of the DPIS, respectively, thereby inducing hyperalgesia and analgesia.

It is obvious that PGE$_2$ is not the sole signal substance in the hypothalamus to mediate pain modulation by peripherally derived inflammatory messages. It remains to be determined whether central modulation of pain involves actions of the other eicosanoids, nitric oxide, classical transmitters (catecholamines and serotonin), peptides (opioids, α-MSH, and CRF), and a number of proinflammatory and antiinflammatory cytokines (interferon-α), IL-1ra, IL-4, and IL-10), and how they are interrelated.

ACKNOWLEDGMENTS

This work is supported by Grant-in-Aid for Scientific Research ((A)10307001 and (B)09557006 to T. Hori) from the Ministry of Education, Science, and Culture, Japan.

REFERENCES

1. KUSHNER, I. 1997. The phenomenon of the acute phase response. Ann. N.Y. Acad. Sci. **389:** 39–48.
2. HORI, T., T. NAKASHIMA, S. TAKE *et al.* 1991. Immune cytokines and regulation of body temperature, food intake and cellular immunity. Brain Res. Bull. **27:** 309–313.
3. FERREIRA, S.H., B.B. LORENZETTI & A.F. BRISTOW. 1988. Interleukin-1β as a potent hyperalgesic agent antagonized by a tripeptide analogue. Nature **334:** 698–700.
4. ROMANOVSKY, A.A., V.A. KULCHITSKY, N.V. AKULICH *et al.* 1996. First and second phases of biphasic fever: two sequential stages of the sickness syndrome? Am. J. Physiol. **271:** R244–R253.
5. MAIER, S.F., E.P. WIERTELAK, D. MARTIN & L.R. WATKINS. 1993. Interleukin-1 mediates the behavioral hyperalgesia produced by lithium chloride and endotoxin. Brain Res. **623:** 321–324.
6. WATKINS, L.R., E.P. WIERTELAK, L.E. GOEHLER *et al.* 1994. Neurocircuitry of illness-induced hyperalgesia. Brain Res. **639:** 283–299.
7. WIERTELAK, E.P., K.P. SMITH, L. FURNESS *et al.* 1994. Acute and conditioned hyperalgesic responses to illness. Pain **56:** 227–234.
8. ABE, M., T. OKA, T. HORI & S. TAKAHASHI. 1998. The preoptic hypothalamus mediates hyperalgesia induced by intravenous injection of lipopolysaccharide. Anesthesiology **89:** A1157.
9. OKA, T., K. OKA, M. HOSOI & T. HORI. 1996. Inhibition of peripheral interleukin-1β-induced hyperalgesia by the intracerebroventricular administration of diclofenac and a-melanocyte-stimulating hormone. Brain Res. **736:** 237–242.
10. WONG, M.L., A. AL-SHEHELEE, P.W. GOLD & J. LICINIO. 1996. Cytokines in the brain. *In* Cytokines and the Nervous System. N.J. Rothwell, Ed.: 3–20. R.G. Landes Co. Austin, TX.
11. ROTHWELL, N.J. 1996. The role of cytokines in neurodegeneration. *In* Cytokines and the Nervous System. N.J. Rothwell, Ed.: 145–162. R.G. Landes Co. Austin, TX.
12. VAN DAM, A.M., M. BROUNS, S. LOUISSE & F. BERKENBOSCH. 1992. Appearance of interleukin-1 in macrophages and in ramified microglia in the brain of endotoxin-treated rats: a pathway for the induction of non-specific symptoms of sickness? Brain Res. **588:** 291–296.
13. COCEANI, F., J. LEES, J. MANCILLA *et al.* 1993. Interleukin-6 and tumor necrosis factor in cerebrospinal fluid: changes during pyrogen fever. Brain Res. **612:** 165–171.

14. BREDER, C.D., C. HAZUKA, T. GHAYUR et al. 1994. Regional induction of tumor necrosis factor α expression in the mouse brain after systemic lipopolysaccharide administration. Proc. Natl. Acad. Sci. USA **91:** 11393–11397.
15. SANNA, P.P., F. WEISS, M.E. SAMSON et al. 1995. Rapid induction of tumor necrosis factor α in the cerebrospinal fluid after intracerebroventricular injection of lipopolysaccharide revealed by a sensitive capture immuno-PCR assay. Proc. Natl. Acad. Sci. USA **92:** 272–275.
16. WONG, M.L, P.B. BONGIOMO, V. RETTORI et al. 1997. Interleukin (IL)-1β, IL-1 receptor antagonist, IL-10, and IL-13 gene expression in the central nervous system and anterior pituitary during systemic inflammation: pathophysiological implications, Proc. Natl. Acad. Sci. USA **94:** 227–232.
17. OKA, T., S. AOU & T. HORI. 1993. Intracerebroventricular injection of interleukin-1β induces hyperalgesia in rats. Brain Res. **624:** 61–68.
18. OKA, T., S. AOU & T. HORI. 1994. Intracerebroventricular injection of interleukin-1β enhances nociceptive neuronal responses of the trigeminal nuiclecus caudalis in rats. Brain Res. **656:** 236–244.
19. WATKINS, L.R., E.P. WIERTELAK, L.E. GOEHLER et al. 1994. Characterization of cytokine-induced hyperalgesia. Brain Res. **654:** 15–26.
20. OKA, T., K. OKA, M. HOSOI & T. HORI. 1995. Intracerebroventricular injection of interleukin-6 induces thermal hyperalgesia in rats, Brain Res. **692:** 123–128.
21. OKA, T., Y. WAKUGAWA, M. HOSOI et al. 1996. Intracerebroventricular injection of tumor necrosis factor-α induces thermal hyperalgesia in rats. Neuroimmunomodulation **3:** 135–140.
22. TONOSAKI, Y. & Y. SUGIURA. 1998. α-MSH modulates Fos expression in the paraventricular nucleus and hyperalgesia induced by intracerebroventricular administration of interleukin-1β in rats. Ann. N.Y. Acad. Sci. **840:** 615–618.
23. NAKAMURA, H., K. NAKANISHI, A. KITA & T. KADOKAWA. 1988. Interleukin-1 induces analgesia in mice by a central action. Eur. J. Pharmacol. **149:** 49–54.
24. BIANCHI, M., P. SACERDOTE, P. RICCIANDI-CASTAGNOLI, P. MANTEGAZZA & A.E. PANERAI. 1992. Central effects of tumor necrosis factor-α and interleukin-1α on nociceptive thresholds and spontaneous locomotor activity. Neurosci. Lett. **148:** 76–80.
25. KITA, A., K. IMANO & H. NAKAMURA. 1993. Involvement of corticotropin-releasing factor in the antinociception produced by interleukin-1 in mice. Eur. J. Pharmacol. **273:** 317–322.
26. BIANCHI, M. & A.E. PANERAI. 1995. CRH and the noradrenergic system mediate the antinociceptive effect of central interleukin-1α in the rat. Brain Res. Bull. **36:** 113–117.
27. ADAMS, J.U., J.L. BUSSIERE, E.B. GELLER & M.W. ADLER. 1993. Pyrogenic doses of intracerebroventricular interleukin-1 did not induce analgesia in the rat hot-plate or cold-water tail flick tests. Life Sci. **53:** 1401–1409.
28. YABUUCHI, K., A. NISHIYORI, M. MINAMI & M. SATOH. 1996. Biphasic effects of intracerebroventricular interleukin-1β on mechanical nociception in the rat. Eur. J. Pharmacol. **300:** 59–65.
29. OKA, T., K. OKA, M. HOSOI et al. 1995. The opposing effects of interleukin-1β microinjected into the preoptic hypothalamus and the ventromedial hypothalamus on nociceptive behavior in rats. Brain Res. **700:** 271–278.
30. SELLAMI, S. & R. DE BEAUREPAIRE. 1995. Hypothalamic and thalamic sites of action of interleukin-1β on food intake, body temperature and pain sensitivity in the rat, Brain Res. **694:** 69–77.
31. OKA, T., S. AOU & T. HORI. 1994. Intracerebroventricular injection of prostaglandin E_2 induces thermal hyperalgesia in rats: the possible involvement of EP3 receptors. Brain Res. **663:** 287–292.
32. SIRKO, S., L. BISHAI & F. COCEANI. 1989. Prostaglandin formation in the hypothalamus in vivo: effect of pyrogens. Am. J. Physiol. **256:** R616–R624.
33. KOMAKI, G., A. ARIMURA & K. KOVES. 1992. Effect of intravenous injection of IL-1β on PGE_2 levels in several brain areas as determined by microdialysis. Am. J. Physiol. **262:** E246–E251.

34. SEHIC, E., M. SZEKELY, A.L. UNGAR *et al.* 1996. Hypothalamic prostaglandin E$_2$ during lipopolysaccharide-induced fever in guinea pigs. Brain Res. Bull. **39:** 391–399.
35. NAVARRA, P., G. POZZOLI, L. BRUNETI *et al.* 1992. Interleukin-1β and interleukin-6 specifically increase the release of prostaglandin E$_2$ from rat hypothalamic explants in vitro. Neuroendocrinology **56:** 61–68.
36. PODDUBIUK, Z.M. 1976. A comparison of the central actions of prostaglandins A$_1$, E$_1$, E$_2$, F$_{1\alpha}$ and F$_{2\alpha}$ in the rat, I. behavioral, antinociceptive and anticonvulsant actions of intraventricular prostaglandins in the rat. Psychopharmacology **50:** 89–94.
37. OHKUBO, T., M. SHIBATA, H. TAKAHASHI & R. INOKI. 1983. Effect of prostaglandin D$_2$ on pain and inflammation. Jpn. J. Pharmacol. **33:** 264–266.
38. BHATTACHARYA, S.K. 1986. The antinociceptive effect of intracerebroventricularly administered prostaglandin D$_2$ in the rat. Psychopharmacology **89:** 121–124.
39. WATANABE, Y., Y. WATANABE & O. HAYAISHI. 1988. Quantitative autoradiographic localization of prostaglandin E$_2$ binding sites in monkey diencephalon. J. Neurosci. **8:** 2003–2010.
40. MATSUMURA, K., Y. WATANABE, K. IMAI-MATSUMURA *et al.* 1992. Mapping of prostaglandin E$_2$ binding sites in rat brain using quantitative autoradiography. Brain Res. **581:** 292–298.
41. SUGIMOTO, Y., R. SHIGEMOTO, T. NAMBA *et al.* 1994. Distribution of the messenger RNA for the prostaglandin E receptor subtype EP3 in the mouse nervous system. Neuroscience **62:** 919–928.
42. MATSUDA, T., T. HORI & T. NAKASHIMA. 1992. Thermal and PGE$_2$ sensitivity of the organum vasculosum lamina terminalis region and preoptic area in rat brain slices. J. Physiol. (London) **454:** 197–212.
43. OKA, T., M. HOSOI, K. OKA & T. HORI. 1997. Biphasic alteration in the trigeminal nociceptive neuronal responses after intracerebroventricular injection of prostaglandin E$_2$ in rats. Brain Res. **749:** 354–357.
44. SUGIMOTO, Y., M. NAMBA, A. HONDA *et al.* 1992. Cloning and expression of a cDNA for mouse prostaglandin E receptor EP3 subtype. J. Biol. Chem. **267:** 6463–6466.
45. FUNK, C.D., L. FURCI, G.A. FITZGERALDO *et al.* 1993. Cloning and expression of cDNA for the human prostaglandin E receptor EP1 subtype. J. Biol. Chem. **268:** 26767–26772.
46. BOIE, Y., R. STOCCO, N. SAWYER *et al.* 1997. Molecular cloning and characterization of the four prostaglanndin E$_2$ prostanoid receptor subtypes. Eur. J. Pharmacol. **340:** 227–241.
47. OKA, T., T. HORI, M. HOSOI *et al.* 1997. Biphasic modulation in the trigeminal nociceptive neuronal responses by the intracerebroventricular prostaglandin E$_2$ may be mediated through different EP receptor subtypes in rats. Brain Res. **771:** 278–284.
48. HOSOI, M., T. OKA & T. HORI. 1997. Prostaglandin E receptor EP3 subtype is involved in thermal hyperalgesia through its actions in the preoptic hypothalamus and the diagonal band of Broca in rats. Pain **71:** 303–311.
49. HOSOI, M., T. OKA, M. ABE *et al.* 1999. Prostaglandin E$_2$ has antinociceptive effect through EP1 receptor in the ventromedial hypothalamus in rats. Pain **83:** 221–227.
50. BATSHAKE, B., C. NILSSON & J. SUNDELIN. 1995. Molecular characterization of the mouse prostanoid EP1 receptor gene. Eur. J. Pharmacol. **231:** 809–814.
51. USHIKUBI, F., M. HIRATA & S. NARUMIYA. 1995. Molecular biology of prostanoid receptors; an overview. J. Lipid Mediat. Cell Signaling **12:** 343–359.
52. HONDA, A., Y. SUGIMOTO, T. NAMBA *et al.* 1993. Cloning and expression of a cDNA for mouse prostaglandin E receptor EP2 subtype. J. Biol. Chem. **268:** 7759–7762.
53. ROBERTSON, R.P. & S.A. LITTLE. 1983. Down-regulation of prostaglandin E receptors and homologous desensitization of isolated adipocytes. Endocrinology **113:** 1732–1738.
54. LIMAS, C. & C.J. LIMAS. 1987. Homologous regulation of prostaglandin E$_2$ receptors in rat renal medulla. Arch. Biochem. Biol. **259:** 89–97.
55. NEGISHI, M., Y. SUGIMOTO, A. IRIE *et al.* 1993. Two isoforms of prostaglandin E receptor EP3 subtype. J. Biol. Chem. **268:** 9517–9521.
56. OKA, T. & T. HORI. 1994. EP1 receptor mediation of prostaglandin E$_2$-induced hyperthermia in rats. Am. J. Physiol. **267:** R289–R294.

57. ANDO, T., T. ICHIJO, T. KATAFUCHI & T. HORI. 1995. Inntracerebroventricular injection of prostaglandin E_2 increases splenic sympathetic nerve activity in rats. Am. J. Physiol. **269:** R662–R668.

58. OKA, K., T. OKA & T. HORI. 1997. Prostaglandin E_2 may induce hyperthrmia through EP1 receptor in the anterior wall of the third ventricle and neighboring preoptic regions. Brain Res. **767:** 92–99.

59. BLATTEIS, C.M. & E. SEHIC. 1997. Prostaglandin E_2: a putative fever mediator. *In* Fever: Basic Mechanisms and Management. P.A. Mackowiak, Ed.: 117–145. Lippincott-Raven. Philadelphia, PA.

60. ELMQUIST, J.K., T.E. SCAMMELL & C.B. SAPER. 1997. Mechanisms of CNS response to systemic immune challenge: the febrile response. Trends Neurosci. **20:** 565–570.

61. LACROIX, S. & S. RIVEST. 1998. Effect of acute systemic inflammatory response and cytokines on the transcription of the genes encoding cyclooxygenase enzymes (COX-1 and COX-2) in the rat brain. J. Neurochem. **70:** 452–466.

62. MATSUMURA, K., K. CAO, M. OZAKI *et al.* 1998. Brain endothelial cells express cyclooxygenase-2 during lipopolysaccharide-induced fever: light and electron microscopic immunocytochemical studies. J. Neurosci. **18:** 6279–6289.

63. JONES, S.L. 1992. Descending control of nociception. *In* Pain and Headache. P.L. Gildenberg, Ed.: 203–295. S. Karger. Basel.

64. RIZVI, T.A., M. ENNIS & M.T. SHIRPLEY. 1992. Reciprocal connections between the medial preoptic area and the midbrain periaqueductal gray in rat: a WGA-HRP and PHA-L study. J. Comp. Neurol. **315:** 1–15.

65. RHODES, D.L. & J.C. LIEBESKIND. 1978. Analgesia from rostral brain stem stimulation in the rat. Brain Res. **143:** 521–532.

66. CARSTENS, E., J.D. MACKINNON & M.J. GUINAN. 1982. Inhibition of spinal dorsal horn neuronal responses to noxious skin heating by medial preoptic and septal stimulation in the cat. J. Neurophysiol. **48:** 981–991.

67. CULHANE, E.S. & E. CARSTENS. 1988. Medial hypothalamic stimulation suppresses nociceptive spinal dorsal horn neurons but not the tail-flick reflex in the rat. Brain Res. **438:** 137–144.

68. DUYSENS, J., R. DOM & J. GUYBELS. 1989. Suppression of the hinlimb flexor reflex by stimulation of the medial hypothalamus and thalamus in the rat. Brain Res. **499:** 131–140.

69. MOHKA, S.S., G.E. GOLDSMITH, R.F. HELLON & R. PURI. 1987. Hypothalamic control of nocireceptive and other neurones in the marginal layer of the dorsal horn of the medulla (trigeminal nucleus caudalis) in the rat. Exp. Brain Res. **65:** 427–436.

70. TAKESHIGE, C., T. SATO, T. MERA *et al.* 1992. Descending pain inhibitory system involved in acupuncture analgesia. Brain Res. Bull. **29:** 617–634.

71. HORI, T., M. SHIBATA, T. NAKASHIMA *et al.* 1988. Effects of interleukin-1 and arachidonate on the preoptic and anterior hypothalamic neurons, Brain Res. Bull. **20:** 75–82.

72. NAKASHIMA, T., T. HORI, T. MORI *et al.* 1989. Recombinant human interleukin-1β alters the activity of preoptic thermosensitive neurons in vitro. Brain Res. Bull. **23:** 209–213.

73. XIN, L. & C.M. BLATTEIS. 1992. Blockade by interleukin-1 receptor antagonist of IL-1β-induced neuronal activity in guinea pig preoptic area slices. Brain Res. **569:** 348–352.

74. KURIYAMA, K., T. HORI, T. MORI & T. NAKASHIMA. 1990. Actions of interferon-α and interleukin-1β on glucose-responsive neurons in the ventromedial hypothalamus. Brain Res. Bull. **24:** 803–810.

Molecular Mechanisms of Fever and Endogenous Antipyresis

WIESLAW KOZAK,[a] MATTHEW J. KLUGER,[a,b] JOHANNES TESFAIGZI,[c]
ANNA KOZAK,[a] KIMBERLY P. MAYFIELD,[c] MACIEJ WACHULEC,[a]
AND KAROL DOKLADNY[c]

[a]Medical College of Georgia, 1120 Fifteenth Street, CJ-3301,
Augusta, Georgia 30912-7620, USA

[c]Lovelace Respiratory Research Institute, P.O. Box 5890,
Albuquerque, New Mexico 87185, USA

ABSTRACT: This review summarizes recent studies on endogenous antipyretic mechanisms. Fever is the result of a balance between pyrogenic and cryogenic cytokines and hormones. Although there is considerable evidence that fever evolved as a host defense response, it is important that the rise in body temperature not be too high. Many endogenous cryogens or antipyretics that limit the rise in body temperature have been identified during the last 25 years. These include α-MSH, arginine vasopressin, glucocorticoids, TNF (under certain circumstances), and IL-10. Most recently, evidence has accumulated that cytochrome P-450 (P-450), part of the alternative pathway for arachidonic acid metabolism, plays an important role in reduction of fever and inflammation. Supporting a role for P-450 in endogenous antipyresis and antiinflammation includes evidence that (1) inducers of P-450 reduce fever, (2) inhibitors of P-450 cause a larger fever, (3) and P-450 arachidonic acid metabolites reduce fever.

INTRODUCTION

In the preface to the *Molecular Mechanisms of Fever*,[1] Kluger suggests that "One reason basic researchers have been attracted to this [fever] area is that fever is an example of a *regulated* change in homeostasis" and that "fever represents a *physiology of change.*" Indeed, since the classic work by Liebermeister in the middle of nineteenth century, it has been known that temperature regulation is not disrupted during fever. Rather, an individual upon contracting a disease associated with fever (e.g., infection, inflammation, trauma, and some tumors) regulates body temperature at a higher level than does a healthy individual. Hence, it is believed that the febrile temperature is a result of the upward resetting of the controlling variables, the setpoint of thermoregulation, presumably in the preoptic-anterior hypothalamus. On the other hand, since a provocative paper by DuBois published in 1949,[2] investigators and clinicians have appreciated that the febrile range has an upper limit,[3] in that

[b]Address for correspondence: Matthew Kluger, Ph.D., Vice President for Research and Dean, School of Graduate Studies, Medical College of Georgia, 1120 Fifteenth Street, CJ-3301, Augusta, GA 30912-2760. Voice: 706-721-6900; fax: 706-721-6478.
mkluger@mail.mcg.edu

the elevation of body temperature during fever does not exceed safe measures. In other words, the process of resetting the thermoregulatory set point upward during disease is controlled and, apparently, must be carefully guarded from reaching a dangerously high level. In this respect, fever appears to be a tightly controlled and regulated response which, on the one hand, reflects the shift of the set point of thermoregulation and, on the other hand, involves mechanisms acting to prevent fever from reaching dangerous heights. These latter mechanisms have been collectively called *endogenous antipyresis*. The study of the mechanisms underlying the generation of fever has a longer history than the investigation of endogenous antipyresis. Accordingly, there is a great deal more knowledge regarding endogenous pyretic than antipyretic mechanisms.[4] This review summarizes recent studies on endogenous antipyretic mechanisms.

MOLECULAR COMPONENTS OF FEVER AND ANTIPYRESIS

Over the past 25 years, evidence has accumulated that the endogenous febrile and antipyretic systems are operating at the level of neuroendocrino-immunomodulation. In fact, studies into the mechanisms underlying fever and endogenous antipyresis have significantly contributed to our understanding of the interaction between the immune system and central nervous system (CNS). Fever is triggered by the release of *endogenous pyrogens* from a large number of various immune types of cells including macrophage-like cells. Endogenous mediators of fever include cytokines, among which interleukin-1 (IL-1) and IL-6 are considered most important.[5,6] Inhibition of the production of one of these cytokines or neutralization of their activity results either in abrogation (e.g., if IL-6 is attenuated) or in substantial reduction (e.g., if IL-1β is attenuated) of fever during systemic or localized experimental inflammation.[7–9]

The search for *endogenous antipyretics* responsible for limiting the height of the febrile response began with studies of periparturient ewes and newborn lambs demonstrating refractoriness to pyrogenic effects of lipopolysaccharide (LPS).[10] Subsequent studies revealed that arginine vasopressin (AVP),[11,12] α-melanocyte-stimulating hormone (αMSH),[13,14] and glucocorticoids[15,16] can act as endogenous antipyretics opposing the effects of pyrogens. This led to the notion that fever is the result of a balance between pyrogenic cytokines and antipyretic hormones modulating the action of cytokines, presumably at the CNS level.[4] Nevertheless, components of the endogenous antipyresis can be also demonstrated within the cytokine network. Studies from our laboratory and others, using various techniques of neutralization of the cytokines (antibodies, inactivating binding proteins and receptors) as well as gene-deletion techniques (cytokine gene knockout mice), revealed that, besides pyrogenic cytokines, there are also cytokines that can be defined as endogenous antipyretics. They include tumor necrosis factor-α (TNF-α) and IL-10.

On the basis of data demonstrating that the injection of TNF-α induced elevation of body temperature in, for example, rabbits and humans,[4–6] this cytokine has been regarded as an endogenous pyrogen. Surprisingly, Long *et al.*[17] reported that pretreatment with TNF-α antiserum, instead of preventing fever, enhanced the febrile response to LPS in rats. In subsequent studies in mice, we observed that TNF-α can cause a drop in body temperature rather than fever.[18] A decrease in temperature induced by injection of TNF-α has also been observed in rats.[19] Furthermore, we observed that TNF-α prevented fever in mice[18] and rats[20] if co-injected with LPS. More interesting, unlike IL-1β and IL-6, inactivation of TNF-α provokes higher LPS-induced fever in mice,[18] the effect previously seen in rats. In support of these data, mice deficient in genes for production of the signaling receptors for TNF-α, p55, and p75 receptors (TNF double receptor-knockout mice) respond with a higher fever to injection of LPS compared to wild-type mice.[21] IL-10 knockout mice also demonstrated a higher fever to LPS than control wild-type mice.[22] Accordingly, injection of a recombinant murine IL-10 into mice does not generate fever. It does prevent, however, the LPS-induced elevation of body temperature in mice.[22] A similar inhibitory effect of IL-10 on fever has also been observed in humans.[23] Thus, one can hypothesize that, in addition to the balance between cytokines and hormones, the height of fever can also be affected and regulated by a balance between pyrogenic and antipyretic cytokines. The cytokine-to-cytokine effects during fever may be accompanied and further supplemented by the interactions of cytokines with a number of cytokine receptor antagonists, inhibitory soluble/shedded cytokine receptors, inhibitory cytokine-binding proteins, and cytokine-chaperon proteins,[5] which are also ascribed to the continuously growing cytokine family. Although this matter needs thorough investigation, the inhibitory effect of IL-1 receptor antagonist on fever in rats has already been demonstrated.[9]

Recently, we and others have reported that endogenous antipyresis may also be operating at the level of arachidonic acid cascade. Prostaglandin (PG) E_2 is considered a key mediator of fever acting downstream of the endogenous pyrogens and ultimately responsible for the upward resetting of the set point of thermoregulation.[24] It seems reasonable, therefore, to postulate that the regulation of the rate of production and/or metabolization of PGE_2 may possibly constitute an additional physiological system, to complement the cytokine–hormones and the cytokine–cytokine interactions in endogenous antipyresis and the regulation of fever. Data presented by Fraifeld *et al.*[25] implicate the involvement of the lipoxygenase pathway in endogenous antipyresis, whereas our data[26–28] and that from Nakashima and coworkers[29] indicate that the cytochrome *P*-450/epoxygenase pathway of the arachidonate metabolism is also part of the endogenous antipyretic system.

ALTERNATIVE PATHWAYS OF ARACHIDONIC ACID METABOLISM

Liberation of arachidonic acid from membrane structural glycerophospholipids is a hallmark for most, if not all, infectious as well as chronic and/or acute inflammatory disorders. Free arachidonic acid can be metabolized by cyclooxygenase and lipoxygenase enzyme systems to generate prostaglandins, thromboxanes, leukotrienes, and hydroperoxyeicosatetraenoic acids. The importance of the cyclooxygenase pathway in generation of fever and in induction of other symptoms of the acute-phase response during disease has been substantially documented.[24] The earliest studies on lipoxygenase, on the other hand, did not support any role for this pathway in fever.[30] However, as mentioned above, data have recently been reported suggesting a role for lipoxygenases in endogenous antipyresis.[25]

A third pathway of the arachidonate metabolism, producing epoxyeicosatrienoic acids (EETs) and mono-hydroxyeicosatetraenoic acids (mono-HETEs), has been described.[31] The pathway is carried out by the cytochrome P-450 (CYP450) monooxygenases, referred to as the epoxygenase pathway (P-450). Specific CYP450 enzymes catalyze monoxygenation of arachidonic acid leading to (a) epoxidation and giving rise to four regioisomers, 5,6-, 8,9-, 11,12-, and 14,15-EETs, which in turn are converted by epoxide hydrolases to corresponding dihydroxyeicosatrienoic acids (DHETs); (b) allylic oxidation to produce six regioisomers, 5-, 8-, 9-, 11-, 12-, and 15-HETEs, and (c) ω/ω-1 hydroxylation to result in 19- and 20-HETEs.[32,33] Among many tissues and organs, P-450 epoxygenase activity has also been detected in brain structures, including hypothalamus.[34] It has been shown that rat astrocytes[35] and isolated brain slices[36] make EET regioisomers from arachidonic acid. A generation of HETE regioisomers in cerebral tissues has also been documented.[37] P-450 arachidonic acid metabolites are currently implicated in a variety of biological functions, including kidney function,[32,33] cerebral blood flow,[36,37] and blood pressure.[38]

Involvement of the cytochrome P-450-dependent epoxygenase pathway of arachidonic acid in inflammation and fever has not been thoroughly investigated. It is known, however, that infections and inflammatory stimuli induce changes in the activities and expression of various forms of CYP in humans and experimental animals.[39] These effects could be a part of the homeostatic mechanisms associated with inflammation and infection. They also could be a part of the pathophysiology of fever. The formation of biologically active metabolites of arachidonic acid via P-450s indicates that pharmacological modulations of these enzymes may have consequences for the inflammatory disorders. Indeed, we have recently found that administration of the compounds that induce P-450 attenuates some histopathological and molecular measures of the LPS-provoked lung inflammation in the rat (unpublished data, manuscript in preparation). Our data have shown that inhibitors of P-450 augment fever in rodents, enhance the LPS-induced increase of plasma IL-6,[26] and exacerbate the elevation of PGE_2 in plasma and cerebrospinal fluid.[27] On the other hand, administration of the inducers of P-450 reduce fever in mice and rats.[28] Furthermore, intracerebral (i.c.v.) infusion of P-450 arachidonic acid metabolites reduce LPS-induced fever in rats.[28] The experimental protocols and data from these experiments are briefly discussed in the following sections of the article.

INDUCERS OF CYTOCHROME P-450
DECREASE FEVER IN MICE AND RATS

The rat P-450 monooxygenase isoforms known to catalyze the epoxidation of arachidonic acid are CYP1A1, CYP1A2, CYP4A1, CYP2B1, CYP2B4, CYP2C9, CYP2C11, CYP2C23, CYP2E1, CYP2G1, and CYP2J3.[40,41] All of these gene families are markedly inducible as a result of the exposure to xenobiotics. The fibrates (oxyisobutyrates) are the largest structurally related group of inducers investigated, and detailed induction protocols have been described for clofibrate, ciprofibrate, clobuzarit, and bezafibrate.[42] Administration of dehydroepiandrosterone (DHEA), a naturally occurring C_{19} steroid found in mammals, is also effective in induction of

TABLE 1. Effect of *P*-450 modulators on acute-phase responses of mice

Strain	*P*-450 Modulator (route of admin)		Acute-phase response[a] (stimulus)	Effect	Reference
	Inducer	Inhibitor			
Swiss Webster		NDGA (i.m.)	Fever (LPS) Motor act. (LPS)	Increase No effect	26
Swiss Webster		SKF-525A (i.p.)	Fever (LPS) Motor act. (LPS)	Increase No effect	26
Swiss Webster		Clotrimazole (i.m.)	Fever (LPS) Motor act. (LPS)	Increase[b] No effect	26
Swiss Webster		Clotrimazole (i.m.)	Fever (turp.) Motor act. (turp.)	Increase Decrease	Unpublished
Swiss Webster	Clofibrate (s.c.)		Fever (turp.) Motor act. (turp.) Food intake (turp.)	Decrease Increase Increase	28
Swiss Webster	Clofibrate (s.c.)		Fever (LPS) Motor act. (LPS) Food intake (LPS)	Decrease Increase Increase	28
Swiss Webster	Clofibrate (s.c.)		High dose of LPS[c] Morbidity Motor act. (LPS)	Decrease Increase	Unpublished
Swiss Webster		SKF-525A (i.p.)	Plasma IL-6 bioactivity (LPS)	Increase	26
Swiss Webster		SKF-525A (i.p.)	Plasma TNF bioactivity (LPS)	Decrease	26

ABBREVIATIONS: LPS, lipopolysaccharide; turp, turpentine; NDGA, nordihydroguaiaretic acid; i.m., intramuscular; i.p., intraperitoneal; s.c., subcutaneous.
[a]Compared to LPS or turpentine-injected animals treated with vehicle (rather than modulator of *P*-450).
[b]Blocked by indomethacin.
[c]10mg/kg.

TABLE 2. Effect of *P-450* modulators on fever in the rat

Strain	P-450 Modulator (route of admin)		Acute-phase response[a] (stimulus)	Effect	Reference
	Inducer	Inhibitor			
Sprague-Dawley		SKF-52A (i.m.)	Fever (LPS)	Increase	27
Sprague-Dawley		SKF-525A (icv)	Fever (LPS)	Increase	27
Sprague-Dawley		Miconazole (i.m.)	Fever (LPS)	Increase	28
Sprague-Dawley		Clotrimazole (i.m.)	Fever (LPS)	Increase	27
Sprague-Dawley		Econazole (i.m.)	Fever (LPS)	Increase	Unpublished
Sprague-Dawley		1-ABT (i.p.)	Fever (LPS)	Increase	Unpublished
Sprague-Dawley		17-ODYA (i.m.)	Fever (LPS)	Increase	28
Sprague-Dawley	Clofibrate (i.m., i.p.)		Fever (LPS)	Decrease	Unpublished
Sprague-Dawley	Bezafibrate (i.m., i.p.)		Fever (LPS)	Decrease	28
Sprague-Dawley	DHEA (i.p.)		Fever (LPS)	Decrease	28
Sprague-Dawley		SKF-525a (i.c.v.); SKF-525A (i.p.)	CSF PGE$_2$ (LPS); Plasma PGE$_2$ (LPS)	Increase	27
Wister		Econazole, clotrimazole	Fever (IL-1)	Increase	29
Sprague-Dawley	8,9-EET; 11,12-EET; 14,15-EET; 12(R)-HETE[b]		Fever (LPS)	Decrease	28

ABBREVIATIONS: LPS, lipopolysaccharide; i.m., intramuscular; i.p., intraperitoneal; i.c.v., intracerebroventricular; CSF, cerebrospinal fluid; 1-ABT, 1-aminobenzotriazole; 17-ODYA, 17-octadecynoic acid; DHEA, dehydroepiandrosterone.
[a]Compared to LPS injected rats treated with vehicle (rather than modulator of *P-450*).
[b]Epoxyeicosatrienoic and hydroxyeicosatetraenoic acids administered i.c.v.

the *P*-450 epoxygenases.[42] To test the effect of *P*-450 inducers on fever in mice and rats, clofibrate, bezafibrate, and DHEA (dehydroisoandrosterone 3-sulfate, all Sigma) were dissolved in a warm sterile corn oil (Sigma) at a stock concentration of 50 mg/ml. Stock solutions were rewarmed (38°C), sonicated, and diluted with warm corn oil to a desired concentration. Inducers of cytochrome *P*-450 were administered at doses 10 and 100 mg/kg (bezafibrate and DHEA), and 0.5 and 5 mg/kg (clofibrate), three times at 24-h intervals before the induction of fever. The routes of administration are indicated in TABLES 1 and 2. Sterile corn oil was used as a control injection.

Specific pathogen-free young adult male Swiss Webster mice (Taconic) and Sprague-Dawley rats (Charles River) were housed individually in plastic cages in temperature-controlled rooms at 25 ± 1°C for rats and 30 ± 1°C for mice, with a 12:12-h light–dark cycle (lights on at 0600). Body temperature and motor activity of each animal were monitored with intra-abdominal implanted temperature-sensitive telemetry transmitters (Dataquest III System, MiniMitter).[18,20,26,27]

Fever in animals was induced by an i.p. injection of a saline-diluted LPS (*E. coli* endotoxin 0111:B4; Sigma, L2630) at doses of 50 and 80 µg/kg for rats and 100 µg/kg and 2.5 mg/kg for mice. In separate experiments, fever in mice was induced by a subcutaneous (s.c.) injection of turpentine (10 µl/mouse). LPS and turpentine were injected 24 h after the third administration of the *P*-450 inducer. Saline was used as control injections.

Pretreatment of mice (TABLE 1) and rats (TABLE 2) with inducers of the cytochrome *P*-450 resulted in reduction of fever. The effect was dose-dependent; the higher the dose of *P*-450 inducer, the larger the inhibition of fever. In mice, fever was reduced in both models, that is, as a result of the i.p. injection of LPS to model a systemic inflammation and as a result of the s.c. administration of turpentine to model a localized inflammation. Furthermore, pretreatment of mice with clofibrate (5 mg/kg) reduced the other LPS-induced components of the acute-phase response, such as decreased motor activity and food intake (TABLE 1).

INHIBITORS OF CYTOCHROME *P*-450 CAUSE LARGER FEVER IN MICE AND RATS

The facts that the CYP monooxygenases exist in many isoforms and that enzyme inducers and inhibitors are frequently nonspecific complicate the task of elucidating the pathophysiological role of these enzymes. As a result, in studies testing the effects of the inhibition of the enzyme on fever, we used two types of the monooxygenase inhibitors. One approach used a "suicide substrate," an acetylenic derivative 17-octadecynoic acid (17-ODYA) designed to resemble the substrate and at the same time to inactivate the enzyme. 17-ODYA inhibits epoxygenation and ω-hydroxylation of arachidonic acid and other fatty acids.[41] Inactivation is irreversible, and activity is restored on *de novo* synthesis of the enzyme.[41] In the other experiments, we used imidazole antimycotics (clotrimazole, econazole, miconazole), nordihydroguaiaretic acid, and aminobenzotriazole, which are the "mechanism-based" reversible inhibitors of a number of *P*-450 monooxygenase isoforms.[43]

Proadifen (SKF-525A) is a water-soluble inhibitor of a broad spectrum of the P-450-dependent oxygenate reactions.

To test the effects of inhibitors of P-450 on fever in mice and rats, doses of the inhibitors were injected twice: one injection 24 h before LPS and/or turpentine, and then at the time of the LPS or turpentine injection. Data presented in TABLES 1 and 2 indicate that, in contrast to the effects of P-450 inducers on fever in mice and rats, treatment with inhibitors of P-450 resulted in augmentation of fever. Amplifying effects of SKF-525A on fever in rats (TABLE 2) have been observed when the drug was administered either peripherally (i.p. or i.m.) or centrally (i.c.v. into the lateral cerebral ventricle). Exacerbation of fever due to pretreatment with P-450 inhibitors was dose-dependent. Clotrimazole, an inhibitor of P-450, amplified a turpentine-induced lethargy in mice (TABLE 1). In a supplementary experiment, we observed that the exacerbation of fever in mice treated with a P-450 inhibitor (clotrimazole; TABLE 1) was abolished by indomethacin,[26] an inhibitor of cyclooxygenases. These data suggest that the amplification of fever using inhibitor(s) of P-450 was associated with a shift into a higher rate of the synthesis of PGE_2, tempting a hypothesis that the exacerbation of fever is associated with the higher levels of PGE_2. This hypothesis was tested on rats.[27]

PROADIFEN (SKF-525A), AN INHIBITOR OF P-450, EXACERBATES PGE_2 LEVELS IN RATS

Two experiments were performed using 44 rats to study the effect of SKF-525A on PGE_2 levels in plasma and cerebrospinal fluid (CSF) during LPS fever.[27] All rats were implanted intra-abdominally with biotelemitters to monitor temperature. In the first experiment, 20 rats were pretreated i.p. with SKF-525A (15 mg/kg) or saline as control and 30 min later were injected with LPS (i.p.; 50 µg/kg) or control saline (four groups, five rats/group). Heparinized blood (cardiac puncture) was taken 3 h after the LPS injection. In the second experiment, 24 rats were also implanted with lateral ventricle cannulae and given artificial cerebrospinal fluid (aCSF, control) or SKF-525A i.c.v. (5 µg/rat) 10 min before LPS (i.p.; 50 µg/kg) or control saline (four groups; six rats/group). Three hours later a 150- to 200-µl CSF sample (cisternal puncture) was collected from each rat.

In the first experiment (SKF-525A given i.p.), the plasma PGE_2 levels in control-injected rats, (i.e., saline/saline and SKF-525A/saline) were, respectively, 14.4 ± 2.5 pg/ml and 33.2 ± 8.6 pg/ml (difference not significant; $p > 0.05$). Injection of LPS triggered a significant elevation of plasma PGE_2 within 3 h to 169.6 ± 37.5 pg/ml. Administration of SKF-525A (15 mg/kg; i.p.) induced an even larger elevation of PGE_2 within that time in LPS-injected rats to 343.4 ± 45.4 pg/ml ($p < 0.05$ between saline/LPS and SKF-525A/LPS groups).

In the second experiment, the concentration of PGE_2 in CSF changed dramatically when SKF-525A was administered i.c.v. into the LPS-injected rats. Injection of LPS (i.p.) induced significant elevation of CSF PGE_2 from 4.5 ± 1.4 pg/ml (aCSF/saline group) to 30.9 ± 5.2 pg/ml ($p < 0.05$ between saline- and LPS-injected groups) in rats infused i.c.v. with aCSF. Administration of SKF-525A (5 µg/rat; i.c.v.)

amplified the effect of LPS about threefold to a CSF PGE_2 of 92.5 ± 21.1 pg/ml in LPS-injected rats ($p < 0.05$ between aCSF/LPS and SKF-525A/LPS groups).

The augmenting effect of the inhibitor of P-450 on LPS-induced elevation of PGE_2 reflected the levels of IL-6 and TNF-α.[26] Generation of these two cytokines is regulated in part by PGE_2; PGE_2 is required for IL-6 synthesis, and it inhibits generation of TNF-α. Accordingly, SKF-525A significantly enhanced the LPS-induced levels of IL-6, whereas it suppressed the increase of TNF-α.[26] These alterations to *in vivo* generation of PGE_2, IL-6, and TNF-α paralleled the effects of SKF-525A on fever in mice and rats.

P-450 ARACHIDONIC ACID METABOLITES REDUCE LPS FEVER IN RATS[28]

Data showing the reduction and/or amplification of fever following treatment with, respectively, inducers and/or inhibitors of P-450 monooxygenases, implicate the involvement of this enzyme system in fever, particularly in the regulation of the height of fever. Several mechanisms involving P-450 can be considered. One possibility is that the modulation of the activity of P-450 affects arachidonate metabolism, in that inhibition of P-450 results in more arachidonic acid to be metabolized via cyclooxygenases and, hence, more PGE_2 can be produced per unit of time, which translates into a higher fever. Another hypothesis is that P-450 itself is engaged in the inactivating metabolism of PGE_2, and that inhibition of the P-450 results in reduction of the rate of neutralization of PGE_2. Data discussed above, showing that proadifen (SKF-525A), an inhibitor of cytochrome P-450, enhances the LPS-induced elevation of PGE_2, support this hypothesis. However, a complementary hypothesis is that some P-450 arachidonic acid metabolites, and possibly P-450 eicosanoid metabolites, can act as endogenous antipyretics. Thus, induction of the P-450 monooxygenase enzyme system might accelerate the rate of the generation of fever-preventing P-450 arachidonate metabolites, resulting in a lower fever. Data from the studies using clofibrate, bezafibrate, and DHEA presented in this report support this hypothesis. To test whether or not the P-450 monooxygenase (epoxygenase) products are antipyretic, we administered various regioisomers of epoxyeicosatrienoic and monohydroxyeicosatetraenoic acids into the rat brain and estimated the changes of fever following the peripheral (i.p.) injection of LPS. This route of EET or HETE isomer administration was applied since (i) the preoptic-anterior hypothalamus is considered the center for thermoregulation as well as regulation of fever,[3,4] (ii) expression of P-450 has been demonstrated in the hypothalamus,[34] and (iii) infusion of SKF-525A, an inhibitor of P-450, into the brain exacerbated the LPS-induced fever in rats.[27]

For the cerebral injections (into the lateral ventricle; i.c.v.), rats were implanted stereotaxically with a 5-mm long, 22-gauge stainless-steel, thin-walled cannula (Plastic Products) into the lateral ventricle, as described elsewhere.[27,28] Ethanol solutions of 12(R)-HETE, 5,6-EET, 8,9-EET, 11,12-EET, and 14,15-EET were purchased from Cayman Chemical. Before i.c.v. infusion, ethanol was evaporated under nitrogen in a cold room (about 10°C), and the specimens were reconstituted with aCSF to a desired concentration. In this study, fever in rats was induced by an i.p. injection of LPS at a dose of 80 µg/kg.

Four of five examined isomers appeared to reduce fever when infused into the lateral ventricle a few minutes before the i.p. administration of LPS.[28] The most potent antipyretic isomers (dosage-wise) in our experiments were 11,12-EET followed by 14,15-EET. They significantly and dose-dependently reduced fever if administered i.c.v. in the range of nanograms per rat. All other tested epoxygenase metabolites except the 5,6-EET isomer, significantly reduced fever when infused i.c.v. in a dose range of micrograms per rat (TABLE 2). The effects observed for these isomers, that is, 8,9-EET, 14,15-EET, and 12(R)HETE, were dose-dependent.

CONCLUDING REMARKS

FIGURE 1 summarizes data presented in this report and illustrates hypotheses regarding the interactions within the arachidonate cascade in the modulation of fever. On the basis of the results just described, on our data earlier published,[26–28] and that from Nakashima et al.[29] and Fraifeld et al.,[25] we conclude that besides interactions among the cytokines and hormones, the process of endogenous antipyresis also operates at the level of the arachidonate cascade, reflecting the interactions among the enzymes, substrates, and metabolites of the cascade.

It is well documented that the metabolism of arachidonic acid via cyclooxygenases and, in turn, production of prostaglandins, particularly PGE_2, is an essential pathway for the generation of fever.[24] Data presented in this report suggest that when arachidonic acid is metabolized via the P-450 pathway, the net result can be antipyresis. This latter conclusion is based in part on the study in which we used pharmacological agents to modulate (induce and/or inhibit) P-450 monooxygenases. It must be stressed, however, that the selectivity and specificity of such an approach is limited due to the magnitude and complexity of the cytochrome P-450 gene superfamily.[41,44] One cannot rule out, therefore, that the drugs used in our study altered not only the expression of the arachidonate epoxygenases, but also might affect other P-450 isoforms, which could result in influencing the LPS fever in rats. More direct data were obtained when we applied the exogenous P-450 arachidonic acid metabolites to test their effects on fever. These results clearly support the hypothesis that metabolization of the arachidonic acid via P-450 can indeed give rise to the antipyretic eicosanoids.

The multiple mechanisms underlying the antipyretic action of epoxyeicosanoids may involve an "endogenously induced" inhibition of the activity of cyclooxygenases. In support of this notion, it has been found that some tested isomers of EET are potent inhibitors of platelet[45] and vascular smooth muscle[46] cyclooxygenases. In the study by Fang et al.,[46] 14,15-EET exerted a potent inhibitory effect on the production of PGE_2, whereas 5,6-EET isomer was ineffective in the inhibition of cyclooxygenases, which is in accordance with our findings that 5,6-EET was not effective in the attenuation of fever in rats. Interestingly, the potency of some EETs examined, that is, 8,9-EET, and 14,15-EET, surpassed that of ibuprofen and aspirin, well-known antiinflammatory agents, in the inhibition of the activity of isolated cyclooxygenase enzyme preparation.[45] It is believed that aspirin inhibits fever and attenuates inflammation by blocking cyclooxygenase activity and, in consequence,

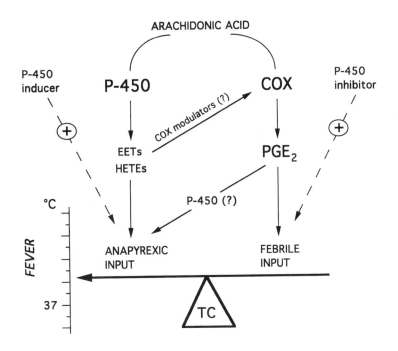

FIGURE 1. Schematic illustrating the summary and interpretation of the data present-ed in this report. We have observed that inducers of *P*-450 reduced, whereas inhibitors exacerbated, fever in the rat. This observation indicates that treatment with inducers of *P*-450 amplified an antipyretic input (anapyrexic input), whereas treatment with inhibitors of *P*-450 enhanced a febrile input into the thermoregulatory center (TC). The underlying mechanisms of the *P*-450-related antipyresis may involve generation of the antipyretic metabolites from arachidonic acid. These metabolites may either act directly on TC or attenuate the activity of cyclooxygenases (COX) to suppress the production of PGE$_2$ and, in turn, diminish a pro-febrile signaling into TC. We have shown that an inhibitor of *P*-450 enhanced the LPS-induced PGE$_2$ level in plasma and cerebrospinal fluid.[27] This finding suggests either a rerouting of the substrate (i.e., arachidonic acid) into the COX pathway as a result of the inhibition of *P*-450 or *P*-450 participation in the metabolization of PGE$_2$ dur-ing inflammation and fever.

the generation of PGE$_2$.[47] It has recently been found, however, that aspirin is a potent inducer of *P*-450, and administration of a single dose of aspirin produces a signifi-cant increase in the activity of CYP2E1 and CYP4A1, the CYP isoforms involved in the metabolism of arachidonic acid.[48,49] Therefore, the possibility arises that aspirin attenuates inflammation and inhibits fever by another mechanism as well, that is, by inducing a cytochrome *P*-450, which metabolizes arachidonic acid. This may result in (1) lowering the concentration of the substrate (i.e., arachidonic acid) for cyclooxy-genases and (2) in a generation of the arachidonic acid metabolites, which can act within a feedback loop to attenuate the activity of cyclooxygenases. This hypothesis is consistent with data reported recently by Node *et al.*,[50] showing that several cyto-chrome *P*-450 epoxygenase-derived metabolites exert antiinflammatory properties.

ACKNOWLEDGMENTS

Research supported by the National Institute of Allergy and Infectious Disease Grant AI-27556 and funds from Lovelace Respiratory Research Institute. The study was conducted in facilities fully accredited by the Association for the Assessment and Accreditation of Laboratory Animal Care International.

REFERENCES

1. KLUGER, M.J. 1998. Preface. *In* Molecular Mechanisms of Fever. Ann. N.Y. Acad. Sci. **856:** xi–xii.
2. DUBOIS, E.F. 1949. Why are fever temperatures over 106°F rare? Am. J. Med. Sci. **217:** 361–368.
3. MACKOWIAK, P.A. & J.A. BOULANT. 1996. Fever's glass ceiling. Clin. Infect. Dis. **22:** 525–536.
4. KLUGER, M.J. 1991. Fever: role of pyrogens and cryogens. Physiol. Rev. **71:** 93–127.
5. DINARELLO, C.A. 1997. Cytokines as endogenous pyrogens. *In* Fever: Basic Mechanisms and Management. P.A. Mackowiak, Ed.: 87–116. Lippincott-Raven. Philadelphia.
6. KLUGER, M.J., W. KOZAK, L.R. LEON *et al.* 1995. Cytokines and fever. Neuroimmunomodulation **2:** 216–223.
7. KOZAK, W., M.J. KLUGER, D. SOSZYNSKI *et al.* 1998. IL-6 and IL-1β in fever: studies using cytokine-deficient (knockout) mice. Ann. N.Y. Acad. Sci. **856:** 33–47.
8. LEMAY, L.G., I. OTTERNESS, S.L. KUNKEL *et al.* 1990. In vivo evidence that the rise in plasma IL-6 following injection of a fever-inducing dose of LPS is mediated by IL-1β. Cytokine **2:** 199–204.
9. LUHESHI, G., A.J. MILLER, S. BROWER *et al.* 1996. Interleukin-1 receptor antagonist inhibits endotoxin fever and systemic interleukin-6 induction in the rat. Am. J. Physiol. **270:** E91–E95.
10. KASTING, N.W., W.L. VEALE & K.E. COOPER. 1978. Suppression of fever at term of pregnancy. Nature **271:** 245–246.
11. VEALE, W.L., N.W. KASTING & K.E. COOPER. 1981. Arginine vasopressin and endogenous antipyresis: evidence and significance. Fed. Proc. **40:** 2750–2753.
12. PITTMAN, Q.J. & M.F. WILKINSON. 1992. Central arginine vasopressin and endogenous antipyresis. Can. J. Physiol. Pharmacol. **70:** 786–790.
13. MURPHY, M.T., D.B. RICHARDS & J.M. LIPTON. 1983. Antipyretic potency of centrally administered α-melanocyte stimulating hormone. Science **221:** 192–193.
14. CATANIA, A. & J.M. LIPTON. 1993. α-Melanocyte stimulating hormone in the modulation of host reactions. Endocrinol. Rev. **14:** 564–576.
15. COELHO, M.M., G.E.P. SOUZA & I.R. PELA. 1992. Endotoxin-induced fever is modulated by endogenous glucocorticoids in rats. Am. J. Physiol. **263:** R423–R427.
16. MORROW, L.E., J.L. MCCLELLAN, C.A. CONN & M.J. KLUGER. 1993. Glucocorticoids alter fever and IL-6 responses to psychological stress and lipopolysaccharide. Am. J. Physiol. **264:** R1010–R1016.
17. LONG, N.C., S.L. KUNKEL, A.J. VANDER & M.J. KLUGER. 1990. Antiserum against TNF enhances LPS fever in the rat. Am. J. Physiol. **258:** R591–R595.
18. KOZAK, W., C.A. CONN, J.J. KLIR *et al.* 1995. TNF soluble receptor and antiserum against TNF enhance lipopolysaccharide fever in mice. Am. J. Physiol. **269:** R23–R29.
19. BIBBY, D.C. & R.F. GRIMBLE. 1989. Temperature and metabolic changes in rats after various doses of tumor necrosis factor α. J. Physiol. **410:** 367–380.
20. KLIR, J.J., J.L. MCCLELLAN, W. KOZAK *et al.* 1995. Systemic but not central administration of tumor necrosis factor-α attenuates LPS-induced fever in rats. Am. J. Physiol. **268:** R480–R486.

21. LEON, L.R., W. KOZAK, J. PESCHON & M.J. KLUGER. 1997. Exacerbated febrile responses to LPS, but not turpentine, in TNF double receptor-knockout mice. Am. J. Physiol. **272:** R563–R569.

22. LEON, L.R., W. KOZAK, K. RUDOLPH & M.J. KLUGER. 1999. An antipyretic role of interleukin-10 in LPS fever in mice. Am. J. Physiol. **276:** R81–R89.

23. PAJKRT, D., L. CAMAGLIO, M.C.M. TIEL-VAN BUUL *et al.* 1997. Attenuation of proinflammatory response by recombinant human IL-10 in human endotoxemia. J. Immunol. **158:** 3971–3977.

24. BLATTEIS, C.M. & E. SEHIC. 1997. Prostaglandin E$_2$: a putative fever mediator. *In* Fever: Basic Mechanisms and Managemant. P.A. Mackowiak, Ed.: 117–146. Lippincot-Raven. Philadelphia.

25. FRAIFELD, V., L. PAUL & J. KAPLANSKI. 2000. The relationship between hypothalamic prostaglandin E$_2$ or leukotrienes and the body temperature response to lipopolysaccharide in different murine strains. J. Thermal Biol. **25:** 17–20.

26. KOZAK, W., I. ARCHULETA, K.P. MAYFIELD *et al.* 1998 Inhibitors of alternative pathways of arachidonate metabolism differentially affect fever in mice. Am. J. Physiol. **275:** R1031–R1040.

27. KOZAK, W., K.P. MAYFIELD, A. KOZAK & M.J. KLUGER. 2000. Proadifen (SKF-525A), an inhibitor of cytochrome P-450, augments LPS-induced fever and exacerbates prostaglandin-E$_2$ levels in the rat. J. Thermal Biol. **25:** 45–50.

28. KOZAK, W., M.J. KLUGER, A. KOZAK, M. WACHULEC & K. DOKLADNY. 2000. Role of cytochrome P-450/epoxygenase in fever in mice and rats. Am. J. Physiol. **279:** R455–R460.

29. NAKASHIMA, T., Y. HARADA, S. MIYATA & T. KIYOHARA. 1996. Inhibitors of cytochrome P-450 augment fever induced by interleukin-1β. Am. J. Physiol. **271:** R1274–R1279.

30. MASHBURN, T.A., JR., J. LLANOS, R.A. AHOKAS & C.M. BLATTEIS. 1986. Thermal and acute-phase protein responses of guinea pigs to intrapreoptic injections of leukotrienes. Brain Res. **376:** 285–291.

31. CAPDEVILA, J.H., & J.R. FALCK. 1989. Cytochrome P-450 and the bioactivation of arachidonic acid. Blood Vessels **26:** 54–57.

32. FITZPATRICK, F.A. & R.C. MURPHY. 1989. Cytochrome P-450 metabolism of arachidonic acid: formation and biological actions of "epoxygenase"-derived eicosanoids. Pharmacol. Rev. **40:** 229–241.

33. MCGIFF, J.C. 1991. Cytochrome P-450 metabolism of arachidonic acid. Annu. Rev. Pharmacol. Toxicol. **31:** 339–369.

34. SCHILTER, B. & C.J. OMIECINSKI. 1993. Regional distribution and expression modulation of cytochrome p-450 and epoxide hydrolase mRNAs in the rat brain. Mol. Pharmacol. **44:** 990–996.

35. ALKAYED, N.J., J. NARAYANAN, D. GEBREMEDHIN *et al.* 1996. Molecular characterization of an arachidonic acid epoxygenase in rat brain astrocytes. Stroke **27:** 971–979.

36. ELLIS, E.F., S.C. AMRUTHESH, R.J. POLICE & L.M. YANCEY. 1991. Brain synthesis and cerebrovascular action of cytochrome P-450/monooxygenase metabolites of arachidonic acid. Adv. Prostaglandin Thromboxane Leukot. Res. **21A:** 201–204.

37. HARDER, D.R., W.B. CAMPBELL & R.J. ROMAN. 1995. Role of cytochrome P450 enzymes and metabolites of arachidonic acid in the control of vascular tone. J. Vasc. Res. **32:** 79–92.

38. MAKITA, K., J.R. FALCK & J.H. CAPDEVILA. 1996. Cytochrome P450, the arachidonic acid cascade, and hypertension: new vistas for an old enzyme system. FASEB J. **10:** 1456–1463.

39. MORGAN, E.T. 1997. Regulation of cytochromes P450 during inflammation and infection. Drug Metab. Rev. **29:** 1129–1188.

40. CAPDEVILA, J.H., D.C. ZELDIN, K. MAKITA *et al.* 1995. Cytochrome P450 and the metabolism of arachidonic acid and oxygenated eicosanoids. *In* Cytochrome P450: Structure, Mechanism, and Biochemistry. P.R. Ortiz de Montellano, Ed.: 443–471. Plenum Press. New York.

41. WANG, M.H., E. BRAND-SCHIEBER, B.A. ZAND et al. 1998. Cytochrome P450-derived arachidonic acid metabolism in the rat kidney: characterization of selective inhibitors. J. Pharmacol. Exp. Ther. **284:** 966–973.
42. GIBSON, G.G. & B.G. LAKE. 1991. Induction protocols for the cytochrome P450IVA subfamily in animals and primary hepatocyte cultures. Methods Enzymol. **206:** 353–364.
43. CAPDEVILA, J., L. GIL, M. ORELLANA et al. 1988. Inhibitors of cytochrome P-450-dependent arachidonic acid metabolism. Arch. Biochem. Biophys. **261:** 257–263.
44. NELSON, D.R., T. KAMATAKI, D.J. WAXMAN et al. 1993. The P450 superfamily: update on new sequences, gene mapping, accesion numbers, early trivial names of enzymes, and nomenclature. DNA Cell Biol. **12:** 1–51.
45. FITZPATRICK, F.A., M.D. ENNIS, M.E. BAZE et al. 1986. Inhibition of cyclooxygenase activity and platelet aggregation by epoxyeicosatrienoic acids. J. Biol. Chem. **261:** 15334–15338.
46. FANG, X., S.A. MOORE, L.L. STOLL et al. 1998. 14,15-Epoxyeicosatrienoic acid inhibits prostaglandin E_2 production in vascular smooth muscle cells. Am. J. Physiol. **275:** H2113–H2121.
47. VANE, J.R. 1971. Inhibition of prostaglandin synthesis as a mechanism of action for aspirin-like drugs. Nature New Biol. **231:** 232–235.
48. DAMME, B., D. DARMER & D. PANKOW. 1996. Induction of hepatic cytochrome P4502E1 in rats by acetylsalicylic acid or sodium salicylate. Toxicology **106:** 99–103.
49. CAI, Y., A.K. SOHLENIUS, K. ANDERSSON et al. 1994. Effects of acetysalicylic acid on parameters related to peroxisome proliferation in mouse liver. Biochem. Pharmacol. **47:** 2213–2219.
50. NODE, K., Y. HUO, X. RUAN et al. 1999. Anti-inflammatory properties of cytochrome P450 epoxygenase-derived eicosanoids. Science **285:** 1276–1279.

CXC Chemokine Receptors Expression during Chronic Relapsing Experimental Autoimmune Encephalomyelitis

ANDRZEJ R. GLABINSKI,[a,b] SAGE O'BRYANT,[c] KRZYSZTOF SELMAJ,[b] AND RICHARD M. RANSOHOFF[c]

[b]Department of Neurology, Medical University of Lodz, Lodz, Poland

[c]Department of Neurosciences, Cleveland Clinic Foundation, Cleveland, Ohio, USA

ABSTRACT: Chemokines are small proinflammatory cytokines that possess the ability to stimulate migration of inflammatory cells towards the tissue site of inflammation. Previous reports showed that several chemokines may be involved in the pathogenesis of experimental autoimmune encephalomyelitis (EAE), an animal model of autoimmune central nervous system (CNS) inflammation. Inflammatory cells respond to chemotactic chemokine gradient through the chemokine receptors (ChRs). The goal of this study was to analyze expression of ChRs belonging to CXC subfamily during different stages of chronic relapsing EAE. We found significantly increased expression of CXCR2 and CXCR4 in the spinal cord during the first and second disease attacks. The kinetics of this expression in CNS and blood suggests that CXCR2 is expressed by leukocytes migrating from the blood, but CXCR4 is expressed mainly by CNS parenchymal cells. Those results support the interpretation that chemokine–chemokine receptor interactions may play an important role in the development of CNS autoimmune inflammation.

INTRODUCTION

Chemokines are proinflammatory cytokines that possess the ability to stimulate migration of inflammatory cells towards the tissue site of inflammation.[1–3] About 40 human chemokines have been described so far, and their number is still growing. Based on their structure, chemokines can be divided into four separate subfamilies. The largest groups are CC chemokines, which have the first two cysteines adjacent to one another, and CXC chemokines, in which those cysteines are separated by one additional amino acid. The well-known CC chemokines are MCP-1 (monocyte chemoattractant protein-1), MIP-1 (macrophage inflammatory protein-1) and RANTES (regulated upon activation T-cell expressed and secreted). Representative of CXC chemokines are interleukin-8 (IL-8); growth-related oncogene-α, -β, -χ (GRO-α, -β, -χ); and γ-interferon-inducible protein, 10 kDa (IP-10). CC chemokines stimulate migration of mononuclear inflammatory cells, whereas CXC chemokines

[a]Address for correspondence: Andrzej Glabinski, M.D., Ph.D., Department of Neurology, Medical University of Lodz, ul. Kopcinskiego 22, 90-153 Lodz, Poland. Voice: +4842-678-7746; fax: +4842-678-2293.

aglabinski@afazja.am.lodz.pl

act mainly on neutrophils. An exception is those CXC chemokines without an ELR (glutaminic acid–leucine–arginine) motif preceding the first two cysteines, which can initiate migration of mononuclear cells.[1–3]

Chemokines exert their functions through a large family of chemokine receptors (ChRs).[4,5] ChRs belong to the class A family of peptides, well known in biology as a group of G-protein-coupled, seven-transmembrane domain receptors (GPCRs). They are designated according to their affinity to chemokine ligands as CCR or CX-CR. Additionally, a receptor to the recently described chemokine fractalkine/neurotactin, the only member of a new CX3C chemokine family, has been identified. ChRs can be classified as shared, specific, viral, and promiscuous.[5] Shared receptors possess the ability to bind several different chemokines from the same subfamily. Specific receptors bind only one known ligand. Some viruses are able to express proteins with a significant homology to chemokines. DARC (Duffy antigen/receptor for chemokines) is the only known promiscuous chemokine receptor that can bind chemokines from both CC and CXC groups, and it is localized mainly on erythrocytes and endothelium.[4,5]

EAE (experimental autoimmune encephalomyelitis) is an autoimmune disease of the central nervous system (CNS) that is considered to be an animal model for human demyelinating disease—multiple sclerosis (MS). The main pathological feature of active phase of EAE is the presence of perivascular inflammatory foci localized randomly within the CNS. They are formed by hematogenous mononuclear leukocytes that have migrated from the blood. This type of pathology suggests that chemokines may play a significant role in its development. Numerous studies have shown increased expression of several different chemokines in acute and chronic EAE.[6–11] Interventional studies demonstrated that some antibodies against chemokines can prevent and ameliorate EAE development.[12,13] Recently, the first studies were published showing increased expression of some chemokines during MS.[14,15] All this informations delivers strong evidence that chemokines are important players in the patomechanism of autoimmune demyelination. Studying ChR expression in EAE and MS may give additional insight into the process of development of those diseases. Here we describe the expression pattern of CXC chemokine receptors in the CNS, blood, and spleen during different stages of ChREAE. We found significantly increased expression of CXCR2 and CXCR4 in the spinal cord during the first and second disease attacks. Kinetics of this expression in CNS and blood suggest that CXCR2 is expressed by migrating from the blood leukocytes, but CXCR4 is expressed mainly by CNS parenchymal cells.

MATERIALS AND METHODS

Induction and Clinical Evaluation of ChREAE

Female (SWRxSJL/J)F1 mice were bred in the animal facility of Cleveland Clinic Foundation. They were immunized between 8 and 10 weeks of age with an encephalitogenic PLP peptide representing residues 139–151 (PLPp:139–151) as previously described.[16] Post-immunization (PI), all mice were weighed and examined daily for clinical signs of EAE. The following clinical scoring scale was used: 0, no disease; 1, decreased tail tone or slightly clumsy gait; 2, tail atony and/or moderately clumsy gait and/or poor righting ability; 3, limb weakness; 4, limb paralysis; 5, morbound state.[9] Relapse onset was defined as the day when new clinical signs appeared, and onset of remission was defined as the day that clinical signs improved. Confirmatory evidence of attack and remission onset was loss or gain of 5–10% of body weight in a single day.[10] Mice were sacrificed by cervical dislocation or anesthetized and perfused via cardiac puncture with PBS, as approved by the Animal Research Committee of the Cleveland Clinic Foundation, in compliance with the Public Health Service policy on humane care and use of laboratory animals.

RNA Extraction

Animals were sacrificed at days 1, 2, 3, 4, and 7 relative to onset of the first attack of the disease, and at days 1, 2, 3, 4, and 6 relative to onset of the second attack (1–3 animals per each time point). Five normal, unimmunized animals were used as controls, and five additional animals were sacrificed during remission between the first and second attacks. Spinal cords, brains, and spleens were frozen in liquid nitrogen, powdered in a chilled mortar and pestle, and total cellular RNA was isolated using TRIZOL (Gibco/BRL). Blood was collected via cardiac puncture. Chemokine receptor mRNA expression was analyzed in animals perfused with PBS. Systemic immune activation was monitored by assay of blood and splenic chemokine receptor mRNA expression.

RNAse Protection Assay for Chemokine Receptors

The RNAse protection assay was performed using Pharmingen's RiboQuant™ Ribonuclease Protection Assay System mCR6 for CXC mouse chemokine receptors according to the manufacturer's instructions (Pharmingen, San Diego, CA). The hybridization signal was quantitated with Storm phosphorimager (Molecular Dynamics, Sunnyville, CA) and normalized to the L32 gene signal.

Statistical Analysis

Results were analyzed using the unpaired, two-tailed t-test; $p < 0.05$, was considered significant.

RESULTS

CXC Receptor Expression in CNS during ChREAE

CXCR2 expression in spinal cord was significantly increased during the first and second disease attacks (1 attack vs. normals: $p = 0.02$; 2 attack vs. normals: $p = 0.03$; 1 attack vs. remission: $p = 0.03$) (see FIGURE 1A). Similarly CXCR4 expression was increased in spinal cords (1 attack vs. normals: $p = 0.003$; 2 attack vs. normals: $p = 0.006$; remission vs. normals: $p = 0.03$) (FIG. 1A). We did not detect BLR1 (CXCR5) in spinal cords.

In brains, CXCR2, CXCR4, and BLR1 were detected in all groups but that expression did not differ significantly between groups ($p > 0.05$) (FIG. 1B).

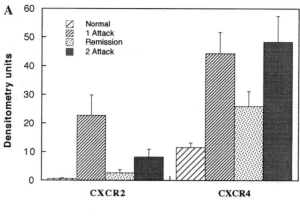

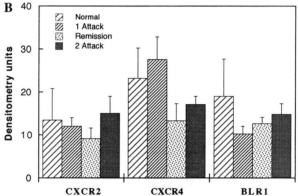

FIGURE 1. Central nervous system CXC chemokine receptor expression during ChREAE: (**A**) spinal cord and (**B**) brain. Animals were sacrificed at predetermined time points: normal, unimmunized control animals; 1 attack, first attack of ChREAE; remission, remission between first and second disease attacks; 2 attack, second disease attack. Each bar represents mean value from a group of 6–7 animals, error bar shows +SE. Expression is shown in densitometry units normalized to L32 as described in MATERIALS AND METHODS.

Peripheral CXC Chemokine Receptor Expression during ChREAE

In the blood of animals with ChREAE, we detected expression of all three CXC receptors studied (CXCR2, CXCR4, and BLR1). Only CXCR2 expression was significantly increased during the first attack (1 attack vs. normals: $p = 0.04$) (see FIGURE 2A).

In spleen, CXCR2 expression was similar in all groups ($p > 0.05$) (FIG. 2B). CXCR4 expression in spleen was significantly lower during remission than in other groups (remission vs. normals: $p = 0.01$; remission vs. 1 attack: $p = 0.005$; remission vs. 2 attack: $p = 0.01$) (FIG. 2B). BLR1 expression was increased in spleen during the second attack (2 attack vs. 1 attack: $p = 0.02$; 2 attack vs. remission: $p = 0.02$) (FIG. 2B).

Kinetics of CXCR Expression during Initial Attack of ChREAE

We analyzed expression of CXCR receptors on days 1, 2, 3, 4, and 7 of the first attack of ChREAE (see FIGURE 3). Expression of CXCR2 and CXCR4 in spinal cords during the initial disease attack was increasing slowly with the peak of expression on days 4 and 3, respectively (FIG. 3A). In blood, the peak of CXCR2 expression was observed earlier (on day 2); CXCR4 and BLR1 did not show any significant peak (FIG. 3B).

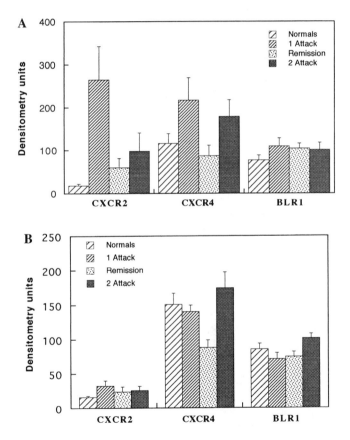

FIGURE 2. Peripheral CXC chemokine receptor expression during ChREAE: (**A**) blood and (**B**) spleen. Animals were sacrificed at predetermined time points: normal, unimmunized control animals; 1 attack, first attack of ChREAE; remission, remission between first and second disease attacks; 2 attack, second disease attack. Each bar represents mean value from a group of 6–7 animals, error bar shows +SE. Expression is shown in densitometry units normalized to L32 as described in MATERIALS AND METHODS.

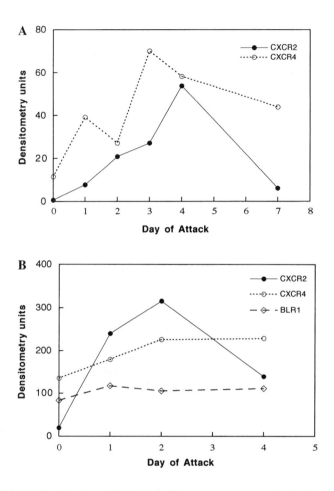

FIGURE 3. The kinetics of CXC chemokine receptors expression during the first attack of ChREAE: (**A**) spinal cord and (**B**) blood. Animals were sacrificed on days 1, 2, 3, 4, and 7 after clinical signs of the disease appeared. Day 0: mean value from the group of unimmunized control animals. Expression is shown in densitometry units normalized to L32 as described in MATERIALS AND METHODS.

Correlation of CXCR Expression in Spinal Cord with Disease Severity

We analyzed CXCRs expression in spinal cords of animals with different clinical scores during the initial attack of ChREAE (see FIGURE 4). Expression of CXCR2 and CXCR4 in spinal cord correlated well with disease severity (FIG. 4). Expression of CXC chemokine receptors in spleen did not show this correlation (data not shown).

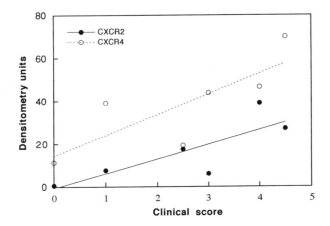

FIGURE 4. Correlation between CXC chemokine receptors expression in spinal cord and disease severity. Animals with different clinical scores of disease intensity (see MATERIALS AND METHODS) were sacrificed during the first attack of ChREAE. Expression is shown in densitometry units normalized to L32 as described in MATERIALS AND METHODS.

DISCUSSION

We report significantly increased expression of two CXC chemokine receptors—CXCR2 and CXCR4—in spinal cords during the first and second attacks of ChRE-AE. The comparison of kinetics of this expression in spinal cord and blood suggest that both receptors have distinct cellular sources.

The interactions between chemokines and their receptors play an important role in the mechanism leading to accumulation of inflammatory cells in CNS parenchyma. Several previous reports showed that many different chemokines can be involved in that process.[6–10,17] It has been reported that transient increase of expression of MCP-1 and IP-10 occurs at the beginning of acute, monophasic EAE.[6,7] Several other chemokines were also found to be overexpressed in spinal cords at the onset of the disease.[8] In ChREAE MCP-1, IP-10, GRO-α, MIP-1α, and RANTES are overexpressed during spontaneous relapse of the disease.[10] Cellular sources of chemokine expression during EAE were astrocytes for some chemokines (MCP-1, IP-10, GRO-α) and inflammatory cells for others (MIP-1α, RANTES).[10] We suggested a role for chemokines in amplification of inflammatory cells' migration to the CNS. According to this concept, the disease is initiated by migration of a small number of antigen-specific inflammatory cells insufficient in number to produce full disease manifestation. The second, antigen-nonspecific wave of inflammatory cells migrating to the CNS leads to CNS tissue destruction and is directed by a chemokine gradient created mainly by CNS parenchymal cells expressing chemokines.[18]

Several different types of ChR have been identified so far, predominantly on inflammatory cells. Studies *in vitro* showed that some CNS parenchymal cells can also express ChRs.[11] Astrocytes were shown to express CCR1[19] and CXCR4[20] in culture. Cultured microglia express CCR3, CCR5, CXCR4, and CX3CR1.[21,22] Cultured neurons can express CCR1, CCR5, CXCR2, and CXCR4.[23] Many ChRs (CCR3, CCR5, CXCR2, CXCR4, CX3CR1, DARC) were detected in normal CNS, and some of them were found to be upregulated in CNS pathologies.[11] CCR3 and CXCR2 were detected on neurons in Alzheimer's disease.[24] CCR3, CCR5, and CXCR4 were upregulated during SIV encephalomyelitis.[25] Increased expression of CCR2, CCR5, CXCR4, and CX3CR1 was reported in one EAE study (acute rat model).[26]

We found significantly increased expression of CXCR2 and CXCR4 during the first attack of ChREAE. The kinetics of this expression is different for both receptors and reveals information suggesting their potential cellular sources in that pathology. The highest expression of CXCR2 and CXCR4 during the first disease attack was observed in spinal cord on days 4 and 3, respectively. Such late expression in relation to attack onset suggests that their main source are late-entry antigen-nonspecific inflammatory cells or endogenous CNS cells. Indeed, monocytes can express CXCR4, and neutrophils are able to express CXCR2.[2] The peak of CXCR2 expression in blood was detected much earlier (on day 2), suggesting that inflammatory cells expressing this receptor are still in circulation at that time point and migrate to the CNS later. Studies of the kinetics of CXCR4 expression in the blood did not show any significant changes, which may suggest that the peak observed in the spinal cord at day 3 of the attack results mainly from increased expression of this receptor by CNS endogenous cells. It was previously shown that cultured astrocytes, microglia,[20,26] and even neurons[23] can express CXCR4.

The observed kinetics of ChR expression is in agreement with the concept that chemokines amplify inflammatory cell migration to the CNS at the beginning of an EAE attack.[18] The expression of GRO-α, the ligand of the CXCR2 receptor, was detected at the beginning of ChREAE.[10] Astrocytes expressing this chemokine can stimulate migration of inflammatory cells bearing CXCR2 across the blood–brain barrier and initiate their accumulation in CNS parenchyma. The role of the CXCR4 ligand SDF-1 in EAE is still unknown, but Jiang and coworkers have previously demonstrated upregulation of CXCR4 during rat EAE.[26] Further in situ hybridization and immunohistochemistry studies need to be done to address directly the cellular source of ChRs.

The level of CXCR2 and CXCR4 expresion during remission was lower than during disease attacks. It may be a result of an active process that downregulates the expression of those receptors in the CNS during the recovery phase of the disease or a result of apoptosis of cells expressing ChRs in that compartment. This expression is again significantly upregulated at the beginning of the second attack. Triggering factors for the initiation of the new attack could be new antigen-specific T cells that may initiate each relapse of the disease. They can be, according to the determinant spreading concept, directed against different autoantigen epitopes at the beginning of each relapse.[27] A new wave of inflammatory cells migrating to the CNS may increase ChR concentration behind the blood–brain barrier, directly bringing receptors on their surfaces or indirectly via stimulation of CNS endogenous cells for ChR expression.

Expression of CXCR2 and CXCR4 in the spinal cord during disease attack correlates with disease severity and suggests a significant role in EAE pathogenesis for those receptors and the cells expressing them. This observation confirms that interactions between chemokines and chemokine receptors can be a promising target for development of therapeutics for the treatment of autoimmune CNS inflammation.

ACKNOWLEDGMENTS

This work was supported by Grants 1RO3 TW00784-01A1 and 2R01NS32151 for RMR and KBN 4P05A05913 for ARG. We thank Ann Chernosky for technical assistance.

REFERENCES

1. BAGGIOLINI, M. *et al.* 1997. Human chemokines: an update. Annu. Rev. Immunol. **15:** 675–705.
2. LUSTER, A. 1998. Chemokines—chemotactic cytokines that mediate inflammation. N. Engl. J. Med. **338:** 436–445.
3. ROLLINS, B.J. 1997. Chemokines. Blood **90:** 909–928.
4. MURPHY, P. 1996. Chemokine receptors: structure, function and role in microbial pathogenesis. Cytokine Growth Factor Rev. **7:** 47–64.
5. PREMACK, B. & T. SCHALL. 1996. Chemokine receptors: gateways to inflammation and infection. Nature Med. **2:** 1174–1178.
6. RANSOHOFF, R.M. *et al.* 1993. Astrocyte expression of mRNA encoding cytokines IP-10 and JE/MCP-1 in experimental autoimmune encephalomyelitis. FASEB J. **7:** 592–600.
7. HULKOWER, K. *et al.* 1993. Expression of CSF-1, c-fms, and MCP-1 in the central nervous system of rats with experimental allergic encephalomyelitis. J. Immunol. **150:** 2525–2533.
8. GODISKA, R. *et al.* 1995. Chemokine expression in murine experimental autoimmune encephalomyelitis. J. Neuroimmunol. **58:** 167–176.
9. GLABINSKI, A.R. *et al.* 1995. Central nervous system chemokine gene expression follows leukocyte entry in acute murine experimental autoimmune encephalomyelitis. Brain Behav. Immun. **9:** 315–330.
10. GLABINSKI, A.R. *et al.* 1997. Synchronous synthesis of α- and β-chemokines by cells of diverse lineage in the central nervous system of mice with relapses of experimental autoimmune encephalomyelitis. Am. J. Pathol. **150:** 617–630.
11. GLABINSKI, A.R. & R. RANSOHOFF. 1999. Chemokines and chemokine receptors in CNS pathology. J. Neurovirol. **5:** 3–12.
12. KARPUS, W.J. *et al.* 1995. An important role for the chemokine macrophage inflammatory protein–1α in the pathogenesis of the T-cell–mediated autoimmune disease, experimental auotimmune encephalomyelitis. J. Immunol. **155:** 5003–5010.
13. KARPUS, W. & K. KENNEDY. 1997. MIP-1 alpha and MCP-1 differentially regulate acue and relapsing autoimmune encephalomyelitis as well as Th1/Th2 lymphocyte differentiation. J. Leuk Biol. **62:** 681–687.
14. MCMANUS, C. *et al.* 1998. MCP-1, MCP-2 and MCP-3 expression in multiple sclerosis lesions: an immunohistochemical and in situ hybridization study. J. Neuroimmunol. **86:** 20–29.
15. SIMPSON, J. *et al.* 1998. Expression of monocyte chemoattractant protein-1 and other β-chemokines by resident glia and inflammatory cells in multiple sclerosis lesions. J. Neuroimmunol. **84:** 238–249.
16. YU, M. *et al.* 1996. Interferon-beta inhibits progression of relapsing-remitting experimental autoimmune encephalomyelitis. J. Neuroimmunol. **64:** 91–100.

17. GLABINSKI, A.R. *et al.* 1998. Expression of chemokines RANTES, MIP-1α and GRO-α correlates with inflammation in acute experimental autoimmune encephalomyelitis. Neuroimmunomodulation **5:** 166–171.
18. GLABINSKI, A.R. *et al.* 1995. Regulation and function of central nervous system chemokines. Int. J. Dev. Neurosci. **13:** 153–165.
19. TANABE, S. *et al.* 1997. Murine astrocytes express a functional chemokine receptor. J. Neurosci. **17:** 6522–6528.
20. HEESEN, M. *et al.* 1997. Alternate splicing of mouse fusin/CXC chemokine receptor-4: stromal cell-derived factor-1alpha is a ligand for both CXC chemokine receptor-4 isoforms. J. Immunol. **158:** 3561–3564.
21. HE, J. *et al.* 1996. CCR3 and CCR5 are co-receptors for HIV-1 infection of microglia. Nature **385:** 645.
22. TANABE, S. *et al.* 1997. Functional expression of the CXC-chemokine receptor-4/fusin on mouse microglial cells and astrocytes. J. Immunol. **159:** 905–911.
23. HESSELGESSER, J. *et al.* 1997. CD4-independent association between HIV-1 gp120 and CXCR4: functional chemokine receptors are expressed in human neurons. Curr. Biol. **7:** 112–121.
24. HORUK, R. *et al.* 1997. Expression of chemokine receptors by subsets of neurons in the central nervous system. J. Immunol. **158:** 2882–2890.
25. WESTMORELAND, S.V. *et al.* 1998. Chemokine receptor expression on resident and inflammatory cells in the brain of macaques with simian immunodeficiency virus encephalitis. Am. J. Pathol. **152:** 659–665.
26. JIANG, Y. *et al.* 1998. Chemokine receptor expression in cultured glia and rat experimental allergic encephalomyelitis. J. Neuroimmunol. **86:** 1–12.
27. YU, M. *et al.* 1996. A predictable sequential pattern of determinant spreading invariably accompanies progression of experimental autoimmune encephalomyelitis: a basis for peptide-specific therapy after onset of clinical disease. J. Exp. Med. **183:** 1777–1788.

Contribution of Differently Localized α_2- and β-Adrenoceptors in the Modulation of TNF-α and IL-10 Production in Endotoxemic Mice

J. SZELÉNYI,[a,c] J.P. KISS,[a] É. PUSKÁS,[b] M. SZELÉNYI,[b] AND E.S. VIZI[a]

[a]*Department of Pharmacology, Institute of Experimental Medicine, Hungarian Academy of Sciences, P.O.B. 67, H-1450 Budapest, Hungary*

[b]*National Institute of Haematology and Immunology, P.O.B. 424, H-1519 Budapest, Hungary*

ABSTRACT: Evidence is presented that the immune response to endotoxemia is under tonic control of the sympathetic nervous system. Adrenergic agents may influence the immune response both directly through α- and β-adrenergic receptors expressed by immunologically competent cells and indirectly via alteration of the endogenous NA level by influencing the activity of release-regulating presynaptic α_2-adrenoceptors located on the sympathetic nerve terminals. In the immunomodulatory effect of NA/adrenergic drugs, their action on β-adrenoceptors was dominant, but the considerable role of α-adrenoceptors on macrophages was also demonstrated. According to our findings, regulation of the ascending wing of the inflammatory response, that is, TNF-α production, is more sensitive to the adrenoceptor effect, whereas modulation of its deregulation by IL-10 production also involves some other determining factors.

INTRODUCTION

Neuroimmune communications are among the mechanisms by which the immune response can be modulated. The primary and secondary immune organs are innervated by the sympathetic nervous system, which provides them with its neurotransmitters both systematically and *in situ*.[1] As immune cells are equipped with various neurotransmitter receptors, their functions can be influenced by these mediators.[2] Expression of both α_2- and β-adrenoceptors were reported on macrophages.[3,4] These receptors can be activated by the endogenous ligand noradrenaline (NA), released from noradrenergic varicosities, and/or by adrenergic drugs used frequently in clinical practice. The adrenergic agents may influence the immune response both directly through the α- and β-adrenergic receptors expressed by immunologically competent cells and indirectly via alteration of the endogenous NA level by influencing the activity of release-regulating presynaptic α_2-adrenoceptors located on the sympathetic nerve terminals.

[c]Author for correspondence. Voice: (36) (1) 210-0819/281; fax: (36) (1) 210-0813.
szelenyi@koki.hu

Various mediators can regulate cytokine responsiveness to endotoxemia. Noradrenaline, adrenaline, and dopamine, the principal transmitters of the sympathetic nervous system, have been shown to regulate cytokine production by interacting with their specific surface receptors.[5–7] The relative weight and significance of differently localized adrenoceptors in the modulation of cytokine production have not yet been clarified. Therefore, our studies were focused on the role of adrenoceptors, located both on the noradrenergic nerve terminals and on the macrophages, in regulating the production of a proinflammatory cytokine, tumor necrosis factor-α (TNF-α), and an anti-inflammatory cytokine, interleukin-10 (IL-10).

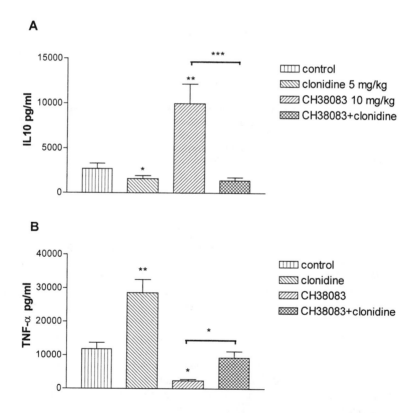

FIGURE 1. Effect of the α_2-adrenergic agonist clonidine (5 mg/kg) on LPS-evoked IL-10 (**A**) and TNF-α (**B**) production in control animals and in animals pretreated with the α_2-adrenergic antagonist CH-38083 (10 mg/kg) 60 minutes before LPS administration. Clonidine was injected i.p. 30 minutes before LPS treatment. Data are expressed as mean ± SEM of 8–10 animals per group.

DIRECT AND INDIRECT EFFECTS OF THE α2-ADRENOCEPTOR AGONIST CLONIDINE ON LPS-INDUCED TNF-α AND IL-10 PRODUCTION

Administration of clonidine, a known α2-adrenoceptor agonist, to mice prior to inducing endotoxemia by bacterial lipopolysaccharide (LPS) treatment, resulted in significantly increased TNF-α production, while it significantly suppressed the formation of the anti-inflammatory cytokine IL-10.

To examine whether the effect of clonidine is mediated via α2-adrenoceptors, the selective α2-adrenoceptor antagonist CH-38083 was administered to mice 30 minutes before clonidine treatment. As expected, CH-38083 alone suppressed LPS-induced TNF-α and enhanced IL-10 production by abolishing the negative feedback control of NA, that is, by increasing the sympathetic outflow.[7] Pretreatment with CH-38083 completely abolished the stimulatory effect of clonidine on TNF-α production, since the TNF-α level returned to the control level. On the contrary, the inhibitory effect of clonidine on IL-10 induction remained unchanged even in the presence of CH-38083 (see FIGURE 1).

The possible site of the action of clonidine on macrophages is the α2-adrenoceptor (direct effect); however, some other targets (e.g., imidazoline receptor) might also contribute. Occupation of α2-adrenoceptors by agonists results in suppression of the intracellular cAMP level, as these receptors are associated with a Gi-type protein. Because of a negative correlation between cAMP level and inflammatory cytokine production as well as a positive correlation between cAMP level and anti-inflammatory cytokine induction in macrophages,[8,9] the lower level of cAMP may explain both the increased TNF-α and the decreased IL-10 production.

The effects of clonidine and CH-38083, on the other hand, can also be explained by their action on the α2-adrenoceptors of sympathetic nerve terminals (indirect effect). Clonidine reduces whereas CH-38083 increases the release of NA by regulating its negative feedback, which in turn influences the function predominantly of the β-adrenoceptors on macrophages. It is well known that, upon stimulation, these receptors cause an increase in the intracellular cAMP level, which leads to decreased inflammatory cytokine production.[10,11] Therefore, if clonidine inhibits the release of NA, the stimulatory effect of this transmitter will be weaker on macrophage β-adrenoceptors, which results in lower cAMP and consequently higher TNF-α and lower IL-10 levels. Because the α2-antagonists increase the release of NA,[12,13] the opposite effects can be expected from CH-38083, which was proved by our experiments (FIG. 1).

Taken together, these results suggest that clonidine has multiple sites of action in contributing to modulate the LPS-induced immune response. It should also be noted that besides the cytokine response, LPS-induced endotoxemia is accompanied by changes in acute-phase protein (APP) levels and in white blood cell (WBC) count. NA/adrenergic drugs might also modulate these latter alterations, as our experiments suggested; therefore, they might also contribute to the observed changes in the cytokine profile. According to these observations, it seems likely that besides the indirect action of clonidine via the NA release-modulating α2B-adrenoceptors on the sympathetic nerve terminals, its direct action on macrophages might have several targets too, among them the α2-adrenoceptors. The effect of clonidine on the acute-phase response and/or on other receptors expressed on immune cells (e.g., imidazo-line receptors) might explain the ineffectiveness of CH-38083 on the clonidine-modulated IL-10 response.

EFFECTS OF THE β-ADRENOCEPTOR AGONIST ISOPROTERENOL ON LPS-INDUCED TNF-α AND IL-10 PRODUCTION

In contrast to α_2-adrenergic compounds, the receptorial influence of β-adrenergic drugs on the immune response is succeeded only directly through β-adrenoceptors located on macrophages. Administration of the β-adrenoceptor agonist isoproterenol significantly decreased LPS-induced TNF-α and increased IL-10 production in mice. Pretreatment with the β-antagonist propranolol blocked the β-adrenoceptors, that is, it prevented the action of endogenous NA and/or isoproterenol, resulting

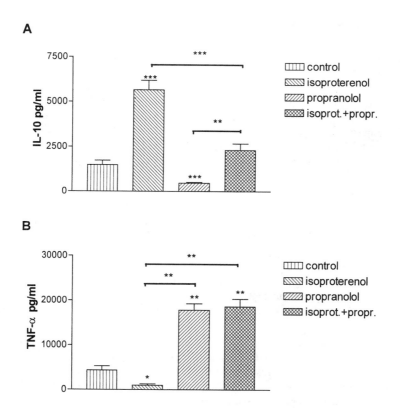

FIGURE 2. Effect of the β-adrenergic agonist isoproterenol (5 mg/kg) on LPS-evoked IL-10 (**A**) and TNF-α (**B**) production in control animals and animals pretreated with the β-adrenergic antagonist propranolol (10 mg/kg) 60 minutes before LPS administration. Iso-proterenol was injected i.p. 30 minutes before LPS treatment. Data are expressed as mean ± SEM of 8–10 animals per group.

in significantly lower IL-10 and higher TNF-α levels (see FIGURE 2). It is noteworthy, however, that the effect of isoproterenol on TNF-α was completely abolished, whereas under the same conditions IL-10 production was only partially inhibited.

Our data with the β-agonist isoproterenol confirm previous findings on the role of β-adrenoceptors in the modulation of cytokine production.[11,14] Isoproterenol elicits its pharmacological actions by stimulating the adenylate cyclase-cAMP system. It is generally assumed that increased cAMP levels participate in the modulation of cytokine production, because elevation in IL-10 and decrease in TNF-α levels were observed due to the *in vitro* or *in vivo* administration of stable cAMP analogues.[15,16] Reduced TNF-α levels were observed under endotoxemic conditions in mice, in which LPS-induced elevation of TNF-α production was suppressed by isoproterenol.[17] Recent findings which show that stimulation of adrenoceptors enhances IL-6 and IL-10 levels and reduces LPS-induced plasma TNF-α, IL-12, MIP-1α, and NO production suggest that *in vivo* stimulation of β-adrenoceptors downregulates the release of the proinflammatory cytokines by augmenting the production of IL-10.[18] However, evidence of other pathways was also reported, demonstrating that isoproterenol can inhibit the production of proinflammatory mediators even in IL-10–deficient mice.[19] This suggests that the effect of isoproterenol on the production of TNF-α, IL-12, MIP-1α, and NO might have other bypasses that are independent of the enhanced production of IL-10.

In our experiments, isoproterenol-mediated suppression of TNF-α could be prevented completely by pretreatment with the β-adrenoceptor antagonist propranolol, whereas enhancement of the IL-10 response was only partially inhibited (FIG. 2). These results demonstrate clearly that receptor-mediated elevation of cAMP enhances IL-10 synthesis and suppresses TNF-α production, whereas they provide further evidence, especially concerning IL-10, for the participation of other regulatory mechanisms too.

CONTRIBUTION OF α_2- AND β-ADRENOCEPTORS TO LPS-INDUCED TNF-α AND IL-10 PRODUCTION IN NORMAL AND MONOAMINE-DEPLETED MICE

Concerning the complex immunomodulatory effects of both α_2- and β-adrenergic agonists, we investigated the contribution of the direct and indirect actions of NA and/or adrenergic drugs on the inflammatory response by differently localized adrenoceptors in reserpinized mice. Reserpine depletes the noradrenergic vesicles; therefore, the sympathetic nervous system will be functionally inactive.[12] Under such conditions the function of adrenoceptors on macrophages can be separately investigated without the disturbing interference of neural adrenoceptors. A major finding of the present study is that reserpine pretreatment itself significantly increased the LPS-evoked production of both TNF-α and IL-10 (see FIGURE 3). TNF-α production is under the tonic control of NA, released from sympathetic varicosities, predominantly via the β- and, to a much lesser extent, the α-adrenoceptors.[4,11,20,21] Therefore, the increase in the TNF-α level after monoamine depletion reflects, first of all, the lack of NA action on the β-adrenoceptors. However, the increased IL-10 production due to reserpine treatment contradicts this and clearly demonstrates that other

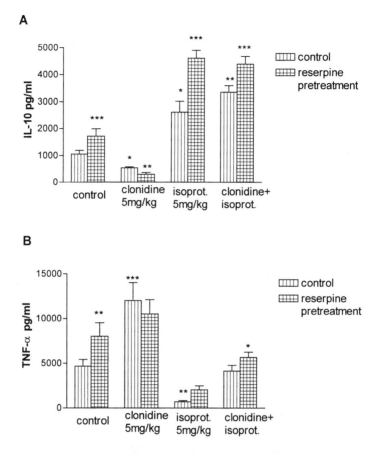

FIGURE 3. Effect of reserpine pretreatment (5 mg/kg reserpine i.p. 48 and 24 hours before the experiment) on LPS-evoked IL-10 (**A**) and TNF-α (**B**) production in animals treated with clonidine, isoproterenol (5 mg/kg each), and their combination. The α_2- and β-agonists were injected i.p. 30 minutes before LPS treatment. Data are expressed as mean ± SEM of 8–10 animals per group.

nonreceptorial effects are also involved in IL-10 regulation. In fact, in our experiments, reserpine also influenced other parameters of the acute-phase response.

Clonidine had only a little additive effect on TNF-α enhancement by reserpine, whereas it suppressed IL-10 production significantly. By contrast, isoproterenol strongly suppressed the production of TNF-α and enhanced that of IL-10 in both normal and reserpinized mice, confirming the presence of functional β-adrenoceptors on the macrophages in both cases. Therefore, these results can be explained so that macrophage β-adrenoceptors remained silent because of the lack of their endogenous ligand, NA, due to reserpinization.

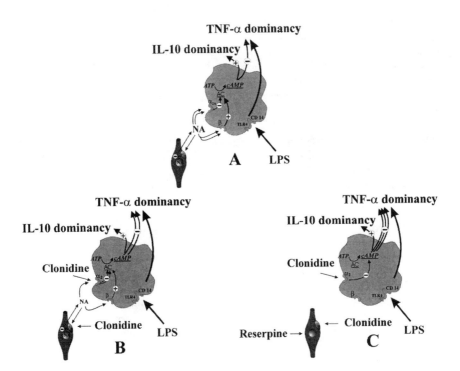

FIGURE 4. Modulation of cytokine production on an LPS-stimulated immune cell by adrenoceptors localized on sympathetic nerve terminals and on immune cells before and after reserpine pretreatment. (**A**) Endogenous NA, released presynaptically from vesicles of the noradrenergic nerve terminals, decreases (−) or increases (+) adenylate-cyclase activity by stimulating α- and β-adrenoceptors on immune cells. Resulting changes in the cAMP level might modulate the proinflammatory (TNF-α)/anti-inflammatory (IL-10) cytokine production in the LPS-activated immune cell; a higher level of cAMP (+) increases IL-10 production, whereas a lower level of cAMP (−) is associated with increased TNF-α production. NA also regulates its own release by a negative feedback mechanism on the α$_{2B}$-adrenoceptors located on the sympathetic nerve terminal. (**B**) The α$_2$-adrenoceptor agonist clonidine decreases the amount of released endogenous NA by activating its negative feedback control by stimulating presynaptic α$_{2B}$-adrenoceptors. The decreased level of NA (represented by *single arrows* rather than the double ones in **A**) results in a decreased cAMP level, because the β-adrenoceptors are less activated, whereas the α-adrenoceptors are kept in a highly stimulated state by their agonist, clonidine. The consequence is the dominance of TNF-α production (represented by doubling the corresponding *arrows* in comparison with the situation in **A**) due to the action of clonidine. (**C**) In reserpine-pretreated mice, presynaptic vesicles are depleted of NA; for this reason, no NA can be released from them, so the β-adrenoceptors on the immune cell remain silent. Clonidine is ineffective on presynaptic α$_{2B}$-adrenoceptors and is restricted to α$_2$-adrenoceptors on the immune cell, resulting in significant TNF-α dominance (represented by *triple arrows*).

When the two adrenoceptor agonists were applied in combination, however, clonidine was able to partially antagonize the TNF-α–suppressing effect of isoproterenol in both normal and monoamine-depleted mice, whereas it was ineffective in preventing the IL-10–enhancing effect of isoproterenol (FIG. 3). As the evidence just presented indicates, IL-10 production might be under more complex control where the effects of LPS on the whole organism superimpose the predominance of the β-adrenoceptor. The LPS-evoked TNF-α production seems, rather, to be under the tonic regulation of the sympathetic outflow. As NA release was prevented by reserpine, the TNF-α modulatory effect of clonidine in the reserpinized mice could only occur on the macrophages (FIG. 4). Consequently, these results clearly show that the macrophages possess α_2-adrenoceptors that contribute to the immune response; therefore, we have provided the first *in vivo* evidence of the presence of functionally active α_2-adrenoceptors on the surface of macrophages.[21]

Our findings may have clinically important implications. Both α- and β-adrenoceptor agonists are widely used in the therapy of different diseases. It is well known from the literature, and our present data also indicate, that these drugs modulate cytokine production in response to pathogenic agents that may affect the immune response. Our data show that α_2-adrenoceptor agonists may counterbalance the unwanted effects of β-agonists by restoring, for example, normal TNF-α production without disturbing their IL-10–enhancing effects. Since α_2-adrenoceptor agonists influence the function of the cardiovascular system (antihypertensive effect) through modulation of sympathetic activity, this therapeutic approach can only be used if subtype selective drugs are developed that exploit the putative diversity of α_2-adrenoceptor subtypes located on nerve terminals and immune cells.

ACKNOWLEDGMENTS

This work was supported by the following grants: the Hungarian Research Fund (OTKA No. T 029233) to J.S. and the Scientific Committee of the Ministry of Health (ETT No. 463/98) and the Hungarian Academy of Sciences (AKP No. 98-112 3,2) to E.S.V. The authors are indebted to Ms. J. Benkö and Ms. V. Gazsi for their excellent technical assistance.

REFERENCES

1. FELTEN, D.L., S.Y. FELTEN, D.L. BELLINGER, S.L. CARLSON, K.D. ACKERMAN, K.S. MADDEN, J.A. OLSCHKOWKI & S. LIVNAT. 1987. Noradrenergic sympathetic neural interactions with the immune system: structure and function. Immunol. Rev. **100:** 225–260.
2. ROSZMAN, T.L. & S.L. CARLSON. 1991. Neurotransmitters and molecular signalling in the immune response *In* Psychneuroimmunology, 2nd edit. R. Ader, D.L. Felten & N. Cohen, Eds.: 311–337. Academic Press. New York.
3. ABRASS, C.K., S.W. O'CONNOR, P.J. SCARPACE & I.B. ABRASS. 1985. Characterization of the β-adrenergic receptor of the rat peritoneal macrophage. J. Immunol. **135:** 1338–1341.
4. SPENGLER, R.N., R.M. ALLEN, D.G. REMICK, R.M. STRIETER & S.L. KUNKEL. 1990. Stimulation of α-adrenergic receptor augments the production of macrophage-derived tumor necrosis factor. J. Immunol. **145:** 1430–1434.

5. DEL REY, A., H.O. BESEDOVSKY, E. SORKIN, M. DA PRADA & S. ARRENBRECHT. 1981. Immunoregulation mediated by the sympathetic nervous system. Cell. Immunol. **63:** 329–336.

6. PASTORES, S.M., G. HASKÓ, E.S. VIZI & V. KVETAN. 1996. Cytokine production and its manipulation by vasoactive drugs. New Horiz. **4:** 252–264.

7. VIZI, E.S. 1998. Receptor-mediated local fine tuning by noradrenergic innervation of neuroendocrine and immune systems. Ann. N.Y. Acad. Sci. **851:** 388–396.

8. HASKÓ, G., C. SZABÓ, Z.H. NÉMETH, A.L. SALZMAN & E.S. VIZI. 1998. Suppression of interleukin-12 production by phosphodiesterase inhibition in murine endotoxaemia is interleukin-10 independent. Eur. J. Immunol. **28:** 468–472.

9. VAN DER POUW-KRAAN, T.C.T.M., L.C.M. BOEIJE, R.J.T. SMEENK, J. WIJDENES & L.A. AARDEN. 1995. Prostaglandin-E2 is a potent inhibitor of human interleukin 12 production. J. Exp. Med. **181:** 775–779.

10. MADDEN, K.S., V.M. SANDERS & D.L. FELTEN. 1995. Catecholamine influences and sympathetic neural modulation of immune responsiveness. Annu. Rev. Pharmacol. Toxicol. **35:** 417–448.

11. SEVERN, A., N.T. RAPSON, C.A. HUNTER & F.Y. LIEW. 1992. Regulation of tumor necrosis factor production by adrenaline and β-adrenergic agonists. J. Immunol. **148:** 3441ëP3445.

12. ELENKOV, I.J. & E.S. VIZI. 1991. Presynaptic modulation of release of noradrenaline from the sympatethic nerve terminals in rat spleen. Neuropharmacology **30:** 1319–1324.

13. KISS, J.P., G. ZSILLA, A. MIKE , T. ZELLES, E. TÓTH, A. LAJTHA. & E.S. VIZI. 1995. Subtype specificity of the presynaptic α_2-adrenoceptors modulating hippocampal norepinephrine release in rat. Brain Res. **674:** 238–244.

14. VAN DER POLL, T., J. JANSEN, E. ENDERT, H.P. SAUERWEIN & S.J.H. VAN DEVENTER. 1994. Noradrenaline inhibits lipopolysaccharide induced tumor necrosis factor and interleukin 6 production in human whole blood. Infect. Immunol. **62:** 2046–2050.

15. PLATZER, C., C.H. MEISEL, K. VOGT, M. PLATZER & H.D. VOLK 1994. Up-regulation of monocytic IL-10 by TNF-α and cAMP elevating drugs. Int. Immunol. **7:** 517–521.

16. ARAI, T., K. HIROMATSU & N.KOBAYASHI. 1995. IL-10 is involved in the protective effect of dibutyryl cyclic adenosine monophosphate on endotoxin-induced inflammatory liver injury. J. Immunol. **155:** 5743–5751.

17. SZABÓ, C., G. HASKÓ, B. ZINGARELLI, Z.H. NÉMETH, A.L. SALZMAN, V. MCCARTHY KVETAN, S. PASTORES & E.S. VIZI. 1997. Isoproterenol regulates tumour necrosis factor, interleukin-10, interleukin-6 and nitric oxide production and protects against the redevlopment of vascular hyporeactivity in endotoxaemia. Immunology **90:** 95–100.

18. BERG, T.J., R. KÜHN, K. RAJEWSKY, W. MÜLLER, S. MENON, N. DAVIDSON, G. GRÜNIG & D. RENNICK. 1995. Interleukin-10 is a central regulator of the response of LPS in murine model of endotoxaemic shock and the Schwartzman reaction, but not endotoxin tolerance J.Clin. Invest. **96:** 2339–2347.

19. HASKÓ, G., C. SZABÓ Z. NÉMETH, A.L. SALZMAN & E.S. VIZI. 1998. Stimulation of β-adrenoceptors inhibits endotoxin-induced IL-12 production in normal and IL-10 deficient mice. J. Neuroimmunol. **88:** 57–61.

20. ELENKOV, I.J., G. HASKÓ, K.J. KOVÁCS. & E.S. VIZI. 1995. Modulation of lipopolysaccharide-induced tumor necrosis factor-α production by selective α- and β-adrenergic drugs in mice. J. Neuroimmunol. **61:** 123–131.

21. SZELÉNYI, J., J.P. KISS & E.S. VIZI. 2000. Differential involvement of sympathetic nervous system and immune system in the modulation of TNF-α production by α_2- and β-adrenoceptors in mice. J. Neuroimmunol. **103:** 34–40.

Regulation of Cytokine Secretion and Amyloid Precursor Protein Processing by Proinflammatory Amyloid Beta (Aβ)

BRUCE D. GITTER,[a] LEONARD N. BOGGS, PATRICK C. MAY,
DAN L. CZILLI, AND CHRISTOPHER D. CARLSON

Neuroscience Diseases Research Division, Lilly Research Laboratories,
Eli Lilly and Co., Lilly Corporate Center, Indianapolis, Indiana 46285, USA

ABSTRACT: Neurodegenerative processes in Alzheimer's disease (AD) are thought to be driven, in part, by the deposition of amyloid beta (Aβ), a 39–43-aminoacid peptide product resulting from an alternative cleavage of amyloid precursor protein (APP). In addition to its neurotoxic properties, Aβ may influence neuropathology by stimulating glial cell cytokine and acute phase protein secretion in affected areas of the brain (e.g., cortex, hippocampus). Using an *in vitro* human astrocyte model (U-373 MG astrocytoma cells), the effects of Aβ treatment on acute phase protein (APP and alpha-1-antichymotrypsin [α_1-ACT]) and interleukin-8 (IL-8) were examined. U-373 MG cells secreted increased levels of α_1-ACT and neurotrophic/neuroprotective alpha-cleaved APP (αAPP) after exposure to interleukin-1β (IL-1β) for 24 hours. Aβ treatment resulted in a similar, but modest increase in α_1-ACT secretion, a two- to threefold stimulation of IL-8 production, and, conversely, a profound reduction in the levels of secreted αAPPs. Aβ inhibited αAPP secretion by U-373 MG cells in a concentration- and conformation-dependent manner. Moreover, the reduction in αAPP secretion was accompanied by an increase in cell-associated APP. Another proinflammatory amyloidogenic peptide, human amylin, similarly affected APP processing in U-373 astrocytoma cells. These data suggest that Aβ may contribute to Alzheimer's-associated neuropathology by lowering the production of neuroprotective/neurotrophic αAPPs. Moreover, the concomitant increase in cell-associated APP may provide increased substrate for the generation of amyloidogenic peptides within astrocytes.

INTRODUCTION

Alzheimer's disease (AD) is a neurodegenerative disorder pathologically characterized by cortical atrophy, neuronal loss, and the presence of neurofibrillary tangles and senile amyloid plaques. These characteristic lesions are localized to regions of the brain important for cognition, learning, and memory, such as the cerebral cortex and hippocampus.[1] The neuropathology of AD, driving the progressive loss of cognitive function and memory, may result from the deposition of Aβ, a 39–43-amino-

[a]Address for correspondence: Dr. Bruce D. Gitter, Neuroscience Diseases Research Division, Lilly Research Laboratories, Lilly Corporate Center, Indianapolis, IN 46285. Voice: 317-276-4271; fax: 317-276-5546.
gitter_bruce_d@Lilly.com

acid peptide product derived from beta- and gamma-secretase cleavages of amyloid precursor protein (APP).[2–5] Thus, Aβ may influence AD pathophysiology by its neurotoxic and proinflammatory activity.[6–13]

Processing of APP by α-secretase within the Aβ domain produces the secreted N-terminal portion, αAPPs, and therefore precludes Aβ formation.[14–16] In contrast to the neurotoxic and proinflammatory properties of Aβ, αAPPs and full-length APP are neuroprotective and neurotrophic.[17–20] Therefore, the beneficial and negative effects of APP and Aβ, respectively, suggest that AD pathology is dependent on APP processing. Any circumstance that would increase intracellular APP levels, enhance β- and γ-secretase activities or inhibit α-secretase activity may lead to increased Aβ production/deposition, neurotoxicity/inflammation, and AD pathology. In addition, inhibition of α-secretase that reduces secretion of neuroprotective αAPPs could enhance AD associated neurotoxicity. Inasmuch as an increase in cell-associated APP immunoreactivity can be detected in degenerating neurons and dystrophic neurites around amyloid deposits in AD brain,[21,22] alterations in APP processing in AD brain lesions may be influenced, at least in part, by an Aβ-driven amplification loop.

In the present study, we investigated the role of Aβ in APP processing. Using our previously characterized *in vitro* human astrocytoma model of Aβ and amylin effects on inflammatory cytokine secretion,[8,23] we determined the effects of amyloidogenic peptides on the secretion of αAPPs and accumulation of cell-associated APP.

MATERIALS AND METHODS

Cell Culture Conditions, Aβ, Amylin, and IL-1β Treatment

U-373 MG human astrocytoma cells (American Type Culture Collection, Rockville, MD) were maintained at 37°C (humidified 5% CO_2/air incubator) in EMEM (Bio-Whitiker, Walkersville, MD) supplemented with 10% heat-inactivated fetal bovine serum, 4 mM glutamine, and 50 mg/ml gentamicin sulfate (Gibco/BRL, Gaithersburg, MD). U-373 MG cells were trypsinized and plated at a density of 2×10^5 cells/cm^2 in serum-containing EMEM the night before peptide or IL-1β treatment. Cells were re-washed twice with serum-free EMEM supplemented with 4 mM glutamine, 50 mg/ml gentamicin sulfate, and 12.5 mg/ml polymyxin B (Sigma Chemical Co., St. Louis, MO) before addition of test samples. Aβ (1–40, lots ZM605, ZN428, and ZN571, $Aβ_{40-1}$, or human and rat amylin [Bachem, King of Prussia, PA]) were prepared as 700 μM solutions in sterile water and used fresh or after aging in a 37°C incubator for various times. Cells were treated in serum-free EMEM and peptides were added to the cultures as a 2× solution. Recombinant human IL-1β was a kind gift of J.L. Bobbitt (Biotechnology Division, Lilly Research Laboratories, Indianapolis, IN). IL-1β was diluted into serum-free medium just prior to the addition to U-373 MG cultures.

Thioflavin-T Fluorescence Assay

Thioflavin-T fluorescence of Aβ peptides was monitored using a modified, previously described protocol.[24] In a 96-well microtiter plate, 75 μl of 100 mM AB (ZN428) peptide samples (in serum-free EMEM) were reacted with 75 μl of a

25-μM stock solution (200 mM Tris-HCl, pH 7.4) of Thioflavin T (Sigma Chemical Co., St. Louis, MO). After a 15-minute incubation at room temperature (in darkness), relative fluorescence was determined using a Cytofluor 2350 multiwell fluorometer (Millipore Corp., Bedford, MA).

Western Blot Hybridization

Conditioned media were prepared for Western blotting by the addition of dithiothreitol (DTT, Sigma Chemical Co., St. Louis, MO) to a final concentration of 200 mM (2×) followed by an equal volume of 2× Tricine-SDS sample buffer (Novex, San Diego, CA). Cell lysates were prepared by adding 1× sample buffer (containing 100 mM DTT) directly to the plate. We saw no change in cell viability following Aβ or amylin treatment as judged by MTT cytotoxicity assay (data not shown). Furthermore, using Coomassie stained gels, the amount and distribution of proteins appeared to be similar in control and peptide-treated cultures. Samples were heated to 100°C for 10 minutes prior to electrophoresis. Proteins were separated on 10% polyacrylamide Tricine/SDS (SDS/PAGE) gels (Novex, San Diego, CA) and transferred to Immobilon P membranes (Millipore Corp., Bedford, MA) in 2× transfer buffer/20% methanol (Novex, San Diego, CA). Samples from control U-373 MG cultures were run on each gel in addition to an APP (purified from 293 cells permanently transfected with the Swedish isoform of full-length APP$_{695}$ or APP$_{751}$) or α1-ACT (Calbiochem, San Diego, CA) standard. Membranes were blocked in 5% nonfat dry milk in TBS/Tween (24 mM Tris, 137 mM NaCl, 5 mM KCl, 0.05% Tween-20, pH 7.5) for one hour at room temperature on a shaker platform. Membranes were incubated with the primary mouse monoclonal antibodies to APP (8E5[25]) or α_1 ACT (Calbiochem, San Diego, CA) prepared in 5% nonfat dry milk in TBS/Tween for one hour at room temperature. Membranes were washed three times for five minutes/wash at room temperature in TBS/Tween. Bound mouse antibodies were detected by incubating the membranes at room temperature for one hour in TBS/Tween:5% nonfat dry milk containing peroxidase-conjugated Affinipure goat-anti-mouse IgG (Jackson ImmunoResearch Labs, West Grove, PA). Membranes were washed as described above, and hybridization of antibody/protein complexes was detected using ECL reagents (Amersham Life Science, Buckinghamshire, England) followed by exposure to Reflection NEF-496 autoradiography film (NEN Life Science Products, Boston, MA). Relative APP levels were quantified using a Molecular Dynamics (Sunnyvale, CA) scanning laser densitometer and analyzed using IPlab Gel software on a Macintosh computer.

IL-8 Measurements

IL-8 was quantified in U-373 MG supernatants using R&D Quantikine human IL-8 ELISA kits (R&D Systems, Minneapolis, MN).

Cytotoxicity Assay

Cellular toxicity was monitored using the CellTiter 96 AQ$_{ueous}$ One Solution Cell Proliferation Assay (Gibco/BRL, Gaithersburg, MD) according to the manufacturer's protocol.

Statistics

Significance between groups was determined by analysis of variance and post-hoc Tukey-Kramer multiple comparison tests. Data are presented as mean ± standard deviation, $n = 3$–6.

RESULTS

U-373 MG human astrocytoma cells were treated overnight with 35 µM (freshly prepared) Aβ (ZM605) and 10 ng/ml recombinant human IL-1β either alone or in combination for 24 hours. Following treatment, the secretion of αAPPs and α_1ACT into the culture supernatant was determined by Western blot analysis. IL-1 predictably stimulated an increase in α_1ACT and αAPP secretion. Aβ modestly stimulated α_1ACT release, but profoundly inhibited secretion of αAPP, even when the cells were co-treated with IL-β (see FIGURE 1). Focusing further on APP processing, we determined whether the effect of Aβ was dependent on the β-sheeted secondary structure and aggregation state of the peptide. Using a peptide lot that required aging-induced conformational changes for biologic (*in vitro* neurotoxic) activity,

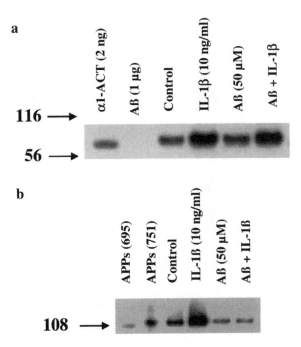

FIGURE 1. Secretion of α_1-ACT and αAPPs by Aβ-treated U-373 MG human astrocytoma cells. U-373 MG cells were treated for 24 hours with 50 µM Aβ (ZM605) or IL-1β. α_1-ACT (**a**) and αAPPs (**b**) were detected in cell culture supernatants by SDS/PAGE and Western blot hybridization.

a

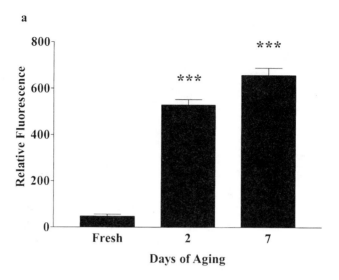

b

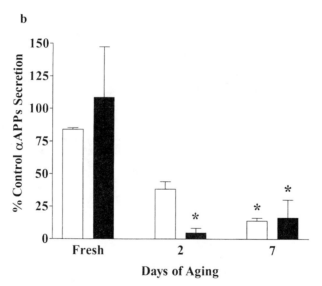

FIGURE 2. Inhibition of αAPP secretion by Aβ-treated U-373 MG human astrocytoma cells is dependent on the peptide aggregation state. (**a**) Thioflavin-T fluorescence of freshly prepared, 2-, and 7-day aged Aβ (ZN428) was monitored as described in *Materials and Methods.* Values represent the mean ± SD of triplicate determinations; ***$p < 0.001$ (vs. freshly prepared peptide). (**b**) U-373 MG cells were treated for 24 hours with 10 μM (□) or 50 μM (■) Aβ (ZN428). After SDS/PAGE and Western blot hybridization, αAPP in cell culture supernatants was quantified by laser densitometry scanning. Values represent the mean ± SD of triplicate determinations; *$p < 0.05$ (vs. control cultures).

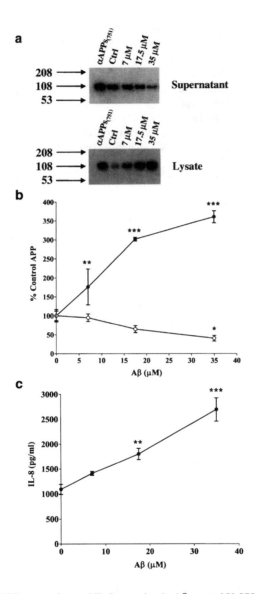

FIGURE 3. APP processing and IL-8 secretion in Aβ-treated U-373 MG human astro-cytoma cells. (**a**) U-373 MG cells were treated with various concentrations of Aβ (ZN571) for 24 hours. APP was detected in cell culture supernatants and cell lysates by SDS/PAGE and Western blot hybridization. (**b**) Secreted αAPP (○) and cell-associated APP (●) levels (following SDS/PAGE and Western blot hybridization) were quantified by laser densitom-etry scanning. The amount of APP in Aβ-treated cultures is expressed as a percentage of APP in control cultures. Values represent the mean ± SD of triplicate determinations. ***$p < 0.001$, **$p < 0.01$, *$p < 0.05$ (vs. control cultures). (**c**) Levels of IL-8 in cell culture supernatants of Aβ-treated U-373 MG cells were determined by ELISA. Values represent the mean ± SD of triplicate determinations. ***$p < 0.001$, **$p < 0.01$ (vs. control cultures).

U-373 cells were treated with freshly prepared, 2-day and 7-day aged Aβ (ZN428). The effect of peptide aging on β-sheeted secondary structure and aggregation state was monitored by thioflavin-T fluorescence. As little as two days of peptide aging produced significant changes in Aβ secondary structure and aggregation state (see FIGURE 2a) along with a strong inhibition of APP secretion (FIG. 2b). In subsequent studies, αAPP levels were compared to the presence of cell-associated APP by Western blot analysis of cell lysates. Aβ (ZN571; 24-hour aged) inhibited αAPP secretion and reciprocally stimulated the accumulation of cell-associated APP in a concentration-dependent manner (see FIGURE 3a and b). To control for nonspecific effects on protein secretion by Aβ in U-373 MG cells, we examined the effect of various concentrations of Aβ on IL-8 secretion. Aβ (ZN571) significantly stimulated IL-8 secretion from U-373 MG cells in a concentration-dependent manner (FIG. 3c). Moreover, stimulation of IL-8 secretion by Aβ showed a similar peptide conformation-dependence (data not shown) as observed with the effects of Aβ on APP processing. In additional experiments to address peptide specificity, we observed no effects of the reverse peptide, $A\beta_{40-1}$, on APP processing or cytokine secretion. These experiments demonstrated that the decrease in αAPP secretion and the increase in cellular APP by $A\beta_{1-40}$ are due to the formation of a beta-sheeted structure specific for the primary sequence of the 1-40 peptide. Furthermore, the decrease in αAPP secretion was not due to a toxic effect of Aβ in U-373 MG cells, because there was no change in cell viability as measured by the MTS cytotoxicity assay following $A\beta_{1-40}$ treatment (data not shown). $A\beta_{40-1}$ was also not toxic to U-373 MG cells after 24 hours of treatment (data not shown).

Additional studies to examine the role of secondary peptide structure on the effects of APP processing in U-373 human astrocytoma cells were conducted using human and rat amylin. After 24 hours of treatment, human, but not rat, amylin strongly inhibited αAPP secretion with a slightly diminishing effect at increasing peptide concentrations (see FIGURE 4a). As observed after Aβ exposure, inhibition of αAPP secretion by human (but not rat) amylin-treated U-373 MG cells was associated with a profound increase in cell-associated APP (FIG. 4b).

DISCUSSION

The close association of inflammatory mediators (cytokines, complement and anti-complement proteins, acute phase reactants) and activated glial cells with compact neuritic plaques suggests a role for immune/inflammatory pathways in the neurodegenerative process.[26–29] Thus, the formation and deposition of fibrillar Aβ may be an integral driver of AD inflammation, acute phase responses, and neurodegeneration. In support of this hypothesis, a variety of studies have linked the *in vitro* neurotoxic and proinflammatory effects of Aβ with the aggregation state and secondary (β-sheet) structure of the peptide.[6–8,30] In addition, similar *in vitro* activities of amyloidogenic peptides, such as human amylin, have also been attributed to aggregation state and secondary structure.[23,31,32] In the present study, the effects of Aβ and human amylin on U-373 MG human astrocytoma cell APP processing are consistent with aggregation state and secondary structure–dependence. In addition, our results compare favorably with previous studies demonstrating an increase in cell-

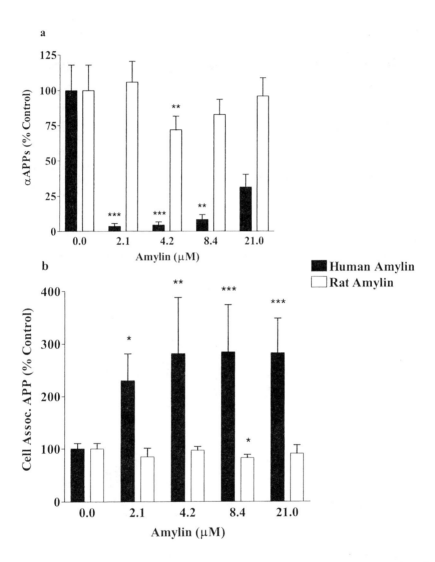

FIGURE 4. Human amylin inhibits secretion of αAPP and stimulates accumulation of cell-associated APP in U-373 MG human astrocytoma cells. U-373 MG cells were treated for 24 hours with various concentrations of human or rat amylin. Secreted αAPPs and cell-associated APP levels were determined in cell culture supernatants (panel **a**) and cell lysates (panel **b**) by SDS/PAGE, Western blot hybridization, and laser densitometry scanning. The amount of APP in amylin-treated cultures is expressed as a percentage of APP in control cultures. Values represent the mean ± SD of triplicate determinations. $***p < 0.001$, $**p < 0.01$, $*p < 0.05$ (vs. control cultures).

associated APP in Aβ-treated neuronal and non-neuronal cells.[33–36] The profound increase in cell-associated APP in Aβ-treated U-373 MG cells may be an *in vitro* correlate of the increase in APP surrounding Aβ deposits in AD brain.[21,22] A consequence of increasing cell-associated APP is the potential for providing additional substrate for amyloidogenic beta and gamma secretase cleavages, resulting in a feed-forward stimulation of Aβ production.[34]

In the present study, Aβ profoundly reduced the secretion of αAPP from U-373 MG human astrocytoma cells (FIGS. 1–3). It is not clear at present whether alpha secretase activity *per se* was inhibited or if alpha-cleaved material was retarded and remained cell-associated. Further analysis of cell-associated APP using antibodies specific for carboxy-terminal APP epitopes should help clarify this point. However, decreasing the production of this neurotrophic/neuroprotective protein may accelerate the progression of AD neuropathology.

Gliosis, a characteristic feature of AD pathology, may be involved in disease progression by the Aβ-induced production of inflammatory mediators and acute phase reactants.[8–10,13] Thus, as an acute phase reactant,[37,38] APP is rapidly induced in glial cells following a variety of CNS injuries, including chemical lesion, trauma, and ischemia.[39–43] It is widely believed that these CNS injuries represent risk and/or potentiating factors in AD. Thus, our further understanding of neuroinflammatory influences of APP processing may lead to new strategies in the hunt for new therapeutic agents.

ACKNOWLEDGMENTS

The authors thank Drs. Sheila Little, Donald McClure, and Gerald Becker for providing purified αAPP. We also thank Dr. Sheila Little for critical review of this manuscript.

REFERENCES

1. HARDY, J. & D. ALLSOP. 1991. Amyloid deposition as the central event in the aetiology of Alzheimer's disease. Trends Pharmacol. Sci. **12:** 383–388.
2. GLENNER, G.G. & C.W. WONG. 1984. Alzheimer's disease: initial report of the purification and characterization of a novel cerebrovascular amyloid protein. Biophys. Res. Commun. **120:** 885–890.
3. SELKOE, D.J. 1994. Cell biology of the amyloid beta-protein precursor and the mechanism of Alzheimer's disease. Annu. Rev. Cell Biol. **10:** 373–403.
4. SCHENK, D., R.E. RYDEL, P. MAY, S. LITTLE, J. PANETTA, I. LIEBERBURB & S. SINHA. 1995. Therapeutic approaches related to amyloid-b peptide and Alzheimer's disease. J. Med. Chem. **38:** 4141–4154.
5. SELKOE, D.J. 1997. Alzheimer's disease: genotypes, phenotype, and treatment. Science **275:** 630–631.
6. SIMMONS, L.K., P.C. MAY, K.J. TOMASELLI, R.E. RYDEL, K.S. FUSON, E.F. BRIGHAM, S. WRIGHT, I. LIEBERBURG, G.W. BECKER, D.N. BREMS & W.Y. LI. 1993. Secondary structure of amyloid-β peptide correlates with neurotoxic activity *in vitro*. Mol. Pharmacol. **45:** 373–379.
7. LORENZO, A. & B.A. YANKNER. 1994. β-amyloid neurotoxicity requires fibril formation. Proc. Natl. Acad. Sci. USA **91:** 12243–12247.

8. GITTER, B.D., L.M. COX, R.E. RYDEL & P.C. MAY. 1995. Amyloid β potentiates cytokine secretion by interleukin-1β-activated human astrocytoma cells. Proc. Natl. Acad. Sci. USA **92:** 10738–10741.

9. ARAUJO, D.M. & C.W. COTMAN. 1992. β-amyloid stimulates glial cells in vitro to produce growth factors that accumulate in senile plaques in Alzheimer's disease. Brain Res. **569:** 141–145.

10. HAGA, S., I. KAZUHIKO, M. SATO & I. TSUYOSHI. 1993. Synthetic Alzheimer amyloid β/A4 peptides enhance production of complement C3 component by cultured microglial cells. Brain Res. **601:** 88–94.

11. LORTON, D., J.-M. KOCSIS, L. KING, K. MADDEN & K.R. BRUNDEN. 1996. β Amyloid induces increased release of interleukin-1β from lipopolysaccharide-activated human monocytes. J. Neuroimmunol. **67:** 21–29.

12. KLEGARIS, A.D., G. WALKER & P.L. MCGEER. 1997. Interaction of Alzheimer β amyloid peptide with the human monocytic cell line THP-1 results in a protein kinase C dependent secretion of tumor necrosis factor-α. Brain Res. **747:** 114–121.

13. JOHNSTONE, M., A.J.H. GEARING & K.M. MILLER. 1999. A central role for astrocytes in the inflammatory response to β-amyloid; chemokines, cytokines and reactive oxygen species are produced. J. Neuroimmunol. **93:** 182–193.

14. ESCH, F.S., P.S. KEIM, E.C. BEATTIE, R.W. BLACHER, A.R. CULWELL, T. OLTERS-DORF, D. MCCLURE & P.J. WARD. 1990. Cleavage of amyloid-β peptide during constitutive processing of its precursor. Science **248:** 1122–1124.

15. SISODIA, S.S., E.H. KOO, K. BEYREUTHER, A. UNTERBECK & D.L. PRICE. 1990. Evidence that β-amyloid protein in Alzheimer's disease is not derived by normal processing. Science **248:** 492–495.

16. WANG, R., J.F. MESCHIA, R.J. COTTER & S.S. SISODIA. 1991. Secretion of the β/A4 amyloid precursor protein: identification of a cleavage site in cultured mammalian cells. J. Biol. Chem. **266:** 16960–16964.

17. MATTSON, M.P., B. CHENG, A.R. CULWELL, F.S. ESCH, I. LIEBERBURG & R.E. RYDEL. 1993. Evidence for excitoprotective and intraneuronal calcium-regulating roles for secreted forms of the β-amyloid precursor protein. Neuron **10:** 243–254.

18. SMITH-SWINTOWSKY, V., L. CREED PETTIGREW, S.D. CRADDOCK, A.R. CULWELL, R.E. RYDEL & M.P. MATTSON. 1998. Secreted forms of β-amyloid precursor protein protect against ischemic brain injury. J. Neurochem. **63:** 781–784.

19. MUCKE, L., C.R. ABRAHAM, M.D. RUPPE, E.M. ROCKSTEIN, S.M. TOGGAS, M. MALLORY, M. ALFORD & E. MASLIAH. 1995. Protection against HIV gp120 induced brain damage by neuronal expression of human amyloid precursor protein. J. Exp. Med. **181:** 1551–1556.

20. OHSAWA, I., C. TAKAMURA & S. KOHSAKA. 1997. The amino-terminal region of amyloid precursor protein is responsible for neurite outgrowth in rat neocortical explant culture. Biochem. Biophys. Res. Commun. **236:** 59–65.

21. SHOJI, M., S. HIRAI, H. YAMAGUCHI, Y. HARIGAYA & T. KAWARABAYASHI. 1990. Amyloid β-protein precursor accumulates in dystrophic neurites of senile plaque in Alzheimer-type dementia. Brain Res. **512:** 164–168.

22. CUMMINGS, B.J., J.H. SU, J.W. GEDDES, W.E. VAN NOSTRAND, S.L. WAGNER, D.D. CUNNINGHAM & C.W. COTMAN. 1992. Aggregation of the amyloid precursor protein within degenerating neurons and dystrophic neurites in Alzheimer's disease. Neuroscience **48:** 763–777.

23. GITTER, B.D., L.M. COX, C.D. CARLSON & P.C. MAY. 2000. Human amylin stimulates inflammatory cytokine secretion from human glioma cells. NeuroImmunoModulation. **7:** 147–152.

24. LEVINE, H., III. 1997. Stopped-flow kinetics reveal multiple phases of thioflavin T binding to Alzheimer β (1-40) amyloid fibrils. Arch. Biochem Biophys. **342:** 306–316.

25. JOHNSON-WOOD, K., M. LEE, R. MOTTER, K. HU, G. GORDON, R. BARBOUR, K. KHAN, M. GORDON, H. TAN, D. GAMES, I. LIEBERBURG, D. SCHENK, P. SEUBERT & L. MCCONLOGUE. 1997. Amyloid precursor protein processing and Aβ$_{42}$ deposition in a transgenic mouse model of Alzheimer disease. Proc. Natl. Acad. Sci. USA **94:** 1550–1555.

26. McGeer, P.L., J. Rogers & E.G. McGeer. 1994. Neuroimmune mechanisms in Alzheimer's disease pathogenesis. Alzheimer Dis. Assoc. Disord. **8:** 149–158.
27. Griffin, W.S.T., L.C. Stanley, C. Ling, L. White, V. Macleod, L.J. Perrot, C.L. White, III & C. Araoz. 1989. Brain interleukin-1 and S-100 immunoreactivity are elevated in Down syndrome and Alzheimer's disease. Proc. Natl. Acad. Sci. USA **86:** 7611–7615.
28. Ishizuka, K., T. Kimura, R. Igata-Yi, S. Katsuragi, J. Takamatsu & T. Miyakawa. 1997. Identification of monocyte chemoattractant protein-1 in senile plaques and reactive microglia of Alzheimer's disease. Psychiatry Clin. Neurosci **51:** 135–138.
29. Griffin, W.S.T., J.G. Sheng, G.W. Roberts & R.E. Mrak. 1995. Interleukin-1 expression in different plaque types in Alzheimer's disease: significance in plaque evolution. J. Neuropathol. Exp. Neurol. **54:** 276–281.
30. Pike, C.J., D. Burdick, A.J. Walencewicz, C.G. Glabe & C.W. Cotman. 1993. Neurodegeneration induced by β-amyloid peptides *in vitro*: the role of peptide assembly state. J. Neurosci. **13:** 1676–1687.
31. May, P.C., L.N. Boggs & K.S. Fuson. 1993. Neurotoxicity of human amylin in rat primary hippocampal cultures. Similarity to Alzheimer's disease amyloid-β neurotoxicity. J. Neurochem. **61:** 2330–2333.
32. Hom, J.T., T. Estridge, P. Pechous & P.A. Hyslop. 1995. The amyloidogenic peptide human amylin augments the inflammatory activities of eosinophils. J. Leukocyte Biol. **58:** 526–532.
33. Cribbs, D.H., J. Davis-Salinas, C.W. Cotman & W.E. Van Nostrand. 1995. Aβ induces increased expression and processing of amyloid precursor protein in cortical neurons. Alzheimer's Res. **1:** 197–200.
34. Davis-Salinas, J., S.M. Saporito-Irwin, C.W. Cotman & W.E. Van Nostrand. 1995. Amyloid β-protein induces its own production in cultured degenerating cerebrovascular smooth muscle cells. J. Neurochem. **65:** 931–934.
35. Schmitt, T.L., E. Steiner, K. Trieb & B. Grubeck-Lobenstein. 1997. Amyloid β-protein$_{25-35}$ increases cellular APP and inhibits the secretion of APPs in human extraneuronal cells. Exp. Cell Res. **234:** 336–340.
36. Moreno-Flores, M.T., O. Salinero & F. Wandosell. 1998. β-amyloid peptide (25-35) induced APP expression in cultured astrocytes. J. Neurosci. Res. **52:** 661–671.
37. Vandenabeele, P. & W. Fiers. 1991. Is amyloidosis during Alzheimer's disease due to an IL-1/IL-6-mediated acute phase response in the brain? Immunol. Today **12:** 217–219.
38. Alstiel, L. & K. Sperber. 1991. Cytokines in Alzheimer's disease. Prog. Neuropsychopharmacol. Biol. Psych. **15:** 481–495.
39. Siman, R., P.J. Card, R.B. Nelson & L.G. Davis. 1989. Expression of β-amyloid precursor protein in reactive astrocytes following neuronal damage. Neuron **3:** 275–285.
40. Otsuka, N., M. Tomonaga & K. Ikeda. 1991. Rapid appearance of β-amyloid precursor protein immunoreactivity in damaged axons and reactive glial cells in rat brain following needle stab injury. Brain Res. **568:** 335–338.
41. Bramlett, H.M., S. Kraydieh, E.J. Green & W.D. Dietrich. 1997. Temporal and regional patterns of axonal damage following traumatic brain injury: a beta-amyloid precursor protein immunohistochemical study in rats. J. Neuropathol. Exp. Neurol. **56:** 1132–1141.
42. Banati, R.B., J. Gehrmann, G. Wiessner, K.-A. Hossmana & G.W. Kreutzberg. 1995. Glial expression of the β-amyloid precursor protein (APP) in global ischemia. J. Cereb. Blood Flow Metab. **15:** 647–654.
43. Palacios, G., G. Mengod, A. Tortsa, I. Ferrer & J.M. Palacios. 1995. Increased β-amyloid precursor protein expression in astrocytes in the gerbil hippocampus following ischaemia: association with proliferation of astrocytes. Eur. J. Neurosci. **7:** 501–510.

Increased Sensitivity of the Baroreceptor Reflex after Bacterial Endotoxin

HEINER ROGAUSCH,[a] NGOC-THINH VO, ADRIANA DEL REY, AND HUGO O. BESEDOVSKY

Institute of Physiology, Philipps-University, Marburg, Germany

ABSTRACT: Lipopolysaccharide (LPS), an endotoxin that elicits the production of several cytokines, induces cardiovascular changes characterized by increased perfusion of immune organs and compensatory sympathetic vasoconstriction in other tissues. We therefore hypothesized that to adapt to altered blood flow distribution following LPS administration, changes in the sensitivity of reflexes that control blood pressure would occur. Our data show that the sensitivity of the baroreceptor reflex increases significantly two and three hours after the intravenous administration of a subpyrogenic dose of the endotoxin. This change in sensitivity that could occur at peripheral or central levels may underlie necessary adjustments of cardiovascular mechanisms during the course of certain immune responses.

INTRODUCTION

Besides their local immunoregulatory functions, endogenously produced cytokines are involved in neuroendocrine and autonomic nervous system feedback interactions.[1] Some mediators of these interactions, such as cytokines, hormones, and neurotransmitters, affect mechanisms that underlie the complex and tight regulation of cardiovascular functions. Evidence indicates that these functions are adjusted during immune processes in which redistribution of the blood flow between different organs occurs. Indeed, endogenously produced interleukin-1 (IL-1), a cytokine that does not exert direct effects on vascular smooth muscle,[2,3] increases blood flow in lymphoid but not in non-lymphoid organs, thus causing a redistribution of the heart minute volume in the body.[4] Particularly in the spleen, this effect is mainly based on local inhibition of sympathetic nerve-mediated vasoconstriction.[3] The increase in blood flow in lymphoid organs following administration of low doses of lipopolysaccharide (LPS) occurs despite the fact that this cytokine causes an increase in catecholamine levels in blood[5] and in sympathetic nerve activity.[6] The coordination of locally induced changes in blood flow with cardiovascular alterations due to systemic neuroendocrine mechanisms may require the re-setting of the quick reflexes that control blood pressure. In the present studies we tested the hypothesis that the sensitivity of the baroreceptor reflex mechanism (BRR), which is essential for the control of cardiovascular functions, is affected by cytokines produced following stimulation with LPS. Because cytokines such as IL-1 are produced within a short

[a]Address for correspondence: Institute of Physiology, Philipps-University, 35037 Marburg, Germany. Voice: +49-6421-2865318; fax: +49-6421-2868925.
rogausch@mailer.uni-marburg.de

time following administration of LPS, we focused on short-term regulation by the baroreceptor reflex.

MATERIAL AND METHODS

Male Wistar rats were anesthetized with sodium pentobarbital, and the femoral vein and artery were cannulated to allow injections and pressure measurements. An ultrasonic flow probe (Transonic Systems Inc., Ithaca, NY 14850, USA, model T 206 with the perivascular flowsensor 1R) was placed at the subdiaphragmatic abdominal aorta. Pressure and flow signals were analyzed for changes per millisecond of heart rate, arterial blood pressure, and peripheral vascular resistance. Phenylephrine injections were used to induce reflex bradycardia, and the slope of changes in arterial pressure versus pulse interval duration was calculated by linear regression analysis and used as a measure of BRR sensitivity.[7] This procedure is a test of the overall performance of the BRR and does not allow differentiation between changes occurring at the level of the baroreceptors or of the central nervous system; however, the procedure has the advantage that the pressure sensory regions remain undisturbed from any preparative manipulations, that the sensors are excited by pulsatile instead of steady stretch, and that the BRR operates under the influence of catecholamines as during pathophysiological conditions. When all cardiorespiratory values were stable for at least 30 minutes, reflex-mediated changes in heart rate following the increase in arterial blood pressure by phenylephrine were determined. The sensitivity of the BRR was measured over three hours following the intravenous application of 10 µg/kg bw LPS (from *Escherichia coli* 026:B6, Sigma, St Louis, MO). A control group received an equal volume of vehicle alone (physiological saline, NaCl 0.9%).

Statistical analysis was performed by Student's *t* test.

RESULTS AND DISCUSSION

Normal Baroreceptor Reflex. An intravenous bolus injection of the alpha sympathicomimetic agent phenylephrine at a dose of 30 µg/kg increased the arterial blood pressure from 105 ± 5 mm Hg to 212 ± 11 mm Hg; concomitantly also the peripheral vascular resistance rose. This step was followed by depression of the onset of heart rate, that is, prolongation of the pulse interval duration, which counterbalanced the high vascular resistance. The injection of 1 mg/kg of the cholinergic blocker atropine interrupted the BRR-mediated inhibition of the heart rate, and both arterial blood pressure and peripheral vascular resistance remained high for up to 10 minutes. This indicates that vagal efferent signals are responsible for the reduced heart rate and that the reflex-induced bradycardia can be taken as a general measure of the sensitivity of the BRR. The data also indicate that the BRR normalizes peripheral vascular resistance. In the following experiments, we investigated whether LPS affects the sensitivity of the BRR.

Influence of the Endotoxin LPS on the Sensitivity of the BRR. The slope of pulse interval duration versus mean arterial blood pressure reflects the sensitivity of the BRR. FIGURE 1 shows that this gain was stable for at least three hours under control

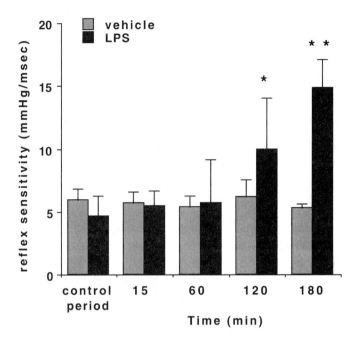

FIGURE 1. Sensitivity of the baroreceptor reflex was determined following phenyl-ephrine administration as described in *Material and Methods.* After a control period, rats received the vehicle alone or LPS ($n = 4$/group), and measures were continued for 180 minutes. Results are expressed as mean ± SD. $*p < 0.05; **p < 0.01$.

conditions in anesthetized animals that received 0.5 ml 0.9% NaCl at the end of the control period. The intravenous injection of LPS increased the sensitivity of the BRR after two hours ($p < 0.05$) and three hours ($p < 0.01$), that is, reflex bradycardia was more sensitive to changes in pressure after LPS than during the control period or when compared in animals that received the vehicle alone.

Several local mechanisms may induce an acutely higher sensitivity of the barore-ceptors, including the possible paracrine influence of prostaglandins released from endothelial cells.[8] These agents favor the excitation of baroreceptors and their response to increases in pressure. Because cytokines induced by LPS increase pros-taglandin synthesis, this possibility should be taken into consideration. We are cur-rently testing the contribution of local factors to the response of a peripheral baroreceptor, using *in situ* isolated carotid preparations. However, it is at present not possible to ascertain whether the higher reflex gain after LPS treatment is only based on an increased sensitivity of the baroreceptors, because CNS structures that control cardiovascular functions could also be involved. These studies should help to under-stand interactions between immune, cardiovascular, and autonomic nervous systems that are expected to be particularly relevant for metabolic and other homeostatic adjustments during the course of infectious diseases.

ACKNOWLEDGMENTS

This work was supported by Deutsche Forschungsgemeinschaft SFB 297.

REFERENCES

1. BESEDOVSKY, H. & A. DEL REY. 1996. Immune-neuro-endocrine interactions: facts and hypotheses. Endocr. Rev. **17:** 64–102.
2. TAKAHASHI, H., M. NISHIMURA, M. SAKAMOTO, I. IKEGATI, T. NAKANISHI & M. YOSHIMURA. 1992. Effects of interleukin-1β on blood pressure, sympathetic nerve activity, and pituitary endocrine functions in anaesthetised rats. Am. J. Hypert. **5:** 224–229.
3. ROGAUSCH, H., A. DEL REY, A. KABIERSCH & H. BESEDOVSKY. 1995. Interleukin-1 increases splenic blood flow by affecting the sympathetic vasoconstrictor tonus. Am. J. Physiol. **268:** R902–R908.
4. ROGAUSCH, H., A. DEL REY, A. KABIERSCH, W. RESCHKE, J. ÖRTEL & H.O. BESEDOVSKY. 1997. Endotoxin impedes vasoconstriction in the spleen: role of endogenous interleukin-1 and sympathetic innervation. Am. J. Physiol. **272:** R2048–R2054.
5. BERKENBOSCH, F., D.E.C. DE GOEIJ, A. DEL REY & H.O. BESEDOVSKY. 1989. Neuroendocrine, sympathetic and metabolic responses induced by interleukin-1. Neuroendocrinology **50:** 570–576.
6. NIIJIMA, A., T. HORI, S. AOU & Y. OOMURA. 1991. The effects of interleukin-1β on the activity of adrenal, splenic and renal sympathetic nerves in the rat. J. Autonom. Nerv. Syst. **36:** 183–192.
7. HAINSWORTH, R. 1991. Reflexes from the heart. Physiol. Rev. **71:** 617–658.
8. CHEN, H., M.W. CHAPLEAU, T.S. McDOWELL & F.M. ABBOUD. 1990. Prostaglandins contribute to activation of baroreceptors in rabbits. Possible paracrine influence of endothelium. Circ. Res. **67:** 1394–1404.

Not All Peripheral Immune Stimuli That Activate the HPA Axis Induce Proinflammatory Cytokine Gene Expression in the Hypothalamus

ADRIANA DEL REY,[a] ANKE RANDOLF,[a] FERNANDO PITOSSI,[b]
HEINER ROGAUSCH,[a] AND HUGO O. BESEDOVSKY[a,c]

[a]Division of Immunophysiology, Institute of Physiology,
Philipps-University, Marburg, Germany

[b]Institute for Biochemical Research, Buenos Aires, Argentina

ABSTRACT: Administration of low doses of lipopolysaccharide (LPS) that do not disrupt the blood–brain barrier (BBB) results in the expression of interleukin-1β (IL-1β), IL-6, and tumor necrosis factor-alpha (TNFα) in the hypothalamus in parallel to stimulation of the hypothalamus–pituitary–adrenal (HPA) axis. This endocrine response is triggered by peripheral cytokines, and we recently obtained evidence that brain-borne IL-1 contributes to its maintenance. LPS preferentially stimulates cells of the macrophage lineage and B lymphocytes. The possibility that primarily stimulation of other types of peripheral immune cells also results in the expression of proinflammatory cytokines in the brain and in the activation of the HPA axis was investigated. Our results showed that, in contrast to LPS, administration of the superantigen staphylococcal enterotoxin B (SEB), which stimulates T cells by binding to appropriate Vβ domains of the T-cell receptor, did not result in induction of IL-1β, IL-6, and TNFα expression in the hypothalamus. Furthermore, although IL-2 transcripts in the spleen were highly increased, expression of this gene was not detected in the brain. However, as with LPS, SEB administration also results in elevated levels of glucocorticoids in blood. Therefore, our data suggest that increased expression of proinflammatory cytokines in the brain is not a necessary step in the stimulation of the HPA axis by SEB.

INTRODUCTION

Microglial cells, astrocytes, and certain neurons can produce cytokines such as interleukin-1β (IL-1β), IL-6, and tumor necrosis factor-alpha (TNFα).[1] It was initially thought that these cytokines are only induced during inflammatory, infectious, and autoimmune processes in association with a massive entrance of immune cells into the brain. It was later shown that peripheral administration of the bacterial endotoxin lipopolysaccharide (LPS)[2,3] and immobilization stress[4] also trigger the

[c]Address for correspondence: Prof. Dr. Hugo O. Besedovsky, Institute of Physiology, Philipps-University, Deutschhausstrasse 2, 35037 Marburg, Germany. Voice: +49-6421-2862174; fax: +49-6421-2868925.

besedovs@mailer.uni-marburg.de

expression of cytokines in the CNS. This effect may be due to disruption of the blood-brain barrier (BBB) by LPS,[5] to nonspecific mechanisms such as cardiovascular and respiratory dysfunctions caused by the endotoxin, or to the procedure used to induce stress. However, we have observed that peripheral administration of a low dose of LPS that does not disrupt the BBB[5] and does not cause overt alterations in animals also results in cytokine induction in the CNS, suggesting that stimulation of certain types of peripheral immune cells triggered this effect.[6]

LPS preferentially affects cells of the macrophage lineage and B lymphocytes and induces the production of cytokines that can stimulate the hypothalamus–pituitary–adrenal (HPA) axis. We have now performed similar studies to analyze the possibility that stimulation of other types of peripheral immune cells also results in the expression of proinflammatory cytokines in the CNS in parallel to the activation of the HPA axis. For this purpose, we compared the effect of staphylococcal enterotoxin B (SEB), a superantigen that stimulates a large proportion of T lymphocytes expressing appropriate Vb domains,[7] with that of a low dose of LPS.

MATERIAL AND METHODS

Animals

BALB/c and C57Bl/6J male mice (nine weeks old) were obtained from Harlan-Winkelmann, Germany. Animals were housed individually for 1 week before experiments were started and kept single-caged throughout. Animals were housed in temperature- and light (12-hour cycles)-controlled rooms and were fed *ad libitum*.

Reagents

SEB from *Staphylococcus aureus* was obtained from Sigma-Aldrich Chemie GmbH, Steinheim, Germany, and LPS from *Escherichia coli* 0111:B4 from Difco Laboratories, Detroit, MI, USA.

Experimental Procedure

SEB (10 mg/mouse) was injected i.p. into BALB/c mice. LPS (0.5 μg/mouse) was injected into C57Bl/6J mice. Physiological saline solution (0.9% NaCl) was simultaneously used in both cases to inject control animals. Groups of mice were killed by cervical dislocation two and four hours later, and blood was collected in EDTA-coated tubes. The spleen and hypothalamus were dissected, immediately frozen in liquid nitrogen, and used for determination of mRNA cytokine expression by right RT-PCR. To block IL-1 receptors in the brain, 50 mg of the IL-1 receptor antagonist (IL-1ra) were injected i.c.v. 30 minutes before LPS administration.

Corticosterone Determinations

Corticosterone plasma levels were determined by radioimmunoassay as previously described.[8]

Cytokine Determinations

IL-1β, IL-2, IL-6, TNFα, IL-4, and interferon-gamma (IFNγ) gene expression was determined by semiquantitative RT-PCR as previously described.[6] The values from SEB probes were obtained from nonradioactive RT-PCR. Data acquisition and integration were performed with a BP-MI Charged Couple Device camera using ONE-Dscan (Scananalytics, Billerica, MA, USA) on 1.5% ethydium bromide-stained agarose gels.

Statistical Analysis

Results are expressed as mean ± SE. Data were analyzed using one-way analysis of variance (ANOVA) followed by Fisher's exact test for multiple comparisons. Differences were considered significant at *p* < 0.05.

RESULTS AND DISCUSSION

Both LPS and SEB have been used as models of septic shock induced by gram-negative and gram-positive bacteria, respectively. However, for our studies, it was necessary to use doses of these bacterial products that do not cause overt disease, as indicated by the fact that the animals do not lose weight for several days after inoculation. Doses of 10 μg/mouse of SEB and 0.5 μg/mouse of LPS into normal mice fulfill this condition. It was previously reported that the HPA axis is stimulated by administration of a relatively large dose of SEB.[9] Thus, we then established that i.p. administration of SEB at a dose of 10 mg/mouse caused an increase in corticosterone blood levels comparable to those of 0.5 μg of LPS (see FIGURE 1).

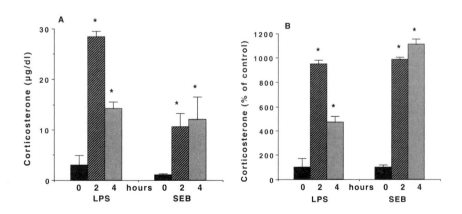

FIGURE 1. LPS and SEB administration results in increased corticosterone blood levels. LPS (0.5 μg) or SEB (10 μg) was injected i.p. into C57Bl/6J and BALB/c mice, respectively. Physiological saline (0.9% NaCl) was used as control in both cases. Groups of animals were killed after 2 and 4 hours. (**A**) Results of corticosterone determinations in plasma. Values obtained for simultaneous controls were pooled and are shown as time 0. For comparison, results are shown in **B** as % of the corresponding controls. Results are expressed as mean ± SE. **p* < 0.05.

The effect of administration of the aforementioned doses of LPS and SEB on gene expression of different cytokines in the spleen was evaluated. Two hours after LPS administration, IL-1β, IL-6, and TNFα were highly expressed in the spleen. The ratio cDNA/c.f. was: for IL-1β: 0.8 ± 0.2 in controls and 28 ± 3 in LPS-treated mice; for IL-6: 0.1 in controls and 62 ± 12 in LPS-treated mice; for TNFα: 0.5 ± 0.1 in controls and 22 ± 1 in LPS-treated mice. Among the cytokines studied, IL-2, IL-4, and IFNγ showed the highest inducibility in the spleen two hours after SEB administration. The ratio cDNA/c.f. was: for IL-2: 1 ± 0.1 in controls and 23 ± 6 in SEB-treated mice; for IL-4: 0.5 ± 0.2 in controls and 10 ± 3 in SEB-treated mice; for IFNγ: 0.80 ± 0.12 in controls and 9 ± 3 in SEB-treated mice. When compared to the effect of LPS, IL-1β gene expression was only modestly increased two hours following SEB administration (controls: 0.4 ± 0.1; SEB-treated mice: 2.5 ± 0.1).

In the hypothalamus, LPS administration caused a clear increase in IL-1 and IL-6 and, at a lower level, also in TNFα mRNA (see FIGURE 2). By contrast, no changes in expression of the genes for these cytokines were detected two and four hours after SEB administration. Because SEB induced a quick expression of IL-2 in the spleen, we explored the possibility that this superantigen causes a similar effect in the brain. However, in neither control nor SEB-treated mice were mRNA transcripts for this cytokine detected in the hypothalamus.

The semiquantitative RT-PCR used in our experiments is a very sensitive technique with a limit of sensitivity of roughly 10 transcripts/100 cells.[6] Using this technique, we expected to find the IL-2 gene expressed in the brain of SEB-treated animals because IL-2 is produced during the process of activation of T cells and evidence exists that activated T cells can penetrate the brain parenchyma. Indeed, injection of in vitro stimulated T lymphocytes to normal animals results in the detection of these cells in the CNS a few hours later.[10,11] Based on these data and on evidence that superantigens stimulate a large proportion of T lymphocytes,[7] some of the cells stimulated in vivo by SEB should have crossed the BBB. If they would continue to produce IL-2, the expression of this cytokine should have been detected with the semiquantitative RT-PCR technique used. This apparent contradiction could be explained if it is considered that IL-2 production following SEB stimulation is transient and therefore that expression of this cytokine may not be an appropriate marker for the penetration of SEB-activated T cells in the CNS.

Another series of experiments was designed to study the contribution of IL-1 expressed in the brain for the stimulation of the HPA axis. Mice received LPS injected i.p. and IL-1 receptor antagonist (IL-1ra) or the vehicle alone, injected i.c.v. Two hours after injection, corticosterone blood levels were comparably increased in both groups of LPS-treated mice (time 0: 2.3 ± 0.8 μg/dl; 2 hours: 12.2 ± 0.8 in vehicle-injected and 11.8 ± 1.0 mg/dl in IL-1ra–injected mice). However, four hours after LPS administration, the levels of corticosterone of animals treated with the cytokine receptor antagonist were significantly lower than those of mice that received the vehicle alone (LPS + vehicle: 13.8 ± 1.0; LPS + IL-1ra: 8.2 ± 0.9; $p < 0.01$). These results suggest that IL-1 endogenously produced in the CNS contributes to maintain the stimulation of the HPA axis following LPS administration; although stimulation of this axis still occurred when IL-1ra was administered i.c.v., it was significantly reduced at a later stage. Since this effect coincides temporally with IL-1 gene expression in the hypothalamus, the data obtained indicate a role of brain-borne IL-1 in the

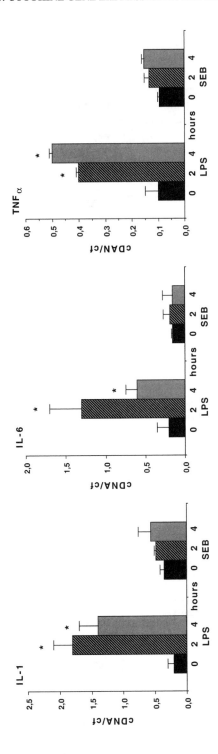

FIGURE 2. LPS, but not SEB, induces increased IL-1β, IL-6, and TNF-α gene expression in the hypothalamus. The hypothalamus of the animals from which the results shown in FIGURE 1 were derived were used to determine cytokine gene expression by semiquantitative RT-PCR. Results are expressed as mean ± SE of the ratio cDNA and the corresponding competitive fragment (cf) for each cytokine. * $p < 0.05$.

maintenance of stimulation of the HPA axis. As shown in FIGURE 1, SEB triggered the stimulation of the HPA axis but, in contrast to the spleen, no induction of IL-1 and of other proinflammatory cytokines was detected in the CNS. This indicates that a mechanism different from the one that maintains the response of the HPA axis to LPS contributes to the sustained increase in corticosterone blood levels induced by SEB. This mechanism seems not to involve centrally produced IL-2, because mRNA transcripts for this cytokine were not detectable in the hypothalamus.

ACKNOWLEDGMENTS

This work was supported by the Volkswagen Stiftung and the Deutsche Forschungsgemeinschaft (SFB 297).

REFERENCES

1. ROTHWELL, N.J. & S.J. HOPKINS. 1995. Cytokines and the nervous system II: actions and mechanisms of action. Trends Neurosci. **18:** 130–136.
2. GATTI, S. & T. BARTFAI. 1993. Induction of tumor necrosis factor-alpha mRNA in the brain after peripheral endotoxin treatment: comparison with interleukin-1 family and interleukin-6. Brain Res. **624:** 291–294.
3. LAYE, S., P. PARNET, E. GOUJON & R. DANTZER. 1994. Peripheral administration of lipopolysaccharide induces the expression of cytokine transcripts in the brain and pituitary of mice. Mol. Brain Res. **27:** 157–162.
4. MINAMI, M., Y. KURAISHI, T. YAMAGUCHI, S. NAKAI, Y. HIRAI & M. SATOH. 1991. Immobilization stress induces interleukin-1 beta mRNA in the rat hypothalamus. Neurosci. Lett. **123:** 254–256.
5. LUSTIG, S., H.D. DANENBERG, Y. KAFRI, D. KOBILER, & D. BEN-NATHAN. 1992. Viral neuroinvasion and encephalitis induced by lipopolysaccharide and its mediators. J. Exp. Med. **176:** 707–712.
6. PITOSSI, F., A. DEL REY, A. KABIERSCH & H.O. BESEDOVSKY. 1997. Induction of cytokine transcripts in the CNS and pituitary following peripheral administration of endotoxin to mice. J. Neurosci. Res. **46:** 287–298.
7. HERMAN, A., J.W. KAPPLER, P. MARRACK & A.M. PULLEN. 1991. Superantigens: mechanism of T-cell stimulation and role in immune responses. Ann. Rev. Immunol. **9:** 745–772.
8. BESEDOVSKY, H.O., A. DEL REY, I. KLUSMAN, H. FURUKAWA, G. MONGE ARDITI & A. KABIERSCH. 1991. Cytokines as modulators of the hypothalamus-pituitary-adrenal axis. J. Steroid Biochem. Molec. Biol. **40:** 613–618.
9. GONZALO, A., A. GONZALEZ-GARCIA, C. MARTINEZ & G. KROEMER. 1993. Glucocorticoid-mediated control of the activation and clonal deletion of peripheral T cells in vivo. J. Exp. Med. **177:** 1239–1246.
10. HICKEY, W.F. 1991. T-lymphocyte entry and antigen recognition in the central nervous system. *In* Psychoneuroimmunology. R. Ader, D.L. Felten & N. Cohen, Eds.: 149–175. Academic Press. New York.
11. WEKERLE, H., D. SUN, R.L. OROPEZA-WEKERLE & R. MEYERMANN. 1987. Immune reactivity in the central nervous system: modulation of T lymphocyte activation by glial cells. J. Exp. Biol. **132:** 43–57.

Mechanisms of Behavioral and Neuroendocrine Effects of Interleukin-1 in Mice

PIERRE J. NEVEU[a] AND STÉPHANE LIÈGE

Neurobiologie Intégrative, INSERM Unit 394, Institut François Magendie, rue Camille Saint-Saëns, 33077 Bordeaux, France

ABSTRACT: Interleukin-1β is a key molecule in brain-immune interactions that, apart from its immune effects, stimulates the hypothalamo–pituitary–adrenal (HPA) axis and induces behavioral alterations. However, its physiological role during stress responses remain to be elucidated. The possible mechanisms involved in IL-1–mediated stimulation of the HPA axis during stress were assessed by using different approaches. They were first studied in mice deficient for the IL-1β-converting enzyme (ICE) gene. Mature IL-1β derives from a precursor, the pro-IL-1β, devoid of any conventional signal sequence that is mainly processed by ICE. After immune or stress stimulation, ICE-deficient mice were shown to have a hyperactive HPA axis and to able to produce immunoreactive IL-1β. This indicates that the greater reactivity of the HPA axis could result from a higher sensitivity to non-ICE-matured IL-1β, as suggested by a higher basal transcription of hypothalamic IL-1 receptor type I (IL-1 RI) in ICE-deficient mice. The biological effects of IL-1β are mediated by IL-1 RI associated with the IL-1 receptor accessory protein (IL-1RAcP). IL-IRAcP is an essential component for IL-1 action at the periphery, but its role in the brain is not well known. Therefore, the effects of i.c.v. IL-1β were studied in IL-1RAcP -deficient mice. In normal mice, i.c.v. IL-1β depresses peripheral immune responses, induces the production of plasma IL-6, and stimulates the HPA axis. None of these effects were observed in IL-1RAcP-deficient mice, indicating that IL-1RAcP is necessary for the induction of the main neuroendocrine and immune effects of central IL-1β. In normal mice, the role of IL-1β was assessed by pretreating the animal with the IL-1 receptor antagonist (IL-1Ra). IL-1Ra did modify the activation of the HPA axis observed during stress, except when the animals were previously sympathectomized. This suggests that the sympathetic nervous system can downregulate the IL-1β-induced stimulation of the HPA axis. Finally, the modulation of the production and physiological activities of IL-1 were studied in normal mice, taking advantage of interindividual differences in brain–immune interactions linked to cerebral lateralization. Behavioral/brain lateralization was shown to be related to behavioral response to peripheral administration of IL-1, and to the production of IL-1 and IL-6 in response to LPS. This suggests that cytokines, and especially IL-1β, may represent one of the factors responsible for interindividual differences in brain–immune interactions.

[a]Address for correspondence. Voice: 33 5 57 57 37 10; fax: 33 5 56 98 90 26.
pierre.neveu@bordeaux.inserm.fr

INTRODUCTION

Cytokines are soluble mediators first identified in the immune system that play an important role in many physiological and pathological processes. They are key molecules, because they mediate the activity of immune cells on neuroendocrine systems,[1,2] brain neurochemistry, and behavior.[3,4] The involvement of these molecules might be more general, as they have been suggested to play a role in the stress response[5] and stress-related disorders including depression.[6–8] Brain cytokines produced during stress, and especially interleukin-1 (IL-1), may be involved in behavioral alterations, activation of the HPA axis, and immunosuppression.[9]

This paper summarizes the results of our research on the mechanisms by which cytokines modulate behavior and HPA axis activity. We first present possible steps intrinsic to the IL-1 system critical in the regulation of endocrine and immune activities of IL-1. We mainly studied the production of mature IL-1β through the activity of IL-1β converting enzyme (ICE) and the functional activity of IL-1 receptor, especially the role of the IL-1 receptor accessory protein (IL-1RAcP). These two mechanisms were studied using ICE- and IL-1RAcP–deficient mice, respectively. In a second section, we discuss extrinsic mechanisms that modulate the endocrine and immune activities of IL-1, taking advantage of interindividual differences in brain–immune interactions linked to lateralization.

MECHANISMS INTRINSIC TO THE IL-1 SYSTEM

Importance of ICE in the Production of IL-1β

Mature IL-1β is processed from a 31-kDa precursor devoid of any conventional signal sequence, the proIL-1β. This precursor is mainly processed by ICE to an active 17-kDa form, the mature IL-1β.[10] Deletion of the gene coding for ICE by homologous recombination was expected to result in the inability to produce mature IL-1β in response to an immune challenge. The first studies with ICE knockout (KO) mice confirmed that lipopolysaccharide (LPS) is unable to induce the production of IL-1β in these mice *in vitro* as well as *in vivo*.[11–13] Based on these findings, it can be predicted that ICE-deficient mice should display attenuated activation of the HPA axis in response to LPS injection and possibly during stress if endogenous IL-1β plays a role in stress-induced activation of the HPA axis. To test this prediction, we measured plasma levels of corticosterone and ACTH in ICE-deficient mice injected with LPS or rat recombinant IL-1β or subjected to restraint stress.[14] Contrary to what was expected, ICE-deficient mice had a hyperreactive HPA axis as demonstrated by an increased production of ACTH especially after IL-1β administration (see FIGURE 1). No difference was observed in plasma levels of corticosterone that reached maximum levels in both wild-type and ICE-KO mice. The hyperreactivity of the HPA axis was not due to an increased production of IL-6, because plasma levels of this cytokine in response to IL-1β administration were similar in ICE-KO and wild-type mice. Furthermore, ICE-KO mice did not differ from their wild-type littermates in terms of plasma levels of immunoreactive IL-1β. These results indicate that pro-IL-1β is processed by non-ICE proteases in ICE-KO mice, as previously suggested.[15] Moreover, the increase in ACTH after restraint was greater in ICE-KO

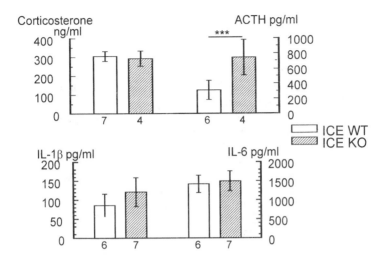

FIGURE 1. Plasma levels of corticosterone, ACTH, IL-1β, and IL-6 in ICE-KO mice injected with rat recombinant IL-1β.

than in wild-type mice, although this stress did not result in any variation in plasma IL-1β and IL-6 (data not shown).

The mechanisms accounting for the HPA axis hyperreactivity of ICE-KO mice to immune and nonimmune stress remain to be elucidated, but the present results do not support a critical role for IL-1β in restraint-induced stimulation of the HPA axis.

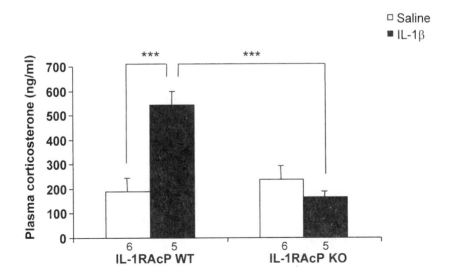

FIGURE 2. Plasma corticosterone in IL-1RAcP KO and WT mice after i.c.v. IL-1β.

Role of IL-1RAcP in the Central Effects of IL-1

IL-1RAcP is a critical component of the IL-1 receptor system. IL-1RAcP alone does not bind IL-1, but it increases IL-1 binding affinity for the type I IL-1 receptor (IL-1RI).[16,17] IL-1RAcP is necessary for the IL-1 signaling pathway.[16,18,19] In IL-1RAcP–deficient mice, peripheral injection of IL-1 fails to induce IL-6 production[16] and a febrile response.[19] Even though IL-1RAcP is highly expressed in the brain, its functional role in the central effects of IL-1 had not been investigated. Mice deficient for the IL-1RAcP gene were used to assess the role of IL-1RAcP in brain activity of IL-1β.[20] In normal mice, i.c.v. IL-1β activates the HPA axis,[21,22] induces the production of peripheral IL-6,[23] and decreases peripheral immune responses.[24] I.c.v. administration of various doses of human recombinant IL-1β did not increase plasma corticosterone levels in IL-1RAcP KO mice (see FIGURE 2). IL-1 administration had no effect on plasma and brain cortex levels of IL-6 (see FIGURE 3). Likewise, the immunosuppressive effects of central IL-1β on mitogen-induced splenocyte proliferation were abrogated in IL-1RAcP KO mice (see FIGURE 4). These results clearly show that IL-1RAcP is necessary for the induction of the main neuroendocrine and immune effects of central IL-1β.

MECHANISMS EXTRINSIC TO THE IL-1 SYSTEM

Interaction of IL-1 and Peripheral Catecholamines in Stress-Induced Stimulation of the HPA Axis

The possible role of catecholamines in the regulation of IL-1–induced corticosterone production was assessed by pretreating animals with IL-1ra in the absence of peripheral catecholamines. The increase in plasma corticosterone and ACTH induced by restraint was not modified by a peripheral injection of IL-1ra. The stress-induced increase in plasma levels of corticosterone was enhanced in mice chemically sympathectomized using 6-hydroxydopamine (6-OHDA), suggesting that catecholamines could depress corticosterone production. Interestingly, the increase in plasma corticosterone induced by 6-OHDA in stressed animals was reversed by IL-1ra. This suggests that catecholamines could inhibit the IL-1β–induced corticosterone production. An alternative explanation is that 6-OHDA induces an inflammatory reaction mediated by IL-1 and responsible for activation of the HPA axis. Further investigation is clearly needed to fully understand the interactions between peripheral catecholamines and cytokines in the stimulation of the HPA axis.

Interindividual Differences, Linked to Lateralization, in the Endocrine and Behavioral Effects of Cytokines

Behavioral lateralization, as assessed by paw preference in a food-reaching task in mice, is associated with brain metabolism asymmetries and immune reactivity.[25] Therefore, each individual may be characterized by a lateralization score in association with a particular pattern of immune reactivity. Because cytokines play a pivotal role in brain-immune interactions, we hypothesized that the production and effects of cytokines depend on behavioral-brain lateralization.

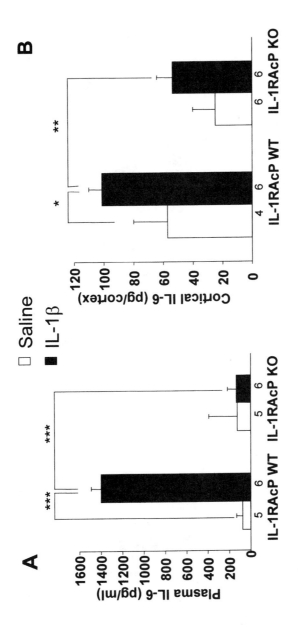

FIGURE 3. Plasma (A) and cortical (B) IL-6 in IL-1RAcP KO and WT mice after i.c.v. IL-1β.

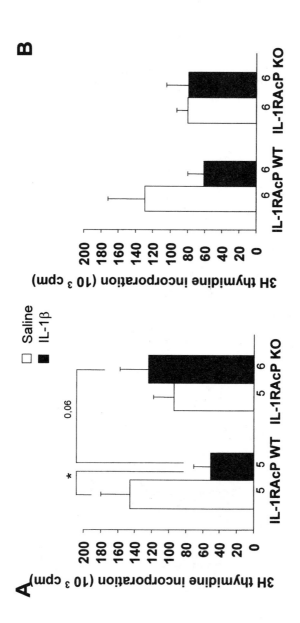

FIGURE 4. Splenocyte mitogenic response to 1 μg/ml ConA in IL-1RAcP KO and WT mice after 750 pg (**A**) or 50 ng (**B**) i.c.v. IL-1β.

Cytokines and especially IL-1 are known to induce sickness behavior character-ized by depressed social interaction, increased immobility, loss of body weight, and reduced food intake.[26] When studying IL-1–induced sickness behavior in mice pre-viously selected for their paw preference, we were able to demonstrate that the behavioral effects of IL-1 depend on lateralization.[27] Depression of social interac-tion was more pronounced in right-pawed than in left-pawed animals. Likewise, immobility was more important in right-pawed mice. There was a similar trend for food intake to be lower and loss of body weight to be higher in right-pawed mice than in left-pawed animals. These experiments confirm previous data[25] and show that interindividual differences may be responsible for the variability among mem-bers of a population in the responses to various insults including psychological stres-sors and infections. They further demonstrate that cytokines are at least partly responsible for interindividual differences in brain-immune interactions. More recently, we observed interindividual variations in exploratory models of anxiety involving interactions between gender and lateralization.[28] This observation may be the first step in studying the link between cytokines, anxiety, and interindividual differences.

The existence of interindividual differences in the activity of the HPA axis, first demonstrated after an immune stress, was also found after a psychological stress. As previously reported, the increase in plasma corticosterone induced by a 1-hour restraint differed in left- and right-pawed animals,[29] but as just discussed, these dif-ferences are unlikely to result in IL-1 functioning differences.

Before studying the mechanisms by which lateralization modulates cytokine–induced activation of the HPA axis, we studied the influence of lateralization on the activity of the HPA axis in normal untreated animals. By means of perifusion exper-iments, we measured the production of ACTH by the pituitary and that of corticos-terone by the adrenals from animals selected for their paw preference.[30] No differences in ACTH and corticosterone production were found in relation to lateralization. Recently, we looked for interindividual differences in HPA axis functioning by measuring the distribution of mineralocorticoid (MR) and glucocor-ticoid (GR) receptors in the hippocampus of animals selected for their lateraliza-tion.[31] The ratio of right/total MR binding was inversely correlated with individual paw preference scores. The affinity of MRs did not depend on lateralization. GR binding capacity was similar in each hemisphere, and no relationship was found between GR binding capacity and paw preference scores. Because IL-1 was shown to decrease the affinity of MRs in the hippocampus,[32] it may be hypothesized that interindividual sensitivity of the HPA axis to cytokines in relation to lateralization results at least partly from differences in hippocampal MR distribution associated to lateralization.

Production of IL-1 and IL-6 and Their Endocrine Effects during Immune and Psychological Stress

In line with our previous observations on the importance of cerebral lateraliza-tion, as assessed by paw preference, in neurochemical, neuroendocrine, and immune effects of LPS in mice,[33] we investigated the role of cerebral lateralization on cytok-ine production in response to LPS. In a first series of experiments, plasma levels of IL-1β and IL-6 were determined in LPS-treated mice previously selected for their paw preference and belonging to two different strains, C3H and BALB/c.[34] Plasma levels of IL-1β and IL-6 increased in response to LPS in both strains, and this increase was dependent on paw preference in BALB/c but not in C3H mice. Increased levels of IL-1β were observed in left-pawed but not in ambidextrous and right-pawed mice. For IL-6, the LPS-induced increase was higher in ambidextrous than in left- and right-pawed animals (see FIGURE 5). These results are in accordance with previous data showing that the link between lateralization and immune reactivity may be evidenced in some but not all strains tested.[35] However, the absence of a link between lateralization and cytokine production in the C3H strain was rather surprising. We had previously shown that LPS activated the HPA axis, as shown by increased plasma levels of ACTH, in right-pawed but not in left-pawed C3H mice.[33] Activation of the HPA axis by LPS is mediated by several cytokines, including IL-1[36] and IL-6.[37] However, the production of both IL-1 and IL-6 was equally increased in right- and left-pawed C3H mice. In contrast to C3H mice, BALB/c mice displayed a link between lateralization and the production of IL-1β and IL-6 in response to LPS. Basal levels of plasma IL-1 were higher in ambidextrous than in strongly lateralized animals. However, in response to LPS, plasma levels of IL-1 increased with time only in right-pawed mice but not in left-pawed and ambidextrous animals. Concerning plasma levels of IL-6, basal levels were similar in the three experimental groups. In response to LPS, IL-6 peaked at two hours, and the increase was higher in ambidextrous than in left- and right-pawed animals. Surprisingly, plasma levels of IL-6 decreased thereafter, whereas levels of IL-1 did not.

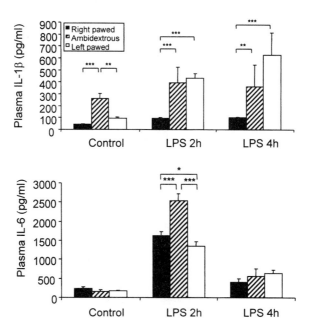

FIGURE 5. Plasma levels of IL-1β and IL-6 in response to LPS in BALB/c mice selected for their paw preference.

Similarly, a link between lateralization and cytokine production has been reported in male BALB/c mice infected by *Listeria monocytogenes*.[38]

The possible production of cytokines during psychological stress was assessed using restraint as a stressor.[39] Restraint for 1–2 hours did not increase plasma levels of IL-1 in C3H mice, adrenalectomized or not, in IL-1RAcP KO mice or in ICE-KO mice. These results suggest that in these strains of mice, stimulation of the HPA axis appears to be independent of IL-1.

CONCLUSION

Present results, using KO mice, show that (1) pro-IL-1β may be processed in mature not only by ICE but also by non-ICE proteases, and (2) IL-1RAcP is necessary for the induction of the main neuroendocrine and immune effects of central IL-1β. Using different experimental approaches, we were unable to demonstrate that IL-1 plays a critical role in the stimulation of the HPA axis by a psychological/physical stress such as restraint. Finally, modulation of the production and physiological activities of IL-1 were studied, taking advantage of interindividual differences in brain-immune interactions linked to cerebral lateralization. Behavioral/brain lateralization is related to behavioral response to peripheral administration of IL-1 and to the production of IL-1 and IL-6 in response to LPS. These results show that the bilateral pathway between the brain and IL-1 is subjected to lateralization even though the mechanisms involved remain unknown.

REFERENCES

1. TURNBULL, A.V. & C. RIVIER. 1995. Regulation of the HPA axis by cytokines. Brain Behav. Immun. **9:** 253–275.
2. SPANGELO, B.L., A.M. JUDD, G.B. CALL, J. ZUMWALT & W.C. GOROSPE. 1995. Role of the cytokines in the hypothalamic-pituitary-adrenal and gonadal axes. Neuroimmunomodulation **2:** 299–312.
3. BESEDOVSKY, H.O. & A. DEL REY. 1996. Immune-neuro-endocrine interactions: facts and hypotheses. Endocrine Rev. **17:** 64–102.
4. KENT, S., R.M. BLUTHÉ, K.W. KELLEY & R. DANTZER. 1992. Sickness behavior as a new target for drug development. Trends Pharm. Sci. **13:** 24–28.
5. SHINTANI, F., T. NAKAKI, S. KANBE, K. SATO, G. YAGI, M. SHIOZAWA, S. AISO, R. KATO & M. ASAI. 1995. Involvement of interleukin-1 in immobilization stress-induced increase in plasma adrenocorticotropic hormone and in the release of hypothalamic monoamines in the rat. J. Neurosci. **15:** 1961–1970.
6. SMITH, R.S. 1991. The macrophage theory of depression. Med. Hypotheses **35:** 298–306.
7. MAES, M. 1995. Evidence for an immune response in major depression: a review and hypothesis. **19:** 11–38.
8. CAPURON, L., A. LIN, A. RAVAUD, N. GUALDE, E. BOSMANS, R. DANTZER, M. MAES & P.J. NEVEU. 2000. Association between immune activation and early depressive symptoms in cancer patients treated with IL-2 and/or IFN-α. Submitted.
9. WEISS, J.M., S.K. SUNDAR, K.J. BECKER & M.A. CIERPAL. 1989. Behavioral and neural influences on cellular immune responses: effects of stress and interleukin-1. J. Clin. Psychiatry **50:** 43–53.
10. DINARELLO, C.A. 1996. Biological basis for interleukin-1 in disease. Blood **87:** 2095–2147.

11. LI, P., H. ALLEN, BANERJEE, S. FRANKLIN, L. HERZOG, C. JOHNSTON, J. MCDOWELL, M. PASKIND, L. RODMAN & J. SALFELD. 1995. Mice deficient in IL-1 beta-converting enzyme are defective in production of mature IL-1 beta and resistant to endotoxic shock. Cell **80:** 401–411.

12. KUIDA, K., J.A. LIPPKE, G. KU, M.W. HARDING, D.J. LIVINGSTON, M.S. SU & R.A. FLAVELL. 1995. Altered cytokine export and apoptosis in mice deficient in interleukin-1 beta converting enzyme. Science **267:** 2000–2003.

13. KUIDA, J.A. LIPPKE, M.S. SU & R.A. FLAVELL. 1998. Mice deficient in interleukin-1beta converting enzyme. *In* Contemporary Immunology: Cytokine Knockouts. S.K.M. Durum, Ed.: 173–188. Humana Press Inc. Totowa, NJ.

14. LIÈGE, S., E. MOZE, P. PARNET, K.W. KELLEY & P.J. NEVEU. 2000. Activation of the hypothalamic-pituitary-adrenal axis in IL-1β- converting enzyme-deficient mice. Neuroimmunomodulation. **7:** 189–194.

15. FANTUZZI, G., G. KU, M.W. HARDING, D.J. LIVINGSTON, J.D. SIPE, K. KUIDA, R.A. FLAVEL & C.A. DINARELLO. 1997. Response to local inflammation of IL-1 beta-converting enzyme-deficient mice. J. Immunol. **158:** 1818–1824.

16. CULLINAN, E.B., L. KWEE, P. NUNES, D.J. SCHUSTER, G. JU, K.W. MCINTYRE, R.A. CHIZZONITE & M.A. LABOW. 1998. IL-1 receptor accessory protein is an essential component of the IL-1 receptor. J. Immunol. **161:** 5614–5620.

17. GREEFEDER, S.A., P. NUNES, L. KWEE, M. LABOW, R.A. CHIZZONITE & G. JU. 1995. Molecular cloning and characterization of a second subunit of the interleukin 1 receptor complex. J. Biol. Chem. **270:** 13757–13765.

18. HOFMEISTER, R., K. WIEGMANN, C. KORHERR, K. BERNARDO, M. KRONKE & W. FALK. 1997. Activation of acid shingomyelinase by interleukin-1 (IL-1) requires the IL-1 receptor accessory protein. J. Biol. Chem. **272:** 27730–27736.

19. ZETTERSTROM, M., J. LUNDKVIST, D. MALINOWSKY, G. ERIKSSON & T. BARTFAI. 1998. Interleukin-1-mediated febrile responses in mice and interleukin-1 beta activation of NfKB in mouse primary astrocytes, involves the interleukin-1 receptor accessory protein. Eur. Cytokine Netw. **9:** 131–138.

20. LIÈGE, S., S. LAYÉ, E. MOZE & P.J. NEVEU. 2000. Interleukin-1 receptor accessory protein (IL-1RAcP) is an essential receptor for IL-1β action in the brain. J. Neuroimmunol. In press.

21. BESEDOVSKY, H., A. DELREY, E. SORKIN, & C.A. DINARELLO. 1986. Immunoregulatory feedback between interleukin-1 and glucocorticoid hormmones. Science **233:** 652–654.

22. SAPOLSKY, R., C. RIVIER, G. YAMAMOTO, P. PLOSKY & W. VALE. 1987. Interleukin-1 stimulates the secretion of hypothalamic corticotropin-releasing factor. Science **238:** 522–524.

23. DE SIMONI, M.G., M. SIRONI, A. DELUIGI, A. MANFRIDI, A. MONTOVANI & P. GHEZZI. 1990. Intracerebroventricular injection of interleukin 1 induces high circulating levels of interleukin 6. J. Exp. Med. **171:** 1773–1778.

24. SUNDAR, S.K., K.J. BECKER, M.A. CIERPIAL, M.D. CARPENTER, L.A. RANKIN, S.L. FLEENER, J.C. RITCHIE, P.E. SIMSON & J.M. WEISS. 1989. Intracerebroventricular infusion of interleukin 1 rapidly decreases peripheral cellular immune responses. Proc. Natl. Acad. Sci. USA **86:** 6398–6402.

25. NEVEU, P.J. 1996. Lateralization and stress responses in mice: interindividual differences in the association of brain, neuroendocrine, and immune responses. Behav. Genet. **26:** 373–377.

26. DANTZER, R., R.M. BLUTHÉ, A. AUBERT, G. GOODALL, J.L. BRET-DIBAT, S. KENT, E. GOUJON, S. LAYÉ, P. PARNET & K.W. KELLEY. 1996. Cytokine actions on behavior. *In* Cytokines and the Nervous System. N.J. Rothwell, Ed.: 117–144. Landes. London.

27. NEVEU, P.J., R.M. BLUTHÉ, S. LIÈGE, S. MOYA, B. MICHAUD & DANTZER. 1998. Interleukin-1-induced sickness behavior depends on behavioral lateralization in mice. Physiol. Behav. **63:** 587–590.

28. MRABET, O., Z. ES-SALAH, A. TELHIQ, A. AUBERT, S. LIÈGE, K. CHOULLI & P.J. NEVEU. 2000. Influence of gender and behavioral lateralization on two exploratory models of anxiety in C3H mice. Behav. Proc. In press.

29. NEVEU, P.J. & S. MOYA. 1997. In the mouse, the corticoid stress response depends on lateralization. Brain Res. **749:** 344–346.

30. BETANCUR, C., C. SANDI, S. VITIELLO, J. BORRELL, C. GUAZA & P.J. NEVEU. 1992. Activity of the hypothalamic-pituitary-adrenal axis in mice selected for left- or right-handedness. Brain Res. **589:** 302–306.

31. NEVEU, P.J., S. LIÈGE & A. SARRIEAU. 1998. Asymmetrical distribution of hippocampal mineralocorticoid receptors depends on lateralization in mice. Neuroimmunomodulation **5:** 16–21.

32. SCHHOBITZ, B., W. SUTANTO, M.P. CAREY, F. HOLSBOER & E.R. DEKLOET. 1994. Endotoxin and interleukin-1 decrease the affinity of hippocampal mineralocorticoid (type I) receptor in parallel to activation of the hypothalamic-pituitary-adrenal axis. Neuroendocrinology **60:** 124–133.

33. DELRUE, C., B. DELEPLANQUE, F. ROUGE-PONT, S. VITIELLO & P.J. NEVEU. 1994. Brain monoaminergic, neuroendocrine and immune responses to an immune challenge in relation to brain and behavioral lateralization. Brain Behav. Immun. **8:** 137–152.

34. GAO, M.X., K.S. LI, J. DONG, S. LIÈGE, B. JIANG & P.J. NEVEU. 2000. Strain-dependent association between lateralization and LPS-induced IL-1β and IL-6 production in mice. Neuroimmunomodulation **8:** 78–82.

35. FRIDE, E., R.L. COLLINS, P. SKOLNICK & P.K. ARORA. 1990. Strain-dependent association between immune function and paw preference in mice. Brain Res. **522:** 246–250.

36. RIVIER, C., R. CHIZZONITE & VALE. 1989. In the mouse, the activation of the hypothalamic-pituitary-adrenal axis by a lipopolysaccharide (endotoxin) is mediated through interleukin-1. Endocrinology **125:** 2800–2805.

37. PERLSTEIN, R.S., M.H. WHITNALL, J.Q.S. ABRAMS, E.H. MOUGEY & R. NETA. 1993. Synergic roles of interleukin-6, interleukin-1 and tumor necrosis factor in the adrenocorticotropin response to bacterial lipopolysaccharide in vivo. Endocrinology **132:** 946–952.

38. KIM, D., J.N. CARLSON, R.F. SEGAL & D.A. LAWRENCE. 1999. Differential immune responses in mice with left- and right-turning preference. J. Neuroimmunol. **93:** 164–171.

39. LI, K.S., S. LIÈGE, E. MOZE & P.J. NEVEU. 2000. Plasma corticosterone and immune reactivity in restrained female C3H mice. Stress. In press.

Genetic Regulation of Nerve Avulsion-Induced Spinal Cord Inflammation

TOMAS OLSSON,[a] CECILIA LUNDBERG, OLLE LIDMAN, AND FREDRIK PIEHL

Neuroimmunology Unit, Department of Medicine, Karolinska Institute, CMM L08;04, Karolinska Hospital, S-171 76 Stockholm, Sweden

ABSTRACT: In the animal model for multiple sclerosis (MS), experimental autoimmune encephalitis (EAE), genetic loci correlating with incidence or severity of disease are located both within and outside of the major histocompatibility complex (MHC). Whereas polymorphisms within MHC class I and II molecules are likely to be a major determinant of MHC gene influence in rat EAE, it is still unclear how non-MHC gene regions influence disease. Genetic control of inflammation can hypothetically be either general or specific for a particular target tissue. For the latter, gene regulation of pathomechanisms in the CNS could affect reactivity of microglia or astrocytes, local cytokine/chemokine production, or even neuronal vulnerability. We have obtained strong support for this notion by observations of rat strain–dependent variation in the inflammatory response after ventral root avulsion, a model in which mainly non-antigen–specific elements of the immune system promote inflammation. A comparison of strains with similar MHC haplotypes on different backgrounds and strains with different MHC haplotypes on the same background, respectively, demonstrates that the inflammatory phenotype is regulated mainly by non-MHC genes. Interestingly, different features of the inflammatory response, such as induction of MHC class II expression, glial activation, cytokine expression, and neuronal vulnerability, varied between rat strains and were largely independent of each other. The genetic control of several basic features of inflammation in the CNS is of great relevance not only for MS/EAE, but also for several other neurological conditions with inflammatory components such as cerebrovascular and neurogenerative dieases and trauma.

GENE REGULATION OF SUSCEPTIBILITY TO EXPERIMENTAL AUTOIMMUNE ENCEPHALITIS

Incidence rates for multiple sclerosis (MS) in different populations and genetic linkage analyses of concordance rates in twins or siblings provide firm evidence for a genetic impact on the susceptibility of this disease.[1,2] Experience from whole genome scans of MS[2] is as follows: (1) No non-HLA region has shown unequivocal linkage to disease. (2) Regions with suggestive linkage largely vary between studies; however, certain regions start to emerge as "hot spots," such as the 17q22-q24 region.[3] (3) Stratification for the risk increasing HLA haplotype reveals HLA DR2-dependent and DR2-nondependent loci.[2] (4) Linkage analysis in MS families will require immensely large materials to localize susceptibility genes, because each

[a]Author for correspondence. Voice: +46-8-51776242; fax: +46-8-51776248.
Tomas.Olsson@cmm.ki.se

gene has only a modest or low impact on MS. These partly frustrating results may be due to genetic heterogeneity in which different genes may predispose for the same phenotype, that is, MS, and these may vary between families and populations. In addition, the disease-predisposing genes may contribute with only small increases to the risk of developing MS. An alternative strategy is to study gene influences in animal models and by synteny comparisons to define candidate genes to be tested by association in human materials. Even if not the same as in MS, genes defined in animals may also unravel pathogenetic pathways with potential impact on MS. Furthermore, the disease gene-regulated pathways are accessible for experimental testing and evaluation of new therapies.

Striking advantages with disease gene-mapping studies in experimental animals are that genetic heterogeneity can be reduced and variation in environmental influences minimized. Thus, great efforts are made to map the gene(s) regulating EAE. However, this has not been achieved to date at a single gene level, but only for larger genetic loci comprising up to several hundred different genes. Gene regions correlating with increased incidence rates have been mapped to both the major histocompatibility complex (MHC) as well as the rest of the genome.[4,5] The current belief is that the MHC gene influence in rat EAE can, at least partially, be attributed to polymorphisms of MHC class I and II molecules, which determine the ability to present particular autoantigenic peptides.[6-8] In both mice[5] and rats,[9-11] non-MHC gene regions influencing disease susceptibility have been mapped. There is currently a scarcity of information on how these non-MHC loci contribute to disease susceptibility. Regulation of cytokine expression may be important, because differences in rat EAE disease evolution can be correlated to the cytokine profiles in susceptible and resistant strains.[8,12-14] Genetic control of organ-specific inflammatory disease may theoretically affect general immunoregulatory events, which would then dispose the animal to different organ-specific inflammatory diseases. Indeed, there is a striking colocalization of genome regions predisposing to different inflammatory diseases.[9,15,16] Conversely, it is also theoretically possible that other disease-regulating genes are target specific. In the CNS, such genes could affect reactivity of microglia or astrocytes, local cytokine or chemokine production, or even neuronal vulnerability. These cell types and inflammatory mediators are implicated in primary inflammatory diseases such as MS, but they also take part in neurodegenerative diseases. Target-specific events may also be important in view of recent experience from magnetic resonance imaging in MS. Thus, the degree of inflammation as measured with a T2 lesion load displays a poor correlation to neurological deficits, suggesting that there may be interindividual differences in vulnerability to inflammatory damage. With this background, we wanted to explore the possibility of genetically determined differences in the susceptibility and regulation of pathomechanisms in a target-selective experimental paradigm with non-antigen–specific inflammatory activation and neuronal degeneration.

VENTRAL ROOT AVULSION AS A MODEL FOR CNS INFLAMMATION

Genetic regulation of different components of target tissue inflammation would thus provide an additional level at which genetic susceptibility loci could be involved. This is not easily addressed in EAE, however, because it is impossible to discriminate between effects of the systemic autoantigen-driven immune response and CNS-specific factors. Instead, peripheral nerve trauma with its subsequent inflammatory reactions around lesioned nerve cells may represent a suitable experimental paradigm. Peripheral nerve trauma is accompanied by a retrograde reaction with changes in axotomized nerve cell bodies.[17–19] There are also several "inflammatory" features shared with autoimmune or infectious conditions, such as activation of surrounding glia, upregulation of major histocompatibility complex (MHC) antigens, and increased production of inflammatory mediators.[20–25] In primarily inflammatory diseases of the nervous system, such as multiple sclerosis and EAE, myelin autoreactive CD4+ T cells are considered to be of great importance in the propagation of disease by the release of proinflammatory cytokines.[26] In contrast, T cells may play only a minor role in the nerve avulsion model, because very few of them were determined to be recruited, and *in vivo* depletion of α/β TCR bearing T cells did not affect the response.[25]

In contrast to more distal nerve transections in the rat, avulsion of ventral roots leads to the loss of a majority of the lesioned cells.[27,28] Although deprivation of neurotrophic factors such as brain-derived neurotrophic factor (BDNF) and ciliary neurotrophic factor is likely to be a major determinant of nerve cell death, long-term treatment *in vivo* with BDNF only saves a fraction of motoneurons after ventral root avulsion in adult rats.[29,30] Therefore, other mechanisms could also cause the death of adult motoneurons after nerve injury. Alhough there may be some consensus that macrophage activation in the peripheral nerve after nerve lesion to some degree facilitates axonal regeneration,[31] the question about the inflammatory response occurring around lesioned nerve cell bodies is more controversial. This can, to a large extent, depend on differences in the experimental models used, but also on the inflammatory response which may have both beneficial and harmful effects depending on the nature of the lesion.[32] We have previously demonstrated that the majority of nerve cells are lost during the second and third postoperative weeks, whereas few

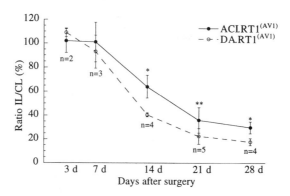

FIGURE 1. Motoneuron survival after ventral root avulsion. Motoneuron numbers as ratios between lesioned and unlesioned sides at different time points after ventral root avulsion. The number of surviving motoneurons on the lesioned side in the DA strain is significantly reduced at 2, 3, and 4 weeks after the lesion as compared to the ACI strain. n is the number of animals for each strain; IL, ipsilateral; CL, contralateral. $*p < 0.05$; $**p < 0.01$ (Mann-Whitney test).

additional cells are lost during the following week (see FIGURE 1).[25] The peak in expression of proinflammatory cytokines that occurs at the very onset of motoneuron death suggests an inflammatory component in this type of neurodegenerative process. This hypothesis is supported by the fact that several cytokines, including gamma interferon (IFN-γ) and tumor necrosis factor-alpha (TNF-α), upregulate the production of potentially cell-toxic compounds such as glutamate agonists[33,34] and NO[35,36] in microglia and astrocytes and that both IFN-γ and TNF-α also display direct cell-toxic effects on some cell types in the nervous system.[37,38] However, evidence so far is only circumstantial, and future studies are needed to demonstrate if and how the neuroinflammatory reaction after mechanical nerve injuries contributes to nerve cell death.

GENETICS OF TARGET TISSUE VULNERABILITY

Despite the role assigned to the local inflammatory response in the brain, there is a relative paucity of studies addressing the genetic regulation of target tissue-specific inflammatory features. In a model of standardized CNS trauma in which ventral roots are avulsed, we examined the response in the two inbred rat strains, DA and ACI.[25] These two strains have similar MHC haplotypes (RT1^{AV1}), but differ considerably in their susceptibility to EAE.[13,39] Interestingly, the DA strain consistently displayed much stronger microglial activation, MHC class II induction, IFN-γ and TNF-α mRNA induction, and a greater degree of motoneuron loss (FIG. 1), demonstrating a genetic regulation of these events. DA rats with a different MHC haplotype (RT1^H) gave a similar result as DA (RT1^{AV1}), providing further evidence for non-MHC gene(s) regulating the phenotypic differences between the strains. To examine the inheritance pattern for the susceptibility to neuronal loss and inflammatory response after nerve root avulsion, an intercross experiment betweenACI and DA was established. F1(DA×ACI) were back-crossed to parental ACI or DA rats, resulting in F2(F1×ACI) and F2(F1×DA) rats. Analyses of nerve cell survival and MHC class II expression (see FIGURE 2) revealed that the F1×ACI and F1×DA groups mounted an intermediate response in comparison with the two parental strains. The continuous distribution pattern of neuronal loss and inflammatory response within the F1×ACI and F1×DA groups suggests that more than one gene is conferring susceptibility to both variables after nerve root avulsion.

Two questions emerged from these experiments: first, whether identical genetic traits regulate susceptibility to both EAE- and nerve avulsion-induced inflammation and, second, whether different aspects of the inflammatory response, such as glial MHC expression and microglial activation, are interconnected or regulated independently of each other. To address these questions we performed a comprehensive characterization of the inflammatory response to ventral root avulsion in a panel of inbred rat strains (BN(RT1^N), DA(RT1^{AV1}), E3(RT1^U), LEW(RT1^{AV1}), LEW(RT1^N), and PVG(RT1^{AV1})) frequently used in autoimmune disease models.[40] Several different parameters, including activation of microglia and astrocytes, MHC class II induction on glia, expression of the cytokine IL-1β, and motoneuron death, were examined. The activation patterns of astrocytes and microglia differed considerably between strains and largely correlated with strain differences in the expression of complement 3 (C3) mRNA (see FIGURE 3). The induction of expression of

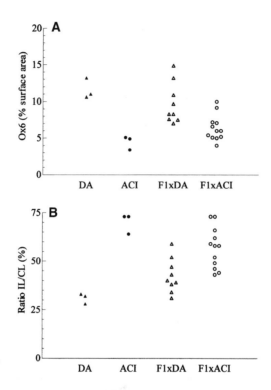

FIGURE 2. A. MHC class II expression as percentage of the surface area occupied by O×6-immunopositive cells and motoneuron numbers as ratios between lesioned and unlesioned sides in parental DA (DA), parental ACI (ACI), F2 (F1×DA), and F2 (F1×ACI) rats two weeks after ventral root avulsion. **B.** Motoneuron survival. Both motoneuron survival and MHC class II expression are distributed relatively continuously within the F2(F1×DA) and F2(F1×ACI) groups and reflect an intermediate response as compared with the parental strains. Differences between F1×DA and F1×ACI concerning motoneuron survival (Kruskal-Wallis, Dunn's post-hoc test; $p < 0.05$) and MHC class II expression (ANOVA, Newman-Keul's post-hoc test; $p < 0.01$) are significant. IL, ipsilateral; CL, contralateral.

MHC class II also displayed a strain-specific pattern. Notably, the BN strain displayed early induction, whereas E3 largely lacked injury-induced MHC class II expression (see FIGURE 4). Interestingly, there was also a strain-specific pattern in the induction of cytokine mRNA. Thus, levels of IL-1β were increased on the side of the lesion in all strains, but this induction was significantly higher in the BN strain. Finally, the degree of neuronal survival was also significantly different between the strains (see FIGURE 5).

These results clearly demonstrate major genetic polymorphisms affecting multiple levels of the regulation of target tissue inflammation in the CNS after mechanical trauma. The characteristic phenotypes of the different strains seem mainly to be regulated by non-MHC genes, because differences between LEW strains with different

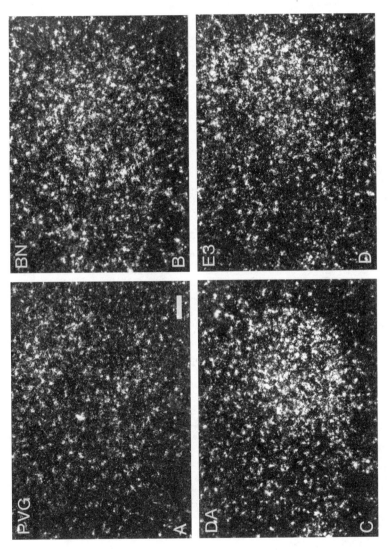

FIGURE 3. Dark-field photomicrographs of the ventral horn showing *in situ* hybridization labeling for C3 mRNA in the PVG (**A**), BN (**B**), DA (**C**), and E3 (**D**) strain one week after ventral root avulsion. The degree of C3 mRNA induction correlated with the degree of glia activation in the different strains. Much stronger labeling is present in the DA rat compared with PVG. Note that E3 displays relatively intense activation despite a relative lack of injury-induced MHC class II expression. *Scale bar*, 0.1 mm.

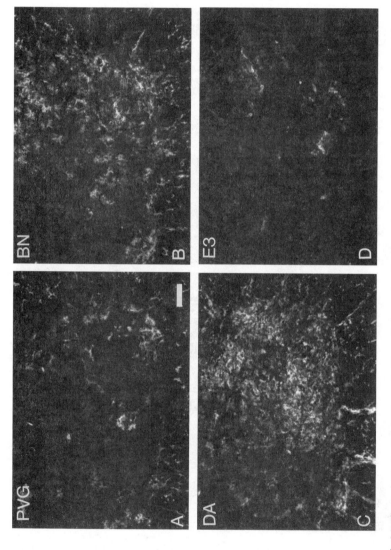

FIGURE 4. MHC class II induction in the ventral horn three weeks after ventral root avulsion in the PVG (**A**), BN (**B**), DA (**C**), and E3 (**D**) rat. Strong immunolabeling for MHC class II (O×6) is seen in the BN and DA strains, whereas E3 displays a conspicuous lack of injury-induced MHC class II expression. *Scale bar*, 0.1 mm.

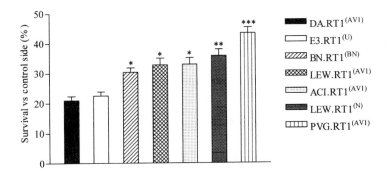

FIGURE 5. Motoneuron survival three weeks after surgery. Survival of avulsed moto-neurons differed considerably between strains and in part correlated with the degree of inflammatory activation. However, differences in survival between the E3 and LEW strains, which both display an intermediate inflammatory response, suggest a variable degree of neuronal vulnerability after this type of lesion. Data are presented as a ratio between lesioned and unlesioned sides three weeks after ventral root avulsion. Statistical signifi-cance was determined against the DA rat (Kruskal-Wallis, Dunn's post-hoc test).

MHC haplotypes were small, whereas the PVG and DA strains (which share the same MHC haplotype) displayed the largest differences. The strain-dependant dif-ferences in nerve avulsion-induced inflammation correlated only partly with EAE susceptibility. The EAE-susceptible DA strain consistently ranked very high in the different inflammatory parameters, whereas the EAE-resistant PVG strain displayed a low degree of inflammation. Interestingly, the E3 strain, which is also resistant to EAE induction,[14] demonstrated a vigorous inflammatory response except for a con-spicuous lack of injury-induced MHC class II expression.

CONCLUDING REMARKS

Glial activation, in particular, microgliosis, is a prominent feature of virtually all pathological conditions in the brain. The functional implications of this activation are not yet determined. However, there is reason to believe that it may have an impor-tant role in the development of pathology. For example, in Alzheimer's disease, microgliosis is prominent and has been suggested to actively participate in the neu-rodegenerative process.[41,42] The implication of the results presented herein is that genetic factors regulating different characteristics of the local inflammatory response and nerve cell survival may be very important in the evolution of pathology also in these conditions.

ACKNOWLEDGMENTS

We thank Associate Professor Robert A. Harris for expert advice. This work was supported by Ake Wibergs, Magn Bergvalls, Tore Nilsons, and David och Astrid Hageléns Stiftelse, NHR, and the Swedish Medical Research Council.

REFERENCES

1. EBERS, G.C., D.E. BULMAN, A.D. SADOVNICK *et al.* 1986. A population-based study of multiple sclerosis in twins. N. Engl. J. Med. **315:** 1638–1642.
2. CHATAWAY, J., R. FEAKES, F. CORADDU *et al.* 1998. The genetics of multiple sclerosis: principles, background and updated results of the United Kingdom systematic genome screen. Brain **121:** 1869–1887.
3. KUOKKANEN, S., M. GSCHWEND, J. RIOUX *et al.* 1997. Genomewide scan of multiple sclerosis in Finnish multiplex families. Am. J. Hum. Genet. **61:** 1379–1387.
4. WILLIAMS, R. & M. MOORE. 1973. Linkage of susceptibility to experimental allergic encephalomyelitis to the major histocompatibility locus in the rat. J. Exp. Med. **138:** 775–783.
5. SUNDVALL, M., J. JIRHOLT, H. YANG *et al.* 1995. Identification of murine loci associated with susceptibility to chronic experimental autoimmune encephalomyelitis. Nat. Genet. **10:** 313–317.
6. MUSTAFA, M., C. VINGSBO, T. OLSSON *et al.* 1994. Protective influences on experimental autoimmune encephalomyelitis by MHC class I and class II alleles. J. Immunol. **153:** 3337–3344.
7. ISSAZADEH, S., P. KJELLÉN, T. OLSSON *et al.* 1997. Major histocompatibility complex-controlled protective influences on experimental autoimmune encephalomyelitis are peptide specific. Eur. J. Immunol. **27:** 1584–1587.
8. WEISSERT, R., E. WALLSTRÖM, M. STORCH *et al.* 1998. MHC haplotype-dependent regulation of MOG-induced EAE in rats. J. Clin. Invest. **102:** 1265–1273.
9. DAHLMAN, I., J. LORENTZEN, K. DE GRAAF *et al.* 1998. Quantitative trait loci disposing for both experimental arthritis and encephalomyelitis in the DA rat; impact on severity of myelin oligodendrocyte glycoprotein-induced experimental autoimmune encephalomyelitis and antibody isotype pattern. Eur. J. Immunol. **28:** 2188–2196.
10. DAHLMAN, I., L. JACOBSSON, J.C. LORENTZEN *et al.* 1999. A genome wide linkage analysis of chronic relapsing experimental autoimmune encephalomyelitis in the rat identifies a major susceptibility locus on chromosome 9. J. Immunol. **162:** 2581–2588.
11. PIEHL, F., C. LUNDBERG, M. KHADEMI, A. BUCHT, I. DAHLMAN, J.C. LORENTZEN & T. OLSSON. 1999. Non-MHC gene regulation of nerve root injury induced by spinal cord inflammation and neuron death. J. Neuroimmunol. **101:** 87–97.
12. ISSAZADEH, S., J.C. LORENTZEN, M.I. MUSTAFA *et al.* 1996. Cytokines in relapsing experimental autoimmune encephalomyelitis in DA rats: persistent mRNA expression of proinflammatory cytokines and absent expression of interleukin-10 and transforming growth factor-beta. J. Neuroimmunol. **69:** 103–115.
13. LORENTZEN, J.C., M. ANDERSSON, S. ISSAZADEH *et al.* 1997. Genetic analysis of inflammation, cytokine mRNA expression and disease course of relapsing experimental autoimmune encephalomyelitis in DA rats. J. Neuroimmunol. **80:** 31–37.
14. KJELLÉN, P., S. ISSAZADEH, T. OLSSON *et al.* 1998. Genetic influence on disease course and cytokine response in relapsing experimental allergic encephalomyelitis. Int. Immunol. **10:** 333–340.
15. VYSE, T. & J. TODD. 1996. Genetic analysis of autoimmune disease. Cell **85:** 311–318.
16. BECKER, K., R. SIMON, J. BAILEY-WILSON *et al.* 1998. Clustering of non-major histocompatibility complex susceptibility candidate loci in human autoimmune diseases. Proc. Natl. Acad. Sci. USA **95:** 9979–9984.
17. LIEBERMAN, A.R. 1971. The axon reaction: a review of the principal features of perikaryal responses to axon injury. Int. Rev. Neurobiol. **14:** 49–124.
18. KREUTZBERG, G.W., M.B. GRAEBER & W.J. STREIT. 1989. Neuron-glial relationship during regeneration of motorneurons. Metab. Brain Dis. **4:** 81–85.
19. ALDSKOGIUS, H. & M. SVENSSON. 1993. Neuronal and glial responses to axon injury. *In* Advances in Structural Biology, Vol. 2. S.K. Malhotra, Ed.: 191–223. JAI Press. Greenwich, CT.
20. MAEHLEN, J., H. SCHRODER, L. KLARESKOG *et al.* 1988. Axotomy induces MHC class I antigen expression on rat nerve cells. Neurosci. Lett. **92:** 8–13.

21. OLSSON, T., K. KRISTENSSON, Å. LJUNGDAHL *et al.* 1989. Gamma-interferon-like immunoreactivity in axotomized rat motor neurons. J. Neurosci. **9:** 3870–3875.

22. STREIT, W.J., M.B. GRAEBER & G.W. KREUTZBERG. 1989. Peripheral nerve lesion produces increased levels of major histocompatibility complex antigens in the central nervous system. J. Neuroimmunol. **21:** 117–123.

23. NEUMANN, H., A. CAVALIE, D.E. JENNE *et al.* 1995. Induction of MHC class I genes in neurons. Science **269:** 549–552.

24. RAIVICH, G., L. JONES, C. KLOSS *et al.* 1998. Immune surveillance in the injured nervous system: T-lymphocytes invade the axotomized mouse facial motor nucleus and aggregate around sites of neuronal degeneration. J. Neurosci. **18:** 5804–5816.

25. DAHLMAN, I., E. WALLSTRÖM, R. WEISSERT, M. STORCH, B. KORNEK, L. JACOBSSON, C. LININGTON, H. LUTHMAN, H. LASSMANN & T. OLSSON. 1999. Linkage analysis of myelin oligodendrocyte glycoprotein–induced experimental autoimmune encephalomyelitis in the rat identifies a locus controlling demyelination on chromosome 18. Hum. Mol. Gen. **8:** 2183–2190.

26. OLSSON, T. 1995. Critical influences of the cytokine orchestration on the outcome of myelin antigen-specific T-cell autoimmunity in experimental autoimmune encephalomyelitis and multiple sclerosis. Immunol. Rev. **144:** 245–268.

27. KOLIATSOS, V.E., W.L. PRICE, C.A. PARDO *et al.* 1994. Ventral root avulsion: an experimental model of death of adult motor neurons. J. Comp. Neurol. **342:** 35–44.

28. PIEHL, F., G. TABAR & S. CULLHEIM. 1995. Expression of NMDA receptor mRNAs in rat motoneurons is down-regulated after axotomy. Eur. J. Neurosci. **7:** 2101–2110.

29. KISHINO, A., Y. ISHIGE, T. TATSUNO *et al.* 1997. BDNF prevents and reverses adult rat motor neuron degeneration and induces axonal outgrowth. Exp. Neurol. **144:** 273–286.

30. NOVIKOV, L., L. NOVIKOVA & J.O. KELLERTH. 1997. Brain-derived neurotrophic factor promotes axonal regeneration and long-term survival of adult rat spinal motoneurons in vivo. Neuroscience **79:** 765–774.

31. PERRY, V., M. BROWN & S. GORDON. 1987. The macrophage response to central and peripheral nerve injury. A possible role for macrophages in regeneration. J. Exp. Med. **165:** 1218–1223.

32. HIRSCHBERG, D.L., E. YOLES, M. BELKIN *et al.* 1994. Inflammation after axonal injury has conflicting consequences for recovery of function: rescue of spared axons is impaired but regeneration is supported. J. Neuroimmunol. **50:** 9–16.

33. PIANI, D., M. SPRANGER, K. FREI *et al.* 1992. Macrophage-induced cytotoxicity of N-methyl-D-aspartate receptor positive neurons involves excitatory amino acids rather than reactive oxygen intermediates and cytokines. Eur. J. Immunol. **22:** 2429–2436.

34. GIULIAN, D., M. CORPUZ, S. CHAPMAN *et al.* 1993. Reactive mononuclear phagocytes release neurotoxins after ischemic and traumatic injury to the central nervous system. J. Neurosci. Res. **36:** 681–693.

35. CHAO, C., S. HU, T. MOLITOR *et al.* 1992. Activated microglia mediate neuronal cell injury via a nitric oxide mechanism. J. Immunol. **149:** 2736–2741.

36. LEE, S.C., D.W. DICKSON, W. LIU *et al.* 1993. Induction of nitric oxide synthase activity in human astrocytes by interleukin-1 beta and interferon-gamma. J. Neuroimmunol. **46:** 19–24.

37. LOUIS, J.C., E. MAGAL, S. TAKAYAMA *et al.* 1993. CNTF protection of oligodendrocytes against natural and tumor necrosis factor-induced death. Science **259:** 689–692.

38. VARTANIAN, T., Y. LI, M. ZHAO & K. STEFANSSON. 1995. Interferon-gamma-induced oligodendrocyte cell death: implications for the pathogenesis of multiple sclerosis. Mol. Med. **1:** 732–743.

39. LORENTZEN, J.C., S. ISSAZADEH, M. STORCH *et al.* 1995. Protracted, relapsing and demyelinating experimental autoimmune encephalomyelitis in DA rats immunized with syngeneic spinal cord and incomplete Freund's adjuvant. J. Neuroimmunol. **63:** 193–205.

40. LUNDBERG, C., O. LIDMAN, R. HOLMDAHL *et al.* Strain-dependent differences in inflammation and neurodegeneration after mechanical nerve injury in the rat; evidence for independent non-MHC gene regulation at several different levels. Submitted.
41. GONZALEZ-SCARANO, F. & G. BALTUCH. 1999. Microglia as mediators of inflammatory and degenerative diseases. Annu. Rev. Neurosci. **22:** 219–240.
42. EIKELENBOOM P. & R.J. VAN MUISWINKEL. 1998. Inflammation and Alzheimer's disease: relationships between pathogenic mechanisms and clinical expression. Exp. Neurol. **154:** 89–98.

C-fos and IL-2 Gene Expression in Rat Brain Cells and Splenic Lymphocytes after Nonantigenic and Antigenic Stimuli

E.A. KORNEVA, S.V. BARABANOVA, O.I. GOLOVKO,
M.A. NOSOV, N.S. NOVIKOVA, AND T.B. KAZAKOVA

Department of General Pathology and Pathophysiology,
Institute of Experimental Medicine, Russian Academy of Medical Sciences,
12 Acad. Pavlov Str., St. Petersburg 197376, Russia

ABSTRACT: Immunostimulatory or immunosuppressive stress models were used: (1) rotation stress (RS) and (2) immobilization (restraint) stress (IS). Intravenous injection of tetanus toxoid (anatoxin) (TT) was chosen as the antigenic stimulus (500 μg/kg weight), and intravenous injection of saline solution was used as the control. Splenic lymphocytes (CBA mice) or different brain structures (Wistar and Sprague-Dawley rats) were analyzed. The c-fos and interleukin-2 (IL-2) mRNA expression was measured using a digoxigenin (Dig)-labeled cDNA probe by spot or *in situ* hybridization. Rotation stress stimulated IL-2 mRNA synthesis in lymphocytes in the presence of ConA and rIL-2 by 40%. IL-2 mRNA synthesis in lymphoid cells obtained from animals after IS and after IS in combination with the administration *in vitro* of the cytotoxic drug CsA to the splenic lymphocytes was inhibited (30% and 99%), accordingly, as compared with control rats. Induction of c-fos mRNA synthesis in rat brain cells was noted 30 minutes after RS in the hypothalamus (lateralis hypothalamic area, LHA), thalamus, corpus collosum, and sensorimotor zone of the brain cortex. IL-2 mRNA synthesis was shown two hours after RS in the same structures. The increased number of c-fos mRNA-positive cells two hours after TT injection was shown in the posterior hypothalamus area (PHA), LHA, dorsomedial nucleus (DMH), ventromedial nucleus (VMH), and anterior hypothalamus area (AHA) as compared to the effect of i.v. saline injection. Moreover, IL-2 mRNA-positive cell induction was noted in the PHA, DMH, and VMH. Six hours after TT injection, c-fos mRNA expression was decreased in the PHA, LHA, and AHA. Activation of c-fos and IL-2 mRNA was detected in the paraventricularis nucleus 6 hours after TT i.v. injection. Thus, inhibition or stimulation of IL-2 gene expression in lymphoid cells depends on the nature of the stressors. RS or antigenic stimuli induce c-fos and IL-2 gene expression in definite structures of the brain. The dynamics of this process are time dependent. The partial correlation between c-fos and IL-2 mRNA expression in localization in brain structures and time dependence was shown.

INTRODUCTION

The identification of molecular-genetic mechanisms of neuroimmune interaction is a significant part of the problem of neuroimmunomodulation. It is well known that different kinds of stress, immunosuppressor drugs, or antigens can influence the activity of nervous and immunocompetent cells. Currently, specific molecular-

197

biological methods for gene expression analysis allow us to investigate the process of neuroimmunological interactions at the genetic level to determine early changes in the mechanisms of cell activation. As the specific markers that reflect changes in cell metabolic processes, the expression of immediate-early genes, such as the protooncogene c-fos, may be analyzed. As one of the cellular immediate-response genes, it can be used for functional anatomical mapping toll to identify the brain cells that become activated in response to various stimuli.[1–4] Basal expression of c-fos is relatively low in the brain cells, but it can be induced rapidly and transiently by depolarizing agents,[5] seizure induction,[6] sensory stimulation,[7] stress,[4] and injection of different substances.[8,9]

c-Fos protein, on the other hand, by dimerization with members of the jun family, forms a transcription factor, activator protein-1 (AP-1), that transactivates other inducible genes,[10,11] such as the cytokine-interleukin-2 (IL-2) gene. IL-2 protein has multiple immunoregulatory functions and is known as T-cell growth factor.[12] Emerging evidence suggests that IL-2 is also a modulator of neuronal and neuroendocrine function. Recent studies have shown the effects of IL-2 on growth and survival of neuronal cells and hormone release.[13,14] The presence of specific IL-2 binding sites, IL-2–like mRNA, and IL-2 receptor in different regions of the brain was reported.[15,16] The role of IL-2 in the brain is not clear, but the ability of IL-2 to penetrate the blood-brain barrier further suggests that it can take part in the communication between the central nervous system (CNS) and the immune system.[17] Nevertheless, some data on the effects of various stimuli on IL-2 gene expression in the brain do exist.

The aim of the present study was to demonstrate immediate-early gene expression in immunocytes as well as their expression and localization in the nervous system after nonantigenic (rotation stress [RS] and immobilization [restraint] stress [IS]) or antigenic stimuli (i.v. injection of tetanus toxoid [anatoxin], TT]) and to determine the possible correlation and difference in the induction of their mRNAs. C-fos and IL-2 genes were used as markers for activated splenic lymphocytes and brain cells.

Expression of the c-fos gene after bacterial endotoxin (lipopolysaccharide, LPS)[18,19] and plateled-derived growth factor[20] application has been reported.

MATERIALS AND METHODS

Reagents. The anti–c-fos polyclonal antibodies used in this study were obtained from Santa Cruz Biotech. Inc. (USA) and the digoxigenin (Dig) kit from Boehringer-Mannheim (Germany). pUC-v-fos plasmid DNA was supplied by Prof. V.A. Pospelov (Institute of Cytology, Russian Academy of Sciences, St. Petersburg) and pPL32IL-2 plasmid DNA by Dr. A.P. Perevozchikov (Institute of Experimental Medicine, Russian Academy of Sciences, St. Petersburg).

Animals. Male mice (CBA, weighing 18–20 g, aged 10–12 weeks) and male Wistar (200 g) and Sprague-Dawley rats (250–300 g) were maintained on a 12-hour light/dark cycle at a constant room temperature. Water and food were given *ad libitum.*

Experimental Models and Splenic Lymphocyte Preparation. By restraint, stress mice were placed in special containers unable to move for eight hours at room temperature without food or water. The procedure was repeated over three days, and then the animals were allowed three days of rest. The mice were then sacrificed, and lymphocytes were isolated by Ficoll-verografin (Pharmacia) gradient ($d = 1.076$) centrifugation ($4,000 \times g$/40 minutes). The $1–2 \times 10^6$ cells were incubated at 37°C, 100% humidity, 5% CO_2 in RPMI 1640 plus 10% fetal bovine serum, 10 mM HEPES, 2 mM glutamine, 50 mM β-mercaptoethanol, 50 U/ml penicillin, and 50 mg/ml streptomycin. Control wells do not or contained 5–20 mg/ml ConA + 30 U/ml rIL-2 (because this combination of mitogen with IL-2 is usually used for T-cell stimulation).[21,22] Incubation time was 2–8 hours.[23] Induced IL-2 mRNA was analyzed by isolation of total RNA and spot hybridization with IL-2 Dig-labeled cDNA. The immunosuppressive effect was obtained by the addition of the cytostatic drug cyclosporin A (CsA) in a concentration of 1 mg/10^6 lymphoid cells.

By rotation, stress mice or male Wistar rats (20 animals) were sitting in a rotation camera at 78 rpm four times for 10 minutes at five-minute intervals. Lymphocytes from stressed animals were isolated after two hours (as just described); brain sections were prepared as mentioned down (using frozen sections).

Experiments with the iv TT injection were made in 20 male Sprague-Dawley rats (Harlan, The Netherlands) weighing 250–300 g.[a]

Analysis of c-fos mRNA Expression by the Spot Hybridization Method. The RNA extracting method employed to obtain total RNA from mouse spleen lymphocytes was based on the method by Chomczynski and Sacchi.[24] Aliquots of total RNA from 2×10^7 lymphoid cells were subjected to spot hybridization with Dig-labeled IL-2 cDNA[25] on Hybond nylon membrane. Intensity of spot color was measured by THE densitometric method on an Ultrascan XL (LKB) densitometer. As a control to IL-2 mRNA synthesis in lymphocytes obtained from stressed animals, lymphoid cells from intact animals were used.

Preparation of Frozen Brain Sections. All rats of two strains were taken from their cages at the same time of day and handled as little as possible. Thirty minutes or two hours after stimulation, they were anesthetized (phenobarbital 60 mg/kg was injected intraperitoneally in the right ileal area), and intracardial perfusion (100 ml, 10–15 ml/minute) with cold saline plus heparin (10 U/ml) followed by 150 ml of 4% paraformaldehyde in PBS buffer (pH 7.4) was done. The isolated brain was stored in 4% paraformaldehyde in PBS with 15% sucrose for the night at +4°C. The tissues were then placed in PBS and stored at −20°C. Frozen tissues were cut in cryostat (30 mm) and placed on pretreated[26] sterile glasses to be processed for *in situ* hybridization. The nearest sections (3×30 mm) from the same brain were used for *in situ* hybridization for c-fos mRNA and IL-2 mRNA The sections correspond to the same level indicated in Swanson's stereotaxic rat brain atlas,[27] NN 26, 27, 28. No double-staining for mRNA and protein was conducted in this case.

Preparation of Paraffin Sections. Animals were anesthetized two or six hours after injection. The isolated brain was washed twice (1 hour) in PBS, and then tissue dehydration was conducted through graded ethanol (50%, 1 hour; 70%, 1 hour; 90%, 40 minutes; 96%, 40 minutes; 100%, twice for 40 minutes) and 1:1 ethanol:chloroform, 40 minutes, and chloroform, 40 minutes. Tissues were incubated in the chloroform–

---

[a]In this series of experiments *in situ* hybridization was made in paraffin section.

paraffin mix and then in paraffin. Cut sections (10 mm) were floated on demineralized water and placed on pretreated slides. Paraffin was removed in xylene 60°C 30 minutes, and sections were washed in fresh xylene for five minutes.

Preparation of Labeled cDNA Fragments. Isolation of plasmid DNA, restriction digestion, electrophoretic analysis, and labeling with nonradioactive label digoxigenin were performed by the methods described by Manniatis *et al.*[25] and the Boehringer Application Manual.[26]

Analysis of c-fos mRNA Expression by the in situ *Hybridization Method.* Sections on glass were hydrated in 99% ethanol for five minutes twice, 96% for five minutes twice, and 70% for five minutes; and in water for five minutes. Then with coverslips, they were placed in a humid chamber, treated with 20–30 ml proteinase K (10 g/ml in 50 mM Tris-HCl, pH 7.4, 10 mM EDTA, and 10 mM NaCl) for 15 minutes at 37°C and washed with 0.2% glycine in PBS for five minutes twice. Sections were fixed with 0.4% paraformaldehyde (30 minutes at room temperature), washed for five minutes in water, and treated with 5–10 ml of the hybridization mixture (60% deionized formamide, 0.3 M NaCl, 0.03 M Na citrate, 10 mM EDTA, 25 mM NaH_2PO_4, pH 7.4, 5% dextran sulfate, 250 ng/ml fragmented chicken erythrocytes DNA and 25 ng/ml c-fos or IL-2 Dig-labeled cDNA for the brain cryostat sections.

For the brain paraffin sections, a probe cocktail was used: 10 ml 50× Denhart's solution, 50 ml dextran sulfate 50%, 10 ml sonicated salmon sperm DNA (10 mg/ml), 100 ml 20× SSC, 500 ng digoxigenin-labeled probe in 50 ml TE, 250 ml water, and 250 ml formamide. Hybridization was made at +37°C for 16 hours. Coverslips were removed in 60% formamide, 0.3 M NaCl, and 0.03 M Na citrate at the RT and washed in 2 × SSC three times, at +37°C in 0.2 × SSC, and for five minutes in PBS. Staining and detection of the labeled cells were done using the antibodies against digoxigenin.[26] The cells were counted and photographed using the Ista-Video-Test System.

Cell Counting and Statistical Analysis. The nomenclature and nuclear boundaries defined in Swanson's stereotaxic rat brain atlas[27] were used in this study.

Each brain section was examined at 100× using light microscopy. The total number of c-fos mRNA or IL-2 mRNA positive cells in each hypothalamic structure were counted in three ocular fields (one ocular field = 25 squares; 1 square = 0.0025 cm^2) for three sections and then divided by the number of sections to provide a mean cell count per section. Results were expressed as the mean value (SE). Statistical analysis was made using Student's *t* test.

RESULTS AND DISSCUSION

Effect of Rotation and Immobilization (Restraint) Stress on c-fos and IL-2 Gene Expression in Mouse Splenic Lymphocytes

It is known that the production of cytokine IL-2 in T lymphocytes does not take place in unstimulated lymphocytes. Only the addition of mitogens or antigens leads to the induction of IL-2 mRNA expression and IL-2 synthesis.[21,22] Therefore, IL-2 mRNA synthesis in isolated lymphocyte cells from stressed animals cells was performed in the presence of ConA and rIL-2.

Analysis of c-fos gene expression in splenic lymphocyte cells shows the high level of c-fos mRNA synthesis in intact lymphocytes without the presence of ConA + rIL-2. Rotation stress (two hours after application) stimulated c-fos gen e expression in lymphocytes 1.5 times compared to controls (see FIGURE 1A).

ConA + rIL-2 stimulation of *in vitro* incubated mice lymphocytes caused IL-2 mRNA synthesis, but the quantity of IL-2 mRNA was 30% less after immobilizing stress (see FIGURE 2) and 40% higher after rotation stress (FIG. 1B). The effect of rotation stress on IL-2 mRNA expression can partially be explained by the increased level of IL-1 as shown by Korneva *et al.*[28]

The inhibitory effect of restraint stress may be compared to a small degree with the influence of cytostatic drugs. The addition of the cytostatic drug CsA to ConA + rIL-2–stimulated lymphocytes from control animals led to 94.6% inhibition of IL-2 mRNA synthesis. A combination of immobilization stress and CsA application caused total repression of IL-2 mRNA expression. It is well known that the cytotoxic effect of CsA is bound with its action on one of intermediate stage in the signal

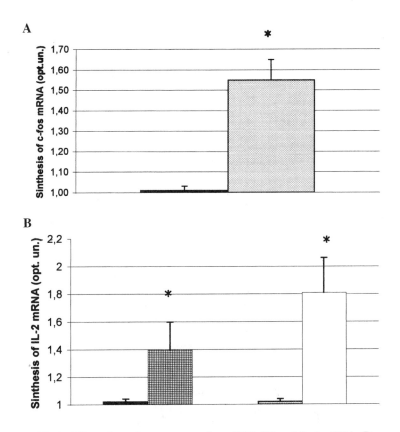

FIGURE 1. Effect of rotation stress on c-fos mRNA (**A**) and IL-2 mRNA (**B**) expression in mouse splenic lymphocytes. Groups of animals: ■, intact animals; ▨, animals after rotation stress; ▦, animals in the presence of ConA + rIL-2; □, animals after rotation stress in the presence of ConA + rIL-2. *$p < 0.05$.

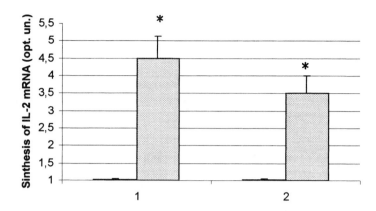

FIGURE 2. Effect of immobilization stress on IL-2 mRNA production in mouse splenic lymphocytes. Groups of animals: **1**, intact animals; **2**, after immobilization stress; ■, control; ▨, animals in the presence of ConA + rIL-2. $*p < 0.05$.

transduction cascade, that is, interaction with the intracellular receptor cyclophilin and then inhibition of calcineurin activity. That is why CsA prevents the activation of two protein trans-factors (AP-1 and NF-AT), which are normally stimulated in IL-2 gene expression.[29]

Effect of Rotation Stress on c-fos and IL-2 Gene Expression in Different Brain Structures

Experiments were performed 30 minutes and two hours after the stress stimuli. This time was chosen because of the difference in the time of c-fos and IL-2 gene expression: c-fos mRNA is induced 5 minutes after stimuli application and achieves maximum in two hours,[3] but IL-2 mRNA synthesis is induced later. The earliest time for IL-2 mRNA induction in lymphocytes is two hours.[23]

The c-fos and IL-2 mRNA expression in rat brain was shown in intact animals at a very low level. C-fos mRNA was tested 30 minutes and two hours after the rotation stress in the hypothalamus (LHA), thalamus, striatum, and sensorimotor region of the brain. The induction of IL-2 mRNA was noted in the same brain structures plus the corpus collosum two hours after stress. Photomicrographs in FIGURE 3 show the number of c-fos–positive cells in LHA after rotation stress.

The testing of immediate-early gene expression as a marker of metabolic processes and neuronal cell activation allows detection of the earliest steps of cell activation. Thus, the nonantigenic stimuli cause the induction of the chains of molecular-genetic reactions in both immunocompetent and nervous cells.

Effect of Antigen Injection on c-fos and IL-2 Gene Expression in Brain Structures

Tetanus toxoid (TT) was selected as a nontoxic and highly purified bacterial antigen. Low levels of c-fos and IL-2 mRNA expression were noted in all investigated

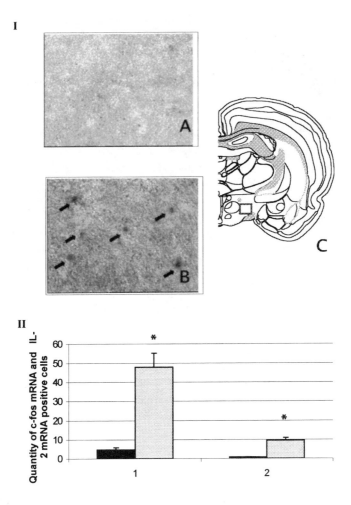

FIGURE 3. Photomicrographs of the lateralis hypothalamic area (LHA) with c-fos mRNA positive cells (*arrows*) in rat brain (**I**) and the quantity of c-fos (**1**) and IL-2 (**2**) mRNA positive cells in the LHA after rotation stress (**II**). Groups of rats: **A**, intact animals; **B**, animals after rotation stress; **C**, scheme of the brain (level 26 according to Swanson's Brain Maps). In a square, analyzed structures. Groups of animals: ■, intact; ▨, animals two hours after rotation stress. *$p < 0.05$.

brain structures of intact animals. Injection of saline did not lead to an increase in the number of c-fos and IL-2 mRNA positive cells in the PHA, LHA, DMH, VMH, AHA, and SO.

The iv TT injection markedly increased the number of c-fos mRNA positive cells in PHA, LHA, DMH, VMH, and AHA and IL-2 mRNA positive cells in PHA, DMH, and VMH two hours after injection.

Six hours after TT injection, activity of c-fos gene expression was decreased in PHA, LHA, and DMH compared with that after two hours. The level of c-fos mRNA positive cells at six hours was increased in PHA, LHA, AHA, and PVH compared to that after saline injection.

Six hours after TT injection, activation of IL-2 mRNA expression was shown only in PVH.

Photomicrographs in FIGURE 4 show c-fos mRNA positive cells in PVH after saline or TT injection in two and six hours. The quantity of c-fos mRNA positive

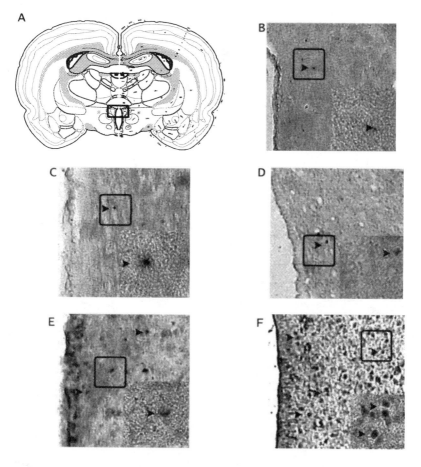

FIGURE 4. Photomicrographs of PVH with c-fos mRNA positive cells (*arrows*) in rat brain (Sprague-Dawley) after iv injection of saline or tetanus toxoid. (**A**) Scheme of the brain (level 26 according to Swanson's Brain Maps). In squares, analyzed structures. Groups of rats: (**B**) intact animals; (**C**) injection of saline in two hours; (**D**) injection of tetanus toxoid in two hours; (**E**) injection of saline in six hours; (**F**) injection of tetanus toxoid in six hours. In squares, part of the structures are shown; magnification ×40.

cells in the different hypothalamic structures of the rat brain after saline or TT injection in two and six hours is presented in FIGURE 5.

Photomicrographs in FIGURE 6 also show IL-2 mRNA positive cells in PVH after saline or TT injection in two and six hours. The quantity of IL-2 mRNA positive cells in the different hypothalamic structures of the rat brain after saline or TT injections in two and six hours is presented in FIGURE 7.

Thus, c-fos mRNA was not synthesized in PVH in two hours or in DMH and VMH in six hours. IL-2 mRNA was not detected in LHA, AHA, and PVH in two hours or in all brain structures besides PVH, in six hours.

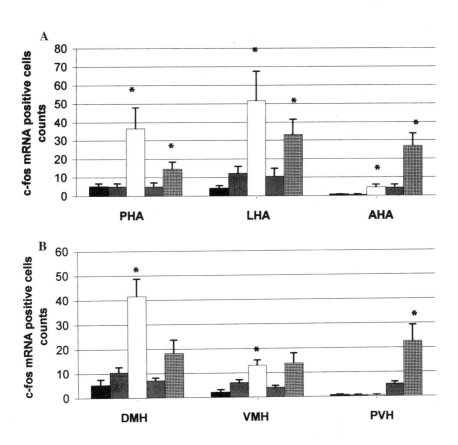

FIGURE 5. The quantity of c-fos mRNA positive cells in the different hypothalamic structures of the rat brain after saline or tetanus toxoid iv injection. Groups of rats: ■, intact; ▨, injection of saline in two hours; ☐, injection of tetanus foxoid in two hours; ▨, injection of saline in six hours; ▦, injection of tetanus toxoid in six hours. *$p < 0.05$ compared to injection of saline.

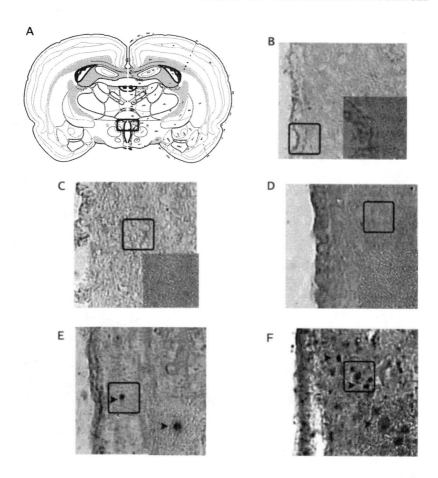

FIGURE 6. Photomicrographs of PVH with IL-2 mRNA positive cells (*arrows*) in rat brain (Sprague-Dawley) after i.v. injection of saline or tetanus toxoid. (**A**) Scheme of the brain (level 26 according to Swanson's Brain Maps). In squares, analyzed structures. Groups of rats: (**B**) intact animals; (**C**) two hours after injection of saline; (**D**) two hours after injection of tetanus toxoid; (**E**) six hours after injection of saline; (**F**) six hours after injection of tetanus toxoid. In squares, part of the structures are shown; magnification ×40.

CONCLUSIONS

The results confirm the earlier data of other investigators about the presence of c-fos mRNA and c-Fos–like immunoreactivity in the brain of intact animals on a low level.[16,29] Nonantigenic and antigenic stimulation resulted in increased c-fos gene expression in brain cells, which is in line with previous findings.[1–11] The induction of c-fos mRNA and IL-2 mRNA synthesis in different structures of the brain by nonantigenic stimuli and by an antigenic agent is shown. As just mentioned, c-Fos

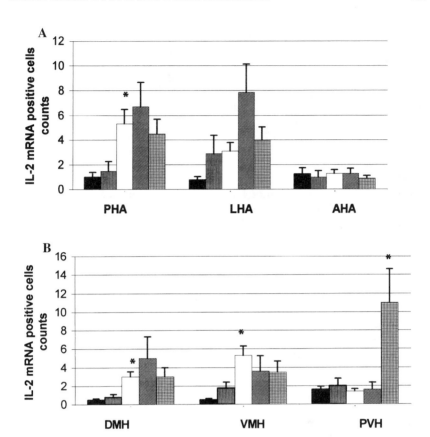

FIGURE 7. The quantity of IL-2 mRNA positive cells in the different hypothalamic structures of the rat brain after saline or tetanus toxoid iv injection. Groups of rats: ■, intact; ▥, two hours after injection of saline; ☐, two hours after injection of tetanus toxoid; ▨, six hours after injection of saline; ▦, six hours after injection of tetanus toxoid. *$p < 0.05$ compared to injection of saline.

protein is known as an transactivater of the IL-2 gene. The correlation of c-fos mRNA and IL-2 mRNA induction in the same structures of the brain after rotation stress or antigen injection can be understood on these grounds.

The increase in c-fos mRNA and IL-2 mRNA expression did not occur in all investigated structures, and higher levels of these mRNAs have been observed in hypothalamic structures (LHA and PVN). The hypothalamic-pituitary-adrenal axis is activated by stress stimuli. High levels of c-fos and IL-2 gene expression in hypothalamic structures after stress application might be expected as evidence of their activation as regulators of the hypothalamic-pituitary-adrenal axis.

The data obtained showed elevated levels of c-fos mRNA expression in definite brain structures two hours after TT injection, and decreased levels in six hours. These results correspond to the data of Riverst[30] who detected maximum levels of c-fos mRNA expression in three hours and degradation of mRNA by 9–12 hours after injection of LPS. The dynamics of activation of c-fos and IL-2 mRNA expression in the hypothalamic structures after antigen injection also corresponded to the dynamics of electrical activity of rat hypothalamic structures after antigen injection.[31] The first wave of electrical activity evaluation in the hypothalamic structures was shown 30 minutes two hours after antigen injection. Intensive changes were observed in PHA. Less intensive activation was found in PVN, VMH, and AHA. The activation of c-fos mRNA expression in two hours after TT injection in PHA, LHA, DMH, VMH, and AHA was shown. The activation of IL-2 mRNA expression was found in PHA, VMH, and DMH two hours after TT application. So, the correlation between the electrical activity of the hypothalamic structures (PHA, AHA, and VMH) and c-fos and IL-2 expression was shown. Interestingly, activation of c-fos and IL-2 expression in PVH appeared only six hours after the influence of antigen. Possibly, "late" activation of PVH is connected with activation of neurohormonal mechanisms of the reaction to antigen.

The data show that induction of c-fos mRNA and IL-2 mRNA takes place in definite structures of the brain; for instance, c-fos mRNA was noted in PHA, LHA, AHA, DMH, and VMH, whereas IL-2 mRNA was not detected in LHA, AHA, and PVH in 2 hours, possibly because c-Fos protein is working as a transactivating factor not only for activation of IL-2 gene expression but also for induction of another inducible gene expression.

It is important to analyze c-fos and IL-2 gene expression after antigen injection combined with stressor stimuli.

REFERENCES

1. GREENBERG, M.E. & E.B. ZIFF. 1984. Nature. **311:** 433–434.
2. CECCATELLI, S., M.J. VILLAR, M. GOLDSTEIN & T. HOKFELT. 1989. Proc. Natl. Acad. Sci. USA **86:** 9569–9573.
3. BULLITT, E. 1990. J. Comp. Neurol. **296:** 517–530.
4. IMAKI, T., T. SHIBASAKI, M. HOTTA & H. DEMURA. 1993. Endocrinology **131:** 240–246.
5. MURPHY, T.H, P.F. WORLEY, Y. NAKABEPPU, B. CHRISTY, J. GASTEL & J.M. BARABAN. 1991. J. Neurochem. **57:** 1862–1872.
6. SCHREIBER, S.S., G. TOCCO, T.J. SHORS & R.F. TOMPSON. 1991. Neuroreport **2:** 17–20.
7. HUNT, S.P, A. PINI & G. EVAN. 1987. Nature **328:** 632–634.
8. CHANG, M.M., S.E. LEEMAN & H.D. NIALL. 1971. Nature **232:** 86–87.
9. RICHARD, D., S. RIVEST & C. RIVIER. 1992. Brain **594:** 131–137.
10. SHENG, M. & M.E. GREENBERG. 1990. Neurons **4:** 477–485.
11. MORGAN, J.I. & T. CURRAN. 1991. Annu. Rev. Neurosci. **14:** 421–451.
12. HATAKEYAMA, M. & T. TANIGUCHI. 1991. *In* Interleukin-2. Peptide Growth Factors and Their Receptors I. M.B. Sporn & A.B. Roberts, Eds.: 523–540. Springer-Verlag. New York.
13. AWATSUJI, H., Y. FURUKAWA, M. NAKAJIMA, S. FURUKAWA & K. HAYASHI. 1993. J. Neurosci. Res. **35:** 305–311.
14. KARANTH, S., L. KRZYSZTOF & S.M. MCCANN. 1993. Proc. Natl. Acad. Sci. USA **90:** 3383–3387.
15. ARAJIO, D.M., P.A. LAPCHAK, B. COLLIER & R. QUIRION. 1989. Brain Res. **498:** 257–266.
16. LAPCHAK, P.A, D.M. ARAJIO, R. QUIRION & A. BEAUDET. 1991. Neuroscience **44:** 173–184.

17. BANKS, W.A., A.J. KASTIN & R.D. BROADWELL. 1995. Neuroimmunomodulation **2:** 241–248.
18. OLADEHINE, A.& C.M. BLATTEIS. 1995. Neuroimmunomodulation **2:** 282–289.
19. GAYKEMA, R.P.A., L.E. GOEHLER, F.J.H. TILDERS, J.G.J.M. BOL, M. McGORRY, M. FLESHNER, S.F. MAIER & L.R. WATKINS. 1998. **5:** 234–240.
20. ORLANDINI, M.. L. MARCONCINI, R. FERRUZZI & S. OLIVIERO. 1996. Proc. Natl. Acad. Sci. USA **93:** 11675–11680.
21. MOUZAKI, A., R. WEIL, L. MUSTER & D. RUNGGER. 1991. EMBO J. **10:** 1399–1406.
22. MOUZAKI, A., Y. DAI, R. WEIL & D. RUNGGER. 1992. Cytokine **4:** 151–160.
23. GOLOVKO, O.I., T.V. GRISHINA, N.S. NOVIKOVA, M.A. NOSOV, A.A. MULBERG, E.A. KORNEVA & T.B. KAZAKOVA. 1996. Neurokhimiya **13:** 194–204 (in Russian).
24. CHOMCZYNSKI, P.& N. SACCHI. 1987. Analyt. Biochem. **162:** 156–159.
25. MANNIATIS, T., E. FRITSCH & J. SAMBROOK. 1993. *In* Molecular Cloning. A Labor Manual. : 1–479. Cold Spring Harbor Laboratory.
26. BOEHRINGER MANHEIM. 1992. *In* Nonradioactive in situ Hybridization. Application Manual. GmbH. Biochemica. : 1-75.
27. SWANSON, L.W. 1992. *In* Brain Maps Computer Graphics Files. Elsevier Sci. B.V., Amsterdam, The Netherlands.
28. DRAGUNOW, M., M.R. PETERSON & H.A. ROBERTSON. 1987. Eur. J. Pharmacol. **135:** 113–114.
29. KORNEVA, E.A., E.G. RYBAKINA, E.E. FOMICHEVA & I.A. KOZINEZ. 1992. Int. J. Tiss. Reac. **14:** 219–224.
30. RIVEST , S., G. TORRES & C. RIVIER. 1992. Brain Res. **587:** 13–23.
31. KORNEVA, E.A., V.A. GRIGORYEV, V.M. KLIMENKO & Y.D. STOLAROV. 1989. *In* Electro-physiological Immune Reactions. : 1–47. Nauka. Leningrad.

Tumor Necrosis Factor-α Induces Neuronal Death by Silencing Survival Signals Generated by the Type I Insulin-Like Growth Factor Receptor

H.D. VENTERS,[a] R. DANTZER,[b] AND K.W. KELLEY[a]

[a]Laboratory of Immunophysiology, Department of Animal Sciences, University of Illinois, Urbana, Illinois 61801, USA

[b]INSERM U394, Integrative Neurobiology, 33077 Bordeaux Cedex, France

ABSTRACT: Within the central nervous system, the proinflammatory cytokine tumor necrosis factor (TNF)-α is best characterized by its ability to directly foment signals of death. However, recent evidence suggests that TNF-α also promotes neurodegeneration through inhibition of a vital survival signal, insulin-like growth factor-I (IGF-I). By inhibiting essential components of the IGF-I survival response, such as phosphatidylinositol 3′-kinase (PI 3-kinase), low nontoxic concentrations of TNF-α indirectly trigger the death of neurons. We suggest that this inhibition of survival signaling is a pathophysiologically relevant action of TNF-α in the brain. This type of cross-talk by which vastly different receptors utilize shared intracellular substrates is potentially applicable to a broad number of receptors that are coexpressed on the same cell. The use of neuronal growth factors in the treatment of neurodegenerative diseases, such as cerebral ischemia and the AIDS dementia complex, may prove much more effective if the elevated expression of TNF-α in these disorders is neutralized.

SILENCING OF DEATH AND SURVIVAL SIGNALS

Tumor necrosis factor-alpha (TNF-α) is a proinflammatory cytokine with a wide range of biological effects, but it is best characterized by its ability to induce death signals. Because TNF receptors have a well-characterized death domain,[1] the cytotoxic property of TNF-α has largely been interpreted as a consequence of a direct effect of this cytokine on its cell targets. Data reported earlier this year established that the death signal induced after activation of the TNF-α receptor can be blocked by an intracellular protein that binds to one of the TNF receptors and is known as the silencer of death domain (SODD).[2] From experiments carried out on neurons, it is now apparent that TNF-α can induce cell death by interfering with important cellular survival signals.[3] This mechanism is more likely than direct cytotoxicity to represent events during pathophysiological conditions and implies the necessity of replacing current linear models of life and death signals with more realistic cross-talk models.

Most of the current literature concerning signaling systems that regulate the life and death of a cell focuses almost exclusively on activation of either a survival or a death receptor. However, the simultaneous activation of both survival and death signals is likely to happen *in vivo*. In primary cultures of granular neurons from the cerebella of mice, low picogram concentrations of TNF-α effectively inhibit survival signals that ensue from activation of the insulin-like growth factor-I (IGF-I) receptor.[3] These data not only provide indirect proof for the expression of a functionally active receptor for TNF-α on neurons, but also offer the unexpected result that very low concentrations of TNF-α can have important effects on normal nontransformed cells.

CYTOKINE SIGNALS OF DEATH AND SURVIVAL IN THE BRAIN

Neurons in the CNS are exposed to a myriad of life and death signals. During nervous system development, approximately one and a half times the final number of neurons are created. Excess, unutilized neurons are culled from the overall population through apoptosis. During this same time, neuronal growth factors, such as nerve growth factor (NGF), the neurotrophins (BDNF, NT-3, NT-4, and NT-5), and IGF-I, promote neuronal growth, differentiation, and survival (reviewed in Ref. 4). Later in life, neuronal cell death may result from pathological causes such as trauma, toxicity, vascular disorder, infection, or genetic diseases. During these events, neuronal death may occur through either apoptosis or necrosis. Contemporary understanding suggests not only that both apoptosis and necrosis may occur in parallel during CNS degeneration (reviewed in Ref. 5), but also that hybrid forms of neuronal death may be observed.[6]

Investigation of the regulation of immune events has led to the concept of cytokines counterbalancing one another to either promote (proinflammatory) or inhibit (anti-inflammatory) inflammation. This balancing system, which is heavily weighted towards anti-inflammatory signals in the normal brain, ultimately controls the life and death of neurons. Conversely, proinflammatory signals likely predominate during neurodegenerative conditions such as Alzheimer's disease.[7] It is widely accepted that pro- and anti-inflammatory cytokines inhibit the synthesis of one another. As early as 1993, Chao and colleagues[8] convincingly demonstrated that interleukin-4 (IL-4) inhibits the synthesis of TNF-α by activated microglia, thereby promoting the survival of neurons.[8] Recent evidence intimates a more subtle, yet physiologically relevant level of regulation between pro- and anti-inflammatory cytokines in the brain.[3] This regulation occurs at the level of two receptors that are coexpressed on the same cell such as receptors for IGF-I and TNF-α. In this view, activation on one receptor affects an intracellular substrate on a second receptor. This effect can be either positive or negative. The receptors for two molecules, IGF-I and TNF-α, provide an apt model for this new concept and its application to neuronal survival.

TNF-α AS A SIGNAL OF DEATH

The pleiotropic cytokine TNF-α exerts a variety of biological actions in different tissues. Within the CNS, TNF-α is known to initiate cascades associated with neuronal apoptosis and neurological impairment.[9,10] TNF-α has been implicated as contributing to neuronal death in brain ischemia and HIV-1 infection. TNF-α expression increases following ischemic insult to brain tissue,[11] which correlates with neuronal death. Interruption of TNF-α signaling through administration of a fragment of the soluble TNF receptor reduces the size of infarct incurred during ischemia.[12] In an *in vitro* model of HIV infection that uses Tat protein-induced neuronal apoptosis, blockade of TNF-α action abrogates cell death.[13,14] In addition to its cytotoxic effects on neurons, TNF-α can promote the apoptotic demise of both normal oligodendrocytes[15] and cancerous gliomas.[16]

Contrary to the preponderance of evidence that TNF-α is toxic to neurons, it has also been reported to be neuroprotective, particularly in conditions of excitotoxic death of neurons caused by glutamate, NMDA, AMPA/kainate activation, and glucose deprivation.[17] The exact factors responsible for shifting the effect of TNF-α from neurotoxicity to neuroprotection are not known, but likely include cell and receptor type, culture conditions, and the concentration of TNF-α used.

Two different receptors for TNF (TNFR) have been identified and are expressed as the p55 kDa (type 1) and p75 (type 2) kDa isoforms. The ability of TNF-α to signal apoptosis has been linked to the association of TNFR1-associated death domain protein (TRADD) to the TNFR1 (p55) death domain. Binding of a second protein, Fas-associated death domain (FADD), to the TRADD-death domain complex initiates the apoptotic signal cascade.[18] This cascade includes caspase-8 (FLICE)-induced activation of acid sphingomyelinase, resulting in cleavage of sphingomyelin to ceramide and phosphorylcholine.[19] Ceramide produced by sphingomyelinases has been recognized as an important second messenger, capable of activating the ceramide-activated protein kinase, ceramide-activated protein phosphatase, and protein kinase Cζ. Signaling through this pathway is known to promote apoptosis in numerous cell types (reviewed in Ref. 20). Interestingly, activation of ceramide pathways using non-apoptotic doses of a ceramide analog (C2) inhibits IGF-I-stimulated proliferation of breast cancer cell lines (MCF-7, T47D) much as non-apoptotic doses of TNF-α can inhibit IGF-I survival promotion in primary neurons.[3,21]

Other proteins, such as TNFR-associated factor 2 (TRAF2) and receptor-interacting protein (RIP) are similarly recruited to TRADD and signal *c-jun* N-terminal kinase/stress-activated protein kinase (JNK/SAPK) and NF-κB activation, respectively.[22,23]

TNF-α–mediated activation of apoptosis is regulated at the level of the p55 receptor itself. A recent report by Jiang *et al.*[2] identifies a protein, SODD, that commonly associates with the p55 death domain and is released upon ligand binding. The release of this inhibitory protein allows for TRADD association. The degree of SODD association with the p55 death domain may therefore constitutively regulate TNF-α–dependent death signaling.

IGF-I AS A SURVIVAL SIGNAL

IGF-I is a well-characterized growth factor for a variety of cells, including those of the hematopoietic system.[24,25] This same antiapoptotic property of IGF-I occurs in neurons.[26] Binding sites for IGF-I are found on numerous types of neurons, including forebrain, midbrain, and cerebellar neurons.[27,28] IGF-I appears to possess the ability to improve neuronal survival in conditions of brain insults that are typically associated with an overexpression of proinflammatory cytokines, such as stroke, brain trauma, multiple sclerosis, Alzheimer's disease, and various neuropathies (reviewed in Ref. 29). Stroke patients exhibit an immediate decrease in plasma IGF-I and IGF-I binding protein (IGFBP)-3 levels, which is sustained throughout 10 days postinfarct.[30] A similar observation has been made with regard to IGF-I and IGFBP mRNA expression after hypoxic-ischemic injury in rat brain.[31] Administration of IGF-I both before[32] and after[33] hypoxic-ischemic injury reduces neuronal death. The use of IGF-I recombinant analogs to occupy IGFBPs, thereby releasing more unbound IGF-I for neuroprotection, diminishes the size of infarct in an experimental model of brain ischemia.[34]

In addition to neurons, microglial cells are known to both express[35] and respond to IGF-I. The rapid proliferation of astrocytes at sites of nerve damage has led to numerous investigations of a role for IGF-I in astroglial scarring. One recent report indicates that continuous infusion of IGF-I to the cerebellum decreases this type of reactive astrogliosis.[36]

The protective effects of IGF-I in the central nervous system do not require the induction of cell death. In a model of fully reversible brain inflammation induced by intracerebroventricular administration of the cytokine inducer lipopolysaccharide (LPS), IGF-I centrally injected attenuated LPS-induced behavioral depression[37] in exactly the same manner as the classical anti-inflammatory cytokine IL-10.[38]

Most IGF-I survival signals are mediated by the type I IGF receptor, a heterotetramer containing tyrosine kinase activity (reviewed in Ref. 39). This receptor has a high affinity for IGF-I (1×10^{-10} M), an approximately 10-fold lower affinity for IGF-II, and an approximately 10- to 100-fold lower affinity for insulin. The IGF-I receptor mediates its effects by signaling through a transmembrane disulfide-linked heterotetramer (βααβ) that shares a high degree of homology to the closely related insulin receptor. The ligand-binding α chains are extracellular, whereas the β chains, essentially tyrosine kinases, are transmembrane. Following binding of IGF-I, β chains of the IGF-I receptor undergo phosphorylation on tyrosine residues at a variety of sites in the juxtamembrane, regulatory, and carboxyl terminal regions. The best characterized substrates of the IGF-I receptor, IRS-1 and IRS-2, are also the major substrates of the insulin receptor (reviewed in Ref. 40). These cytosolic substrates have multiple tyrosine residues located in YMXM or YXXM motifs. IRS-1 and IRS-2 act as docking proteins that regulate the activities of other intracellular proteins containing src homology 2 (SH2) and src homology 3 (SH3). The IRS-1 and IRS-2 proteins have been reported to differentially regulate cellular responses, such as those that occur in brown fat in response to insulin and IGF-I.[41]

The phosphorylation of IRS proteins on tyrosine residues leads to their association with the 85-kDa regulatory subunit of phosphatidylinositol-3′ kinase (PI 3-kinase). PI 3-kinase is a lipid and serine kinase consisting of an 85-kDa regulatory subunit containing two SH2 domains. The p110 kDa subunit of PI 3-kinase catalyzes the phosphorylation of membrane bound PI, PI 4-phosphate, and PI 4,5-biphosphate on the 3′ position of the inositol ring. The products of the PI 3-kinase reaction are D-3 phosphorylated phosphoinositides, which signal downstream events involved in regulating cell growth and metabolism (reviewed in Ref. 42). A recent report using rat hypothalamic GT1-7 cells observed a PI 3-kinase-dependent induction of NF-κB that was associated with neuronal cell survival.[43]

IGF-I inhibits the actions of TNF-α in a variety of cells, including oligodendrocytes.[44] The oncogenic properties of *c-myc*, which promotes apoptosis through the FAS (also known as CD95 and APO-1) receptor-ligand pathway, are inhibited by IGF-I. IGF-I acts on the *c-myc* pathway downstream of Fas in reducing apoptosis.[45] This antagonism of apoptosis is observed in neonatal rat islets of Langerhans, where treatment with TNF-α and gamma interferon (IFN-γ) induce Fas-mediated apoptosis. and pretreatment with IGF-I eliminates Fas-mediated killing.[46]

TNF-α INHIBITION OF SURVIVAL SIGNALING

Recent evidence suggests that in a proinflammatory cytokines inhibit the actions of anti-inflammatory cytokines. Examples include IFN-γ inhibition of IL-4 receptor expression[47] and IL-4–induced STAT6 acting as an antagonist of NFκβ binding.[48]

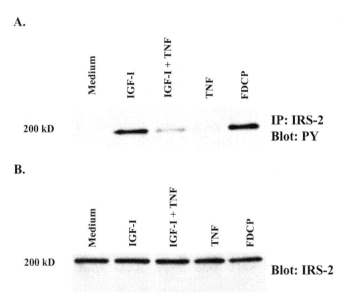

FIGURE 1. TNF-α reduces tyrosine phosphorylation of IRS-2 in murine cerebellar granule neurons. (**A**) Tyrosine phosphorylation (PY) of IRS-2 in neurons. Neurons were cultured and treated with IGF-I (100 ng/ml), TNF-α (10 pg/ml), or both. Whole cell lysates were precipitated with an anti–IRS-2 antibody, separated by SDS-PAGE electrophoresis, transferred to vinylidene difluoride membranes, and blotted with an antibody to phosphotyrosine. Addition of IGF-I to cerebellar neurons or the positive control FDCP myeloid progenitor cells led to substantial phosphorylation on tyrosine of the IRS-2 protein. Pretreatment with TNF-α potently inhibited the ability of IGF-I to tryosine phosphorylate IRS-2, whereas TNF-α alone had no effect. (**B**) IRS-2 protein expression. The IRS-2 protein, as assessed by Western blotting with an anti-IRS-2 antibody, was uniformly expressed in granule neurons regardless of treatment. Adapted from Venters *et al.*[3]

Best characterized is the ability of TNF-α to inhibit insulin signaling in hepatic and adipose cells.[49,50] In these experiments, TNF-α inhibited both insulin receptor auto-phosphorylation and downstream signaling such as IRS recruitment and PI 3-kinase activation. TNF-α–induced cleavage of sphingomyelin to ceramide and choline by sphingomyelinase appears to be the postreceptor mechanism for this phenomenon. Beyond receptor substrates, TNF-α has also been observed to inhibit insulin-induced activation of the transcription factor STAT5 in mouse muscle cells[51] and IGF-I–induced protein synthesis in human muscle cells.[52]

Within the CNS, TNF-α has recently been identified as a potent inhibitor of IGF-I signaling in cerebellar granule neurons.[3] These observations were made using doses of TNF-α that were sufficiently low as to not directly cause neurodegeneration. In these experiments, IRS-2 was identified as the primary form of IRS in murine

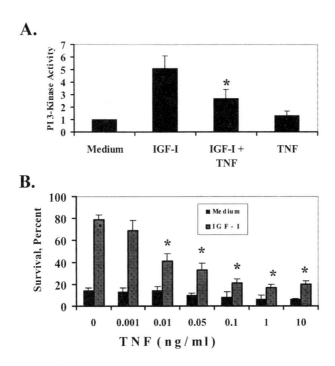

FIGURE 2. TNF-α inhibits the ability of IGF-I to increase PI 3-kinase enzymatic activity in IRS-2 immunoprecipitates and to subsequently promote neuronal survival. (**A**) IRS-2 precipitable PI 3-kinase activity in neurons. TNF-α (10 pg/ml) inhibits (*$p < 0.005$) the ability of IGF-I to activate PI 3-kinase in lysates from cerebellar granule neurons immunoprecipitated with an anti-IRS-2 antibody. (**B**) Neuronal survival. TNF-α causes neuronal degeneration by blocking the ability of IGF-I to promote neuronal survival. Cerebellar granule neurons were treated with concentrations of TNF-α ranging from 1 to 10,000 pg/ml in the presence or absence of IGF-I (100 ng/ml), and cell survival was measured 24 hours later. The survival-promoting ability of IGF-I was inhibited (*$p < 0.05$) by 50% with as little as 10 pg/ml TNF-α and almost fully blocked at a concentration of 100 pg/ml. Adapted from Venters *et al.*[3]

cerebellar granule neurons. Pretreatment with TNF-α at 10 pg/ml for 40 minutes was able to effectively block tyrosine phosphorylation of IRS-2 that resulted from a 3-minute incubation with IGF-I (see FIGURE 1A). This effect of TNF-α occurred without reducing IRS-2 protein expression (FIG. 1B). The same experimental conditions revealed that TNF-α (10 pg/ml) also inhibited IGF-I promotion of IRS-2 precipitable PI 3-kinase activity (see FIGURE 2A). Each of these signaling events constitutes essential components of IGF-I survival promotion.[40,42] Most significantly, however, 10 pg/ml of TNF-α dramatically inhibited the ability of IGF-I to promote neuronal survival (FIG. 2B). In these experiments, the effects of TNF-α survival-promotion were achieved without a direct contribution of TNF-α to cell toxicity.

The appearance of both TNF-α and IGF-I in perivascular tissue during ischemia supports some sort of interaction between these two proteins. The ability of a soluble form of the p55 TNF-α receptor[11] as well as a specific antibody to TNF-α[10] to assuage neuronal death during ischemia may result as much from enabling IGF-I survival signaling as from inhibition of TNF-α neurotoxicity. Inhibition of both IRS-2 phosphorylation and PI 3-kinase activation allows TNF-α to dampen the otherwise vigorous anti-inflammatory signaling pathway initiated by IGF-I binding to its receptor.

These observations create an interesting question with respect to sites of receptor interaction. Given the ability of TNF-α to inhibit insulin and IGF-I at the level of receptor activation, one might suppose that this is the sole site of interaction between TNF-α and these survival factors. However, the ability of TNF-α to induce serine phosphorylation of IRS proteins suggests that TNF-α may interfere with more than one signaling event within an individual survival pathway.

Another cytokine known to induce resistance to insulin and IGF-I signaling is IL-1. Both IL-1 and TNF-α are potent proinflammatory cytokines known to often exert similar effects in the periphery and CNS.[53] It is therefore possible that the inhibition of survival signaling caused by TNF-α will be applicable to IL-1.

CONCLUDING REMARKS

Overexpression of TNF-α and other proinflammatory cytokines in the brain has been implicated in a variety of neuropathologies, including the AIDS dementia complex and stroke. The emerging concept is that the clinical outcome of inflammatory events in the central nervous system is dependent upon the balance of proinflammatory cytokines and anti-inflammatory cytokines. The molecular character of crosstalk between receptors for proinflammatory cytokines and neuronal survival factors is more complex than previously thought. In cerebellar granule neurons, low, picogram amounts of TNF-α act to potently inhibit both the IRS-2 phosphorylation and PI 3-kinase activation that play a pivotal role in IGF-I signaling. This mechanism of action appears to apply to different cell types during inflammation and may be of greater pathological significance than direct cytotoxicity, which requires much higher concentrations of TNF-α. These data support a new model for neurodegeneration whereby a proinflammatory cytokine inhibits the activation of receptors for anti-inflammatory cytokines (see FIGURE 3).[54] We term this phenomenon the silencing

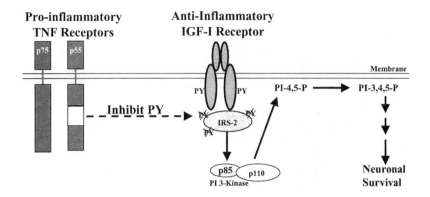

FIGURE 3. Molecular basis for the silencing of survival signals (SOSS) as a new concept in neurodegeneration. TNF-α (10 pg/ml) inhibition of IGF-I survival signaling in neurons is accompanied by a significant impairment in the ability of IGF-I to tyrosine phosphorylate (PY) IRS-2, which is the major IRS docking protein in murine granule neurons. Reduced tyrosine phosphorylation of IRS-2 leads to inhibition in the ability of this large docking protein to activate the survival enzyme PI 3-kinase. By inhibiting key IGF-I survival signals such as PI 3-kinase, TNF-α promotes neurodegeneration without directly inducing neurotoxicity. From Venters *et al.*[60]

of survival signals (SOSS). This model may help to explain the mechanism by which IGF-I protects neurons in various neurodegenerative conditions associated with overexpression of proinflammatory cytokines.[29] This model also suggests that targeting neurons with exogenous IGF-I during neurodegeneration may prove to be much more efficient when matched with efforts to inhibit TNF-α signaling.

REFERENCES

1. WEISS, T., M. GRELL, K. SIEMIENSKI, F. MUHLENBECK, H. DURKOP, K. PFIZENMAIER, P. SCHEURICH & H. WAJANT. 1998. TNFR80-dependent enhancement of TNFR60-induced cell death is mediated by TNFR-associated factor 2 and is specific for TNFR60. J. Immunol. **161:** 3136–3142.
2. JIANG, Y., J.D. WORONICZ, W. LIU & D.V. GOEDDEL. 1999. Prevention of constitutive TNF receptor 1 signaling by silencer of death domains. Science **283:** 543–546.
3. VENTERS, H.D., Q. TANG, Q. LIU, R.W. VANHOY, R. DANTZER & K.W. KELLEY. 1999. A new mechanism of neurodegeneration: a proinflammatory cytokine inhibits receptor signaling by a survival peptide. Proc. Natl. Acad. Sci. USA **96:** 9879–9884.
4. CONNOR, B. & M. DRAGUNOW. 1998. The role of neuronal growth factors in neurodegenerative disorders of the human brain. Brain. Res. Brain. Res. Rev. **27:** 1–39.
5. LEE, J.M., G.J. ZIPFEL & D.W. CHOI. 1999. The changing landscape of ischaemic brain injury mechanisms. Nature **399:** A7–A14.
6. MACMANUS, J.P., I. RASQUINHA, U. TUOR & E. PRESTON. 1997. Detection of higher-order 50- and 10-kbp DNA fragments before apoptotic internucleosomal cleavage after transient cerebral ischemia. J. Cereb. Blood Flow Metab. **17:** 376–387.
7. COTTER, R.L., W.J. BURKE, V.S. THOMAS, J.F. POTTER, J. ZHENG & H.E. GENDELMAN. 1999. Insights into the neurodegenerative process of Alzheimer's disease: a role for mononuclear phagocyte-associated inflammation and neurotoxicity. J. Leuk. Biol. **65:** 416–427.

8. CHAO, C.C., T.W. MOLITOR & S. HU. 1993. Neuroprotective role of IL-4 against activated microglia. J. Immunol. **151:** 1473–1481.

9. PERRY, S.W., J.A. HAMILTON, L.W. TJOELKER, G. DBAIBO, K.A. DZENKO, L.G. EPSTEIN, Y. HANNUN, J.S. WHITTAKER, S. DEWHURST & H.A. GELBHARD. 1998. Platelet-activating factor receptor activation: an initiator step in HIV-1 neuropathogenesis. J. Biol. Chem. **273:** 17660–17664.

10. KNOBLACH, S.M., L. FAN & A.I. FADEN. 1999. Early neuronal expression of tumor necrosis factor-α after experimental brain injury contributes to neurological impairment. J. Neuroimmunol. **95:** 115–125.

11. BARONE, F.C., B. ARVIN, R.F. WHITE, A. MILLER, C.L. WEBB, R.N. WILLETTE, P.G. LYSKO & G.Z. FEUERSTEIN. 1997. Tumor necrosis factor-α. A mediator of focal ischemic brain injury. Stroke **28:** 1233–1244.

12. NAWASHIRO, H., D. MARTIN & J.M. HALLENBECK. 1997. Neuroprotective effects of TNF binding protein in focal cerebral ischemia. Brain Res. **778:** 265–271.

13. NEW, D.R., S.B. MAGGIRWAR, L.G. EPSTEIN, S. DEWHURST & H.A. GELBARD. 1998. HIV-1 Tat induces neuronal death via tumor necrosis factor-α and activation of non-N-methyl-D-aspartate receptors by a NFκB-independent mechanism. J. Biol. Chem. **273:** 17852–17858.

14. SHI, B., J. RAINA, A. LORENZO, J. BUSCIGLIO & D. GABUZDA. 1998. Neuronal apoptosis induced by HIV-1 Tat protein and TNF-α: potentiation of neurotoxicity mediated by oxidative stress and implications for HIV-1 dementia. J. Neurovirol. **4:** 281–290.

15. SELMAJ, K., C.S. RAINE, M. FAROOQ, W.T. NORTON & C.F. BROSNAN. 1991. Cytokine cytotoxicity against oligodendrocytes: apoptosis induced by lymphotoxin. J. Immunol. **147:** 1522–1529.

16. ASHLEY, D.M., J.H. SAMPSON, G.E. ARCHER, L.P. HALE & D.D. BIGNER. 1998. Local production of TGF beta 1 inhibits cerebral edema, enhances TNF-α induced apoptosis and improves survival in a murine glioma model. J. Neuroimmunol. **86:** 46–52.

17. CHENG, B., S. CHRISTAKOS & M.P. MATTSON. 1994. Tumor necrosis factors protect neurons against metabolic-excitotoxic insults and promote maintenance of calcium homeostasis. Neuron **12:** 139–153.

18. HSU, H., J. XIONG & D.V. GOEDDEL. 1995. The TNF receptor 1-associated protein TRADD signals cell death and NF-κB activation. Cell **81:** 495–504.

19. SCHWANDNER, R., K. WIEGMANN, K. BERNARDO, D. KREDER & M. KRONKE. 1998. TNF receptor death domain-associated proteins TRADD and FADD signal activation of acid sphingomyelinase. J. Biol. Chem. **273:** 5916–5922.

20. MATHIAS, S., L.A. PENA & R.N. KOLESNICK. 1998. Signal transduction of stress via ceramide. Biochem. J. **335:** 465–480.

21. PERKS, C.M., Z.P. GILL, P.V. NEWCOMB & J.M. HOLLY. 1999. Activation of integrin and ceramide signalling pathways can inhibit the mitogenic effect of insulin-like growth factor I (IGF-I) in human breast cancer cell lines. Br. J. Cancer **79:** 701–706.

22. LIU, Z.G., H. HSU, D.V. GOEDDEL & M. KARIN. 1996. Dissection of TNF receptor 1 effector functions: JNK activation is not linked to apoptosis while NF-κB activation prevents cell death. Cell **87:** 565–576.

23. NATOLI, G., A. COSTANZO, A. IANNI, D.J. TEMPLETON, J.R. WOODGETT, C. BALSANO & M. LEVRERO. 1997. Activation of SAPK/JNK by TNF receptor 1 through a noncytotoxic TRAF2-dependent pathway. Science **275:** 200–203.

24. TSARFATY, G., D.L. LONGO & W.J. MURPHY. 1994. Human insulin-like growth factor I exerts hematopoietic growth-promoting effects after in vivo administration. Exp. Hematol. **22:** 1273–1277.

25. MINSHALL, C., S. ARKINS, J. STRAZA, J. CONNERS, R. DANTZER, G.G. FREUND & K.W. KELLEY. 1997. IL-4 and insulin-like growth factor-I inhibit the decline in Bcl-2 and promote the survival of IL-3-deprived myeloid progenitors. J. Immunol. **159:** 1225–1232.

26. DUDEK, H., S.R. DATTA, T.F. FRANKE, M.J. BIRNBAUM, R. YAO, G.M. COOPER, R.A. SEGAL, D.R. KAPLAN & M.E. GREENBERG. 1997. Regulation of neuronal survival by the serine-threonine protein kinase Akt. Science **275:** 661–665.

27. GARCIA-SEGURA, L.M., J.R. RODRIGUEZ & I. TORRES-ALLEMAN. 1997. Localization of the insulin-like growth factor I receptor in the cerebellum and hypothalamus of adult rats: an electron microscopic study. J. Cytol. **26:** 479–490.

28. KAR, S., J.G. CHABOT & R. QUIRION. 1993. Quantitative autoradiographic localization of [^{125}I]insulin-like growth factor I, [^{125}I]insulin-like growth factor II, and [^{125}I]insulin receptor binding sites in developing and adult rat brain. J. Comp. Neurol. **333:** 375–397.

29. DORE, S., S. KAR & R. QUIRION. 1997. Rediscovering an old friend, IGF-I: potential use in the treatment of neurodegenerative diseases. Trends Neurosci. **20:** 326–331.

30. SCHWAB, S., M. SPRANGER, S. KREMPIEN, W. HACKE & M. BETTENDORF. 1997. Plasma insulin-like growth factor I and IGF binding protein 3 levels in patients with acute cerebral ischemic injury. Stroke **28:** 1744–1748.

31. LEE, W.H., G.M. WANG, L.B. SEAMAN & S.J. VANNUCCI. 1996. Coordinate IGF-I and IGFBP5 gene expression in perinatal rat brain after hypoxia-ischemia. J. Cereb. Blood Flow Metab. **16:** 227–236.

32. TAGAMI, M., K. IKEDA, Y. NARA, H. FUJINO, A. KUBOTA, F. NUMANO & Y. YAMORI. 1997. Insulin-like growth factor-I attenuates apoptosis in hippocampal neurons caused by cerebral ischemia and reperfusion in stroke-prone spontaneously hypertensive rats. Lab. Invest. **76:** 613–617.

33. GUAN, J., S.J. SKINNER, E.J. BEILHARZ, K.M. HUA, S. HODGKINSON, P.D. GLUCKMAN & C.E. WILLIAMS. 1996. The movement of IGF-I into the brain parenchyma after hypoxic-ischaemic injury. Neuroreport **7:** 632–636.

34. LODDICK, S.A., X.J. LIU, Z.X. LU, C. LIU, D.P. BEHAN, D.C. CHALMERS, A.C. FOSTER, W.W. VALE, N. LING & E.B. DE SOUZA. 1998. Displacement of insulin-like growth factors from their binding proteins as a potential treatment for stroke. Proc. Natl. Acad. Sci. USA **95:** 1894–1898.

35. ARKINS, S., N. REBEIZ, A. BIRAGYN, D.L. REESE & K.W. KELLEY. 1993. Murine macrophages express abundant insulin-like growth factor-I class I Ea and Eb transcripts. Endocrinology **133:** 2334–2343.

36. FERNANDEZ, A.M., J. GARCIA-ESTRADA, L.M. GARCIA-SEGURA & I. TORRES-ALEMAN. 1997. Insulin-like growth factor I modulates c-Fos induction and astrocytosis in response to neurotoxic insult. Neuroscience **76:** 117–122.

37. DANTZER, R., G. GHEUSI, R.W. JOHNSON & K.W. KELLEY. 1999. Central administration of insulin-like growth factor-1 inhibits lipopolysaccharide-induced sickness behavior in mice. Neuroreport **10:** 289–292.

38. BLUTHE, R.M., N. CASTANON, F. POUSSET, A. BRISTOW, C. BALL, J. LESTAGE, B. MICHAUD, K.W. KELLEY & R. DANTZER. 1999. Central injection of IL-10 antagonizes the behavioural effects of lipopolysaccharide in rats. Psychoneuroendocrinology **24:** 301–311.

39. WERNER, H., C. HERNANDEZ-SANCHEZ, E. KARNIELI & D. LEROITH. 1995. The regulation of IGF-I receptor gene expression. Int. J. Biochem. Cell Biol. **27:** 987–994.

40. WHITE, M.F. 1998. The IRS-signaling system: a network of docking proteins that mediate insulin and cytokine action. Recent Prog. Horm. Res. **53:** 119–138.

41. VALVERDE, A.M., M. LORENZO, S. PONS, M.F. WHITE & M. BENITO. 1998. Insulin receptor substrate (IRS) proteins IRS-1 and IRS-2 differential signaling in the insulin/insulin-like growth factor-I pathways in fetal brown adipocytes. Mol. Endocrinol. **12:** 688–697.

42. TOKER, A. & L.C. CANTLEY. 1997. Signalling through the lipid products of phosphoinositide-3-OH kinase. Nature **387:** 673–676.

43. HECK, S., F. LEZOUALCH, S. ENGERT & C. BEHL. 1999. Insulin-like growth factor-1-mediated neuroprotection against oxidative stress is associated with activation of nuclear factor kappa β. J. Biol. Chem. **274:** 9828–9835.

44. YE, P. & A.J. D'ERCOLE. 1999. Insulin-like growth factor I protects oligodendrocytes from tumor necrosis factor-α-induced injury. Endocrinology **140:** 3063–3072.

45. HUEBER, A.O., M. ZORNIG, D. LYON, T. SUDA, S. NAGATA & G.I. EVAN. 1997. Requirement for the CD95 receptor-ligand pathway in c-Myc-induced apoptosis. Science **278:** 1305–1309.

46. HARRISON, M., A.M. DUNGER, S. BERG, J. MABLEY, N. JOHN, M.H. GREEN & I.C. GREEN. 1998. Growth factor protection against cytokine-induced apoptosis in neonatal rat islets of Langerhans: role of Fas. FEBS Lett. **435:** 207–210.

47. SERPIER, H., P. GILLERY, V. SALMON-EHR, R. GARNOTEL, N. GEORGES, B. KALIS & F.X. MAQUART. 1997. Antagonistic effects of interferon-gamma and interleukin-4 on fibroblast cultures. J. Invest. Dermatol. **109:** 158–162.

48. BENNETT, B.L., R. CRUZ, R.G. LACSON & A.M. MANNING. 1997. Interleukin-4 suppression of tumor necrosis factor α-stimulated E-selectin gene transcription is mediated by STAT6 antagonism of NF-κB. J. Biol. Chem. **272:** 10212–10219.

49. PERALDI, P., G.S. HOTAMISLIGIL, W.A. BUURMAN, M.F. WHITE & B.M. SPIEGELMAN. 1996. Tumor necrosis factor (TNF)-α inhibits insulin signaling through stimulation of the p55 TNF receptor and activation of sphingomyelinase. J. Biol. Chem. **271:** 13018–13022.

50. PAZ, K., R. HEMI, D. LEROITH, A. KARASIK, E. ELHANANY, H. KANETY & Y. ZICK. 1997. A molecular basis for insulin resistance. Elevated serine/threonine phosphorylation of IRS-1 and IRS-2 inhibits their binding to the juxtamembrane region of the insulin receptor and impairs their ability to undergo insulin-induced tyrosine phosphorylation. J. Biol. Chem. **72:** 29911–29918.

51. STORZ, P., H. DOPPLER, A. WERNIG, K. PFIZENMAIER & G. MULLER. 1998. TNF inhibits insulin induced STAT5 activation in differentiated mouse muscle cells pmi28. FEBS Lett. **440:** 41–45.

52. FROST, R.A., C.H. LANG & M.C. GELATO. 1997. Transient exposure of human myoblasts to tumor necrosis factor-α inhibits serum and insulin-like growth factor-I stimulated protein synthesis. Endocrinology **138:** 4153–4159.

53. LUHESHI, G.N., A. STEFFERL, A.V. TURNBULL, M.J. DASCOMBE, S. BROUWER, S.J. HOPKINS & N.J. ROTHWELL. 1997. Febrile response to tissue inflammation involves both peripheral and brain IL-1 and TNF-α in the rat. Am. J. Physiol. **272:** R862–R868.

54. VENTERS, H.D., R. DANTZER & K.W. KELLEY. 2000. A new concept in neurodegeneration: TNFα is a silencer of survival signals (SOSS). Trends Neurosci. **23:** 175–180.

The Neuroimmunomodulatory Peptide α-MSH

TAKASHI ICHIYAMA,[a,b,e] SOICHIRO SATO,[d] KUNIYUKI OKADA,[a,b]
ANNA CATANIA,[c] AND JAMES M. LIPTON[a]

[a]*Department of Physiology, University of Texas Southwestern Medical Center at Dallas,
5323 Harry Hines Blvd., Dallas, Texas 75235, USA*

[b]*Department of Pediatrics, Yamaguchi University School of Medicine,
Yamaguchi 755-8505, Japan*

[c]*3rd Division of Internal Medicine, Ospedale Maggiore di Milano IRCCS,
Milan 20122, Italy*

[d]*Department of Internal Medicine, Keio University School of Medicine, Tokyo 160, Japan*

ABSTRACT: Alpha-melanocyte-stimulating hormone (α-MSH), a neuroimmunomodulatory peptide of ancient origin, is known to be involved in the control
of host responses. In inflammatory cells, in the periphery and within the central nervous system, α-MSH modulates the production and action of proinflammatory cytokines. This broad influence occurs via endogenous α-MSH
(melanocortin) receptors. The key to this anti-inflammatory influence is inhibition of NF-κB. Indeed α-MSH inhibits activation of this nuclear factor
through preservation of IκBα, which binds to NF-κB and prevents its migration to the nucleus. Cells transfected with α-MSH plasmid vector are resistant
to challenge with bacterial lipopolysaccharide. The peptide also act on central
melanocortin receptors to modulate inflammation in the periphery. In brief, α-
MSH and certain of its fragments such as α-MSH [11–13] KPV modulate
inflammation via three general actions: direct actions on peripheral host cells;
actions on inflammatory cells within the brain to modulate local reactions; and
descending neural anti-inflammatory pathways that control inflammation in
peripheral tissues.

INTRODUCTION

Alpha-melanocyte-stimulating hormone (α-MSH) is a 13-amino-acid peptide
with potent neuroimmunomodulatory properties derived from proopiomelanocortin
(POMC). α-MSH modulates the production and actions of proinflammatory agents
in the brain, pituitary, peripheral tissues, and phagocytes. The endogenous peptide is
increased in inflammatory diseases, presumably as a natural countermeasure to
inflammation. Administration of α-MSH modulates inflammatory responses in animal models and human cells. α-MSH and certain of its fragments such as α-MSH
[11–13] KPV modulate inflammation via three general actions: direct actions on
peripheral host cells; actions on inflammatory cells within the brain to modulate
local reactions; and descending neural anti-inflammatory pathways that control
inflammation in peripheral tissues.

[e]Author for correspondence. Voice: 214-648-2357.
James.Lipton@email.swmed.edu

Receptors that underlie the effects of α-MSH and related melanocortins have been identified and cloned. Five G-protein–linked receptors (MC-1R through MC-5R) are currently recognized. When transfected into carrier cells, these receptors increase intracellular cAMP upon stimulation with melanocortin molecules.

The potent and broad anti-inflammatory actions of α-MSH, coupled with its extremely low toxicity and its effectiveness when administered centrally, raise the possibility that it might be useful in the treatment of inflammatory and neurodegenerative brain disorders.

INFLUENCE OF α-MSH TREATMENT ON
BRAIN AND CIRCULATING TNF-α

TNF-α occurs in abundance in lesions of multiple sclerosis (MS) and in other neurodegenerative disorders such as Alzheimer's disease. The capacity of TNF-α to promote myelin destruction and to increase adhesion molecule expression makes it a prime suspect in the etiology of MS lesions. Therefore, we determined if α-MSH inhibits production of brain TNF-α *in vivo* and *in vitro* and which cells might be involved.

To test for this potential influence of the peptide, TNF-α was induced centrally by local injection of bacterial lipopolysaccharide (LPS) in mice. α-MSH given intracerebroventricularly (i.c.v.), intraperitoneally (i.p.), or both i.p. and i.c.v. inhibited production of TNF-α within brain tissue.[1] Inhibition of TNF-α protein formation by α-MSH was confirmed by inhibition of TNF-α mRNA. Plasma TNF-α concentration was markedly elevated after central LPS, indicative of an augmented peripheral host response induced by the CNS signal. The increase was inhibited by α-MSH treatments in relation to inhibition of central TNF-α. The presence within normal mouse brain of mRNA for the α-MSH receptor MC-1 suggests that the inhibitory effects of α-MSH on brain and plasma TNF-α might be mediated by this receptor subtype. The inhibitory effect of α-MSH on brain TNF-α did not depend upon circulating factors, because the effect also occurred in brain tissue *in vitro*. This indicates that α-MSH can act directly on brain cells to inhibit their production of TNF-α. Because central TNF-α contributes to pathology in CNS disease and injury and promotes inflammation in the periphery, agents that act upon brain α-MSH receptors should decrease the pathological TNF-α reaction and promote tissue survival.

INFLUENCES OF α-MSH ON ASTROCYTE AND
MICROGLIAL INFLAMMATORY PRODUCTS *IN VITRO*

Damage to oligodendrocytes and Schwann cells is caused by nonspecific mediators of inflammation such as reactive oxygen and nitrogen-free radicals, proinflammatory cytokines, and proteases produced by activated microglia, macrophages, and astrocytes. Evidence already exists that α-MSH reduces production of such mediators by macrophages. Research has been extended to include observations on astrocytes and microglia.

We tested the capacity of α-MSH and the COOH-terminal tripeptide fragment KPV to inhibit TNF-α production induced by bacterial endotoxin in cells of a human glioma line (A-172, anaplastic astrocytoma cells).[2] Both peptides were effective, although the α-MSH [1–13] sequence was more potent. The anticytokine effect of α-MSH in glioma cells may be mediated by human melanocortin-1 receptors; mRNA for this receptor subtype was expressed by the glioma cells.

In further experiments, we tested the effects of the melanocortin peptides α-MSH [1–13], α-MSH [11–13], and ACTH [1–24] on the production of tumor necrosis factor-α (TNF-α), interleukin-6 (IL-6), and nitric oxide (NO) in a cultured murine microglial cell line (N9) stimulated with lipopolysaccharide (LPS) plus interferon-γ (IFN-γ). Melanocortin peptides inhibited the production of these cytokines and NO in a concentration-related fashion, likely by increasing intracellular cAMP. When stimulated with LPS + IFN-γ, microglia increased the release of α-MSH. Production of TNF-α, IL-6, and NO was greater in activated microglia after immunoneutralization of endogenous α-MSH. The results suggest that α-MSH is an autocrine anti-inflammatory factor in microglia.[3] In related experiments, α–MSH and KPV inhibited TNF-α and NO production by murine microglia stimulated with β-amyloid and interferon-γ.[4] These data suggest that α-MSH peptides could be beneficial in the treatment of Alzheimer's disease.

The results of these experiments complement those of the *in vivo* studies and provide an explanation for any salutary influence of α-MSH in terms of its anticytokine and anti-NO activities.

α-MSH AND ITS RECEPTORS IN REGULATION OF TUMOR NECROSIS FACTOR-α PRODUCTION BY HUMAN MONOCYTE/MACROPHAGES

The hypothesis that central and peripheral phagocytes contain an autocrine circuit based on α-MSH has major implications for therapy of inflammatory disorders. To extend our observations on this autocrine circuit, cells of the human monocyte/macrophage line THP-1 were stimulated with LPS in the presence or absence of α-MSH. Consistent with our previous observations, the peptide inhibited the production of TNF-α in relation to peptide concentration.[5] Nuclease protection assays with a probe for the human melanocortin receptor MC-1R indicated that expression of this receptor subtype occurs in THP-1 cells; RT/PCR studies revealed that MC-3R and MC-5R are also expressed in these cells. Incubation of resting macrophages with an antibody to MC-1R promoted TNF-α production and reduced the inhibitory influence of α-MSH on TNF-α production by macrophages stimulated with endotoxin. These data demonstrate an autocrine circuit in macrophages based on melanocortin peptides and their receptors. Targeting of this neuroimmunomodulatory circuit should be therapeutically beneficial in inflammatory disorders.

EFFECT OF α-MSH ON NF-κB ACTIVATION AND IκBα DEGRADATION IN HUMAN GLIOMA CELLS AND EXPERIMENTAL BRAIN INFLAMMATION

As just reported, α-MSH modulates production of proinflammatory cytokines in brain tissue and peripheral inflammatory cells. Transcription of the genes for these proinflammatory cytokines is regulated by the nuclear factor κB (NF-κB). Recent research indicates that activation of NF-κB in the CNS promotes neurodegenerative processes. NF-κB likely contributes to the onset or acceleration of neuronal dysfunction and degeneration in many neurological diseases, including Parkinson's disease, Alzheimer's disease, and CNS viral infections. Therefore, molecules that modulate NF-κB activity could be a novel pharmacological approach to several neurological diseases.[6] We examined whether α-MSH limits degradation of IκBα inhibitor protein and inhibits activation of NF-κB induced by LPS in human glioma cells and mouse brain.[7] Electrophoretic mobility shift assays of nuclear extracts from glioma cells and whole mouse brains stimulated with LPS showed that α-MSH preserved expression of IκBα protein *in vitro* (glioma cells) and *in vivo* (brain tissue) and inhibited NF-κB activation. Chloramphenicol acetyltransferase assay indicated that α-MSH suppresses NF-κB–dependent reporter gene expression induced by LPS. The findings are consistent with the possibility that the anti-inflammatory action of α-MSH in CNS inflammation occurs via modulation of NF-κB activation by peptide-induced inhibition of degradation of IκBα protein.

Because in clinical therapeutics treatment should be given peripherally, we examined whether systemic α-MSH also inhibits activation of NF-κB in experimental murine brain inflammation induced by LPS. Data demonstrated that similar to its central administration, α-MSH given systemically inhibited NF-κB activation by reducing IκBα degradation.[8]

INHIBITION OF PERIPHERAL NF-κB ACTIVATION BY CENTRAL ACTION OF α-MSH

Previous research has shown that central α-MSH inhibits inflammation in peripheral tissues via descending neural anti-inflammatory pathways.[9] In further experiments, we demonstrated that centrally administered α-MSH inhibited NF-κB activation and IκBα degradation induced by TNF-α injected into the footpad of the mouse.[7] These effects were reversed by intraperitoneal injection of a nonspecific β-adrenergic receptor blocker and a specific β2-adrenergic receptor antagonist in mice with spinal cord transection. These findings indicate that α-MSH can act centrally to inhibit NF-κB activation in peripheral acute inflammation via a descending neural pathway involving β2-adrenergic receptors.

AUTOCRINE α-MELANOCYTE–STIMULATING HORMONE INDUCED BY GENE CONSTRUCT INSERTION INHIBITS NF-κB ACTIVATION IN HUMAN GLIOMA CELLS

Using a plasmid vector encoding α-MSH, we examined whether autocrine α-MSH inhibits activation of NF-κB in human glioma cells. Electrophoretic mobility shift assays of nuclear extracts demonstrated that NF-κB activation induced by LPS was inhibited in glioma cells transfected with the α-MSH vector. Western blot analysis revealed that this inhibition was linked to preservation of the expression of I-κBα protein. Chloramphenicol acetyltransferase assay indicated that NF-κB–dependent reporter gene expression was suppressed in cells transfected with the α-MSH vector. Finally, fluorescence staining confirmed that glioma cells bear α-MSH receptors. The findings are consistent with the idea that in CNS inflammation, autocrine α-MSH exerts anti-inflammatory actions via modulation of NF-κB activation by preservation of I-κBα protein. Based on this action of the peptide, it should be possible to treat neurodegenerative diseases, stroke, encephalitis, trauma, and other CNS disorders that have an inflammatory component through gene therapy with the α-MSH vector.[8]

ACKNOWLEDGMENTS

This work was supported by National Institutes of Health grant NS10046 and Progetto Sclerosi Multipla, grant 96/J/T9, Istituto Superiore di Sanità, Italy.

REFERENCES

1. Rajora, N., G. Boccoli, D. Burns, S. Sharma, A.P. Catania & J.M. Lipton. 1997. α-MSH modulates local and circulating TNFα in experimental brain inflammation. J. Neurosci. **17:** 2181–2186.

2. Wong, K.Y., N. Rajora, A.P. Catania & J.M. Lipton. 1997. A mechanism of anti-inflammatory action of α-MSH peptides within the brain: modulation of TNFα production by human glioma cells. Neuroimmunomodulation **4:** 37–41.

3. Delgado, R., A. Carlin, L. Airaghi, M.T. Demitri, L. Meda, D. Galimberti, P.L. Baron, J.M. Lipton & A. Catania. 1998. Melanocortin peptides inhibit production of proinflammatory cytokines and nitric oxide by activated microglia. J. Leuk. Biol. **63:** 740–745.

4. Galimberti, D., P.L. Baron, L. Meda, E. Prat, E., Scarpini, R. Delgado, A. Catania & J.M. Lipton. 1999. α-MSH peptides inhibit production of nitric oxide and TNF-α by microglial cells activated with β-amyloid and interferon γ. Biochem. Biophys. Res. Commun. In press.

5. Taherzadeh, S., S. Sharma, V. Chhajlani, I. Gantz, N. Rajora, M.T. Demitri, L. Kelly, H. Zhao, A. Catania & J.M. Lipton. 1999. α-MSH and its receptors in regulation of inflammatory tumor necrosis factor-α (TNFα) by human monocyte/macrophages. Am. J. Physiol. **276:** R1289–R1294.

6. Grilli, M. & M. Memo. 1999. Nuclear factor-κB/Rel proteins: a point of convergence of signaling pathways relevant in neuronal function and dysfunction. Biochem. Pharmacol. **57:** 1–7.

7. Ichiyama, T., H. Zhao, A. Catania, S. Furukawa & J.M. Lipton. 1999. α-Melanocyte-stimulating hormone inhibits NF-κB activation and IκBα degradation in human glioma cells and in experimental brain inflammation. Exp. Neurol. **157:** 359–365.

8. ICHIYAMA, T., T. SAKAI, A. CATANIA, S. BARSH, S. FURUKAWA & J.M. LIPTON. 1999. Systemically administered α-melanocyte-stimulating peptides inhibit NF-κB activation in experimental brain inflammation. Brain Res. In press.
9. MACALUSO, A., D. McCOY, G. CERIANI, T. WATANABE, J. BILTZ, A. CATANIA & J.M. LIPTON. 1994. Anti-inflammatory influences of alpha-MSH molecules: central neurogenic and peripheral actions. J. Neurosci. **14:** 2377–2382.

The Neuropeptide α-MSH in Host Defense

ANNA CATANIA,[a,b] MARIAGRAZIA CUTULI,[b] LETIZIA GAROFALO,[b] ANDREA CARLIN,[b] LORENA AIRAGHI,[b] WILMA BARCELLINI,[c] AND JAMES M. LIPTON[d]

[b]Division of Internal Medicine, Ospedale Maggiore di Milano IRCCS, 20122 Milan, Italy

[c]Division of Hematology, Ospedale Maggiore di Milano IRCCS, 20122 Milan, Italy

[d]Department of Physiology, University of Texas Southwestern Medical Center at Dallas, Dallas, Texas 75235, USA

ABSTRACT: The presence of the ancient peptide α-melanocyte–stimulating hormone (α-MSH) in barrier organs such as gut and skin suggests that this potent anti-inflammatory molecule may be a component of the innate host defense. In tests of antimicrobial activities, α-MSH and its fragment KPV showed inhibitory influences against the gram-positive bacterium *Staphylococcus aureus* and the yeast *Candida albicans*. Anti-tumor necrosis factor and antimicrobial effects of α-MSH suggest that the peptide might likewise reduce replication of human immunodeficiency virus (HIV). Treatment with α-MSH reduced HIV replication in chronically and acutely infected human monocytes. At the molecular level, α-MSH inhibited activation of the transcription factor NF-κB known to enhance HIV expression. α-MSH that combines antipyretic, anti-inflammatory, and antimicrobial effects could be useful in the treatment of disorders in which infection and inflammation coexist.

INTRODUCTION

Production of natural antimicrobial peptides by phagocytes and epithelia has been recognized for a long time.[1,2] Components of the innate host defense system initiate the response to microbial penetration before time-consuming adaptive immunity starts. Natural antimicrobial peptides are generally effective against bacteria, fungi, and viruses,[1,2] and some of these peptides might be used as therapeutic agents. Indeed, one of them, a synthetic homolog of bactericidal/permeability-increasing protein (BPI), has been used successfully to treat children with severe meningococcal sepsis.[3]

α-Melanocyte stimulating hormone (α-MSH) is a 13-amino-acid peptide with potent anti-inflammatory properties.[4,5] It is produced by posttranslational processing of the larger precursor molecule proopiomelanocortin (POMC).[6] α-MSH reduces production of proinflammatory mediators by host cells *in vitro*[7,8] and local and systemic reactions in animal models of inflammation.[9] The active message sequence resides in the C-terminal tripeptide α-MSH ([11–13], KPV) which has

[a]Address for correspondence: Dr. Anna Catania, 3rd Division of Internal Medicine, Padiglione Granelli, Ospedale Maggiore di Milano IRCCS, Via F. Sforza 35, 20122 Milano, Italy. Voice/fax: +39-02-5503-3318.

Anna.Catania@unimi.it

anti-inflammatory influences *in vivo* and *in vitro* that parallel those of the parent molecule.[10,11] α-MSH is produced by many cell types including peripheral[7] and central[12] phagocytes and by keratinocytes.[13] Immunoreactive α-MSH is also found in the mucosal barrier of the gastrointestinal tract in intact and hypophysectomized rats[14] and in humans.[15] The presence in barrier organs of this ancient peptide suggests that it might have a role in host defense. To test this possibility, we determined whether α-MSH has antimicrobial and anti-HIV influences.

α-MSH PEPTIDES HAVE ANTIMICROBIAL PROPERTIES

To determine if α-MSH peptides have antimicrobial influences, we tested their capacity to inhibit colony forming units (cfu) of two representative infectious agents: the gram-positive bacterium *Staphylococcus aureus* and the yeast *Candida albicans*. In experiments on *S. aureus,* α-MSH and its C-terminal tripeptide KPV inhibited *S. aureus* colony formation over a wide range of concentrations, including the picomolar concentrations that naturally occur in human plasma.[16] *C. albicans* cfu were likewise greatly reduced by concentrations of both α-MSH (1–13) and (11–13) from 10^{-12} to 10^{-4} M. Flow cytometry tests confirmed the *C. albicans* killing activity of α-MSH peptides. Indeed, in α-MSH–treated yeast, the propidium iodide incorporation was markedly increased.

The pathogenesis of *C. albicans* infection involves adhesion to host epithelial and endothelial cells and morphologic switching of yeast cells from the ellipsoid blastospore to various filamentous forms: germ tubes, pseudohyphae, and hyphae.[17] Coincubation of *C. albicans* with α-MSH (1–13) and (11–13) inhibited germ tube formation induced by horse serum. Therefore, α-MSH reduces not only *C. albicans* viability, but also germ tube formation, which is associated with increased virulence of the yeast.

Many of the effects of α-MSH are known to be mediated by induction of cAMP.[6] Melanocortin receptors are G-protein–linked receptors whose signal transduction occurs through induction of adenylyl cyclase and an increase in cAMP.[18] Therefore, we measured the effects of α-MSH on cAMP accumulation in *C. albicans* and found that both α-MSH (1–13) and (11–13) enhanced cAMP content in the yeast. Because previous observations showed that cAMP-enhancing agents inhibit mRNA and protein synthesis in *C. albicans,*[19] it is likely that the antimicrobial effect of α-MSH was caused by enhancement of this mediator. It may be that microorganisms express one or more so far unrecognized melanocortin receptors that, like those present in higher species, bind α-MSH and its fragments and induce adenylyl cyclase.

α-MSH PEPTIDES INHIBIT HIV EXPRESSION IN CHRONICALLY INFECTED U1 CELLS AND ACUTELY INFECTED MONOCYTES

Replication of HIV is dependent on the state of activation of infected cells and is regulated by interactions between viral and host factors.[20] Among the latter, proinflammatory cytokines have a prominent enhancing effect on HIV replication.[21] Tumor necrosis factor-alpha (TNF-α)[22] and other cytokines such as interleukin-1

(IL-1)[22] and IL-6[23] promote HIV replication and have detrimental influences on HIV disease progression.[24] Inhibition of such proinflammatory cytokines is therefore a target for adjunctive therapies of HIV infection. α-MSH is known to inhibit all these cytokines[4,25,26] and is a candidate as an adjunctive treatment for HIV infection. Therefore, we investigated the effects of α-MSH peptides on HIV expression in chronically infected promonocytic U1 cells and in acutely infected human monocytes.

α-MSH [1–13] and the tripeptide KPV significantly inhibited p24 release from TNF-α–stimulated U1 cells. Similar to the aforementioned antimicrobial effects, the anti-HIV influences of α-MSH also occurred over a broad range of peptide concentrations, including physiological picomolar concentrations. These low concentrations significantly inhibited p24 release by approximately 35%, suggesting that the small amounts of endogenous α-MSH present in the circulation can inhibit HIV expression. Greater concentrations caused more pronounced HIV inhibition, with the most effective concentration for both peptides being 10^{-5} M. In this concentration, α-MSH [1–13] and KPV caused approximately 50% inhibition of p24 release. The inhibitory activity of KPV on HIV expression was confirmed by the reduction of both spliced and unspliced HIV RNA.

U1 cells are an *in vitro* model of latent HIV infection in which induction of viral replication does not lead to production of the infecting virus.[27] Therefore, we investigated the effects of KPV also in acutely infected monocyte-derived macrophages (MDM), which are a more realistic model of productive HIV infection.[28] Treatment with the tripeptide significantly inhibited RT release in these acutely infected cells.

Because NF-κB is a central mediator in cytokine activation of HIV transcription,[22] we determined the effect of KPV on NF-κB DNA binding in U1 cells. TNF-α treatment greatly enhanced NF-κB DNA binding activity, and coincubation of cells with the tripeptide significantly reduced NF-κB activation. These observations suggest that inhibition of HIV replication in infected cells is likely exerted through reduction of NF-κB activation.

CONCLUSIONS

The ancient anti-inflammatory peptide α-MSH, produced by cells with a primary role in host defense such as phagocytes and keratinocytes, clearly has direct antimicrobial effects. The endogenous peptide likely contributes to a reduction in the microbial burden. However, concentrations of the peptide greater than those found in human plasma were much more effective in killing bacteria and yeast and in reducing HIV expression in monocytes. This suggests that α-MSH peptides given in pharmacological concentrations should be tested as adjunctive therapy for infections.

ACKNOWLEDGMENTS

This research was supported by grants 980.1.14 Progetto Terapia Antivirale AIDS from Istituto Superiore di Sanità and 100.08 from Ospedale Maggiore di Milano; and grant NS10046 from the National Institutes of Health, National Institute of Neurological Diseases and Stroke.

REFERENCES

1. MARTIN, E., T. GANZ & R.I. LEHRER. 1995. Defensins and other endogenous peptide antibiotics of vertebrates. J. Leukoc. Biol. **58:** 128–136.
2. GANZ, T. & J. WEISS. 1997. Antimicrobial peptides of phagocytes and epithelia. Sem. Hematol. **34:** 343–354.
3. GIROIR, B.P., P.A. QUINT, P. BARTON, E.A. KIRSH, L. KITCHEN, B. GOLDSTEIN, B.J. NELSON, N.I. WEDEL, S.F. CARROL & P.J. SCANNON. 1997. Preliminary evaluation of recombinant amino-terminal fragment of human bactericidal/permeability-increasing protein in children with severe meningococcal sepsis. Lancet **350:** 1439–1443.
4. CATANIA, A. & J.M. LIPTON. 1993. α-Melanocyte stimulating hormone in the modulation of host reactions. Endocr. Rev. **14:** 564–576.
5. LIPTON, J.M. & A. CATANIA. 1997. Anti-inflammatory actions of the neuroimmunomodulator α-MSH. Immunol. Today **18:** 140–145.
6. EBERLE, A.N. 1988. The Melanotropins. Karger. Basel, Switzerland.
7. RAJORA, N., G. CERIANI, A. CATANIA, R.A. STAR, M.T. MURPHY & J.M. LIPTON. 1996. α-MSH production, receptors and influence on neopterin in a human monocyte/macrophage cell line. J. Leukoc. Biol. **59:** 248–253.
8. STAR, R.A., N. RAJORA, J. HUANG, R.C. STOCK, A. CATANIA & J.M. LIPTON. 1995. Evidence of autocrine modulation of macrophage nitric oxide synthase by α-MSH. Proc. Natl. Acad. Sci. USA **92:** 8016–8020.
9. LIPTON, J.M., G. CERIANI, A. MACALUSO, D. MCCOY, K. CARNES, J. BILTZ & A. CATANIA. 1994. Anti-inflammatory effects of the neuropeptide α-MSH in acute, chronic, and systemic inflammation. Ann. N.Y. Acad. Sci. **741:** 137–148.
10. RICHARDS, D.B. & J.M. LIPTON. 1984. Effect of α-MSH (11–13) (lysine-proline-valine) on fever in the rabbit. Peptides **5:** 815–817.
11. HILTZ, M.E. & J.M. LIPTON. 1989. Anti-inflammatory activity of a COOH-terminal fragment of the neuropeptide α-MSH. FASEB J. **3:** 2282–2284.
12. DELGADO, R., A. CARLIN, L. AIRAGHI, M.T. DEMITRI, L. MEDA, D. GALIMBERTI, P.L. BARON, J.M. LIPTON & A. CATANIA. 1998. Melanocortin peptides inhibit production of proinflammatory cytokines and nitric oxide by activated microglia. J. Leukoc. Biol. **63:** 740–745.
13. LUGER, T.A., E. SCHAUER, F. TRAUTINGER, J. KRUTMANN, J. ANSEL, A. SCHWARZ & T. SCHWARTZ. 1993. Production of immunosuppressing melanotropins by human keratinocytes. Ann. N.Y. Acad. Sci. **680:** 567–570.
14. FOX, J.A.E.T. & J. KRAICER. 1981. Immunoreactive α-melanocyte stimulating hormone, its distribution in the gastrointestinal tract of intact and hypophysectomized rats. Life Sci. **28:** 2127–2132.
15. LARSSON, L.-I. 1981. Adrenocorticotropin-like and α-melanotropin-like peptides in a subpopulation of human gastrin cell granules: bioassay, immunoassay, and immunocytochemical evidence. Proc. Natl. Acad. Sci. USA **78:** 2990–2994.
16. CATANIA, A., L. AIRAGHI, L. GAROFALO, M. CUTULI & J.M. LIPTON. 1998. The neuropeptide α-MSH in AIDS and other conditions in humans. Ann. N.Y. Acad. Sci. **840:** 848–856.
17. GOW, N.A. 1997. Germ tube growth of *Candida albicans*. Curr. Topics Med. Mycol. **8:** 43–55.
18. TATRO, J.B. 1996. Receptor biology of the melanocortins, a family of neuroimmunodulatory peptides. Neuroimmunomodulation **3:** 259–284.
19. BHATTACHARYA, A. & A. DATTA. 1977. Effect of cyclic AMP on RNA and protein synthesis in *Candida albicans*. Biochem. Biophys. Res. Commun. **77:** 1483–1484.
20. FAUCI, A.S. 1996. Host factors in the pathogenesis of HIV-induced disease. Nature **384:** 529–534.

21. POLI, G. & A.S. FAUCI. 1993. Cytokine modulation of HIV expression. Semin. Immunol. **5:** 165–173.
22. OSBORN, L., S. KUNKEL & G.J. NABEL. 1989. Tumor necrosis factor α and interleukin 1 stimulate the human immunodeficiency virus enhancer by activation of the nuclear factor κB. Proc. Natl. Acad. Sci. USA **86:** 2336–2340.
23. POLI, G., P. BRESSLER, A. KINTER, E. DUH, W.C. TIMMER, A. RABSON, J.S. JUSTEMENT, S. STANLEY & A.S. FAUCI. 1990. Interleukin 6 induces human immunodeficiency virus expression in infected monocytic cells alone and in synergy with tumor necrosis factor by transcriptional and post-transcriptional mechanism. J. Exp. Med. **172:** 151–158.
24. ROSEMBERG, Z.F. & A.S. FAUCI. 1991. Immunopathogenesis of HIV infection. FASEB J. **5:** 2382–2390.
25. RAJORA, N., G. BOCCOLI, D. BURNS, S. SHARMA, A. CATANIA & J.M. LIPTON. 1997. α-MSH modulates local and circulating tumor necrosis factor α in experimental brain inflammation. J. Neurosci. **17:** 2181–2186.
26. CATANIA, A., L. GAROFALO, M. CUTULI, A. GRINGERI, E. SANTAGOSTINO & J.M. LIPTON. 1998. Melanocortin peptides inhibit production of proinflammatory cytokines in blood of HIV-infected patients. Peptides **19:** 1099–1104.
27. FOLKS, T.M., J.S. JUSTEMENT, A. KINTER, S. SCHNITTMAN, J. ORENSTEIN, G. POLI & A.S. FAUCI. 1988. Characterization of a promonocyte clone chronically infected with HIV and inducible by 13-phorbol-12-myristate acetate. J. Immunol. **140:** 1117–1122.
28. POLI, G., A.L. KINTER, J.S. JUSTEMENT, P. BRESSLER, J.H. KEHRL & A.S. FAUCI. 1991. Transforming growth factor β suppresses human immunodeficiency virus expression and replication in infected cells of the monocyte/macrophage lineage. J. Exp. Med. **173:** 589–597.

The Role of α-MSH as a Modulator of Cutaneous Inflammation

T.A. LUGER,[a,b] T. BRZOSKA,[a] T.E. SCHOLZEN,[a] D.-H. KALDEN,[a]
C. SUNDERKÖTTER,[a] C. ARMSTRONG,[c] AND J. ANSEL[c]

[a]Department of Dermatology and Ludwig Boltzmann Institute for Cell Biology and
Immunobiology of the Skin, University of Münster, Münster, Germany

[c]Department of Dermatology, Emory University, Atlanta, Georgia, USA

ABSTRACT: Among various neuropeptides such as substance P, calcitonin gene-related peptide and others, α-melanocyte-stimulating hormone (α-MSH) was found to be produced in the skin. Moreover, melanocortin receptor 1 (MC-1R), which is specific for α-MSH and ACTH, is expressed in the skin on keratinocytes, dendritic cells, macrophages and endothelial cells. In monocytes, macrophages and dendritic cells α-MSH inhibits the production and activity of immunoregulatory and proinflammatory cytokines such as IL-2, IFN-γ, TNF-α and IL-1. It downregulates the expression of costimulatory molecules such as CD86 and CD40 and induces the production of suppressor factors such as the cytokine synthesis inhibitory factor IL-10. On endothelial cells α-MSH is capable of downregulating the LPS-induced expression of adhesion molecules such as vascular cell adhesion molecule (VCAM) and E-selectin. Moreover, the LPS-induced activation of transcription factors such as NFκB is downregulated by α-MSH. In a mouse model i.v. or topical application of α-MSH was found to inhibit the induction phase as well as the effector phase of contact hypersensitivity (CHS) reactions and to induce hapten-specific tolerance. These findings indicate that the production of immunosuppressing neuropeptides such as α-MSH by epidermal cells may play an essential role during the pathogenesis of immune and inflammatory reactions in the skin.

INTRODUCTION

Melanocortins such as melanocyte-stimulating hormones (α-, β-, γ-MSH) are generated from the precursor hormone proopiomelanocortin (POMC) by proteolytic cleavage, conducted by specific prohormone convertases.[1] POMC-derived peptide hormones such as α-MSH, adrenocorticotropin (ACTH) and β-endorphin (β-EP) were originally described in the pituitary gland. However, there is evidence from several studies that POMC-peptides are produced by many different cells and tissues including the immune system and the skin. Accordingly, all major constituents of the epidermis such as keratinocytes, Langerhans cells and melanocytes were found to express POMC mRNA and to release POMC-peptides.[2] Under normal conditions neither POMC synthesis nor release of α-MSH by keratinocytes are detectable at a

[b]Address for correspondence: Thomas A. Luger, Department of Dermatology, University of Münster, Von-Esmarch Str. 56, 48149 Münster, Germany. Voice: +49-251-8356504; fax: +49-251-8356522.
luger@uni-muenster.de

significant level. However, upon exposure to noxious stimuli, such as endotoxins (LPS) or irradiation with ultraviolet (UV) light, keratinocytes *in vitro* and *in vivo* express increased amounts of POMC mRNA and release α-MSH, ACTH and β-EP.[3,4]

Melanocortins and ACTH exert their activities via a group of five melanocortin receptors (MC-R) belonging to the family of G-protein-coupled receptors with seven transmembrane domains.[5,6] In addition to the central nervous system and melanocytes, MC-R have been detected recently on adipocytes, keratinocytes, endothelial cells, fibroblasts and immunocompetent as well as inflammatory cells. Among the five MC-Rs, MC-1R and MC-5R were the main ones found to be expressed in the skin, whereas immunocompetent cells almost exclusively express MC-1R, which is specific for α-MSH but with a lower affinity also binds ACTH.[7] There is accumulating evidence from several recent studies that melanocortins and their receptors are responsible for a variety of other important functions in addition to their well-known pigment-inducing capacity.[2,8] Most interestingly, MC-4R appears to be crucially involved in food intake and body weight control, since MC-4R knockout mice develop obesity.[9,10] In humans POMC mutations resulting in melanocortin deficiency have been reported to be associated with a severe early onset of obesity, adrenal insufficiency and red hair.[11] Similarly, mice deficient for POMC develop altered pigmentation, hyperphagia and obesity as well as defective adrenal gland development causing corticosteroid and aldosterone deficiency.[12] In addition, POMC peptides in the skin were found to stimulate keratinocyte proliferation, fibroblast collagenase activity and cytokine production.[2] Finally, there is strong evidence from many investigations that among POMC-peptides α-MSH exerts a variety of immunomodulating and anti-inflammatory activities, mainly, by affecting functions of monocytes, dendritic cells and endothelial cells.[13] Therefore, this review will briefly summarize our current view on the role of α-MSH as a mediator of skin inflammation.

EFFECT OF α-MSH ON MONOCYTES AND DENDRITIC CELLS

In view of the crucial role distinct antigen-presenting cells play during the initiation of immune responses several investigations focused on the potential role of α-MSH to modulate monocyte functions. Studies addressing the question whether any of the MC-Rs are detectable on monocytes provided clear evidence that peripheral blood-derived monocytes after treatment with LPS, which promotes the differentiation into macrophages, significantly express MC-1R at the protein as well as at the mRNA level.[14] Moreover, macrophages, monocytic cell lines (THP1, U937) and dendritic cells generated from peripheral blood derived monocytes were also found to express MC-1R.[14,15] These data indicate that MC-1R is upregulated irrespective of whether differentiation occurs into macrophages or dendritic cells. Among other MC-Rs, there is some evidence that MC-3R and MC-5R are expressed on a monocytic cell line (THP-1),[16] whereas other MC-Rs have so far not been detected on these cells.

The expression of MC-1R on different monocyte-derived cell lineages implies a possibly important role of POMC peptides such as α-MSH in modulating biological functions of these cells. Accordingly, α-MSH has been shown to regulate the migration of monocytes possibly via modulating the secretion of chemokines such as IL-8 and Gro-α.[17] The production of nitric oxide and neopterin by macrophages is inhibited by α-MSH.[18,19] Moreover, α-MSH was found to upregulate the LPS-mediated mRNA expression and release of the cytokine synthesis inhibitor IL-10 in monocytes in a dose-dependent manner, whereas IL-10 production by T-lymphocytes was not affected by α-MSH.[20] On the other hand, the synthesis and release of proinflammatory cytokines such as IL-1, IL-6 and TNF-α is downregulated by α-MSH.[21] In addition, α-MSH turned out to be a potent inhibitor of IL-1–mediated effects such as thymocyte proliferation and fever induction.[22] Thus, by inducing suppressor factors and inhibiting the production and activity of pro-inflammatory cytokines and other mediators α-MSH may have a central role in the downregulation of inflammation.

Other studies have addressed the question whether α-MSH exerts its immunomodulatory potential by altering the expression of accessory molecules on immunocompetent cells. There is evidence that α-MSH downregulates MHC class I molecules on monocytes[2] and the expression of CD86 on LPS-stimulated monocytes in a dose-dependent manner, whereas CD80 expression was not substantially affected.[14] Similar findings were obtained when peripheral blood–derived DCs were treated with α-MSH.[15] Thus, α-MSH significantly suppressed the expression of the co-stimulatory molecules CD86 and CD40. Taken together, these findings indicate that α-MSH is capable of modifying functions of immunocompetent cells including monocytes, macrophages and DCs. Since α-MSH blocks accessory signals such as CD86, CD40 and induces additional suppressor factors (IL-10) this molecule may be one of the signals required for the downregulation of an immune response and possibly the induction of tolerance.

The molecular mechanisms responsible for the alteration of the function of immunocompetent cells by α-MSH still are poorly understood. The activation of the transcription factor NFκB appears to be a crucial event in immune and inflammatory responses. NFκB is activated by proinflammatory cytokines such as IL-1, TNF-α as well as endotoxin and other stimuli. It controls the expression of many genes involved in inflammation including cytokines, MHC-class I, adhesion molecules, and nitric oxide synthetase.[23] Upon treatment with α-MSH the TNF-α, IL-1, LPS and ceramide-mediated activation of NFκB was significantly suppressed in a dose- and time-dependent manner.[24,25] Moreover, the TNF-α mediated degradation of the inhibitory subunit IκBα and the nuclear translocation of the p65 subunit of NFκB was inhibited. α-MSH–mediated inhibition of NFκB activation was found to be dependent on cAMP. Suppression of NFκB activation was not cell-specific and could be observed in monocytes, monocytic cell lines (U937), keratinocytes, fibroblasts and endothelial cells.[24–26] These data suggest that α-MSH appears to function as a general inhibitor of NFκB activation and thereby exerts its anti-inflammatory and immunomodulating effects.

EFFECT OF α-MSH ON VASCULAR ENDOTHELIAL CELLS

Endothelial cells play a crucial role in inflammation and immune reactions. The multiple steps ultimately leading to adherence and transmigration of inflammatory cells are regulated by a distinct set of adhesion molecules such as vascular adhesion molecule (VCAM-1), intercellular adhesion molecule (ICAM), integrins and

E-selectins which upon stimulation are expressed on both endothelial cells and inflammatory cells.[27] Accordingly, proinflammatory stimuli such as LPS, IL-1, TNF-α and others upregulate the expression of adhesion molecules and thus allow for inflammatory cells to adhere and migrate into the surrounding tissue. The down-regulation of endothelial cell adhesion molecule expression thus appears to be an important event in the control of inflammation. Therefore, recent investigations focused on the capacity of α-MSH to modulate the expression of adhesion molecules on human dermal microvascular endothelial cells as well as melanocortin receptor expression in these cells. Accordingly, human dermal microvascular endothelial cells (HDMEC) constitutively express only low amounts of MC-1R that were significantly upregulated upon stimulation with proinflammatory cytokines such as IL-1 and α-MSH[28] itself.

The functional relevance of MC-1R expression on HDMECs was supported by the observation that α-MSH in a dose-dependent manner was capable of downregulating the LPS-induced expression of ICAM-1, VCAM and E-selectin on mRNA and protein level.[26] The importance of this finding was further documented by *in vitro* adhesion assays, demonstrating that α-MSH significantly suppresses the LPS-mediated adhesion of lymphocytes to monolayers of HDMECs.[26] Since the signaling pathway involved in the regulation of adhesion molecule expression is mediated by NF?B, it was examined whether α-MSH affects NFκB-activation in endothelial cells. As in monocytes, α-MSH completely downregulated the LPS-mediated activation of NFκB in HDMECs.[26] In addition, α-MSH treatment of HDMECs blocked the LPS-mediated NFκB mRNA expression, but upregulated the IκB mRNA expression. These findings indicate that α-MSH via modulating the expression of different adhesion molecules is capable of preventing adhesion and transmigration of inflammatory cells and thus contributes to the downregulation of an inflammatory response.

IN VIVO EFFECT OF α-MSH ON APC AND ENDOTHELIAL CELLS

There is evidence from several studies that α-MSH *in vivo* affects immune and inflammatory reactions.[13] It has been demonstrated in a murine model of contact hypersensitivity (CHS) that systemic as well as topical application of α-MSH downregulates the elicitation phase as well as the sensitization phase of CHS.[29] Moreover, α-MSH, when applied before epicutaneous sensitization with haptens, was capable of inducing hapten-specific tolerance since animals could be sensitized with other antigens .[29] Tolerance induction by α-MSH appears to be mediated at least in part by the induction of cytokines such as IL-10 since subcutaneous administration of IL-10 antibodies partially could block inhibitory effects of α-MSH.[29] The crucial role of MC-R expression for α-MSH–mediated tolerance induction was further supported by studies using the artificial α-MSH antagonist HS-024. Preliminary studies indicate that this α-MSH antagonist inhibits the α-MSH effects on contact hypersensitivity and tolerance induction in a dose-dependent manner.[30]

Since α-MSH *in vitro* downregulates the expression of adhesion molecules on vascular endothelial cells, the *in vivo* relevance of this observation was investigated using a mouse model of leukocytoclastic vasculitis, the local Shwartzman reaction.

This model consists of a preparatory phase initiated by local subcutaneous low-dose injection of LPS followed by the challenge phase elicited by systemic application of LPS after 24 hours. When mice were injected i.v. with α-MSH prior to the preparatory phase a marked reduction of vascular hemorrhage following systemic application of LPS in the challenge phase was observed.[31] This reduction was also associated with a diminished expression of E-selectin and VCAM-1[31] indicating that α-MSH may reduce the vasculitic response in the local Shwartzman reaction by downregulating endothelial cell adhesion molecules.

CONCLUSION

The POMC-derived peptide α-MSH, which is produced in the skin following injury such as UV-irradiation, appears to function as a potent mediator involved in the downregulation of immune and inflammatory reactions.[3] Since α-MSH has been shown to block CHS and to induce tolerance, UV-induced epidermal cell–derived α-MSH may be responsible for the UV-mediated immunosuppression as well as tolerance induction. α-MSH exerts its immunosuppressing effects mostly via affecting the function of antigen-presenting cells. Accordingly, it induces the production of interleukin-10, inhibits the production of IL-1 and IL-12, and downregulates the expression of accessory molecules such as CD86 and CD40.[2] There is further evidence that α-MSH may interfere with the initiation of the immune response by inhibiting the chemokine-mediated migration of antigen-presenting cells. Therefore, α-MSH in several ways appears to perturb the function of antigen-presenting cells and possibly direct the outcome of an immune response towards tolerance. The inhibitory effect of α-MSH on the effector phase of CHS and the local Shwartzman reaction, however, seems to mainly involve its effect on vascular endothelial cells. Since the expression of adhesion molecules including ICAM-1, VCAM-1 and E-selectin are downregulated by α-MSH, inflammatory cells are prevented to adhere to endothelial cells and to transmigrate through the vessel wall. These findings suggest that the inhibitory effect of α-MSH on inflammatory reactions mainly appears to be due to the downregulation of adhesion molecule expression on vascular endothelial cells.

The major binding site of α-MSH on immunocompetent cells as well as endothelial cells appears to be MC-1R.[14,28] Under normal noninflammatory conditions MC-1R expression on both monocytic cells and endothelial cells is not detectable. However, upon exposure to proinflammatory signals MC-1R expression is significantly upregulated. There is evidence from several *in vitro* studies that α-MSH significantly affects the function of monocytes and endothelial cells after stimulation with LPS or proinflammatory cytokines such TNF-α or IL-1.[14,28] In contrast, in the absence of proinflammatory stimuli α-MSH has no effect. Thus, α-MSH appears to function as an important mediator required for the downregulation of inflammation but has no effect on cells which have not been activated during the course of inflammation. This is further supported by the observation that α-MSH is able to suppress the LPS-, TNF-α– or IL-1–induced NFκB activation which is required for most types of inflammation. These findings as well as the observation that an N-terminal tripeptide of α-MSH is responsible for most of the *in vitro* and *in vivo* anti-inflammatory effects of α-MSH suggest a potential use of these compounds for the treatment of inflammatory diseases.

ACKNOWLEDGMENTS

This work was supported by the Deutsche Forschungsgemeinschaft (SFB 293), the Volkswagenstiftung (I/74 582) and Interdisziplinäres Zentrum für Klinische Forschung (C7).

REFERENCES

1. SEIDAH, N.G., S. BENJANNET, J. HAMELIN, A.M. MARMABACHI, A. BASAK, J. MARCINKIEWICZ, M. MBIKAY, M. CHRETIEN & M. MARCINKIEWICZ. 1999. The subtilisin/kexin family of precursor convertases: emphasis on PC1, PC2/7B2, POMC and the novel enzyme SKI-1. Ann. N. Y. Acad. Sci. **885:** 57–74.

2. LUGER, T.A., T. SCHOLZEN & S. GRABBE. 1997. The role of alpha- melanocyte-stimulating hormone in cutaneous biology. J. Invest. Dermatol. Symp. Proc. **2:** 87–93.

3. SCHAUER, E., F. TRAUTINGER, A. KOCK, A. SCHWARZ, R. BHARDWAJ, M. SIMON, J.C. ANSEL, T. SCHWARZ & T.A. LUGER. 1994. Proopiomelanocortin-derived peptides are synthesized and released by human keratinocytes. J. Clin. Invest. **93:** 2258–2262.

4. WINTZEN, M., M. YAAR, J.P. BURBACH & B.A. GILCHREST. 1996. Proopiomelanocortin gene product regulation in keratinocytes. J. Invest. Dermatol. **106:** 673-678.

5. CONE, R.D., D. LU, S. KOPPULA, D.I. VAGE, H. KLUNGLAND, B. BOSTON, W. CHEN, D.N. ORTH, C. POUTON & R.A. KESTERSON. 1996. The melanocortin receptors: agonists, antagonists, and the hormonal control of pigmentation. Rec. Progr. Hormone Res. **51:** 287–317.

6. TATRO, J.B. 1996. Receptor biology of the melanocortins, a family of neuroimmunomodulatory peptides. Neuroimmunomodulation **3:** 259–284.

7. BRZOSKA, T., T. SCHOLZEN, E. BECHER & T.A. LUGER. 1997. Effect of UV light on the production of proopiomelanocortin-derived peptides and melanocortin receptors in the skin. *In* Skin Cancer and UV Irradiation. P. Altmeyer, K. Hoffmann & M. Stuecker, Eds.: 227–237. Springer Verlag. Berlin.

8. REES, J.L. & E. HEALY. 1997. Melanocortin receptors, red hair, and skin cancer. J. Invest. Dermatol. Symp. Proc. **2:** 94–98.

9. HUSZAR, D., C.A. LYNCH, V. FAIRCHILD-HUNTRESS, J.H. DUNMORE, Q. FANG, L.R. BERKEMEIER, W. GU, R.A. KESTERSON, B.A. BOSTON, R.D. CONE, F.J. SMITH, L.A. CAMPFIELD, P. BURN & F. LEE. 1997. Targeted disruption of the melanocortin-4 receptor results in obesity in mice. Cell **88:** 131–141.

10. JORDAN, A. & I.J. JACKSON. 1998. Melanocortin receptors and antagonists regulate pigmentation and body weight. Bioessays **20:** 603–606.

11. KRUDE, H., H. BIEBERMANN, W. LUCK, R. HORN, G. BRABANT & A. GRUTERS. 1998. Severe early-onset obesity, adrenal insufficiency and red hair pigmentation caused by POMC mutations in humans. Nat. Genet. **19:** 155–157.

12. YASWEN, L., N. DIEHL, M.B. BRENNAN & U. HOCHGESCHWENDER. 1999. Obesity in the mouse model of pro-opiomelanocortin deficiency responds to peripheral melanocortin. Nat. Med. **5:** 1066–1070.

13. LUGER, T.A., T. SCHOLZEN, T. BRZOSKA, E. BECHER, A. SLOMINSKI & R. PAUS. 1998. Cutaneous immunomodulation and coordination of skin stress responses by alpha-melanocyte-stimulating hormone. Ann. N.Y. Acad. Sci. **840:** 381–394.

14. BHARDWAJ, R., E. BECHER, K. MAHNKE, M. HARTMEYER, T. SCHWARZ, T. SCHOLZEN & T.A. LUGER. 1997. Evidence for the differential expression of the functional alpha-melanocyte-stimulating hormone receptor MC-1 on human monocytes. J. Immunol. **158:** 3378–3384.

15. BECHER, E., K. MAHNKE, T. BRZOSKA, D.-H. KALDEN, S. GRABBE & T.A. LUGER. 1999. Human peripheral blood-derived dendritic cells express functional melanocortin receptor MC-1R. Ann. N.Y. Acad. Sci. **885:** 188–195.

16. TAHERZADEH, S., S. SHARMA, V. CHHAJLANI, I. GANTZ, N. RAJORA, M.T. DEMITRI, L. KELLY, H. ZHAO, T. ICHIYAMA, A. CATANIA & J.M. LIPTON. 1999. alpha-MSH and its receptors in regulation of tumor necrosis factor-alpha production by human monocyte/macrophages. Am. J. Physiol. **276:** R1289–R1294.

17. GENEDANI, S., M. BERNARDI, M.G. BALDINI & A. BERTOLINI. 1992. Influence of CRF and alpha-MSH on the migration of human monocytes in vitro. Neuropeptides **23:** 99–102.

18. LIPTON, J.M., A. CATANIA & R. DELGADO. 1998. Peptide modulation of inflammatory processes within the brain. Neuroimmunomodulation **5:** 178–183.

19. RAJORA, N., G. CERIANI, A. CATANIA, R.A. STAR, M.T. MURPHY & J.M. LIPTON. 1996. alpha-MSH production, receptors, and influence on neopterin in a human monocyte/macrophage cell line. J. Leukoc. Biol. **59:** 248–253.

20. BHARDWAJ, R.S., A. SCHWARZ, E. BECHER, K. MAHNKE, Y. ARAGANE, T. SCHWARZ & T.A. LUGER. 1996. Pro-opiomelanocortin-derived peptides induce IL-10 production in human monocytes. J. Immunol. **156:** 2517–2521.

21. LIPTON, J.M. & A. CATANIA. 1998. Mechanisms of anti-inflammatory action of the neuroimmunomodulatory peptide alpha-MSH. Ann. N.Y. Acad. Sci. **840:** 373–380.

22. HUANG, Q.H., M.L. ENTWISTLE, J.D. ALVARO, R.S. DUMAN, V.J. HRUBY & J.B. TATRO. 1997. Antipyretic role of endogenous melanocortins mediated by central melanocortin receptors during endotoxin-induced fever. J. Neurosci. **17:** 3343–3351.

23. BAEUERLE, P.A. & D. BALTIMORE. 1996. NF-kappa B: ten years after. Cell **87:** 13–20.

24. MANNA, S.K. & B.B. AGGARWAL. 1998. Alpha-melanocyte-stimulating hormone inhibits the nuclear transcription factor NF-kappa B activation induced by various inflammatory agents. J. Immunol. **161:** 2873–2880.

25. BRZOSKA, T., D.-H. KALDEN, T.E. SCHOLZEN & T.A. LUGER. 1999. Molecular basis of the α-MSH/IL-1 antagonism. Ann. N.Y. Acad. Sci. **885:** 230–238.

26. KALDEN, D.-H., M. FASTRICH, T. BRZOSKA, T. SCHOLZEN, M. HARTMEYER, T. SCHWARZ & T.A. LUGER. 1999. Alpha-melanocyte-stimulating hormone reduces endotoxin-induced activation of nuclear factor NF-κB in endothelial cells. Ann. N.Y. Acad. Sci. **885:** 254–261.

27. BUTCHER, E.C. 1991. Leukocyte-endothelial cell recognition: three (or more) steps to specificity and diversity. Cell **67:** 1033–1036.

28. HARTMEYER, M., T. SCHOLZEN, E. BECHER, R.S. BHARDWAJ, T. SCHWARZ & T. LUGER. 1997. Human dermal microvascular endothelial cells express the melanocortin receptor type 1 and produce increased levels of IL-8 upon stimulation with alpha-melanocyte-stimulating hormone. J. Immunol. **159:** 1930-1937.

29. GRABBE, S., R.S. BHARDWAJ, K. MAHNKE, M.M. SIMON, T. SCHWARZ & T.A. LUGER. 1996. alpha-Melanocyte-stimulating hormone induces hapten-specific tolerance in mice. J. Immunol. **156:** 473-478.

30. BRZOSKA, T., B. ALTMANN, M. FASTRICH, M. MÖLLER, D. H. KALDEN, T. SCHOLZEN, H.B. SCHIÖTH, A. SKOTTNER, J.E.S. WIKBERG & T.A. LUGER. 2000. New agonists and antagonists for the Melanocortin receptors: evaluation of the efficiency of synthetic α-MSH analogues. Arch. Dermatol. Res. **252:** 85.

31. SUNDERKÖTTER, C., D.-H. KALDEN, T. BRZOSKA, C. SORG & T.A. LUGER. 1999. α-MSH reduces vasculitis in the local Shwartzman reaction. Ann. N.Y. Acad. Sci. **885:** 414–418.

Neuropeptide Regulation of Immunity

The Immunosuppressive Activity of Alpha-Melanocyte–Stimulating Hormone (α-MSH)

A.W. TAYLOR,[a] D.G. YEE, T. NISHIDA, AND K. NAMBA

Schepens Eye Research Institute and the Department of Ophthalmology, Harvard Medical School, Boston, Massachusetts 02114, USA

ABSTRACT: The ocular microenvironment is an extreme example of regional immunity. Within its microenvironment, expression of delayed type hypersensitivity (DTH) is suppressed. This immunosuppression is mediated in part by the constitutive expression of α-MSH. Previously we have found that α-MSH suppresses the production of IFN-γ by activated effector T cells. Recently we have found that α-MSH can mediate induction of TGF-β–producing T cells that act as regulatory T cells. This has encouraged us to further examine the potential for α-MSH to suppress T cell–mediated inflammation (autoimmune disease) and to regulate lymphokine production by effector T cells. When α-MSH was injected i.v. into mice at the time of peak retinal inflammation, the severity of experimental autoimmune uveitis (EAU) was significantly suppressed. Effector T cells activated *in vitro* in the presence of α-MSH proliferated and produced IL-4 and enhanced levels of TGF-β while their IFN-γ and IL-10 production was suppressed. The α-MSH-treated T cells functioned as regulatory T cells by suppressing *in vitro* IFN-γ production by other inflammatory T cells. This regulatory activity was the function of α-MSH–treated CD4+ CD25+ T cells. Therefore, α-MSH mediates immunosuppression by inducing a differential expression of lymphokine production and by inducing activation of regulatory functions in T cells. This implies that α-MSH may take part in regional mechanisms of immunosuppression and possibly peripheral tolerance. Thus, α-MSH can be used to suppress autoimmune disease and possibly reestablish tolerance to autoantigens.

INTRODUCTION

The activation, type, and intensity of an effector T cell response is not limited to antigen sensitivity alone, but also to local immunoregulatory mechanisms to which neurologically derived factors can contribute. This regional regulation insures that the most effective immune defense is mounted in proportion with preserving the unique functionality of the infected tissue. An extreme example of regional immunity is the immune-privileged microenvironment of the ocular anterior chamber.[1,2] Within this microenvironment, delayed type hypersensitivity–mediating T cells are suppressed.[3] This suppression is mediated by factors constitutively produced within

[a]Address for correspondence and reprint requests: Andrew W. Taylor, Ph.D., Schepens Eye Research Institute, 20 Staniford Street, Boston, MA 02114. Voice: 617-912-7452; fax: 617-912-0113. awtaylor@vision.eri.harvard.edu

the anterior chamber.[4–8] Specific neuropeptides are present within the ocular microenvironment that help to maintain immunosuppression.[9] Changes in neuropeptide expression by neurons that innervate ocular tissues are associated with loss of immune privilege.[10] Recently we have found that the neuropeptide α-MSH suppresses IFN-γ production, but not proliferation by activated effector T cells.[11] This has suggested that α-MSH may regulate regional induction of specific effector T cell responses.

The thirteen amino acid–long (1.6 kD) α-MSH is encoded within the proopiomelanocortin hormone (POMC) gene and released from the POMC protein through two endoproteolytic cleavage steps.[12,13] It has a fundamental role in modulating host defense mechanisms in mammals differing from its original description as an amphibian melanin-inducing factor.[14,15] Systemic and central injections of α-MSH suppress innate inflammatory responses induced by endotoxin, IL-1 and TNF such as suppression of macrophage reactive oxygen intermediates and nitric oxide generation as well as production of inflammatory cytokines.[16–21] In addition, α-MSH induces its own production and receptor expression on the macrophages promoting autocrine suppression of inflammatory-macrophage activities. Also, α-MSH suppresses macrophage and neutrophil chemotactic responses to chemokines and microbial chemoattractants.[19,22] Macrophages, keratinocytes, CNS-derived neurons, and possibly any cell that can synthesize POMC are sources of α-MSH.[21,23,24] In normal mammalian aqueous humor (fluid filling the ocular anterior chamber) there is constitutively expressed on average 30 pg/ml of α-MSH.[7]

Besides its suppression of innate-mediated inflammation, α-MSH may also suppress adaptive immune-mediated inflammation. α-MSH suppresses IFN-γ production by activated primed T cells, but not proliferation, suggesting that α-MSH may selectively regulate specific effector T cell activities.[11] Recently we have found that α-MSH mediates the induction of TGF-β–producing T cells that suppress the activation of other inflammatory T cells.[25] These findings suggest that α-MSH suppresses T cell–mediated inflammation and mediates selective production of T cell lymphokines.

METHODS

Reagents

The experiments used synthetic α-MSH (Peninsula Laboratories, Belmont, CA); recombinant TGF-β2 and soluble TGF-β receptor type II (R&D Systems, Minneapolis, MN); anti-CD4 (RM4-4), anti-CD25 (IL-2-receptor-α; 7D4) and anti-CD3ε (145-2C11) (Pharmingen, San Diego, CA). B10.RIII (Jackson Laboratories Bar Harbor, ME) and BALB/c (Institute breeding program) female mouse strains four to eight weeks old were treated with approval by the institutional animal care and use committee in accordance with the U.S. Animal Welfare Act.

α-MSH Treatment of in Vivo Primed T Cells

In vivo primed T cells were obtained from the draining popliteal lymph node of BALB/c mice immunized via a cutaneous foot injection with 0.5 mg desiccated

Mycobacterium tuberculosis (Difco, Detroit, MI). The T cells were enriched, 99% $CD3^+$ by flow cytometry analysis, using a mouse T cell enrichment column (R&D Systems). Into the wells of a 96-well plate were added 100 μl of T cells (4×10^6 cells/ml), 50 μl of diluted α-MSH and 50 μl of anti-CD3ε (1 μg/ml) in serum-free culture media. The cultures were incubated for 48 hours and the culture supernatants were assayed using sandwich enzyme linked immunosorbent assays (ELISA) for IFN-γ, IL-4 and IL-10.[25] Total TGF-β was assayed using the standard CCL-64 bioassay.[26] The *serum-free* culture media[7] was RPMI 1640 (BioWittaker, Walkerville, MD), 1/75 dilution of sterile 7.5% BSA solution (Sigma Chemical, St. Louis, MO), 1/500 dilution of "ITS+" solution (Collaborative Biomedical Products, Bedford, MA). To assay proliferation the T cell cultures were initially incubated for 24 hours and 20 μl of 50 μCi/ml of ^{3}H-thymidine (NEM, Boston, MA) was added to the wells, and the cultures were incubated for an additional 24 hours. The cells were collected onto glass-wool filter paper using a Tomtec Plate Harvester 96 and radiolabel was measured using a Wallac 1205 Betaplate Liquid Scintillation Counter.

Fluorescence-Activated Cell Sorting

For immunostaining and flow cytometry, T cells (2×10^6 cells) from 24-hour cultures of the α-MSH-treated activated T cells were used. The cells were centrifuged and washed once in PBS/BSA buffer (10 mM PBS, 3% BSA). The cells were resuspended in 50 μl of PBS/BSA buffer containing 2 μg of PE-conjugated anti-CD4 and FITC-conjugated anti-CD25 antibodies and incubated for 30 minutes at room temperature. The cells were centrifuged, resuspended in 1 ml of PBS/BSA buffer, and washed two times. The stained cells were sorted by a Coulter ELITE cell sorter calibrated for two-color fluorescence. The cells were sorted into two populations, $CD25^+$ $CD4^+$ cells and the remaining cells ($CD4^-$ plus $CD25^-CD4^+$ cells). Sorted cells were used immediately in culture experiments.

Assay for in Vitro Regulatory T Cell Activity

The α-MSH–treated, TCR-stimulated T cells, as described above, were cultured for 48 hours. The cells were collected and added (2×10^5 cells) to cultures of freshly isolated enriched inflammatory T cells (2×10^5 cells) activated with anti-CD3ε (1 μg/ml). The mixed cell cultures were incubated 48 hours and the culture supernatants were assayed for IFN-γ by sandwich ELISA.

α-MSH Treatment of Experimental Autoimmune Uveitis (EAU)

EAU was induced by immunizing B10.RIII mice with 50 μg of human interphotoreceptor retinoid binding protein peptide (161–180; IRBPp) emulsified in complete Freund's adjuvant containing 2.0 mg/ml of *Mycobacterium tuberculosis* H37RA.[27] The retinal inflammation was clinically assessed every three days starting six days after the immunization. Some mice received an i.v. injection of 50 μg of α-MSH 10 days and 12 days after the immunization. Funduscopic examinations of the retina were done on eyes topically treated with 0.5% Tropicamide and Neo-Synephrine saline to dilate the pupil. The severity of inflammation was clinically graded on a 0 to 5 scale. No inflammation was scored 0, only white focal lesions of vessels were scored 1, linear lesions of vessels within the half of retina were scored as 2, linear lesions of vessels over half of retina were scored as 3, severe chorioretinal exudates or retinal hemorrhages in addition to the vasculitis were scored as 4, and subretinal hemorrhage or retinal detachments were scored as 5.

RESULTS

α-MSH Suppression of EAU

Previously, Lipton and colleagues showed that systemic injections of α-MSH suppressed localized inflammation mediated by innate immune responses induced by IL-1 and endotoxin.[15,17–19] Since we have previously found that α-MSH suppresses the activation of inflammatory T cells and promotes the activation of TGF-β–producing T cells in the ocular microenvironment,[25] we examined the possibility whether systemic injections of α-MSH could suppress experimental autoimmune uveitis (EAU) in the mouse eye. Mice were immunized to induce EAU as described in the methods and at the peak of retinal inflammation (day 11) mice received two injections of α-MSH (50 μg/mouse) on day 10 and 12 (see Figure 1). The mean uveitis score was markedly suppressed in the mice injected with α-MSH in comparison to mice that were untreated. In one case (Fig. 1, Δ) where the uveitis was mild (score 2 on day 11) the injection of α-MSH completely resolved the inflammation (score 0 on day 17). This demonstrates that by elevating the systemic levels of α-MSH, localized T cell–mediated inflammation can be suppressed.

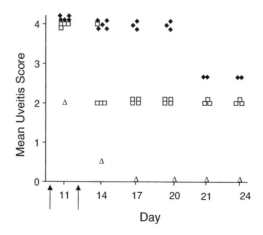

FIGURE 1. Suppression of EAU by intravenous injections of α-MSH. B10.R111 mice were immunized with IRBPp to induce EAU. Five mice were injected with 50 μg of α-MSH i.v. on Days 10 and 12 (□, △) and five mice did not receive α-MSH injections (◆). The data are presented as the mean uveitis score of each mouse.

α-MSH Regulates T Cell Lymphokine Production

Since we have previously found that α-MSH mediates induction of TGF-β–producing T cells while suppressing induction of IFN-γ,[11,25] we examined the lymphokine profile of T cells activated in the presence of α-MSH to see if α-MSH influences production of other lymphokines (TABLE 1). Enriched Primed T cells were stimulated with anti-CD3ε in the presence of 30 pg/ml of α-MSH and incubated for 48 hours. The concentration of α-MSH used in these experiments is the concentration of α-MSH in the fluids of aqueous humor and cerebral spinal fluid of mammals.[7,28] The culture supernatants were assayed for IFN-γ, IL-4, IL-10, and TGF-β. α-MSH significantly suppressed IFN-γ production; however, enhanced TGF-β production and had no effect on proliferation (TABLE 1). In addition, α-MSH suppressed IL-10 but not IL-4 production by the activated primed T cells (TABLE 1). This lymphokine profile favored by α-MSH suggests that α-MSH induces activation of regulatory T cells,[29–33] while suppressing inflammatory T cell activity.

α-MSH Induces Regulatory T Cells

If α-MSH induces the activation of regulatory T cells, then these T cells in turn should suppress the activity of other inflammatory T cells. To test this possibility, we mixed α-MSH–treated cells with freshly activated T cells, which normally produce IFN-γ, and assayed the cultures for IFN-γ production (TABLE 2). The freshly activated T cells were significantly suppressed in their production of IFN-γ by unsorted α-MSH-treated T cells (TABLE 2). This corresponds with our previous findings that α-MSH–treated T cells can suppress DTH.[25] The addition of soluble TGF-β receptor type II (sTGF-βRII) significantly neutralized the unsorted α-MSH–induced regulatory T cell suppression of IFN-γ production by freshly activated T cells (TABLE 2). Therefore, the TGF-β produced by α-MSH–induced regulatory T cells is sufficient to suppress IFN-γ production by other T cells.

TABLE 1. Effects of α-MSH on primed T cells activated with anti-CD3ε

Treatment	Cytokine (pg/ml)[a]				Proliferation (CPM)[c]
	IFN-γ	IL-4	IL-10	TGF-β	
anti-CD3ε only	1262 ± 132	267 ± 22	61 ± 14	49 ± 14	40171 ± 899
anti-CD3ε + α-MSH[b]	809 ± 44*	214 ± 63	21 ± 9*	248 ± 73*	38526 ± 1224
−anti-CD3ε	206 ± 1*	155 ± 78	1 ± 1*	7 ± 3*	864 ± 235*

[a]Culture supernatant (48 h after treatment) were assayed for cytokines by ELISA for IFN-γ, IL-4, IL-10, and by bioassay for TGF-β. Data presented as mean ± SEM of 4 independent experiments each.

[b]Primed T cells were stimulated with anti-CD3ε in the presence of 30 pg/ml of α-MSH.

[c]Cell cultures were treated with ^{3}H-thymidine 24 h after start of assay and incubated for an additional 24 hours before scintillation counting of the cells. Data presented as counts per minute (CPM) ± SEM of 4 independent experiments.

*Significantly ($p \leq 0.05$) different to primed T cells treated with only anti-CD3ε.

TABLE 2. Effects of adding α-MSH–treated T cells into cultures of freshly activated primed T cells

Added α-MSH–treated cells[a]	IFN-γ (pg/ml)[b]
None	153 ± 3
Unsorted cells	43 ± 7[*,**]
Unsorted cells + sTGF-βRII[c]	130 ± 47[**]
CD25[+] CD4[+] cells[d]	46 ± 30[*]
CD4[−] and CD25[−] CD4[+] cells[d]	175 ± 5

[a]Cells were added to cultures containing fresh primed T cells and anti-CDε.

[b]Supernatants were assayed for IFN-γ 48 h after addition of α-MSH treated cells. Data presented as mean ± SEM of 4 independent experiments.

[c]Soluble TGF-β receptor type II (sTGF-βRII; 0.5 μg/ml) was added to the culture with the unsorted α-MSH–treated T cells.

[d]Primed T cells anti-CD3ε stimulated in the presence of α-MSH for 24 h were stained and sorted by fluorescent activated cell sorting.

[*]Significantly ($p \leq 0.05$) different to cultures with no added cells (None). [**]Significantly ($p \leq 0.05$) different.

To see if a specific subtype of primed T cells are induced by α-MSH to express regulatory activity, the α-MSH–treated T cells were stained for CD4 and IL-2 receptor-alpha (CD25) a marker of T cell activation. The CD25-expressing CD4 cells were sorted out by fluorescent-activated cell sorting and added to cultures of freshly activated primed T cells. The immunosuppressive activity was associated with the CD25-expressing CD4 cells and not with other cells in the primed T cell population (TABLE 2). This indicates that α-MSH induces activation of regulatory CD4[+] T cells that suppress inflammation mediated by other T cells.

DISCUSSION

The neuropeptide α-MSH mediates the induction of TGF-β–producing T cells. The lymphokine profile of α-MSH-treated primed T cells is immunosuppressive instead of pro-inflammatory. Therefore, the suppression of autoimmune uveitis is possibly due to α-MSH suppressing production of inflammatory lymphokines by activated autoreactive T cells while inducing activation of regulatory T cells. Previously we have demonstrated that such α-MSH–treated T cells suppress antigen-specific DTH *in vivo* through bystander suppression.[25] This suggested that regulation is mediated though non-antigen–specific mechanisms, such as a cytokine. Our present results demonstrate that it is at least through the production of TGF-β that α-MSH–treated T cells mediate immunosuppression. Therefore, α-MSH induces activation of regulatory T cells that can mediate regional immunosuppression by producing soluble immunosuppressive factors.

Our results also indicate that if the concentration of α-MSH is sufficiently elevated either systemically or regionally, then immunogenic inflammation should be suppressed. Along with mediating the suppression of inflammatory T cells and inducing immunosuppressive lymphokine production, α-MSH is also antagonizing IL-1, TNF, and IFN-γ inflammatory activities. In addition, the lymphokines produced by the α-MSH–induced regulatory T cells have the potential to suppress inflammatory macrophage activities.[34,35] Therefore, the suppression of autoimmune disease seen in FIGURE 1 must include the general anti-inflammatory activity of α-MSH along with the effects of α-MSH on activated T cells. There is also the potential that regulatory T cells have been induced by systemic injections of α-MSH.

Our results further suggest that α-MSH has a physiological role in regulating inflammatory immune responses. Its activity within a localized tissue site can regulate the intensity and duration of an inflammatory response, and possibly, through induction of regulatory T cells whether immunogenic inflammation can occur at all, i.e., tolerance. In immune-privileged eyes, there is normally a constitutive presence of α-MSH.[7] Since the ocular microenvironment has adapted several mechanisms to prevent induction of inflammation, α-MSH may potentially affect immune cells more so then seen in other tissue sites. It is likely that within the normal ocular microenvironment α-MSH mediates induction of regulatory T cells that in turn mediate peripheral tolerance to ocular autoantigens. Therefore, the ability of α-MSH to selectively regulate the expression of lymphokines in activated T cells means that α-MSH can regulate the induction, intensity and type of immune responses in a regional tissue site.

The suppression of DTH by adoptively transferring α-MSH–induced regulatory T cells[25] suggests that if these cells were autoreactive regulatory T cells they would suppress induction of inflammatory autoimmune disease. Such regulatory T cells would only be activated in sites where their antigen is presented and through their production of immunosuppressive lymphokines would suppress the activation of nearby autoreactive inflammatory T cells. This could occur either in the periphery or within a draining lymph node. It is to be seen where α-MSH–induced regulatory T cells migrate.

We have demonstrated the importance of the neuropeptide α-MSH in regulating the adaptive immune response. α-MSH selectively regulates the production of lymphokines by activated effector T cells. This selective immunoregulation by α-MSH has an important role in maintaining immunogenic homeostasis through suppression of inflammation and possibly tolerance to autoantigens. It also suggests the potential to exploit α-MSH immunosuppressive activities for the purposes of treating autoimmune diseases.

REFERENCES

1. STREILEIN, J.W. 1999. Immunoregulatory mechanisms of the eye. Prog. Retin. Eye Res. **18:** 357–370.
2. TAYLOR, A.W. 1999. Ocular immunosuppressive microenvironment. Chem. Immunol. **73:** in press.
3. COUSINS, S.W., W.B. TRATTLER & J.W. STREILEIN. 1991. Immune privilege and suppression of immunogenic inflammation in the anterior chamber of the eye. Curr. Eye Res. **10:** 287–297.
4. COUSINS, S.W., M.M. MCCABE, D. DANIELPOUR & J.W. STREILEIN. 1991. Identification of transforming growth factor-beta as an immunosuppressive factor in aqueous humor. Invest. Ophthalmol. Vis. Sci. **32:** 33–43.

5. GRANSTEIN, R., R. STASZEWSKI, T.L. KNISELY, E. ZEIRA, R. NAZARENO, M. LATINA & D.M. ALBERT. 1990. Aqueous humor contains transforming growth factor-β and a small (less than 3500 daltons) inhibitor of thymocyte proliferation. J. Immunol. **144:** 3021–3026.

6. JAMPEL, H.D., N. ROCHE, W.J. STARK & A.B. ROBERTS. 1990. Transforming growth factor-β in human aqueous humor. Curr. Eye Res. **9:** 963–969.

7. TAYLOR, A.W., J.W. STREILEIN & S.W. COUSINS. 1992. Identification of alpha-melanocyte stimulating hormone as a potential immunosuppressive factor in aqueous humor. Curr. Eye Res. **11:** 1199–1206.

8. TAYLOR, A.W., J.W. STREILEIN & S.W. COUSINS. 1994. Immunoreactive vasoactive intestinal peptide contributes to the immunosuppressive activity of normal aqueous humor. J. Immunol. **153:** 1080–1086.

9. TAYLOR, A.W. 1996. Neuroimmunomodulation in immune privilege: role of neuropeptides in ocular immunosuppression. Neuroimmunomodulation **3:** 195–204.

10. FERGUSON, T.A., S. FLETCHER, J. HERNDON & T.S. GRIFFITH. 1995. Neuropeptides modulate immune deviation induced via the anterior chamber of the eye. J. Immunol. **155:** 1746–1756.

11. TAYLOR, A.W., J.W. STREILEIN & S.W. COUSINS. 1994. Alpha-melanocyte-stimulating hormone suppresses antigen-stimulated T cell production of gamma-interferon. Neuroimmunomodulation **1:** 188–194.

12. LEE, T.H., A.B. LERNER & V. BUETTNER-JANUSCH. 1961. The isolation and structure of α- and β-melanocyte-stimulating hormones from monkey pituitary glands. J. Biol. Chem. **236:** 1390–1394.

13. NAKANISHI, S., A. INOUE, T. KITA, M. NAKAMURA, A. C.Y. CHANG, S.N. COHEN & S. NUMA. 1979. Nucleotide sequence of cloned cDNA for bovine corticotropin-β-lipotropin precursor. Nature **278:** 423–427.

14. LIPTON, J.M. 1990. Modulation of host defense by the neuropeptide α-MSH. Yale J. Biol. Med. **63:** 173–182.

15. LIPTON, J.M. & A. CATANIA. 1997. Anti-inflammatory actions of the neuroimmunomodulator α-MSH. Immunol. Today **18:** 140–145.

16. HOLDEMAN, M., O. KHORRAM, W.K. SAMSON & J.M. LIPTON. 1985. Fever-specific changes in central MSH and CRF concentrations. Am. J. Physiol. **248:** R125–R129.

17. WATANABE, T., M.E. HILTZ, A. CATANIA & J.M. LIPTON. 1993. Inhibition of IL-1β-induced peripheral inflammation by peripheral and central administration of analogs of the neuropeptide α-MSH. Brain Res. Bull. **32:** 311–314.

18. MARTIN, L.W., A. CATANIA, M.E. HILTZ & J.M. LIPTON. 1991. Neuropeptide alpha-MSH antagonizes IL-6- and TNF-induced fever. Peptides **12:** 297–299.

19. CHIAO, H., S. FOSTER, R. THOMAS, J. LIPTON & R.A. STAR. 1996. α-Melanocyte stimulating hormone reduces endotoxin-induced liver inflammation. J. Clin. Invest. **97:** 2038–2044.

20. RAJORA, N., G. CERIANI, A. CATANIA, R.A. STAR, M.T. MURPHY & J.M. LIPTON. 1996. α-MSH production, receptors, and influence on neopterin in a human monocyte/macrophage cell line. J. Leuk. Biol. **59:** 248–253.

21. STAR, R.A., N. RAJORA, J. HUANG, R. CHAVEZ, A. CATANIA & J.M. LIPTON. 1995. Evidence of autocrine modulation of macrophage nitric oxide synthase by α-MSH. Proc. Natl. Acad. Sci. USA **90:** 8856–8860.

22. CATANIA, A., N. RAJORA, F. CAPSONI, F. MINONZIO, R.A. STAR & J.M. LIPTON. 1996. The neuropeptide α-MSH has specific receptors on neutrophils and reduces chemotaxis in vito. Peptides **17:** 675–679.

23. CHAKRABORTY, A.K., Y. FUNASAKA, A. SLOMINSKI, G. ERMAK, J. HWANG, J.M. PAWELEK & M. ICHIHASHI. 1996. Production and release of proopiomelanocortin (POMC) derived peptides by human melanocytes and keratinocytes in culture: regulation by ultraviolet B. Biochim. Biophys. Acta **1313:** 130–138.

24. O'DONOHUE, T.L. & D.M. DORSA. 1982. The opiomelanotropinergic neuronal and endocrine systems. Peptides **3:** 353–395.

25. NISHIDA, T. & A.W. TAYLOR. 1999. Specific aqueous humor factors induce activation of regulatory T cells. Invest. Ophthalmol. Vis. Sci. **40:** 2268–2274.

26. TAYLOR, A.W., P. ALARD, D.G. YEE & J.W. STREILEIN. 1997. Aqueous humor induces transforming growth factor-beta (TGF-beta)-producing regulatory T-cells. Curr. Eye Res. **16:** 900–908.
27. SILVER, P.B., L.V. RIZZO, C.C. CHAN, L.A. DONOSO, B. WIGGERT & R.R. CASPI. 1995. Identification of a major pathogenic epitope in the human IRBP molecule recognized by mice of the H-2r haplotype. Invest. Ophthalmol. Vis. Sci. **36:** 946–954.
28. TAYLOR, A.W. & J.W. STREILEIN. 1996. Inhibition of antigen-stimulated effector T cells by human cerebrospinal fluid. Neuroimmunomodulation **3:** 112–118.
29. CHEN, Y., V.K. KUCHROO, J.I. INOBE, D.A. HAFLER & H.L. WEINER. 1994. Regulatory T cell clones induced by oral tolerance: suppression of autoimmune encephalomyelitis. Science **265:** 1237–1240.
30. CASPI, R., L. STIFF, R. MORAWENTZ, N. MILLER-RIVERO, C. CHAN, B. WIGGERT, R. NUSSENBLATT, H. MORSE & L. RIZZO. 1996. Cytokine-dependent modulation of oral tolerance in a murine model of autoimmune uveitis. Ann. N.Y. Acad. Sci. **778:** 315–324.
31. WEINER, H.L. 1997. Oral tolerance: immune mechanisms and treatment of autoimmune diseases. Immunol. Today **18:** 335–343.
32. SHI, F.D., H. LI, H. WANG, X. BAI, P.H. VAN DER MEIDE, H. LINK & H.G. LJUNGGREN. 1999. Mechanisms of nasal tolerance induction in experimental autoimmune myasthenia gravis: identification of regulatory cells. J. Immunol. **162:** 5757–5763.
33. INOBE, J., A.J. SLAVIN, Y. KOMAGATA, Y. CHEN, L. LIU & H.L. WEINER. 1998. IL-4 is a differentiation factor for transforming growth factor-beta secreting Th3 cells and oral administration of IL-4 enhances oral tolerance in experimental allergic encephalomyelitis. Eur. J. Immunol. **28:** 2780–2790.
34. TAKEUCHI, M., M.M. KOSIEWICZ, P. ALARD & J.W. STREILEIN. 1997. On the mechanisms by which transforming growth factor-β2 alters antigen-presenting abilities of macrophages on T cell activation. Eur. J. Immunol. **27:** 1648–1656.
35. TSUNAWAKI, S., M. SPORN, A. DING & C. NATHAN. 1988. Deactivation of macrophages by transforming growth factor-β. Nature **334:** 260–262.

Natural Immunity and Neuroimmune Host Defense

ISTVAN BERCZI,[a,b] LÓRÁND BERTÓK,[c] AND DONNA A. CHOW[a]

[a]*Department of Immunology, Faculty of Medicine, University of Manitoba, Winnipeg, Manitoba, R3E 0W3, Canada*

[c]*"Fodor Jozsef" National Center for Public Health, "Frederic Joliot-Curie" National Research Institute of Radiobiology and Radiohygiene, Budapest, Hungary*

ABSTRACT: Innate resistance is mediated by non-immune defense and by natural immunity. Non-immune defense includes diverse mechanisms (e.g., physico-chemical defense by bile acids). Natural killer (NK) cells, $\gamma\delta$ T lymphocytes and CD5[+] B lymphocytes are key mediators of natural immunity. These cells utilize germ-line coded receptors that recognize highly conserved, homologous epitopes (homotopes). Typically, it is not the antigen, but cytokines and hormones that regulate the level of NK-mediated cytotoxicity. These include interleukin-2, interferons, prolactin and growth hormone. Less is known about $\gamma\delta$ T lymphocytes. CD5[+] B lymphocytes produce germ-line coded antibodies (predominantly IgM) that are polyspecific, and able to recognize a great variety of microorganisms, cancer cells and self-components. Antigen is not an effective stimulus for natural antibody (NAb), but bacterial lipopolysaccharide (LPS) is. During the acute phase response (febrile illness) the T-cell–regulated adaptive immune response is switched off and natural immune mechanisms are amplified several hundred to a thousand times within 24–48 hours (immunoconversion). This immunoconversion is initiated by immune-derived cytokines, and involves profound neuroendocrine and metabolic changes, all in the interest of host defense. Immune recognition is assured by natural antibodies and by some liver-derived acute phase proteins, such as C-reactive protein or endotoxin-binding protein, the level of which is elevated in the serum. Thus, natural immunity is essential for a first and last line of defense and the neuroendocrine system is an important promoter of this activity.

THE NATURAL IMMUNE SYSTEM

Innate resistance may be divided into host defense mediated by non-immune mechanisms and natural immune defense. Non-immune defense mechanisms include behavioral defense (e.g., avoidance, aversion, cough, vomiting, diarrhea, etc.); skin defense mechanisms (for instance the reaction to UV irradiation); non-immune mucosal defense (the secretion of mucus, antimicrobial proteins, enzymes, low pH in the stomach, etc.); defense by exocrine secretions by the salivary, lacrimal and sweat glands, the liver, mammary gland and male exocrine glands; and

[b]Address for correspondence: Dr. I. Berczi, Department of Immunology, University of Manitoba, 795 McDermot Avenue, Winnipeg, Manitoba, R3E 0W3, Canada. Voice: 204-789-3320; fax: 204-789-3921.

berczii@ms.umanitoba.ca

TABLE 1. Natural immunity

Non-immune defense	Immune defense
Behavioral neural: avoidance, cough, vomiting, diarrhea	Natural killer cells Tγδ cells CD5⁺ B lymphocytes: producing natural antibody (NAb)
Skin: pigmentation, vitamin-D, sweat-gland and keratinocyte-derived mediators, etc.	T lymphocytes: after activation by superantigens, chemokines, cytokines, etc.
Mucosal exocrine: mucus, enzymes, defensins and other antimicrobial substances, bile acids, HCl in stomach, cytokines, hormones, neuropeptides, etc.	B lymphocytes: activated by LPS, superantigens, cytokines, etc.
	Mast cells: triggered by physical, chemical factors and by neuropeptides
	Phagocytes: reacting to bacterial substances, NAb, opsonins, etc.
Systemic: nitric oxide, oxygen radicals, heat shock proteins, non-immune interferons, enzymes, properdin, prostaglandins, leukotrienes, chemokines, blood clotting, species-related resistance	Complement: activated by natural antibodies and by the alternate pathway
	Acute phase proteins: C-reactive protein, endotoxin-binding protein, mannose-binding protein

non-immune systemic host defense, which includes oxygen radicals, nitric oxide, heat-shock proteins, non-immune interferons, inductive enzyme synthesis, properdin, chemokines, prostaglandins and leukotrienes, blood clotting and species-related natural resistance.[1–6,35] The natural immune system comprises highly specialized cells, such as NK[d] cells, γδ T lymphocytes, and B cells secreting NAb. However, antigen-specific T and B lymphocytes may also be activated by alternate

[d]ABBREVIATIONS: ACTH, adrenocorticotropic hormone; ANP, atrial natriuretic peptide; APP, acute-phase proteins; APR, acute phase response; AVP, arginine vasopressin; B, lymphocyte; C', complement; CAT, catecholamines; CNS, central nervous system; CRF, corticotropin-releasing factor; CRP, C-reactive protein; DHEA, dehydroepiandrosterone; E_2 estradiol; EDT, endothelium; β-END, β-endorphin; FSH, follicle-stimulating hormone; GC, glucocorticoid; GH, growth hormone; GLH, growth and lactogenic hormones; GLU, glucagon; HPA, hypothalamus-pituitary-adrenal axis; IGF-I, insulin-like growth factor-I; IL-1, interleukin-1; INS, insulin; LBP, lipopolysaccharide endotoxin binding protein; LH, luteinizing hormone; LPS, lipopolysaccharide; MBP, mannose-binding protein; MEL, melatonin; MF, macrophage; α-MSH, α-melanocyte-stimulating hormone; NAb, natural antibody; NK, natural killer cell; PLT, platelet; PMN, polymorphonuclear leukocyte; PRL, prolactin; PS, progesterone; SP, substance P; T, T lymphocyte; T_3, thyroxin; T_4, triiodothyronine; TNF, tumor necrosis factor; TRH, thyrotrophin-releasing hormone; TS, testosterone; TSH, thyroid-stimulating hormone; VD3, vitamin D3.

TABLE 2. Examples of homotopes, their receptors and their functions

Homotope	Source	Homotope receptor	Immune activation
Lipid-A of LPS	Gram negative bacteria	LBP	B, MF, C', PLT, EDT, CNS, ENG
Phosphoryl choline, galactose, cationic proteins	Microbes, degraded cells	CRP	B, T, MF, C' PMN, NK, PLT
Diverse carbohydrates	Microbes	MBP	MF, PMN, C'
Diverse epitopes; charged molecules, carbohydrates, superantigens	Microbes, cancer cells, self components	Natural antibodies	B, T, MF, C' PMN, NK
Superantigens ("toxins")	Microbes, self components?	TcR, BcR (sIg)	T, B Inflammatory cells
Lipid, glycolipid, peptides	Microbes, self?	CD1	T
Phosphate-containing nonpeptides	Microbes, self?	$\gamma\delta$ TcR	T$\gamma\delta$

pathways during natural immune reactions where specific antigen does not play a role. Neutrophilic, eosinophilic and basophilic leukocytes and mast cells also are integrated in the natural immune system[5,7–9] (see TABLE 1). As is indicated in the table the entire immune system may be activated by natural immune mechanisms.

Natural immune reactions are based on the recognition of evolutionarily preserved homologous epitopes (homotopes) by serum proteins and germ-line encoded cellular receptors that belong to several molecular families (see TABLE 2). Homotopes are associated with microorganism, cancer cells, degenerated cells and with other cell components. Serum proteins, such as lipopolysaccharide endotoxin–binding protein (LBP), C-reactive protein (CRP),[10] mannose-binding protein (MBP)[11] or NAb,[12,13] serve as recognition molecules of homotopes. After combination with the appropriate homotope these soluble receptors acquire the capacity to activate various cells within the immune system and elsewhere. Other homotopes act directly on cell surface receptors, such as CD1,[14] or the antigen receptor of T[15,16] and B[17] lymphocytes. Most, if not all, of these homotope receptors are polyspecific and allow the recognition of a vast variety of molecular structures associated with pathogens and abnormal cell components with the aid of relatively few germ line–encoded molecules. There is evidence to indicate that microbial homotopes are stable because they are essential for the survival or for the pathogenicity of the microorganism.[4,5,7,9]

NATURAL IMMUNITY AND HOST DEFENSE

Natural immune mechanisms represent the first line of host defense against infectious disease, tissue injury and against a variety of noxious agents. In addition, evidence is increasing that natural immune mechanisms are part of normal physiological regulation of various bodily functions. As is obvious from TABLE 3, LPS is capable of activating the entire immune system after complexing with LBP, which in turn will be recognized by the CD14 cell surface molecule on macrophages and on some other cells. Alternate LPS receptors also exist. It is remarkable that LPS is capable of acting on numerous other targets in the body that include platelets, endothelium, peritoneum, adipocytes, the central nervous system, the vagus and possibly other peripheral nerves, and endocrine glands.[5,9,18–23] It seems very remarkable that systemically LPS activates multiple targets in concert, all of which play essential roles in neuroimmune host defense. CRP also is capable of complete immune activation, similarly to NAb. Therefore, CRP may be considered at least as good as NAb in host defense. Clearly CRP, LBP and MBP are capable of directing immune reactions against well defined targets, just as antibodies do. Once target identification has been achieved, the immune effector mechanisms (e.g., inflammation, phagocytosis, cytotoxicity) are shared with adaptive immune mechanisms and, consequently are equally effective.[5]

TABLE 3. Immune activation by LPS, CRP and NAb

Cells/systems activated	Lipopolysaccharide (LBP)	C-reactive protein	Natural antibody
1. Complement	+	+	+
2. Monocyte/macrophage, Kupfer cells in liver, etc.	+	+	+
3. T cells	+ (T$\gamma\delta$)	+ (CTL)	+
4. B-cells	+	+	+
5. Mast cells discharge	+ (via C3a, C5a)	+ (via C3a, C5a)	+ (via C3a, C5a)
6. Polymorphonuclear cells	+ (via C3a, C5a)	+	+ (via C3a, C5a)
7. NK cells	−	+	+
8. Platelets	+	+	+?
9. Endothelium	+		
10. Peritoneum	+		
11. Adipocyte	+		
12. CNS (astrocytes, glia cells)	+		
13. Vagus nerve	+		
14. Endocrine glands ("Resident Mf" follicular stellate cells)	+		

NOTE: +, action and/or stimulation; −, no effect

Most cells in the body are capable of producing interferons-α and -β after viral infections and secreting chemotactic and proinflammatory cytokines (chemokines) after injury. Moreover, sensory nerve fibers are capable of triggering inflammation in response to irritation which does not involve tissue injury. Thus neurogenic inflammation does not only function as a potent defense reaction, but in some cases it may be regarded as a preemptive response.[10,24,25] Mucosal secretions take this preemptive response one step further (e.g. defending the host outside the body) on mucosal surfaces. Natural immune defense is fundamental to mucosal defense, although adaptive immune reactions also play a role. For instance, the submandibular gland in rodents produces non-immune resistance factors, such as enzymes, antimicrobial proteins and mucus, in addition to C-reactive protein and natural antibodies belonging mainly to the IgA class. Because immune reactions take place on mucosal surfaces, self-nonself discrimination by the immune system is of limited value. Current evidence indicates that mucosal immune and inflammatory reactions are under strict neuroendocrine control. In rodents the submandibular gland plays a key role in the regulation of mucosal immunity and in the coordination of mucosal defense with systemic immune reactions.[4,26]

One may suggest on the basis of current evidence that natural immune mechanisms are in the frontline of host defense at all times. The natural immune system is capable of detecting instantaneously pathogenic agents, infected and injured cells by genetically preserved polyspecific cellular receptors and serum recognition proteins, and, via the nervous system, it even reacts to irritants. The entire immune system may be activated by natural immune pathways. The polyspecificity of recognition molecules mediating natural immunity is a distinct advantage as they are capable of providing a wide spectrum of host defense with minimal usage of the genome. The prerequisite for adaptive immunity is prior exposure to the pathogenic agent. This is not necessary for natural immunity because of its innate characteristics.

Bacteria, such as mycobacteria in Freund's adjuvant, killed gram-negative bacteria, corynebacterium, etc., have been used as immunological adjuvants for decades. Some bacterial products, such as LPS and its "detoxified" forms, are being applied to therapy to boost host defense under various situations. Sublethal doses of endotoxin or its detoxified forms increase resistance against infectious agents and injury, protect against X-irradiation, enhance the antibody response, exert an antitumor effect, stimulate bone marrow function, activate the complement system and blood clotting, promote regeneration and healing in the liver and possibly even in the central nervous system.[2,3,5] LBP provided defense against gram-negative bacterial infection in mice.[27] Mice transgenic for human CRP showed increased resistence against infection with staphylococci.[28] Finally, experimental superantigen-based immunotherapy of human pancreatic and colorectal cancer is already under way, using monoclonal antibody-staphylococcal enterotoxin A fusion protein.[29]

Host Defense in Febrile Illness

Fever is the unmistakable hallmark of an acute phase response (APR), which is a polyspecific defense reaction capable of increasing host resistance to infectious disease and insults within hours via the rapid elevation of liver-derived recognition proteins and natural antibodies. Acute febrile disease may be elicited by infection, trauma or injury. It is associated with a profound suppression of the adaptive immune response and the rapid elevation of natural immune defense mechanisms, which may be amplified several hundred to a thousand times within 24-48 hours. Immune-derived cytokines, primarily IL-1, IL-6 and TNF-α, initiate APR. These cytokines activate leukocytes and also act on the central nervous system and on numerous organs and tissues in the body, which leads to a neuroendocrine and metabolic response. IL-1 is a major mediator of fever and also activates the HPA axis and affects other endocrine organs. TNF has a similar function to IL-1. It is a powerful proinflammatory cytokine and also mediates catabolism during APR.[3,5,6,30,31]

The major neuroendocrine changes induced by bacterial endotoxin are summarized in TABLE 4. Cytokine production is under tight control during APR primarily by the elevation of hormones of the HPA axis: e.g., CRF, ACTH (stimulating gluco-corticoids), α-MSH and β-END. This axis suppresses the adaptive immune response and regulates fever and inflammation by acting on the nervous, endocrine and immune systems. Circulating GH and PRL levels rise at the beginning of febrile illness returning to normal within a few hours and may become subnormal in cases of prolonged illness. The immunostimulatory function of growth and lactogenic hormones is suppressed during APR, and the IGF-I response to GH is impaired. The levels of insulin (INS) and glucagon (GLU) are consistently elevated and insulin resistance is present. The conversion of T4 to T3 in the tissues is also impaired (euthyroid sick syndrome). Sex hormone levels are suppressed and testosterone (TS) levels may stay subnormal for lengthy periods.[3,5,6,32]

IL-6 is a multifunctional cytokine which stimulates the production of acute phase proteins (APP) in the liver. Catecholamines and glucocorticoids amplify the production of APP, the serum level of which could rise from several hundred to a thousand times within 1–2 days. By this conversion the production of polyspecific defense

TABLE 4. **Major neuroendocrine changes induced by endotoxin**

The HPA Axis	Response	Immunostimulatory hormones	Response	Gonadotropins and steroid hormones	Response
CRF	↑	TRH	↓	LH	↑↓
AVP	↑	TSH	0↓	FSH	↓
ACTH	↑	T4	↓	E2	↑↓
GC	↑	T3	↓	TS	↑↓
α-MSH	↑	PRL	↑↓	DHEA	↓?
β-END	↑	GH	↑↓	PS	↑↓
CAT	↑	IGF-I	↓		
		INS	↑		
		GLU	↑		
		leptin	↑		

NOTE: ↑, increase; ↓, decrease; ↑↓, variable effect; 0, no effect; ?, predicted change.

molecules such as LBP and CRP is increased enormously. Leukocyte generation in the bone marrow, the metabolic activity of leukocytes, and the production of natural antibodies are also enhanced. Likewise, complement and fibrinogen production are elevated. All these changes are consistent with the rapid enhancement of polyspecific host resistance to infection and various other insults. A number of APPs function as enzyme inhibitors and inhibitors of inflammation, which is likely to provide damage control during APR.[3,5,6,31]

Febrile illness may be regarded as an emergency defense reaction which takes over the task of host defense in situations when local defense mechanisms, including adaptive immunity, have failed to control the pathogenic agent. Under these conditions a systemic immune activation results in the elevation of cytokines in the circulation which leads to neuroendocrine and metabolic changes. The adaptive immune response is suppressed by hormones of the HPA axis to which the suppression of growth and lactogenic hormone function and of thyroid hormone function is likely to contribute. Current evidence indicates that interleukin-6 is likely to function as an emergency growth hormone and insulin may be the principal growth factor fueling elevated leukocyte production and activity under these circumstances. It is clear from studies with endotoxin that anti-inflammatory cytokines, such as the IL-1 receptor antagonist, the TNF synthesis inhibitor, IL-10, and leukemia inhibitory factor, all participate in the regulation of immune inflammatory processes during APR. Interferon-γ acts as an antagonist to these cytokines.[5] The end result of the profound immune, neuroendocrine and metabolic changes during acute febrile illness is that the immune system is removed from T lymphocyte–mediated control and is placed under the control of natural antibodies and liver-derived serum proteins. This immunoconversion assures that host defense during acute illness is rapidly increased to the highest level possible at the expense of muscles and of other tissues and organs. This reaction protects the host polyspecifically not only against infectious disease, but also against tissue injury, toxic and other noxious agents, all through the rapid activation of the natural immune system and the cytokine production that results. On this basis one may conclude that the natural immune system plays an essential role in host defense during health and it takes over host defense to a large extent, if not entirely, during acute febrile illness.

Neuroimmune Host Defense in Health and Disease

It is very well known from neonatal immunobiology that infants/newborn animals fall victim to facultative pathogenic organisms very easily if immune transfer from mother to offspring could not take place. Such animals/infants must rely on their natural immune system for the initial handling of pathogenic agents and may develop febrile illness as the result. If natural immunity is able to control the infection long enough, the infants/animals will mount a specific immune response and will be protected completely against re-infection as a rule. A similar scenario may occur if adult animals/humans are exposed to a new pathogenic agent for which there is no adaptive immunity. New strains of influenza virus or the continuously mutating HIV could be examples. Again it is the natural immune system that must hold the line until specific immunity develops. In these situations adaptive immunity could not possibly develop without initial protection by natural immunity.

In healthy individuals natural and adaptive immune reactions provide continuous protection hand in hand under physiological conditions. In this situation the cells mediating natural immunity fall under the regulatory effect of neuroendocrine mediators, as shown in TABLE 5. The general rule here is that growth and lactogenic hormones, insulin-like growth factor, insulin and thyroid hormones stimulate immune activity, hormones of the HPA axis are permissive or suppressive, and steroid hormones other than GC are immunomodulatory.[10,33]

The adaptive immune system fails gradually due to aging, and may also fail during disease or as the result of various other stressful insults to the body. Here it is interesting to note that stressful insults initially mobilize the adaptive immune system to enhance immune reactivity in peripheral tissues, which are likely sites of penetration by infectious agents.[34] Should the pathogenic insult continue, it signifies

TABLE 5. Neuroendocrine regulation of natural immunity

Hormone/Mediator	NK	CD5+B/NAb	Phacogytosis	APP
GLH hormones				
GH	↑		↑	
PRL	↑		↑	
IGF-I	↑		↑	
INS			↑	
GLU				↑
T3	↑	↑		↓
HPA axis				
ACTH			↓	
GC	↓	↑	0 ↓	↑
α-MSH		↑		↓
β-END	↑↓		↑	
CAT				↑
Steroid hormones				
E2	↓	↑	↑	
DHEA	↑	↑		
PS			↓	
VD3	↑			
Other mediators				
SP				↑
ANP				↑
MEL				↑

NOTE: ↑, increase; ↓, decrease; ↑↓, variable effect; 0, no effect; ?, predicted change.

that the adaptive immune defense system has failed. Under these conditions, the only alternative that remains is to rely fully on the natural immune system for survival. The neuroendocrine and metabolic alterations during the acute phase response lead to a complete switch of the entire immune system to the natural mode of reactivity. This is achieved by the sudden and gross elevation in the serum of polyspecific natural antibodies and liver-derived recognition molecules. At the same time the adaptive immune response is rendered non-functional, primarily by the profound inhibition of the thymus/T cell immunoregulatory system.[3,5,6,9,10] These changes lead to total immunoconversion.

Practical observations in medicine indicate that febrile illness is followed by recovery in the vast majority of the cases, and that upon recovery, adaptive immunity is also induced as a rule. This again points to the complementary nature of the natural and adaptive protective functions of the immune system. There is a lot to be learned about the neuroimmune biology of host defense, so that we could take full advantage in therapy of this astonishingly complex, yet remarkably functional and effective system.

REFERENCES

1. ROITT, I. 1997. Innate immunity. *In* Essential Immunology, ninth edition. I. Roitt, Ed. :3-21. Blackwell Scientific.
2. BERTOK, L. 1983. Stimulation of nonspecific resistance by radio-detoxified endotoxin. *In* Beneficial Effects of Endotoxins. A. Nowotny, Ed. :213–226. Plenum Press. New York.
3. BERCZI, I. 1993. Neuroendocrine defence in endotoxin shock. Acta Microbiol. Hung. **40:** 265–302.
4. SABBADINI, E.R. & I. BERCZI. 1985. The submandibular gland: a key organ in the neuro-immunoregulatory network? Neuroimmunomodulation **2:** 184–202.
5. BERCZI, I. 1998. Neurohormonal host defence in endotoxin shock. Ann. N.Y. Acad. Sci. **840:** 787–802.
6. BERCZI, I. & E. NAGY. 1995. Neurohormonal control of cytokines during injury. *In* Brain Control of the Response to Injury. N.J. Rothwell & F. Berkenbosch, Eds. :32–107. Cambridge University Press.
7. MEDZHITOV, R. & C.A. JANEWAY. 1997. Innate immunity: impact on the adaptive immune response. Curr. Opin. Immunol. **9:** 4–9.
8. BOISMENU, R. & W.L. HAVRAN. 1997. An innate view of γδT cells. Curr. Opin. Immunol. **9:** 57–63.
9. BERCZI, I., D.A. CHOW & E.R. SABBADINI. 1998. Neuroimmunoregulation and natural immunity. Domestic Animal Endocrin. **15:** 273–281.
10. BERCZI, I. & E. NAGY. 1997. Hormones as immune modulating agents. *In* Handbook of Immune Modulating Agents. T. Krezina, Ed. :75-120. Marcel Dekker, New York.
11. TURNER, M.W. 1996. Mannose-binding lectin: the pluripotent molecule of the innate immune system. Immunol. Today **17:** 532–539.
12. CHOW, D.A., H. WANG & Z. ZHANG. 1999. Natural antibody surveillance of neoplastic and activated cells. Biotecnologia Aplicada **16:** 18–19.
13. WANG, H. & D.A. CHOW. 1999. Protein kinase C expression links natural antibody binding with surveillance of activated and preneoplastic cells. Scand. J. Immunol. **49:** 381–390.
14. HUGHES, A.L., M.YEAGER, A.E. ELSHOF & M.J. CHORNEY. 1999. A new taxonomy of mammalian MHC class I molecules. Immunol. Today **20:** 22–26.
15. HERMAN, A., J.W. KAPPLER, P. MARRACK & A.M. PULLEN. 1991. Superantigens—mechanism of T-cell stimulation and role in immune responses. Annu. Rev. Immunol. **9:** 745–772.

16. CHIEN, Y., R. JORES & M.P. CROWLEY. 1996. Recognition by γδ T cells. Annu. Rev. Immunol. **14:** 511–532.
17. SILVERMAN, G.J. 1997. B-cell superantigens. Immunol. Today **18:** 379–386.
18. WHITESIDE, M.B., N. QUAN & M. HERKENHARN. 1999. Induction of pituitary cytokine transcripts by peripheral lipopolisaccharide. J. Neuroendocrinol. **11:** 115–120.
19. GOEHLER, L.E., R.P. GAYKEMA, K.T. NGUYEN, J.E. LEE, F.J. TILDERS, S.F. MAIER & L.R. WATKINS. 1999. Interleukin-1-beta in immune cells of the abdominal vagus nerve: a link between the immune and the nervous system? J. Neurosci. **19:** 2799–2806.
20. FAGGIONI, R., G. FANTUZZI, C. GABAY, A. MOSER, C.A. DINARELLO, K.R. FEINGOLD & C. GUNFELD. 1999. Leptin deficiency enhances sensitivity to endotoxin induced lethality. Am. J. Physiol. **276:** R136–142.
21. HAUPT, W., J. RIESE, C. DENZEL, M. ZOWE, J. GUSINDE, M. SIASSI & W. HOHENBERGER. 1998. Culture of human peritoneum—a new method to measure the local cytokine response and the effect of immunomodulators. Infection **26:** 345–348.
22. LAHN, M., H. KALATARADI, P. MITTELSTADT, E. PFLUM, M. WOLLNER, C. CADY, A. MUKASA, A.T. WELLA, D. IKLE, R. HARBECK. R. O'BRIEN & W. BORN. 1998. Early preferential stimulation of gamma delta T cells by TNF-alpha. J. Immunol. **160:** 5221–5230.
23. LECLERCQ, G. & J. PLUM. 1995. Stimulation of TCR Vγ3 cells by gram-negative bacteria. J. Immunol. **154:** 5313–5319.
24. LOCATI, M., & P.M. MURPHY. 1999. Chemokines and chemokine receptors: biology and clinical relevance in inflammation and AIDS. Annu. Rev. Med. **50:** 425–440.
25. JANCSO, N. 1964. Neurogenic inflammation. Acta Physiol. Acad. Sci. Hung. **23:** 3.
26. RUEDL, C. & H. WOLF. 1995. Features of oral immunization. Int. Arch. Allergy Immunol. **108:** 334–339.
27. LAMPING, M., R. DETTMER, N.W. SCHRODER, D. PFEIL, W. HALLATSCHEK, R. BURGER & R.R. SCHUMANN. 1998. LPS binding protein protects mice from septic shock caused by LPS or gram-negative bacteria. J. Clin. Invest. **101:** 2065–2071.
28. SZALAI, A.J., D.E. BRILES & J.E. VOLANTAKIS. 1996. Role of complement in C-reactive protein-mediated protection of mice from *Streptococcus pneumoniae*. Infect. Immun. **64:** 4850–4853.
29. GIANTONIO, B.J., R.K. ALPAUGH, J. SCHULTZ, C. MCALEER, D.W. NEWTON, B. SHANNON, Y. GUEDEZ, M. KOTB, L. VITEK, R. PERSSON, P.O. GUNNARSON, T. KALLAND, M. DOHLSTEN, B. PRESSON & L.M. WEINER. 1997. Superantigen based immunotherapy: a phase I trial of PNU-214565, a monoclonal antibody-staphylococcal enterotoxin A recombinant fusion protein, in advanced pancreatic and colorectal cancer. J. Clin. Oncol. **15:** 1994–2007.
30. MCCANN, S.M., S. KARANTH, A. KAMAT, W.L. DEES, K. LYSON, M. GIMENO & V. RETTORI. 1994. Induction by cytokines of the pattern of pituitary hormone secretion in infection. Neuroimmunomodulation **1:** 2–13.
31. TORPY, D.J., S.R. BORNSTEIN & G.P. CHROUSOS. 1998. Leptin and interleukin-6 in sepsis. Horm. Metab. Res. **30:** 726–729.
32. BERCZI, I. 1988. Neuroendocrine response to endotoxin. Ann. N.Y. Acad. Sci. **851:** 411–415.
33. BERCZI, I. 1986. Immunoregulation by pituitary hormones. *In* Pituitary Function and Immunity. I. Berczi, Ed. :227–240. CRC Press. Boca Raton, FL.
34. DHABHAR, F.S. & B.S. MCEWEN. 1996. Stress induced enhancement of antigen specific cell-mediated immunity. J. Immunol. **156:** 2608–2615.
35. BERTÓK, L. 1977. Physico-chemical defense of vertebrate organisms: role of bile acids in defense against bacterial endotoxins. Perspect. Biol. Med. **21:** 70–76.

Control of Salivary Secretion by Nitric Oxide and Its Role in Neuroimmunomodulation

V. RETTORI,[a,b] A. LOMNICZI,[c] J.C. ELVERDIN,[c] A. SUBURO,[d] A. FALETTI,[a] A. FRANCHI,[a] AND S.M. McCANN[e]

[a]Centro de Estudios Farmacológicos y Botánicos (CONICET), Buenos Aires, Argentina

[c]Facultad de Odontologia UBA, [d]Facultad de Medicina, Universidad Austral, Buenos Aires, Argentina

[e]Pennington Biomedical Research Center, Louisiana State University, Baton Rouge, Louisiana, USA

ABSTRACT: In many *in vivo* systems exposure to endotoxins (LPS) leads to the co-induction of inducible nitric oxide synthase (iNOS) and cyclooxygenase-2 (COX-2), which is important to the regulation of the function of different systems during infection. In submandibular glands (SMG) neural (n)NOS is localized in neural terminals and in striated, granular convoluted and excretory ducts, endothelial (e)NOS in vascular endothelium and ducts, and iNOS in macrophages and in tubules and ducts. In normal adult male rats, injection of an inhibitor of NOS decreased the stimulated salivary secretion and a donor of NO potentiated it, indicating that NO exerts a stimulatory role. A single high dose of LPS (5 mg/kg, i.p.) induced an increase in NOS activity measured by the ^{14}C-citrulline method, increased PGE content almost 100% as measured by RIA, and blocked stimulated salivary secretion. The administration of a specific iNOS inhibitor, aminoguanidine (AG), with LPS not only decreased NOS activity but significantly decreased PGE content, indicating that NO triggered the activation of COX-2. LPS increased conversion of labeled arachidonate to prostaglandins (PGs) showing that COX was induced. Since a PGE_1 analogue blocked stimulated salivation, the LPS-induced inhibition of salivation is probably due to release of PGs. Therefore, the use of inhibitors of iNOS and COX-2 could be very useful to increase salivation during infection since saliva has antimicrobial actions.

INTRODUCTION

The submandibular gland is one of the major salivary glands together with the parotid and sublingual glands. The initial saliva is secreted by acini into the terminal end of the ducts and drains into the intercalated ducts that are succeeded by granular convoluted tubules (GCT). The cells in GCTs are characterized by numerous serous-type secretory granules in their cytoplasm. These granules are the repositories of a variety of bioactive substances, including both nerve growth factor and epidermal growth factor and the peptidases, kallikrein and renin. In the rat these GCTs are

[b]Address for correspondence: V. Rettori, M.D., Centro de Estudios Farmacológicos y Botánicos (CONICET), Serrano 669, Ciudad de Buenos Aires (1414), Argentina. Voice: 54-11-4855-7204; fax: 54-11-4963-4473.
rettori@connmed.com.ar

succeeded by striated ducts, the appearance of which is due to vertically oriented mitochondria alternating with highly folded plasma membranes. In the rat the principal cells of these ducts are filled with granules. Finally the striated ducts empty into the excretory ducts.[1]

The secretion of saliva is controlled by the autonomic nervous system. The parasympathetic nervous system is the main controller of this secretion via impulses in the chorda tympani nerve that innervates it and releases acetylcholine and substance P (SP). Both can evoke copious salivary secretion by activating muscarinic and tachykinin-1 receptors, respectively. The sympathetic nervous system also controls salivary secretion by acting on α- and β-adrenergic receptors.

Nitric oxide (NO) controls the function of many organs of the body. Nitric oxide synthase (NOS) is present in nerve terminals that are widely distributed in various parts of the submandibular gland (SMG). Therefore, we hypothesized that NO would play a role in control of salivary secretion. Indeed, we found that inhibition of NOS activity by L-nitro-arginine-methyl-ester (L-NAME) or monomethyl-L-arginine (L-NMMA) injected i.v. to rats prior to stimulation of salivary secretion with methacholine (MC) or SP inhibited significantly the secretion of saliva.[2] The SMG contains all three isoforms of NOS: calcium-dependent neural (n)NOS and endothelial (e)NOS and also a calcium-independent NOS (iNOS) as visualized by immunohistochemistry.[2]

Since the salivary glands are a major portal of entry of bacteria and viruses into the body, we wished to evaluate the effects of infection, as mimicked by injection of bacterial lipopolysaccharides (LPS), on salivary secretion and on the activity of NOS in the SMG. It is well known that prostaglandins also play a very important role in inflammation and are induced by NO, which activates cyclooxygenase (COX). Therefore, we also evaluated the role of PGs in the response of the gland to LPS. LPS was found to decrease salivary secretion in response to secretogogues. Since saliva contains a number of substances involved in mediating the defense of the body against pathogens entering the mouth, the decrease in salivary secretion during endotoxemia could be detrimental.

MATERIAL AND METHODS

Salivary Secretion Studies

Male Wistar rats (250–300 g) were used and were housed under standard conditions (12h light/12h dark cycle, at 22–25°C) and with free access to rat chow and tap water. Food was removed 14 h prior to experimental procedures in order to decrease variation in salivary secretion. Salivary responses were determined in anesthetized rats (chloralose 100 mg/kg i.v.). The ducts of the SMG were cannulated and dose-response curves were obtained through the sequential injection, via the right femoral vein, of increasing doses of various secretagogues as described previously.[3]

In order to investigate the role of NO on saliva secretion, rats were injected i.v. with NOS inhibitors, L-NAME or L-NMMA, 1 h prior to injection of increasing doses of sialogogue, to calculate the same dose-response curves in the presence of one of the NOS inhibitors. In another series of experiments one of the sialogogues was injected at the same dose every 5 min. MC was injected at a dose of 10 μg/kg and noradrenaline (NA) at a dose of 30 μg/kg. In order to evaluate whether NO donors would increase the salivary secretion, nitroglycerin was injected (100 mg/kg) i.v. alone or just prior to injection of the second pulse of MC or NA. All the results are expressed as mean volume of saliva secreted ± SEM (assuming saliva density of 1.0 g/ml).

Determination of NOS Activity

A modification of the method of Bredt and Snyder that measures the conversion of [^{14}C]arginine into [^{14}C]citrulline was used.[4] The method indirectly measures NO production, an index of NOS activity. Since the SMG has an active urea cycle in the tissue, arginine will also be converted to citrulline by this cycle, thereby giving false high values for NOS activity. This problem was obviated by addition of L-valine (25 mM) to the HEPES buffer for homogenization and incubation that blocks the arginase of the urea cycle. The details of the method used were published previously.[2]

Measurements of PGE Content in SMG

PGE content of the SMG was measured by specific radioimmunoassay as a determinant of COX activity as described elsewhere.[5]

Measurements of Radioconversion of [^{14}C] Arachidonic Acid (AA) to Prostanoids in SMG

This was performed by chromatography of ethylacetate extracts and counting of the labeled prostanoids as previously reported.[6] The area of each of the radioactive peaks corresponding to authentic prostanoids was calculated and expressed as a percentage of the total radioactivity of the plates.

Measurements of Plasma Nitrite (NO$_2$)/Nitrate (NO$_3$)

NO$_2$/NO$_3$ serum concentration (as a marker for endogenous NO production) was determined by colorimetric assay with a nitrate/nitrite assay kit (Cayman Chemical Co., Cat. # 780001, Ann Arbor, MI 48108).

Immunohistochemical Localization of NOS

The antisera used in this study were raised in rabbits against different NOS isoenzymes and immunocytochemical studies were performed by the method of Julia Polak.[7]

RESULTS

Distribution of NOS in SMG

nNOS immunoreactivity was demonstrated in several segments of the duct system of the SMG but was absent from the acini. This activity was massive when we compare it to NOS activity of nerve fibers (nNOS) or macrophages (iNOS) in the gland. Within the ducts, we could differentiate between a membrane-associated and a cytoplasmic NOS immunoreactivity. Membrane-associated NOS was greater for iNOS than nNOS (see FIGURES 1 and 2 and TABLE 1). eNOS was not studied but has been localized to vascular endothelium and salivary ducts.[8]

Effect of NO on Salivary Secretion

Since there is little or no spontaneous salivary secretion in the rat in our conditions, salivary secretion could only be studied after injection of various secretogogues. Prior injection of L-NAME or L-NMMA, (as described above) inhibited significantly the response to MC or SP.[2] In the present study we evaluated the response to isoproterenol (a β-adrenergic receptor agonist) and NA before and after the injection of L-NMMA. There was a decrease in salivary secretion after inhibition of NOS which became significant with the highest dose of isoprotenerol or NA (see FIGURE 3).

In order to determine if NO itself stimulates salivary secretion, we injected a NO donor, nitroglycerin (100 mg/kg) i.v. The injection of nitroglycerin alone had no significant effect on salivary secretion. Therefore, we used MC or NA as sialogogues. MC was injected at the high dose (10 μg/kg) every 5 min during 20 minutes. Nitroglycerin (100 mg/kg) was injected one minute before the second injection of MC. There was a significant potentiation of salivary outflow after administration of MC

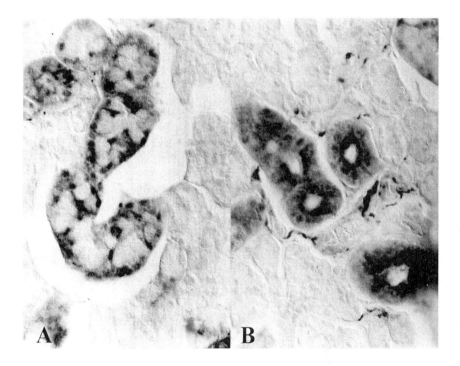

FIGURE 1. Immunohistochemical localization of nNOS in SMG. **A:** a granular convoluted tubule and **B:** striated ducts (1200×).

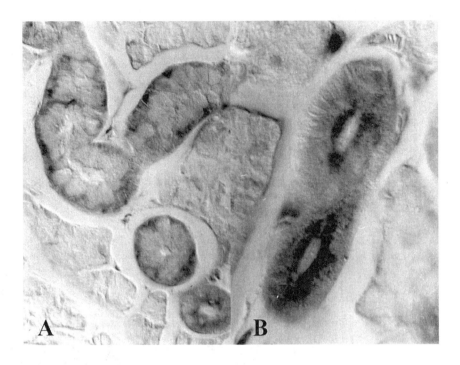

FIGURE 2. Immunohistochemical localization of iNOS in SMG. **A:** a granular convoluted tubule and **B:** striated ducts (1200×).

that was of very short duration and was not significant by the next stimulation. The same pattern of effect was observed with NA (see FIGURE 4). Therefore, we can conclude that NO exerts a stimulatory action on salivary secretion in normal male rats.

Effect of LPS on Salivary Secretion

Injection of LPS (5 mg/kg i.p.) to induce endotoxemia, 6 h before the measurement of salivary secretion stimulated with MC or NA as described above for the

TABLE 1. Relative levels of NOS immunoreactivity in SMG slices

Distribution	nNOS	iNOS
Nerve fibers	++	−
Apical membrane of excretory and striated ducts	++	+++
Cytoplasm of excretory and striated ducts	+	+
Cytoplasm of granular convoluted tubules	++	++
Macrophages	−	+

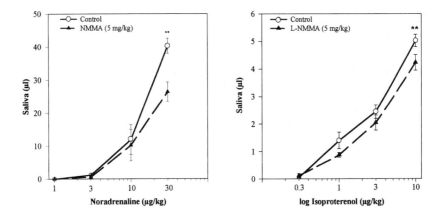

FIGURE 3. The effect of L-NMMA on salivary secretion induced by NA and isoproterenol. Values are means ± SEM of six experiments. $^{**}p < 0.01$ vs. the respective control.

nitroglycerin experiments, produced an almost total block of salivary secretion (data not shown).

Activity of NOS after L-NMMA, LPS and LPS Plus Aminoguanidine (AG)

By using the method of the conversion of [^{14}C]arginine to citrulline by NOS, we have shown previously that the activity of NOS after administration of L-NMMA

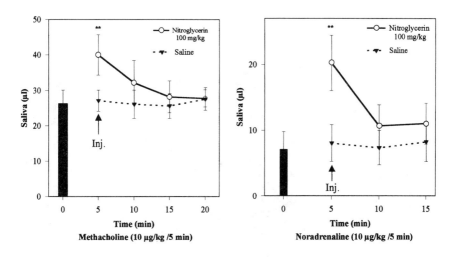

FIGURE 4. The effect of nitroglycerin on salivary secretion induced by MC or NA. Values are means ± SEM of six experiments. $^{**}p < 0.01$ vs. the respective control.

(5mg/kg) i.v. 1 h prior to sacrifice was highly significantly ($p < 0.001$) reduced.[2] Administration of LPS (5mg/kg) 6 h prior to sacrifice induced a 20% increase ($p < 0.05$) of NOS activity in the SMG. Since AG has been shown to be a specific inhibitor of iNOS *in vitro*[9] and *in vivo*,[10] we injected AG (20 mg/kg) i.p. 2 min prior to injection of LPS and measured the activity of NOS in the SMG at the same time (6 h) as for LPS alone. The administration of LPS together with AG prevented the increase of NOS as elicited with LPS alone ($p < 0.05$) as compared to the LPS group. These results suggest that the increased NOS activity after LPS could be due to the induction of iNOS in the SMG.

Effect of LPS on Immunoreactivity of iNOS in SMG

LPS was injected at the same dose and same time as for other experiments. SMGs were obtained at 6 h and immunohistochemical studies performed as described above. There was an increase in the number of macrophages stained with iNOS, but no other observable changes (see FIGURE 5).

Effect of LPS and LPS plus AG on NO₂/NO₃ in Plasma

Plasma levels of NO_2/NO_3 were almost undetectable in control animals. Six hours after injection of LPS there was a dramatic increase in plasma NO_2/NO_3 concentration ($p < 0.001$). When AG was administrated just prior to LPS the increase in

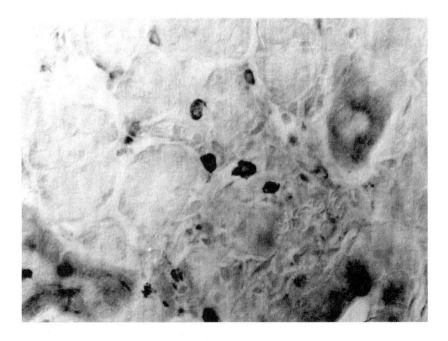

FIGURE 5. Immunohistochemical localization of iNOS in SMG showing macrophage-like cells after LPS injection. (400×)

plasma NO_2/NO_3 was significantly lower ($p < 0.001$), but still highly significantly greater than in control rats ($p < 0.001$).

Effect of LPS and LPS plus AG on PGE Content in SMG

Injection of LPS also dramatically increased PGE content at 6 h by 100% ($p < 0.001$). The injection of AG just prior to LPS blocked completely the effect of LPS as PGE content of control was identical to that of the LPS + AG group.

Effect of LPS and LPS plus AG on COX as Measured by Radioconversion of [^{14}C]-AA to Prostanoids by SMG

The radioconversion assay of [^{14}C]-AA that indirectly measures COX activity by measuring arachidonate metabolites such as 6-keto $PGF_1\alpha$, $PGF_2\alpha$ and PGE_2 gave similar results to those observed when PGE content of the SMG was measured by RIA. The results were expressed as percentage of total cpm of a particular prostanoid on plate/100 mg wet weight of the SMG. The PGE_2 values were (mean ± SEM): Control group = 7.3 ± 1, LPS = 12.2 ± 1, and LPS ± AG = 8.11 ± 0.8. The increase induced by LPS was significant ($p < 0.05$) versus the other two groups. Similar results were obtained for 6-keto-$PGF_2\alpha$ and $PGF_1\alpha$ .The increased COX activity after LPS probably represents COX2 induction by LPS, and its blockade by the inhibitor of iNOS, AG, suggests that it was induced by NO.

Effect of a PGE₁ Analogue on Salivary Secretion

Since we have found that NO has a stimulatory effect on salivary secretion and that the administration of LPS that increases NOS activity with higher production of NO paradoxically produced an almost total abolition of stimulated salivary secretion, we hypothesized that this inhibition could be caused by an inhibitory effect of PGs. Therefore, we stimulated salivary secretion by NA as previously described, and injected the PGE_1 analogue (Alprostadil, 3 µg/kg). The injection of the analogue inhibited dramatically ($p < 0.01$) the stimulated salivary secretion.

DISCUSSION

The results of our previously reported research[2] and that reported here establish the control of salivary secretion by NO. Inhibition of NOS by L-NAME or L-NMMA inhibits the secretion induced by muscarinic cholinergic agonists, SP, noradrenaline and the β-adrenergic agonist, isoproterenol. Conversely, nitroglycerin, a releaser of NO, increased stimulated salivation. NO has a relatively small role, at least in the anesthetized rat, since the effect of nitroglycerin is relatively small and NOS inhibitors only partially reduced the effects of secretogogues. There was no NOS in the acini that form the original secretion of the gland. Since NO would have to diffuse some distance to reach these cells, we hypothesize that this initial secretion is unaffected by NO. iNOS was frequently seen in macrophages within the gland. The content of this "constitutive" iNOS in the salivary gland was much higher than that seen in other organs, such as the pituitary gland,[11] perhaps because of constant exposure of the gland to pathogens entering the oral cavity that would induce iNOS by releasing LPS or other bacterial and viral toxins.

Since saliva contains many compounds important to combat invading organisms, it was important to study the effect of LPS on salivary secretion. The same dose of LPS shown previously to produce a massive increase in iNOS mRNA in the anterior pituitary and pineal glands and to increase iNOS content,[11] increased the number of iNOS-containing macrophages in the SMG and increased the total NOS activity. This induction of iNOS by LPS was accompanied by a complete block of salivation in response to potent secretagogues.

In our previous studies, it was demonstrated that NO not only activates guanylyl cyclase leading to cGMP production that modulates secretion in glands, for example stimulating the release of FSH and LH[12] and inhibiting release of prolactin[13] from the anterior pituitary. It is probable that cGMP also mediates the stimulation of salivation evoked by NO. NO also activates another Fe^{++}-containing enzyme, cyclooxygenase, leading to production of PGs.[14] LPS induces iNOS in the SMG that directly induces NO release that should activate COX. Indeed, PGE content in the gland was elevated and we showed here that there was a markedly increased conversion of labeled arachidonate to PGs in the SMG of LPS-injected rats at the time that iNOS was increased. Furthermore, the PGE_1 analogue tested inhibited salivation produced by NA, confirming previous results.[15]

Therefore, our results are consistent with the following chain of events: LPS induces iNOS, which induces COX2, causing PG release that inhibits salivation.

If this chain of events is correct it should be possible to reduce the inhibitory effect of LPS on salivation with a specific inhibitor of iNOS or COX. Indeed, AG, a highly selective inhibitor of iNOS, decreased NOS in the gland and reduced the increase in plasma NO_2/NO_3 induced by LPS. If a dose of AG can be found to increase salivation during infection, it might be therapeutically useful by decreasing the hyposialosis induced by infection. Saliva has many useful effects in counteracting infection. For example, the NO secreted has antibacterial action in the mouth but is rapidly reduced to NO_2/NO_3, which then arrives at the acid environment of the stomach that rapidly converts NO_3 back to NO, generating antibacterial action there.[16] In addition a number of other antibacterial compounds are present in saliva, aiding in its antibacterial action.

ACKNOWLEDGMENTS

This work was supported by BID 802-OC-AR-PICT 00353, PIP 955/98, Consejo Nacional de Investigaciones Científicas y Técnicas and TO 04, Facultad Odontología UBA.

REFERENCES

1. TANDLER, B. & C.J. PHILLIPS. 1998. Microstructure of mammalian salivary glands and its relationship to diet. *In* Glandular Mechanisms of Salivary Secretion. Oral Frontiers on Biology. J.R. Garret, J. Ekström & L.C. Anderson, Eds. **10:** 21–35. Karger. Basel.

2. LOMNICZI, A., A.M SUBURO, J.C. ELVERDIN, C.A. MASTRONARDI, S. DIAZ, V. RETTORI & S.M. MCCANN. 1998. Role of nitric oxide in salivary secretion. Neuroimmunomodulation **5:** 226–233.

3. BIANCIOTTI, L., J.C. ELVERDIN, M. VATTA, C. COLATRELLA & B. FERNÁNDEZ. 1994. Atrial natriuretic factor enhances induced salivary secretion in the rat. Regul. Pept. **49:** 195–202.

4. CANTEROS, G., V. RETTORI, A. GENARO, A. SUBURO, M. GIMENO & S.M. MCCANN. 1996. Nitric oxide synthase content of hypothalamic explants: increased by norepinephrine and inactivated by NO and cGMP. Proc. Natl. Acad. Sci. USA. **93:** 4246–4250.

5. FALETTI, A., J.M. VIGGIANO & M. GIMENO. 1995. Beta-endorphin inhibits prostaglandin synthesis in rat ovaries and blocks induced ovulation. Prostaglandins **49:** 93–103.

6. FRANCHI, A.M., M. CHAUD, V. RETTORI, A. SUBURO, S.M. MCCANN & M. GIMENO. 1994. Role of nitric oxide in eicosanoid synthesis and uterine motility in estrogen-treated rat uteri. Proc. Natl. Acad. Sci. USA **91:** 539–543.

7. SPRINGALL, D.R., V. RIVEROS-MORENO, L. BUTTERY, A. SUBURO, A.F. BISHOP, M. MERRET, S. MONCADA & J.M. POLAK. 1992. Immunological detection of nitric oxide synthase(s) in human tissues using heterologous antibodies suggesting different isoforms. Histochemistry **98:** 259–266.

8. BENTZ, B.G., G.K. HAINES, D.G. HANSON & J.A. RADOSEVICH. 1998. Endothelial constitutive nitric oxide synthase (ecNOS) localization in normal and neoplastic tissue. Head & Neck **July:** 304–309.

9. GRIFFITHS, M.J., M. MESSENT, R.J. MACALLISTER & T.W. EVANS. 1993. Aminoguanidine selectively inhibits inducible nitric oxide synthase. Br. J. Pharmacol. **110:** 963–968.

10. WU, C.C., S.Y. CHEN, C. SZABÓ, C. THIEMERMANN & J.R. VANE. 1995. Aminoguanidine attenuates the delayed circulatory failure and improves survival in rodent models of endotoxic shock. Br. J. Pharmacol. **114:** 1666–1672.

11. WONG, M.L., V. RETTORI, A. AL-SHEKHLEE, P.B. BONGIORNO, G. CANTEROS, S.M. MCCANN, P.W. GOLD & J. LUCINIO. 1996. Inducible nitric oxide synthase gene expression in the brain during systemic inflammation. Nature Med. **2:** 581–584.

12. MCCANN, S.M., M. KIMURA, A. WALCZEWSKA, S. KARANTH, V. RETTORI & W.H. YU. 1998. Hypothalamic control of FSH and LH by FSH-RF, LHRH, cytokines, leptin and nitric oxide. Neuroimmunomodulation **5:** 193–202.

13. DUVILANSKI, B.H., C. ZAMBRUNO, A. SEILICOVICH, D. PISERA, M. LASAGA, M.C. DÍAZ, N. BELOVA, V. RETTORI, & S.M. MCCANN. 1992. Role of nitric oxide in control of prolactin release by the adenohypophysis. Proc. Natl. Acad. Sci. USA **92:** 170–174.

14. RETTORI, V., M. GIMENO, K. LYSON & S.M MCCANN. 1992. Nitric oxide mediates norepinephrine-induced prostaglandin E_2 release from the hypothalamus. Proc. Natl. Acad. Sci. USA **89:** 115432–11546.

15. YU, Y.H. 1986. Modulating effects of prostaglandins on parasympathetic-mediated secretory activity of rat salivary glands.Prostaglandins **31:** 1087–1097.

16. WEITZBERG, E. & J.O.N. LUNDBERG. 1998. Nonenzymatic nitric oxide production in humans. *In* Nitric Oxide: Biology and Chemistry. L. Ignarro, Y.R. Lancaster, Jr. & U. Förstermaun, Eds. **2:** 1–7. Academic Press.

Nerve Growth Factor and Neuroimmune Interactions in Inflammatory Diseases

ANDREW M. STANISZ[a,b] AND JOLANTA A. STANISZ[c]

[a]*Department of Pathology and Molecular Medicine, McMaster University, Hamilton, Ontario L8N 3Z5, Canada*

[c]*AJBioCom, Dundas, Canada*

ABSTRACT: Discovered almost 50 years ago, nerve growth factor (NGF) has been extensively studied in various biological systems. NGF has recently been suggested to play an important role in mediating and/or regulating immune response, in addition to its trophic and tropic effects on nerve growth and regeneration It is clear that in complex interactions between immune cells and nervous system NGF plays a central role. We have only just begun to identify and understand the direct mechanisms by which NGF activates target cells, the precise identity of the target cells, and the particular factors released from target cells. Nerve growth factor together with possibly other neurotrophins such as BDNF (brain-derived nerve growth factor), GDNF (glial-derived nerve growth factor) or NT3 are important modulators of immunity. More detailed studies are needed at the receptor, mediator and cellular levels to better understand the neuroimmunomodulatory properties of neurothrophins and NGF. The nature of the involvement of NGF in inflammation and inflammatory diseases remains a particularly interesting question. By blocking NGF or mediators released upon NGF activation, we are able to control the progress of inflammation, thereby opening many therapeutic opportunities for the future.

INTRODUCTION

Since its discovery almost 50 years ago nerve growth factor (NGF) has been extensively studied in number of biological systems. In addition to its trophic and tropic effects on nerve growth and regeneration NGF has been recently suggested to play an important role in mediating and/or regulating immune response. For a more detailed review of the field the reader is referred to the excellent, recently published papers by L. Aloe *et al.*,[1] A. Braun *et al.*,[2] and J. Bienenstock.[3] Our previous research concentrated on the effects of neuropeptides on immunity with particular interest focused on tachykinin, substance P (SP).[4,5] Combined with the known effects of NGF on SP synthesis and release[6] it led us to believe that NGF also might be an important factor affecting immune cell.

Here, we will discuss briefly the immunomodulatory properties of NGF which directly relate to our own work. Over several years we have been studying the role NGF plays in activating lymphocytes and mast cells in health and disease. In

[b]Address for correspondence: Dr. Andrew M. Stanisz, Department of Pathology and Molecular Medicine, HSC Room 3N5C, 1200 Main Street West, Hamilton, Ontario L8N 3Z5, Canada. Voice: 905-525-9140 ext. 22592; fax: 905-522-3454.

stanisz@fhs.mcmaster.ca

particular, we have been interested in NGF function in both acute and chronic inflammatory diseases.

NGF AND IMMUNE CELLS

From the anatomical observations (particularly in skin and mucosa) it is clear that SP-containing nerves and immune cells such as mast cells or lymphocytes are in very close proximity.[7,8] It has also been documented that NGF can be synthesized by various cells of the immune system such as T cells,[9] B cells,[10] macrophages,[11] mast cells,[12] and eosinophils[13] as well as connective tissue cells such as fibroblast[14] or keratinocytes.[15] In addition to its neuronal source, NGF is therefore readily available in the microenvironment surrounding immune cells.

Similarly, two distinct receptors, p75 and/or trkA, have been found on T-cells,[16] B-cells,[17] macrophages[18,19] or mast cells.[20] Nerve growth factor was found to have a profound autocrine effects on immune cells. It has mastopoietic effects in rodents[21] and is also a potent mast cell degranulator[22] with often-differential properties. For example, NGF increases IL-6 production, whereas TNF-α production is decreased in mast cells in the presence of NGF.[23]

In earlier studies NGF has been shown to increase lymphocyte proliferation,[24] IL-2 receptor expression[25] and immunoglobulin synthesis.[26] However, effects of NGF on lymphocyte function appear to be much more complex. In our own work the NGF affected murine lymphocytes by altering the levels of cAMP and cGMP. At the same time it has a marginal effects on lymphocyte proliferation, and immunoglobulin synthesis was virtually not affected.[27] In addition the effects of NGF were seen only after prolonged time (over 96 h), suggesting either the involvement of a (several) intermediate cell(s) and their products or activation of a small subpopulation of lymphocytes. This has been further supported by the observation that both trkA and p75 receptors for NGF are found on B cells, but T lymphocytes have only trkA receptors. It is also possible, that NGF receptor expression on lymphocytes is cell cycle–dependent and various subpopulations of T and B cells react differentially to NGF. For example, whereas NGF promotes growth and differentiation of B-lymphocytes,[26] it increases IgG4 synthesis preferentially and has no effect on other IgG subclasses.[28] The same group has reported inhibitory effects of NGF on immunoglobulin production by plasma cells.[29]

NGF AND DISEASES

Nerve growth factor has been associated with a variety of autoimmune and inflammatory diseases in which elevated levels in circulating plasma have been found.[30] For example, increased levels of NGF are found in multiple sclerosis,[31] systemic lupus erythematous,[32] and arthritis.[33] Our own observations suggest that both SP and NGF are elevated in rheumatoid arthritis but not in patients with osteoarthritis.[34] Moreover, in the animal model of arthritis, NGF upregulates release and/or synthesis of SP and therefore contributes directly to inflammation.[6] NGF has been associated with hyperalgesia[35] and bronchial smooth muscle hyperreactivity, contributing to asthma[36] and its animal model.[37] In our recent studies patients with allergic rhinitis have significantly increased levels of NGF in nasal lavages as compared to control patients. NGF levels correlated well with the severity of the disease. In addition, basal levels of NGF were further elevated upon challenging the patients with antigen delivered in aerosol after only 10 minutes. These effects were antigen-specific and local—NGF was elevated only in challenged nostrils. In those patients elevated levels of NGF mRNA have been found in nasal biopsies. Control patients remain unresponsive to antigen challenge.[38] In separate experiments, administration of neutralizing anti-NGF antibody to sensitized animals resulted in inhibition of their response to allergen. These results are in agreement with recent data obtained by Braun and colleagues.[37] In yet another model of inflammation (this time induced in murine intestinal mucosa by infection with *Trichinella spiralis*) elevated levels of both SP and NGF have been found and correlated well with the degree of inflammatory response.[39] Furthermore, administration of neutralizing antibody against SP or NGF significantly inhibited the development of inflammation, suggesting the direct role that NGF can play in this disease. It was shown by Aloe *et al.*[40] in a similar animal model that NGF was increased in *Schistosoma mansoni* infection.

One can not dispute the effects of stress on chronic inflammatory diseases. Although postulated, the role of NGF here is much more indirect, complex and not fully understood owing to the multifactorial nature of stress. However, early observations suggest that NGF is elevated in fighting animals.[41] Interestingly, blood levels of NGF in parachute jumpers and expression of NGR receptors on peripheral lymphocytes obtained during the jump are also significantly increased.[42] On the other hand, in our preliminary experiments administration of anti-NGF antibody to animals increases stress-related response by means of increased gut permeability.

CONCLUSIONS

It is clear that in complex interactions between immune cells and the nervous system NGF plays a central role. The direct mechanisms by which NGF activates target cells, precise identity of the target cells, and particular factors released from target cells are only just beginning to be identified and understood. Nerve growth factor together with possibly other neurotrophins such as BDNF (brain-derived nerve growth factor), GDNF (glial-derived nerve growth factor) or NT3 are important modulators of immunity. Indeed, more detailed studies are needed at the receptor, mediator and cellular levels to better understand the neuroimmunomodulatory properties of neurothrophins and NGF. In particular, how NGF is involved in inflammation and inflammatory diseases remains a very interesting question. By blocking NGF or mediators released upon NGF activation, we are able to control the progress of inflammation. This opens numerous therapeutic opportunities for future study.

REFERENCES

1. ALOE, L. *et al.* 1997. The expanding role of nerve growth factor: from neurotrophic activity to immunologic diseases. Allergy **52:** 883–894.
2. BRAUN, A. *et al.* 2000. Role of neurotropins in allergic bronchial asthma. In press.

3. BIENENSTOCK, J. 1999. Mast cell–nerve interactions: possible significance of nerve growth factor. In press.
4. STANISZ, A.M. 1994. Neuronal factors modulating immunity. Neuroimmunomodulation **1:** 217–230.
5. STANISZ, A.M. *et al.* 1986. Differential effects of vasoactive intestinal peptide, substance P and somatostatin on immunoglobulin synthesis and proliferation by lymphocytes from Peyer's patches, mesenteric lymph nodes and spleen. J. Immunol. **136:** 152–156.
6. DONNERER, J. *et al.* 1993. Upregulation, release and axonal transport of substance P and calcitonine gene–related peptide in adjuvant inflammation and regulatory function of nerve growth factor. Regul. Pept. **46:** 150–154.
7. STEAD, R.H. *et al.* 1989. Mast cells are closely apposed to nerves in the human gastrointestinal mucosa. Gastroenterology **97:** 575–585.
8. STEAD, R.H. *et al.* 1987. Intestinal mucosal mast cells in normal and nematode-infected rat intestine are in intimate contact with peptinergic nerves. Proc. Natl. Acad. Sci. USA **84:** 2975-2979.
9. LAMBIASE, A. *et al.* 1997. Human CD4[+] T cell clones produce and release nerve growth factor and express high-affinity nerve growth factor receptors. J. Allergy Clin. Immunol. **100:** 408–414.
10. TORCIA, M. *et al.* 1996. Nerve growth factor is an autocrine survival factor for memory B-lymphocytes. Cell **85:** 345–356.
11. TORII, H. *et al.* 1997. Expression of neurotrophic factors and neuropeptide receptors by Langerhans cells and Langerhans cell-like cell line XS52: further support for a functional relationship between Langerhans cells and epidermal nerves. J. Invest. Dermatol. **109:** 586–591.
12. LEON, A. *et al.* 1994. Mast cell synthesize, store and release nerve growth factor. Proc. Natl. Acad. Sci. USA **91:** 3739–3743.
13. SOLOMON, A. *et al.* 1998. Nerve growth factor is preformed in and activates human peripheral blood eosinophils. J. Allergy Clon. Immunol. **102:** 454–460.
14. YOUNG, M. *et al.* 1974. Secretion of a nerve growth factor by primary chick fibroblast cultures. Science **187:** 361–362.
15. TRON, V.A. *et al.* Expression and modulation of nerve growth factor in murine keratinocytes (PAM 212). J. Clin. Invest. **85:** 1085–1089.
16. EHRHARD, P.B. *et al.* 1993. Expression of nerve growth factor and nerve growth factor receptor tyrosine kinase Trk in activated CD4 positive T-cell clones. Proc. Natl. Acad. Sci. USA **90:** 10984–10988.
17. MELAMED, I. *et al.* 1996. Nerve growth signal transduction in human B lymphocytes is mediated by gp140 trk. Eur. J. Immunol. **26:** 1985–1992.
18. EHRHARD, P.B. *et al.* 1993. Expression of functional trk protooncogene in human monocytes. Proc. Natl. Acad. Sci. USA **90:** 5423–5427.
19. PEZZATI, P. *et al.* Expression of nerve growth factor receptor immunoreactivity on follicular dendritic cells from human mucosa associated lymphoid tissue. Immunology **76:** 485–490.
20. NILSSON, G. *et al.* 1997. Human mast cells express functional TrkA and are a source of nerve growth factor. Eur. J. Immunol. **27:** 2295–2301.
21. ALOE, L. *et al.* 1977. Mast cells increase in tissues of neonatal rats injected with nerve growth factor. Brain Res. **133:** 358–366.
22. HORIGOME, K. *et al.* 1994. Effects of nerve growth factor on rat peritoneal mast cells. J. Biol. Chem. **269:** 2695–2701.
23. MARSHALL, J.S. *et al.* 1990. The role of mast cell degranulation products in mast cell hyperplasia.1. Mechanisms of action of nerve growth factor. J. Immunol. **144:** 1886–1892.
24. THORPE, L.W. *et al.* 1987. The influence of nerve growth factor on the in vitro proliferative response of rat spleen lymphocytes. J. Neurosci. Res. **18:** 134–139.
25. THORPE, L.W. *et al.* 1987. Effects of nerve growth factor expression on interleukin-2 receptors on cultured human lymphocytes. Ann. N.Y. Acad. Sci. **496:** 310–311.
26. OTTEN, U. *et al.* 1989. Nerve growth factor induces growth and differentiation of human B lymphocytes. Proc. Natl. Acad. Sci. USA **86:** 10059–10063.

27. STEPIEN, H. *et al.* 1991. The effect of nerve growth factor on DNA synthesis, cyclic AMP and cyclic GMP accumulation by mouse spleen lymphocytes. Int. J. Immunopharmacol. **13:** 51–56.
28. KIMATA, H. *et al.* 1991. Nerve growth factor specifically induces human IgG4 production. Eur. J. Immunol. **21:** 137–141.
29. KIMATA, H. *et al.* 1991. Nerve growth factor inhibits immunoglobulin production but not proliferation of human plasma cell lines. Clin. Immunol. Immunopathol. **69:** 145–151.
30. ALOE, L. *et al.* 1994. Nerve growth factor and autoimmune diseases. Autoimmunity **19:** 141-150.
31. BRACCI-LAUDIERO, L. *et al.* 1992. Multiple sclerosis patients express increased levels of B-nerve growth factor in cerebrospinal fluid. Neurosci. Lett. **147:** 9–12.
32. BRACCI-LAUDIERO, L. *et al.* 1993. Increased levels of NGF in sera of systemic lupus erythematous patients. NeuroReport **5:** 563–565.
33. ALOE, L. *et al.* 1992. Nerve growth factor in the synovial fluid of patients with chronic arthritis. Arthritis Rheum. **35:** 351–355.
34. AGRO, A. *et al.* Are lymphocyte a target for substance P modulation in arthritis. Semin. Arthritis Rheum. **21:** 252–258.
35. WOOLF, C.J. *et al.* 1997. Cytokines, nerve growth factor and inflammatory hyperalgesia: the contribution of tumor necrosis factor alpha. Br. J. Pharmacol. **121:** 417–424.
36. BONINI, S. *et al.* 1996. Circulating nerve growth factor levels are increased in humans with allergic diseases and asthma. Proc. Natl. Acad. Sci. USA **93:** 10955–10960.
37. BRAUN, A. *et al.* 1998. Role of nerve growth factor in a mouse model of allergic airway inflammation and asthma. Eur. J. Immunol. **28:** 3240–3251.
38. SANICO, A.M. *et al.* Nerve growth factor expression and release is dysregulated in allergic inflammatory disease of upper airways. Submitted.
39. AGRO, A. *et al.* 1993. Inhibition of murine intestinal inflammation by anti-substance P antibody. Reg. Immunol. **5:** 120–126.
40. ALOE, L. *et al.* 1994. *Schistosoma mansoni* infection enhances the levels of NGF in the liver and hypothalamus. NeuroReport **5:** 1030–1032.
41. ALOE, L. *et al.* 1986. Aggressive behavior induces release of nerve growth factor from mouse salivary gland into the bloodstream. Proc. Natl. Acad. Sci. USA **83:** 6184–6187.
42. ALOE, L. *et al.* 1994. Emotional stress induced by parachute jumping enhances blood nerve growth factor levels and distribution of nerve growth factor receptors on lymphocytes. Proc. Natl. Acad. Sci. USA **91:** 10440–10444.

Role of Neurotransmitter Autoantibodies in the Pathogenesis of Chagasic Peripheral Dysautonomia

LEONOR STERIN-BORDA[a] AND ENRI BORDA

Centro de Estudios Farmacológios y Botánicos (CEFYBO), Consejo Nacional de Investigaciones Científicas y Técnicas de la República Argentina (CONICET) and Pharmacology Department, School of Medicine and Dentistry, Buenos Aires University, Buenos Aires, Argentina

ABSTRACT: Chagas' disease is caused by a parasite, *Trypanosoma cruzi*, which is widely distributed in South and Central America. Dysautonomias, derangements of sympathetic and parasympathetic nervous system function, are seen fairly often during the chronic course of Chagas' disease. Many infected subjects developed, in the course of the disease, neurogenic cardiomyopathy or digestive damage. Our investigations show the existence of circulating antibodies in Chagas' disease that bind to β-adrenergic and muscarinic cholinergic receptor (mAChR). The neurotransmitter receptor–autoantibody interaction triggers in the cells intracellular signal transductions that alter the physiological behavior of the target organs, leading to tissue damage. Moreover, the deposit of autoantibodies behaving as agonists induces desensitization and/or down regulation of the receptors. This in turn can lead to a progressive blockade of them with sympathetic and parasympathetic denervation. Using synthetic peptides for immunoblotting and enzyme immunoassay, we demonstrated that these autoantibodies reacted against the second extracellular loop of the human heart β_1 adrenoceptor and M_2 cholinoceptor. Also, the corresponding affinity-purified antipeptide antibodies displayed an agonist-like activity associated with specific receptor activation. A strong association between circulating antipeptide M_2 mAChR autoantibodies and the presence of patients' low heart rate variablity index, bradycardia and cardiac or esophageal autonomic dysfunction in chronic chagasic patients was verified. This fact make these antipeptide antibodies a proper marker of cardiac neuromyopathy and achalasia.

Chagas' disease, one of the most common determinants of congestive heart failure and sudden death in the world, is caused by a parasite, *Trypanosoma cruzi* (*T. cruzi*), which is widely distributed in South and Central America.[1] In the chronic state of Chagas' disease, up to 30% of the infected subjects developed at least one of the clinical forms of the disease, namely cardiomyopathy, neuropathy, or digestive damage (achalasia and megacolon). Dysautonomic derangements of sympathetic and parasympathetic nervous system function are seen fairly often during chronic chagasic cardiac and digestive damage. However, chronic manifestations of Chagas' disease are extraordinarily complex processes with a poorly understood pathophysiology.

[a]Address for correspondence: Leonor Sterin-Borda, M.D., CEFYBO, Serrano 669, 1414 Buenos Aires, Argentina. Fax: 54-11-4856-2751.

The paradoxical severe involvement of the organs in the absence of any intracellular form of the parasite has prompted many investigators to propose involvement of autoimmune mechanisms in the pathogenesis of the disease.[2-4]

Why do the myocardium and gastrointestinal tract fail during the evolution of chronic Chagas' disease? Borrowing from basic science, we postulated a molecular-specific mechanism that may be abnormal and comprise the intrinsic function responsible for contraction and relaxation of the active or resting state of muscle in the presence of neural or hormonal influence. So, the ability of the muscle to rapidly increase or decrease its performance in response to various physiological or physical stimuli could be altered. This adaptive response is modulated by endogenous bioactive compounds, including neurotransmitters, cytokines, and autocrine and paracrine hormones. Continuous chronic use of these compensatory mechanisms to support the failing organ, contribute to cellular necrosis and apoptosis. When cell loss occurs, a remodeling process takes place, which is one of the major determinants of muscle hypertrophy or dilation.[5]

Among the specific abnormalities that modulated function, we could include changes in β-adrenergic and muscarinic cholinergic signal transduction.[6] Thus, the ability of the autonomic nervous system to modulate the function of heart and esophagus is altered in the failing of these organs because of multiple changes at the level of receptors, G proteins, and adenylate and guanylate cyclases.[7]

Thus, chronic Chagas' heart disease and achalasia belongs to the category of peripheral autonomic dysfunction in which the modulated function is primarily affected. Therefore, the chronic hyperactivation at the level of postsynaptic neurotransmitter receptors and their cellular signaling induces organ failure. As can be seen in FIGURE 1, the molecular mechanism involved in chagasic peripheral dysautonomia is induced by hyperactivation of neurotransmitter receptors including

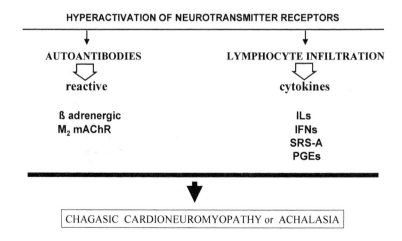

FIGURE 1. Molecular mechanisms involved in chagasic peripheral dysautonomia. Central role of neurotransmitter-reactive autoantibodies and cytokines in production of adverse biological effects that lead to progressive dysautonomia in Chagas' disease.

autoreactive antibodies to β-adrenergic and M_2 mAChR and cell-mediated reactivity through cytokines release. The antibody-receptor recognition triggers signal transduction, which alters normal function inducing physiological, biochemical and pharmacological alteration of the target organs.[3,4] On the other hand, in chagasic-infected organs the mononuclear cell infiltration causes the release of cytokines and biologically active lipid metabolites.[8] These factors (ILs, IFNs, SRS-A, PGE) may alter normal function either directly or indirectly via sympathetic and/or parasympathetic activation.[9–13] Therefore, both the reactive autoantibodies and the cell-mediated reactivity can alter the autonomic nervous system modulation triggering organ failure. Furthermore, we have reported that the myocardial β-adrenergic action of chagasic autoantibodies was highly enhanced by human lymphocytes.[14]

Studies from our laboratory on chagasic cardiomyopathy have demonstrated that chagasic sera can react *in vitro* with the plasma membrane of living heart cells inducing morphologic and functional changes and modifying their β-adrenergic and cholinergic receptor activity.[15,16] Immunofluorescent and ultrastructural immuno-histochemical studies of myocardial cells contracting in the presence of chagasic sera showed widely distributed sarcolemmal deposits of immunoglobulins and C3. Transmission electron microscopy demonstrated sarcolemmal damage. Fixation of the antibody to the sarcolemma occurs concomitantly with alteration of physiologic and pharmacologic function of the isolated myocardium. These effects were prevented by β-adrenergic and cholinergic blocking agents.[3,17] The deposit of an antibody on the myocardial neurotransmitter receptors, which behaves like an agonist, could induce desensitization and/or downregulation of the receptor. This, in turn, could lead to a progressive blockade of myocardial neurotransmitter receptors, with sympathetic and parasympathetic denervation, a phenomenon that has been described in the course of Chagas' cardioneuromyopathy.

Adequate proof has been presented supporting the existence of autoantibodies against β_1[18–22] and muscarinic cholinergic[23–27] receptors in the sera of chagasic patients, which are able to activate the signal transduction system coupled to these receptors and reflect the biological effect of the antibodies.

In the case of the interaction of chagasic IgG with muscarinic cholinergic receptors of myocardium we determined a molecular approach:

1. chagasic sera but not normal sera quantitatively precipitated the muscarinic cholinergic receptor of the heart;
2. by cardiac membrane protein solubilization and electrophoretical fractionation, chagasic sera recognized a protein fraction of 78–80 kD, similar to the molecular weight of the atria muscarinic cholinergic receptor;[23] and
3. chagasic but not normal IgGs are able to immunoprecipitate the human M_2 muscarinic cholinergic receptor and to induce internalization of those receptors in M_2 CHO cells in a concentration- and time-dependent manner.

Chagasic antibodies induced the phosphorylation of M_2 mAChR from Sf9 cells.[28] These results point to a role for these autoantibodies in rapid receptor desensitization events, given the possibility that these antibodies could impair cardiac function by desensitization of receptors *in vivo*. It is important to note that either the binding assay or the intracellular signal transduction events induced by chagasic IgG are specific since they were exerted by the F(ab')2 fraction.

Circulating autoantibodies are present previous to the development of the cardiomyopathy. This could be explained by the fact that the peak of serum immunoglobulin with sympathetic and parasympathetic activity precedes the impairment of heart neurotransmitter receptor-mediated activity,[29] indicating that these antibodies may be an early marker of heart autonomic dysfunction. In this sense, we have observed, in human and experimental models of chagasic disease,[30] that circulating β-adrenergic and muscarinic cholinergic antibodies increase with the time of infection. At least in chagasic mice, the increase in circulating antibodies is coincident with the increase in myocarditis index.[30]

A very important issue for the understanding of the immune pathology of chronic chagasic neuromycardiopathy is the fact that, using an experimental autoimmune myocarditis model very similar to chronic Chagas' myocarditis on the basis of immunopathologic and histologic data, we have detected circulating autoantibodies against myocardial β-adrenergic and M_2 mAChR.[29,30] Moreover, we have detected an anti T. cruzi monoclonal antibody which recognizes a 150-kD antigen of T. cruzi and reacts with both adrenoceptors and cholinoceptors of myocardium.[31]

It is known that mAChRs and β-adrenergic receptors belong to members of the G protein–coupled receptor family and undergo desensitization upon persistent stimulation by their specific agonists. The whole process includes a phosphorylation reaction by either second messenger-dependent kinases or G protein–coupled receptor kinases that precedes uncoupling of receptors from G proteins and, subsequently, sequestration and downregulation of receptors can occur. We observed that chagasic antibodies induce uncoupling of receptors from G proteins and a rapid sequestration of receptors away from membrane environment,[28] using purified M_2 mAChRs (CHO cells stably transfected with M_2 receptors) to assess the ability of chagasic IgG to bind and desensitize those receptors. The in vivo situation during the course of Chagas' disease can be described as that of a persistent stimulus-circulating antibodies acting on cardiac mAChRs and therefore the possibility that a desensitization process is set up appears plausible.

The molecular interaction between autoreactive antibodies and neurotransmitter receptors was demonstrated using a synthetic peptide on immunoblotting and enzyme immmunoassays. We reported that chagasic autoantibodies react against the second extracellular loop of the human heart muscarinic receptor and $β_1$-adrenergic receptor in patients with Chagas' disease. Furthermore, the affinity-purified antipeptide antibodies were able not only to interact with the second extracellular loop of the human M_2 mAChR, but they also displayed an "agonist-like" activity modifying the intracellular events associated with specific muscarinic receptor activation; that is, decreased contractility, increased cGMP and decreased cAMP production in atria. All of the biological effects on rat atria triggered by chagasic antipeptide antibodies were blunted by atropine and resembled the effects of the authentic agonist, confirming the participation of cardiac mAChR activation. Not only did antipeptide autoantibodies behave as cholinergic agonists, but they also diminished the reaction of myocardium to exogenous carbachol, suggesting that, while in an early step they were able to activate mAChR, they might ultimately bind irreversibly to those receptors.[32]

The real clinical relevance of these findings is the demonstration, of a strong association between the existence of circulating anti-peptide antibodies in chagasic

TABLE 1. Distribution of antibodies from chagasic sera directed against peptide corresponding to the second extracellular loop of human neurotransmitter receptors tested by ELISA and CONTRACTILITY

Chagasic Groups	Methods			
	Biological		Serological	
	dF/dt	%	ELISA	%
Asymptomatic with dysautonomia	504/520	97	509/520	98
Asymptomatic without dysautonomia	109/420	26	105/420	25
Cardiopathy with dysautonomia	245/250	98	247/250	99
Cardiopathy without dysautonomia	9/230	4	11/230	5
Control (non-chagasic)	1/500	1	2/500	1

Microtiter wells were coated with 1 μg peptide and enzyme immunoassay (ELISA) was carried out in the presence of sera from different chagasic groups and controls. Values of O.D. above two SD of those of normal individuals were taken as positive. Contractility (dF/dt) was measured in isolated atria; 5×10^{-7} M of different sera were used during 15 min of exposition.

patients and the presence of dysautonomic symptoms, making these autoantibodies proper markers of cardiac autoimmune neurocardiomyopathy and achalasia.[32]

So, as can be seen in TABLE 1, an association between the existence of the circulating antipeptide M_2 mAChR autoantibodies and the presence of dysautonomic syndrome in chagasic patients (asymptomatic and cardiopathic) was observed. A strong association between ELISA and biological data was found ($\alpha < 0.001$).

The seropositive patients without myocardial autonomic dysfunction with detectable anti-peptide autoantibodies must be evaluated sequentially in order to ascertain the prognostic value of this test as an early marker of heart autonomic dysfunction. Moreover, analyzing the prevalence of antipeptide antibodies, we observed differences in their distribution in asymptomatic patients dependent on the heart rate variability (HRV) index. TABLE 2 shows an association of the presence of M_2 antipeptide mAChR autoantibodies in chagasic patients and parasympathetic HRV index. Thus, lower HRV indexes are associated with the presence of antipeptide antibodies. On the contrary, the HRV indexes of chagasic patients without circulating antipeptide

TABLE 2. Distribution of antipeptide antibodies in sera of chagasic patients correlated with heart rate variability (HRV) index

Groups	Methods	
	HRV Index	n
Chagasic antipeptide Ab-positive	0.59 ± 0.04	14
Chagasic antipeptide Ab-negative	2.32 ± 0.15	12
Control (non-chagasic)	2.46 ± 0.16	12

HRV index values are mean ± SEM of n: number of chagasic antipeptide mAChR autoantibodies (Ab) positive or negative. Normal control values are also shown.

antibodies did not differ from those of normal subjects. As data were obtained from asymptomatic patients, they confirm the value of the antipeptide antibody as an early marker of the disease evolution.

Chagasic achalasia has been described as a dysautonomia-related dysfunction in which excitatory neuronal influence of esophageal motility appears to be unopposed by the impaired inhibitory neural influence that governs smooth muscle relaxation. On this basis, we have considered the possibility that autoantibodies against mAChRs participate in the pathogenesis of chagasic achalasia by modulating the muscarinic effector response in the lower esophagus.[33] Thus, we reported the presence of circulating IgG autoantibodies against mAChRs in chagasic achalasia able to increase the contractile tone and decrease cAMP accumulation of the lower esophageal sphincter. Moreover, those autoantibodies inhibit the relaxant contractile effect of the β agonist and the accumulation of cAMP triggered by isoproterenol. TABLE 3 shows the prevalence of circulating antipeptide M_2 mAChRs autoantibodies in chagasic patients with or without achalasia. It can be seen that in patients with achalasia the prevalence of autoantibodies is significantly higher than in other groups. These results suggest that the presence of mAChR autoantibodies that exert a stimulatory effect on esophageal tone could contribute to the predominantly excitatory unbalance characteristic of chagasic achalasia.

It is important to note that the biological activity of the M_2 muscarinic agonistic circulating autoantibodies, present in both chagasic cardioneuromyopathy and achalasia, could be neutralized by short synthetic peptides corresponding to the functional epitopes in the antigenic extracellular loops and that this could be of possible therapeutic use in preventing the development of cardiac and esophageal chagasic dysautonomia. Preliminary studies show that chronic treatment *in vivo* with M_2 synthetic peptide substantially improved the cardiac dysfunction of chronic chagasic mice at the time that the titers of circulating autoantibodies against M_2 mAChR-peptide decreased.

These results suggested that treatment with synthetic peptide neutralized circulating autoantibodies, preventing their fixation on the myocardial mAChR. The use of synthetic peptides from neurotransmitter receptors may be useful as a tool for therapy, diagnosis and prognosis of chagasic cardioneuromyopathy and achalasia.

TABLE 3. Distribution of antipeptide antibodies from sera of chagasic patients with or without achalasia

Groups	Methods			
	Biological		Serological	
	tone	%	ELISA	%
Chagasic with achalasia	26/28	93	25/28	89
Chagasic without achalasia	6/26	23	7/26	27
Control (non-chagasic)	1/30	3	0/20	0

Microtiter wells were coated with 1 μg peptide and enzyme immunoassay (ELISA) was carried out in the presence of sera from different chagasic groups and controls. Values of O.D. above two S.D. of those of normal individuals were taken as positive. Tone was measured on low esophageal sphincter; 5×10^{-7} M of different sera were used during 15 min of exposition.

REFERENCES

1. WHO EXPERT COMMITEE. 1991 Control of Chagas' disease. Technical Report Series **811:** 1–10.
2. COSSIO, P.M., C. DIEZ, A. SZARFMAN, E. KREUTZER, B. CANDIOLO & R.M. ARANA. 1991. Chagasic cardiopathy: demonstration of a serum globulin factor which reacts with endocardium and vascular structures. Circulation **49:** 13–18.
3. STERIN-BORDA, L., M. CANTORE, J. PASCUAL et al. 1986. Chagasic IgG binds and interacts with β adrenoceptor coupled adenylate cyclase system. Int. J. Immunopharmacol. **8:** 581–588.
4. BORDA, E.S., J. PASCUAL, P.M. COSSIO, M. VEGA, R.M. ARANA & L. STERIN-BORDA. 1984. A circulating IgG in Chagas' disease which binds to β adrenoceptor of myocardium and modulates its activity. Clin. Exp. Immunol. **57:** 679–686.
5. BRISTOW, M.R. 1998. Why does the myocardium fail? Insights from basic science. Lancet **352**(Suppl. I): 8–14.
6. BRISTOW, M.R., W. NINOBE & R. RUSMUSSEL. 1992. Beta adrenergic neuroeffector abnormalities in the failing human heart are produced by local, rather than systemic mechanisms. J. Clin. Invest. **89:** 803–815.
7. BRISTOW, M.R., R. GINSBURG & W. MINOBE. 1982. Decreased catecholamines sensitivity and beta adrenergic receptor density in failing human heart. N. Engl. J. Med. **307:** 205–211.
8. BRACCO, M.M., L. STERIN-BORDA, S. FINK, M. FINIASZ & E.S. BORDA. 1984. Stimulatory effect of lymphocytes from Chagas' patients on spontaneously beating rat atria. Clin. Exp. Immunol. **55:** 405–412.
9. BORDA, E., C. PEREZ LEIROS, L. STERIN-BORDA & M.M. BRACCO. 1991. Cholinergic response of isolated rat atria to IFN-γ. J. Neuroimmunol. **32:** 53–59.
10. STERIN-BORDA, L., C. PEREZ LEIROS, M.M. BRACCO & E. BORDA. 1996. Effect of IL-2 on the myocardium. Participation of the sympathetic system. J. Mol. Cell. Cardiol. **28:** 2457–2465.
11. PEREZ LEIROS, C., L. STERIN-BORDA, P.M. COSSIO, O. BUSTOABAD & E.S. BORDA. 1996. Potential role of mononuclear cells infiltration on the autoimmune myocardial dysfunction. Clin. Exp. Immunol. **63:** 648–655.
12. PEREZ LEIROS, C., L. STERIN-BORDA & E.S. BORDA. 1988. Lymphocytes infiltration induces dysfunction in autoimmune myocarditis: role of SRS-A. J. Mol. Cell. Cardiol. **20:** 149–158.
13. GORELIK, G., E. BORDA, S. GONZALEZ CAPPA & L. STERIN-BORDA. 1992. Lymphocyte from *T.cruzi* infected mice altered heart contractility. Participation of arachidonic acid metabolites. J. Mol. Cell. Cardiol. **24:** 9–20.
14. STERIN-BORDA, L., C. DIEZ, P.M. COSSIO & M.M. BRACCO. 1982. β adrenergic effect of antibodies from chagasic patients and normal human lymphocytes on isolated rat atria. Clin. Exp. Immunol. **50:** 534–540.
15. STERIN-BORDA, L., P.M. COSSIO, M.F. GIMENO, C. DIEZ, R. LAGUENS, P. CABEZA-MECKER & R. ARANA. 1976. Effect of chagasic sera on the isolated rat atrial preparation. Cardiovasc. Res. **10:** 613–622.
16. STERIN-BORDA, L., G. GORELIK & E.S. BORDA. 1991. Chagasic IgG binding with cardiac muscarinic cholinergic receptors modifies cholinergic-mediated cellular transmembrane signals. Clin. Immunol. Immunopathol. **61:** 387–397.
17. GOIN, J.C., E. BORDA, C. PEREZ LEIROS, R. STORINO & L. STERIN-BORDA. 1994. Identification of antibodies with muscarinic cholinergic activity in human Chagas' disease: pathological implications. J. Aut. Nerv. System **47:** 45–52.
18. PASCUAL, J., E.S. BORDA, P.M. COSSIO, R.M. ARANA & L. STERIN-BORDA. 1987. Modification of sarcolemmal enzymes of chagasic IgG and its effect on cardiac contractility. Biochem. Pharmacol. **35:** 3839-3845.
19. PASCUAL, J., E.S. BORDA & L. STERIN-BORDA. 1987. Chagasic IgG modifies the activity of sarcolemmal ATPases through a β adrenergic mechanisms. Life Sci. **40:** 313–319.

20. STERIN-BORDA, L., L. CANGA, E.S. BORDA, P.M. COSSIO & R.M. ARANA. 1981. Chagasic sera alter the effect of ouabain on isolated rat atria. Eur. J. Pharmacol. **69:** 1–10.
21. BORDA, E. & L. STERIN-BORDA. 1996. Anti adrenergic and muscarinic receptor antibodies in Chagas' cardiomyopathy. Int. J. Cardiol. **154:** 149–156.
22. GOIN, J.C., E.S. BORDA, A. SEGOVIA & L. STERIN-BORDA. 1991. Distribution of antibodies against β adrenoceptors in the course of human *Trypanosoma cruzi* infection. Proc. Soc. Exp. Biol. Med. **197:** 186–192.
23. GOIN, J.C., C. PEREZ LEIROS, E. BORDA & L. STERIN-BORDA. 1994. Modification of cholinergic-mediated cellular transmenbrane signals by the interaction of human chagasic IgG with cardiac muscarinic receptors. Neuroimmunomodulation **1:** 284–291.
24. STERIN-BORDA, L., G. GORELIK, A. GENARO, J.C. GOIN & E. BORDA. 1990. Human chagasic IgG interacting with lymphocyte neurotransmitter receptors triggers intracellular signal transduction. FASEB J. **4:** 1661–1667.
25. STERIN-BORDA, L., C. PEREZ LEIROS, M. WALD, G. CREMASCHI & E.S. BORDA. 1988. Antibodies to β_1 and β_2 adrenoceptors in Chagas' disease. Clin. Exp. Immunol. **74:** 349–354.
26. STERIN-BORDA, L., G. CREMASCHI, A.M. GENARO, A. VILA ECHAGUE, J.C. GOIN & E. BORDA. 1986. Involvement of nitric oxide synthase and protein kinase C activation on chagasic antibodies action upon cardiac contractility. Mol. Cell. Biochem. **160/161:** 75–82.
27. STERIN-BORDA, L., C. PEREZ LEIROS, J.C. GOIN, G. CREMASCHI, A. GENARO, A. VILA ECHAGUE & E. BORDA. 1997. Participation of nitric oxide signaling system in the cardiac muscarinic cholinergic effect of human chagasic IgG. J. Mol. Cell. Cardiol. **29:** 1851–1865.
28. PEREZ LEIROS, C., L. STERIN-BORDA, E. BORDA, J.C. GOIN & M. HOSEY. 1997. Desensitization and sequestration of human M_2 mAChRs by autoantibodies from patients with Chagas' disease. J. Biol. Chem. **272:** 12989–12993.
29. PEREZ LEIROS, C., N. GOREN, L. STERIN-BORDA, L. LUSTIG & E. BORDA. 1994. Alterations in cardiac muscarinic acetylcholine receptors in mice with autoimmune myocarditis and association with circulating muscarinic receptor-related autoantibodies. Clin. Aut. Res. **4:** 249–255.
30. STERIN-BORDA, L., G. GORELIK, M. POSTAN, S. GONZALEZ CAPPA & E. BORDA. 1999. Alterations in cardiac beta adrenergic receptor in chagasic mice and their association with circulating beta adrenoceptor related antibodies. Cardiovasc. Res. **41:** 116–125.
31. CREMASCHI, G., N.W. ZWIRNER, G. GORELIK, E.L. MALCHIODI, M.G. CHIARIMONTE, C.A. FOSSATI & L. STERIN-BORDA. 1995. Modulation of cardiac physiology by an anti-*Trypanosoma cruzi* monoclonal antibody after interaction with myocardium. FASEB J. **9:** 1482–1488.
32. GOIN, J.C., C. PEREZ LEIROS, E. BORDA & L. STERIN-BORDA. 1997. Interaction of human chagasic IgG with the second extracellular loop of the human heart mAChRs. Functional and Pathological Implications. FASEB J. **10:** 77–83.
33. GOIN, J.C., L. STERIN-BORDA, C. BILDER, L. MONASTRA, M. IANTORNO, R. CASTRO & E. BORDA. 1999. Pathological implications of circulating mAChR antibodies in chagasic patients with achalasia. Gastroenterology. **117:** 798–805.

Nuclear Factor-κB is Involved in the Catecholaminergic Suppression of Immunocompetent Cells

JONAS BERGQUIST,[a,d,e] BERTIL OHLSSON,[b] AND ANDREJ TARKOWSKI[c]

[a]Institute of Clinical Neuroscience, Department of Neurochemistry,
Göteborg University, Sahlgrenska University Hospital, Göteborg, Sweden

[b]Wallenberg Laboratory, Göteborg University,
Sahlgrenska University Hospital, Göteborg, Sweden

[c]Department of Rheumatology, Göteborg University,
Sahlgrenska University Hospital, Göteborg, Sweden

[d]Department of Analytical Chemistry, Uppsala University, SE-751 21 Uppsala, Sweden

ABSTRACT: Catecholamines are known to exert a powerful impact on the immune system by downregulation of proliferation and differentiation, and induction of apoptosis. However, the mechanism for this regulatory route is still unclear. Therefore well established human monocytic cell-lines and non-transformed human monocytes, obtained from peripheral blood, were incubated with an optimal concentration of LPS and varying concentrations of the catecholamine dopamine. The proliferative response to LPS was determined by [^{3}H]thymidine incorporation, and a significant suppressive effect by dopamine was obtained. LPS-induced binding of NF-κB to DNA, determined by electrophoretic mobility shift assay, was inhibited by extrinsic dopamine, leading to a decreased proliferation and cytokine expression. In contrast, the intracellular ceramide concentration was not affected by incubation of peripheral blood lymphocytes with dopamine. Our findings suggest that the NF-κB–I-κB transcription machinery may well be involved in the catecholaminergic regulation of the immune system, while the ceramide–SAPK/JNK cascade appears not to play a significant role in this suppression.

INTRODUCTION

Immunocompetent cells (human peripheral blood mononuclear cells—PBMCs, T cells, B cells, mouse splenocytes, macrophages, and hybridoma cell lines) have all been shown both to produce and to be suppressed by exogenous catecholamines (dopamine and norepinephrine)[1–5] and by acetylcholine.[6,7] This has been found both in proliferative responses (analyzed by [^{3}H]thymidine incorporation) and differentiation assays (analyzed by cytokine release of IL-1, IL-2, IL-4, IL-6, IL-8, IFN-γ, and TNF-α, as well as by immunoglobulin production). Furthermore, an induction of apoptosis involving the Bcl-2/Bax and Fas/FasL systems has been found to be

[e]Address for correspondence: J. Bergquist, Department of Analytical Chemistry, Uppsala University, SE-751 21 Uppsala, Sweden. Voice: +46-18-471-3695; fax: +46-18-471-3692.
jonas.bergquist@kemi.uu.se

triggered by increasing concentration of exogenous catecholamines.[2,4] Adrenergic and cholinergic receptors are known to exist on the surface of both T and B cells as well as mRNA expression of α1A, α2A, α2B, and β2 adrenergic, the muscarinic m3, and the nicotinic cholinergic receptors in lymphocytes.[8–12] Previous studies demonstrated receptor-mediated effects on migration and activation of lymphocytes. However, other mechanisms may be involved, including direct uptake of catecholamines across the cellular membrane and the nucleus envelope via specific transporter proteins.[3] Catecholamines appear to regulate the activity of immunocompetent cells, which is possibly a part of the explanation of the immunological privilege of the CNS. This represents a novel mechanism for catecholamines as messengers in the neuroimmune axis, but the exact details of the regulatory mechanism have yet to be determined.

The transcription factor nuclear factor-κB (NF-κB) has been shown to be involved in the regulation of mitogen-stimulated cytokine and Ig synthesis. NF-κB is bound to I-κB in the cytoplasm until a mitogen (e.g. LPS) is introduced and a phosphorylation of I-κB occurs.[13] When this happens NF-κB is released from I-κB and can be transported into the nucleus, where it binds to specific promotor domains in the genome.[14] This binding initiates the transcription of the downstream genes. NF-κB is an important regulator of cell death, as shown in a variety of experimental settings. The function of NF-κB in the apoptotic cell death seems to be very dependent on the system and type of stimulus examined.[15] Recently, the regulation of HIV-1 expression by dopamine in Jurkat T cells and in peripheral blood mononuclear cells has been investigated.[16] HIV-1 replication was increased by dopamine, which correlated with the increased levels of HIV-1 transactivation. The data revealed that dopamine stimulated transcription through the NF-κB element present in the long terminal repeat.

Apoptosis is also known to be induced by ceramide.[17] Ceramide is an initiator of the activation of mitogen-activated protein (MAP) kinase family members in the SAPK/JNK signaling pathway. This pathway has been implicated in TNF-α or stress-induced apoptosis in, for example, human monoblastic leukemia cells.[18] However, the context of the signaling events may be important, since activation of the ceramide-SAPK/JNK cascade has been reported to lead to proliferation and differentiation rather than apoptosis in some systems.[18] Ceramide has been suggested as the secondary messenger mediating the apoptotic signal for Fas engagement, but this has recently been debated.[19–21] It is also interesting to notice that there is a structural homology between LPS and ceramide.[22] Ceramide has also been reported to inhibit TNF-α production following activation of NF-κB.[23]

The aim of this study was to investigate whether binding of NF-κB to DNA could be inhibited by catecholamines. This would subsequently lead to a decreased proliferative response and a decreased cytokine expression by immunocompetent cells. If so, this would be a possible mechanism for the catecholaminergic regulation of the immune system. In this experiment we have used non-transformed human monocytes and human monocytic cell lines. In parallel, we have studied the expression of intracellular ceramide by peripheral blood mononuclear cells during catecholamine-induced apoptosis to assess whether the ceramide-SAPK/JNK cascade plays a role in the catecholaminergic regulatory mechanism of the immune system.

MATERIALS AND METHODS

Preparation of Monocytes and Isolation of Nuclei

Peripheral blood mononuclear cells were separated using gradient centrifugation (see below). The mononuclear cells were washed three times in cold PBS. The concentration of mononuclear cells was adjusted to 10^7 cell/mL in RPMI containing 5% FCS. The cells were incubated for 2 h at 37°C, 3 mL/well in a 6-well Nunc microtiter plate. The wells were then washed three times with warm RPMI to remove nonadherent cells. Adherent cells were cultured in RPMI containing 10% FCS and different concentrations of dopamine for 24 h at 37°C. The cells were rinsed three times with warm RPMI, and then cultured in complete medium containing LPS (10 ng/mL) for 1 h at 37°C. The monocytes were detached by incubation for 10 min at 37°C in PBS containing 0.5 mM EDTA and using a rubber policeman. They were then washed twice in PBS and frozen until nuclei were isolated (see below).

Monocytic cell line THP-1 was plated at 10^6 cell/mL in 24-well plate together with the dopamine (0, 10 nM, 1 μM, or 100 μM respectively) for 24 h. Cells were washed with PBS and incubated in complete endotoxin-free medium containing LPS (10 ng/mL) for 1 hour. Thereafter, the cells were rinsed and harvested into tubes and pellets were frozen (−80°C) until isolation of nuclei occurred. The monocyte pellets were lysed by adding 250 μL of distilled water and vortexing. The tubes were left on ice for 15 min; then 250 μL of the 2.0 M sucrose with buffers (1 mM EDTA, 10 mM Hepes, 1 mM DTT) were added. These samples were layered over 800 μL of the buffered sucrose solution in ultracentrifuge tubes. After centrifugation for 1 h (30,000 rpm, 75,000 × *g*, 4°C, Optima™ TLX ultracentrifuge [Beckman]), the sucrose layer was carefully removed. With the tubes tipped slightly downwardly over ice, the insides of the tubes were carefully washed with a syringe filled with distilled water (to avoid spraying the pellet). The nuclei were pelleted in the bottom of the tube and appeared as a fine whitish film. The pellets were then frozen (−80°C) until extraction.

Preparation of Human Peripheral Blood Mononuclear Cells

One fresh SAGMAN buffy coat unit was diluted to 160 mL with 0.9% NaCl. Then, 20 mL of this mixture was layered carefully over 15 mL Lymphoprep (Nycomed) in 50-mL Sarstedt tubes. The tubes were centrifuged at 800 × *g* for 25 min and the mononuclear cell fraction was harvested into new tubes. It was diluted with 0.9% NaCl to 25 mL and washed at 400 × *g* for 15 min. The lymphocytes were pelleted, whereas the platelets remained in the supernatant. The supernatant was removed and complete cell culture medium (Iscoves) was added to the lymphocyte pellet with various concentrations of dopamine. After the incubation, the lymphocytes were pelleted by centrifugation at 200 × *g* for 10 min and washed twice with 0.9% NaCl.

Preparation of Nuclear Protein Extract

Nuclear pellets were resuspended in the smallest volume possible (50 μL) of extraction buffer (20 mM Hepes, pH 7.9 at 4°C, 25% glycerol, 0.42 M NaCl, 1 mM EDTA, 1mM EGTA, 1mM DTT + proteinase inhibitors [Boehringers Complete™ Mini Tablets, 1 tablet/10 mL]). After extraction at 4°C for 45 min on a mixer, the extract was transferred to a small Eppendorf tube. After sedimentation at $35,000 \times g$ at 4°C for 30 min, the supernatant was stored at −80°C in aliquots until the analysis of NF-κB could be performed.

Proliferative Responses of Human Monocytes and Peripheral Blood Mononuclear Cells

Proliferation of leukocytes was induced by LPS stimulation. The cells were incubated with 10 ng/mL of LPS (GIBCO) at a concentration of 1×10^6 mononuclear cells/mL in 96-well flat-bottomed microtiter plates (Nunc, Roskilde, Denmark) in 0.1 mL culture medium at 37°C in 5% CO_2 and 95% humidity. To these cultures 0–2,000 μM dopamine was added. The cells were either preincubated with the compounds at 37°C for 24 h, then washed, recounted and resuspended in culture medium, before stimulation with mitogens, or cultured with the mentioned compounds throughout the mitogen stimulation. The cells were cultured for 72 h; during the final 18 h of culture 1 μCi [^{3}H]thymidine (Radiochemical Centre, Amersham, UK) was included in each well. The cultures were harvested on glass fiber filters, processed and counted in a β-counter. The cultures were set up in triplicates and results expressed as percentage of control mean counts/min.

Analysis of NF-κB

For electrophoretic mobility shift assay (EMSA) a double-stranded oligonucleotide, corresponding to a part of the TNF-α promoter containing a binding site for NF-κB, was labeled with $α[^{32}P]$-labeled deoxynucleotide using Klenow polymerase. This oligonucleotide was used in the binding reaction with the nuclear protein extracts.

The protein-DNA binding reaction was carried out in a volume of 20 μL containing 20 mM Tris-HCl, pH 7.9, 60 mM NaCl, 0.1 mM EGTA, 1 mM DTT, 5% glycerol, 5 μg of poly(dI-dC)poly(dI-dC) (Pharmacia Biotech). Approximately 80,000 Cerenkov cpm corresponding to 2 ng of the probe was added to each reaction, which proceeded at room temperature for 20 min after the same amount of protein nuclear extracts was added to every reaction.

In one protein-DNA binding reaction experiment, rabbit polyclonal IgG towards the p65 subunit of NF-κB was added to the binding reactions to identify NF-κB.

Optional: to one binding reaction purified recombinant p50, the subunit of NF-κB that form the homodimer form of the human transcription factor NF-κB was added to the protein-DNA binding reaction instead of nuclear protein extracts to localize the retarded protein-DNA band corresponding to the NF-κB-DNA complex.

The reaction mixtures were electrophoretically separated through a native 5% polyacrylamide gel containing $0.25 \times$ TBE (2.2 mM Tris borate, 2.2 mM boric acid, 0.5 mM EDTA) and 3% glycerol to separate DNA-protein complexes from unbound DNA-probe. The gel was vacuum-dried.

The dried gel was put into a Phospho Imager and the amount of NF-κB was estimated. The amount of NF-κB per μg nuclear protein extract in each binding reaction could be expressed; where the amount shifted, labeled oligonucleotide with the human recombinant NF-κB could be used as a reference.

The Phospho Imager of the electrophoretic gel could also be shown to illustrate the electrophoretical pattern. Antibodies against NF-κB will supershift the band corresponding to the NF-κB-DNA complex. The results were expressed as percentage of control mean counts/lane.

Analysis of Ceramide

The frozen peripheral blood mononuclear cell pellets were resuspended in 500 μL ultrapure water (Millipore, Bedford, MA, USA). The suspensions were refrozen on dry-ice and ethanol, thawed in cold water and sonicated for 1 min (Bransonic B-2200-E, Germany). This procedure was repeated four times. The protein levels were determined using the bicinchoninic acid protein assay reagent method (Pierce, Rockford, IL, USA), and ultrapure water was added to a final volume of 700 μL. For the lipid extraction, 2000 μL of methanol and 1000 μL of chloroform ($C/M/H_2O$ 4:8:3 by volume) were added. The extractions were made end-over-end for 1 h in room temperature and the suspensions were centrifuged at $1500 \times g$ for 15 min. The supernatants were transferred to clean tubes and the pellets were re-extracted as

TABLE 1. **Proliferation, nuclear factor-κB and ceramide expression in human monocytes and mononuclear cells following incubation with dopamine**[a]

	Dopamine						
	10 nM	1 μM	10 μM	100 μM	500 μM	1,000 μM	2,000 μM
Proliferative responses[b]							
Peripheral blood monocytes 24 h	105	98	75	19	—	—	—
Monocyte cell line 24 h	—	—	102	24	—	2	0.8
Monocyte cell line 72 h	—	—	100	89	—	0.2	0.1
Nuclear factor-κB[c]							
Peripheral blood monocytes	50	20	20	—	—	—	—
Monocyte cell line	—	—	—	55	46	38	33
Ceramide[d]							
Human PBMCs	—	—	103	95	88	—	—

[a]All experiments, expressed as % of control, were performed in triplicate (ceramide $n = 5$), and in all cases the relative standard deviation was less than 10%.

[b]Proliferative responses were measured by incorporation of [^{3}H]thymidine. Monocytes were incubated with 10 ng/mL of LPS, together with the listed concentration of dopamine for the time indicated.

[c]Nuclear factor-κB binding to DNA were measured by electrophoretic mobility shift assay. Monocytes were incubated with 10 ng/mL of LPS, together with the listed concentration of dopamine for 24 h before the nuclei were isolated and extracted for the analysis of NF-κB.

[d]The intracellular concentration of ceramide was measured by thin layer chromatography. The isolated peripheral blood mononuclear cells were incubated with the listed concentration of dopamine for 24 h prior to the analysis of ceramide.

described above. Supernatants were pooled and dried. Intracellular levels of ceramide in the cell extract was determined using the thin layer chromatography method earlier described.[24,25] The results were expressed as percentage of control ceramide in pmol/mg protein.

RESULTS

TNF-α is a potent activator of expression for genes encoding for several cytokines. The expression of the TNF-α gene is mainly regulated by the transcription factor NF-κB. Several binding sites for this transcription factor have been found on the TNF-α promoter.[26] We were interested in studying the effect of catecholamines on an LPS-induced activation of NF-κB in human monocytes, isolated both from peripheral blood and transfected cell lines. A significant suppressive effect on proliferation was seen already with 10 μM dopamine in peripheral blood monocytes and with 100 μM dopamine in the monocyte cell line after 24 h (see TABLE 1). The dopamine concentration needed to obtain similar results after 72-h incubation was higher, most likely owing to degradation of dopamine in the cell medium. The results obtained after EMSA showed that LPS induced binding of NF-κB to the TNF-α promoter. However, the LPS-induced binding of NF-κB to the TNF-α promoter was dose-dependently decreased in cell cultures incubated with dopamine (see FIG. 1, TABLE 1). These results indicate that the regulatory mechanism of dopamine in the immune system may involve inhibition of the binding of NF-κB to specific promoter regions in the genome. The sensitivity to dopamine was more pronounced in ex vivo–obtained monocytes compared to hybridoma cells, as observed earlier.[1–4] The ceramide content of peripheral blood mononuclear cells was not affected upon incubation with dopamine (TABLE 1).

DISCUSSION

In this study we have found that dopamine suppresses LPS-mediated activation of NF-κB. These observations agree with results obtained from earlier studies indicating that the transcription factor families NF-κB/Rel are of importance in the regulation of cytokine production.[26–31] T cells from c-Rel knock-out mice fail to respond to activation and proliferation signals mediated by the TCR and mitogens.[32] The mechanism behind the decreased LPS activation of NF-κB in cells incubated with catecholamines is not yet clear. However, similar results to ours have been obtained in macrophages incubated with glucocorticoids.[33,34] The glucocorticoids increased the expression of I-κB. When macrophages were exposed to LPS, the NF-κB–I-κB complex dissociated after I-κB was phosphorylated, but NF-κB was then bound to another unphosphorylated I-κB. The excess of I-κB in comparison to NF-κB inhibited the translocation of NF-κB from the cytoplasm to the nucleus.

Our results suggest that catecholamines may inhibit the translocation of NF-κB from the cytoplasm to the nucleus. The lack of effect of dopamine on the intracellular ceramide in mononuclear cells, known to dramatically suppress proliferation and

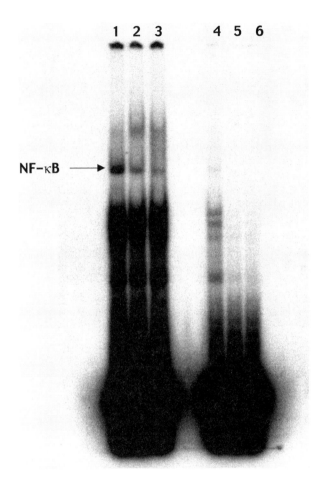

FIGURE 1. A representative Phospho Image of an electrophoretic mobility shift assay (EMSA) gel for the analysis of NF-κB expression in monocytes that have been incubated with dopamine for 24 h. *Lane 1* is control (10 ng/mL LPS, no dopamine); *lane 2*: 10 ng/mL LPS, 100 μM dopamine; *lane 3*: 10 ng/mL LPS, 500 μM dopamine; *lane 4*: 10 ng/mL LPS, 1000 μM dopamine; *lane 5*: 10 ng/mL LPS, 2000 μM dopamine; and *lane 6* is negative control (no LPS and no dopamine). The results can also be found in TABLE 1.

differentiation as well as induce apoptosis, suggests that the TNF-α-ceramide signaling pathway[17] may not be involved.

The transcription factor NF-κB has been found to be involved in several inflammatory diseases like rheumatic arthritis and arteriosclerosis. In this and earlier studies we have found that catecholamines decreased the inflammatory response. Molecules with similar properties could in the future be developed to be potential immunosuppressive drugs to immunomodulate these diseases.

ACKNOWLEDGMENTS

We like to acknowledge Rita Persson and Margareta Verdreng for excellent technical assistance and Lone Bovin at the Institute of Inflammatory Research, Rigshospitalet, Copenhagen, Denmark, for performing the ceramide analysis. This work was supported by the Fredrik and Ingrid Thuring Foundation, the Wilhelm and Martina Lundgren Foundation, the Magnus Bergvall Foundation, the Swedish Alzheimer Foundation, the Syskonen Svensson Foundation, the Gamla Trotjänarinnor Foundation, the Knut and Alice Wallenberg foundation, the Swedish Lundbeck Foundation, the Swedish Society for Medical Research, the Swedish Natural Science Research Council (Grant K-AA/KU 12003-300) and the Swedish Medical Research Council (Grant 13123).

REFERENCES

1. BERGQUIST, J., A. TARKOWSKI, R. EKMAN & A. EWING. 1994. Discovery of endogenous catecholamines in lymphocytes and evidence for catecholamine regulation of lymphocyte function via an autocrine loop. Proc. Natl. Acad. Sci. USA **91:** 12912–12916.
2. BERGQUIST, J., E. JOSEFSSON, A. TARKOWSKI, R. EKMAN & A. EWING. 1997. Measurements of catecholamine-mediated apoptosis of immunocompetent cells by capillary electrophoresis. Electrophoresis **18:** 1760–1766.
3. BERGQUIST, J., A. TARKOWSKI, A. EWING & R. EKMAN. 1998. Catecholaminergic suppression of immunocompetent cells. Immunol. Today **19:** 562–567.
4. JOSEFSSON, E., J. BERGQUIST, R. EKMAN & A. TARKOWSKI. 1996. Catecholamines are synthesized by mouse lymphocytes and regulate function of these cells by induction of apoptosis. Immunology **88:** 140–146.
5. BERGQUIST, J. & J. SILBERRING. 1998. Identification of catecholamines in the immune system by electrospray ionization mass spectrometry. Rapid Commun. Mass Spectrom. **12:** 683–688.
6. SCHAUENSTEIN, K., I. RINNER, P. FELSNER, P. LIEBMANN, H.S. HASS, D. HOFER & A. WOLFLER. 1997. The role of the autonomous nervous system in the dialogue between the brain and immune system. *In* Current Update Psychoneuroimmunology. G. Wieselmann, Ed.: 13–21. Springer, Wien.
7. RINNER, I., K. KAWASHIMA & K. SCHAUENSTEIN. 1998. Rat lymphocytes produce and secrete acetylcholine independent of differentiation and activation. J. Neuroimmunol. **81:** 31–37.
8. BLALOCK, J.E. 1992. Production of peptide hormones and neurotransmitters by the immune system. *In* Neuroimmunoendocrinology, 2 edit. J.E. Blalock, Ed. **52:** 1–24. Karger. Basel.
9. RICCI, A., J.A. VEGA, D. ZACCHEO & F. AMENTA. 1995. Dopamine D1-like receptors in the thymus of aged rats: a radioligand binding and autoradiographic study. J. Neuroimmunol. **56:** 155–160.
10. SANTAMBROGIO, L., M. LIPARTITI, A. BRUNI & R. DAL TOSO. 1993. Dopamine receptors on human T- and B-lymphocytes. J. Neuroimmunol. **45:** 113–120.
11. PLAUT, M. 1987. Lymphocyte hormone receptors. Annu. Rev. Immunol. **5:** 621–669.
12. RINNER, I. & K. SCHAUENSTEIN. 1998. Expression of adrenergic and cholinergic receptor mRNA in immune cells of the rat. Psychoneuroimmunomodulation **5:** 39.
13. GHOSH, S. & D. BALTIMORE. 1990. Activation in vitro of NF-kappa B by phosphorylation of its inhibitor I kappa B. Nature **344:** 678–682.
14. SEN, R. & D. BALTIMORE. 1986. Inducibility of kappa immunoglobulin enhancer-binding protein NF-kappa B by a posttranslational mechanism. Cell **47:** 921–928.
15. BAICHWAL, V.R. & P.A. BAEUERLE. 1997. Activate NF-kappa B or die? Curr. Biol. **7:** R94–R96.

16. ROHR, O., B.E. SAWAYA, D. LECESTRE, D. AUNIS & E. SCHAEFFER. 1999. Dopamine stimulates expression of the human immunodeficiency virus type 1 via NF-kappa B in cells of the immune system. Nucleic Acids Res. **27:** 3291–3299.

17. OBEID, L.M., C.M. LINARDIC, L.A. KAROLAK & Y.A. HANNUN. 1993. Programmed cell death induced by ceramide. Science **259:** 1769–1771.

18. VERHEIJ, M., R. BOSE, X.H. LIN, B. YAO, W.D. JARVIS, S. GRANT, M.J. BIRRER, E. SZABO, L.I. ZON, J.M. KYRIAKIS, A. HAIMOVITZ-FRIEDMAN, Z. FUKS & R.N. KOLESNICK. 1996. Requirement for ceramide-initiated SAPK/JNK signalling in stress-induced apoptosis. Nature **380:** 75–79.

19. HSU, S.C., C.C. WU, T.Y. LUH, C.K. CHOU, S.H. HAN & M.Z. LAI. 1998. Apoptotic signal of Fas is not mediated by ceramide. Blood **91:** 2658–2663.

20. GULBINS, E., R. BISSONNETTE, A. MAHBOUBI, S. MARTIN, W. NISHIOKA, T. BRUNNER, G. BAIER, G. BAIER-BITTERLICH, C. BYRD, F. LANG *et al.* 1995. FAS-induced apoptosis is mediated via a ceramide-initiated RAS signaling pathway. Immunity **2:** 341–351.

21. COCK, J.G., A.D. TEPPER, E. DE VRIES, W.J. VAN BLITTERSWIJK & J. BORST. 1998. CD95 (Fas/APO-1) induces ceramide formation and apoptosis in the absence of a functional acid sphingomyelinase. J. Biol. Chem. **273:** 7560–7565.

22. MACKICHAN, M.L. & A.L. DEFRANCO. 1999. Role of ceramide in lipopolysaccharide (LPS)-induced signaling. LPS increases ceramide rather than acting as a structural homolog. J. Biol. Chem. **274:** 1767–1775.

23. GAMARD, C.J., G.S. DBAIBO, B. LIU, L.M. OBEID & Y.A. HANNUN. 1997. Selective involvement of ceramide in cytokine-induced apoptosis. Ceramide inhibits phorbol ester activation of nuclear factor kappa B. J. Biol. Chem. **272:** 16474–16481.

24. PREISS, J., C.R. LOOMIS, W.R. BISHOP, R. STEIN, J.E. NIEDEL & R.M. BELL. 1986. Quantitative measurement of sn-1,2-diacylglycerols present in platelets, hepatocytes, and ras- and sis-transformed normal rat kidney cells. J. Biol. Chem. **261:** 8597–8600.

25. VAN VELDHOVEN, P.P., W.R. BISHOP, D.A. YURIVICH & R.M. BELL. 1995. Ceramide quantitation: evaluation of a mixed micellar assay using E. coli diacylglycerol kinase. Biochem. Mol. Biol. Int. **36:** 21–30.

26. COLLART, M.A., P. BAEUERLE & P. VASSALLI. 1990. Regulation of tumor necrosis factor alpha transcription in macrophages: involvement of four kappa B-like motifs and of constitutive and inducible forms of NF-kappa B. Mol. Cell. Biol. **10:** 1498–1506.

27. SHAKHOV, A.N., M.A. COLLART, P. VASSALLI, S.A. NEDOSPASOV & C.V. JONGENEEL. 1990. Kappa B-type enhancers are involved in lipopolysaccharide-mediated transcriptional activation of the tumor necrosis factor alpha gene in primary macrophages. J. Exp. Med. **171:** 35–47.

28. HINZ, M., D. KRAPPMANN, A. EICHTEN, A. HEDER, C. SCHEIDEREIT & M. STRAUSS. 1999. NF-kappa B function in growth control: regulation of cyclin D1 expression and G0/G1-to-S-phase transition. Mol. Cell. Biol. **19:** 2690–2698.

29. KALTSCHMIDT, B., C. KALTSCHMIDT, S.P. HEHNER, W. DROGE & M.L. SCHMITZ. 1999. Repression of NF-kappa B impairs HeLa cell proliferation by functional interference with cell cycle checkpoint regulators. Oncogene **18:** 3213–3225.

30. GUTTRIDGE, D.C., C. ALBANESE, J.Y. REUTHER, R.G. PESTELL & A.S. BALDWIN, JR. 1999. NF-kappa B controls cell growth and differentiation through transcriptional regulation of cyclin D1. Mol. Cell. Biol. **19:** 5785–5799.

31. GUERRINI, L., A. MOLTENI & F. BLASI. 1998. Possible stage-specific function of NF-kappa B during pre-B cell differentiation. FEBS Lett. **434:** 140–144.

32. LIOU, H.C., Z. JIN, J. TUMANG, S. ANDJELIC, K.A. SMITH & M.L. LIOU. 1999. c-Rel is crucial for lymphocyte proliferation but dispensable for T cell effector function. Int. Immunol. **11:** 361–371.

33. AUPHAN, N., J.A. DIDONATO, C. ROSETTE, A. HELMBERG & M. KARIN. 1995. Immunosuppression by glucocorticoids: inhibition of NF-kappa B activity through induction of I kappa B synthesis. Science **270:** 286–290.

34. SCHEINMAN, R.I., P.C. COGSWELL, A.K. LOFQUIST & A.S. BALDWIN, JR. 1995. Role of transcriptional activation of I kappa B alpha in mediation of immunosuppression by glucocorticoids. Science **270:** 283–286.

The Peripheral CRH/Urocortin System

CHRISTOPH M. BAMBERGER[a,b] AND ANA-MARIA BAMBERGER[c]

[a]*Department of Medicine, University Hospital Eppendorf, 20246 Hamburg, Germany*

[c]*Institute for Pathology, University Hospital Eppendorf, 20246 Hamburg, Germany*

ABSTRACT: The hypothalmus-pituitary-adrenal (HPA) axis and the immune system communicate at multiple levels: On the one hand, immune system–derived substances, such as interleukin-1, interleukin-6, tumor necrosis factor alpha, and leukemia inhibitory factor can stimulate the HPA axis. On the other hand, HPA axis-derived substances, most importantly glucocorticoids, can modulate the immune response. Furthermore, factors that were originally thought to be restricted to the HPA axis have been found to be expressed by immune cells. Proteins belonging to the CRH (corticotropin-releasing hormone) family represent important examples of such hormones. In the early 1990s, it was shown that immunoreactive CRH was present at sites of chemically induced inflammation. Administration of anti-CRH antibodies reduced the degree of inflammation, pointing to a pro-inflammatory role of "peripheral" CRH. We and others could show that lymphocytes are one source of immunoreactive CRH; however, the antiserum used in our study as well as in previous reports crossreacted with urocortin, a newly discovered member of the CRH family. Using RT-PCR, we could clearly demonstrate that human lymphocytes expressed urocortin but not CRH mRNA. These results were confirmed by immunocytochemistry, employing urocortin- and CRH-specific antibodies, respectively. The possible functional roles of urocortin expression in the immune system are discussed.

CRH, UROCORTIN, AND THE HPA AXIS

Corticotropin-releasing hormone (CRH) is the principal regulator of the hypothalamus pituitary adrenal (HPA) axis in mammals.[1–5] By stimulating adrenocorticotropic hormone (ACTH) and, thus, cortisol secretion, centrally produced CRH exerts numerous peripheral effects including immunosuppression.[5] Moreover, CRH activates the sympathetic system, the end products of which (i.e., catecholamines) can also suppress certain immune responses.[6] Other effects of CRH within the central nervous system (CNS) include the induction of anxiety and motor activity as well as the inhibition of food intake and sexual behavior. All these *central* effects of CRH are usually referred to as the *stress response*.

Most of the CRH extracted from body fluids is bound to a specific binding protein, termed CRH-binding protein.[7] It is believed that this protein regulates the concentration of free, biologically active CRH. The effects of CRH are mediated by two types of receptors called CRH receptor 1 (CRH-R1) and CRH-R2.[8–13] The latter

[b]Address for correspondence: Christoph M. Bamberger, M.D. University Hospital Eppendorf, Department of Medicine, Martinistr. 52, 20246 Hamburg, Germany. Voice: 49-40-42803-3907; fax: 4-40-42803-5470.
bamberger@uke.uni-hamburg.de

comes in at least three different splice variants which may have distinct biological functions. Both receptors are expressed at numerous sites within the CNS. CRH-R1 is the main receptor subtype expressed by anterior pituitary corticotrophs and, thus, mediates the principal functions of CRH, that is, activation of the HPA axis.

Urotensin-1, sauvagine, and the recently discovered 40 aminoacid peptide urocortin share a considerable degree of homology with CRH, and are, therefore, considered to be members of one protein family. Of this family, only CRH and urocortin have been found to be expressed in mammals and humans, whereas urotensin-1 and sauvagine were identified in fish and amphibia, respectively.[14–16] Urocortin shares 45% sequence homology with CRH and can bind to the CRH-binding protein, to CRH-R1 and, with even higher affinity than CRH itself, to CRH-R2.[15,16] The functional role of urocortin cannot easily be concluded from its expression pattern within the CNS. The highest urocortin concentrations are found in the Edinger-Westphal nucleus, which does not project to any of the known stress centers.[17] When administered intracerebroventricularly or systemically, urocortin can evoke most of the responses of CRH, including activation of the HPA axis.[15,18–24] However, if it does so *in vivo* is questionable. On the one hand, stress can still lead to increased ACTH and cortisol release in CRH knock-out mice, and this response is blocked by an CRH-R1 antagonist.[25] On the other hand, anti-urocortin antibodies do not block activation of the HPA axis in intact animals.[26] It is therefore conceivable that CRH regulates ACTH release under normal conditions and urocortin—following the principle of redundancy—takes over when CRH is absent.

THE HPA IMMUNE AXIS

In recent years, it has become widely accepted that the HPA axis and the immune system can interact at multiple levels. This has led some authors to use the term HPA immune axis.[5,27,28] Firstly, glucocorticoids, the main endproducts of the HPA axis, are potent modulators of the immune response.[5,27–29] By binding to and activating the intracellular glucocorticoid receptor, glucocorticoids inhibit the transcription rates of many important immune genes, such as the interleukin-2 and the leukemia inhibitory factor (LIF) gene.[30,31] This results in immunosupression in most circumstances. Secondly, immune system–derived substances (e.g., interleukin-1, interleukin-6, tumor necrosis factor alpha, and LIF) can activate the HPA axis at the level of the hypothalamus, the pituitary, and the adrenal gland.[5,28,32–37] Finally, substances that were originally believed to be restricted to the HPA axis have been found to be-expressed in immune cells and vice versa. One important example of such substances are proteins belonging to the CRH family.

PERIPHERAL EXPRESSION OF CRH AND UCN

In 1989, Hargreaves *et al.* demonstrated that fluid from sites of caragheenin-induced inflammation could stimulate the release of β-endorphin in rat pituitary cell cultures. Karalis *et al.* confirmed in 1991 that the CRH-like activity of such fluid did indeed contain immunoreactive CRH.[39] Subsequently, the presence of immunoreactive CRH in inflamed rat and human tissues (e.g., in experimental uveitis)[40] in the synovia of patients with rheumatoid arthritis,[41] in inflammatory thyroid lesions,[42] and in colonic mucosa of patients with ulcerative colitis,[43] was reported by several investigators. In addition to its expression at sites of inflammation, peripheral CRH was found to be present in the human placenta,[44,45] the ovary,[46] the endometrium,[47] and in peripheral nerves.[48]

The peripheral expression pattern of urocortin is less well studied. So far, it was found to be expressed in the human placenta and fetal membranes,[49,50] in rat cardiac myocytes,[51] and in myenteric plexus of the rat gastrointestinal mucosa.[52]

Despite the obvious pathophysiological relevance of "immune" CRH, there are few data concerning the exact source of CRH and the actual expression levels of the CRH gene at inflammatory sites. Several studies suggested that lymphocytes may be an important source of immunoreactive CRH.[53,54] However, the presence of CRH mRNA in lymphocytes had never been proven unequivocally. Expression studies in mice revealed that the CRH gene is actively transcribed in splenic T lymphocytes,[55] indicating that immune cells might be an important source of CRH production during the immune/inflammatory response. However, Karalis et al. could not demonstrate CRH mRNA expression in acute inflammatory sites,[39] while Crofford et al. only detected it in chronic inflammatory responses.[41] Furthermore, the expression of urocortin in human lymphocytes had not been investigated before we initiated the study that is summarized here. Using a conventional CRH-RIA and employing an anti-CRH1-41 antibody we could confirm previous results showing release of immunoreactive CRH by cultured human lymphocytes.[56] However, when we tested purified urocortin we could demonstrate that it was also detected by this assay, indicating a considerable degree of crossreactivity of the employed antibody. RT-PCR experiments using CRH- and urocortin-specific primers, clearly showed that only urocortin mRNA, but not CRH mRNA was expressed by unstimulated and stimulated normal human lymphocytes.[56] These results were confirmed by Northern blot experiments using CRH- and urocortin-specific probes, respectively (unpublished results). We could extend these results to the protein level by showing that immunoreactive urocortin, but not CRH was expressed by human lymphocytes.[56] For this experiment, we used antibodies that could distinguish between CRH and urocortin. In summary, we could demonstrate that normal human lymphocytes (and Jurkat T lymphoma cells) express urocortin mRNA and peptide. Furthermore, we showed that neither CRH mRNA nor peptide were expressed by these cells. Since the conventional anti-CRH1-41 antiserum can detect both human CRH and human urocortin, part of the previously described peripheral CRH-like immunoreactivity may have been produced by other cell types, such as peripheral nerves, and/or may have been urocortin.

FUNCTIONAL ROLE OF "IMMUNE" CRH AND UCN

What is the functional role of immune CRH expressed by peripheral nerves and urocortin produced by lymphocytes? Few studies suggest an anti-inflammatory role of peripheral CRH/urocortin. Systemic administration of CRH reduced the degree of edema in thermal, cold, or acid injury.[57–59] In the rat carageenin model, systemic administration of urocortin also caused a reduction of edema, however, similar effects could be achieved by the administration of dihydralazine, a well-known blood pressure lowering agent.[60] Since urocortin was also shown to lower the blood pressure to a significant extent, the observed "anti-inflammatory" effects could well be due a reduced perfusion pressure in the inflamed tissue. In addition, systemic administration of CRH or urocortin stimulates the HPA axis, and, thus, includes the (confounding) immunsuppressive effects of glucocorticoids. For these reasons, *systemic* administration of CRH or urocortin would not reflect their true *local* functions. Most studies point to direct proinflammatory effects of local CRH/urocortin. In support of this concept, Karalis *et al.* demonstrated that the inflammatory response in the rat carageenin model could be markedly inhibited by administration of anti-CRH antibodies.[39] Similar results were obtained with the CRH-R1 antagonist antialarmin.[61] Furthermore, urocortin has been shown to be one of the most potent mast cell degranulators.[62]

REFERENCES

1. VALE, W.W., J. SPIESS, C. RIVIER & J. RIVIER. 1981. Characterization of a 41 residue ovine hypothalamic peptide that stimulates the secretion of corticotropin and β-endorphin. Science 213: 1394–1397.
2. RIVIER, J., J. SPIESS & W.W. VALE. 1983. Chemical and biological characterization of rat hypothalamic corticotropin-releasing factor. Proc. Natl. Acad. Sci. USA 80: 4851–4855.
3. SHIBAHARA, S., Y. MORIMOTO, Y. FURUTANI *et al.* 1983. Isolation and sequence analysis of the human corticotropin-releasing factor precursor gene. EMBO J. 5: 775–779.
4. SCHULTE, H.M., G.P. CHROUSOS, P.W. GOLD *et al.* 1985. Continuous administration of synthetic ovine corticotropin-releasing factor in man: physiological and pathophysiological implications. J. Clin. Invest. 75: 1781–1785.
5. CHROUSOS, G.P. 1995. The hypothalamic-pituitary-adrenal axis and immune-mediated inflammation. N. Engl. J. Med. 332: 1351–1362.
6. MADDEN, K.S., V.M. SANDERS & D.L. FELTEN. 1995. Catecholamine influences and sympathetic neural modulation of immune responsiveness. Ann. Rev. Pharmacol. Toxicol. 35: 417–448.
7. ZHAO, X.J., G. HOHEISEL, J. SCHAUER & S.R. BORNSTEIN. 1997. Corticotropin-releasing hormone-binding protein and its possible role in neuroendocrinological research. Horm. Metab. Res. 29: 373–378.
8. CHEN, R., K.A. LEWIS, M.H. PERRIN & W.W. VALE. 1993. Expression and cloning of a human corticotropin-releasing factor receptor. Proc. Natl. Acad. Sci. USA 90: 8967–8971.
9. KOSTICH, W.A., A. CHEN, K. SPERLE & B.L. LARGENT. 1998. Molecular identification and analysis of a novel human corticotropin-releasing factor (CRF) receptor: the CRF2gamma receptor. Mol. Endocrinol. 12: 1077–1085.
10. VALDENAIRE, O., T. GILLER, V. BREU, J. GOTTOWIK & G. KILPATRICK. 1997. A new functional isoform of the human CRF2 receptor for corticotropin-releasing factor. Biochim. Biophys. Acta 1352: 129–132.
11. CHANG, C.P., R.V. PEARCE, S. O'CONNELL & M.G. ROSENFELD. 1993. Identification of a seven transmembrane helix receptor for corticotropin-releasing factor and sauvagine in mammalian brain. Neuron 11: 1187–1195.
12. LIAW, C.W., T.W. LOVENBERG, G. BARRY, T. OLTERDORF, D.E. GRIGORIADIS & E.B. DE SOUZA. 1996. Cloning and characterization of the human corticotropin-releasing factor-2 receptor complementary desoxyribonucleic acid. Endocrinology 137: 72–77.
13. LOVENBERG, T.W., C.W. LIAW, D.E. GRIGORIADIS, C. CLEVENGER, D.T. CHALMERS & E.B. DE SOUZA. 1995. Cloning and characterization of a functionally distinct corticotropin-releasing factor receptor subtype from rat brain. Proc. Natl. Acad. Sci. USA 92: 836–840.

14. BARSYTE, D., D.R. TIPPING, D. SMART, J.M. CONLON, B.I. BAKER, D.A. LOVEJOY. 1999. Rainbow trout (*Oncorhynchus mykiss*) urotensin-I: structural differences between urotensins-I and urocortins [In Process Citation]. Gen. Comp. Endocrinol. **115:** 169–177.
15. VAUGHAN, J., C. DONALDSON, J. BITTENCOURT et al. 1995. Urocortin, a mammalian neuropeptide related to fish urotensin I and to corticotropin-releasing factor [see comments]. Nature **378:** 287–292.
16. DANALDSON, C.J., S.W. SUTTON, M.H. PERRIN et al. 1996. Cloning and characterization of human urocortin. Endocrinology **137:** 3896.
17. IINO, K., H. SASANO, Y. OKI et al. 1999. Urocortin expression in the human central nervous system. Clin. Endocrinol. (Oxf) **50:** 107–114.
18. ASAKAWA, A., A. INUI, N. UENO, S. MAKINO, M.A. FUJINO & M. KASUGA. 1999. Urocortin reduces food intake and gastric emptying in lean and ob/ob obese mice [see comments]. Gastroenterology **116:** 1287–1292.
19. ASABA, K., S. MAKINO & K. HASHIMOTO. 1998. Effect of urocortin on ACTH secretion from rat anterior pituitary in vitro and in vivo: comparison with corticotropin-releasing hormone. Brain Res. **806:** 95–103.
20. SAJDYK, T.J., D.A. SCHOBER, D.R. GEHLERT & A. SHEKHAR. 1999. Role of corticotropin-releasing factor and urocortin within the basolateral amygdala of rats in anxiety and panic responses. Behav. Brain Res. **100:** 207–215.
21. JONES, D.N., R. KORTEKAAS, P.D. SLADE, D.N. MIDDLEMISS & J.J. HAGAN. 1998. The behavioural effects of corticotropin-releasing factor-related peptides in rats. Psychopharmacology (Berl) **138:** 124–132.
22. OZAWA, M., Y. OKI, F. WATANABE et al. 1998. Effect of urocortin and its interaction with adrenocorticotropin (ACTH) secretagogues on ACTH release.Peptides **19:** 513–518.
23. SPINA, M., E. MERLO-PICH, R.K. CHAN et al. 1996. Appetite-suppressing effects of urocortin, a CRF-related neuropeptide. Science **273:** 1561–1564.
24. MOREAU, J.L., G. KILPATRICK & F. JENCK. 1997. Urocortin, a novel neuropeptide with anxiogenic-like properties. NeuroReport **8:** 1697–1701.
25. WENINGER, S.C., A.J. DUNN, L.J. MUGLIA et al. 1999. Stress-induced behaviors require the corticotropin-releasing hormone (CRH) receptor, but not CRH [In Process Citation]. Proc. Natl. Acad. Sci. USA **96:** 8283–8288.
26. TURNBULL, A.V., J. VAUGHAN, J.E. RIVIER, W.W. VALE & C. RIVIER. 1999. Urocortin is not a significant regulator of intermittent electrofootshock-induced adrenocorticotropin secretion in the intact male rat. Endocrinology **140:** 71–78.
27. CHROUSOS, G.P. & P.W. GOLD. 1992. The concepts of stress and stress system disorders. Overview of physical and behavioral homeostasis [published erratum appears in JAMA 1992 Jul 8; **268**(2): 200]. JAMA **267:** 1244–1252.
28. ELENKOV, I.J., E.L. WEBSTER, D.J. TORPY & G.P. CHROUSOS. 1999. Stress, corticotropin-releasing hormone, glucocorticoids, and the immune/inflammatory response: acute and chronic effects. Ann. N.Y. Acad. Sci. **876:** 1–11; discussion 11–13.
29. BAMBERGER, C.M., H.M. SCHULTE & G.P. CHROUSOS. 1996. Molecular determinants of glucocorticoid receptor function and tissue sensitivity to glucocorticoids. Endocr. Rev. **17:** 245–261.
30. BAMBERGER, C.M., T. ELSE, A.M. BAMBERGER, F.U. BEIL & H.M. SCHULTE. 1997. Regulation of the human interleukin-2 gene by the alpha and beta isoforms of the glucocorticoid receptor. Mol. Cell. Endocrinol. **136:** 23–28.
31. BAMBERGER, A.M., I. ERDMANN, C.M. BAMBERGER, S.S. JENATSCHKE & H.M. SCHULTE. 1997. Transcriptional regulation of the human 'leukemia inhibitory factor' gene: modulation by glucocorticoids and estradiol. Mol. Cell. Endocrinol. **127:** 71–79.
32. BERNARDINI, R., T.C. KAMILARIS, A.E. CALOGERO et al. 1990. Interactions between tumor necrosis factor-alpha, hypothalamic corticotropin-releasing hormone, and adrenocorticotropin secretion in the rat. Endocrinology **126:** 2876–2881.
33. MASTORAKOS, G., G.P. CHROUSOS & J.S. WEBER. 1993. Recombinant interleukin-6 activates the hypothalamic-pituitary-adrenal axis in humans. J. Clin. Endocrinol. Metab. **77:** 1690–1694.

34. AKITA, S., J. MALKIN & S. MELMED. 1996. Disrupted murine leukemia inhibitory factor (LIF) gene attenuates adrenocorticotropic hormone (ACTH) secretion. Endocrinology **137:** 3140–3143.

35. AKITA, S., J. WEBSTER, S.G. REN, H. TAKINO, J. SAID & S. MELMED. 1995. Human and murine pituitary expression of leukemia inhibitory factor. Novel intrapituitary regulation of adrenocorticotropin hormone synthesis and secretion. J. Clin. Invest. **95:** 1288–1298.

36. WANG, Z., S.-G. REN & S. MELMED. 1996. Hypothalamic and pituitary leukemia inhibitory factor gene expression in vivo: a novel endotoxin-inducible neuro-endocrine interface. Endocrinology **137:** 2947–2953.

37. EHRHART-BORNSTEIN, M., J.P. HINSON, S.R. BORNSTEIN, W.A. SCHERBAUM & G.P. VINSON. 1998. Intraadrenal interactions in the regulation of adrenocortical steroidogenesis. Endocr. Rev. **19:** 101–143.

38. HARGREAVES, K.M., A.H. COSTELLO & J.L. JORIS. 1989. Release from inflamed tissue of a substance with properties similar to corticotropin-releasing factor. Neuroendocrinology **49:** 476–482.

39. KARALIS, K., H. SANO, J. REDWINE, S. LISTWAK, R.L. WILDER & G.P. CHROUSOS. 1991. Autocrine or paracrine inflammatory actions of corticotropin-releasing hormone in vivo. Science **254:** 421–423.

40. MASTORAKOS, G., E.A. BOUZAS, P.B. SILVER *et al.* 1995. Immune corticotropin-releasing hormone is present in the eyes of and promotes experimental autoimmune uveoretinitis in rodents. Endocrinology **136:** 4650–4658.

41. CROFFORD, L.J., H. SANO, K. KARALIS *et al.* 1993. Corticotropin-releasing hormone in synovial fluids and tissues of patients with rheumatoid arthritis and osteoarthritis. J. Immunol. **151:** 1587–1596.

42. SCOPA, C.D., G. MASTORAKOS, T.C. FRIEDMAN, M. MELACHRINOU, M.J. MERINO & G.P. CHROUSOS. 1994. Presence of immunoreactive corticotropin releasing hormone in thyroid lesions. Am. J. Pathol. **145:** 1159–1167.

43. KAWAHITO, Y., H. SANO, S. MUKAI *et al.* 1995. Corticotropin releasing hormone in colonic mucosa in patients with ulcerative colitis. Gut **37:** 544–551.

44. CHALLIS, J.R.G., S.G. MATTHEWS, C. VAN MEIER & M.M. RAMIREZ. 1995. The placental corticotrophin-releasing hormone-adrenocorticotrophin axis. Placenta **16:** 481–502.

45. GRINO, M., G.P. CHROUSOS & A.N. MARGIORIS. 1987. The corticotropin-releasing hormone gene is expressed in human placenta. Biochem. Biophys. Res. Commun. **148:** 1208–1214.

46. MASTORAKOS, G., E.L. WEBSTER, T.C. FRIEDMAN & G.P. CHROUSOS. 1993. Immunoreactive corticotropin-releasing hormone and its binding sites in the rat ovary. J. Clin. Invest. **92:** 961–968.

47. MASTORAKOS, G., C.D. SCOPA, L.C. KAO *et al.* 1996. Presence of immunoreactive corticotropin-releasing hormone in human endometrium. J. Clin. Endocrinol. Metab. **81:** 1046–1050.

48. BILEVICIUTE, I., M. AHMED, J. BERGSTROM, A. ERICSSON-DAHLSTRAND, A. KREICBERGS & T. LUNDEBERG. 1997. Expression of corticotropin-releasing factor in the peripheral nervous system of the rat. NeuroReport **8:** 3127–3130.

49. PETRAGLIA, F., P. FLORIO, R. GALLO *et al.* 1996. Human placenta and fetal membranes express human urocortin mRNA and peptide. J. Clin. Endocrinol. Metab. **81:** 3807–3810.

50. WATANABE, F., Y. OKI, M. OZAWA *et al.* 1999. Urocortin in human placenta and maternal plasma [In Process Citation]. Peptides **20:** 205–209.

51. OKOSI, A., B.K. BRAR, M. CHAN *et al.* 1998. Expression and protective effects of urocortin in cardiac myocytes. Neuropeptides **32:** 167–171.

52. HARADA, S., T. IMAKI, M. NARUSE, N. CHIKADA, K. NAKAJIMA & H. DEMURA. 1999. Urocortin mRNA is expressed in the enteric nervous system of the rat [In Process Citation]. Neurosci. Lett. **267:** 125–128.

53. EKMAN, R., B. SERVENIUS, M.G. CASTRO *et al.* 1993. Biosynthesis of corticotropin-releasing hormone in human T-lymphocytes. J. Neuroimmunol. **44:** 7–13.

54. KRAVCHENCO, I.V. & V.A. FURALEV. 1994. Secretion of immunoreactive corticotropin releasing factor and adrenocorticotropic hormone by T- and B-lymphocytes in response to cellular stress factors. Biochem. Biophys. Res. Commun. **204:** 828–834.

55. MUGLIA, L.J., N.A. JENKINS, D.J. GILBERT, N.G. COPELAND & J.A. MAJZOUB. 1994. Expression of the mouse corticotropin-releasing hormone gene in vivo and targeted inactivation in embryonic stem cells. J. Clin. Invest. **93:** 2066–2072.

56. BAMBERGER, C.M., M. WALD, A.M. BAMBERGER, S. ERGUN, F.U. BEIL & H.M. SCHULTE. 1998. Human lymphocytes produce urocortin, but not corticotropin-releasing hormone. J. Clin. Endocrinol. Metab. **83:** 708–711.

57. KIANG, J.G. & E.T. WEI. 1987. Corticotropin-releasing factor inhibits thermal injury. J. Pharmacol. Exp. Ther. **243:** 517–520.

58. SERDA, S.M. & E.T. WEI. 1991. Corticotropin-releasing factor inhibits the acute inflammatory response of rat pawskin to cold injury. Cryobiology **28:** 185–190.

59. TIAN, J.Q. & E.T. WEI. 1989. Acute inflammatory response of rat pawskin to acid injury is attenuated by corticotropin-releasing factor. Drug Chem. Toxicol. **12:** 61–66.

60. TORPY, D.J., E.L. WEBSTER, E.K. ZACHMAN, G. AGUILERA & G.P. CHROUSOS. 1999. Urocortin and inflammation: confounding effects of hypotension on measures of inflammation. Neuroimmunomodulation **6:** 182–186.

61. WEBSTER, E.L., D.B. LEWIS, D.J. TORPY, E.K. ZACHMAN, K.C. RICE & G.P. CHROUSOS. 1996. In vivo and in vitro characterization of antalarmin, a nonpeptide corticotropin-releasing hormone (CRH) receptor antagonist: suppression of pituitary ACTH release and peripheral inflammation. Endocrinology **137:** 5747–5750.

62. SINGH, L.K., W. BOUCHER, X. PANG *et al.* 1999. Potent mast cell degranulation and vascular permeability triggered by urocortin through activation of corticotropin-releasing hormone receptors. J. Pharmacol. Exp. Ther. **288:** 1349–1356.

Neural Control of Ocular Immune Privilege

J. WAYNE STREILEIN,[a] SHIGEKI OKAMOTO, YOICHIRO SANO,
AND ANDREW W. TAYLOR

*Schepens Eye Research Institute, Department of Ophthalmology,
Harvard Medical School, Boston, Massachusetts 02114, USA*

ABSTRACT: Ocular immune privilege arises from interactions between the
immune apparatus and the eye itself, thereby providing immune protection for
the eye that is devoid of sight-threatening inflammation. On the one hand, antigens injected intraocularly elicit deviant systemic immune responses that are
devoid of immunogenic inflammation (Anterior Chamber–Associated Immune
Deviation, ACAID). On the other hand, the ocular microenvironment (aqueous
humor, secreted by cells that surround this chamber) suppresses intraocular
expression of immunogenic inflammation. Several lines of evidence indicate
that ocular immune privilege is under neural control. First, aqueous humor
contains neuropeptides (α-MSH, VIP, CGRP) that inhibit and alter the functional properties of T lymphocytes and macrophages. Second, when corneal
nerves are severed, the tissues surrounding the anterior chamber cease secreting immunosuppressive factors and ACAID fails—until the nerves regrow.
Third, light deprivation abolishes the capacity of the anterior chamber to support ACAID induction, a process that is sensitive to neuropeptides and melatonin. The photoreceptor(s) responsible for ACAID are connected to the nervous
system and may reside in the anterior segment and/or the retina. Thus, neural
elements from the central nervous system and within the eye help to shape both
the induction and the expression of ocular immunity, thereby promoting
immune privilege.

INTRODUCTION

Immune privilege, a distinctive, physiologic feature of several organs and sites,[1]
was described more than 100 years ago by van Dooremal,[2] who observed that human
tumor cells grew when implanted into the anterior chamber, but not when placed
elsewhere, in adult rabbits. In the 1940s and '50s Sir Peter Medawar discovered the
immunologic basis of organ transplant rejection,[3] and shortly thereafter determined
that the unexpected growth of foreign tumors in the eye had an immunologic explanation.[4] Medawar appreciated that immune privilege can be a property of a particular
tissue (such as the cornea) or a particular site (anterior chamber of the eye, brain).
Immune-privileged tissues, defined experimentally, experience extended survival as
foreign grafts placed at conventional body sites. Immune privileged sites exist where
foreign grafts of conventional tissues experience extended survival.

[a]Address for correspondence and reprint requests: J. Wayne Streilein, M.D. Schepens Eye
Research Institute, 20 Staniford St., Boston, MA 02114. Voice: 617-912-9422; fax: 617-912-0115
waynes@vision.eri.harvard.edu

HOW IMMUNE PRIVILEGE WORKS

When Medawar determined that privilege was "immune," he was aware that the eye and the brain reside behind blood:tissue barriers, and it was thought that both organs lacked lymphatic drainage pathways. He postulated that immune privilege was caused by immunologic ignorance, because the blood:ocular and blood:brain barriers served to isolate these organs from circulating immune cells and molecules. This passive view of immune privilege has largely been supplanted over the past 30 years by experimental evidence that active, regulatory mechanisms contribute to immune privilege.[6,7]

Immune privilege arises from site-specific regulation of induction and expression of systemic immunity to tissue-restricted/derived antigens. On the one hand, injection of antigenic material into privileged sites evokes systemic immune responses that are deviant, i.e., the spectrum of immune effector cells and molecules is different from that evoked by immunization with antigen via non-privileged sites.[8] On the other hand, immune effectors that penetrate beyond blood:tissue barriers at immune-privileged sites or tissues are inhibited locally from carrying out certain effector functions.[9]

THE EYE AS A MODEL IMMUNE-PRIVILEGED SITE

Kaplan and Streilein[10,11] in the 1970s, then Niederkorn, Shadduck and Streilein[12] in the 1980s performed classical experiments that launched modern research on ocular immune privilege. Kaplan and Streilein discovered that injection of allogeneic lymphoid cells into the anterior chamber (AC) of rat eyes produced a deviant systemic response in which high levels of serum alloantibodies co-existed with a blunted capacity to reject orthotopic skin grafts bearing the same alloantigens. Niederkorn and his colleagues injected allogeneic tumor cells into the AC of mouse eyes and generated progressively growing tumors—confirming the existence of immune privilege. More important, mice bearing these intraocular tumors were unable to reject orthotopic donor-specific skin grafts, in part because they failed to develop donor-specific delayed hypersensitivity. More important, sera of tumor-bearing mice contained high titers of donor-specific antibodies. The term Anterior Chamber–Associated Immune Deviation (ACAID) designates this distinctive response to eye-derived antigens.[8,13,14]

ACAID can be induced by a wide variety of antigens placed in the eye—whether AC, vitreous cavity, or subretinal space. Once induced, ACAID is long-lasting, and can be imposed on pre-sensitized individuals. ACAID has been induced in a wide variety of mammals, including cynomolgous monkeys.[15] The essential elements of ACAID are

(a) that antigen be injected into a distinct ocular compartment,
(b) that the eye remain anatomically intact for 3–4 days,
(c) that an antigen-specific signal can be identified in the blood within 24–48 hours,
(d) that an intact spleen is essential (at least for the first 7 days), and
(e) that the spleen acquires antigen-specific T cells that suppress both the induction and the expression of delayed hypersensitivity to the eliciting antigen.

In ACAID the eye provides indigenous antigen-presenting cells (APC) that capture injected antigen, carry it across the trabecular meshwork into the venous drainage of the eye,[16–18] and migrate via the blood to the spleen. This so-called ACAID-induction can be generated *in vitro* by exposing conventional antigen-presenting cells to aqueous humor (AqH).[19] When APCs exposed to AqH are pulsed with antigen and then injected i.v. into naive mice, the recipients acquire ACAID. A similar situation applies to the brain and the fetoplacental unit since conventional APCs first exposed to amniotic fluid or cerebrospinal fluid and then pulsed with antigen also induce ACAID when injected into recipient mice.[20]

LOCAL FACTORS THAT CONTRIBUTE TO ADAPTIVE OCULAR IMMUNE PRIVILEGE

During the past 30 years, the local factors that confer immune privilege on the eye are coming into focus. Three categories exist: structural features of the eye, soluble immunosuppressive factors, and cell surface modifiers of immune effectors. Structural features include

1. strict blood:ocular barriers (blood vessels of the iris and the retina; tight junctions among pigment epithelial cells of ciliary body and retina);
2. absence of lymph vessels; and
3. drainage of aqueous humor directly into the circumferential veins around the limbus.

Absence of lymphatics combined with the direct drainage of AqH into the venous system dictates that antigens escaping the eye must follow the intravenous route—a route long known for promoting tolerance (unresponsiveness) rather than immunity.

The AC is filled with AqH, a clear fluid that contains an amazing array of immunosuppressive and modulatory factors (see TABLE 1). AqH suppresses activation of primed T cells and their differentiation down the pathway toward the immunodestructive Th1 phenotype.[21] More important, AqH converts T cells into regulators that

TABLE 1. Local soluble factors that contribute to ocular immune privilege

Factor	Effects
Transforming growth factor-β_2	Inhibits T cell activation, proliferation and effector function
	Alters APC function $\rightarrow$ immune deviation
	Inhibits NK-cell mediated lysis (18 h *in vitro*)
α-Melanocyte-stimulating hormone	Inhibits IFN-γ production by activated T cells
	Converts effector into regulatory T cells
Vasoactive intestinal peptide	Inhibits T cell activation (proliferation)
Calcitonin gene-related peptide	Inhibits effector functions of activated macrophages (NO)
Migration inhibitory factor	Inhibits NK cell-mediated lysis (4 h *in vitro*)

suppress the activation of bystander T cells with the potential to trigger immunogenic inflammation.[22] AqH also suppresses macrophage and neutrophil effector functions, thereby limiting these potential sources of destructive inflammation.[22,23]

The cells that line the AC (pigment epithelium of iris and ciliary body, corneal endothelium) and the subretinal space (retinal pigment epithelium, RPE) display surface molecules that alter T cells. Ocular parenchymal cells express CD95 ligand (CD95L),[24] a molecule whose receptor (CD95) triggers programmed cell death among cells that express it. CD95L expression by ocular cells promotes apoptosis among CD95$^+$ effector T cells, and activates CD95$^+$ neutrophils.[23] Interestingly, AqH inhibits both of these effects. RPE cells inhibit T cell activation and promote T cell apoptosis through CD95 triggering,[25] although RPE cells secrete a soluble molecule that causes T cells to undergo programmed cell death.[26] Pigment epithelial cells of iris and ciliary body inhibit T cell activation by two pathways: via secretion of soluble factors, one of which is TGF-β_2,[27] and via direct cell-to-cell contact mechanism.[28] T cells whose surfaces directly encounter pigment epithelial cells of iris and ciliary body failed to proliferate in response to a mitogenic signal and converted into regulatory cells, similar to those exposed to AqH.

WHY OCULAR IMMUNE PRIVILEGE EXISTS

The strategies which the eye has devised to shape immune responses to eye-derived antigens are elaborate, effective, and make immune privilege possible. However, why is immune privilege necessary? Investigators in this field believe that immune privilege is an experimentally derived expression of an important physiologic mechanism. Immune privilege represents the consequence of interactions between the immune system and specialized tissues in which local protection is provided by immune effectors that do not disrupt differentiated tissue function. In the case of the eye, where a precise microanatomy must be maintained in order for vision to be preserved, immune privilege allows for immune protection that is devoid of immunogenic inflammation. Inflammation can be tolerated in most tissues, and is typically needed for elimination of pathogens and wound repair. In the eye, inflammation is simply unacceptable to the visual axis. Trace amounts deviate the visual image away from the retina, and blindness results. In nature, blindness (unless prepared for by evolutionary adaptation) is a death sentence!

INFLUENCE OF NEUROPEPTIDES ON OCULAR IMMUNE PRIVILEGE

The list of ocular factors that contribute to immune privilege (TABLE 1) contains a hint that neural influences are likely to be involved: α-MSH, VIP and CGRP in AqH are neuropeptides that are typically released from nerve termini. In addition to their role as neurotransmitters, these peptides are immunomodulatory. Normal AqH prevents T cells stimulated *in vitro* with antigen or mitogens from becoming activated and proliferating. Although TGF-β_2 is present at high levels in normal AqH,[29] the vast majority is latent, and can not be responsible for AqH's endogenous immunosuppression. Taylor and his collaborators[22] demonstrated that α-MSH and VIP enable AqH to suppress T cell activation. Whereas α-MSH does not prevent T cell proliferation, it does inhibit activated T cells from producing IFN-γ. This is relevant to ocular immune privilege since intracameral IFN-γ rapidly degrades the local immunosuppressive microenvironment and abolishes immune privilege. In addition, T cells exposed to α-MSH acquire the capacity to regulate the activation of bystander T cells, in part through the production of TGF-β.[28] VIP is a potent inhibitor of T cell proliferation, and it modifies T cell migration—although this effect on immune privilege is yet obscure. CGRP in AqH acts on macrophages, preventing cells activated by endotoxin and IFN-γ from secreting large amounts of nitric oxide (NO). Treatment of activated macrophages with CGRP abruptly terminates NO production, and neutralization of CGRP removes the inhibitory activity from AqH. The presence of these neuropeptides (and probably others as well) in AqH raises questions as to their origin. The cornea is abundantly supplied with afferent sensory nerves whose termini contain a variety of neuropeptides. However, the cornea is isolated from the rest of the eye (no lymph or blood vessels), and therefore the contents of nerve termini in the cornea probably do not contribute to AqH. Iris and ciliary body are directly immersed in AqH, with the secretory epithelium of the ciliary body being the primary source of this fluid. Both iris and ciliary body are supplied by efferent sympathetic nerves (from the superior cervical ganglion), parasympathetic nerves (from the ciliary ganglion), and autonomic afferents.

INFLUENCE OF NEURAL PATHWAYS ON OCULAR IMMUNE PRIVILEGE

While studying orthotopic corneal allografts in mice, Streilein and his collaborators stumbled on a previously unsuspected neural influence on ocular immune privilege.[30] As an expression of ocular immune privilege, upwards of 50% of orthotopic allogeneic corneal grafts are accepted indefinitely by mice.[31] Many of these grafts look perfectly healthy at four weeks after grafting and remain so indefinitely. Impressed with graft vitality, as well as the quiet clinical appearance of the grafted eye, Streilein *et al.* injected antigen into the AC of graft-bearing eyes at four weeks in an effort to induce ACAID.[30] To their surprise, no ACAID was observed. Even when tested at eight weeks after grafting, ACAID was not observed. Moreover, iris and ciliary body tissues removed from these grafted eyes failed to suppress T cell activation *in vitro*—a property usually displayed by iris and ciliary body tissues removed from normal eyes.[27] Only at 12 weeks after grafting, did injection of antigen into the anterior chamber of grafted eyes induce ACAID.

In clinical ophthalmology, denervation of grafted corneas is well recognized, and clinicans know that it takes many weeks for sensation to be restored in healthy grafts. To test the possibility that denervation of the cornea might be responsible for the loss of ACAID in eyes bearing cornea allografts, the cornea of one eye of BALB/c mice was wounded in one of two ways: (a) a circumferential partial-thickness incision of the cornea very near the limbus; or (b) six radial incisions reaching from the center of the cornea to the limbus. When wounded corneas were removed and examined immunohistochemically for evidence of nerve re-growth, no nerves were observed beyond the circumferential wounds during the first eight weeks. Between 8 and 12 weeks nerve fibers were observed to sprout into the central corneal epithelium. By contrast, nerve fibers were readily detected at all time points after radial incisions of the corneal surface. When tested for ACAID, mice with radial corneal wounds displayed ACAID at all time points examined, whereas mice with circumferential corneal wounds displayed ACAID only when tested at 12 weeks after wounding.

The capacity of the normal eye to support ACAID induction is dependent upon integrity of afferent nerves from the cornea, as is the ability of iris and ciliary body to secrete an immunosuppressive ocular microenvironment. We suspect that tonic signals arise from the corneal surface. These signals are propagated through the trigeminal ganglion to the central nervous system, where they promote, via connections to the nervous supply of the iris and ciliary body, the intraocular secretion of immunomodulatory neuropeptides. These neuropeptides play a central role in ocular immune privilege, in part by rendering the eye capable of supporting ACAID induction, and in part by suppressing immunogenic inflammation locally.

EFFECTS OF LIGHT IN THE VISUAL SPECTRUM ON ACAID

More than a decade ago, Ferguson, Hiyashi, and Kaplan made the extraordinary observation that ambient light is an important factor in ACAID induction.[32] They showed that injection of antigen into the AC of eyes of mice raised from birth in complete darkness failed to induce ACAID. If mice raised in this manner were exposed to ambient light for 48 hours or more, the capacity of their eyes to support ACAID was restored. Moreover, if mice raised in the light were subjected to absolute darkness for 48 hours or more, their eyes lost the capacity to support ACAID induction. Ferguson et al. found that green light (500–510 nm) within the visual spectrum was the relevant photic energy.[33] Although these investigators anticipated that light falling on the retina would be the ACAID-permitting signal, to their surprise they found that severance of the optic nerve had no effect on ACAID induction. Circumstantial evidence pointed to the existence of the relevant photoreceptor in the anterior segment of the eye. In subsequent experiments, Ferguson and his colleagues[34] reported that nerve termini in the iris and ciliary body contain VIP when harvested from eyes in the light, whereas nerve termini of iris and ciliary body contain substance P when harvested from eyes in the dark. Since VIP is immunosuppressive, whereas substance P is immune enhancing, they hypothesized that exposure of the dark-adapted eye to light triggers (perhaps through pupil constriction) the release of substance P, and that this neuropeptide inhibits ACAID.

There is another pathway by which light in the visual spectrum could promote ACAID. Melatonin is a neurohormone that is produced by the pineal gland (systemically) and by the retina and ciliary body (intraocularly).[35] Melatonin is normally produced in the light-deprived retina and light exposure abruptly terminates melatonin secretion. Melatonin has been found to be a potent immunoenhancing agent, acting as an adjuvant when antigens are administered systemically.[36] Okamoto and Streilein have explored the influence of melatonin on ACAID induction in mice (unpublished observations). As mentioned above, antigen presenting cells exposed *in vitro* to AqH or TGF-β2 acquire ACAID-inducing properties. Okamoto and

Streilein treated APCs *in vitro* with TGF-β2 and melatonin under three different conditions. APCs were treated:

   (a) simultaneously with TGF-β_2 and melatonin;
   (b) with TGF-β_2, then exposed 6 h later to melatonin; and
   (c) with melatonin, then exposed 6 h later to TGF-β_2.

Following treatment the cells were washed, pulsed with bovine serum albumin (a heterologous protein antigen) and injected into naive mice that were subsequently immunized with BSA plus adjuvant. When delayed hypersensitivity was assessed thereafter (see TABLE 2), recipients of BSA-pulsed APC treated with TGF-β_2 alone displayed ACAID. Recipients of BSA-pulsed APC treated simultaneously with melatonin and TGF-β_2 failed to acquire ACAID. Similarly, recipients of BSA-pulsed APC treated with melatonin prior to exposure to TGF-β_2 failed to acquire ACAID. However, mice that received BSA-pulsed APC treated first with TGF-β_2 and then melatonin still displayed ACAID. These results indicate that melatonin can prevent APC from acquiring ACAID-inducing properties unless the APCs first encounter TGF-β_2. On the basis of these findings we propose that light deprivation abolishes ACAID as follows: In the normal eye, there is a constant turnover of APCs, and light suppresses retinal melatonin production. The constitutive presence of TGF-β_2 confers ACAID-inducing properties on indigenous APCs. As darkness descends on the diurnal cycle, the retina begins to produce melatonin, but since the effect of TGF-β_2 on APCs is long-lasting and dominant over melatonin, APCs retain their ACAID-promoting qualities. However, in prolonged darkness (beyond 48 h), ocular APCs constitutively turn over, newly immigrant cells encounter progressively higher levels of melatonin, and the eye becomes repopulated with melatonin-influenced, rather than TGF-β_2, APC. Unless melatonin production is terminated by light, injection of antigen at this point no longer induces ACAID.

TABLE 2. **Influence of melatonin on ACAID induction**

APC incubation		Immunization	Ear swelling response
0 h	6 h	BSA + Adjuvant	mm^{-3}
—	—	—	35 (negative control)
PBS	PBS	+	97[*] (positive control)
TGF-β_2	PBS	+	15
TGF-β_2	Melatonin	+	16
Melatonin	TGF-β_2	+	100[*]
TGF-β_2 + Melatonin	—	+	70[*]

NOTE: Peritoneal exudate cells (APCs) were harvested from BALB/c mice. Adherent cells were plated in culture dishes in serum free medium (1×10^5/well), then incubated with melatonin (5 ng/ml) at the same time, before or after incubation with TGF-β_2 (5 ng/ml), washed, then pulsed with bovine serum albumin (100 µg/ml), washed and injected intravenously (2×10^3) into naive BALB/c mice. The recipients were immunized with BSA (200 µg) plus adjuvant 7 days later, and one week later their ear pinnae were challenged with 200 µg/10µl BSA. Ear swelling was measured with an engineer's micrometer 24 h later. Mean ear swelling responses were calculated for groups of 5 animals. [*] indicates values significantly higher than negative control.

SUMMARY AND CONCLUSIONS

Immune privilege in the eye is dependent upon interactions between the immune system and the eye, with the eye providing local factors that profoundly influence both the induction and the expression of immunity to eye-derived antigens. Included among the ocular factors that influence immunity are neural elements. The ocular microenvironment constitutively expresses neuropeptides, presumably derived from nerve termini in the iris and ciliary body. These neuropeptides suppress activation and differentiation of T cells and they inhibit effector functions of activated macrophages. In this manner, immunogenic inflammation within ocular compartments (anterior chamber, vitreous cavity, subretinal space) is avoided, and the integrity of the visual axis is preserved. Sensory input from the ocular surface (corneal afferents) and from the iris and ciliary body (photoreceptors) provides tonic stimulation that empowers the iris and ciliary body to maintain an immunosuppressive local microenvironment. Interruption of this tonic influence (by severing corneal nerves, or by dark-adapting the eyes) leads to collapse of immune privilege and the abolition of ACAID. Thus, the nervous system makes a critical contribution to ocular immune privilege.

REFERENCES

1. BARKER, C.F. & R.E BILLINGHAM. 1977. Immunologically privileged sites. Adv. Immunol. **25:** 1–54.
2. VAN DOORMAL, J.C. 1873. Die Entwicklung der in fremden Grund versetzten lebenden Gewebe. Albrecht Van Graefes Arch. Ophthalmol. **18:** 358–373.
3. MEDAWAR, P.B. 1945. A second study of the behavior and fate of skin homografts in rabbits. J. Anat. (Lond.) **79:** 157–176.
4. MEDAWAR, P.B. 1948. Immunity to homologous grafted skin. III. The fate of skin homografts transplanted to the brain, to subcutaneous tissue, and to the anterior chamber of the eye. Br. J. Exp. Pathol. **29:** 58–74.
5. STREILEIN, J.W. 1995. Unraveling immune privilege. Science **270:** 1158–1159.
6. STREILEIN, J.W. 1993. Immune privilege as the result of local tissue barriers and immunosuppressive microenvironments. Curr. Opinion Immunol. **5:** 428–432.
7. NIEDERKORN, J.Y. 1990. Immune privilege and immune regulation in the eye. Adv. Immunol. **48:** 199–208.
8. STREILEIN, J.W. 1987. Immune regulation and the eye: a dangerous compromise. FASEB J. **1:** 199–208.
9. STREILEIN, J.W., G.A. WILBANKS & S.W. COUSINS. 1992. Immunoregulatory mechanisms of the eye. J. Neuroimmunol. **39:** 185–200.
10. KAPLAN, H.J. & J.W. STREILEIN. 1977. Immune response to immunization via the anterior chamber of the eye. I. F1 lymphocyte-induced immune deviation. J. Immunol. **118:** 809–814.
11. KAPLAN, H.J. & J.W. STREILEIN. 1978. Immune response to immunization via the anterior chamber of the eye. II. An analysis of F1 lymphocyte-induced immune deviation. J. Immunol. **120:** 689–693.
12. NIEDERKORN, J., J.W. STREILEIN & J.A. SHADDUCK. 1980. Deviant immune responses to allogeneic tumors injected intracamerally and subcutaneously in mice. Invest. Ophthalmol. Vis. Sci. **20:** 355–363.
13. STREILEIN, J.W., J.Y. NIEDERKORN & J.A. SHADDUCK. 1980. Systemic immune unresponsiveness induced in adult mice by anterior chamber presentation of minor histocompatibility antigens. J. Exp. Med. **152:** 1121–1125.
14. STREILEIN, J.W., B.R. KSANDER & A.W. TAYLOR. 1997. Immune deviation in relation to ocular immune privilege. J. Immunol. **158:** 3557–3560.

15. EICHORN, M., M. NOREBER, J.W. STREILEIN & E. LUTJEN-DRECOLL. 1993. Anterior chamber associated immune deviation elicited via primate eyes. Invest. Ophthal. Vis. Sci. **34:** 2926–2930.

16. WILLIAMSON, J.S.P., D. BRADLEY & J.W. STREILEIN. 1989. Immunoregulatory properties of bone marrow derived cells in the iris and ciliary body. Immunology **67:** 96–102.

17. WILBANKS, G.A. & J.W. STREILEIN. 1991. Studies on the induction of anterior chamber associated immune deviation (ACAID). I. Evidence that an antigen-specific ACAID-inducing, cell-associated signal exists in the peripheral blood. J. Immunol. **146:** 2610–2617.

18. WILBANKS, G.A., M. MAMMOLENTI & J.W. STREILEIN. 1991. Studies on the induction of anterior chamber associated immune deviation (ACAID). II. Eye-derived cells participate in generating blood-borne signals that induce ACAID. J. Immunol. **146:** 3018–3024.

19. WILBANKS, G.A., M. MAMMOLENTI & J.W. STREILEIN. 1992. Studies on the induction of Anterior Chamber-Associated Immune Deviation (ACAID) III. Induction of ACAID depends upon intraocular transforming growth factor-β. Eur. J. Immunol. **22:** 165–173.

20. WILBANKS, G.A. & J.W. STREILEIN. 1992. Fluids from immune privileged sites endow macrophages with capacity to induce antigen specific immune deviation via a mechanism involving transforming growth factor-beta. Eur. J. Immunol. **22:** 1031–1036.

21. KAISER, C., B.R. KSANDER & J.W. STREILEIN. 1989. Inhibition of lymphocyte proliferation by aqueous humor. Regional Immunol. **2:** 42–49.

22. TAYLOR, A.W. 1999. Ocular Immunosuppressive Microenvironment. *In* Immune Responses and the Eye. J.W. Streilein, Ed. Chem. Immunol. **73:** 72–89. Karger, Basel.

23. CHEN, H.H., Y. SUN & G.J. NABEL. 1998. Regulation of the proinflammatory effects of Fas ligand (CD95L). Science **282:** 1714–1717.

24. GRIFFITH, T.S., T. BRUNNER, S.M. FLETCHER, D.R. GREEN & T.A. FERGUSON. 1995. Fas ligand-induced apoptosis as a mechanism of immune privilege. Science (Wash DC) **270:** 1189–1192.

25. JORGENSON, A., A.K. WIENCKE, M. LA COUR, C.G. KOESTEL, H.O. MADSON, S. HAMANN, G.M. LUI, E. SCHERFIG, J.U. PRAUSE. A. SVEJGAARD, N. ODUM, M.H. NISSEN & C. ROPKE. 1998. Human retinal pigment epithelial cell-induced apoptosis in activated T cells. Invest. Ophthal. Vis. Sci. **39:** 1590–1599.

26. FARROKH-SIAR, W.L., K.A. REZAI, R.T. SEMNANI, S.C. PATEL, J.R. ERNEST, E.J. PETERSON., G.A. KORETZKY & G.A. VAN SEVENTER. 1999. Human fetal retinal pigment epithelial cells induce apoptosis in the T-cell line Jurkat. Invest. Ophthal. Vis. Sci. **40:** 1503–1511.

27. STREILEIN, J.W. & D. BRADLEY. 1991. Analysis of immunosuppressive properties of iris and ciliary body cells and their secretory products. Invest. Ophthal. Vis. Sci. **32:** 2700–2710.

28. YOSHIDA, M., M. TAKEUCHI & J.W. STREILEIN. 2000. Participation of pigment epithelium of iris and ciliary body in ocular immune privilege. I. Inhibition of T cell activation in vitro by direct cell to cell contact. Invest. Ophthal. Vis. Sci. **41:** 811–821.

29. COUSINS, S., M. MCCABE, R. DANIELPOUR & J.W. STREILEIN. 1991. Identification of transforming growth factor-beta as an immunosuppressive factor in aqueous humor. Invest. Ophthalmol. Vis. Sci. **32:** 2201–2211.

30. STREILEIN, J.W., D. BRADLEY, Y. SANO & Y. SONODA. 1996. Immunosuppressive properties of tissues obtained from eyes with experimentally manipulated corneas. Invest. Ophthal. Vis. Sci. **37:** 413–424.

31. SONODA, Y. & J.W. STREILEIN. 1992. Orthotopic corneal transplantation in mice. Evidence that the immunogenetic rules of rejection do not apply. Transplantation **54:** 694–703.

32. FERGUSON, T.A., J.D. HAYASHI & H.J. KAPLAN. 1988. Regulation of the systemic immune response by visible light and the eye. FASEB J. **2:** 3017-3021.

33. FERGUSON, T.A., S.L. MAHENDRA, P. HOOPER & H.J. KAPLAN. 1992. The wavelength of light governing intraocular immune reactions. Invest. Ophthal. Vis. Sci. **33:** 1788–1795.
34. FERGUSON, T.A., S. FLETCHER, J. HERNDON & T.S. GRIFFITH. 1995. Neuropeptides modulate immune deviation induced via the anterior chamber of the eye. J. Immunol. **155:** 1746–1756.
35. MARTIN, X.D., H.Z. MALINA, M.C. BRENNAN, P.D. HENDRICKSON & P.R. LICHTER. 1992. The ciliary body—the third organ found to synthesize indoleamines in humans. Eur. J. Ophthal. **2:** 67–72.
36. MAESTRONI, G.J.M. & A. CONTI. 1990. The pineal neurohormone melatonin stimulates activated $CD4^+$ $Thy-1^+$ cells to release opioid agonist(s) with immunoenhancing and anti-stress properties. J. Neuroimmunol. **28:** 167–176.

Nerve-Driven Immunity

The Direct Effects of Neurotransmitters on T-Cell Function

MIA LEVITE[a]

Department of Immunology, The Weizmann Institute of Science, Rehovot 76100, Israel

ABSTRACT: We carried out studies to explore whether neurotransmitters can directly interact with their T-cell–expressed receptors, leading to either activation or suppression of various T-cell functions. Human and mouse T cells were thus exposed directly to neurotransmitters in the absence of any additional molecule, and various functions were studied, among them cytokine secretion, proliferation, and integrin-mediated adhesion and migration. In this review, I describe the effects of four neuropeptides: somatostatin (SOM), calcitonin-gene-related-peptide (CGRP), neuropeptide Y (NPY), and substance P (Sub P), and one non-peptidergic neurotransmitter—dopamine. We found that SOM, NPY, CGRP, and dopamine interact directly with T cells, leading to the activation of β_1 integrins and to the subsequent integrin-mediated T-cell adhesion to a component of the extracellular matrix. In contrast, Sub P had a reverse effect—full blockage of integrin-mediated T-cell adhesion triggered by a variety of signals. Each of these neurotransmitters exerted its effect through direct interaction with its specific receptor on the T-cell surface, since the effect was fully blocked by the respective receptor-antagonist. Taken together, this set of findings indicates that neurotransmitters can directly interact with T cells and provide them with either positive (integrin-activating, pro-adhesive) or negative (integrin-inhibiting, anti-adhesive) signals. We further found that the above neurotransmitters, by direct interaction with their specific receptors, drove T cells (of the Th0, Th1, and Th2 phenotypes) into the secretion of both typical and atypical ("forbidden") cytokines. These results suggested that neurotransmitters can substantially affect various cytokine-dependent T-cell activities. As a whole, our studies suggest an important and yet unrecognized role for neurotransmitters in directly dictating or modulating numerous T-cell functions under physiological and pathological conditions.

INTRODUCTION

The concept that the immune system, the nervous system and the endocrine system are functionally interconnected is gaining support,[1–3] although the detailed mechanisms of this intercommunication remain to a great extent unknown. The anatomical basis of this assumed neuroimmune interplay is likely to be formed by the recently discovered autonomic and sensory peptidergic innervation of lymphoid tissues,[1,2] yet its functional importance is still unrecognized and probably underestimated. On these grounds, it is a challenge to unveil the possible influence of direct neuronal signals (as

[a]Address for correspondence: Dr. Mia Levite, Department of Immunology, The Weizmann Institute of Science, Rehovot 76100, Israel. Voice: 972-8-9343556; fax: 972-8-9344173.
mia.levite@weizmann.ac.il

opposed to indirect neuroendocrine signaling) on the function of the immune system. In particular, an intriguing critical question is whether specific nerve-secreted neurotransmitters can directly turn on/off T-cell function and if so, by which mechanisms.

The scientific rationale behind this question lies on a few basic and often forgotten facts:

(a) All the primary and secondary lymphoid organs (including the thymus, spleen, lymph nodes bone marrow and others) are massively innervated by nerves using various neuropeptides and small molecules (dopamine among others) as neurotransmitters.[1,2] Thus, T-cell populations are most probably exposed to a variety of signals secreted from nerve terminals under the phasic or tonic conditions dictated by the electrical activity patterns of the direct innervation.

(b) Neurotransmitters (both peptidergic and non-peptidergic) are released from nerve terminals at various extravascular targets to which T cells are attracted under conditions of inflammation, foreign body invasion and/or disease. Moreover, both fenestrated and non-fenestrated blood capillaries are innervated by nerves secreting such molecules, thus enabling a direct signaling with blood-borne T-cells.[4–8]

(c) T-lymphocytes (as well as other cells of the immune system) express specific receptors for various neurotransmitters on their surface.[9–13]

The presence of neurotransmitters in loci where T-cells reside or pass through in conjunction with the occurrence of neurotransmitter-receptors on lymphocytes strongly suggests a functional correlation.

SPECIFIC NEUROTRANSMITTERS OF INTEREST

Neurotransmitters seen as likely to directly affect T-cell function should be secreted from nerve terminals that are in close association with T cells under normal and/or pathological conditions, and T lymphocytes should harbor specific receptors for these neurotransmitters.

Among the candidates that appear to meet these criteria are the four peptidergic neurotransmitters: substance P (Sub P), neuropeptide Y (NPY), somatostatin (SOM) and calcitonin gene-related peptide (CGRP), and one classical non-peptidergic neurotransmitter—the catecholamine dopamine.

All these neurotransmitters are localized in the central and peripheral nervous system, where they exert a broad spectrum of activities including the modulation of motor and sensory neuron activity and the regulation of endocrine functions.[1,4–8] These neurotransmitters appear also in nerve terminals innervating blood capillaries, where they act as vasodilators and affect the vascular permeability as well as the behavior of various cell types including lymphocytes.

Lymphoid organs and tissues from a large variety of mammals have been shown to be innervated by nerves that contain the above mentioned neurotransmitters in the nerve terminals.[1,2] Specific receptors for SOM, CGRP Sub P and NPY, as well as for dopamine, have been suggested on different immunocytes, primarily on the basis of binding and gene expression methodologies.[9–13]

In this paper, I review some of the results obtained in my laboratory pertaining to two specific questions:

1. Can neurotransmitters, by direct interaction with their cognate receptors, and in the absence of any additional stimulatory effectors, trigger or inhibit T-cell function?

2. Is the neurotransmitter-evoked T-cell function quantitatively and qualitatively similar to that evoked by a "classical" antigen acting via the TCR?

THE EFFECTS OF NEUROTRANSMITTERS ON T-CELL β_1 INTEGRIN FUNCTION

To investigate whether neurotransmitters can directly affect T-cell integrin functions, we studied their effects on β_1-integrin-mediated adhesion of resting human T-cells to fibronectin (FN), a major glycoprotein component of the extracellular matrix (ECM). Binding of T cells to ECM components such as FN is required in a broad spectrum of normal and diseased conditions and is in fact a prerequisite for the extravasation and subsequent migration of T-cells from the blood vessels into extravascular tissues in general, and into inflamed stressed or diseased tissues in particular.[14–16]

The adhesion of T-cells to FN is mediated by the β_1 integrins, a subclass of specific cell-surface adhesion receptors within the large versatile integrin superfamily. The activation of the β_1 integrins is absolutely required for the T-cell/FN interactions[14–16] since resting T-cells cannot adhere. The activation of the integrin moieties and the subsequent adhesion to ECM components are very dynamic, rapid and tightly regulated processes, since cells convert rapidly and transiently (within seconds to minutes) from a non-adherent to an adherent phenotype. It is this dynamic cycling between adhesive and non-adhesive states that endows the cell with the ability to regulate rapidly its adhesion to ligands on opposing cell surfaces and matrices, a prerequisite for extravasation and subsequent migration to target tissue.[14–16]

Can neuropeptides, in the absence of any additional stimuli, activate the T-cell β_1-integrins, resulting in the subsequent adhesion of the cells to FN?

Studying five neurotransmitters—SOM, CGRP, NPY, Sub P and dopamine—we found[21] that physiological concentrations of the former three neuropeptides, as well as of dopamine induced high levels of adhesion of resting human and murine T-cells to FN (see FIGURE 1, A–D). The levels of T-cell adhesion induced by SOM, CGRP, NPY and dopamine were comparable in magnitude and often even higher than those induced by the very potent phorbol ester PMA.

By a procedure of preincubations and washings of either the T-cells or the immobilized FN, we concluded that the adhesion triggered by SOM, CGRP and dopamine was mediated by their direct interaction with the T-cells, rather than with the FN glycoprotein (data not shown). Furthermore, by the use of specific receptor-antagonists or agonists, we obtained evidence that SOM, CGRP and dopamine directly interacted with their T-cell–expressed receptors, subsequently leading to integrin-mediated adhesion to FN (see FIGURE 2, A,B). These experiments also shed light on some of the receptor subtypes involved. Thus, the results (FIG. 2, A,B) demonstrate that the pro-adhesive effects of SOM and CGRP on T cells were specifically and significantly

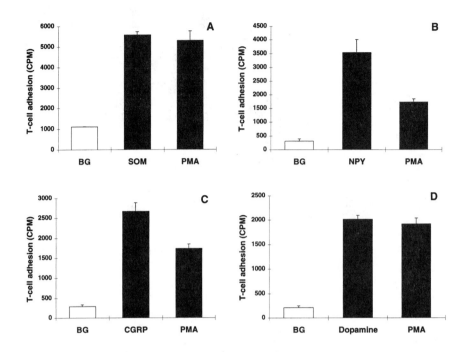

FIGURE 1. SOM, CGRP, NPY and dopamine induce T-cell adhesion to FN. Human T-cells, purified from fresh blood samples, were labeled with ^{51}[Cr], washed, resuspended in adhesion medium, pretreated (30 min 37°C) with either SOM [**A**], CGRP [**B**], NPY [**C**] or dopamine [**D**] (10^{-8} M), and added to the FN-coated wells. Non-adherent T cells were removed by washing. After incubation, the adherent T cells were lysed, and the radioactivity in the resulting supernatants was determined. Neurotransmitter-treated T-cell adhesion to BSA-coated (rather than FN-coated) wells, and the adhesion to FN of untreated T cells was less than 6%. One representative experiment out of five is depicted. BG: background, representing untreated groups of T cells.[21]

($p < 0.05$) inhibited by the presence of their respective receptor antagonists: Cyclo-[7-aminoheptanoyl-phe-trp-lys-thr (bzl)] (cyclo-SOM)[17] and CGRP (8–37) suppressing preferentially specific receptor subtypes.[18]

Dopamine-induced T-cell adhesion was mediated by direct interaction with its D3 receptor, since the specific D3 receptor agonist 7-OH-DPAT (DPAT)[19] induced, like dopamine, a marked T-cell adhesion to FN, while a specific D3 receptor antagonist, U-maleate (U-Mal), completely inhibited dopamine and DPAT-induced effects (FIG. 2D) (unpublished data).

In the absence of commercially available NPY receptor antagonists, we utilized NPY (18–36) C-terminal fragment, a selective NPY receptor-agonist for the Y2 receptor subtype,[20] to study whether NPY triggers T-cell adhesion via its specific receptor. We found that NPY (18–36) induced, like the intact NPY, a marked adhesion of T-cells to FN (FIG. 2C), implying that T-cells express a functional NPY receptor of the Y2 subtype, which upon activation may provide the T-cells with a pro-adhesive signal.

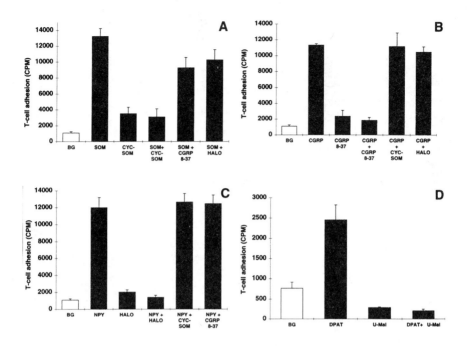

FIGURE 2. Neurotransmitters induce T-cell adhesion via direct interaction with their T-cell expressed receptors. Purified human T-cell were treated with SOM [**A**], CGRP [**B**], NPY [**C**] or dopamine [**D**] (10^{-8}M), following a brief (2 min.) incubation with their specific receptor antagonists, and T-cell adhesion to FN was measured as described in FIGURE 1. The receptor antagonists included: cyclo-[7-aminoheptanoyl-phe-trp-lys-thr (bzl)] (CYC-SOM), CGRP (8–37), Haloperidol (HALO) and U-Maleate (U-Mal). One experiment out of three is presented.

By the use of specific anti-integrin monoclonal antibodies and specific signal transduction blockers we observed that the T-cell adhesion induced by SOM, CGRP, NPY and dopamine was mediated specifically by the $\alpha_4\beta_1$ and $\alpha_5\beta_1$ integrins, as well as by diverse intracellular signaling pathways including G-proteins, tyrosine protein kinase (TPK), protein kinase C (PKC) and phosphoinositol 3 kinase (PI-3).[21]

In contrast to the four neurotransmitters discussed above, substance P failed to induce T-cell adhesion to FN. In fact, Sub P exerted exactly the opposite effect: it blocked the adhesion of T-cells to FN triggered by a variety of signals including neurotransmitters, chemokines (such as MIP 1β) and phorbol esters.[21] Representative results are shown in FIGURE 3A. Sub P is thus endowed with a unique property, since, to the best of our knowledge, no other physiological molecule was reported to block T-cell adhesion to ECM components, in contrast to the numerous molecules able to promote this process.

Sub P–induced inhibition was mediated through its NK1 receptor expressed on T cells, since spantide 1, a specific antagonist of the Sub P NK1 type receptor, abolished the Sub P–induced effect (FIG. 3B).

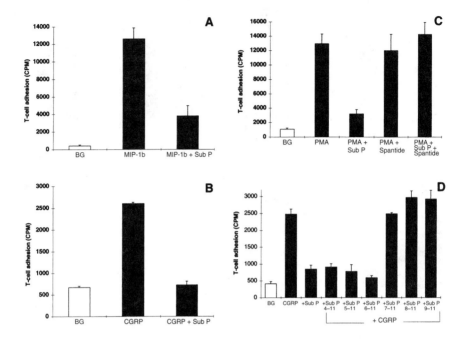

FIGURE 3. Substance P and its fragments inhibit T-cell adhesion to FN via the NK1 receptor subtype. Purified T-cells were preincubated (5 min.) with Sub P (10^{-8}M), and then exposed to either MIP-1β (20 ng/ml) [**A**], CGRP (10^{-8}M) [**B**], or PMA [**C**]. The adhesion to FN-coated wells was then assayed as described in FIGURE 1. Alternatively, T cells were pre-treated with Spantide 1 (10^{-6}M), the Sub P NK1 receptor antagonist, then with Sub P, and finally with PMA [**C**]. [**D**] Analysis of Sub P amino acid sequences required for optimal inhibition of T-cell adhesion. The adhesion to FN-coated surfaces of T-cells, treated with either intact or C-terminal amino acid fragments of Sub P (10^{-10}M), was determined as described above. One experiment representative of three is shown.[21]

Since the 11-amino-acid-long substance P exerts some of its effects through its C-terminus portion, and others through its NH$_2$-terminal portion,[13] we investigated which fragment is responsible for Sub P inhibitory effect on T-cell adhesion. We found that C-terminus Sub P fragments [4–11], [5–11] and [6–11] were as efficient as the full-length Sub P in blocking the T-cell adhesion, while the shorter fragments, at concentrations as high as 10^{-3}M, were inactive (FIG. 3C). Interestingly, the N-terminal Sub P fragment [1–4] was also a very strong inhibitor of T-cell adhesion to FN, active at a concentration as low as 10^{-10}M (comparable to the parent intact Sub P) (data not shown). The inhibitory effects of all the above Sub P fragments were mediated through the SP NK1 receptor subtype, since they were completely abrogated by spantide-1 (data not shown). These observations indicate that Sub P can inhibit integrin-mediated T-cell adhesion either through its C-terminal fragment [6–11] or through its N-terminal [1–4] fragment.[21]

Taken together, these studies showed:

1. that T-cells carry functional receptors for SOM, CGRP, NPY, Sub P and dopamine, and

2. that direct interaction with a neurotransmitter can provide T-cells with either positive (integrin-activating, pro-adhesive) or negative (integrin-inhibiting, anti-adhesive) signals that regulate β_1 integrin–mediated functions.

These observations suggest that neurotransmitters may directly and rapidly influence T-cell integrin-mediated processes, such as adhesion migration and extravasation, in numerous physiological and pathological conditions.

THE EFFECTS OF NEUROTRANSMITTERS ON T-CELL CYTOKINE SECRETION

To investigate whether neuropeptides can directly stimulate T-cells to secrete cytokines, and if so, to compare quantitatively and qualitatively neuropeptide-induced versus antigen-induced cytokine secretion, four neuropeptides, SOM, CGRP, NPY, and Sub P, were applied (with no additional molecules) to antigen-specific mouse T-cell lines, and their cytokine secretion determined.[22] Several T-cell lines, differing in their cytokine secretion profile, were used. Upon "classical" antigenic stimulation the Th1 lines typically secreted IL-2 and IFN-γ, the Th2 cells secreted primarily IL-4 and IL-10, while the Th0 cells had the potential to secrete the whole repertoire of T-cell cytokines.

The representative experiment presented in FIGURE 4 shows that CGRP at a physiological concentration of 10^{-8}M, and in the absence of any additional stimulatory factors, induced a significant secretion of cytokines from a Th0 anti-MBP 87–99 T-cell line. The level of CGRP-induced cytokine secretion was comparable in magnitude to that measured upon antigenic-stimulation.

TABLE 1 shows that the other neuropeptides tested, SOM, Sub P and NPY, could also by themselves induce the secretion of various cytokines from different T-cell lines.

Comparing neuropeptide-driven versus classical antigen-driven cytokine secretion from the Th0, Th1, Th2 mouse T-cell populations, it was found,[22] that some neuropeptides drove the distinct Th1 and Th2 populations to a "forbidden" cytokine secretion: secretion of Th2 cytokines from a Th1 T-cell line, and vice versa. Such a phenomenon could not be induced by classical antigenic stimulation. Representative results are shown in FIGURE 5, A and B. This observation suggests that the distinction between Th0/Th1/Th2 T-cell subtypes, based on their cytokine secretion profile, refers only to an antigen-driven stimulation. Neuropeptide-induced cytokine secretion may require the creation of a new classification.

Other conclusions emerging from these studies are the following:

1. Neuropeptides can directly affect the cytokine secretion of naïve T-cells.

2. Some neuropeptides can induce cytokine secretion of resting T-cells, while others can only affect the cytokine secretion of already activated (i.e., antigen-stimulated) T-cells.

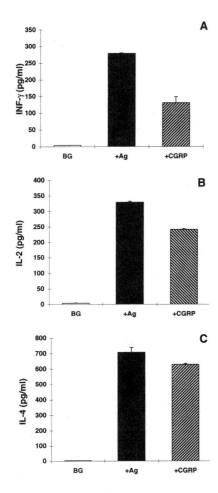

FIGURE 4. The direct exposure of T-cells to CGRP leads to cytokine secretion. A Th0 type anti-MBP 87–99 T-cell line was stimulated either with its antigen (10 μg/ml) and syngeneic antigen-presenting cells (APCs), or only with CGRP (10^{-8}M), and 20 h post incubation the supernatants were collected and the levels of IFN-γ (**A**), IL-2 (**B**), and IL-4 (**C**) measured by ELISA.[22] The results represent mean ± SD concentration of duplicate culture supernatants, measured in duplicate wells in the ELISA plates. Results of control cultures are expressed as background (BG).

3. The effect of a given neuropeptide on a given T-cell population can be either stimulatory or inhibitory, depending on:

    (i)   the cytokine in question;
    (ii) the activation state of the cells;
    (iii) the T-cell Th phenotype (Th0/Th1/Th2); and
    (iv) the lymphoid organ from which the T-cells derive (spleen, thymus, etc.)

4. The effect of a given neuropeptide on the cytokine secretion of a given T-cell population can be either synergistic with the antigen-induced cytokine secretion, or antagonistic, or simply neutral.

5. The relationship between a neuropeptide-induced effect and an antigen-induced effect can vary with respect to the secretion of the same cytokine from

TABLE 1.

| | T-cell line/clone | | | | |
| | Th0 | Th1 | Th2 | | |
	Anti-MBP 87–99	Anti-MBP 87–99	Anti-MBP 87–99	Anti Cop-1	Anti-Hsp 65
SOM	IL-2	IL-2	IL-2	0	0
	IFN-γ	0	IFN-γ	IFN-γ	IFN-γ
	IL-4	0	IL-4	0	ND
	IL-10	0	IL-10	IL-10	ND
CGRP	IL-2	0	IL-2	IL-2	0
	IFN-γ	0	IFN-γ	0	0
	TNF-α	ND	ND	ND	ND
	IL-4	IL-4	ND	0	ND
	IL-10	0	IL-10	IL-10	ND
NPY	0	IL-2	0	IL-2(?)	IL-2
	0	IFN-γ	IFN-γ	IFN-γ	0
	0	IL-4	0	0	ND
	0	0	0	0	ND
Sub P	0	0	0	IL-2	0
	0	0	IFN-γ	IFN-γ	0
	0	0	0	0	ND
	0	0	0	0	ND

ND = Not done.

different cell Th populations, as well as for different cytokines secreted from the same cell population.

The above conclusions suggest that T-cells possess variable pathways controlling the pattern of cytokine secretion, and that within a T-cell, there is a cross talk between messages transmitted via the T-cell receptor (TCR) and via the specific neurotransmitter-receptors.

Taken together, the main suggestion emerging from this study is that the nervous system, through neuropeptides interacting with their specific T-cell–expressed receptors, can lead to the secretion of both typical and atypical cytokines; that may result in a potentially altered function and destiny of T-cells *in vivo*.

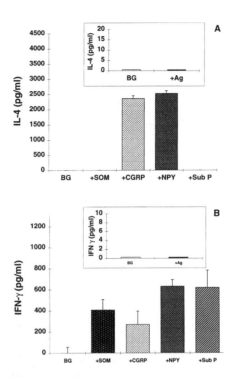

FIGURE 5. Neuropeptides drive T-cells to "forbidden" cytokine secretion. [A] Neuropeptides induce the secretion of IL-4 from a Th1 type T-cell line, while the antigen fails to do so (*insert*). The antigen induced a high secretion only of IL-2 and IFN-γ from these cells (data not shown). [B] Neuropeptides induce the secretion of IFN-γ from a Th2 type T-cell line, while the antigen fails to do so (*insert*). The antigen induced a high secretion only of IL-4 and IL-10 from these cells (data not shown). The Th1- and Th2-type anti-MBP 87–99 T-cell lines were stimulated either with their antigen (MBP 87–99) and syngeneic APCs, or only with CGRP, SOM, NPY or Sub P (10^{-8} M). Following 18 h incubation, supernatants were collected and the levels of IL-2, IFN-γ, IL-4 and IL-10 were measured by ELISA, of which only the IL-4 secretion of the Th1 line, and the IFN-γ secretion of the Th2 line, are shown. The results represent mean ± SD of duplicate culture supernatants, measured in duplicate wells in the ELISA plates.[22]

THE EFFECTS OF NEUROTRANSMITTERS ON T-CELL PROLIFERATION

Do SOM, CGRP, NPY and Sub P augment the proliferation of T-cells in the absence of any additional stimulatory molecules? Using mouse antigen-specific T-cell lines and human Jurkat T-cells, the answer emerging from our studies is in most cases negative. Thus, the neuropeptide-induced T-cell cytokine secretion described above is not correlated with increased cell proliferation. This is in contrast to the effects of the antigen, which induces both proliferation and cytokine secretion. Representative experiments are shown in FIGURE 6A.

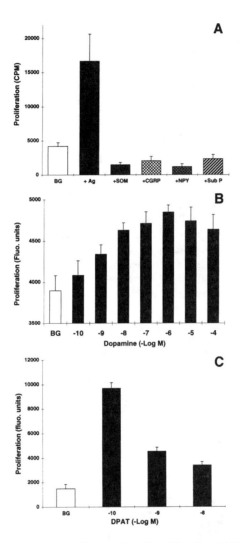

FIGURE 6. Neurotransmitter effects on T-cell proliferation. [**A**] The direct effects of neuropeptides on T-cell cytokine secretion is not correlated with an augmented proliferation. A Th1 type T-cell line was stimulated either with its antigen and syngeneic APCs, or only with CGRP, SOM, NPY or Sub P (10^{-8}M). The level of cell proliferation following 72 hours was determined as described.[22] Results are expressed as mean ± SD cpm thymidine incorporation for 6 replicate wells. [**B,C**] Dopamine and its D3 agonist trigger T-cell proliferation. [**B**] Human cultured Jurkat cells were incubated with increasing concentrations of dopamine (in the absence of any additional factors), and the level of proliferation following 48 hours was determined with the CyQuant cell proliferation assay kit (Molecular Probes). [**C**] Normal human T-cells purified from fresh blood samples (as described in FIG. 1) were incubated with increasing concentrations of 7-Hydroxy-DPAT hydrobromide (DPAT), a specific dopamine D3 agonist. The proliferation assay (48 hours) was performed as described in [**A**]. Results are expressed as mean ± SD fluorescence intensity, and one out of three experiments is shown.

However, in contrast to the neuropeptides (SOM, CGRP, NPY and Sub P), dopamine, in the absence of any additional stimuli, does promote T-cell proliferation (unpublished data). Representative results are shown in FIGURE 6B. The dopamine-induced T-cell proliferation is mediated through its D3 receptor, since the effect is reproduced by the highly specific D3 receptor agonist 7-OH-DPAT, as shown in FIGURE 6C.

DIRECT EFFECTS OF NEUROTRANSMITTERS ON OTHER T-CELL PROPERTIES AND FUNCTIONS

SOM, CGRP, NPY, Sub P and dopamine directly affect not only integrin-mediated functions, cytokine secretion and proliferation, but also additional T-cell activities and properties, such as the T-cell membrane potential (data not shown, study in progress). Such a neurotransmitter-induced shift in the T-cell membrane potential is likely to affect various T-cell reactivities, since a series of downstream intracellular elements (such as voltage-gated ion channels, various kinases) and processes (such as IL-2 production and proliferation), as well as the overall functional state of the cell, were either reported or suggested to be associated with changes of the membrane potential.[23,24]

Other T-cell properties affected by the direct interaction with some neurotransmitters are the cell cycle and programmed cell death. This is manifested either by "pushing" the cells from the Sub G1 phase (associated with apoptosis) towards proliferation, or vice versa, depending on the nature of the given neurotransmitter, the age of the cells and their activation state (M. Levite, L. Abel & A. Globerson, study in progress). Furthermore, the *in vitro* ability of thymocytes to reconstitute a lymphoid-depleted fetal thymus can be significantly affected by a short-term exposure to neurotransmitters (M. Levite, L. Abel & A. Globerson, study in progress).

DISCUSSION

The results emerging from these studies suggest that the nervous system has the potential to directly and rapidly trigger or silence various T-cell functions: The neurotransmitters secreted from nerve terminals, under the 'instructions' of the central or peripheral nervous system, may directly interact with their respective receptors on T-cells and convey thereby functional and important messages.

Clearly, such messages transmitted directly to lymphocytes through nerve-secreted neurotransmitters may be quantitatively, qualitatively, kinetically and contextually different from those conveyed by the "classical" immunological signaling processes (i.e., through encounter with an antigen, cytokine, etc.), and as such deserve a thorough investigation and characterization.

Our findings so far show that the neuropeptides SOM, CGRP, NPY and Sub P, and one of the important CNS neurotransmitters, dopamine, can directly interact with their respective receptors on the T-cell surface, and either stimulate or silence key immunological functions such as cytokine secretion and integrin-mediated activities. One may suggest that such direct neurotransmitter-T-cells interactions can play an important role in shaping T-cell activities under numerous normal and pathological conditions.[4,25–29]

In principal, nerve-secreted neurotransmitters may encounter T-cells in both lymphoid and non-lymphoid tissues in which T-cells reside or patrol through.[1,2,29] Furthermore, since the nervous system interacts with peripheral organs in a bi-directional mode, i.e. by emitting and receiving signals,[3,30] the neurotransmitters may be secreted at a given location (by descending nerves) in response to changes in environmental conditions that are sensed by, and reported to, the nervous system (by ascending sensory nerves). The sensory nerves themselves may be involved in local neuroimmune transactions, as in the case of the axon reflex.[31] Thus, neuroimmune contacts may serve for the exchange of reciprocal information between the nervous system and the immune system.

One may further speculate that nerve-evoked signaling may serve not only for passing information from and to the nervous system, but also for communications within the immune system compartments. This might be an especially intriguing mechanism when bearing in mind that the neuronal networks are highly branched, complexed and widely spread and that a nerve-evoked signal can be conveyed either simultaneously or gradually to several cell populations within the same organ, or even to another organ. Such a network might clearly contribute to a wide, rapid and efficient spread of information which may be important for an orchestrated operation of the immune system.

ACKNOWLEDGMENTS

The studies described in this review were supported by grants from the Volkswagen-Stiftung foundation, and the Rochlin Foundation to M. Levite.

REFERENCES

1. WEIHE, E., D. NOHR, S. MICHEL, S. MULLER, H.J. ZENTEL, T. FINK & J. KREKEL. 1991. Molecular anatomy of the neuro-immune connection. Int. J. Neurosci. **59:** 1–23.

2. FINK, T. & E. WEIHE. 1988. Multiple neuropeptides in nerves supplying mammalian lymph nodes: messenger candidates for sensory and autonomic neuroimmunomodulation? Neurosci. Lett. **90:** 39–44.

3. STERNBERG, E.M. 1997. Emotions and disease: from balance of humors to balance of molecules. Nat. Med. **3:** 264–267.

4. WILDER, R.L. 1995. Neuroendocrine-immune system interactions and autoimmunity. Annu. Rev. Immunol. **13:** 307–338.

5. PAYAN, D.G., D.R. BREWSTER, A. MISSIRIAN BASTIAN & E.J. GOETZL. 1984. Substance P recognition by a subset of human T lymphocytes. J. Clin. Invest. **74:** 1532–1539.

6. GOEBELER, M., U. HENSELEIT, J. ROTH & C. SORG. 1994. Substance P and calcitonin gene-related peptide modulate leukocyte infiltration to mouse skin during allergic contact dermatitis. Arch. Dermatol. Res. **286:** 341–346.

7. NIO, D.A., R.N. MOYLAN & J.K. ROCHE. 1993. Modulation of T lymphocyte function by neuropeptides. Evidence for their role as local immunoregulatory elements. J. Immunol. **150:** 5281–5288.

8. JOHNSTON, J.A., D.D. TAUB, A.R. LLOYD, K. CONLON, J.J. OPPENHEIM & D.J. KEVLIN. 1994. Human T lymphocyte chemotaxis and adhesion induced by vasoactive intestinal peptide. J. Immunol. **153:** 1762–1768.

9. HIRUMA, K., T. KOIKE, H. NAKAMURA, T. SUMIDA, T. MAEDA, H. TOMIOKA, S. YOSHIDA & T. FUJITA. 1990. Somatostatin receptors on human lymphocytes and leukaemia cells. Immunology **71:** 480–485.

10. SREEDHARAN, S.P., K.T. KODAMA, K.E. PETERSON & E.J. GOETZL. 1989. Distinct subsets of somatostatin receptors on cultured human lymphocytes. J. Biol. Chem. **264:** 949–952.

11. MCGILLIS, J.P., S. HUMPHREYS & S. REID. 1991. Characterization of functional calcitonin gene-related peptide receptors on rat lymphocytes. J. Immunol. **147:** 3482–3489.

12. WIEDERMANN, C.J., K. SERTL & C.B. PERT. 1986. Substance P receptors in rat spleen: characterization and autoradiographic distribution. Blood **68:** 1398–1401.

13. REGOLI, D., A. BOUDON & J.L. FAUCHERE. 1994. Receptors and antagonists for substance P and related peptides. Pharmacol. Rev. **46:** 551–599.

14. SPRINGER, T.A. 1994. Traffic signals for lymphocyte recirculation and leukocyte emigration: the multistep paradigm. Cell **76:** 301–314.

15. LLOYD, A.R., J.J. OPPENHEIM, D.J. KELVIN & D.D. TAUB. 1996. Chemokines regulate T cell adherence to recombinant adhesion molecules and extracellular matrix proteins. J. Immunol. **156:** 932–938.

16. SHIMIZU, Y. & S. WR. HUNT. 1996. Regulating integrin-mediated adhesion: one more function for PI 3-kinase? Immunol. Today **17:** 565–573.

17. FRIES, J.L., W.A. MURPHY, J. SUEIRAS-DIAZ & D.H. COY. 1982. Somatostatin antagonist analog increases GH, insulin, and glucagon release in the rat. Peptides **3:** 811–814.

18. CHIBA, T., A. YAMAGUCHI, T. YAMATANI, A. NAKAMURA, T. MORISHITA, T. INUI, M. FUKASE, T. NODA & T. FUJITA. 1989. Calcitonin gene-related peptide receptor antagonist human CGRP-(8–37). Am. J. Physiol. **256:** E331–E335.

19. RICCI, A., E. BRONZETTI, L. FELICI, S. GRECO & F. AMENTA. 1998. Labeling of dopamine D3 and D4 receptor subtypes in human peripheral blood lymphocytes with [^{3}H]7-OH-DPAT: a combined radioligand binding assay and immunochemical study. J. Neuroimmunol. **92:** 191–195.

20. MOUSLI, M., A. TRIFILIEFF, J.T. PELTON, J.P. GIES & Y. LANDRY. 1995. Structural requirements for neuropeptide Y in mast cell and G protein activation. Eur. J. Pharmacol. **289:** 125–133.

21. LEVITE, M., L. CAHALON, R. HERSHKOVIZ, L. STEINMAN & O. LIDER. 1998. Neuropeptides, via specific receptors, regulate T cell adhesion to fibronectin. J. Immunol. **160:** 993–1000.

22. LEVITE, M. 1998. Neuropeptides, by direct interaction with T cells, induce cytokine secretion and break the commitment to a distinct T helper phenotype. Proc. Natl. Acad. Sci. USA **95:** 12544–12549.

23. FREEDMAN, B.D., M.A. PRICE & C.J. DEUTSCH. 1992. Evidence for voltage modulation of IL-2 production in mitogen-stimulated human peripheral blood lymphocytes. J. Immunol. **149:** 3784–3794.

24. MALTSEV, V.A. 1990. Oscillating and triggering properties of T cell membrane potential. Immunol. Lett. **26:** 277–282.

25. KHACHATRYAN, A., S. GUERDER, F. PALLUAULT, G. COTE, M. SOLIMENA, K. VALENTIJN, I. MILLET, R.A. FLAVELL & A. VIGNERY. 1997. Targeted expression of the neuropeptide calcitonin gene-related peptide to beta cells prevents diabetes in NOD mice. J. Immunol. **158:** 1409–1416.

26. NAGAI, Y., S. UENO, Y. SAEKI, F. SOGA, M. HIRANO & T. YANAGIHARA. 1996. Decrease of the D3 dopamine receptor mRNA expression in lymphocytes from patients with Parkinson's disease. Neurology **46:** 791–795.

27. LAFAILLE, J.J., F.V. KEERE, A.L. HSU, J.L. BARON, W. HAAS, C.S. RAINE & S. TONEGAWA. 1997. Myelin basic protein-specific T helper 2 (Th2) cells cause experimental autoimmune encephalomyelitis in immunodeficient hosts rather than protect them from the disease. J. Exp. Med. **186:** 307–312.

28. MERRILL, J.E. & E.N. BENVENISTE. 1996. Cytokines in inflammatory brain lesions: helpful and harmful. Trends Neurosci. **19:** 331–338.
29. FELTEN, D.L., S.Y. FELTEN, D.L. BELLINGER & D. LORTON. 1992. Noradrenergic and peptidergic innervation of secondary lymphoid organs: role in experimental rheumatoid arthritis. Eur. J. Clin. Invest. **22**(Suppl. 1): 37–41.
30. BALLIEUX, R.E. 1992. Bidirectional communication between the brain and the immune system. Eur. J. Clin. Invest. **22**(Suppl. 1): 6–9.
31. MAGGI, C.A. 1995. Tachykinins and calcitonin gene-related peptide (CGRP) as cotransmitters released from peripheral endings of sensory nerves. Prog. Neurobiol. **45:** 1–98.

Cytokines and Neurotrophins Interact in Normal and Diseased States

U. OTTEN,[a,b] P. MÄRZ,[c] K. HEESE,[d] C. HOCK,[e] D. KUNZ,[a] AND S. ROSE-JOHN[c]

[a]Department of Physiology, University of Basel, CH-4051 Basel, Switzerland

[c]Department of Medicine, Section Pathophysiology,
University of Mainz, D-55101 Mainz, Germany

[d]BF Research Institute, c/o National Cardiovascular Center, Osaka, Japan

[e]Department of Psychiatry Research, University of Zürich, CH-8029 Zürich, Switzerland

ABSTRACT: Neurotrophins (NTs) such as nerve growth factor (NGF) as well as cytokines, for example, interleukin-6 (IL-6), are communicators between the nervous and immune systems. There is evidence for mutual interactions between NTs and cytokines. Strategies are being developed to elucidate the molecular mechanism/s of interactions and to understand how cytokines are involved in health and disease. Analysis of underlying signaling pathways in glial cells indicates that different transcription factors, such as NF-κB, cAMP–responsive-element binding protein (CREB), and activator protein 1 (AP-1), are involved in NT induction. IL-6 and NTs of the NGF family are coexpressed at sites of nerve injury. Interactions of these factors could modulate both neuronal de- and regeneration: IL-6 in conjunction with its soluble IL-6 receptor induces a specific pattern of NTs in astrocytes in defined brain regions. This indicates that the IL-6 system mediates a local supply of NTs that participate in diverse CNS functions, such as protection of neurons from insults, neuronal survival, and neuroimmune responses.

One family of specific neurotrophic factors that participates in nervous system development, maintenance, and response to trauma is the neurotrophin family, which includes nerve growth factor (NGF), brain-derived neurotrophic factor (BDNF), neurotrophin-3 (NT-3), NT-4/5, and NT-6.[1] Two types of cell-surface receptors are involved in these neurotrophin-mediated effects:[2] the low-affinity receptor p75, a member of the tumor necrosis factor receptor family, which binds to all neurotrophins with similar, but low affinity; and the high-affinity trk tyrosine kinases. TrkA is the receptor for NGF, trkB for BDNF, and NT-4/5 and trkC for NT-3. Ligand activation of these two receptor types can elicit opposite actions, in particular the prevention or promotion of neuronal apoptosis.

Increasing evidence indicates that neurotrophins participate in the inflammatory response.[3,4] NGF and the trkA receptor are expressed in activated CD4-positive T-cell clones.[5] NGF is also produced in a variety of other immune cells.[6–8] Functional

[b]Address for correspondence: U. Otten, Department of Physiology, University of Basel, Vesalgasse 1, CH-4051 Basel, Switzerland. Voice: +41-61-2673548; fax: +41-61-2673582.
uwe.otten@unibas.ch

trkA receptors are expressed by human monocytes, T and B cells, mast cells, and basophils.[5,6,8–10]

Recent studies have demonstrated that activated human T cells, B cells, and monocytes produce neurotrophins including BDNF *in vitro* and in inflammatory brain lesions.[11] In addition, stimulated human peripheral blood mononuclear cells express trkB and trkC receptors.[12] Thus, the fact that activated immune cells similar to neurons coexpress neurotrophins and their receptors strongly suggests that neurotrophins such as NGF act in an autocrine or paracrine fashion in the immune as well as in the nervous systems. This neurotrophin cross talk between immune cells and neurons is of importance for neuronal survival and protection against damaging signals. In fact, local release of NGF from engineered T cells drastically interferes with the development of the demyelinating inflammatory changes evoked by neurtogenic T lymphocytes during the course of experimental allergic neuritis.[13] Thus, neurotrophins, including NGF, may exert anti-inflammatory effects, opening up new ways in the specific treatment of degenerative or inflammatory disorders.

Interleukin-6 (IL-6), a member of the neuropoietic cytokine family, was initially characterized in terms of its activities in the immune system and during inflammation.[14] Increasing evidence also supports a key role of IL-6 in neuronal survival, differentiation, regeneration, and degeneration in the peripheral and central nervous system (CNS)(for references, see Ref. 15). Major sites of IL-6 production are neurons and glial cells. IL-6 functions are mediated by a specific receptor system composed of a binding site (IL-6R) and a signal-transducing component, gp130, leading to cytoplasmic signaling cascades that activate components of the JAK/STAT pathway, particularly the activation of the transcription factor STAT-3. An intriguing fact is that besides the membrane-bound IL-6R, a soluble form of the IL-6R (sIL-6R) can be generated by shedding of the membrane-bound receptor or alternatively by splicing of the IL-6R pre-mRNA (see FIGURE 1). The sIL-6R can form a complex with its ligand, IL-6, with similar affinity to the cognate membrane-bound receptor, and associates with gp130, thereby activating the IL-6 signal transduction pathway. This ability of sIL-6R to confer IL-6 responsiveness to cells devoid of the membrane-bound IL-6R, but expressing gp130, has been named *transsignaling*.[16] The potential biological importance of the sIL-6R is underlined by its presence in serum, urine, synovial fluid, and cerebrospinal fluid (CSF) of normal individuals and augmented serum levels in various autoimmune diseases.

IL-6 can promote completely opposite actions on neurons triggering either neuronal survival after injury or causing neuronal degeneration and death in disorders such as Alzheimer's disease (AD).[15] At present the mechanisms contributing either to the physiological or pathophysiological functions of IL-6 in the CNS are not solved. Because IL-6 and neurotrophins are coexpressed at sites of nerve injury, it is an attractive hypothesis that neurotrophin–cytokine cross talk is involved in both physiological and pathophysiological processes in the CNS. Strategies are being developed to elucidate the molecular mechanisms of interactions and to understand how cytokines are involved in health and disease.

Microglial cells are the principal immune cells resident in the CNS and the major source of brain immune mediators.[17] Activated microglia generally are regarded as cytotoxic effector cells, which release several potentially cytotoxic substances, implicating these microglia-derived factors to neuronal death in stroke, trauma, and

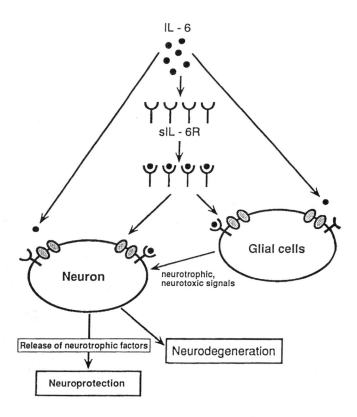

FIGURE 1. IL-6: a molecule with benefical and destructive potentials. The IL-6 can act either directly on neurons or indirectly via glial cells, such as astrocytes and microglia, stimulating them to produce and release secondary mediators. Thus, IL-6 can either protect neurons against injury or can be neurotoxic, causing neurodegeneration and neuronal death. A soluble form of the ligand-binding receptor subunit (sIL-6R) generated by one cell type in complex with IL-6 can directly stimulate target cells that express gpl30 but lack membrane-bound IL-6R.[15]

neurodegenerative disorders.[18,19] Activated microglia also release neurotrophins, such as NGF. This led us to investigate the signaling mechanisms involved in neurotrophin synthesis in human microglial cells that express neurotrophins, such as NGF, BDNF, NT-3, and NT-4/5, as well as the NGF receptor trkA and the low-affinity neurotrophin receptor p75.[20]

Using reverse transcription-polymerase chain reaction (RT-PCR), competitive RT-PCR, Southern blot, and ELISA techniques, the effects of various inflammatory stimuli and their potency in modulating neurotrophin expression in microglial cells were analyzed. We found that the cytokines interleukin-1β (IL-1) and tumor necrosis factor-α (TNF-α) synergistically stimulate microglial NGF transcription and protein release (see FIGURE 2 A and B). Moreover, exposure of microglial cells to complement factor 3a (C3a) induces expression of all neurotrophins, including NGF (FIG. 2

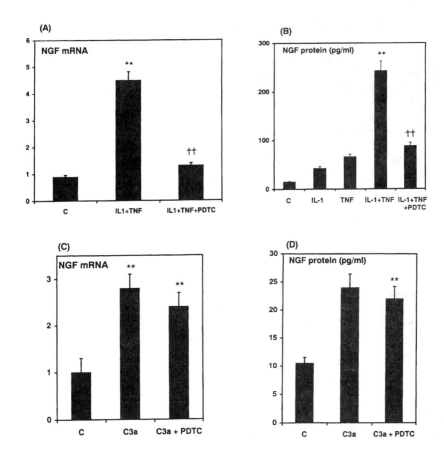

FIGURE 2. Stimulation of NGF expression in human microglial cells by inflammatory stimuli: NF-κB–dependent and –independent mechanisms. Human microglial cells were stimulated for 4 h (mRNA) or 24 h (protein) with cytokines (both at 1 nM, **A** and **B**) or complement 3a (5 nM, **C** and **D**) in absence or presence of PDTC (100 μM). Values are the ratios of densitometric scores for NGF and S12 PCR products. NGF protein was determined in the supernatants by ELISA. Data are means ± SEM of three independent experiments, each done in duplicate. **C**, control. ∗∗ $p < 0.01$, compared with unstimulated controls; ††$p < 0.01$, compared with cytokine-activated cells.[20]

C and D). To assess the role of the transcription factor, nuclear factor-κB (NF-κB), known to be upregulated in microglial cells at sites of inflammation, in inflammatory mediator-induced microglial NGF expression, the effect of the NF-κB inhibitor, pyrrolidine dithiocarbamate (PDTC), was analyzed. In the presence of PDTC, a dose-dependent inhibition of cytokine-activated NGF expression occurred (FIG. 2 A and B). By contrast, the C3a-dependent induction of NGF synthesis does not involve an NF-κB–dependent pathway (FIG. 2 C and D). This suggests that other transcription factors involved in microglial activation, such as AP-1 (activator protein 1) and CREB (cAMP–responsive-element binding protein), contribute to complement-stimulated neurotrophin synthesis in human microglial cells. Our recent observation that the ATP metabolite adenosine, a potent activator of microglial cells, induces microglial NGF mRNA expression and NGF protein release via stimulation of adenosine A2a-receptors indicates that a CREB-sensitive mechanism contributes to adenosine modulation of microglial neurotrophin expression.[21]

In conclusion, our results provide new evidence for a cytokine-NGF cascade involved in inflammatory mediator-induced microglial activation that is modulated by NF-κB–dependent and –independent mechanisms. Intervention in intracellular signaling pathways for microglial neurotrophin production could be a new rational basis for treatment of CNS injury. Preliminary experiments suggest that immunophilin ligands, such as cyclosporin A and FK506, known to elicit neuroprotective actions, enhance microglial neurotrophin expression.

In addition, CSF levels of NGF were found to be significantly elevated in AD patients and to a lesser extent in patients with major depression (DE) (unpublished observations) (see FIGURE 3). We hypothesize that inflammatory-mediated induction of neurotrophins in microglial cells may contribute to elevated NGF levels in the AD brain. This assumption is supported by the abundance of reactive microglia in direct association with neuritic plaques in the AD brain.[22]

As stated above, IL-6 exerts specific effects in the nervous system.[15] IL-6 and IL-6R mRNAs are detected in certain regions of the rat brain, where both genes are developmentally regulated and localized in specific neuronal subtypes. IL-6 neuronal effects are importantly modulated by sIL-6R. Cultured sympathetic and sensory neurons as well as PC12 cells require IL-6 and its soluble receptor for survival, and morphological and biochemical differentiation (for references, see Maerz et al.[23]).

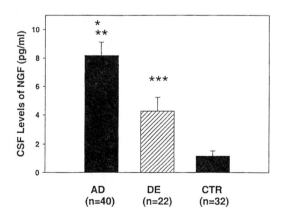

FIGURE 3. NGF levels in the cerebrospinal fluid (CSF) of patients with Alzheimer's disease (AD), major depression in the elderly (DE), and nondemented control subjects (CTR). Levels (pg/ml) are given in means ± SEM. Asterisks (★, ★★, ★★★) indicate significance ($p < 0.05$) (Mann-Whitney U-test). ★, AD vs. DE, $p < 0.02$; ★★, AD vs. CTR, $p < 0.001$; ★★★, DE vs. CTR, $p < 0.01$.

Furthermore, accelerated nerve regeneration occurred in transgenic mice, which had high plasma levels of human IL-6 and sIL-6R.[24] In addition, in wobbler mice, the coadministration of IL-6 and sIL-6R delayed the progression of motor neuron disease.[25]

Similarly, sIL-6R can modulate the responsiveness of astrocytes to IL-6, leading to diverse responses such as region-specific morphological differentiation and neurotrophin production.[26] Treatment of astrocytes from various brain regions of newborn rats with IL-6 and sIL-6R induced expression of neurotrophins of the NGF family in a region-specific manner (see FIGURE 4). NGF is maximally induced in hippocampus and cortex, NT-3 in hippocampus, and NT-4/5 in cortex and cerebellum (not shown). Thus, we propose that elevated IL-6 levels, together with sIL-6R, occurring at sites of inflammation, not only stimulate neurons directly but also act on glial cells, leading to the induction of neurotrophins that promote CNS neuron regeneration (FIG. 1). Our results are of interest with respect to the findings that IL-6 functions as an immune-suppressive cytokine by inhibiting TNF-α–induced astroglia VCAM-1 expression.[27] Because it has been shown that neurotrophins such as NGF and NT-3 inhibit interferon-γ–mediated MHC class II expression in isolated microglia,[28] it can be hypothesized that the IL-6/sIL-6R complex modulates immune responses in the CNS also via neurotrophins.

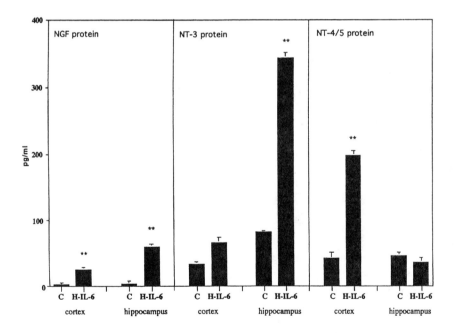

FIGURE 4. Stimulation of neurotrophin release from rat astroglia by hyper-IL-6 (H-IL-6). Rat astroglial cultures were treated for 24 h with medium alone (C = control) or stimulated with H-IL-6 (10 ng/mL). NGF, NT-3, and NT-4/5 protein were determined in the supernatant by ELISA and expressed as mean ± SEM of two independent experiments, each done in duplicate (★★ $p < 0.01$).[26]

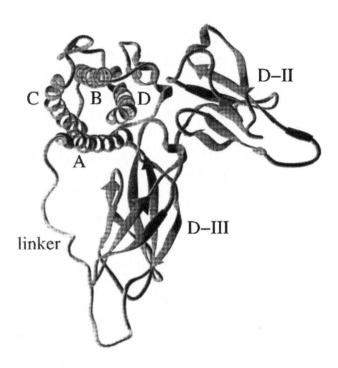

FIGURE 5. Hyper-IL-6: a highly active designer cytokine consisting of IL-6 and soluble IL-6R. Molecular model of the fusion protein of IL-6 and sIL-6R (Hyper-IL-6) consisting of IL-6 and sIL-6R fused by a flexible peptide linker. A, B, C, and D denote the four helices of IL-6; D-II and D-III are the two cytokine-binding receptor domains of the sIL-6R, which were used for the construction of the fusion protein.[23]

However, future studies will have to define whether IL-6/sIL-6R is causative to neurodegenerative events, reflects an ongoing inflammation, or is even a beneficial mediator of an anti-inflammatory response leading to neuroprotection.

Our strategy was to design a highly active fusion protein of IL-6 and sIL-6R, hyper-IL-6R (H-IL-6), in which IL-6 is covalently linked to sIL-6R (see FIGURE 5).[23]

This designer cytokine opens up the possibility of studying the mechanisms of neuroprotective and neuropathological actions of IL-6 in the CNS. Furthermore, such a tool might have considerable therapeutic potential in the treatment of neurodegenerative diseases.

ACKNOWLEDGMENTS

This study was supported by the Swiss National Science Foundation (Grant No. 3100-049397.96-1), by the Deutsche Forschungsgemeinschaft (SFB 505/B5) to U.O., and by grants from the Deutsche Forschungsgemeinschaft (Bonn, Germany) and the Stiftung Innovation Rheinland-Pfalz (Mainz, Germany) to S.R.-J.

REFERENCES

1. BARBACID, M. 1995. Neurotrophic factors and their receptors. Curr. Opin. Cell Biol. **7:** 148–155.
2. CHAO, M.V. & B.L. HEMPSTEAD. 1995. p75 and Trk: a two-receptor system. Trends Neurosci. **18:** 321–326.
3. OTTEN, U. & R.A. GADIENT. 1995. Neurotrophins and cytokines—intermediaries between the immune and nervous systems. Int. J. Dev. Neurosci. **13:** 147–151.
4. LEVI-MONTALCINI, R. *et al.* 1996. Nerve growth factor: from neurotrophin to neurokine. Trends Neurosci. **19:** 514–520.
5. EHRHARD, P.B. *et al.* 1993. Expression of nerve growth factor and nerve growth factor receptor tyrosine kinase Trk in activated CD4-positive T-cell clones. Proc. Natl. Acad. Sci. USA **90:** 10984–10988.
6. LEON, A. *et al.* 1994. Mast cells synthesize, store, and release nerve growth factor. Proc. Natl. Acad. Sci. USA **91:** 3739–3743.
7. BRAUN, A. *et al.* 1998. Role of nerve growth factor in a mouse model of allergic airway inflammation and asthma. Eur. J. Immunol. **28:** 3240–3251.
8. TORCIA, M. *et al.* 1996. Nerve growth factor is an autocrine survival factor for memory B lymphocytes. Cell **85:** 345–356.
9. EHRHARD, P.B. *et al.* 1994. Expression of functional trk protooncogene in human monocytes. Proc. Natl. Acad. Sci. USA **90:** 5423–5427.
10. BURGI, B., U.H. OTTEN, B. OCHENSBERGER, S. RIHS, K. HEESE, P.B. EHRHARD, C.F. IBANEZ & C.A. DAHINDEN. 1996. Basophil priming by neurotrophic factors. Activation through the trk receptor. J. Immunol. **157**(12): 5582–5588.
11. KERSCHENSTEINER, M. *et al.* 1999. Activated human T cells, B cells and monocytes produce brain-derived neurotrophic factor *in vitro* and in inflammatory brain lesions: a neuroprotective role of inflammation? J. Exp. Med. **189:** 865–870.
12. BESSER, M. & R. WANK. 1999. Cutting edge: clonally restricted production of the neurotrophins brain-derived neurotrophic factor and neurotrophin-3 mRNA by human immune cells and Th1/Th2-polarized expression of their receptors. J. Immunol. **162:** 6303–6306.
13. KRAMER, R. *et al.* 1995. Gene transfer through the blood-nerve barrier: nerve growth factor engineered neuritogenic T lymphocytes attenuate experimental autoimmune neuritis. Nature Med. **1:** 1162–1166.
14. TAGA, T. & T. KISHIMOTO. 1997. gp130 and the interleukin-6 family of cytokines. Annu. Rev. Immunol. **15:** 797–819.
15. GADIENT, R.A. & U. OTTEN. 1997. Interleukin-6—a molecule with both beneficial and destructive potentials. Prog. Neurobiol. **52:** 379–390.
16. ROSE-JOHN, S. & P.C. HEINRICH. 1994. Soluble receptors for cytokines and growth factors: generation and biological function. Biochem. J. **300:** 281–290.
17. KREUTZBERG, G.W. 1996. Microglia: a sensor for pathological events in the CNS. Trends Neurosci. **19:** 312–318.
18. GIULIAN, D. 1992. Microglia and disease of the nervous system. Curr. Neurol. **12:** 23–54.
19. MCGEER, P.L. & E.G. MCGEER. 1995. The inflammatory response system of the brain: implications for therapy of Alzheimer and other neurodegenerative diseases. Brain Res. Rev. **21:** 195–218.
20. HEESE, K., C. HOCK & U. OTTEN. 1998. Inflammatory signals induce neurotrophin expression in human microglial cells. J. Neurochem. **70:** 699–707.
21. HEESE, K. *et al.* 1997. Nerve growth factor (NGF) expression in rat microglia is induced by adenosine A_{2a}-receptors. Neurosci. Lett. **231:** 83–86.
22. EIKELENBOOM, P. & R. VEERHUIS. 1996. The role of complement and activated microglia in the pathogenesis of Alzheimer's disease. Neurobiol. Aging **17:** 673–680.
23. MAERZ, P., U. OTTEN & S. ROSE-JOHN. 1999. Neural activities of IL-6-type cytokines often depend on soluble cytokine receptors. Eur. J. Neurosci. **11:** 2995–3004.
24. HIROTA, H. *et al.* 1996. Accelerated nerve regeneration in mice by upregulated expression of IL-6 and IL-6 receptor after trauma. J. Exp. Med. **183:** 2627–2634.

25. IKEDA, K. *et al.* 1996. Coadministration of interleukin-6 (IL-6) and soluble IL-6 receptor delays progression of wobbler mouse motor neuron disease. Brain Res. **726:** 91–97.

26. MAERZ, P. *et al.* 1999. Role of interleukin-6 and soluble IL-6 receptor in region-specific induction of astrocytic differentiation and neurotrophin expression. Glia **26:** 191–200.

27. OH, J.W. *et al.* 1998. Role of IL-6 and soluble IL-6 receptor in inhibition of VCAM-1 gene expression. J. Immunol. **161:** 4992–4999.

28. NEUMANN, H. *et al.* 1998. Neurotrophins inhibit major histocompatibility class II inducibility of microglia: involvement of the p75 neurotrophin receptor. Proc. Natl. Acad. Sci. USA **95:** 5779–5784.

Overproduction of IFN-γ and TNF-α from Natural Killer (NK) Cells Is Associated with Abnormal NK Reactivity and Cognitive Derangement in Alzheimer's Disease

S.B. SOLERTE,[a] L. CRAVELLO, E. FERRARI, AND M. FIORAVANTI

*Department of Internal Medicine, Geriatrics and Gerontology Clinic,
Postgraduate School of Geriatrics, University of Pavia, 27100 Pavia, Italy*

ABSTRACT: Alterations of natural killer (NK) function can be involved in the neuroimmune mechanism of neurodegeneration in dementia of the Alzheimer's type (DAT). NK cell cytotoxicity (NKCC) and the generation and release of IFN-γ and TNF-α (spontaneous and modulated by IL-2) from pure NK cells (CD 16+, CD 56+, CD 3–) were studied together with circulating IFN-γ and TNF-α levels and cognitive function in 22 old patients with DAT and 15 healthy old subjects. Higher ($p < 0.001$) IL-2 modulated NKCC (with IL-2 50 U/mL and 100 U/mL) was demonstrated in DAT patients (+35% and +99% from baseline) than in healthy subjects (+6% and +76% from baseline). Increased spontaneous and IL-2–induced release of IFN-γ and TNF-α from NK cells were found in DAT patients compared to healthy subjects ($p < 0.001$), whereas no difference of serum IFN-γ and TNF-α was demonstrated between DAT and control groups. Significant negative correlations among the spontaneous release of IFN-γ and TNF-α from NK and the decrease of the score of cognitive function (MMSE) were found in patients with DAT. In conclusion, alterations of NKCC control and NK-derived cytokine release in DAT could be involved in the neuroinflammatory mechanism related to the progression of neurodegeneration and dementia.

INTRODUCTION

Neuroimmune-inflammatory components have been associated with the pathogenesis of neurodegeneration in Alzheimer's disease (AD).[1–5] Humoral and cellular immune factors could interact with astrocytes and microglial cells also inducing changes of blood brain barrier (BBB) integrity and permeability.

Among the immune factors, natural killer cells (NK) have been considered with some interest. In fact, it has been suggested that these cells, involved in non-major histocompatibility complex (MHC)–restricted cytotoxic activity against tumoral and viral targets,[6,7] represent a biological marker associated with pathophysiology and diagnosis of AD.[8] We have previously found that NK cells could be abnormally

[a]Address for correspondence: Dr. B. Solerte, Department of Internal Medicine, Geriatrics and Gerontology Clinic, Postgraduate School of Geriatrics, University of Pavia, Piazza Borromeo 2, 27100 Pavia, Italy. Voice: 0039 382 27769; fax: 0039 382 28827.
bsolerte@libero.it

activated in old patients with dementia of the Alzheimer's type (DAT), suggesting a link between NK dysregulation and the neuroimmune mechanism of neurodegeneration.[9–14]

Our hypothesis concerns the possibility that NK functional and molecular alterations found in DAT could also be responsible for changes in the generation and release of TNF-α and IFN-γ from these cells.[15] This suggested evidence could have important consequences because these cytokines may have a role in the development of AD neuropathology[16] by enhancing the production of β–amyloid peptides[17] or by a direct neurotoxic effect against neuronal cells.[18] Moreover TNF-α and IFN-γ may be involved in the impairment of brain glucose metabolism[19] and in the disruption of LTP (long-term potentiation)-dependent learning and memory.[20]

Within this context, we have specifically examined the association of NK cytotoxic activity (NKCC) with circulating and NK-related (spontaneous and modulated by IL-2 and cortisol) release of TNF-α and IFN-γ in old patients with DAT and healthy matched old subjects. The possible correlation between cytokines and the cognitive pattern of DAT patients was also evaluated.

SUBJECTS AND METHODS

Our investigation was approved by the Ethical Committee of the Department of Internal Medicine of the University of Pavia, and written informed consent was obtained from all subjects and patients or, where appropriate, from their caregivers. Fifteen healthy old subjects (9 women and 6 men) and 22 old patients (12 women and 10 men) with dementia of the Alzheimer's type (DAT) were included in the study. Healthy old subjects fulfilled the criteria of the SENIEUR protocol in order to exclude clinical and immunological alterations.[21] The diagnosis of probable or possible DAT was conducted according to the criteria of DSM III-R[22] and confirmed for probable DAT with the diagnostic standards of NINCDS-ADRDA criteria.[23] All patients with DAT had a Hachinski ischemic score of less than 4.[24] Diagnosis of DAT was also supported by clinical and neurological exhamination, by brain imaging (MRI or CT scan), and by the analysis for APOE genotype by DNA genomic extraction of whole blood, amplified by polymerase chain reaction (PCR):[25] three patients had the ε3/ε3 type, 12 had the ε3/ε4 type, and 7 had the ε4/ε4 type. Cognitive status and the severity of dementia were assessed by using the Minimum Mental State Examination test (MMSE);[26] the score of MMSE ranged from 6 to 16 in patients with DAT, and therefore their dementia was classified as moderate to severe. Finally, patients with DAT were free of any medication and of diseases known to affect immune function.

Whole blood was drawn and anticoagulated with 2Na-EDTA for blood count of total lymphocytes, hemoglobin, and hematocrit.

Serum proteins (albumin, prealbumin, transferrin, and retinol binding protein) were determined by immunonephelometry with specific antisera, calibrators, and quality controls (BNA-Nephelometer; Dade Behring, Milano, Italy).

Immunological procedures were conducted in a completely sterile manner by using a class II biological safety cabinet (Microflow 51426, MDH Ltd., Andover, UK). After an overnight fast, peripheral blood mononuclear cells (PBMC) were obtained from heparinized venous blood samples of healthy subjects and patients with DAT. The separation of NK cells was obtained as previously described.[13,14] PBMC were isolated by Ficoll-Hypaque density gradient, and plastic adherent cells and B cells were removed by incubation at 37°C in Petri-culture dishes for 1 hour. The remaining nonadherent cells were passed through nylon wool columns preincubated for 1 h with RPMI 1640 supplemented with 10% heat-inactivated autologous serum (RPMI/AS) at 37°C (% CO_2 in air). T/NK cells were obtained by rinsing the columns with tissue culture medium, which leaves B cells and remaining monocytes attached to the nylon wool. The enriched fraction of PBMC containing T/NK cells was used for the magnetic cell separation procedure (MACS, Miltenyi Biotech GmbH, Bergisch, Gladbach, Germany). The negative unlabeled fraction represents the enriched non-magnetic NK cell fraction (CD 16+, CD 56+, CD 3– cells), whereas the magnetic labeled fraction recognized the non–NK cells (CD 3+, CD 4+, CD 19+, CD 33+ cells). The efficiency of the separation was measured with flow cytometry by using Anti-Leu 11b (anti-CD 16+) and Anti-Leu 19 (anti-CD 56+) antibodies purchased from Becton Dickinson and FACScan (Becton Dickinson, Mountain View, CA, USA). The purity of the NK cell population was of $97 \pm 1\%$, whereas viability was more than 95% (Trypan blue uptake). After magnetic separation, NK cells were washed three times (with 0.9% saline and complete RPMI medium), finally resuspended in complete RPMI 1640 medium (with 10% of heat inactivated fetal calf serum, 1% of glutamine, and 100 µg/mL of gentamycin), and concentrated to a measured density of 7.75×10^6 cells/mL of complete medium. These cells were incubated for 20 h at 37°C in a humidified atmosphere of 95% air and 5% CO_2 (Heraeus incubator BB 6220, Hanau, Germany), without modulators (spontaneous conditions), with IL-2 (50 and 100 U/mL/cells of recombinant human IL-2, Proleukin, Chiron Corporation, Emeryville, USA), cortisol (10^{-6} M/mL/cells of Hydrocortisone, SIGMA Chimica, Milano, Italy), and cortisol coincubated with IL-2 (100 U/mL/cells) in order to measure IL-2–modulated NKCC against tumoral targets K562[13,14,27,28] and to determine the concentrations of TNF-α and IFN-γ released in the supernatant fluids of NK cells. A 500 µL volume of the supernatant fluids of NK cells was centrifuged, and 300 µL of volume was frozen at $-80°C$ until the assay of cytokines. The fluid was resuspended at 4°C and analyzed for TNF-α and IFN-γ content by a standard ELISA procedure (Bender MedSystems Diagnostics GmbH, Wien, Austria). The sensitivity of the method was 0.5 pg/mL for TNF-α and 0.3 pg/mL for IFN-γ; the intraassay precision was below 6%, and the interassay variations were within 5%–8%.

One-way analysis of variance (ANOVA, F-test), paired Student's *t* test, and linear regression analysis with parametric Pearson's correlation coefficient determination were employed for statistical analysis. The threshold of statistical significance was $p < 0.05$ (two-tailed). All the analyses were run with the SPSS, Inc./PC+ version 3.0 statistical package (SPSS, Inc., Chicago, IL, USA).

RESULTS

Clinical and biochemical parameters, serum TNF-α and IFN-γ levels, and NKCC (spontaneous and IL-2–modulated) of healthy old subjects and patients with DAT are summarized in TABLE 1. No differences concerning body weight and the total

TABLE 1. Mean variations of clinical, biochemical, and immunological parameters in healthy old subjects and patients with DAT[a]

	Healthy old subjects	Old patients with DAT	ANOVA F test
n	15.0	22	—
Age (years)	77.0 (6)	76.5 (5.5)	ns
BMI (kg/m^2)	22.2 (1.5)	21.6 (1.2)	ns
Hb, (g/dL)	13.7 (1.2)	13.5 (1.2)	ns
Total lymphocytes (cells/mm^3)	1,949.0 (64)	1,953.0 (56)	ns
Blood glucose (mmol/L)	4.37 (0.58)	4.79 (0.4)	ns
Albumin (g/L)	42.7 (2.9)	41.9 (2.8)	ns
Transferrin (g/L)	3.12 (0.3)	3.13 (0.4)	ns
Prealbumin (g/L)	0.33 (0.05)	0.31 (0.03)	ns
Retinol-binding protein (g/L)	0.042 (0.007)	0.040 (0.006)	ns
NKCC after IL-2, 50 U (% increase)	6.1 (1.3)	35.2 (2.1)	$p < 0.001$
NKCC after IL-2, 100 U (% increase)	76.4 (4.6)	99.1 (6.2)	$p < 0.001$
Serum TNF-α (pg/mL)	3.19 (1.3)	2.36 (1.1)	ns
Serum IFN-γ (pg/mL)	6.43 (2.9)	6.11 (2.7)	ns

ABBREVIATIONS: BMI, body mass index; NKCC, natural killer cell cytotoxicity.
[a]Data are expressed as mean value (standard deviation between brackets).

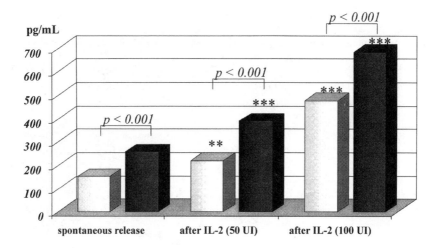

FIGURE 1. Mean variations (±SD) of spontaneous and IL-2–modulated (50 U and 100 U/mL) release of TNF-α in the supernatant fluids of NK cells in healthy old subjects (open bars) and in old patients with dementia of the Alzheimer's type (DAT: closed bars). **$p < 0.01$; ***$p < 0.001$ vs. spontaneous release.

number of lymphocytes, nutritional parameters, and of serum cytokines were found between healthy subjects and DAT patients. In particular, serum TNF-α and IFN-γ levels were similar in the two groups. On the contrary, higher IL-2–modulated NKCC was found in patients with DAT than in healthy old subjects ($p < 0.001$).

FIGURE 1 shows the mean variations of TNF-α release from NK cells (levels in the supernatant fluids of NK) in healthy subjects and in patients with DAT. Higher spontaneous and IL-2–modulated (with 50 and 100 U/mL/cells) TNF-α levels were found in DAT patients than in healthy old subjects ($p < 0.001$).

FIGURE 2 shows the mean variations of IFN-γ release from NK cells (levels in the supernatant fluids of NK) in healthy subjects and in patients with DAT. Higher spontaneous and IL-2–modulated (with 50 and 100 U/mL/cells) IFN-γ levels were found in DAT patients than in healthy old subjects ($p < 0.001$).

FIGURE 3 shows the mean variations of TNF-α and IFN-γ release from NK cells after exposure with cortisol and cortisol plus IL-2 in healthy old subjects and DAT patients. A lower decrease of TNF-α and IFN-γ release from NK after incubation with cortisol and cortisol plus IL-2 was found in patients with DAT (paired Student's *t* test: $p < 0.005$ vs. spontaneous release) than in healthy old subjects. The decrease of TNF-α and IFN-γ release in patients with DAT was completely abolished when cortisol was coincubated with IL-2, 100 U/mL, whereas in healthy subjects the release of cytokines was significantly reduced even during exposure with cortisol plus IL-2 (paired Student's *t* test: $p < 0.001$ vs. spontaneous release).

Significant negative correlations among the spontaneous TNF-α and IFN-γ release from NK and the MMSE score were found in patients with DAT ($y = 31.9 - 0.3x$, $r = -0.85$, $p < 0.001$ for TNF-α; and $y = 31.6 - 0.3x$, $r = -0.74$, $p < 0.001$ for IFN-γ).

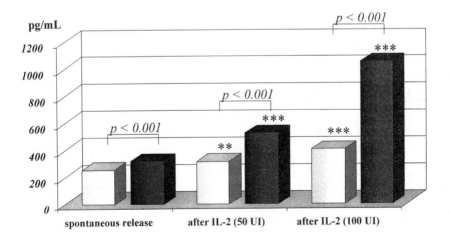

FIGURE 2. Mean variations (±SD) of spontaneous and IL-2–modulated (50 U and 100 U/mL) release of IFN-γ in the supernatant fluids of NK cells in healthy old subjects (open bars) and in old patients with dementia of the Alzheimer's type (DAT: closed bars). **$p < 0.01$; ***$p < 0.001$ vs. spontaneous release.

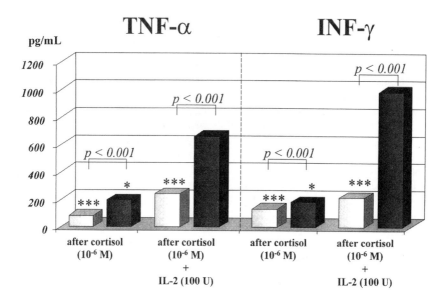

FIGURE 3. Mean variations (±SD) of TNF-α and IFN-γ release in the supernatant fluids of NK cells after exposure with cortisol (10^{-6} M/mL) and cortisol + IL-2 (100 U/mL) in healthy old subjects (open bars) and in old patients with dementia of the Alzheimer's type (DAT: closed bars). $*p < 0.05$; $***p < 0.001$ vs. spontaneous release.

DISCUSSION

Our data have clearly demonstrated an abnormal autocrine production of TNF-α and IFN-γ by pure NK immune cells of patients with moderate to severe DAT. The increased generation of cytokines from NK has been associated with high IL-2–modulated NKCC and with an impairment of the cognitive pattern. Data on NKCC are in agreement with previous studies, indicating an increased cytokine-dependent NK cytotoxic activity in old patients with DAT.[9–14] In these studies the alteration of the NK immune compartment has been suggested to be linked to a dysregulation of transmembrane signaling regulating NK cytotoxic function and dependent on altered downregulation of protein kinase C (PKC)–system activity.[29] On the other hand, the dysregulation of the PKC system has been widely reported in neuronal and nonneuronal cells, suggesting a common molecular defect in the pathophysiology of DAT.[8]

We suggest that the abnormal functional response of NK cells in DAT could also have implications on the autocrine generation and release of inflammatory cytokines, such as TNF-α and IFN-γ directly from NK cells, in particular during IL-2 modulation. In fact, NK activation has been recognized to trigger the release of TNF-α and IFN-γ and of other cytokines with important effects on neuroimmunity, inflammation, and immune response towards viral and tumoral antigens.[7,15,30] Within this context, PKC dysregulation might be responsible for both abnormal NKCC[13] and cytokine generation from NK.[31] Moreover, TNF-α and IFN-γ autocrine overproduction by NK might sustain the increased NKCC response to cytokines arising from the neuroimmune system.[4,15,20] This hypothesis would seem to be confirmed in the present study, since an increased generation of TNF-α and IFN-γ from NK cells has been found in DAT patients either in spontaneous conditions or after IL-2 exposure, whereas the release of TNF-α and IFN-γ was not physiologically suppressed during cortisol incubation. All these experimental observations would seem to introduce new relevant aspects on the neurodegenerative mechanism of DAT. Our hypothesis concerns the possibility that TNF-α and IFN-γ autocrine overproduction by activated NK cells, or by other immune effectors, could induce an enhancer mechanism for AD neurodegeneration involving multiple pathogenetic aspects (see FIGURE 4): neuroimmune-induced alterations,[1–5,20,32,33] increased amyloidogenesis,[17,18] immunovascular and cerebromicrovascular-related alterations,[16,32–35] changes of BBB integrity and permeability with immune infiltration of activated mononuclear and NK cells into the brain,[18,32,33] metabolic disorders (e.g., of glucose delivery and insulin activity) affecting the cholinergic pathway[36–38] regulating learning and memory, and the mechanisms of long-term potentiation (LTP) in the hippocampus.[20] Therefore multiple factors could be linked to the AD neurodegenerative process during exposure of brain parenchyma to TNF-α and IFN-γ produced by peripheral immune cells. The development of diffuse deposits of β-amyloid peptides in brain areas might finally have a feedback role in a vicious cycle to maintain or increase the secretion of proinflammatory cytokines by NK or mononuclear cells migrating across the BBB,[18] so contributing to extend the neuroimmune damage and cognitive impairment.

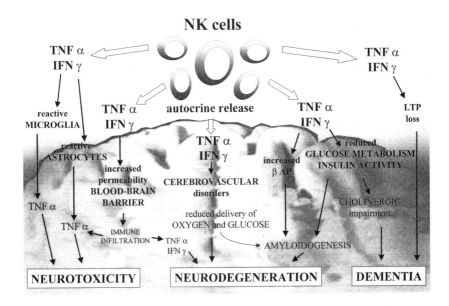

FIGURE 4. Autocrine production of cytokines by NK cells hypothesized as responsible for the enhancer mechanism of Alzheimer's disease neuropathology.

ACKNOWLEDGMENTS

We wish to thank Drs. S. Severgnini and N. Pezza for technical assistance with the immunological and statistical procedures; the work was fully supported by a grant from the University of Pavia (F.A.R. 1998/1999, Comitato 6 and Progetto Ateneo, 2000) .

REFERENCES

1. DICKINSON, D.W. & J. ROGERS. 1992. Neuroimmunology of Alzheimer's disease: a conference report. Neurobiol. Aging **13:** 793–798.
2. AISEN, P.S. & K.L. DAVIS. 1994. Inflammatory mechanisms in Alzheimer's disease: implications for therapy. Am. J. Psychiatry **151:** 1105–1113.
3. HUBERMAN, M., F. SHALIT, I. ROTH-DERI, B. GUTMAN, C. BRODIE, H.E. KO & B. SREDINI. 1994. Correlation of cytokine secretion by mononuclear cells of Alzheimer patients and their disease stage. J. Neuroimmunol. **52:** 147–152.
4. MCGEER, P.L., J. ROGERS & E.G. MCGEER. 1994. Neuroimmune mechanisms in Alzheimer's disease pathogenesis. Alzheimer Dis. Assoc. Disord. **8:** 149–158.
5. SINGH, V.K. 1997. Neuroautoimmunity: pathogenetic implications for Alzheimer's disease. Gerontology **43:** 79–94.
6. ORTALDO, J.R. & R.B. HERBERMAN. 1984. Heterogeneity of natural killer cells. Annu. Rev. Immunol. **2:** 359–373.
7. TRINCHIERI, G. 1989. Biology of natural killer cells. Adv. Immunol. **47:** 187–386.
8. GASPARINI, L., M. RACCHI, G. BINETTI, M. TRABUCCHI, S.B. SOLERTE, D. ALKON, R. ETCHEBERRIGARAY, B. GIBSON, J. BLASS, R. PAOLETTI & S. GOVONI. 1998. Peripheral markers in testing pathophysiological hypotheses and diagnosing Alzheimer's disease. FASEB J. **12:** 17–34.
9. SOLERTE, S.B., M. FIORAVANTI, S. SEVERGINI, M. LOCATELLI, M. RENZULLO, N. PEZZA, N. CERUTTI & E. FERRARI. 1996. Enhanced cytotoxic response of natural killer cells to IL-2 in Alzheimer's disease. Dementia **7:** 343–348.
10. SOLERTE, S.B., M. FIORAVANTI, S. SEVERGNINI, N. CERUTTI, N. PEZZA, M. LOCATELLI, F. TERENZI & E. FERRARI. 1997. Excitatory pattern of γ-interferon on natural killer cell activity in senile dementia of the Alzheimer type. Dement. Geriatr. Cogn. Disord. **8:** 308–313.
11. SOLERTE, S.B., M. FIORAVANTI, S. SEVERGNINI, N. CERUTTI, M. LOCATELLI & E. FERRARI. 1997. Variability of natural killer (NK) cell immune function in normal aging and senile dementia: pathophysiological implications. Aging Clin. Exp. Res. **9**(S4): 32–33.
12. SOLERTE, S.B., N. CERUTTI, S. SEVERGNINI, M. RONDANELLI, E. FERRARI & M. FIORAVANTI. 1998. Decreased immunosuppressive effect of cortisol on natural killer cytotoxic activity in senile dementia of the Alzheimer's type. Dement. Geriatr. Cogn. Disord. **9:** 149–156.
13. SOLERTE, S.B., M. FIORAVANTI, A. PASCALE, E. FERRARI, S. GOVONI & F. BATTAINI. 1998. Increased natural killer cell cytotoxicity in Alzheimer's disease may involve protein kinase C dysregulation. Neurobiol. Aging **19:** 191–199.
14. SOLERTE, S.B., M. FIORAVANTI, N. SCHIFINO, G. CUZZONI, I. FONTANA, G. VIGNATI, S. GOVONI & E. FERRARI. 1999. Dehydroepiandrosterone sulfate decreases the interleukin-2–mediated overactivity of the natural killer cell compartment in senile dementia of the Alzheimer type. Dement. Geriatr. Cogn. Disord. **10:** 21–27.
15. JEWETT, A. & B. BONAVIDA. 1993. Pivotal role of endogenous TNF-α in the IL-2 driven activation and proliferation of the functionally immune NK "free" subset. Cell. Immunol. **151:** 257–263.
16. BUEE, L., P.R. HOF & A. DELACOURTE. 1997. Brain microvascular changes in Alzheimer's disease and other dementias. Ann. N.Y. Acad. Sci. **826:** 7–24.

17. BLASKO, I., F. MARX, F. STEINER, T. HARTMAN & B. GRUBECK-LOEBENSTEIN. 1999. TNFα plus IFNγ induce the production of Alzheimer β-amyloid peptides and decrease the secretion of APPs. FASEB J. **13:** 63–68.

18. FIALA, M., L. ZHANG, X. GAN, M.C. GRAVES, S. HAMA, B. SHERRY, D. TAUB, D. WAY, M. WEINAND, M. WITTE, D. LORTON, Y.-M. KUO & A.E. ROHER. 1998. Amyloid-β induces chemokine secretion and monocyte migration across a blood-brain barrier model. Mol. Med. **4:** 480–489.

19. BOADO, R.J., L. WANG & W.M. PARDRIGE. 1994. Enhanced expression of the blood-brain barrier GLUT1 glucose transporter gene by brain-derived factors. Mol. Brain Res. **22:** 259–267.

20. SEI, Y., L. VITKOVIC & M.M. YOKOYAMA. 1995. Cytokines in the central nervous system: regulatory roles in neuronal function, cell death and repair. Neuroimmunomodulation **2:** 121–133.

21. LIGHTHART, G.J., J.X. CORBERAND, C. FOURNIER, P. GALANAUD, W. HIJMANS, B. KENNES, H.F. MULLER-HERMELINK & G.C. STEINMAN. 1984. Admission criteria for immunogerontological studies in man: the SENIEUR protocol. Mech. Aging Dev. **28:** 47–55.

22. AMERICAN PSYCHIATRIC ASSOCIATION. 1987. Diagnostic and Statistical Manual of Mental Disorders. Third Edition. Revised. Washington DC: American Psychiatric Association.

23. MCKHANN, G., D. DRACHMAN, M. FOLSTEIN, R. KATZMANN, D. PRICE & E.M. STADLAN. 1984. Clinical diagnosis of Alzheimer's disease: report of the NINCDS-ADRDA Workgroup under the auspices of Department of Health and Human Services Task Force on Alzheimer's disease. Neurology **34:** 939–944.

24. HACHINSKI, V.C., N.A. LASSEN & J. MARSHALL. 1974. Multiinfarct dementia: a cause of mental deterioration in the elderly. Lancet **ii:** 207–210.

25. WEHHAM, P.R., W.H. PRICE & G. BLUNDELL. 1991. Apolipoprotein E genotyping by one-stage PCR. Lancet **ii:** 1158–1159.

26. FOLSTEIN, M., S. FOLSTEIN & P.R. MCHUGH. 1975. Mini Mental State. A practical method for grading the cognitive state of patients for the clinician. J. Psychiatr. Res. **12:** 189–198.

27. KORZENIEWSKI, C. & D.M. CALLEWAERT. 1983. An enzyme-release assay for natural cytotoxicity. J. Immunol. Methods **64:** 313–320.

28. PROSS, H. & M. BAYNES. 1977. Spontaneous human lymphocyte mediated cytotoxicity against tumor target cells. A short review. Cancer Immunol. Immunother. **3:** 75–85.

29. LEIBSON, P.J., D.E. MIDTHUN, K.P. WINDEBANK & R.T. ABRAHAM. 1990. Transmembrane signaling during natural killer cell-mediated cytotoxicity. Regulation by protein kinase C activation. J. Immunol. **145:** 1498–1504.

30. CUTURI, M.C., I. ANEGON, F. SHERMAN, R. LOUDON, S.C. CLARK, B. PERUSSIA & G. TRINCHIERI. 1989. Production of hematopoietic colony-stimulating factor by human natural killer cells. J. Exp. Med. **169:** 569–583.

31. KLEGERIS, A., D.G. WALKER & P.L. MCGEER. 1997. Interaction of Alzheimer β-amyloid peptide with the human monocytic cell line THP-1 results in a protein kinase C-dependent secretion of tumor necrosis factor-α. Brain Res. **747:** 114–121.

32. MUNOZ-FERNANDEZ, M.A. & M. FRESNO. 1998. The role of tumor necrosis factor, interleukin 6, interferon-γ and inducible nitric oxide synthase in the development and pathology of the nervous system. Prog. Neurobiol. **56:** 307–340.

33. HARDY, J.A., D.M.A. MANN, P. WESTER & B. WINBLAD. 1986. An integrative hypothesis concerning the pathogenesis and progression of Alzheimer's disease. Neurobiol. Aging **7:** 489–502.

34. SOLERTE, S.B., G. CERESINI, E. FERRARI & M. FIORAVANTI. 2000. Hemorheologic changes and overproduction of cytokines in mild to moderate dementia of the Alzheimer's type: adverse effects on cerebrovascular system and therapeutic approach with pentoxifylline. Neurobiol. Aging. **21:** 271–281.

35. DE LA TORRE, J.C. 1997. Cerebromicrovascular pathology in Alzheimer's disease compared to normal aging. Gerontology **43:** 26–43.

36. KALARIA, R.N. & S.I. HARIK. 1989. Reduced glucose transporter at the blood-brain barrier in cerebral cortex in Alzheimer's disease. J. Neurochem. **53:** 1083–1088.
37. MARCUS, D.L., M. DE LEON, J. GOLDMAN, J. LOGAN, D. CHRISTMAN, A. WOLF, J. FOWLER, K. HUNTER, J. TSAI, J. PEARSON & M.L. FREEDMAN. 1989. Altered glucose metabolism in microvessels from patients with Alzheimer's disease. Ann. Neurol. **26:** 91–94.
38. MEIER-RUGE, W.A. & C. BERTONI-FREDDARI. 1999. Mitochondrial genome lesions in the pathogenesis of sporadic Alzheimer's disease. Gerontology **40:** 246–252.

Beneficial Autoimmune T Cells and Posttraumatic Neuroprotection

MICHAL SCHWARTZ[a]

Department of Neurobiology, The Weizmann Institute of Science, 76100 Rehovot, Israel

ABSTRACT: Injuries of the central nervous system (CNS) lead to an inevitable and irreversible loss of function because of the lack of neurogenesis, poor regeneration, and the spread of degeneration. In most tissues, protection and repair are the function of the immune system. It has long been thought that this does not apply to the CNS, where—because of its immune-privileged character—any immune activity was assumed to be detrimental. We have recently proposed, however, that provided care is taken to avoid the attendant risks, both repair and protection of injured CNS neurons can benefit from immune intervention. In the following I will summarize the data that led to this concept and describe the evidence supporting it.

BACKGROUND

Central Nervous System Injuries

Injuries in the central nervous system (CNS) often lead to an irreversible loss of function. If the primary site of an injury is the cell body, then the loss of function is inevitable, as functional recovery would necessitate neurogenesis, which does not occur in the CNS of adult mammals. If the primary injury is to the nerve fiber, then poor axonal regeneration and the spread of degenerative damage both anterogradely (towards the target organ) and retrogradely (to the cell body) will eventually end in cell body death.[1]

Recovery after axonal injury is theoretically possible if we could find a way to facilitate regeneration.[2–10] Studies have shown that some regeneration does occur spontaneously after axonal injury, but to an extent that is far from achieving any recovery of function. In many nerve injuries, some neurons are directly affected by the primary insult and immediately undergo degeneration, whereas others—which escaped the primary injury—are affected by the toxic environment created by the degenerating neurons and therefore eventually degenerate as well. Thus, the loss of function after traumatic injury is the outcome of a self-propagating process of degeneration. The question then arises: Can this process of degeneration be halted, allowing the rescue of at least some function?

In most tissues, the spread of injury-induced damage is an outcome of cytotoxicity and subsequent phagocytosis, both of which are integral parts of the healing process that occurs in response to the injury. Tissues that undergo irreparable damage in

[a]Address for correspondence: Michal Schwartz, Department of Neurobiology, The Weizmann Institute of Science, 76100 Rehovot, Israel. Voice: 972-8-9342467; fax: 972-8-9344131. bnschwartz@wiccmail.weizmann.ac.il

the course of this aggressive recovery process are readily replaced. In the injured CNS, however, such an aggressive course of recovery would probably do more harm than good, as any nervous tissue that was irreparably damaged in the process would be irreplaceable.

Attempts are now being made to identify the mediators of cytotoxicity that contribute to the secondary degeneration of neurons in the injured CNS, and to minimize their effects by neutralizing them, competing with them, or increasing tissue resistance to them.[11–15]

The Immune-Privileged Character of the CNS

The phenomenon of immune privilege in the mammalian CNS is thought to derive from an evolutionary adaptation that restricts immune responses within the CNS.[16] Several mechanisms contribute to the status of the CNS as a site of immune activity of unique and possibly autonomous character. The most prominent of these mechanisms is the blood–brain barrier, an anatomical and physiological barrier that keeps intruders from entering the CNS.[17] Another mechanism is an immunological barrier, manifested by (1) the reduced expression of major histocompatibility complex class I and class II antigens on certain cells in the CNS,[18,19] and (2) an immunosuppressive microenvironment that contains, for example, astrocytes that suppress or anergize invading T cells,[20] as well as locally produced factors that suppress and regulate immune responses in the CNS.[21–23] These two barriers, which limit both the entry of immune cells into the CNS and their activity there, are thought to protect against remodeling of the dynamic and complex neural network of the brain.

In tissues other than the CNS, immune responses have a pivotal role in protection and repair. This raises the following questions: Does the CNS, like other tissues, depend on immune responses for its protection and repair, particularly after injury? If so, is the restricted activity of CNS-resistant immune cells sufficient for this purpose? The data presented in this article suggest that the injured CNS does indeed require immune intervention in order to limit damage and activate healing but that under normal circumstances such intervention is limited in the CNS, possibly because of the restrictions imposed by its immune-privileged character.[1,24] Specifically, I will show that in spite of the fact that the CNS is a site of restricted immune activity, its recovery from traumatic axonal injury is promoted by autoimmune T cells directed against CNS-associated proteins, such as myelin basic protein.

RECENT FINDINGS CONCERNING IMMUNE ACTIVITY IN THE CNS

Attempts to minimize the spread of degeneration after axonal injury, using the rat optic nerve or the rat spinal cord as a model, have yielded some insights into the mechanisms involved in degeneration and have led to the identification of specific molecules with neuroprotective properties.[11,25,26] With regard to the role played by the immune system in the spread of posttraumatic damage, there are opposing observations. Some data appear to support the notion that at least the innate arm, represented by the activity of macrophages, is destructive.[27–29] For regrowth, however, active macrophages/microglia appear to be important.[6,7,10,30] This would support our contention that there could be a conflict between the inflammation that interferes with CNS protection and the inflammation required for CNS repair.[24,29] With regard to the adaptive arm of the immune response, represented by T-cell activity, the general belief until recently was that injury awakens an autoimmune response, which is likely to be detrimental. We provide evidence that in the context of CNS axonal injury, autoimmune T cells can be beneficial.

Passive Transfer of Autoimmune T Cells Specific to CNS Antigen(s) Limits Secondary Degeneration

When activated, T cells can kill their target cells or produce signaling molecules that activate or suppress the growth, movement, or differentiation of other cells. Thus, T cells are involved in protecting the individual against foreign invaders as well as in maintaining body function. The blood–brain barrier of the CNS is normally impermeable to resting T cells, but memory T cells do patrol the CNS. They do not, however, accumulate in the healthy CNS, unless they recognize and are able to react to their specific antigen there.[31]

Comparative studies of the T-cell response at the sites of injury of optic nerve and sciatic nerve (used as models for injury of the CNS and of the peripheral nervous system (PNS), respectively), using T-cell immunocytochemistry, have revealed a significantly greater accumulation of endogenous T cells in the injured PNS than in the injured CNS.[32,33] Moreover, the CNS shows a marked propensity for elimination of T cells via apoptosis, whereas this mechanism is less effective in the PNS and is almost absent in other tissues such as muscle and skin. These findings suggest that the T-cell response in the traumatized CNS is both restricted and tightly regulated. Is this limitation in T-cell response disadvantageous for the CNS?

To determine whether the accumulation of T cells is beneficial or harmful to the injured CNS, we used an experimental model of a partial lesion of the rat optic nerve, in which maintenance of the nerve after traumatic axonal injury can be assessed. Axonal injury was followed by a transient accumulation of endogenous T cells at the site of the lesion. Passive administration of activated syngeneic T cells specific to a CNS self-antigen, such as myelin basic protein (MBP), as well as of T cells specific to the foreign antigen ovalbumin (OVA), resulted in an increased local accumulation of T cells.[33–35] Although both T-cell lines accumulated at the site of the lesion, there was a clear difference in their effects on the neuroprotection of the damaged tissue in terms of their ability to affect the progression of secondary degeneration. Two weeks after injury, rats injected with the anti-MBP T cells showed significantly less secondary degeneration than rats injected with phosphate-buffered saline (PBS) or with T cells specific to OVA. This was demonstrated using criteria derived from morphometric and electrophysiological studies.[34] Thus, both the numbers of viable retinal ganglion cells and the degree of optic nerve conduction (measured by its compound action potential) were significantly higher in the rats injected with anti-MBP T cells than in the other groups of rats.[34] This neuroprotective effect was discernible despite the transient induction by the anti-MBP T cells of a monophasic paralytic disease known as experimental autoimmune encephalomyelitis (EAE).

Interestingly, the protection of neurons from secondary degeneration was not related to the intrinsic pathogenicity of the anti-MBP T cells. The disease induced by T cells specific to a cryptic epitope of MBP, p51-70, was significantly milder, if seen at all, than the EAE induced by the highly pathogenic anti-MBP T-cell line, but the T cells directed against the cryptic epitope were as effective as those against the encephalitic epitope in reducing secondary degeneration.[34] Thus, induction of clinical autoimmune disease was not a prerequisite for the protection against secondary degeneration mediated by the anti-MBP T cells.

It is not yet fully understood how the anti-MBP T cells arrest the progression of secondary degeneration, although it is known that T cells can synthesize cytokines and neurotrophic factors.[36–38] Myelin in the crushed nerves undergoes degeneration, and its exposure could therefore stimulate the anti-MBP T cells to secrete an array of neurotrophic factors.[25] Using K252a, a compound that inhibits the signal transduction pathway associated with neurotrophic activation, we have shown that immune neuroprotection by the autoimmune T cells indeed involves neurotrophic factors.[35]

The results of our studies on the rat spinal cord were similar to those we obtained in the rat optic nerve. The autoimmune anti-MBP T cells, in spite of causing a transient paralytic response when passively transferred, were found to be capable of protecting against the devastating outcome of spinal contusion. The observed protection coincided with the phase of peak accumulation of the cells, and thus with the peak severity of the experimental disease. Protection was manifested by a significantly lower functional motor deficit after spinal cord contusion (at the level of T7-T8 or T8-T9) in rats treated by passive transfer of anti-MBP T cells than in untreated rats. The beneficial effect of the T cells in protecting the contused spinal cord from the spread of damage was evident not only according to behavioral criteria, but also morphologically, as indicated by retrograde labeling of the relevant brain cells by a dye applied below the site of the lesion. It was further confirmed by diffusion MRI and by immunocytochemistry.[39]

Endogenous Autoimmunity following CNS Injury

A pertinent question arises from our findings: Is the injury-induced physiological response of T cells to MBP beneficial in its effect but insufficient for significant neuroprotection, or is it harmful and in need of modulation? Popovich and his colleagues showed that spinal cord injury in rats awakens a systemic T-cell response directed against MBP.[40–42] More recently, anti-MBP T cells were detected in patients with spinal cord injury, much like the finding in patients with multiple sclerosis.[43] It therefore seems that autoimmunity is awakened in response to CNS injury, and may even have a beneficial effect on the damaged nerve despite the long-held belief that potentially pathogenic T cells are not likely to be found in healthy individuals.[44,45] In fact, anti-MBP T cells do exist in healthy individuals, not only in patients suffering from multiple sclerosis.[46–48] Indeed, myelin components appear to be prominent among the limited set of self-antigens to which autoimmunity naturally exists.[49]

Recent evidence suggests that inflammation in the CNS is associated with an altered presentation of endogenous MBP, resulting in the activation of T cells directed to cryptic epitopes that may be hidden in intact nerves. Epitopes that are not accessible in the intact CNS might become sufficiently accessible after injury to be detected by receptor-bearing T cells. This might explain the similarity in the neuroprotective effects induced by the anti-p51-70 T cells and the anti-MBP T cells, despite their different effects in the intact CNS. Accordingly, it might be worth seeking ways to augment a beneficial autoimmune response therapeutically without triggering a persisting autoimmune disease. Such boosting might be achieved, for example, by employing T cells specific to the self-antigenic epitopes normally sequestered in the intact CNS. These autoimmune T cells would not accumulate in or interact with undamaged sites, and thus would not induce disease, yet they might be able to assist in the repair of injured CNS tissue if the covert epitope is exposed by the injury.

CONCLUDING REMARKS

Until recently, autoimmune T cells were considered to be detrimental only, but the experiments described here show that they can be neuroprotective. Our results suggest that the dialogue between the immune and the nervous system should be re-examined. The findings, beyond their implications for CNS trauma and its treatment, may have a wider significance in the context of nonpathogenic tissue damage. It is conceivable that tissue damage awakens a T-cell response that, in the absence of pathogens, is directed against self-antigens associated with the tissue at the lesion site. Such a response may represent a physiological response that is beneficial for the organism and which can be controlled exogenously so as to avoid any side effects of the benign autoimmunity in the form of autoimmune disease.

REFERENCES

1. SCHWARTZ, M., G. MOALEM, R. LEIBOWITZ-AMIT & I.R. COHEN. 1999. Innate and adaptive immune responses can be beneficial for CNS repair. Trends Neurosci. 22(7): 295–299.
2. CARONI, P. & M.E. SCHWAB. 1988. Antibody against myelin-associated inhibitor of neurite growth neutralizes nonpermissive substrate properties of CNS white matter. Neuron 1(1): 85–96.
3. CHENG, H., Y. CAO & L. OLSON. 1996. Spinal cord repair in adult paraplegic rats: partial restoration of hind limb function [see comments]. Science 273(5274): 510–513.
4. KALB, L. & YARG. 1995. Recovery from spinal cord injury: New approaches. The Neuroscientist 1(6): 321–327.
5. NEUMANN, S. & C.J. WOOLF. 1999. Regeneration of dorsal column fibers into and beyond the lesion site following adult spinal cord injury [In Process Citation]. Neuron 23(1): 83–91.
6. PREWITT, C.M., I.R. NIESMAN, C.J. KANE & J.D. HOULE. 1997. Activated macrophage/microglial cells can promote the regeneration of sensory axons into the injured spinal cord. Exp. Neurol. 148(2): 433–443.
7. RABCHEVSKY, A.G & W.J. STREIT. 1997. Grafting of cultured microglial cells into the lesioned spinal cord of adult rats enhances neurite outgrowth. J. Neurosci. Res. 47(1): 34–48.
8. REIER, P.J., B.T. STOKES, F.J. THOMPSON & D.K. ANDERSON. 1992. Fetal cell grafts into resection and contusion/compression injuries of the rat and cat spinal cord. Exp. Neurol. 115(1): 177–188.
9. WANG, X.M., J.R. TERMAN & G.F. MARTIN. 1998. Regeneration of supraspinal axons after transection of the thoracic spinal cord in the developing opossum, *Didelphis virginiana*. J. Comp. Neurol. 398(1): 83–97.
10. RAPALINO, O., O. LAZAROV-SPIEGLER, E. AGRANOV et al. 1998. Implantation of stimulated homologous macrophages results in partial recovery of paraplegic rats. Nature Med. 4: 814–821.

11. YOLES, E. & M. SCHWARTZ. 1998. Degeneration of spared axons following partial white matter lesion: Implications for optic nerve neuropathies. Exp. Neurol. **153**(1): 1–7.

12. WAXMAN, S.G. 1993. Molecular and cellular organization of the central nervous system: implications for new therapeutics. Res. Publ. Assoc. Res. Nerv. Ment. Dis. **71**(3): 1–21.

13. THIO, C.L., S.G. WAXMAN & H. SONTHEIMER. 1993. Ion channels in spinal cord astrocytes *in vitro*. III. Modulation of channel expression by coculture with neurons and neuron-conditioned medium. J. Neurophysiol. **69**(3): 819–831.

14. SANNER, C.A., T.J. CUNNINGHAM & M.E. GOLDBERGER. 1994. NMDA receptor blockade rescues Clarke's and red nucleus neurons after spinal hemisection. J. Neurosci. **14**(11 Pt 1): 6472–6480.

15. PANTER, S.S., S.W. YUM & A.I. FADEN. 1990. Alteration in extracellular amino acids after traumatic spinal cord injury [see comments]. Ann. Neurol. **27**(1): 96–99.

16. STREILEIN, J.W. 1995. Unraveling immune privilege [comment]. Science **270**(5239): 1158–1159.

17. REESE, T.S. & M.J. KARNOVSKY. 1967. Fine structural localization of a blood-brain-barrier to exogenous peroxidase. J. Cell Biol. **34**(1): 207–217.

18. MATSUMOTO, Y., N. HARA, R. TANAKA & M. FUJIWARA. 1986. Immunohistochemical analysis of the rat central nervous system during experimental allergic encephalomyelitis, with special reference to Ia-positive cells with dendritic morphology. J. Immunol. **136**(10): 3668–3676.

19. WUCHERPFENNIG, K.W. 1994. Autoimmunity in the central nervous system: mechanisms of antigen presentation and recognition. Clin. Immunol. Immunopathol. **72**(3): 293–306.

20. HAILER, N.P., F.L. HEPPNER, D. HAAS & R. NITSCH. 1997. Fluorescent dye prelabelled microglial cells migrate into organotypic hippocampal slice cultures and ramify. Eur. J. Neurosci. **9**(4): 863–866.

21. WILBANKS, G.A. & J.W. STREILEIN. 1992. Fluids from immune privileged sites endow macrophages with the capacity to induce antigen-specific immune deviation via a mechanism involving transforming growth factor-beta. Eur. J. Immunol. **22**(4): 1031–1036.

22. STREILEIN, J.W. 1993. Immune privilege as the result of local tissue barriers and immunosuppressive microenvironments. Curr. Opin. Immunol. **5**(3): 428–432.

23. STREILEIN, J.W. 1995. Unraveling immune privilege. Science **270**: 1158–1159.

24. LOTAN, M. & M. SCHWARTZ. 1994. Cross talk between the immune system and the nervous system in response to injury: implications for regeneration. FASEB J. **8**(13): 1026–1033.

25. YOLES, E. & M. SCHWARTZ. 1998. Elevation of intraocular glutamate levels in rats with partial lesion of the optic nerve. Arch. Ophthalmol. **116**(7): 906–910.

26. YOLES, E. & M. SCHWARTZ. 1997. *N*-methyl-D-aspartate-receptor antagonist protects neurons from secondary degeneration after partial optic nerve crush. J. Neurotrauma **14**: 665–675.

27. CONSTANTINI, S. & W. YOUNG. 1994. The effects of methylprednisolone and the ganglioside GM1 on acute spinal cord injury in rats. J. Neurosurg. **80**(1): 97–111.

28. POPOVICH, P.G., Z. GUAN, P. WEI, I. HUITINGA, N. VAN ROOIJEN & B.T. STOKES. 1999. Depletion of hematogenous macrophages promotes partial hindlimb recovery and neuroanatomical repair after experimental spinal cord injury. Exp. Neurol. **158**(2): 351–365.

29. HIRSCHBERG, D.L. & M. SCHWARTZ. 1995. Macrophage recruitment to acutely injured central nervous system is inhibited by a resident factor: a basis for an immune-brain barrier. J. Neuroimmunol. **61**(1): 89–96.

30. LAZAROV-SPIEGLER, O., A.S. SOLOMON, A.B. ZEEV BRANN, D.L. HIRSCHBERG, V. LAVIE & M. SCHWARTZ. 1996. Transplantation of activated macrophages overcomes central nervous system regrowth failure. FASEB J. **10**(11): 1296–1302.

31. HICKEY, W.F., B.L. HSU & H. KIMURA. 1991. T-lymphocyte entry into the central nervous system. J. Neurosci. Res. **28**(2): 254–260.

32. HIRSCHBERG, D.L., G. MOALEM, J. HE, F. MOR, I.R. COHEN & M. SCHWARTZ. 1998. Accumulation of passively transferred primed T cells independently of their antigen specificity following central nervous system trauma. J. Neuroimmunol. **89:** 88–96.

33. MOALEM, G., A. MONSONEGO, Y. SHANI, I.R. COHEN & M. SCHWARTZ. 1999. Differential T cell response in central and peripheral nerve injury: connection with immune privilege. FASEB J. **13**(10): 1207–1217.

34. MOALEM, G., R. LEIBOWITZ-AMIT, E. YOLES, F. MOR, I.R. COHEN & M. SCHWARTZ. 1999. Autoimmune T cells protect neurons from secondary degeneration after central nervous system axotomy. Nature Med. **5**(1): 49–55.

35. MOALEM, G., A. GDALYAHU, R. LEIBOWITZ-AMIT et al. 2000. Autoimmune T cells retard the loss of function in injured rat optic nerves: possible role of T cell–derived neurotrophins. J. Autoimmunity. In press.

36. EHRHARD, P.B., P. ERB, U. GRAUMANN & U. OTTEN. 1993. Expression of nerve growth factor and nerve growth factor receptor tyrosine kinase Trk in activated CD4-positive T-cell clones. Proc. Natl. Acad. Sci. USA **90**(23): 10984–10988.

37. LAMBIASE, A., L. BRACCI LAUDIERO, S. BONINI et al. 1997. Human CD4+ T cell clones produce and release nerve growth factor and express high-affinity nerve growth factor receptors. J. Allergy Clin. Immunol. **100**(3): 408–414.

38. SANTAMBROGIO, L., M. BENEDETTI, M.V CHAO, R. MUZAFFAR, K. KULIG, N. GABELLINI & G. HOCHWALD. 1994. Nerve growth factor production by lymphocytes. J. Immunol. **153:** 4488–4495.

39. HAUBEN, E., U. NEVO, E. YOLES et al. 1999. Autoimmune T cells as potential neuroprotective therapy for spinal cord injury. Lancet **355:** 286–287.

40. POPOVICH, P.G., B.T. STOKES & C.C. WHITACRE. 1996. Concept of autoimmunity following spinal cord injury: possible roles for T lymphocytes in the traumatized central nervous system. J. Neurosci. Res. **45**(4): 349–363.

41. POPOVICH, P.G., P. WEI & B.T. STOKES. 1997. Cellular inflammatory response after spinal cord injury in Sprague-Dawley and Lewis rats. J. Comp. Neurol. **377**(3): 443–464.

42. POPOVICH, P.G., C.C. WHITACRE & B.T. STOKES. 1998. Is spinal cord injury an autoimmune disease? Neuroscientist **4**(2): 71–76.

43. KIL, K., Y.C. ZANG, D. YANG et al. 1999. T cell responses to myelin basic protein in patients with spinal cord injury and multiple sclerosis. J. Neuroimmunol. **98**(2): 201–207.

44. BURNET, F.M. 1971. "Self-recognition" in colonial marine forms and flowering plants in relation to the evolution of immunity. Nature **232**(5308): 230–235.

45. BURNET, M. 1959. The clonal selection theory of acquired immunity.

46. BURNS, J., A. ROSENZWEIG, B. ZWEIMAN & R.P. LISAK. 1983. Isolation of myelin basic protein-reactive T-cell lines from normal human blood. Cell. Immunol. **81**(2): 435–440.

47. PETTE, M., K. FUJITA, D. WILKINSON et al. 1990. Myelin autoreactivity in multiple sclerosis: recognition of myelin basic protein in the context of HLA-DR2 products by T lymphocytes of multiple-sclerosis patients and healthy donors. Proc. Natl. Acad. Sci. USA **87**(20): 7968–7972.

48. SCHLUESENER, H.J. & H. WEKERLE. 1985. T lymphocyte lines recognizing the encephalitogenic region of myelin basic protein: in vitro selection from unprimed rat T lymphocyte populations. J. Immunol. **135**(5): 3128–3133.

49. COHEN, I.R. 1992. The cognitive paradigm and the immunological homunculus. Immunol. Today **13**(12): 490–494.

Feedsidewards: Intermodulation (Strictly) among Time Structures, Chronomes, in and around Us, and Cosmo-vasculo-neuroimmunity

About Ten-yearly Changes: What Galileo Missed and Schwabe Found

FRANZ HALBERG,[a,b] GERMAINE CORNÉLISSEN,[a] GEORGE KATINAS,[a] YOSHIHIKO WATANABE,[c] KUNIAKI OTSUKA,[c] CRISTINA MAGGIONI,[d] FEDERICO PERFETTO,[e] ROBERTO TARQUINI,[e] OTHILD SCHWARTZKOPFF,[a] AND EARL E. BAKKEN[f]

[a]University of Minnesota, Minneapolis, Minnesota 55455, USA

[c]Tokyo Women's Medical University, Tokyo, Japan

[d]University of Milan, Milan, Italy

[e]University of Florence, Florence, Italy

[f]North Hawaii Community Hospital Inc., Kamuela, Hawaii, USA

ABSTRACT: The spectrum of biological rhythms is extended far beyond circadians, circannuals, and ultradians, such as 1.5-hourly melatonin and 8-hourly endothelin-1 (ET-1) rhythms by statistics of natality, growth, morbidity, and mortality, some covering decades or centuries on millions of individuals. These reveal infradian cycles to be aligned with half-weekly rhythms in ET-1, weekly and half-yearly ones in melatonin, and even longer—about 50-, about 20-, and about 10-year cycles found in birth statistics. About daily, weekly, yearly, and ten-yearly patterns are also found in mortality from myocardial infarctions; the 10-yearly ones are also in heart rate and its variability; in steroid excretion, an aspect of resistance, for example, to bacteria; and in the genetic changes of the bacteria themselves. Automatic physiological measurements cover years and, in one case, cover a decade; the latter reveal an about 10-year (circadecennial) cycle. ECGs, covering months beat-to-beat, reveal circaseptans, gaining prominence in response to magnetic storms or after coronary artery bypass grafting. A spectrum including cycles from fractions of 1 Hz to circasemicentennians is just one element in biological time structures, chronomes. Chaos, trends, and any unresolved variability are the second to fourth elements of chronomes. Intermodulations, feedsidewards, account for rhythmically and thus predictably recurring quantitative differences and even for opposite treatment effects of the same total dose(s) of (1) immunomodulators inhibiting or stimulating DNA labeling of bone in health or speeding up versus slowing down a malignant growth and thus shortening or lengthening survival time, or

[b]Address for correspondence: Dr. Franz Halberg, Professor of Laboratory Medicine and Pathology, Physiology, Biology, Bioengineering and Oral Medicine, Director, Halberg Chronobiology Center, University of Minnesota, 715 Mayo Building, Mayo Mail Code 8609, 420 Delaware St. S.E., Minneapolis, MN 55455. Voice: 612- 624-6976; fax: 612- 624-9989.
halbe001@tc.umn.edu

(2) raising or lowering blood pressure or heart rate in the vascular aspect of the body's defense. Latitude-dependent competing photic and nonphotic solar effects upon the pineal are gauged by alternating yearly (by daylight) and half-yearly (by night) signatures of circulating melatonin at middle latitudes and by half-yearly signatures at noon near the pole. These many (including novel near 10-yearly) changes, for example, in 17-ketosteroid excretion, heart rate, heart rate variability, and myocardial infarction in us and those galactic, solar, and geophysical ones around us have their own special signatures and contribute to a cosmo-vasculo-immunity and, if that fails, to a cosmo(immuno?) pathology.

CHRONOMES: FEEDSIDEWARDS AND MODULATION IN A STRICT SENSE

In a rhythmic system, modulating effects can be exerted upon the mean, the extent of change, and upon its timing. Accordingly, we may quantify, respectively, mean (superposition) and amplitude- or frequency-modulations, the latter two along a multitude of frequencies. Cyclic environmental magnetic pulsations are found in the approximate ranges of EEG and ECG frequencies at one extreme and at the other extreme in relatively low frequency phenomena, such as a near 10-year cycle, that corresponds at least numerically to the sunspot cycle that Galileo, Scheinert, Fabricius, and Harriot missed, but that the pharmacist Samuel Heinrich Schwabe found. Another environmental infradian is the 21-year Hale cycle of bipolar solar activity. The more cycles with different frequencies are found and optimized for prevention and if needed for therapy, the greater is the gain in studies of neuroimmunomodulation, as indicated on the Internet in an Introduction to Chronobiology,[1] succinctly stating the principles (Table 1 and Fig. 20 in Ref. 1) of this discipline and method (Figs. 4–6 in Ref. 1), and defining and documenting intermodulations, the feedsidewards,[1–3] FIGURES 1–3, encountered at different levels of organization, including that of nucleic acid[4] (see also Ref. 5). The cited monograph[1] as a whole introduces a time structure found in any one variable, its chronome (see FIGURE 4). The heretofore hardly appreciated sources of variation in the spectral element of chronomes, current misleaders or at least confounders, become reference standards in a biological periodic system.

Melatonin ultradians can have periods of 1.5 and 3.43 hours;[6] eight-hour cycles are particularly prominent in the endothelin-1 (ET-1) circulating in human blood, also revealing a 3.5-day cycle,[7–9] as does the population density of endotheliocytes, the cells producing ET-1 in mouse ear (see FIGURES 5 and 6). Changes with periods of about 24 hours have long been known,[10,11] but even foremost scholars of biological clocks can perhaps miss not only the rhythms but altogether the presence of melatonin as such[12] in the mouse pineal, because of its spikiness, shown in FIGURE 7[13] (see also Refs. 14–19). Cosine fitting (FIG. 7) is certainly not appropriate for a spike but with transformations can be used for quantification until better methods are developed.[20] A report confirming spikes in the mouse pineal[17] states: "Whether these very small peaks, which may be related to the deficience of *N*-acetyl transferase activity reported by others, have a physiological meaning remains to be determined." Feedsidewards, such as those in FIGURE 1, provide an answer in the affirmative concerning the efficacy of these spikes, notably if focus is extended from

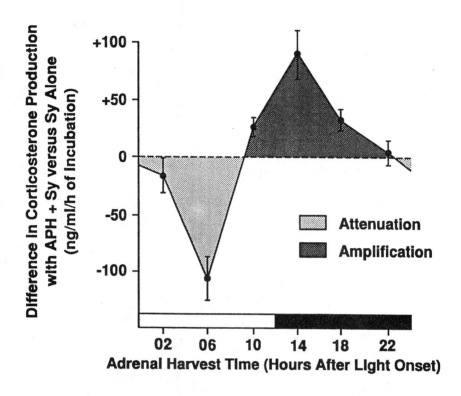

FIGURE 1. Lack of effect, attenuation, or amplication by aqueous pineal homogenate (APH) of corticosterone production by bisected adrenals in response to Sy; mean of 5 isophasic studies is illustrating a feedsideward. Feedsideward: circadian rhythmic pineal interaction with ACTH 1-17 (Sy) effect upon the bisected adrenal. For a study, we may single out a hypothetical spontaneous α rhythm, such as that in the changes in serum corticosterone of undisturbed mice.[1] Again, for a study only, we may turn to the change of serum corticosterone when ACTH is given at different times along the 24-hour scale to separate groups of comparable mice. We now assess a response or β rhythm. In fact, in such studies, even if they are done, as they were *in vitro,* thus removing a gland from the dynamics of the nervous system and the circulation, one ignores an often sizeable effect of the cosmos.[1,2] It is more difficult, but most rewarding, to then proceed in order to study the effect of interactions by more than two periodic entities at different rhythm stages. Thus one entity, the modulator, may influence, in a predictable insofar as rhythmic fashion, the effect of another entity, the actor, upon a third entity, the reactor. Predictable sequences of attenuation, no effect, and amplification can then be found. A case in point is corticosterone production by bisected adrenals stimulated by ACTH 1-17, in the presence versus absence of pineal homogenate. The outcome of 5 studies is shown in this figure, as an example of three interacting circadian rhythms. Chronomodulations involving rhythms at one or several frequencies are known as γ- or δ-rhythms, respectively. These multiple entity interactions usually involve more than one frequency; this is the case for the effect of the immunostimulator cefodizime (HR221) on corticosterone production by the adrenals stimulated by ACTH 1-17.[1]

the 24-hour to the 168-hour scale.[15] FIGURE 8 shows that in the superfused pike pineal, the change along the scale of a week can be greater than that along the scale of 24 hours.[21,22]

Infradian changes are revealed in statistics of natality, morphology, morbidity, and mortality, some covering decades or centuries, some on many thousands or even millions of people. These statistics show clearly the nonrandomness of patterns in various endpoints. An about half-yearly change characterizes the height estimated in 101,044 girls in Berlin and Leipzig, Germany.[23] The circannual pattern of height at birth can be approximated by the fit of two components with periods of 6 and 12 months. The about half-yearly pattern in birth height contrasts with the clear circannual pattern in birth weight in data from South African children.[24] The circannual and circasemiannual patterns are, in part, influenced by the environment, but they can also be accounted for, in part, by genetic features. This is illustrated by data from La Coruña, Spain, where the height and weight of infants was recorded monthly for the first 16 months of life.[25] The data were analyzed in two ways, in relation to either calendar month or as a function of age, that is, time from birth. The larger prominence of the circannual pattern as a function of age, as time elapsed from birth, as compared to the prominence of the pattern as a function of calendar month, illustrates the prominence of the genetic over the environmental aspects of growth, although both influences are present.

In addition to these circannual changes in birth characteristics, a circadian variation is prominent. This is also illustrated in data describing natality statistics of babies of different birth weight in Switzerland. Between 1979 and 1987, these statistics were derived on the basis of 670,013 births.[26] An about weekly pattern also characterizes births as well as stillbirths and perinatal mortality.[26]

Circaseptan patterns in morbidity and mortality are also found in adulthood, as shown in FIGURE 9, where the circaseptan pattern of cardiovascular events (myocardial infarctions, strokes, cardiac arrhythmias, and hypertensive crises) all exhibit nonrandom patterns along the scale of the week, some patterns differing according to the condition investigated.[27,28]

The results in FIGURE 9 stem from a large database of over 6,300,000 calls for an ambulance recorded in Moscow between 1979 and 1981. These circaseptan patterns are not specific to Moscow, because for the case of myocardial infarctions, both 7-day and 3.5-day components are prominently seen in the meta-analysis summarizing data from 47 time series published in nine different papers and covering 104,412 patients.[28] New is the demonstration of nonrandom patterns in several variables along the scale of about 10.5 years, corresponding to the average length of the wobbly solar activity cycle. This is seen, after detrending, for instance, for the mortality from myocardial infarction in Minnesota between 1968 and 1996 (see FIGURE 10). The about 10.5-year variation is statistically significant and accounts for an excess of 220 deaths per year at times of solar maxima, as compared to times of solar minima ($p = 0.023$).[2]

Variations with periods corresponding numerically to those seen in solar activity and other cosmo-, helio-, and geophysical phenomena characterize not only mortality from myocardial infarction, but also different birth statistics, as shown in FIGURE 11. These data stem from a large data base in Moscow[29–32] on body length, head circumference, and birth weight. These variations are found both in boys and

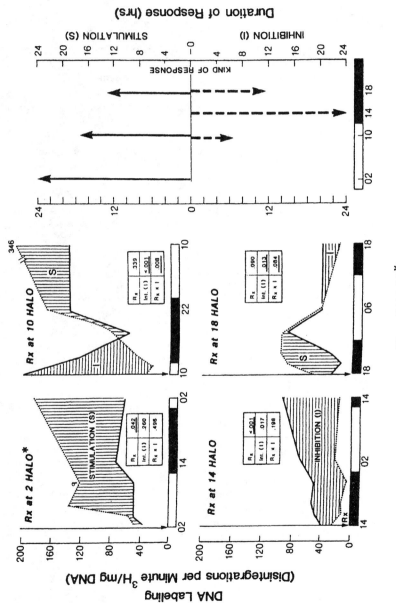

girls and characterize both babies measured in Moscow and in Alma-Ata (not shown), whether these babies were Russians or Kazaks in the same locality, and these low-frequency changes are also found in statistics of neonatal weight from Minnesota.[2]

An influence of geomagnetic disturbance on morbidity and mortality is particularly interesting in the case of epilepsy, which shows an about half-yearly component much more prominent than the about yearly component[27] (see FIGURE 12). This spectral signature resembles that of the geomagnetic disturbance index, K_p, that is also characterized by a prominent and very stable half-yearly component.

Automatic physiological measurements cover years and ECG months beat-to-beat. One example of physiological monitoring over 11 years is shown in Figures 6–8 of Reference 2. Changes in heart rate and heart rate variability, the latter assessed by the standard deviation, over consecutive monthly intervals, in data collected mostly at 15- to 30-minute intervals around the clock for 11 years by a healthy cardiologist, are aligned with the changes in solar activity gauged by Wolf number. There is a positive correlation between heart rate and solar activity, whereas the relation between heart rate variability and solar activity is negative. The negative correlation between heart rate variability and solar activity is further substantiated by the decrease in heart rate variability at times of magnetic storms.[2] The decrease in heart rate variability may be a mechanism also underlying the increased incidence of myocardial infarction following a magnetic storm, as shown in Figure 22 of Reference 2.

Indeed, the incidence of myocardial infarction has shown cross-spectral coherence with both the geomagnetic index, K_p, and the vertical component of the interplanetary magnetic field, B_z.[1,27] The cross-spectral coherence is found at a frequency of about 1 cycle in 3.16 days, that is in a frequency range close to the circasemiseptan region of the spectrum. A similarity of periods has also been found between an 81-hour spectral component in K_p and in human heart rate in isolation from society.[33] A circaseptan component, with a period slightly shorter than seven days, is also detectable in the spectrum of K_p, as a harmonic perhaps of the solar rotation cycle.[27,34,35] Again, at an about weekly period, an association was found by product-moment correlation between the sets of periods revealed by linear-nonlinear least-squares analyses, on the one hand, in newborns' heart rates and blood pressures and, on the other hand, local geomagnetic disturbance at the time of the recording.[36] Although little reliance is placed on product-moment correlations in themselves, much evidence documented by cross-spectral coherence and results from superposed epochs carries greater weight, and is indeed available.[2,27]

FIGURE 2. Chronomodulation by feedsideward is also observed for the effect of ACTH 1-17 upon metaphyseal DNA labeling in the rat. Stimulation is found at one time, inhibition at another time, stimulation preceded by inhibition and inhibition preceded by stimulation at two other times, all in the same post-℞ time span investigated. The original data consist of DNA labeling in CD2F$_1$ mice during 24 hours after treatment by placebo or ACTH 1-17, on the left; the duration of response is shown on the right. The statistical significance of the findings was established by three-way ANOVA of all data (not shown) and by two-way ANOVA for data at each treatment time. ———, placebo; · · · · ·, 20 IU/kg ACTH 1-17; *, *h*ours *a*fter *l*ight *o*nset for mice (♀CD2F$_1$); †, results of two-way analysis of variance at each circadian stage in boxes: main effects are kind of ℞ (placebo vs. ACTH 1-17) and ℞-to-kill interval (2, 4, 8, 12, and 24 hrs); ¶, outlier (that would raise mean to 338) removed.

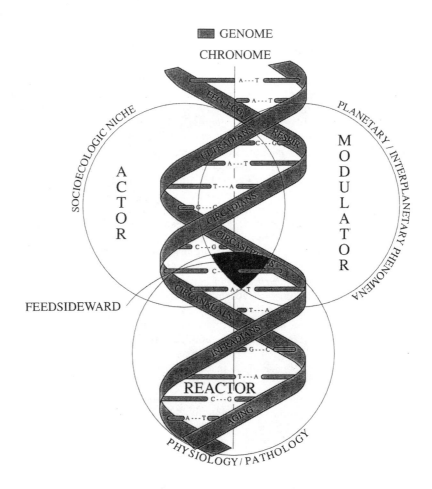

FIGURE 3. Left: Chronomodulation at different levels: in the **left** half, interplanetary solar and galactic factors (**top right**) are conceived as modulating socioecological conditions in the habitat (**top left**), acting upon the healthy or sick organism as a whole. **Right** (opposite page): The results shown in FIGURE 1 are summarized on top; those in the second diagram from the top refer to the effect of the suprachiasmatic nuclei (SCN) on circadian amplitude and acrophase. The finding of a lacking rhythm as a zero amplitude is the result of SCN removal in the case of locomotor activity and water drinking but not in a vast majority of other rhythms sampled at 4-hour or shorter intervals for 24 hours or longer spans and analyzed by inferential statistical means. The third diagram from the top refers to FIGURE 2, and intermodulations in the case of an invading microorganism of sufficient virulence to elicit a host response are sketched at the bottom. Feedsideward: Multiple interactions among several rhythmic entities resulting in a predictable rhythmic sequence of attenuation, no effect, and amplification, implemented by a modulator acting on the interaction between the actor and reactor. As shown in the diagrams, the role played by the modulator, the actor, and the reactor can vary among the interacting entities, and these systems can be exposed to different influences and an integrator. ▨ actor ↔ reactor; ▨ modulator ↔ actor; ▨ modulator ↔ reactor; ▪ feedsideward; ☐ integrator; → influencers.

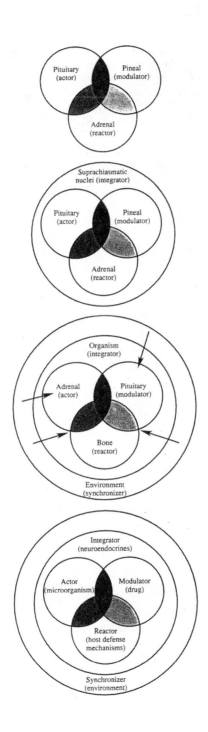

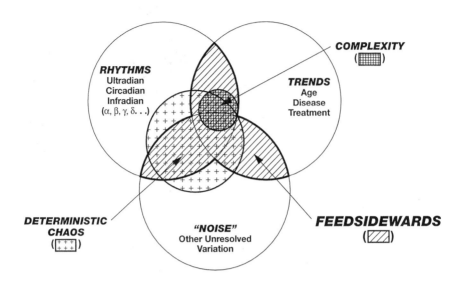

FIGURE 4. Measurable time structure (chronome) of a variable. More and more components in the spectrum of physiological variation are found to have numerical physical environmental counterparts and, vice versa, environmental counterparts have been found for some unusual physiological cycles, believed to be purely societal, such as the week. These physical or biological spectra, organizing irregular chaotic and complex variations and trends in endpoints of rhythms, chaos, and complexity constitute time structures, chronomes. The mapping of physical and biological chronomes proceeds as yet opportunistically in a project on the Biosphere and the Cosmos (BIOCOS), with a systematic Asian Chronome Ecologic Study of Heart Rate Variability (ACEHRV) by Dr. Kuniaki Otsuka, now extended to an international project, focusing on the human electrocardiogram. A data base of reference values thus accumulates with a target length of at least 7 days beat-to-beat for the electrocardiogram and again for at least 7 days at intervals from 15–60 minutes, in the case of human blood pressure. Such mapping is critical for a quantification of health in the range of otherwise neglected physiological variation. Chronome maps are the invaluable and indispensable reference values for the detection of disease risk syndromes. "Measure what is measurable and render meaningfully measurable in time what as yet is not" is what chronomes are all about.

In a clinically healthy individual, an about 9.28-year cycle is found in the daily urinary excretion of 17-ketosteroids, the breakdown products of the adrenal cortex and the male gonad, during a 15-year span (see FIGURE 13). The 95% confidence interval of this cycle does not overlap that of the circadecennian Schwabe sunspot cycle during the corresponding span. This finding is in keeping with the possibility that circadecennians, like circadians, have been coded in the genome by an integrative rather than purely adaptive evolution.[37,38] Circadecennians also characterize mutations and/or other genetic changes in microbes,[39] and the heart rate and its variability[2] and myocardial infarctions as well,[2] perhaps as a feedsideward intermodulation among the foregoing circadecennian cycles.

The phase relations of these cycles are of particular interest, although they are averaged over just one or a few cycles. They are discussed to indicate the need for more extensive systematic study. Thus, the circadecennian trough in heart rate

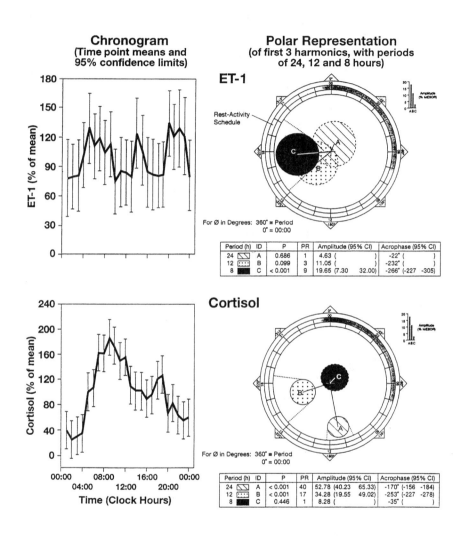

Chronogram
(Time point means and
95% confidence limits)

Polar Representation
(of first 3 harmonics, with periods
of 24, 12 and 8 hours)

ET-1

Rest-Activity
Schedule

For Ø in Degrees: 360° = Period
0° = 00:00

Period (h)	ID	P	PR	Amplitude (95% CI)	Acrophase (95% CI)
24	A	0.686	1	4.63 ( )	-22° ( )
12	B	0.099	3	11.05 ( )	-232° ( )
8	C	< 0.001	9	19.65 (7.30 32.00)	-266° (-227 -305)

Cortisol

For Ø in Degrees: 360° = Period
0° = 00:00

Period (h)	ID	P	PR	Amplitude (95% CI)	Acrophase (95% CI)
24	A	< 0.001	40	52.78 (40.23 65.33)	-170° (-156 -184)
12	B	< 0.001	17	34.28 (19.55 49.02)	-253° (-227 -278)
8	C	0.446	1	8.28 ( )	-35° ( )

00:00   08:00   16:00   00:00
  04:00   12:00   20:00
Time (Clock Hours)

FIGURE 5. Circaoctohoran endothelin-1 (ET-1) versus circadian cortisol in seven clinically healthy students (2 women and 7 men, 22–27 years of age); note that 8-h component (C) is most significant for ET-1 ($p < 0.001$), but it is not detected for cortisol ($p > 0.4$). Time-macroscopic plot of three nearly similar peaks in the vasoconstrictor ET-1 in the human circulation (**top left**) and cosinor validation only of 8-hour component (*black confidence ellipse*) in the case of ET-1 (**top right**). By contrast, one major and a secondary peak are seen for cortisol (**bottom left**); the zero-amplitude assumption is rejected both for a 24-hour and a 12-hour component, but an 8-hour component (*black ellipse*) is not statistically significant for cortisol (**bottom right**).

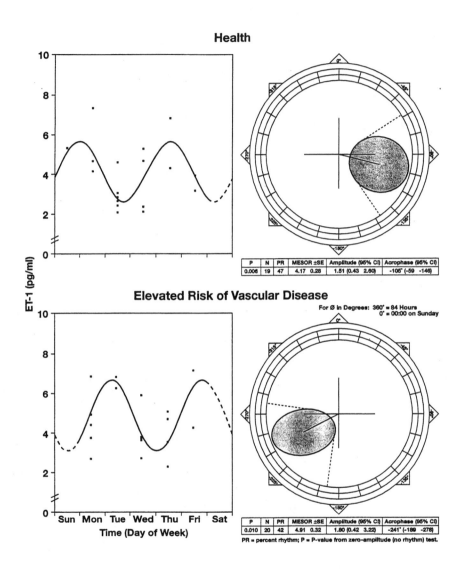

FIGURE 6. Timing of about half-weekly plasma endothelin-1 (ET-1) rhythm in non-diabetic subjects at low (**top**) or high (**bottom**) vascular disease risk. About half-weekly (circasemiseptan) component modulates circadian MESOR (rhythm-adjusted mean) of circulating endothelin-1 of healthy subjects and nondiabetic subjects at high vascular disease risk. There is a large, statistically significant ($p < 0.05$) intergroup difference in the circasemiseptan timing of overall high values (acrophase) of etiopathogenetic interest. $p < 0.05$ from test of equality of MESOR and acrophase between the two groups, each dot represents an individual's circadian MESOR assessed from data at 4-h intervals for 24 hours on different days of the week. A 3.5-day component is not demonstrated in 20 subjects with diabetes, of whom 16 were also at high vascular disease risk (not shown).

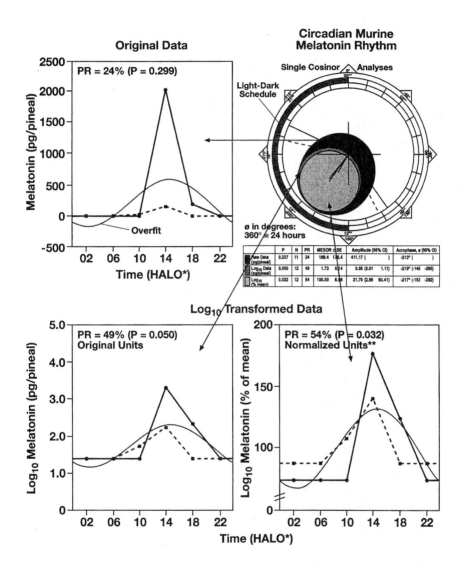

FIGURE 7. Two spiky series (**top left**) can be approximated by single consinor after log transformation (**bottom**) and preferably added normalization of data (**bottom right**). The spiky nature of pineal melatonin along the 24-h scale and inadequacy of cosinor to approximate a spike, a limitation somewhat reduced by data transformations. *, hours after light onset; **, by eliminating interseries difference in average.

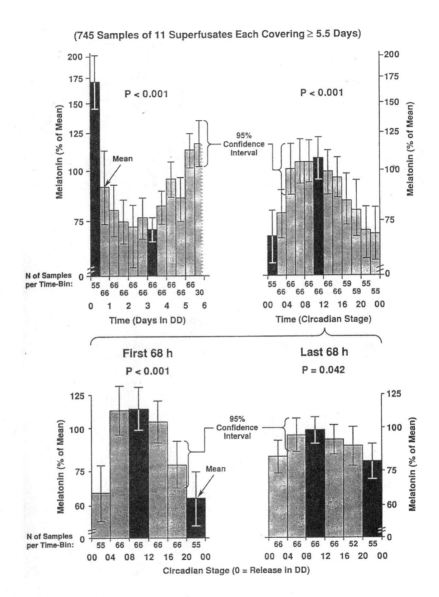

FIGURE 8. Persisting damped circadian rhythm of melatonin release from superfused pike pineals in continuous darkness (DD) and fixed environmental temperature documented by 745 samples of 11 perfusates, each covering about 5.5 days. The extent of change along the scale of a week can more than match the circadian one *in vitro*—in this graph on the secretion of a fish pineal *in vitro* (and in the murine pineal *in vivo* as well, not shown).

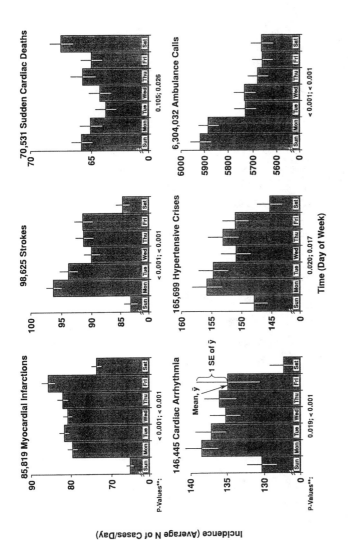

FIGURE 9. The biologic week: nature as well as culture. The weekend can be peak or trough as a function of internal and external interactions. Circaseptan patterns of chronoepidemiologic data are from ambulance calls in Moscow between 1979 and 1981; data are from T. Breus *et al.* (1992). The "Monday phenomenon" (a misnomer) in the distribution of strokes, cardiac arrhythmias, and hypertensive crises becomes (another misnomer) a "weekend phenomenon" for sudden cardiac deaths and for a total of 6,304,032 calls for an ambulance. The underlying circaseptan rhythm is the basic phenomenon. The difference in the internal interaction and/or socioecological synchronizers of these phenomena constitutes another major problem in its own right. Timing can differ further for the same condition, myocardial infarction, as a function of geographic site and/or morbidity versus mortality (cf. FIG. 10). **, one-way ANOVA; cosinor.

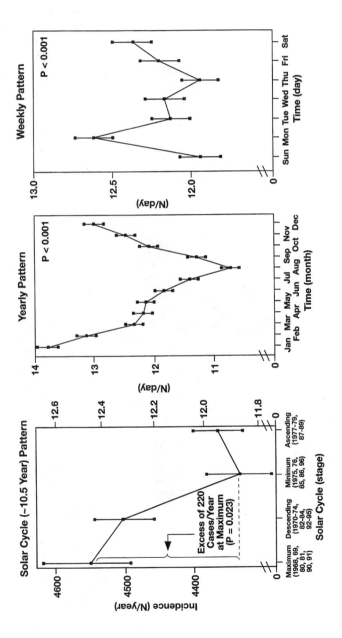

FIGURE 10. Mortality from myocardial infarction in Minnesota (1968–1996). Nonrandom patterns of the incidence of mortality from myocardial infarction in Minnesota along the scales of the week (**right**), year (**middle**), and the about 10.5-year sunspot activity cycle (**left**). By comparison to times of solar minimum, at times of solar maximum there is an excess of 220 deaths per year from myocardial infarction. Note also that there is a (misnamed) "Monday phenomenon" in Minnesota for mortality, whereas there is a "Friday phenomenon" in Moscow for morbidity (cf. FIG. 9). Means ± SE (N = 129,205 deaths from myocardial infarction).

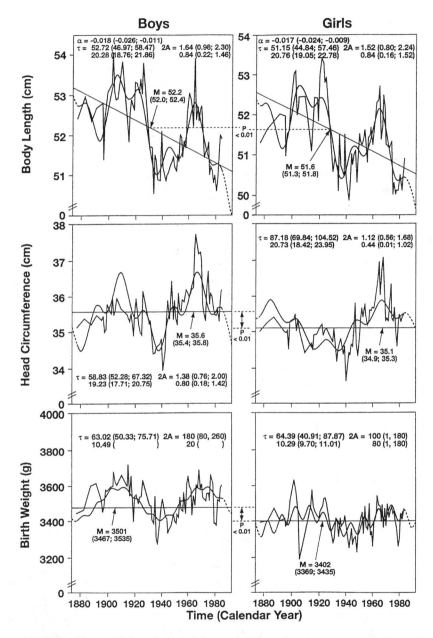

FIGURE 11. Are birth statistics in Moscow influenced by the solar cycle? About 50-year cycles in body length (**top**), about 20-year cycles in head circumference (**middle**), and about 10-year cycles in birth weight (**bottom**) of girls in Moscow. Data from Moscow of 25–100 newborns/year for over a century. Statistics were recorded over 112 years (1874–1985). Nonlinear analysis yields estimate of period (τ, years), double amplitude (2A), MESOR (chronome-adjusted mean, M), and slope (α) with 95% confidence limits.

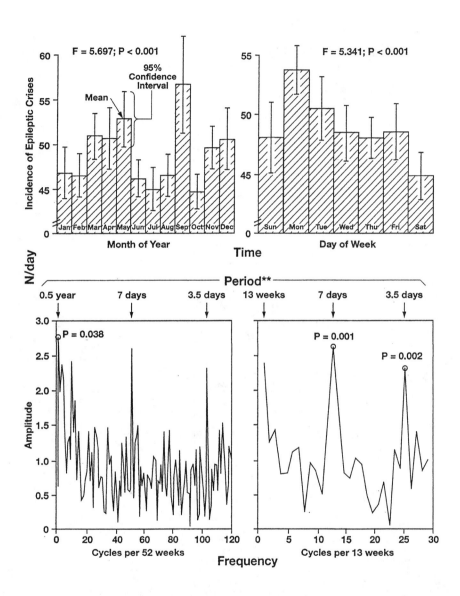

FIGURE 12. Circasemiannual and circaseptan-circasemiseptan patterns of status epilepticus incidence from 53,616 cases recorded in Moscow, Russia between 1 Jan 1979 and 31 Dec 1981. Epilepsy of a severity requiring an ambulance shows two peaks/year (**top**). Accordingly, no spectral peak at one year, but a spectral peak at about a half-year is seen (**bottom**), along with spectral components with periods of 7 and 3.5 days.[27] **, p values from population-mean cosinor on three yearly estimates (**left**) or 12 three-monthly estimates (**right**). Overall least squares spectrum finds 0.5-year, 1.0-, and 0.5-week components statistically significant ($p < 0.001$) (in addition to about 33.1- and 28.0-day components).

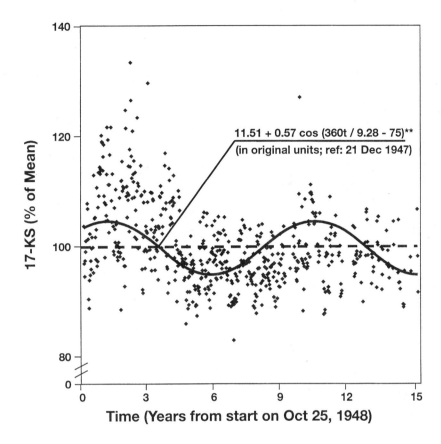

FIGURE 13. Circadecennian cycle in the excretion of urinary 17-ketosteroids by a clinically healthy man, 44–59 years old (weekly averages). **, The model was validated nonlinearly with a period of 9.28 years, with a 95% confidence interval (CI) extending from 8.72 to 9.95 years, nonoverlapping the CIs of the nearest periods in geomagnetic disturbance (K_p) or in solar activity (Wolf number).

variability, which may relate to cardiac vulnerability, immediately follows (if it does not coincide with) the solar maximum, as do the circadecennian peaks in heart rate and blood pressure. The peak of myocardial infarctions lags the solar maxima by just 1.72 years, whereas the peak in the circadecennian changes of human 17-ketosteroid excretion, reflecting the adrenal cortex and the gonads, lags the solar maximum by two years. Nonphotic solar activity may raise human blood pressure and heart rate and the secretion of steroid-producing endocrine glands, whereas it depresses heart rate variability, the latter almost certainly an undesirable effect, as is the increase in the incidence of myocardial infarctions. Genetic changes of air bacteria, which like heart rate variability show a near-antiphase with circadecennian solar activity, lag in relation to the circadecennian trough in Wolf numbers. The aforementioned phase

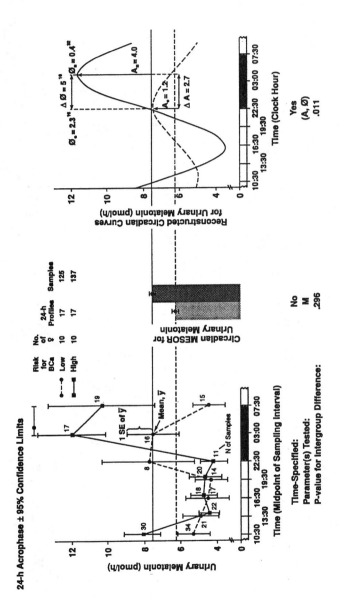

FIGURE 14. Discrimination of high and low familial risk of developing breast cancer (BCa) on the basis of urinary melatonin excretion requires chronobiologic approach. The study used Minnesotan women, 15–59 year of age, providing 4–12 urine samples over a single 24-h span in 1–4 seasons. Spotchecks at a single clock-hour can show an intergroup difference in either direction. Around-the-clock profiles reveal the larger circadian amplitude of urinary melatonin in women at a high versus low familial risk of developing breast cancer, in the absence of a difference in the chronome-adjusted average. Summary by chronogram (**left**), bar diagram (**middle**), best fitting 24-h cosine curve (**right**). Rhythm characteristics: MESOR (M), amplitude (A), and acrophase (φ), tested for difference between low- and high-risk subjects. *p* values compare (1) equivalent of 24-h urine pools (circadian M) failing to discriminate (**bottom middle**) or (2) circadian (A, φ) succeeding in discriminating (**bottom right**).

relations to solar activity are computed, whenever there are data over several cycles, over the series as a whole, rather than for each cycle separately as another limitation. Nonetheless, associations with solar activity, at least for myocardial infarctions, are independently supported by other approaches, and in this light the timing of the physiological circadecennian cycles as a minimum, and perhaps that of the bacterial ones, that may be considered to be involved in pathways to cardiac pathology,[40–42] could provide hints of mechanisms.

SIGNIFICANCE

Melatonin, as a function of circadian stage, inhibits or accelerates a malignant growth,[16,43,44] as does another immunomodulator,[45] in a way reminiscent of the original feedsideward phenomena of FIGURES 1–3, where the pineal stimulates, leaves unaffected or dampens, for example, adrenal corticosterone production *in vitro*, directly or via the pituitary.[1,13,15,16] Melatonin may be a mediator of photic and any nonphotic effects from the sun and the latter also from the galaxies.[46,47]

The circadian amplitude of urinary melatonin is elevated in women with a high familial breast cancer risk (see FIGURE 14)[48] and dampened in patients with actual cancer, (see FIGURE 15)[49] (see also Ref. 50). In the circulation as well, the effect of an intervention can raise the blood pressure and heart rate in the morning and lower it in the afternoon (see FIGURE 16).[51–53] The mechanisms involved in vascular disease risk elevation, that is, in disease risk syndromes,[53–57] are of major interest in the prevention of strokes and other catastrophic vascular diseases and broaden the scope of neuroimmunity to become vasculoimmunity.

The role of melatonin in growth may relate not only to extrauterine but also to intrauterine growth. In the case of pregnant women with intrauterine growth retardation, in contrast to a yearly signature presumably of sunshine and environmental temperature in health, the geomagnetic half-yearly signature is found in circulating melatonin.[58] In health as well, birth weight, height, and chest and abdominal circumference reveal cycles of about 10.5 and 21 years and much longer ones. A view of melatonin in body defense and growth will gain from the perspective of chronomes, feedsidewards, and the influences of the cosmos (see Table 1 in Ref. 2). We are continuously under the influence of the cosmos, acting, perhaps, at specific frequencies, circasemiseptans and circaseptans[2,27,33,36] and, perhaps, circadecennians, in relation to growth, the circulation, and pathology, such as myocardial infarctions and epilepsy. The heart and the brain are closely communicating organs in any event,[59] and both respond to remote chronomes.[27,60–67] These aspects of a cosmopathology deserve follow-up.

The BIOSPHERE and the COSMOS (BIOCOS), an as-yet informal international chronome-mapping endeavor, invites the participation of interested individuals. The aim of BIOCOS is to enable the differentiation, against available maps, of rhythms that account for the difference between life and death by timing in response to the same physical, chemical, or other biological stimulus given in the same total single or overall weekly dose.[1,3–5,45,68–71] Mapping reference standards for rhythms, notably when the periods are of about 10-, 20-, and 50-year lengths, including life spans and their variabilities in populations, is a community affair. So is action on the now-

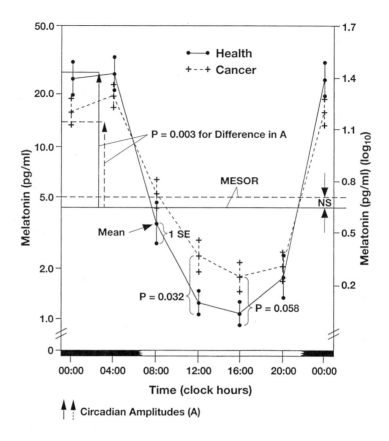

FIGURE 15. Circadian pattern of serum melatonin in health versus cancer differs overall by the circadian amplitude but not by the MESOR, whereas unwarranted inferences may be drawn from spotchecks limited to samplings at one or two single time points. Published studies limited to single clock hours have controversially claimed both a higher and a lower concentration of circulating melatonin in cancer patients. Around-the-clock profiles reveal that spurious differences result from the smaller circadian melatonin amplitude in cancer versus health. In combination with the results in FIG. 14, an increase in circadian amplitude is found with risk elevation and a decrease in actual malignancy. The degrees of generality and the specificity for cancer are questions yet to be resolved.

documented highest risk of catastrophic vascular disease associated with too much blood pressure and too little heart rate variability.[53–57] These are steps toward preventive risk lowering, that is, prehabilitation,[2] to reduce the need for rehabilitation, a task to be implemented across the board, including, with vascular disease, cancer and other conditions.

Conventionally, "modulation" is something that may (or may not) take place, that, if it occurred, may (or may not) be statistically significant, and its outcome (unpredictably) can be an increase, no effect, or a decrease in whatever is measured,

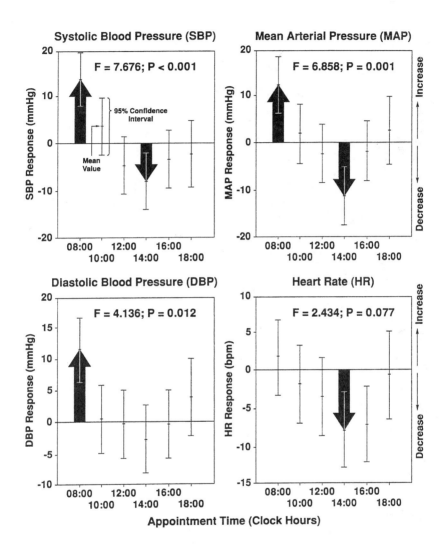

FIGURE 16. Timing clarifies and quantifies tension (stress) effect as pressor or depressor (arrows). White-coat hypertension in the morning may be white-coat hypotension in the afternoon, if the same oral surgery carried out by the surgeon in a white coat raises or lowers blood pressure as a function of clock hour. Effect evaluated in the light of data on 8 control days for each of 23 subjects at the time corresponding to the appointment with the dental surgeon. Circadian stage determines predictable increase or decrease of human blood pressure and heart rate during surgery; assessed as the difference, corrected for posture, between the mean value during the appointment and the value predicted from the circadian profile provided by each patient; results from ambulatory monitoring at 5- to 15-minute intervals for three days bracketing surgery on 23 patients ($N = 254$ sets of measurements per patient; total $N = 5,849$; including monitoring on two previous occasions: total $N = 17,758$).

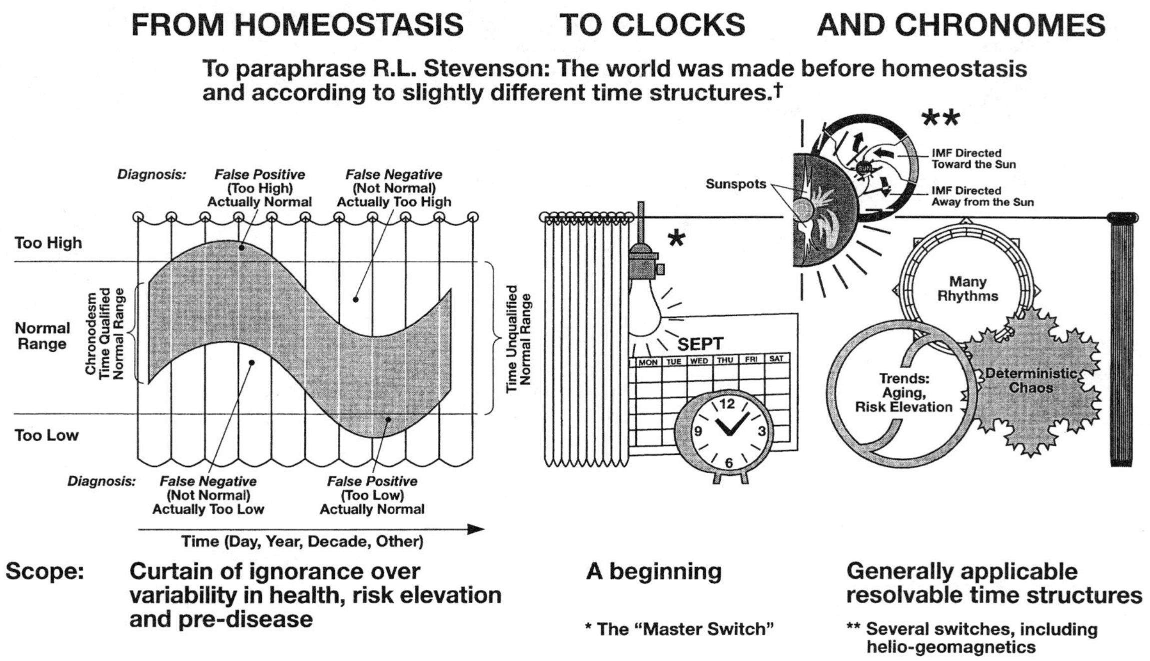

FIGURE 17. Circadian systems and circannual calendars are important beginnings if it is realized that they supersede an imaginary homeostasis and constitute steps on the road toward recognizing much more complex chronomes that cannot be simplified further, without a great loss of information. Disease risk syndromes may be left unrecognized unless chronomes are resolved; and so are effects of the cosmos, that relate to amplitudes, which may be neglected in exclusive focus upon biological time measurement. † Inferential statistical methods map chronomes as molecular biology maps genomes; biological chronomes await resolution of their interactions in us and around us, for example, with magnetic storms in the interplanetary magnetic field (IMF).

in response to the same stimulus. This situation can be remedied if first the rhythmic nature of the organism and its habitats near and far, and second the intermodulations of rhythmic variables in us and around us, can be accounted for, rather than ignored. Many major contributions have been made without chronobiology; the discoveries of insulin and of penicillin were made in homeostatic research, and their consequences have kept innumerable millions of people alive.

Nonetheless, when modulations are considered, however, the postulation and testing of feedsidewards, replacing time-unqualified feedbacks, may allow us to recognize and use the same seemingly contradictory results as features of a recurring sequence in a rhythmic, and to that extent predictable, cycle. Critically for basic and clinical endeavors, alternating opposite outcomes can be assessed by inferential statistical tests as amplitude or phase modulation or superposition in the strict physical sense. The scope of chronomes and of intermodulations among chronomes by far transcends that of biological time measurement (see FIGURE 17).[15]

To conclude in the sense of Einstein, we must keep things simple, but not simpler than they are. Unfortunately for Einstein's other often-used quotation and for those many who refrain from inferential statistical chronome mapping, for example, in the study of conventional modulation, God does play dice. Hence the complete understanding of chronomes cannot be made simpler than it is.

REFERENCES

1. CORNÉLISSEN, G. & F. HALBERG. 1994. Introduction to Chronobiology. Medtronic Chronobiology Seminar #7, April 1994, 52 pp. (Library of Congress Catalog Card #94-060580; <http://revilla.mac.cie.uva.es/chrono>).

2. CORNÉLISSEN, G., F. HALBERG, O. SCHWARTZKOPFF, P. DELMORE, G. KATINAS, D. HUNTER, B. TARQUINI, R. TARQUINI, F. PERFETTO, Y. WATANABE & K. OTSUKA. 1999. Chronomes, time structures, for chronobioengineering for "a full life." Biomed. Instrum. Technol. **33:** 152–187.

3. HALBERG, F. 1983. *Quo vadis* basic and clinical chronobiology: promise for health maintenance. Am. J. Anat. **168:** 543–594.

4. WALKER, W.V., J.E. RUSSELL, D.J. SIMMONS, L.E. SCHEVING, G. CORNÉLISSEN & F. HALBERG. 1985. Effect of an adrenocorticotropin analogue, ACTH 1-17, on DNA synthesis in murine metaphyseal bone. Biochem. Pharmacol. **34:** 1191–1196.

5. HALBERG, F. 1969. Chronobiology. Annu. Rev. Physiol. **31:** 675–725.

6. SALTI, R., F. GALLUZZI, G. BINDI, F. PERFETTO, R. TARQUINI, F. HALBERG & G. CORNÉLISSEN. 2000. Nocturnal melatonin patterns in children. J. Clin. Endocrinol. Metab. **85:** 2137–2144.

7. TARQUINI, B., F. PERFETTO, R. TARQUINI, G. CORNÉLISSEN & F. HALBERG. 1997. Endothelin-1's chronome indicates diabetic and vascular disease chronorisk. Peptides **18:** 119–132.

8. TARQUINI, B., G. CORNÉLISSEN, F. PERFETTO, R. TARQUINI & F. HALBERG. 1997. About-half-weekly (circasemiseptan) component of the endothelin-1 (ET-1) chronome and vascular disease risk. Peptides **18:** 1237–1241.

9. HEROLD, M., G. CORNÉLISSEN, A. LOECKINGER, D. KOEBERLE, P. KOENIG & F. HALBERG. 1998. About 8-hourly variation of circulating human endothelin-1 (ET-1) in clinical health. Peptides **19:** 821–825.

10. QUAY, W.B. 1974. Pineal Chemistry in Cellular and Physiological Mechanisms. Charles C. Thomas. Springeld, Illinois.

11. DOLLINS, A.B., I.V. ZHDANOVA, R.J. WURTMAN, H.J. LYNCH & M.H. DENG. 1994. Effect of inducing nocturnal serum melatonin concentrations in daytime on sleep, mood, body temperature, and performance. Proc. Natl. Acad. Sci. USA **91:** 1824–1828.

12. EBIHARA, S., T. MARKS, D.J. HUDSON & M. MENAKER. 1986. Genetic control of melatonin synthesis in the pineal gland of the mouse. Science **231:** 491–493.

13. BROWN, G.M., L.J. GROTA, S. SÁNCHEZ DE LA PEÑA, F. HALBERG & E. HALBERG. 1983. Circadian melatonin rhythm: part of stimulatory feed-sideward in pineal modulation of adrenal response to ACTH 1-17? Abstracts of papers, Minn. Acad. Sci. 51st Annual Spring Meeting, University of Minnesota-Duluth, April 29–30, 1983: 12.

14. MAESTRONI, G.J.M., A. CONTI & W. PIERPAOLI. 1986. Role of the pineal gland in immunity: circadian synthesis and release of melatonin modulates the antibody response and antagonizes the immunosuppressive effect of corticosterone. J. Neuroimmunol. **13:** 19–30.

15. SÁNCHEZ DE LA PEÑA, S., F. HALBERG, F. UNGAR & D. LAKATUA. 1988. *Ex vivo* hierarchy of circadian-infradian rhythmic pineal-pituitary-adrenal intermodulations in rodents. *In* Biorhythms and Stress in the Physiopathology of Reproduction, P. Pancheri & L. Zichella, Eds.: 177–214. Hemisphere. New York.

16. SÁNCHEZ DE LA PEÑA, S. 1993. The feedsideward of cephalo-adrenal immune interactions. Chronobiologia **20:** 1–52.

17. CONTI, A. & G.J.M. MAESTRONI. 1996. HPLC validation of a circadian melatonin rhythm in the pineal gland of inbred mice. J. Pineal Res. **20:** 138–144.

18. VIVIEN-ROELS, B., A. MALAN, M.C. RETTORI, P. DELAGRANGE, J.P. JEANNIOT & P. PEVET. 1998. Daily variations in pineal melatonin concentrations in inbred and outbred mice. J. Biol. Rhythms **13:** 403–409.

19. HALBERG, F., G. CORNÉLISSEN, A. CONTI, G.J.M. MAESTRONI, C. MAGGIONI, F. PERFETTO, R. SALTI, R. TARQUINI, G.S. KATINAS & O. SCHWARTZKOPFF. 2000. Pineal and chronobiologic history: mind and spirit as feedsidewards in time structures, chronomes, for prehabilitation. *In* The Pineal Gland and Cancer: Neuroimmunoendocrine Mechanisms in Malignancy. C. Bartsch, H. Bartsch, D.E. Blask, D. Cardinali, W. Hrushesky & D. Mecke, Eds. Springer. Heidelberg. In press.

20. CORNÉLISSEN, G. & F. HALBERG. 1998. Chronomedicine. *In* Encyclopedia of Biostatistics. P. Armitage & T. Colton, editors-in-chief: **1:** 642–649. John Wiley & Sons Ltd. Chichester, UK.

21. CORNÉLISSEN, G., A. PORTELA, F. HALBERG, V. BOLLIET & J. FALCÓN. 1995. Toward a chronome of superfused pike pineals: about-weekly (circaseptan) modulation of circadian melatonin release. In Vivo **9:** 323–329.

22. FALCÓN, J., J.-P. RAVAULT, G. CORNÉLISSEN & F. HALBERG. 1996. Circaseptan-modulated circadian rhythmic melatonin release from isolated pike pineal in alternating light and darkness. 4° Convegno Nazionale, Società Italiana di Cronobiologia, Gubbio (Perugia), Italy, June 1–2, 1996: 39–40.

23. OTTO, W. & G. REISSIG. 1963. Zur Anthropologie der Neugeborenen. 4. Mitteilung. Länge und Gewicht der Neugeborenen in den verschiedenen Monaten. Monatsber. Dtsch. Akad. Wiss. Berl. **5:** 549–559.

24. HENNEBERG, M. & G.J. LOUW. 1993. Further studies on the month-of-birth effect on body size: rural schoolchildren and an animal model. Am. J. Phys. Anthropol. **91:** 235–244.

25. GARCIA ALONSO, L., D. HILLMAN, G. CORNÉLISSEN, X. GARCIA PENALTA, Z.R. WANG & F. HALBERG. 1993. Nature, not solely nurture: chronome as well as season governs growth patterns of infants. *In* Chronocardiology and Chronomedicine: Humans in Time and Cosmos, K. Otsuka, G. Cornélissen, F. Halberg, Eds.: 71–75. Life Science Publishing. Tokyo.

26. MARAZZI, A., C. RUFFIEUX, G. CORNÉLISSEN, E.V. SYUTKINA, D. JOHNSON & F. HALBERG. 2000. Circadian and circaseptan patterns of natality and perinatal mortality of infants with different birth weights. Int. J. Prenat. Perinat. Psychol. Med. In press.

27. HALBERG, F., T.K. BREUS, G. CORNÉLISSEN, C. BINGHAM, D.C. HILLMAN, J. RIGATUSO, P. DELMORE, E. BAKKEN & INTERNATIONAL WOMB-TO-TOMB CHRONOME INITIATIVE GROUP. 1991. Chronobiology in space. Keynote, 37th Ann Mtg Japan Soc for Aerospace and Environmental Medicine, Nagoya, Japan, November 8-9, 1991. University of Minnesota/Medtronic Chronobiology Seminar Series, #1, December 1991: 21 pp. of text, 70 figures.

28. CORNÉLISSEN, G., T.K. BREUS, C. BINGHAM, R. ZASLAVSKAYA, M. VARSHITSKY, B. MIRSKY, M. TEIBLOOM, B. TARQUINI, E. BAKKEN, F. HALBERG & INTERNATIONAL WOMB-TO-TOMB CHRONOME INITIATIVE GROUP. 1993. Beyond circadian chronorisk: worldwide circaseptan-circasemiseptan patterns of myocardial infarctions, other vascular events, and emergencies. Chronobiologia **20:** 87–115.

29. NIKITYUK, B., M. BALAKIREVA, G. CORNÉLISSEN & F. HALBERG. 1998. Similarities and differences in the 112-year time course of birth weight between boys and girls. Reports of Vinnitsa State Medical University **2:** 332–333.

30. NIKITYUK, B., M. BALAKIREVA, G. CORNÉLISSEN & F. HALBERG. 1998. Similarities and differences in the 112-year time course of neonatal body length between boys and girls. Reports of Vinnitsa State Medical University **2:** 331.

31. NIKITYUK, B., M. BALAKIREVA, G. CORNÉLISSEN & F. HALBERG. 1998. Similarities and differences in the 112-year time course of neonatal head circumference between boys and girls. Reports of Vinnitsa State Medical University **2:** 334.

32. HALBERG, F., G. CORNÉLISSEN, K. OTSUKA, E.V. SYUTKINA, A. MASALOV, T. BREUS, A. VIDUETSKY, A. GRAFE & O. SCHWARTZKOPFF. 2000. Chronoastrobiology: neonatal numerical counterparts to Schwabe's 10.5 and Hale's 21-year sunspot cycles. In memoriam Boris A. Nikityuk (Sept. 10, 1933–Sept. 30, 1998). Int. J. Prenat. Perinat. Psychol. Med. In press.

33. HALBERG, F., G. CORNÉLISSEN, R.P. SONKOWSKY, C. LANZONI, A. GALVAGNO, M. MONTALBINI & O. SCHWARTZKOPFF. 1998. Chrononursing (chronutrics), psychiatry and language. New Trends Exp. Clin. Psychiatry **14:** 15–26.

34. ROEDERER, J.G. 1995. Are magnetic storms hazardous to your health? Eos, Transactions, American Geophysical Union **76:** 441, 444–445.

35. VLADIMIRSKII, B.M., V.YA. NARMANSKII & N.A. TEMURIANTZ. 1995. Global rhythmics of the solar system in the terrestrial habitat. Biophysics **40:** 731–736.

36. SYUTKINA, E.V., G. CORNÉLISSEN, A.E. GRIGORIEV, M.D. MITISH, T. TURTI, G.V. YATSYK, K. PIMENOV, T.K. BREUS, M.Y. STUDENIKIN, J. SIEGELOVA, B. FISER, J. DUSEK, D. JOHNSON & F. HALBERG. 1997. Neonatal intensive care may consider associations of cardiovascular rhythms with local magnetic disturbance. Scr. Med. **70:** 217–226.

37. HALBERG, F. & A. AHLGREN. 1980. Prologue: puzzles regarding biologic rhythms and their implications for self-help in health care. *In* Chronobiology: Principles and Applications to Shifts in Schedules. L.E. Scheving & F. Halberg, Eds.: v–xxiii. Sijthoff and Noordhoff, Alphen aan den Rijn. the Netherlands.

38. HALBERG, F., N. MARQUES, G. CORNÉLISSEN, C. BINGHAM, S. SÁNCHEZ DE LA PEÑA, J. HALBERG, M. MARQUES, J. WU & E. HALBERG. 1990. Circaseptan biologic time structure reviewed in the light of contributions by Laurence K. Cutkomp and Ladislav Dérer. Acta Entomol. Bohemoslov. **87:** 1–29.

39. FARAONE, P., G. CORNÉLISSEN, G.S. KATINAS, F. HALBERG & J. SIEGELOVA. 1999. Astrophysical influences on sectoring in colonies of microorganisms. Abstract 17, MEFA, Brno, Czech Rep., Nov. 3–6, 1999.

40. SCHUSSHEIM, A.E. & V. FUSTER. 1999. Antibiotics for myocardial infarction? A possible role of infection in atherogenesis and acute coronary syndromes. Drugs **57:** 283–291.

41. VERCELLOTTI, G. 1999. Infectious agents that play a role in atherosclerosis and vasculopathies. What are they? What do we do about them? Can. J. Cardiol. **15**(Suppl. B): 13B–15B.

42. SESSA, R., M. DI PIETRO, I. SANTINO, M. DEL PIANO, A. VARVERI, A. DAGIANTI & M. PENCO. 1999. *Chlamydia pneumoniae* infection and atherosclerotic coronary disease. Am. Heart J. **137:** 1116–1119.

43. BARTSCH, H. & C. BARTSCH. 1981. Effect of melatonin on experimental tumors under different photoperiods and times of administration. J. Neural. Transm. **52:** 269–279.

44. LANGEVIN, T., W. HRUSHESKY, S. SÁNCHEZ & F. HALBERG. 1983. Melatonin (M) modulates survival of CD2F$_1$ mice with L1210 leukemia. Chronobiologia **10:** 173–174.

45. HALBERG, E. & F. HALBERG. 1980. Chronobiologic study design in everyday life, clinic and laboratory. Chronobiologia **7:** 95–120.

46. TARQUINI, B., G. CORNÉLISSEN, F. PERFETTO, R. TARQUINI & F. HALBERG. 1997. Chronome assessment of circulating melatonin in humans. In Vivo **11:** 473–484.

47. WETTERBERG, L., T. BRATLID, L.V. KNORRING, G. EBERHARD & A. YUWILER. 1999. A multinational study of the relationships between nighttime urinary melatonin production, age, gender, body size, and latitude. Eur. Arch. Psychiatr. & Clin. Neurosci. **249:** 256–262.

48. WETTERBERG, L., F. HALBERG, E. HALBERG, E. HAUS, T. KAWASAKI, M. UENO, K. UEZONO, G. CORNÉLISSEN, M. MATSUOKA & T. OMAE. 1986. Circadian characteristics of urinary melatonin from clinically healthy women at different civilization disease risk. Acta Med. Scand. **220:** 71–81.

49. TARQUINI, B., G. CORNÉLISSEN, R. TARQUINI, F. PERFETTO & F. HALBERG. 1999. General and unspecific damping by malignancy of the circadian amplitude of circulating human melatonin? Neuroendocrinol. Lett. **20:** 25–28.

50. CORNÉLISSEN, G., F. HALBERG, F. PERFETTO, R. TARQUINI, C. MAGGIONI & L. WETTERBERG. 2000. Melatonin involvement in cancer: methodological considerations. In The Pineal Gland and Cancer: Neuroimmunoendocrine Mechanisms in Malignancy. C. Bartsch, H. Bartsch, D.E. Blask, D. Cardinali, W. Hrushesky & D. Mecke, Eds. Springer. Heidelberg. In press.

51. RAAB, F., E. SCHAFFER, G. CORNÉLISSEN & F. HALBERG. 1993. More on the dentist's role in the prevention of high blood pressure. Chronobiologia **20:** 245–250.

52. RAAB, F.J., E. SCHAFFER, G. GUILLAUME-CORNÉLISSEN & F. HALBERG. 1998. Interpreting vital sign profiles for maximizing patient safety during dental visits. J. Am. Dent. Assoc. **129:** 461–469.

53. HALBERG, F., G. CORNÉLISSEN, INTERNATIONAL WOMB-TO-TOMB CHRONOME INITIATIVE GROUP. 1995. Resolution from a meeting of the International Society for Research on Civilization Diseases and the Environment (New SIRMCE Confederation), Brussels, Belgium, March 17–18, 1995: Fairy tale or reality? Medtronic Chronobiology Seminar #8, April 1995: 12 pp. text, 18 figures. URL <http://revilla.mac.cie.uva.es/chrono>.

54. OTSUKA, K., G. CORNÉLISSEN & F. HALBERG. 1996. Predictive value of blood pressure dipping and swinging with regard to vascular disease risk. Clin. Drug Invest. **11:** 20–31.

55. OTSUKA, K., G. CORNÉLISSEN, F. HALBERG & G. OEHLERT. 1997. Excessive circadian amplitude of blood pressure increases risk of ischemic stroke and nephropathy. J. Med. Eng. & Technol. **21:** 23–30.

56. HALBERG, F., G. CORNÉLISSEN, J. HALBERG, H. FINK, C-H. CHEN, K. OTSUKA, Y. WATANABE, Y. KUMAGAI, E.V. SYUTKINA, T. KAWASAKI, K. UEZONO, Z.Y. ZHAO & O. SCHWARTZKOPFF. 1998. Circadian Hyper-Amplitude-Tension, CHAT: a disease risk syndrome of anti-aging medicine. J. Anti-Aging Med. **1:** 239–259. (Editor's Note by M. FOSSEL, p. 239.)

57. OTSUKA, K., Ed. 1998. Chronome & Janus-medicine: Heart Rate Variability (HRV) and BP Variability (BPV) from a viewpoint of chronobiology and ecology. Medical Review. Tokyo.

58. MAGGIONI, C., G. CORNÉLISSEN, R. ANTINOZZI, M. FERRARIO, A. GRAFE & F. HALBERG. 1999. A half-yearly aspect of circulating melatonin in pregnancies complicated by intrauterine growth retardation. Neuroendocrinol. Lett. **20:** 55–68.

59. HALBERG, F., E. BAKKEN, G. CORNÉLISSEN, J. HALBERG, E. HALBERG & P. DELMORE. 1989. Blood pressure assessment with a cardiovascular summary, the sphygmochron, in broad chronobiologic perspective. In Heart & Brain, Brain & Heart. H. Refsum, J.A. Sulg & K. Rasmussen, Eds.: 142–162. Springer-Verlag. Berlin.

60. VILLORESI, G., T.K. BREUS, N. IUCCI, L.I. DORMAN & S.I. RAPOPORT. 1994. The influence of geophysical and social effects on the incidences of clinically important pathologies (Moscow 1979–1981). Physica Medica **10:** 79–91.

61. VILLORESI, G., Y.A. KOPYTENKO, N.G. PTITSYNA, M.I. TYASTO, E.A. KOPYTENKO, N. IUCCI & P.M. VORONOV. 1994. The influence of geomagnetic storms and man-made magnetic field disturbances on the incidence of myocardial infarction in St. Petersburg (Russia). Physica Medica **10:** 107–117.
62. ROEDERER, J.G. 1996. Effects of natural magnetic field disturbances on biota. Space Medicine & Medical Engineering (Chn.) **9:** 7–16.
63. MENDOZA, B. & R. DIAZ-SANDOVAL. A preliminary study of the relationship between solar activity and myocardial infarctions in Mexico City. Geofisica Internacional 1999. In press.
64. FEIGIN, V.L., YU.P. NIKITIN & T.E. VINOGRADOVA. 1997. Solar and geomagnetic activities: are there associations with stroke occurrence? Cerebrovas. Dis. **7:** 345–348.
65. MIKULECKY, M., Ed. The Moon and Living Matter. Kosice, Slovakia, September 23–25, 1993. Slovak Medical Society. Bratislava.
66. MIKULECKY, M., Ed. 1994. Sun, Moon and Living Matter. Bratislava, Slovakia, June 28–July 1, 1994. Slovak Medical Society. Bratislava.
67. MIKULECKY, M., Ed. 1997. Chronobiology & Its Roots in the Cosmos. High Tatras, Slovakia, September 2–6, 1997. Slovak Medical Society. Bratislava.
68. HAUS, E. 1964. Periodicity in response and susceptibility to environmental stimuli. Ann. N.Y. Acad. Sci. **117:** 281–291.
69. SCHEVING, L.E. 1976. The dimension of time in biology and medicine: chronobiology. Endeavour **35:** 66–72.
70. REINBERG, A. & M.H. SMOLENSKY. 1983. Biological rhythms and medicine. Cellular, metabolic, physiopathologic, and pharmacologic aspects. Springer. New York.
71. TOUITOU, Y. & E. HAUS, Eds. 1992. Biological Rhythms in Clinical and Laboratory Medicine. Springer-Verlag. Berlin.

Melatonin and Its Relation to the Immune System and Inflammation

RUSSEL J. REITER,[a] JUAN R. CALVO, MALGORZATA KARBOWNIK, WENBO QI, AND DUN XIAN TAN

Department of Cellular and Structural Biology,
The University of Texas Health Science Center, San Antonio, Texas 78229-3900, USA

ABSTRACT: Melatonin (*N*-acetyl-5-methoxytryptamine) was initially thought to be produced exclusively in the pineal gland. Subsequently its synthesis was demonstrated in other organs, for example, the retinas, and very high concentrations of melatonin are found at other sites, for example, bone marrow cells and bile. The origin of the high level of melatonin in these locations has not been definitively established, but it is likely not exclusively of pineal origin. Melatonin has been shown to possess anti-inflammatory effects, among a number of actions. Melatonin reduces tissue destruction during inflammatory reactions by a number of means. Thus melatonin, by virtue of its ability to directly scavenge toxic free radicals, reduces macromolecular damage in all organs. The free radicals and reactive oxygen and nitrogen species known to be scavenged by melatonin include the highly toxic hydroxyl radical ($\cdot$OH), peroxynitrite anion ($ONOO^-$), and hypochlorous acid (HOCl), among others. These agents all contribute to the inflammatory response and associated tissue destruction. Additionally, melatonin has other means to lower the damage resulting from inflammation. Thus, it prevents the translocation of nuclear factor-kappa B (NF-κB) to the nucleus and its binding to DNA, thereby reducing the upregulation of a variety of proinflammatory cytokines, for example, interleukins and tumor neurosis factor-alpha. Finally, there is indirect evidence that melatonin inhibits the production of adhesion molecules that promote the sticking of leukocytes to endothelial cells. By this means melatonin attenuates transendothelial cell migration and edema, which contribute to tissue damage.

INTRODUCTION

A few milligrams of a novel indoleamine were initially extracted from 250,000 ovine pineal glands, and the extracted molecule was structurally identified as *N*-acetyl-5-methoxytryptamine in 1958.[1] It was given the common name melatonin because it is a methoxy derivative of sero*tonin* and, in amphibians, it has a regulatory influence on *mela*nin dispersion in epidermal melanocytes. In mammals, it was initially widely investigated for its effects in determining annual fluctuations in reproductive competence in seasonally breeding mammals.[2] In the last two decades,

[a]Address for correspondence: Russel J. Reiter, Department of Cellular and Structural Biology, Mail Code 7762, The University of Texas Health Science Center, 7703 Floyd Curl Drive, San Antonio, TX 78229-3900. Voice: 210-567-3859; fax: 210-567-6948.
reiter@uthscsa.edu

however, the documented functional implications of this secretory product have expanded markedly. It is possible, considering its known receptor and nonreceptor mediated actions, that melatonin may well influence the physiology of every cell in the organism.

MELATONIN SYNTHESIS, SECRETION, AND METABOLISM

Virtually everything that is known of melatonin synthesis has been determined by examining its production in the mammalian pineal gland.[3] As will be seen below, however, it is by no means the only organ in which melatonin is produced.

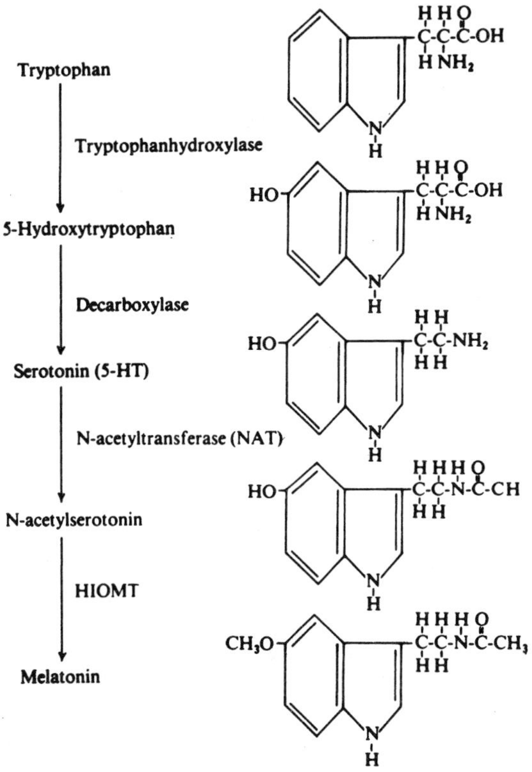

FIGURE 1. Metabolic pathway by which the amino acid tryptophan is converted to melatonin. The first two enzymes in this pathway, that is, the hydroxyase and decarboxylase, have a wide distribution, so serotonin is produced in a number of tissues, most noteworthy in neural tissues. The two enzymes that convert serotonin to melatonin have a more limited distribution. The pineal gland is a primary site of melatonin production, but other organs that produce or possibly produce melatonin include the retina, lens, ovary, gut, and several blood elements. Additionally, some sites, for example, bone marrow cells and bile, contain very high levels of melatonin of unknown origin.

Melatonin is a product of the amino acid tryptophan (see FIGURE 1). After its uptake into cells, tryptophan is first hydroxylated and then decarboxylated, resulting in the formation of 5-hydroxytryptamine (serotonin). The enzymes required for this conversion are widely distributed in neural and other tissues. The metabolism of serotonin to melatonin is likely more restricted due to the limited number of organs that contain the necessary enzymatic machinery to do so, although the list of cells known to contain/produce melatonin is increasing substantially. In organs that produce melatonin, serotonin is N-acetylated, with the resulting formation of N-acetylserotonin (FIG. 1). The final enzyme in the production of melatonin, hydroxyindole-O-methyltransferase (HIOMT), seems to be the most restrictive in terms of organ distribution. It O-methylates N-acetylserotonin to form N-acetyl-5-methoxytryptamine, melatonin.

In the pineal gland in particular, but also in the retina, melatonin generation is strictly photoperiod phase dependent. Thus, during the day pineal melatonin production is curtailed by mechanisms that involve a circuitous route for the transmission of neural messages from the eyes, via the suprachiasmatic nuclei (the biological clock) and the peripheral sympathetic nervous system, to the gland.[4] Conversely, at night pineal melatonin production proceeds unabated.

The nocturnal synthesis of melatonin, however, is interrupted by exposure of animals (and humans) to light of appropriate intensity and wavelength.[5] Considering this, only humans have the capability of determining the quantity of melatonin they produce with the use (or misuse) of artificial light.

Once melatonin is synthesized in the pineal, it is quickly released, generating a blood melatonin rhythm reminiscent of that seen in the gland. Being an amphiphilic molecule, melatonin is capable of entering every cell in the organism; additionally, it readily crosses all morphophysiological barriers, including, as examples, the blood–brain barrier[6] and the placenta.[7] Melatonin is enzymatically degraded in the liver to 6-hydroxymelatonin;[3] however, the indoleamine, in the process of scavenging free radials and reactive species, generates other metabolites, as well, including cyclic 3-hydroxymelatonin (when it scavenges two highly toxic hydroxyl radicals).[8] In the process of scavenging the activated form of peroxynitrous acid, melatonin is reportedly converted to 6-hydroxymelatonin, the same degradation product enzymatically produced in the liver.[9] Besides its direct free radical scavenging activities, which are accomplished without interaction with a receptor, melatonin modifies cell physiology via the membrane and possibly nuclear receptors as well.[10]

MELATONIN IN BODILY FLUIDS AND TISSUES

In all mammalian species, the pineal gland is a major source of circulating melatonin, inasmuch as, after surgical removal of this organ, blood melatonin concentrations are uniformly low during both the day and night.[3] Tissues that take up melatonin from the blood may differentially distribute it intracellularly. Although the number of studies related to the subcellular distribution of melatonin is limited, evidence suggests that highest concentrations are in the nuclei of cells.[6,11] Sufficient quantities of melatonin get into other organelles, however, as indicated by their actions at these sites, for example, cellular membranes[12] and mitochondria.[13]

The synthesis of melatonin in nonpineal organs certainly occurs; it is only a question of how many different organs actually produce the indoleamine. Extra-pineal sites of melatonin production in mammals should not be unexpected considering that it is also produced in plants, unicellular organisms, bacteria, and invertebrates, all of which lack a pineal gland.[14] The retinas of mammals are accepted as being a site of melatonin formation, but it may also be synthesized by the gut, lymphocytes, monocytes, other bone marrow cells, ovary, and the lens of the eye. Recently, melatonin has been identified in very high concentrations in the bile of a variety of mammals, including humans.[15] The levels in this fluid are two to three orders of magnitude higher than in the blood at night, and its origin remains unknown. Other bodily fluids that are known to contain melatonin include saliva, cerebrospinal fluid, ovarian follicular fluid, and the fluid from the anterior chamber of the eye.[3]

Recently, high melatonin levels were also found in the bone marrow.[16,17] This is particularly noteworthy because this tissue gives rise to many cells that are functionally related to the immune system. Melatonin was identified in bone marrow tissue using a variety of techniques, including radioimmunoassay, immunocytochemistry, high-performance liquid chromatography, and mass spectrometry. The immunocytochemical studies revealed melatonin in roughly 50% of the cells in bone marrow smears;[17] the cells that contained immunoreactive melatonin could not be specifically identified as to their type, but it was usually present in the smallest cells in rat bone marrow. Also, considering the high nuclear to cytosol ratio of the immunoreactive cells, they may be lymphocytes, cells that have already been shown to possess membrane and possibly nuclear receptors for melatonin.[10,16] In general, the immunoreactive product in these cells appeared to be located primarily in the cytosol.

A study of the activities of the enzymes, that is, *N*-acetyltransferase (NAT) and HIOMT, which convert serotonin to melatonin, led Conti *et al.*[17] to suggest that melatonin is formed in bone marrow elements. They also reported that some bone marrow cells also express mRNA encoding HIOMT. These findings are consistent with our own observations, which show that long-term pinealectomy diminished but certainly did not eliminate melatonin from the bone marrow.[18] The levels of melatonin in bone marrow, even in animals lacking their pineal gland, are much higher than those normally measured at night in the blood of pineal intact animals. This strongly suggests that much of the melatonin in bone marrow is from nonpineal sources. We also showed that supplementing rats with melatonin by injecting it peripherally significantly increased its concentration in bone marrow tissue, proving that these cells are able to concentrate melatonin against a gradient.[18] This indicates the presence of intracellular binding molecules that assist in retaining the indoleamine intracellularly. The ability of selected cells to concentrate melatonin is not restricted to bone marrow, because it has been shown that neural tissue and human breast cancer cells (especially estrogen receptor–positive breast cancer cells) also can have higher levels of melatonin than those present in the blood.[6,11,19]

MECHANISMS BY WHICH MELATONIN INFLUENCES
THE IMMUNE SYSTEM

It has already been mentioned that at least some immunocompetent cells possess either membrane and/or nuclear receptors for the indoleamine.[10,16] Membrane receptors for melatonin have been well characterized, and they likely mediate some of the many actions of melatonin.[20,21] Additionally, however, nuclear binding sites/receptors for melatonin have been identified (see FIGURE 2), and an interaction of melatonin with these receptors presumably relates to its ability to modify immune function.[22] Although less well characterized than the membrane receptors,[20,21] physiological and pharmacological evidence supports their existence[23,24] and melatonin-nuclear receptor interactions in the regulation of immune function.[10,25]

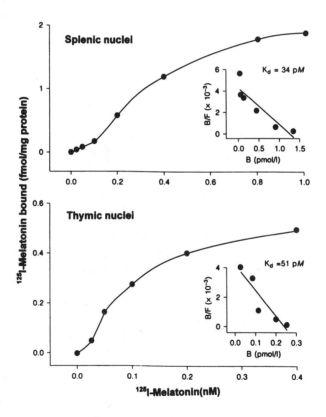

FIGURE 2. A summary of high-affinity binding of melatonin to purified cell nuclei from rat spleen (*top*) and thymus (*bottom*). Diagrammatically represented in the figure are the saturation isotherms and, as shown in the inserts, the Scatchard plots of 2[^{131}I]melatonin binding to these nuclei. In this study, nuclei were incubated with increasing concentrations of 2[^{131}I]melatonin; the incubation was carried out at 15°C for 45 minutes. (Reprinted by permission from Guerrero et al.[10])

Besides its obvious interactions with membrane and nuclear receptors in immune cells, melatonin has non-receptor-mediated actions in all systems, including the immune system. These effects are a consequence of melatonin's ability to directly scavenge free radicals.[26,27] In 1993 it was shown that melatonin directly neutralizes the highly toxic hydroxyl radical (·OH).[28] The ·OH is one of several by-products formed during the metabolism of molecular oxygen (O_2) (see FIGURE 3). Any metabolite that possesses an unpaired electron in its outer orbital is identified as a free radical, whereas the metabolic intermediates whose electrons are paired are referred to as reactive intermediates. Radicals and their intermediates are all differentially reactive and often toxic.

Only a small percentage (1–4%) of the O_2 that aerobic organisms use is converted to reactive intermediates and free radicals. Despite this small percentage, over the course of a lifetime, because of their toxic nature, they gradually destroy tissue, which leads to cellular and eventually organ dysfunction. Even the longevity of

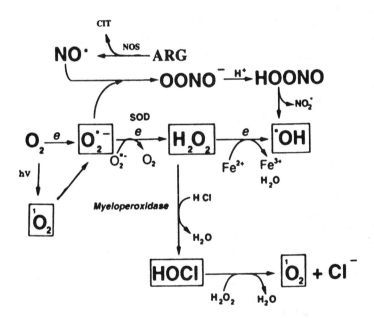

FIGURE 3. Molecular oxygen (O_2) is reduced metabolically to a variety of free radicals (molecules with an unpaired electron and therefore highly reactive) and reactive intermediates. A single electron reduction of O_2 produces the superoxide anion radical (O_2^-), which is either dismutated to hydrogen peroxide (H_2O_2) in the presence of superoxide dismutase (SOD) or is coupled with nitric oxide (NO·) to produce the peroxynitrite anion (ONOO⁻). H_2O_2, via the Fenton reaction, generates the highly toxic hydroxyl radical (·OH). In activated neutrophils and monocytes, myeloperoxidase activity generates hypochlorous acid (HOCl). Many of these reactive agents are produced at sites of inflammation. Because melatonin has the ability to scavenge a number of these reactive products, that is, ·OH, H_2O_2, HOCl, singlet oxygen ($^1O_2$), and the ONOO⁻, it reduces tissue damage during inflammatory reactions. As summarized in the text, melatonin has other anti-inflammatory actions as well.

aerobic organisms has been theoretically linked to the quantity of tissue destruction caused by free radicals. This is referred to as the free radical theory of aging, and free radical scavengers and antioxidants, that is, molecules that scavenge free radicals and their reactive intermediates, have likewise been implicated in preserving longevity and reducing pathophysiology due to their ability to prevent molecular damage.[29,30] Besides melatonin, there are a number of other molecules that effectively reduce the biomolecular destruction caused by oxygen metabolites, for example, ascorbic acid, α-tocopherol, and glutathione.[31]

MELATONIN AND INFLAMMATION

In the immune system, phagocytes play a critical role in warding off bacterial infections by engulfing these agents and destroying them via free radical mechanisms.[32] This process is part of what is known as the inflammatory reaction, and in the extreme it leads to extensive tissue injury mediated by the generated reactive species. The immune cells, which generate these oxidizing agents, include a variety of phagocytes and leukocytes, for example, neutrophils, monocytes, macrophages, and eosinophils. Phagocytes are normally activated by proinflammatory mediators of bacterial products that have receptors on the plasma membrane of the leukocytes. Following interaction with a receptor, the phagocytic cell assembles the multicomponent flavoprotein NADPH oxidase that catalyzes the formation of the superoxide anion radical ($O_2^{\cdot-}$):

$$NADPH + O_2 \rightarrow NADP^+ + O_2^{\cdot-}$$

$O_2^{\cdot-}$ has rather low reactivity toward most biological substrates. The major portion of this free radical is quickly dismutated to hydrogen peroxide (H_2O_2) (FIG. 3). H_2O_2, via the Fenton reaction, interacts with Fe^{2+} (or Cu^{1+}) to yield the very highly reactive and destructive ·OH. H_2O_2 has another fate in certain immune cells. Thus, activated neutrophils and monocytes secrete the hemoprotein myeloperoxidase (MPO) (FIG. 3) into the extracellular fluid where it catalyzes the oxidation of Cl^- by H_2O_2 to produce hypochlorous acid (HOCl):

$$H_2O_2 + Cl^- + H^+ \rightarrow HOCl + H_2O$$

HOCl possesses the two oxidizing equivalents of H_2O_2, and as a result it is roughly 100 to 1,000 times more toxic than either $O_2^{\cdot-}$ or H_2O_2.

Besides its dismutation to H_2O_2, $O_2^{\cdot-}$ couples with nitric oxide (NO·) to generate the peroxynitrite anion ($ONOO^-$):[33]

$$O_2^{\cdot-} + NO· \rightarrow ONOO^-$$

$ONOO^-$ and/or the products it subsequently generates, that is, peroxynitrous acid and the ·OH or a facsimile thereof,[34] participate in the tissue destruction induced by free radicals. Neutrophils are generally believed to produce both $O_2^{\cdot-}$ and NO· and thereby promote the formation of $ONOO^-$ and other destructive species.

In addition to directly scavenging the ·OH and a variety of other agents that cause macromolecular damage during inflammation, melatonin also scavenges both HOCl[35] and $ONOO^-$.[36] In so doing, melatonin has been shown to be a powerful anti-inflammatory agent in several experimental models.[37–39]

It is now accepted that, in addition to causing direct toxicity to biomolecules, the reactive species produced by phagocytic cells may also initiate, as well as exaggerate, the inflammatory response by virtue of their ability to stimulate a number of genes involved in inflammation. The stimulation of inflammation-related genes may occur, for example, by the activation of the transcription factor nuclear factor-kappa B (NF-κB). NF-κB is a wide-spread transcription factor that regulates a number of genes involved in immune and inflammatory responses.[40] Cytosolic NF-κB is activated by a variety of mediators, including oxidants and viral proteins, that enhance reactive oxygen species generation. This allows NF-κB to translocate to the nucleus and bind to DNA, thereby upregulating the production of a variety of enzymes and proinflammatory cytokines, including interleukin-2 (IL-2), IL-6, tumor necrosis factor-alpha (TNF-α), and inducible nitric oxide synthase (iNOS) (see FIGURE 4).

Melatonin was recently shown to reduce NF-κB binding to DNA, probably by preventing its translocation to the nucleus.[41,42] This curtails the production of the proinflammatory cytokines referred to above. Additionally, because melatonin has been shown to reduce leukocyte-endothelial adhesion and leukocyte transendothelial cell migration,[43] it may also inhibit the production of adhesion molecules that are also upregulated by NF-κB. Finally, melatonin has been shown to reduce recruitment of polymorphonuclear leukocytes to inflammatory sites.[44]

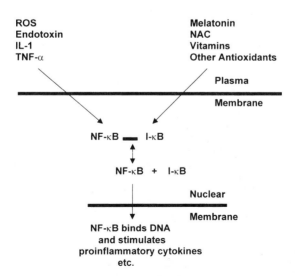

FIGURE 4. A summary of some aspects of the regulation of NF-κB translocation and inflammation. The proinflammatory cytokines produced, when NF-κB binds DNA, include several interleukins, tumor neurosis factor-α, and β-interferon. Melatonin and other free radical scavengers reduce the translocation of NF-κB to the nucleus, thereby reducing the induction of proinflammatory cytokines.

CONCLUDING REMARKS

From this brief discussion, it is obvious that melatonin may reduce tissue destruction during inflammatory responses via a number of means including direct free radical scavenging and indirectly by lowering the production of agents (cytokines and adhesion molecules) that contribute to cellular damage. It is anticipated that in the next decade these interactions will be clarified in greater detail and that melatonin will be experimentally and clinically exploited as an antioxidant and as an anti-inflammatory agent.

REFERENCES

1. LERNER, A.B., J.D. CASE, Y. TAKAHASLKI, T.H. LEE & W. MORI. 1958. Isolation of melatonin, the pineal factor that lightens melatonocytes. J. Am. Chem. Soc. **80:** 2587.
2. REITER, R.J. 1974. Comparative physiology: pineal gland. Annu. Rev. Physiol. **35:** 305–328.
3. REITER, R.J. 1991. Pineal melatonin: cell biology of its synthesis and of its physiological interactions. Endocr. Rev. **12:** 151–180.
4. TECLEMARIAM-MESBAH, R., A. KALSBEEK & P. PEVET. 1994. Afferent projections on preganglionic neurons projecting to the superior cervical ganglion: implications in transmission of photoperiodic information from the SCN to the pineal. Adv. Pineal Res. **8:** 51–56.
5. REITER, R.J. 1985. Action spectra, does-response relationships, and temporal aspects of light's effects on the pineal gland. Ann. N.Y. Acad. Sci. **453:** 215–230.
6. MENENDEZ-PELAEZ, A., B. POEGGELER, R.J. REITER, L. BARLOW-WALDEN, M.I. PABLOS & D.X. TAN. 1993. Nuclear localization of melatonin in different mammalian tissues: Immunocytochemical and radioimmunoassay evidence. J. Cell. Biochem. **53:** 373–382.
7. OKATANI, Y., K. YAMAMOTO, A. HAYASHI, Y. WAKATSUKI & Y. SAGARA. 1998. Maternal-fetal transfer of melatonin in human pregnancy near term. J. Pineal Res. **25:** 129–134.
8. TAN, D.X., L.C. MANCHESTER, R.J. REITER, B.F. PLUMMER, L.J. HARDIES, S.T. WEINTRAUB, VIJAYALAXMI & A.M.M. SHEPHERD. 1998. A novel melatonin metabolite, cyclic 3-hydroxymelatonin: a biomarker of *in vivo* hydroxyl radical generation. Biochem. Biophys. Res. Commun. **253:** 614–620.
9. ZHANG, H., G.L. SQUADRITO, R. UPPER & W.A. PRYOR. 1999. Reaction of peroxynitrite with melatonin: a mechanistic study. Chem. Res. Toxicol. **12:** 526–534.
10. GUERRERO, J.M., M. RAFII-EL-IDRISSI, A. GARCIA-PERGAÑEDA, S. GARCIA-MAURINO, M. GIL-HABA, D. POZO & J.R. CALVO. 1997. *In* Therapeutic Potential of Melatonin. G.J.M. Maestroni, A. Conti & R. J. Reiter, Eds.: 43–51. Karger. Basel.
11. MENENDEZ-PELAEZ, A. & R.J. REITER. 1993. Distribution of melatonin in mammalian tissues: relative importance of nuclear verses cytosolic localization. J. Pineal Res. **15:** 59–69.
12. REITER, R.J., L. TANG, J.J. GARCIA & A. MUÑOZ-HOYOS. 1997. Pharmacological actions of melatonin in free radical pathophysiology. Life Sci. **60:** 2255–2271.
13. MARTIN, M., M. MACIAS, G. ESCAMES, R.J. REITER, M.T. AGAPITO, G.G. ORTIZ & D. ACUÑA-CASTROVIEJO. 2000. Melatonin-induced increased activity of the respiratory chain complex I and IV can prevent mitochondrial damage by ruthenium red *in vivo*. J. Pineal Res. **28**(4): 242–248.
14. HARDELAND, R., I. BALZER, B. POEGGELER, H. FUHRBERG, H. URIA, G. BEHRMANN, R. WOLF, T.J. MEYER & R.J. REITER. 1995. On the primary functions of melatonin in evolution: mediation of photoperiodic signals in a unicell, photooxidation and scavenging of free radicals. J. Pineal Res. **18:** 104–111.

15. TAN, D.X., L.C. MANCHESTER, R.J. REITER, W. QI, M.A. HANES & N.J. FARLEY. 1999. High physiological levels of melatonin in the bile of mammals. Life Sci. **65:** 2523–2529.

16. GONZALEZ-HABA, M.G., S. GARCIA-MAURIÑO, J.R. CALVO, R. GOBERNA & J.M. GUERRERO. 1995. High-affinity binding of melatonin by human circulating T lymphocytes (CD4+). FASEB J. **9:** 1331–1335.

17. CONTI, A., S. CONCONI, E. HERTENS, K. SKWARLO-SONTA, M. MARKOWSKA & G.J.M. MAESTRONI. 2000. Evidence for melatonin synthesis in mouse and human bone marrow cells. J. Pineal Res. **28:** 193–202.

18. TAN, D.X., L.C. MANCHESTER, R.J. REITER, W. QI, M. ZHANG, S.T. WEINTRAUB, J. CABRERA, R.M. SAINZ & J.C. MAYO. 1999. Identification of extremely high levels of melatonin in bone marrow: its origin and significance. Biochem. Biophys. Acta **1472:** 206–214.

19. MAESTRONI, G.J.M. & A. CONTI. 1997. Association of melatonin with nuclear grade and estrogen receptor status in human breast cancer. *In* Therapeutic Role of Melatonin. G.J.M. Maestroni, A. Conti & R.J. Reiter, Ed.: 125–131. Karger. Basel.

20. REPPERT, S.M., D.R. WEAVER & T. EBISAWA. 1994. Cloning and characterization of a mammalian melatonin receptor that mediates reproductive and circadian responses. Neuron **13:** 1177–1185.

21. SHIU, S.Y.W., N. NG & S.F. PANG. 1996. A molecular perspective of the genetic relationships of G-protein coupled melatonin receptor subtypes. J. Pineal Res. **20:** 198–204.

22. GUERRERO, J.M. & R.J. REITER. 1992. A brief survey of pineal gland–immune system interrelationships. Endocr. Res. **18:** 91–113.

23. ACUÑA-CASTROVIEJO, D., R.J. REITER, A. MENENDEZ-PELAEZ, M.I. PABLOS & A. BURGOS. 1994. Characterization of high-affinity melatonin binding sites in purified cell nuclei of liver. J. Pineal Res. **16:** 110–112.

24. CARLBERG, C. & I. WIESSENBERG. 1997. Nuclear signaling of melatonin. *In* Therapeutic Potential of Melatonin, G.J.M. Maestroni, A. Conti & R.J. Reiter, Eds.: 25–35. Karger. Basel.

25. POZO, D., M. DELGADO, J.R. CALVO, A. GARCIA-PERGAÑEDA & J.M. GUERRERO. 1997. Expression of membrane melatonin receptor mRNA in rat thymus and spleen. *In* Therapeutic Potential of Melatonin. G.J.M. Maestroni, A. Conti & R.J. Reiter, Eds.: 36–42. Karger. Basel.

26. REITER, R.J., D. MELCHIORRI, E. SEWERYNEK, B. POEGGELER, L.R. BARLOW-WALDEN, J.I. CHUANG, G.G. ORTIZ & D. ACUÑA-CASTROVIEJO. 1995. A review of the evidence supporting melatonin's role as an antioxidant. J. Pineal Res. **18:** 1–11.

27. REITER, R.J. 1998. Oxidative damage in the central nervous system: protection by melatonin. Prog. Neurobiol. **56:** 359–364.

28. TAN, D.X., L.D. CHEN, B. POEGGELER, L.C. MANCHESTER & R.J. REITER. 1993. Melatonin: a potent endogenous hydroxyl radical scavenger. Endocr. J. **1:** 57–60.

29. HARMAN, D. 1993. Free radical involvement in aging: pathophysiology and functional implications. Drugs & Aging **3:** 60–80.

30. REITER, R.J., M.I. PABLOS, T.T. AGAPITO & J.M. GUERRERO. 1996. Melatonin in the context of the free radical theory of aging. Ann. N.Y. Acad. Sci. **786:** 362–378.

31. CHAPPLE, I.L.C. 1997. Reactive oxygen species and antioxidants in inflammatory diseases. J. Clin. Periodontol. **24:** 287–296.

32. HOFFELD, J.T. 1982. Oxygen radicals in inflammation and immunity. *In* Host-Parasite Interactions in Periodontal Disease. R.J. Genco & S.E. Mergenhagen, Eds.: 343–353. American Society for Microbiology. Washington.

33. BECKMAN, J.S., T.W. BECKMAN, J. CHEN, P.A. MARSHALL & B.A. FREEMAN. 1990. Apparent hydroxyl radical production by peroxynitrite: implications for endothelial injury from nitric oxide and superoxide. Proc. Natl. Acad. Sci. USA **87:** 1620–1624.

34. PRYOR, W. & G. SQUADRITO. 1995. The chemistry of peroxynitrite: a product from the reaction of nitric oxide and superoxide. Am. J. Physiol. **268:** L699–L722.

35. MARSHALL, K.A., R.J. REITER, B. POEGGELER, O.I. ARUOMA & B. HALLIWELL. 1996. Evaluation of the antioxidant activity of melatonin *in vitro*. Free Radical Biol. Med. **41:** 391–395.

36. GILAD, E., S. CUZZOCREA, B. ZINGARELLI, A.L. SALZMAN & C. SZABO. 1997. Melatonin is a scavenger of peroxynitrite. Life Sci. **60:** PL169–PL174.
37. CUZZOCREA, S., B. ZINGARELLI, G. COSTANTINO & A.P. CAPUTI. 1998. Protective effect of melatonin in a non-septic shock model induced by zymosan in the rat. J. Pineal Res. **25:** 24–33.
38. CUZZOCREA, S., G. COSTANTINO, E. MAZZON & A.P. CAPUTI. 1999. Regulation of prostaglandin production in carrageenan-induced pleurisy by melatonin. J. Pineal Res. **27:** 9–14.
39. EL-SOKKARY, G.H., R.J. REITER, S. CUZZOCREA, A.P. CAPUTI, A.F. HASSANEIN & D.X. TAN. 1999. Role of melatonin in reduction of lipid peroxidation and peroxynitrite formation in non-septic shock induced by zymosan. Shock **12**(5): 402–408.
40. SIEBENLIST, U., G. FRANZOSO & K. BROWN. 1994. Structure, regulation and function of NFκB. Annu. Rev. Cell Biol. **10:** 405–431.
41. MOHAN, N., K. SADEGHI, R.J. REITER & M.L. MELTZ. 1995. The neurohormone melatonin inhibits cytosine, mitogen and ionizing radiation induced NF-κB. Biochem. Mol. Biol. Int. **37:** 1063–1070.
42. CHUANG, J.I., N. MOHAN, M.L. MELTZ & R.J. REITER. 1996. Effect of melatonin of NF-κB DNA–binding activity in rat spleen. Cell Biol. Int. **20:** 687–692.
43. BERTUGLIA, S., P.L. MARCHIAFAVA & A. COLANTUONI. 1996. Melatonin prevents ischemia reperfusion injury in the hamster cheek pouch. Cardiovasc. Res. **31:** 947–952.
44. SEWERYNEK, E., R.J. REITER, D. MELCHIORRI, G.G. ORTIZ & A. LEWINSKI. 1996. Oxidative damage in the liver induced by ischemia-reperfusion: protection by melatonin. Hepato-Gastroenterology **43:** 898–905.

Gene Regulation by Melatonin

CARSTEN CARLBERG[a]

Institut für Physiologische Chemie I, Heinrich-Heine-Universität, Düsseldorf, Germany

ABSTRACT: The physiological and neuroendocrine functions of the pineal gland hormone, melatonin, and its therapeutic potential critically depend on the understanding of its target sites and its mechanisms of action. This has progressed considerably in the last few years through the cloning of G protein–coupled seven-transmembrane melatonin receptors (Mel_{1a} and Mel_{1b}) as well as of nuclear receptors (RZR/RORα and RZRβ) that are associated with melatonin signaling. The transcription factor RZR/RORα appears to mediate a direct gene regulatory action of the hormone, and specific binding sites have been identified in promoter regions of a variety of genes, such as 5-lipoxygenase (5-LO), $p21^{WAF1/CIP1}$, and bone sialoprotein (BSP). The membrane signaling pathway clearly shows higher ligand sensitivity than the nuclear signaling pathway, but details of its signal transduction cascade, and target genes are presently unknown. Membrane melatonin receptors are expressed mainly in the central nervous system, whereas RZR/RORα is prominently expressed both in the periphery and the brain. The action of membrane melatonin receptors and their specific agonists have been associated with circadian rhythmicity, whereas direct effects of melatonin in the periphery, such as immunomodulation, cellular growth, and bone differentiation, mainly appear to be mediated by RZR/RORα. It is hypothesized in this review that, in some cases, RZR/RORα may be a primary target of membrane melatonin receptors.

INTRODUCTION

Melatonin (N-acetyl-5-methoxytryptamine) was identified as the skin-lightening ingredient of the pineal gland[1] and is the major hormone of this gland.[2] Melatonin appears to have an important role in the regulation of circadian rhythms, sleep and mood, but there is also various evidence that the pineal gland hormone is important in immunomodulation, reproduction, tumor growth, and aging.[3] The mammalian pineal gland acts as a neuroendocrine transducer for photic information from the retina via the suprachiasmatic nucleus (SCN). Melatonin appears to be a mediator of light and dark information and day length, but the circadian rhythm of melatonin secretion is directed by the SCN, that is, it is of endogenous origin.[4] Melatonin is synthesized in the pineal gland from serotonin under the control of the enzymes arylalkylamine N-acetyltransferase (NAT) and hydroxyindole-O-methyltransferase (HIOMT) (see FIGURE 1).[5] NAT gene expression is regulated by the SCN via β-adrenergic innervation of the pineal, which increases the cAMP level and activates the transcription factor cAMP response element (CRE) binding protein (CREB). The

[a]Address for correspondence: Dr. Carsten Carlberg, Institut für Physiologische Chemie I, Heinrich-Heine-Universität Düsseldorf, Postfach 10 10 07, D-40001 Düsseldorf, Germany. Voice: +49-211-8115358; fax: +49-211-208399.
carlberg@uni-duesseldorf.de

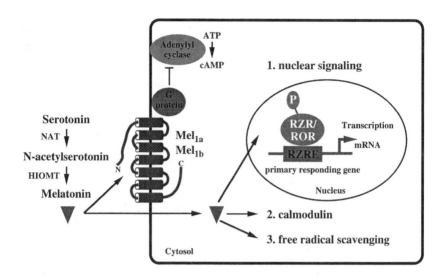

FIGURE 1. Melatonin signaling. The pineal gland hormone, melatonin, shows various molecular actions. Melatonin is synthesized in the pineal gland from serotonin. The hormone binds with high affinity in the picomolar range to the membrane receptors, Mel$_{1a}$ and Mel$_{1b}$, and/or in the nanomolar range to the nuclear receptor RZR/ROR as well as to calmodulin. At even higher concentrations melatonin has also a free radical scavenging function.

NAT promoter contains several CREs that are also bound by members of the CRE modulator (CREM) family, such as the dominant repressor inducible cAMP early repressor (ICER). The diurnal regulation of NAT depends on the interplay between CREB and ICER and finally results in synthesis and release of melatonin in darkness and its inhibition by daylight. Because the biological half-life of the hormone is short, serum levels of melatonin display a clear circadian rhythm with peak levels of approximately 0.4 nM at night time.[3] However, peak serum melatonin concentrations vary considerably between individuals and depend very much on age. Standard oral doses of melatonin (1 to 5 mg), which are taken daily by hundreds of thousands of Americans, result in 10 to 100 times higher serum melatonin concentrations than the usual nighttime peak one hour after ingestion, followed by a decline within four to eight hours. Although no serious side effects have been reported with the ingestion of melatonin, in Europe melatonin has been classified as a medicine and was therefore withdrawn from general sale.

MEMBRANE MELATONIN RECEPTORS

Two membrane-associated melatonin binding sites, referred to as ML1 and ML2, can be distinguished pharmacologically by their high affinity in the picomolar range and their lower affinity in the nanomolar range, respectively (TABLE 1).[6] ML1 receptors are coupled to pertussis toxin–sensitive G proteins and belong to the family of seven-transmembrane receptors (FIG. 1). In mammals, two types of high-affinity membrane melatonin receptors, referred to as Mel_{1a} (also named mt_1) and Mel_{1b} (also named MT_2), have now been cloned.[7,8] Both receptors show 60% homology at the amino acid level. A third membrane melatonin receptor, called Mel_{1c}, was found in amphibians but not in mammals.[9] The Mel_{1a} receptor is expressed in the pars tuberalis of the pituitary and the SCN, that is, in the presumed sites of the reproductive and circadian actions of melatonin, respectively, whereas the Mel_{1b} receptor is mainly expressed in the retina (TABLE 1). *In situ* hybridization and RT-PCR experiments suggest that the Mel_{1a} receptor appears to represent more than 99% of all melatonin membrane binding sites in the brain.[10] The Mel_{1a} receptor appears to mediate the inhibitory action of melatonin on the SCN, whereas the Mel_{1b} receptor may be involved in the phase-shifting response of melatonin.[10]

Not many details on the targets and mediators of their transduction pathways of the membrane melatonin receptors are known yet, but it appears that stimulation of these receptors decreases the intracellular level of cAMP, which then results in the change of the phosphorylation status of target proteins such as CREB.[9] In addition to the inhibition of adenylyl cyclase activity, high-affinity melatonin receptors also regulate cGMP levels through proteins upstream of the guanylyl cyclase such as NO synthase.[11] In mammals, the latter function appears to be specific for the Mel_{1a} receptor.[12] In the pars tuberalis, membrane melatonin receptors modulate the expression of the tuberalin gene, which in turn stimulates the release of prolactin from these cells.[13] Mel_{1a} receptor levels were found to be downregulated by protein kinase C (PKC).[14] Moreover, it has been suggested that second messengers, other than cAMP and cGMP, might be modulated by melatonin via Mel_{1a} receptors,[15] but a clear picture of the spectrum of biochemical signals elicited by melatonin is still lacking. Despite the insight into possible functions of melatonin membrane receptors, little is known about the molecular structure of the receptor or receptor-ligand interactions. However, elucidation of the primary structures of melatonin receptors has allowed construction of a three-dimensional rhodopsin-based model for melatonin recognition at its receptor.[16] According to this model, melatonin is recognized by specific amino acid residues in a binding pocket formed by transmembrane helices. The amino acids suggested to interact with melatonin are highly conserved within the family but are not present in other G protein–coupled receptors.

TABLE 1. Melatonin binding sites and receptors

Binding sites	Receptors	Location	Expression	Function
ML1 (high affinity)	Mel_{1a}(mt1)	Membrane	Pars tuberalis SCN	Reproduction circadian rhythm
	Mel_{1b}(mt2)	Membrane	Retina	?
ML2 (low affinity)	Calmodulin	Cytosol	Ubiquitous	Calcium signaling
	RZR/RORα (NR1F1)	Nucleus	Ubiquitous	Various
	RZRβ (NR1F2)	Nucleus	Retina, SCN pineal	Circadian rhythm?

INTRACELLULAR ACTIONS OF MELATONIN

The small lipophilic structure of melatonin suggests that it may also have intracellular binding sites and actions. Melatonin was shown to act as an intracellular scavenger of hydroxyl and peroxyl radicals and appears to protect against oxidative damage[17] (FIG. 1). In humans, the antioxidant effect probably occurs only at pharmacological melatonin concentrations, but the decrease of nighttime serum melatonin concentration that occurs with aging suggests an antiaging potential of the pineal gland hormone.[18] Melatonin was also found to bind cytosolic calmodulin and thus appears to modulate calcium signaling[19] (FIG. 1).

Most interestingly, the pineal gland hormone was also shown to bind and activate two closely related nuclear receptors, referred to as RZR/RORα[20,21] and RZRβ[22] (FIG. 1; according to the unified nomenclature of the nuclear receptor superfamily, they are now called NR1F1 and NR1F2, respectively[23]) in the low nanomolar range.[24,25] The nuclear receptor superfamily is a family of approximately 100 transcription factors that all contain a highly conserved DNA binding domain of 66 to 70 amino acids forming two zinc finger structures.[26] A further characteristic structure of nuclear receptors is a moderately conserved, carboxy-terminal ligand-binding domain that also contains dimerization and transactivation subdomains.

RZR/RORα and RZRβ show distinct spaciotemporal expression patterns, suggesting that both receptor subtypes have different functions related to cell-specific gene control mechanisms in the context of different biological processes. At least one of the four RZR/RORα isoforms is found in every tissue, but highest expression was found in peripheral blood lymphocytes (B cells, T cells, and neutrophils)[20] and skin.[27] RZR/RORα is expressed during embryonic and postnatal development of the brain in Purkinje cells of the cerebellum, in the olfactory bulb, in the dorsal root ganglia, and in the thalamus and the hippocampus.[28] Moreover, RZR/RORα upregulation was found during the differentiation of embryonic P19 cells into neurons.[29] By contrast, RZRβ is expressed only in the retina and the brain, with highest expression in the pineal gland, the SCN, the pars tuberalis of the pituitary, the hypothalamus, the thalamus, and the spinal cord.[24,30,31] The receptor shows the tendency to be expressed in regions of the brain that are involved in sensory pathways rather than in those involved in motor control.[31,32] Moreover, during embryonic development RZRβ expression in the SCN changes,[30] and in the pineal gland the expression of RZRβ was found to be regulated by cAMP in a day–night rhythm.[33] Interestingly, the RZRβ knockout mouse model shows effects on circadian rhythmicity.[34]

Nuclear receptors regulate gene transcription through the binding to specific DNA sequences, called response elements, which are located in the promoter region of their target genes.[35] Therefore, for each nuclear receptor the characterization of its response elements provides important information. RZR/RORα and RZRβ belong to the minority of the members of the nuclear receptor superfamily that are able to bind as monomers to DNA. They require the typical hexameric core-binding site RGGTCA (R = A or G) and an A/T-rich sequence 5'-flanking to this site; in particular, a T in the -1 position and an A in the -4 position appear to be crucial.[21,22] In theory, the consensus sequence for RZREs should be found every 33 kB, that is, approximately one in ten genes should, on average, carry an RZRE. Therefore, it is not surprising that RZREs have been identified in a broad variety of promoter regions.[36,37] Apparently, the most interesting candidate genes are the proinflammatory enzyme 5-LO,[38] the cell-cycle inhibitor p21$^{WAF1/CIP1}$,[36] and BSP.[36]

RZR/ROR SIGNALING

A constitutive transcriptional activity is well known for a variety of transcription factors, such as NF-κB, AP1, or CREB. Regulation of these transcription factors is mainly achieved through phosphorylation and/or dissociation of repressor proteins. The constitutive activity of RZR/RORα and RZRβ was found to be clearly reduced by the depletion or omission of serum, indicating that serum components may either directly (as true ligands) or indirectly activate RZR/ROR.[22,24,25] Under such conditions of low constitutive activity, it was found that the thiazolidinedione CGP52608 (1-[3-allyl-4-oxo-thiazolidine-2-ylidene]-4-methyl-thiosemicarbazone)[25] and structurally related compounds[39] show, at low nanomolar concentrations (1 to 5 nM), specific activation of RZR/RORα. Those thiazolidinediones that were able to activate RZR/RORα, exhibited potent antiarthritic activity,[39] whereas close analogues were pharmacologically inactive and did not exhibit receptor activation properties. As for thiazolidinediones, low nanomolar concentrations of melatonin were sufficient for RZR/RORα and RZRβ activation. However, at high constitutive activity of RZR/RORα, a significant ligand activation has not yet been observed.[25,40,41] This suggests that RZR/RORα and RZRβ may only be mediators of nuclear melatonin signaling under restricted conditions. However, studies with melatonin responding genes that carry a RZR/ROR binding site in their promoter[38] indicated that these restrictions may only apply under artificial conditions using overexpressed receptors and heterologous promoter constructs.

Ligand binding assays with 2-[^{125}I]-iodomelatonin demonstrated specific binding to nuclear extracts of RZR/ROR-overexpressing cells and in vitro–translated RZR/ROR.[24,25] The thiazolidinedione CGP52608 also showed specific binding to nuclear extracts and appeared to compete with melatonin for the same binding site.[25] Interestingly, CGP52608 does not bind to membrane preparations that contain membrane melatonin receptors.[25] The K_d values of melatonin and CGP52608 binding to nuclear extracts were determined in the low nanomolar range.[24,25] Interestingly, melatonin concentrations are approximately fivefold higher in children than in adults, reaching concentrations averaging 1.4 nM,[42] which may suggest that the nuclear receptors may play a more prominent role in children than in adults.

IMMUNOMODULATORY EFFECTS OF MELATONIN

Melatonin is being considered as playing a fundamental role in immunomodulation, such as an increase of IL-2 and IL-4 production in T lymphocytes.[43] In accordance with that, melatonin receptors with a K_d value of 0.27 nM have been described in CD4$^+$ T cells[44] and monocytes.[45] Mel$_{1a}$ receptors were initially assumed to be expressed exclusively in the brain, but sensitive RT-PCR techniques allowed the detection of the receptors also in lymphocytes.[46] However, the RZR ligand CGP52608 was shown to displace melatonin from spleen and thymus cell nuclei,[47] and in CD4$^+$

T cells, CGP52608 enhanced the production of IL-2, IL-6, and interferon-γ,[48] which suggests that these genes are regulated by melatonin via RZR/RORα. Moreover, melatonin was reported to downregulate the expression of 5-LO in cells that exclusively contain RZR/RORα.[38] In support of this finding, 5-LO mRNA expression levels were increased in the hippocampus of pinealectomized rats as compared with the sham-operated controls.[49] The enzyme 5-LO has a key role in the synthesis of leukotrienes, which mediate allergic and inflammatory reactions.[50] Inflammatory reactions are known to be associated with the generation of a large number of free radicals. Because melatonin inhibits 5-LO activity, it would tend to reduce inflammatory reactions as well as the free radical damage.

ANTIPROLIFERATIVE EFFECTS OF MELATONIN

Melatonin was shown to influence the growth of tumors and was found, in most cases, to have a protective effect. The pineal gland hormone has proved to suppress tumor growth in a number of experimental models, including undifferentiated neoplasms, sarcomas, and carcinomas. The exact mechanisms of the oncostatic action of melatonin are not known. MCF-7 breast carcinoma cells express RZR/RORα,[38] and several important proteins that regulate the cell cycle, such as p21$^{WAF1/CIP1}$, contain an RZRE within their gene promoter regions.[36] The expression of p21$^{WAF1/CIP1}$ was observed to be repressed through a dominant negative RZR/RORα mutant,[51] suggesting that RZR/RORα is an important regulator of the p21$^{WAF1/CIP1}$ gene. Moreover, the RZR/RORα ligand CGP52608 was shown to cause antiproliferative effects.[52] This evidence suggest that RZR/RORα may be the mediator of the antiproliferative effect of the pineal gland hormone. Moreover, a very interesting experimental model is the mouse mutation *staggerer*. Homozygous staggerer mice show severe cerebellar ataxia, immune defects, and reduced size. It had been shown that this mutation caries a disrupted RZR/RORα gene, that is, *staggerer* mice express an RZR/RORα protein that lacks its ligand-binding domain.[53] The *staggerer* phenotype was confirmed by the RZR/RORα knockout.[27,54] Until now, the effects of melatonin on *staggerer* mice have not yet been investigated, but such experiments may help to define the physiological role of RZR/RORα in the context of the pineal gland hormone.

Melatonin was also shown to downregulate the estrogen receptor (ER) expression[55] and to block ER activation.[56] These antiestrogenic effects appear to be mediated by membrane melatonin receptors, as the ER promoter does not contain an RZRE, and RZR/RORα was excluded as mediating antiestrogenic effects of melatonin.[56] Moreover, also TGFβ and the protooncogene c-*myc* have been shown to be upregulated by melatonin in MCF-7 cells.[57] Finally, an indirect, neuroendocrine effect of melatonin on the growth of hormone-responsive cancers may be mediated via the hypothalamic-pituitary axis through an inhibition of the release of the peptide hormones GnRH from the hypothalamus and of LH, FSH, and prolactin from the pituitary, which in turn would have repressive effects on steroid hormone production.

MELATONIN AND BONE

Melatonin has recently been shown to be capable of promoting osteoblast differentiation and mineralization of matrix in culture,[58] which suggests that the pineal gland hormone may play an essential role in regulation of bone growth. As one of the major secretory proteins of osteoblasts, BSP functions to regulate mineralization possibly by its direct interaction with cell surface integrin receptors and/or by initiating nucleation of the bone mineral, hydroxyapatite. Therefore, increased expression of BSP along with other bone marker proteins is required to induce mineralization. There is evidence that the effects of melatonin on BSP expression appear to be initiated by Mel_{1b} receptors, which were found to be expressed in osteoblasts.[58] Melatonin membrane receptors are known to reduce the cAMP levels, and the expression of RZR/RORs were found to be regulated by cAMP, at least in the pineal gland.[33] This suggests that RZR/RORα, as a primary responding gene of membrane melatonin receptors, may regulate BSP gene expression through the strong RZRE in the BSP promoter. The decreasing melatonin levels during the aging process therefore suggests that melatonin may have a significant influence on the rate of synthesis and/or maintenance of bone in the elderly.

CONCLUDING HYPOTHESIS:
MEMBRANE MELATONIN SIGNALING VIA NUCLEAR RECEPTORS?

It has been postulated that, at least in mammals, direct effects of melatonin via membrane receptors are restricted to the brain.[4] The brain-specific expression of Mel_{1a} and Mel_{1b} receptors, as initially reported, supported this view. In fact, melatonin binding sites were found primarily in various regions of the brain, but in the meantime also in peripheral tissues. This would allow three cases for melatonin signaling through nuclear and membrane receptors to be distinguished: cells that express (1) membrane melatonin receptors and RZR/ROR in parallel, (2) only membrane melatonin receptors, or (3) only RZR/ROR. Inasmuch as RZR/ROR is rather ubiquitously expressed, the first case may apply to various structures of the central nervous system (SCN, retina, pars tuberalis, and the pineal gland). Until now, a tissue that only expresses membrane melatonin receptors is not known. RZR/ROR is a phosphoprotein (like, for example, CREB), and its high constitutive activity is likely to be modulated by a change of its phosphorylation status. The role of covalent modifications for the function of RZR/ROR is not yet studied, but it is tempting to speculate that it may be as important as ligand-induced activation. This leads to the idea that the phosphorylation status of RZR/ROR, that is, its constitutive activity, may be modulated by a membrane melatonin receptor, so that RZR/ROR may be a primary target gene of membrane melatonin signaling.

REFERENCES

1. LERNER, A.B., J.D. CASE, Y. TAKAHASHI, T.H. LEE & W. MORI. 1958. Isolation of melatonin, the pineal factor that lightens melanocytes. J. Am. Chem. Soc. **80:** 2587–2595.

2. REITER, R.J. 1991. Pineal melatonin: cell biology of its synthesis and of its physiological interactions. Endocr. Rev. **12:** 151–180.
3. BRZEZINSKI, A. 1997. Melatonin in humans. N. Engl. J. Med. **336:** 186–195.
4. REPPERT, S.M., D.R. WEAVER, S.A. RIVKEES & E.G. STOPA. 1988. Putative melatonin receptors in a human biological clock. Science **242:** 78–81.
5. BORJIGIN, J., X. LI & S.H. SNYDER. 1999. The pineal gland and melatonin: molecular and pharmacologic regulation. Annu. Rev. Pharmacol. Toxicol. **39:** 53–65.
6. KRAUSE, D.N. & M.L. DUBOCOVICH. 1991. Melatonin receptors. Annu. Rev. Pharmacol. Toxicol. **31:** 549–568.
7. REPPERT, S.M., D.R. WEAVER & T. EBISAWA. 1994. Cloning and characterization of a mammalian melatonin receptor that mediates reproductive and circadian responses. Neuron **13:** 1177–1185.
8. REPPERT, S.M., C. GODSON, C.D. MAHLE, D.R. WEAVER, S.A. SLAUGENHAUPT & J.F. GUSELLA. 1995. Molecular characterization of a second melatonin receptor expressed in human retina and brain: the Mel$_{1b}$ melatonin receptor. Proc. Natl. Acad. Sci. USA **92:** 8734–8738.
9. EBISAWA, T., S. KARNE, M.R. LERNER & S.M. REPPERT. 1994. Expression cloning of a high-affinity melatonin receptor from *Xenopus* dermal melanophores. Proc. Natl. Acad. Sci. USA **91:** 6133–6137.
10. LIU, C., D.R. WEAVER, X. JIN, L.P. SHEARMAN, R.L. PIESCHL, V.K. GRIBKOFF & S.M. REPPERT. 1997. Molecular dissection of two distinct actions of melatonin on the suprachiasmatic circadian clock. Neuron **19:** 91–102.
11. JOCKERS, R., L. PETIT, I. LACROIX, P. DE COPPET, P. BARRETT, P.J. MORGAN, B. GUARDIOLA, P. DELAGRANGE, S. MARULLO & A.D. STROSBERG. 1997. Novel isoform of Mel$_{1c}$ melatonin receptors modulating intracellular cyclic guanosine 3',5'-monophosphate levels. Mol. Endocrinol. **11:** 1070–1081.
12. PETIT, L., I. LACROIX, P. DE COPPET, A.D. STROSBERG & R. JOCKERS. 1999. Differential signaling of human Mel$_{1a}$ and Mel$_{1b}$ melatonin receptor through the cyclic guanosine 3'-5'-monophosphate pathway. Biochem. Pharmacol. **15:** 633–639.
13. MORGAN, P., C.A. WEBSTER, J.G. MERCER, A.W. ROSS, D.G. HAZLERIGG, A. MACLEAN & P. BARRETT. 1996. The ovine *pars tuberalis* secretes a factor(s) that regulates gene expression in both lactotrophic and nonlactotrophic pituitary cells. Endocrinology **137:** 4018–4026.
14. BARRETT, P., G. DAVIDSON, D.G. HAZLERIGG, M.A. MORRIS, A.W. ROSS & P.J. MORGAN. 1998. Mel$_{1a}$ melatonin receptor expression is regulated by protein kinase C and an additional pathway addressed by the protein kinase C inhibitor Ro 31-8220 in ovine pars tuberalis cells. Endocrinology **139:** 163–171.
15. GODSON, C. & S.M. REPPERT. 1997. The Mel$_{1a}$ melatonin receptor is coupled to parallel signal transduction pathways. Endocrinology **138:** 397–404.
16. NAVAJAS, C., T. KOKKOLA, A. POSO, N. HONKA, J. GYNTHER & J.T. LAITINEN. 1996. A rhodopsin-based model for melatonin recognition at its G protein-coupled receptor. Eur. J. Pharmacol. **304:** 173–183.
17. REITER, R.J., D. MELCHORRI, E. SEWERYNEK, B. POEGGELER, L. BARLOW-WALDEN, J. CHUANG, G.G. ORTIZ & D. AÇUNA-CASTROVIEJO. 1995. A review of the evidence supporting melatonin's role as an antioxidant. J. Pineal Res. **18:** 1–11.
18. REITER, R.J., D.-X. TAN, B. POEGGELER, A. MENENDEZ-PELAEZ, L.-D. CHEN & S. SAARELA. 1994. Melatonin as a free radical scavenger: implications for aging and age-related diseases. Ann. N.Y. Acad. Sci. **719:** 1–12.
19. ROMERO, M.P., A. GARCIA-PERGADENA, J.M. GUERRERO & C. OSUNA. 1998. Membrane-bound calmodulin in *X. laevis* oocytes as a novel binding site for melatonin. FASEB J. **12:** 1401–1408.
20. BECKER-ANDRÉ, M., E. ANDRÉ & J.F. DELAMARTER. 1993. Identification of nuclear receptor mRNAs by RT-PCR amplification of conserved zinc-finger motif sequences. Biochem. Biophys. Res. Commun. **194:** 1371–1379.
21. GIGUÈRE, V., M. TINI, G. FLOCK, E. ONG, R.M. EVANS & G. OTULAKOWSKI. 1994. Isoform-specific amino-terminal domains dictate DNA-binding properties of RORα, a novel family of orphan hormone nuclear receptors. Genes & Dev. **8:** 538–553.

22. CARLBERG, C., R. HOOFT VAN HUIJSDUIJNEN, J. STAPLE, J.F. DELAMARTER & M. BECKER-ANDRÉ. 1994. RZRs, a novel class of retinoid related orphan receptors that function as both monomers and homodimers. Mol. Endocrinol. **8:** 757–770.

23. NUCLEAR RECEPTOR COMMITTEE. 1999. A unified nomenclature system for the nuclear receptor superfamily. Cell **97:** 161–163.

24. BECKER-ANDRÉ, M., I. WIESENBERG, N. SCHAEREN-WIEMERS, E. ANDRÉ, M. MISSBACH, J.-H. SAURAT & C. CARLBERG. 1994. Pineal gland hormone melatonin binds and activates an orphan of the nuclear receptor superfamily. J. Biol. Chem. **269:** 28531–28534.

25. WIESENBERG, I., M. MISSBACH, J.-P. KAHLEN, M. SCHRÄDER & C. CARLBERG. 1995. Transcriptional activation of the nuclear receptor RZRα by the pineal gland hormone melatonin and identification of CGP52608 as a synthetic ligand. Nucleic Acids Res. **23:** 327–333.

26. FREEDMAN, L.P. 1992. Anatomy of the steroid receptor zinc finger region. Endocrine Rev. **13:** 129–145.

27. STEINMAYR, M., E. ANDRE, F. CONQUET, L. RONDI-REIG, N. DELHAYE-BOUCHAUD, N. AUCLAIR, H. DANIEL, F. CREPEL, J. MARIANI, C. SOTELO & M. BECKER-ANDRE. 1998. *Staggerer* phenotype in retinoid-related orphan receptor alpha-deficient mice. Proc. Natl. Acad. Sci. USA **95:** 3960–3965.

28. SASHIHARA, S., P.A. FELTS, S.G. WAXMAN & T. MATSUI. 1996. Orphan nuclear receptor RORα gene: isoform-specific spatiotemporal expression during postnatal development of brain.

29. MATSUI, T., S. SASHIHARA, Y. OH & S.G. WAXMAN. 1995. An orphan nuclear receptor, mRORα, and its spacial expression in adult mouse brain. Mol. Brain Res. **33:** 217–226.

30. PARK, H.T., S.Y. BAEK, B.S. KIM, J.B. KIM & J.J. KIM. 1996. Developmental expression of "RZRβ, a putative nuclear-melatonin receptor" mRNA in suprachiasmatic nucleus of the rat. Neuroscience Lett. **217:** 17–20.

31. PARK, H.T., Y.J. KIM, S. YOON, J.B. KIM & J.J. KIM. 1997. Distributional characteristics of the mRNA for retinoid Z receptor β (RZRβ), a putative nuclear melatonin receptor, in the rat brain and spinal cord. Brain Res. **747:** 332–337.

32. SCHAEREN-WIEMERS, N., E. ANDRE, J.P. KAPFHAMMER & M. BECKER-ANDRE. 1997. The expression pattern of the orphan nuclear receptor RORβ in the developing and adult rat nervous system suggests a role in the processing of sensory information and in the circadian rhythm. Eur. J. Neurosci. **9:** 2687–2701.

33. BALER, R., S. COON & D.C. KLEIN. 1996. Orphan nuclear receptor RZRβ: cyclic AMP regulates expression in the pineal gland. Biochem. Biophys. Res. Commun. **220:** 975–978.

34. ANDRE, E., K. GAWLAS, M. STEINMAYR & M. BECKER-ANDRE. 1998. A novel isoform of the orphan nuclear receptor RORβ is specifically expressed in pineal gland and retina. Gene **216:** 277–283.

35. GLASS, C.K. 1994. Differential recognition of target genes by nuclear receptor monomers, dimers, and heterodimers. Endocr. Rev. **15:** 391–407.

36. SCHRÄDER, M., C. DANIELSSON, I. WIESENBERG & C. CARLBERG. 1996. Identification of natural monomeric response elements of the nuclear receptor RZR/ROR: they also bind COUP-TF. J. Biol. Chem. **271:** 19732–19736.

37. CARLBERG, C., I. WIESENBERG & M. SCHRÄDER. 1997. Nuclear signalling of melatonin. Front. Horm. Res. **23:** 25–35.

38. STEINHILBER, D., M. BRUNGS, O. WERZ, I. WIESENBERG, C. DANIELSSON, J.-P. KAHLEN, S. NAYERI, M. SCHRÄDER & C. CARLBERG. 1995. The nuclear receptor for melatonin represses 5-lipoxygenase gene expression in human B lymphocytes. J. Biol. Chem. **270:** 7037–7040.

39. MISSBACH, M., B. JAGHER, I. SIGG, S. NAYERI, C. CARLBERG & I. WIESENBERG. 1996. Thiazolidine diones: specific ligands of the nuclear receptor RZR/ROR with potent anti-arthritic activity. J. Biol. Chem. **271:** 13515–13522.

40. TINI, M., R.A. FRASER & V. GIGUÈRE. 1995. Functional interactions between retinoic acid receptor-related orphan nuclear receptor (RORα) and the retinoic acid receptors in the regulation of the γF-crystallin promoter. J. Biol. Chem. **270:** 20156–20161.

41. GREINER, E.F., J. KIRFEL, H. GRESCHIK, U. DÖRFLINGER, P. BECKER, A. MERCEP & R. SCHÜLE. 1996. Functional analysis of the brain-specific nuclear orphan receptor RZRβ. Proc. Natl. Acad. Sci. USA **93:** 10105–10110.

42. WALDHAUSER, F., G. WEISZENBACHER, H. FRISCH, U. ZEITLHUBER, M. WALDHAUSER & R.J. WURTMAN. 1984. Fall in nocturnal serum melatonin during prepuberty and pubescence. Lancet **1:** 362–365.

43. MAESTRONI, G.J.M. 1993. The immunoneuroendocrine role of melatonin. J. Pineal Res. **14:** 1–10.

44. GONZALEZ-HABA, M.G., S. GARCIA-MAURINO, J.R. CALVO, R. GOBERNA & J.M. GUERRERO. 1995. High-affinity binding of melatonin by human circulating T lymphocytes (CD4+). FASEB J. **9:** 1331–1335.

45. BARJAVEL, M.J., Z. MAMDOUH, N. RAGHBATE & O. BAKOUCHE. 1998. Differential expression of the melatonin receptor in human monocytes. J. Immunol. **160:** 1191–1197.

46. POZO, D., M. DELGADO, J.M. FERNANDEZ-SANTOS, J.R. CALVO, R.P. GOMARIZ, I. MARTIN-LACAVE, G.G. ORTIZ & J.M. GUERRERO. 1997. Expression of the Mel$_{1a}$-melatonin receptor mRNA in T and B subsets of lymphocytes from rat thymus and spleen. FASEB J. **11:** 466–473.

47. RAFII-EL-IDRISSI, M., J.R. CALVO, A. HARMOUCH, S. GARCIA-MAURINO & J.M. GUERRERO. 1998. Specific binding of melatonin by purified cell nuclei from spleen and thymus of the rat. J. Neuroimmunol. **15:** 190–197.

48. GARCIA-MAURINO, S., M.G. GONZALES-HABA, J.R. CALVO, M. RAFII-IDRISSI, V. SANCHEZ-MARGALET, R. GOBERNA & J.M. GUERRERO. 1997. Melatonin enhances IL-2, IL-6, and IFN-γ production by human circulating CD4+ cells: a positive nuclear receptor-mediated mechanism involving T helper type 1 lymphocytes and monocytes. J. Immunol. **159:** 574–581.

49. UZ, T., P. LONGONE & H. MANEV. 1997. Increased hippocampal 5-lipoxygenase mRNA content in melatonin-deficient, pinealectomized rats. J. Neurochem. **69:** 2220–2223.

50. SAMUELSSON, B., S.-E. DAHLEN, J.-A. LINDGREN, C.A. ROUZER & C.N. SERHAN. 1987. Leukotrienes and lipoxins: structures, biosynthesis, and biological effects. Science **237:** 1171–1176.

51. LAU, P., P. BAILEY, D.H. DOWHAN & G.E.O. MUSCAT. 1999. Exogenous expression of a dominant negative RORα1 vector in muscle cells impairs differentiation: RORα1 directly interacts with p300 and MyoD. Nucleic Acids Res. **27:** 411–420.

52. KARASEK, M., K. WINCZYK, J. KUNERT-RADEK, I. WIESENBERG & M. PAWLIKOWSKI. 1998. Antiproliferative effects of melatonin and CGP52608 on the murine colon 38 adenocarcinoma *in vitro* and *in vivo*. Neuroendocrinol. Lett. **19:** 71–78.

53. HAMILTON, B.A., W.N. FRANKEL, A.W. KERREBROCK, T.L. HAWKINS, W. FITZHUGH, K. KUSUMI, L.B. RUSSELL, K.L. MUELLER, V. VAN BERKEL, B.W. BIRREN, L. KRUGLYAK & E.S. LANDER. 1996. Disruption of the nuclear hormone receptor RORα in *staggerer* mice. Nature **379:** 736–739.

54. DUSSAULT, I., D. FAWCETT, A. MATTHYSSEN, J.-A. BADER & V. GIGUÈRE. 1998. Orphan nuclear receptor RORα-deficient mice display the cerebellar defects of *staggerer*. Mech. Dev. **70:** 147–153.

55. MOLIS, T.M., L.L. SPRIGGS & S.M. HILL. 1994. Modulation of estrogen receptor mRNA expression by melatonin in MCF-7 human breast cancer cells. Mol. Endocrinol. **8:** 1681–1690.

56. RATO, A.G., J.G. PEDRERO, M.A. MARTINEZ, B. DEL RIO, P.S. LAZO & S. RAMOS. 1999. Melatonin blocks the activation of estrogen receptor for DNA binding. FASEB J. **13:** 857–868.

57. MOLIS, T.M., L.L. SPRIGGS, Y. JUPITER & S.M. HILL. 1995. Melatonin modulation of estrogen-regulated proteins, growth factors, and proto-oncogenes in human breast cancer. J. Pineal Res. **18:** 93–103.

58. ROTH, J.A., B.-G. KIM, W.-L. LIN & M.-I. CHO. 1999. Melatonin promotes osteoblast differentiation and bone formation. J. Biol. Chem. **274:** 22041–22047.

Involvement of Nuclear Receptors in the Enhanced IL-2 Production by Melatonin in Jurkat Cells

JUAN M. GUERRERO,[a] DAVID POZO, SOFÍA GARCÍA-MAURIÑO,
C. OSUNA, P. MOLINERO, AND JUAN R. CALVO

Department of Medical Biochemistry and Molecular Biology,
The University of Seville School of Medicine and Virgen Macarena Hospital,
41009-Seville, Spain

ABSTRACT: This report shows that melatonin enhances IL-2 production by Jurkat cells via a nuclear receptor-mediated mechanism. Jurkat cells express nuclear (RZRα, RORα1, and RORα2) and membrane (mt1) melatonin receptors, and melatonin binds to Jurkat nuclei and membranes with the same affinity described for human peripheral blood mononuclear cells (PBMCs). Melatonin enhances IL-2 production by Jurkat cells activated by either phytohemagglutinin (PHA) or phorbol myristate acetate (PMA). PHA activation of Jurkat cells does not change the profile of melatonin receptor expression; on the contrary, PMA activation negatively regulates the mt1 receptor. In the absence of the membrane receptor, melatonin still activates the IL-2 production. These results show that the expression of the nuclear melatonin receptor is sufficient for melatonin to activate IL-2 production by Jurkat cells.

INRODUCTION

Melatonin, the main secretory product of the pineal gland, exhibits a remarkable functional versatility: transmission of photoperiodic information,[1] control of reproductive physiology,[2] antiaging effects,[3] modulation of immune physiology,[4] and antioxidant activity as a free radical scavenger.[5]

Many functional studies show that melatonin plays a fundamental role in neuroimmunomodulation.[6,7] A regulatory role of melatonin on the immune system is supported by the existence of specific binding sites for melatonin in lymphoid cells.[8,9] We have reported the presence of high-affinity binding sites for melatonin in human circulating T lymphocytes, with an affinity ($K_d = 0.27$ nM) suggesting that they may recognize the physiological concentration of melatonin in serum.[10]

Melatonin could exert at least some of its effects on the immune system by modulating cytokine production. Melatonin is able to activate human Th1 lymphocytes by increasing IL-2 and IFN-γ production *in vitro,* and to enhance IL-6 and IL-12

[a]Address for correspondence: Juan M. Guerrero, Department of Medical Biochemistry and Molecular Biology, The University of Seville School of Medicine and Virgen Macarena Hospital, Avda Sanchez-Pizjuan 4, 41009-Seville, Spain. Voice: +34 95 455 9851; fax: +34 95 490 7048.

guerrero@cica.es

production by PBMCs[11,12] and by cultured monocytes.[12,13] Melatonin has been shown to activate human monocytes inducing their cytotoxic properties[14] and increasing IL-1, IL-6, and TNF production.[15]

Two different mechanisms of action of melatonin in the immune system have been suggested: (1) binding to mt1-membrane receptors,[16,17] and (2) binding to the RZR/ROR nuclear receptor family.[18] By using S 20098, a membrane receptor agonist,[19] and CGP 52608, a nuclear receptor agonist, we have shown the involvement of a nuclear mechanism in the melatonin effects on IL-2 and IL-6 production by human PBMCs, and IL-6 production by cultured monocytes.[13]

While duplicating as closely as possible physiological conditions, a culture of PBMCs is a complex system, with many possible interactions among the different cell populations. For this reason, we have used Jurkat cells, a T-cell acute lymphoblastic leukemia-derived cell line. In this paper we characterize the melatonin effects in these cells, showing melatonin binding to isolated nuclei and membranes, melatonin effect on IL-2 production, and the RNA analysis of melatonin membrane and nuclear receptor expression.

MATERIALS AND METHODS

Melatonin was obtained from the Sigma Chemical Company (St. Louis, MO, USA). CGP 52608 (1-(3-allyl-4-oxothiazolidine-2-ylidene)-4-methyl-thiosemicarbazone) and S 20098 (Servier; N-acetyl-2-(7-methoxynaphthalin-1-yl) ethylamine) were synthesized by Dr. M. Missbach (Chemical Research, Novartis Pharma Inc.) and were kindly provided by Dr. I. Wiesenberg (Pharma Research, Novartis Pharma Inc., Basel, Switzerland).

Jurkat cells were maintained in culture in RPMI-1640 supplemented with 25 mM HEPES, 10% FSC, 2 mM L-glutamine, 100 U/mL penicillin, and 0.1 mg/mL streptomycin in a 5% CO_2/95% air humidified atmosphere at 37°C. When used for cytokine determinations, cells were resuspended in fresh media at 0.2×10^6/mL and cultured for 48 h in 96-well microtiter plates before collecting cell-free culture supernatants.

Purified cell nuclei and membranes were isolated according to the method of Blum.[21] Binding assay conditions were essentially as previously described for PBMCs studies.[13] Data are reported as specific binding, that is, total tracer bound minus the amount of the tracer that was not displaced by 10 μM melatonin.

IL-2 concentrations in the cell-free supernatants were determined by specific ELISA kits according to the manufacturer's guidelines. All kits were purchased from Immunotech International (Immunotech SA, Marseille, France). Ten micrograms of high-quality total RNA from different experimental conditions were reverse transcribed, and 5 μL of cDNA were amplified with specific primers previously described.[22]

Results are expressed as mean ± SEM. Data were statistically analyzed using paired Student's t test.

RESULTS

To determine whether Jurkat cells bind melatonin, binding studies to membranes and nuclei were performed using [^{125}I]melatonin as a radioactive tracer. Both membranes and nuclei were able to bind melatonin. Scatchard[23] analysis of the data disclosed the affinity of the receptors with K_d values of 0.18 nM and 0.19 nM for nuclei and membranes, respectively.

The pharmacological characterization of [^{125}I]melatonin binding was carried out with a tracer concentration of radioligand (100 pM), and with nuclear and membrane receptor agonists, CGP 52608 and S 20098, respectively. FIGURE 1 shows that CGP 52608 was as effective as melatonin in inhibiting [^{125}I]melatonin binding to Jurkat nuclei. As expected, no effect of S 20098 on [^{125}I]melatonin binding to cell nuclei, or CGP 52608 on [^{125}I]melatonin binding to membranes, was observed. However, S 20098 effectively displaced the radioactive tracer in Jurkat cell membranes, suggesting mt1 expression in these cells.

To determine whether melatonin binding to Jurkat cells caused a functional effect of melatonin on these cells, experiments related to melatonin's action on cytokine production were performed. FIGURE 2 shows the effect of increasing concentrations of melatonin on IL-2 production by Jurkat cells stimulated with 0.5 µg/mL PHA. The nuclear receptor agonist, CGP 52608, also increased IL-2 production in a dose-dependent manner; meanwhile, the membrane receptor agonist S 20098 was ineffective.

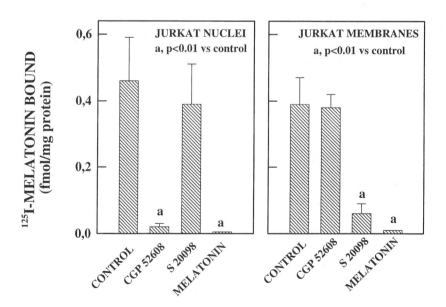

FIGURE 1. Effect of melatonin, CGP 52608, and S 20098 on [^{125}I]melatonin binding to cell nuclei or membranes. Purified cell nuclei or membranes were incubated with [^{125}I]melatonin (100 pM) and in the absence (control) or presence of 10 µM melatonin, CGP 52608, or S 20098. Data are means ± SEM of four experiments performed in triplicate.

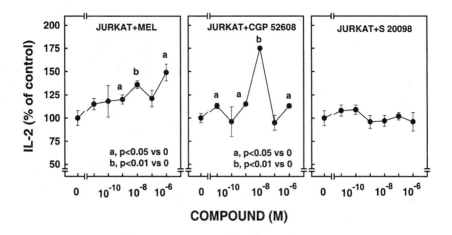

FIGURE 2. Effect of melatonin, CGP 52608, and S 20098 on IL-2 production by Jurkat cells. Cells were stimulated with PHA 0.5 μg/mL and cultured for 48 h with the indicated concentrations of each compound. Data are means ± SEM of four experiments performed in duplicate. Control IL-2 production: 293 ± 25 pg/10^6 cells.

Binding and functional studies supported the concept that activation of the nuclear receptors is involved in the regulation of IL-2 production by melatonin in Jurkat cells. Indeed, the melatonin membrane receptor seems not to play an important role in modulating IL-2 production by Jurkat cells. To confirm these findings, studies of melatonin receptor expression in Jurkat cells were performed. The ability of Jurkat cells to express the RZR/RORα and mt1 genes was determined by RT-PCR analysis of total cellular RNA. Total RNA isolated from Jurkat cells was reverse transcribed and amplified with specific primers. A single amplified band was obtained from RZRα, RORα1, RORα2, and mt1 cDNAs from Jurkat cells; no such band was obtained from amplified RORα3 (TABLE 1).

Trying to find a correlation between melatonin receptor expression and enhanced cytokine production, we stimulated Jurkat cells with different activators and, in each condition established, we assayed the melatonin effect on cytokine production and analyzed the melatonin receptor mRNA expression. PMA has been reported to cause a reduction in the levels of mt1 mRNA and protein expression in ovine pars tuberalis

TABLE 1. Correlation between the expression of nuclear and membrane receptors for melatonin in Jurkat cells and the ability of the compound to activate IL-2 production[a]

	RZRα	RORα1	RORα2	RORα3	mt1	IL-2
PHA	+	+	+	−	+	+
PMA	+	+	+	−	−	+

[a]Cells were cultured in the presence of 10^{-6} M melatonin and 0.5 μg/mL PHA or 1 ng/mL PMA.

cells, indicating an inhibitory role for PKC in regulating melatonin membrane receptors.[25] TABLE 1 shows that PMA-stimulated Jurkat cells did respond to melatonin by increasing IL-2 production, although there was no expression of mt1 receptor. Thus, melatonin activation of the RZR/ROR receptor seems to be the only event required to explain the enhancement in IL-2 production caused by melatonin.

CONCLUDING REMARKS

The results presented in this paper clearly demonstrate a fundamental role of the RZR/RORα receptor activation in the modulation of IL-2 in a human lymphocytic cell line. Binding data in Jurkat cells with the effects of CGP 52608 and S 2098 on melatonin binding to isolated nuclei, and membranes, and on IL-2 production by PHA-activated cells, are in agreement with a nuclear mechanism being primarily involved in the enhancement of cytokine production in this cell line. Results in PMA-activated Jurkat cells, in which the mt1 melatonin receptor is lost, confirms that the melatonin membrane receptor does not play a role in the modulation of IL-2 production in Jurkat cells.

Although the human cell lines used are leukemic cells, the results confirm previous work with cells obtained from healthy donors that have suggested a nuclear receptor-mediated action of melatonin on the immune system.[11,13] We do not rule out a role for the melatonin membrane receptor in modulating some aspects of the immune response, but melatonin binding to the nuclear receptor alone appears to be sufficient for the stimulatory effect of the agent on IL-2 in Jurkat cells.

ACKNOWLEDGMENTS

This study was supported by a research grant from the Spanish Health Ministry (FIS 98/0335) and by Consejería de Educación de la Junta de Andalucia (CTS 0160).

REFERENCES

1. WURTMAN, R.J., J. AXELROD & J.E. FISCHER. 1964. Melatonin synthesis in the pineal gland: effects of light mediated by the sympathetic nervous system. Science **143:** 1328–1330.
2. REITER, R.J. 1998. Melatonin and human reproduction. Ann. Med. **30:** 103–108.
3. PIERPAOLI, W. & W. REGELSON. 1994. Pineal control of aging: effect of melatonin and pineal grafting on aging mice. Proc. Natl. Acad. Sci. USA **91:** 787–791.
4. GUERRERO, J.M. & R.J. REITER. 1992. A brief survey of pineal gland-immune system interrelationships. Endocr. Res. **18:** 91–113.
5. REITER, R.J. 1995. Oxidative processes and antioxidative defense mechanisms in the aging brain. FASEB J. **9:** 526–533.
6. MAESTRONI, G.J.M. 1998. The photoperiod transducer melatonin and the immune-hematopoietic system. J. Photochem. Photobiol. B. **43:** 186–192.
7. NELSON, R.J., G.E. DEMAS, S.L. KLEIN & L.J. KRIEGSFELD. 1995. The influence of season, photoperiod, and pineal melatonin on immune function. J. Pineal Res. **19:** 149–165.

8. LOPEZ-GONZALEZ, M.A., J.R. CALVO, C. OSUNA & J.M. GUERRERO. 1992. Interaction of melatonin with human lymphocytes: evidence for binding sites coupled to potentiation of cyclic AMP stimulation by vasoactive intestinal peptide and activation of cyclic GMP. J. Pineal Res. **12:** 97–104.

9. RAFII-EL-IDRISSI, M., J.R. CALVO, D. POZO, A. HARMOUCH & J.M. GUERRERO. 1995. Specific binding of 2-[^{125}I]iodomelatonin by rat splenocytes: characterization and its role on regulation of cyclic AMP production. J. Neuroimmunol. **57:** 171–178.

10. GONZALEZ-HABA, M.G., S. GARCÍA-MAURIÑO, J.R. CALVO, R. GOBERNA & J.M. GUERRERO. 1995. High-affinity binding of melatonin by human circulating T lymphocytes (CD4$^+$). FASEB J. **9:** 1331–1335.

11. GARCÍA-MAURIÑO, S., M.G. GONZALEZ-HABA, J.R. CALVO, M. RAFII-EL-IDRISSI, V. SANCHEZ-MARGALET, R. GOBERNA & J.M. GUERRERO. 1997. Melatonin enhances IL-2, IL-6 and IFN-γ production by human circulating CD4$^+$ cells: a possible nuclear-receptor mediated mechanism involving Th1 lymphocytes and monocytes. J. Immunol. **159:** 574–581.

12. GARCÍA-MAURIÑO, S., D. POZO, A. CARRILLO-VICO, J.R. CALVO & J.M. GUERRERO. 1999. Melatonin activates Th1 lymphocytes by increasing IL-12 production. Life Sci. **55:** 2143–2150.

13. GARCÍA-MAURIÑO, S., M.G. GONZALEZ-HABA, J.R. CALVO, R. GOBERNA & J.M. GUERRERO. 1998. Involvement of nuclear binding sites for melatonin in the regulation of IL-2 and IL-6 production by human blood mononuclear cells. J. Neuroimmunol. **92:** 76–84.

14. MORREY, K.M., J.A. MCLACHAN, C.D. SERKIN & O. BAKOUCHE. 1994. Activation of human monocytes by the pineal hormone melatonin. J. Immunol. **153:** 2671–2680.

15. BARJAVEL, M.J., Z. MAMDOUH, N. RAGHBATE & O. BAKOUCHE. 1998. Differential expression of the melatonin receptor in human monocytes. J. Immunol. **160:** 1191–1197.

16. GARCÍA-PERGAÑEDA, A., D. POZO, J.M. GUERRERO & J.R. CALVO. 1997. Signal transduction for melatonin in human lymphocytes. Involvement of a pertussis toxin-sensitive G protein. J. Immunol. **159:** 3774–3781.

17. POZO, D., M. DELGADO, J.M. FERNANDEZ-SANTOS, J.R. CALVO, R.P. GOMARIZ, I. MARTIN-LACAVE, G.G. ORTIZ & J.M. GUERRERO. 1997. Expression of the mt1-melatonin receptor mRNA in T and B subsets of lymphocytes from rat thymus and spleen. FASEB J. **11:** 466–473.

18. RAFII-EL-IDRISSI, M., J.R. CALVO, A. HARMOUCH, S. GARCÍA-MAURIÑO & J.M. GUERRERO. 1998. Specific binding of melatonin by purified cell nuclei from spleen and thymus of the rat. J. Neuroimmunol. **86:** 190–197.

19. DEPREUX, P., D. LESIEUR, H.A. MANSOUR, P. MORGAN, H.E. HOWELL, P. RENARD, D.H. CAIGNARD, B. PFEIFFER, P. DELAGRANGE, B. GUARDIOLA, S. YOUS, A. DEMARQUE, G. ADAM & J. RIEUX. 1994. Synthesis and structure-activity relationships of novel naphthalenic and bioisosteric related amidic derivatives as melatonin receptor ligands. J. Med. Chem. **37:** 3231–3239.

20. WIESENBERG, I., M. MISSBACH, J.P. KAHLEN, M. SCHRÄDER & C. CARLBERG. 1995. Transcriptional activation of the nuclear receptor RZRα by the pineal gland hormone melatonin and identification of CGP 52608 as a synthetic ligand. Nucleic Acids Res. **23:** 327–333.

21. BLUM, M., B.S. MCEWEN & J.L. ROBERTS. 1987. Transcriptional analysis of the tyroxine hydroxylase gene expression in the tuberoinfundibular dopaminergic neurons of the rat arcuate nucleus after estrogen treatment. J. Biol. Chem. **262:** 817–821.

22. GARCÍA-MAURIÑO, S., D. POZO, J.R. CALVO & J.M. GUERRERO. 2000. Correlation between nuclear melatonin receptor expression and enhanced cytokine production in human lymphocytic and monocytic cells lines. J. Pineal Res. In press.

23. SCATCHARD, G. 1949. The attractions of proteins for small molecules and ions. Ann. N.Y. Acad. Sci. **51:** 660–672.

24. WEISS, A., R.L. WISKOCIL & J.D. STOBO. 1984. The role of T3 surface molecules in the activation of human T cells: a two-stimulus requirement for IL-2 production reflects events ocurring at a pre-translational level. J. Immunol. **133:** 123–128.

25. BARRET, P., G. DAVIDSON, D.G. HAZLERIGG, M.A. MORRIS, A.W. ROSS & P.J. MORGAN. 1998. Mt1 melatonin receptor expression is regulated by protein kinase C and an additional pathway addressed by the protein kinase C inhibitor Ro 31-8220 in ovine pars tuberalis cells. Endocrinology **139**: 163–171.

Melatonin Mediates Seasonal Changes in Immune Function

RANDY J. NELSON[a] AND DEBORAH L. DRAZEN

Behavioral Neuroendocrinology Group, Departments of Psychology, Neuroscience, and Biochemistry, Reproductive Biology Division, The Johns Hopkins University, Baltimore, Maryland 21218-2686, USA

ABSTRACT: Field studies indicate that immune function is compromised and the prevalence of many diseases are elevated during winter when energetic stressors are extensive. Presumably, individuals would enjoy a survival advantage if seasonally recurring stressors could be anticipated and countered by shunting energy reserves to bolster immune function. The primary environmental cue that permits physiological anticipation of season is daily photoperiod, a cue that is mediated by melatonin. However, other environmental factors, including low food availability and ambient temperatures, may interact with photoperiod to affect immune function and disease processes. This paper will review laboratory studies that consistently report enhanced immune function in short day lengths. Prolonged melatonin treatment mimics short days, and both *in vitro* and *in vivo* melatonin treatment enhances various aspects of immune function, especially cell-mediated immune function, in nontropical rodents. Reproductive responsiveness to melatonin appears to affect immune function. In sum, melatonin may be part of an integrative system to coordinate reproductive, immunologic, and other physiological processes to cope successfully with energetic stressors during winter.

INTRODUCTION

Individuals of species inhabiting the temperate and boreal zones often display marked seasonal changes in morphology, reproduction, metabolism, and other physiological functions. Photoperiod (day length) is the principal proximate factor regulating the timing of seasonal adaptations in rodents.[1,2] For example, melatonin appears to affect body mass regulation, gut efficiency, metabolic rate, pelage development, and nonshivering thermogenesis (NST).[3,4] Melatonin also affects several energy-saving behaviors, including nest-building, torpor, and food intake.[5–7] Central among the suite of winter-coping adaptations thus far identified is the inhibition of reproduction. Exposure to short-day lengths evokes gonadal atrophy in small mammals.[8] Presumably, reproductive regression reflects the energetic incompatibility of breeding (e.g., mating, lactating, and resource defense) and thermoregulatory activities during winter. However, the existence of winter breeding in virtually every population studied indicates that this energetic incompatibility can be resolved.[9,10]

[a]Address for correspondence: Randy J. Nelson, Department of Psychology, Ohio State University, Columbus, OH 43210.

Photoperiodic information is used to initiate or terminate specific seasonal adaptations, including reproduction, in order to maintain a positive energy balance.[4,5,8,11] The annual cycle of changing photoperiod is a very precise temporal cue for determining the time of year. Ambient photoperiodic information is transduced by the pineal gland into a melatonin signal; peak melatonin concentrations occur during the dark portion, and basal levels occur during the light portion of the day.[1,2] The secretory pattern of melatonin allows individuals to ascertain the time of year and thus anticipate predictable seasonal environmental changes.[5,12]

SEASONAL AND PHOTOPERIODIC INFLUENCES ON IMMUNE FUNCTION

In addition to its regulatory effects on breeding, we and others have hypothesized that photoperiodic information may be used to bolster immune function in anticipation of winter.[13–15] Enhanced immune function is another component of the complex web of winter-coping adaptations.

TABLE 1. **Short-day increases in immune function**

Immune parameter	Species	Reference
Splenic mass	Norway rats (*Rattus norvegicus*)	Wurtman & Weisel, 1969
	Deer mice (*Peromyscus maniculatus*)	Vriend & Lauber, 1973
	Syrian hamsters (*Mesocricetus auratus*)	Brainard et al., 1985 Vaughan et al., 1987
Thymic mass	Norway rats	Mahmoud et al., 1994
Lymphocyte count	Deer mice	Blom et al., 1994
Splenocyte proliferation	Deer mice	Demas et al., 1997 Demas & Nelson, 1998
in vitro PBMC proliferation	Rhesus monkeys (*Macaca mulatta*)	Mann et al., 2000
NK cell cytotoxicity	Siberian hamsters (*Phodopus sungorus*)	Yellon et al., 1999
Sponteous blastogenesis	Siberian hamsters	Yellon et al., 1999
Neutrophil count	Deer mice	Blom et al., 1994
White blood cell count	Deer mice	Blom et al., 1994
	Common voles (*Microtus arvalis*)	Dobrowolska & Gromadzka-Ostrowska, 1984
Antibody levels	Deer mice	Nelson & Blom, 1994 Demas & Nelson, 1996
Wound healing rates	Deer mice	Nelson & Blom, 1994

Most laboratory studies of photoperiodic effects on immune function to date have reported enhanced immune function in short-day lengths (see TABLE 1). Although many field studies support this hypothesis with data suggesting enhanced immune function and decreased disease prevalence during the winter as compared to the summer, a substantial number of studies have reported the opposite pattern of results;[13,14] that is, immune function is compromised by the short days of winter. These conflicting results can be resolved by considering additional environmental factors, not usually manipulated in laboratory studies. For example, winter-associated stressors (e.g., restricted food and low ambient temperatures) appear to counteract short-day enhancement of immune function in the lab.[13] Thus, we predict enhanced immune function should be observed during mild winters, whereas compromised immune function should be expected during challenging winters. Long-term field studies are required to test this hypothesis. Although the effects of melatonin on immunity are well established,[13,16] an ecological context is useful to understand the effects of melatonin upon immune function, and to appreciate why this relationship might be adaptive and functional, rather than merely a physiological oddity. Knowledge of the adaptive and functional significance of seasonal fluctuations in immune function may help to provide an improved understanding of the possibilities, as well as the constraints, of melatonin immunotherapy.

If immune function requires substantial energy, then any perturbation at either end of the energy balance equation should influence the immune system. In general, studies have established that either nutritional restriction or intense caloric expenditure compromises immune function during energy shortages.[17] Depending on the state of the individual in question, energy and other nutrients will be (1) diverted from growth in young, infected individuals, (2) diverted from reproductive function in sexually mature individuals, or (3) deflected away from fetal or placental development in pregnant, infected individuals.[18]

The cascade of cellular events during the acute phase immune response and inflammation, and the elevation of body temperature in response to cytokine activation, presumably requires substantial energy, although precise quantification is lacking.[17,19,20] Cytokine activation elevates body temperature, and the energy requirements of inflammation and acute phase immune responses may increase metabolic rates > 10% per degree of body temperature elevation.[17,19,20] In a study of the energetic costs of mounting an immune response,[21] house mice (*Mus musculus*) were injected with a specific antigen, keyhole limpet hemocyanin (KLH). This substance induces an antibody response without inducing prolonged fever or making the treated animal sick.[22] Both oxygen consumption (mL/kg) and metabolic heat production (kcal/kg) increased in KLH-injected animals.

Similarly, the role of energy availability in immune function was examined in female deer mice that were housed in either long (16:8-h light-dark (LD) cycle) or short (8:16-h LD cycle) days for eight weeks and then injected with either saline or 2-deoxy-D-glucose (2-DG), a glucose analogue that inhibits cellular utilization of glucose and induces energetic stress.[23] Stress compromises immune function.[24] Prolonged or severe food shortages may evoke secretion of glucocorticoid hormones;[25,26] glucocorticosteroids actively compromise aspects of immune function.[27–29] Long-day mice injected with 2-DG exhibited elevated corticosterone concentrations and reduced splenocyte proliferation compared with control mice.

Short days buffered the animals against glucoprivation stress. Neither corticosterone concentrations nor splenocyte proliferation differed between 2-DG injected and control mice housed in short days. These data are consistent with the hypothesis that short days provide a buffer against metabolic stress.

TEMPERATURE AND IMMUNE FUNCTION

Given the assumption that immune function requires substantial energy, immune function should be compromised in animals maintained in low as compared to high temperatures. Recently, the interaction between photoperiod and temperature was examined on immunoglobulin (IgG) levels and splenic mass in male deer mice (*Peromyscus maniculatus*).[30] Animals were maintained in LD 16:8 or LD 8:16 photoperiods and either in 20° or 8°C temperatures. Serum IgG levels were elevated in short-day mice maintained at normal room temperature (i.e., 20°), as compared to long-day animals housed at either 20° or 8°C (see FIGURE 1). Long-day deer mice kept at 8°C temperatures had reduced IgG levels as compared to long-day mice maintained at 20°, whereas mice exposed to short days and low temperatures had IgG levels comparable to long-day mice maintained at 20°C. In other words, short days elevat-

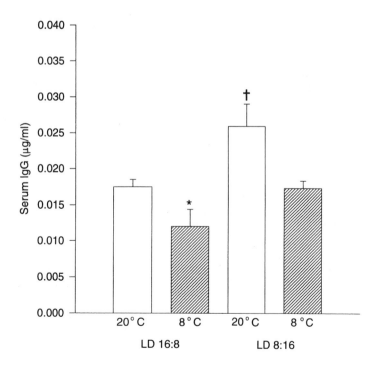

FIGURE 1. Mean (± SEM) immunoglobulin G levels (µg/ml) of male deer mouse housed in long (LD 16:8) days and mild (20°C) or low (8°C) temperatures. Columns with different symbols are significantly different at *p* < 0.05.

ed IgG levels over long days. Low temperatures caused a significant reduction in IgG levels. The net effect of short-day enhancement and low-temperature reduction of IgG levels is no appreciable difference from baseline (i.e., long-day mice kept at 20°C).[30] This adaptive system may help animals cope with seasonal stressors and ultimately increase reproductive fitness. In order to enhance immune function in anticipation of demanding winter conditions, animals must initiate these adaptations well in advance of the demanding conditions. Again, the most reliable environmental cue for time of year is the annual pattern of changing photoperiod, which is encoded by melatonin.

MELATONIN AND IMMUNE FUNCTION

Melatonin treatment of both normal and immunocompromised house mice elevates *in vitro* and *in vivo* antibody responses.[31] Impaired T-helper cell activities in immunocompromised mice are restored by melatonin treatment.[31] Antigen presentation by splenic macrophages to T cells is also enhanced by melatonin; furthermore, this enhancement is coincident with an increase in MHC class II molecules, as well as IL-1 and TNF$_\alpha$ production.[32]

The effects of melatonin on immune function remain controversial. For example, in one early paper, neonatal pinealectomy was reported to be ineffective at evoking immune function change.[33] More recently, neonatal pinealectomy has been reported to affect immune parameters; murine antibody-dependent cellular cytotoxicity (ADCC) was reduced in adults that were pinealectomized before seven days of age.[34] ADCC is a lytic process that occurs when lymphocytes bind to specific antibody-coated target cells through receptors for the Fc portion of the IgG molecule expressed on their membrane. The impairment in ADCC appears peripubertally, around 60 days of age, suggesting an involvement of sex steroid hormones.[34] Pinealectomy also seems to ameliorate collagen II–induced arthritis in mice[35] and has been reported to inhibit humoral immune function and depress bone marrow progenitors for granulocytes and macrophages in mice.[36] Additionally, natural killer (NK) cell activity and IL-2 production are reduced in mice after pinealectomy.[37]

Tonsillar lymphocyte subsets were determined in children ($n = 35$) with recurrent, acute tonsillitis before and after culture using flow cytometry in a tonsillar mononuclear suspension.[38] B lymphocyte numbers were reduced after culture; this decrease was restored in the presence of melatonin or phytohemagglutinin, and even increased above control values when cultured in the presence of both substances. This process was specific for B cells; there was no effect on T lymphocytes or natural killer cells.[38]

The circadian synthesis and release of melatonin modulate antibody response and alter tumorigenesis.[39] At the normal cellular level, melatonin is believed to affect antimitotic processes, as well as cytotoxic activity.[40–42] In mice, the circadian synthesis and release of melatonin plays a significant immunomodulatory role. When the synthesis of endogenous melatonin is blocked, antibody production is depressed; by contrast, transplantation immunity is not affected by pinealectomy.[43,44] Pharmacological and surgical pinealectomy also modulate other immune parameters, including plaque-forming cells and blastogenic responses of spleen cells and thymus cells to various mitogens.[36,45] Furthermore, elimination of melatonin synthesis by pinealectomy profoundly decreased the proliferation of bone marrow progenitors for granulocytes and macrophages (CFU-MG); the night-time peak of melatonin completely abolished CFU-MG proliferation.[36] In summary, melatonin appears to enhance immune function in most cases. In common with reproductive responses mediated by melatonin, there may be a temporal component to the biological actions of melatonin.

The role of melatonin on immune function was tested recently in adult, male Syrian hamsters (*Mesocricetus auratus*) that received daily melatonin injections or vehicle injections at either 0800 or 1700 h for 11 weeks.[46] Presumably, injected melatonin at 1700 h combines with endogenous melatonin to mimic a long-night pattern that evokes winter-type adaptations. The morning melatonin treatment does not combine with the endogenous melatonin and a long-day response should be obtained. Body weights were measured weekly throughout the experiment, and testes weights, spleen weights, and serum were collected at the end of the experiment. Melatonin injections at 1700 h, but not at 0800 h, increased body weights, decreased testes weights and serum testosterone concentrations, and had no effect on immunoglobulin G content in the spleen. Similarly, melatonin injections at 1700 h, but not at 0800 h, increased serum interferon-γ levels, had no effect on interleukin-2 levels, and appeared to increase interleukin-4 levels. Because melatonin injections at 0800 h were ineffective in altering immune measurements and the relationship between reproductive measures and immune measures was high, one parsimonious explanation for these results is that melatonin treatment at 1700 h depressed reproductive hormone concentrations and these depressed concentrations altered immune function.[46] There are many examples of sex steroid hormones and prolactin effects on immune function.

However, melatonin appears to have direct enhancing effects on immune function. This can be stated on both logical and empirical grounds. Because androgens tend to be immunosuppressant and estrogens are immunoenhancing,[47–49] photoperiodic inhibition of steroid production should produce opposite effects on immune function between the sexes. Both sexes, however, display enhanced immune function in short days or after melatonin treatment.[50,51] Furthermore, the combined and separate effects of photoperiod and steroid hormones on immune function were assessed in male and female deer mice (*Peromyscus maniculatus*).[52] Both males and females were either gonadectomized and given steroid replacement, or sham-operated. Mice from each experimental group were subsequently housed in either long (LD 16:8) or short days (LD 8:16) for 10 weeks. Short-day male and female deer mice underwent reproductive regression and displayed reduced serum testosterone or estradiol concentrations, respectively, and elevated lymphocyte proliferation in response to concanavalin A, as compared to long-day mice. Surgical manipulation had no effect on lymphocyte proliferation in either sex. Neither photoperiod nor surgical manipulation affected serum corticosterone concentrations. These results confirm that both male and female deer mice housed in short days enhance immune function relative to long-day animals.[52] Additionally, short-day elevation in splenocyte proliferation appears to be independent of the influence of steroid hormones in this species.

Although the exact role of melatonin in mediating photoperiodic changes in immune function is unknown, it has been hypothesized that enhanced immune function in short days is due to the increase in the duration of melatonin secretion.[46,53,54] Melatonin can act both directly and indirectly on target tissue within the immune system. For example, melatonin receptors have been identified directly on circulating lymphocytes, splenocytes, and thymocytes in rodents.[38,55,56] In addition, treatment of animals with exogenous melatonin enhances both cell-mediated and humoral immune function in species that are, in general, reproductively unresponsive to melatonin (i.e., rats and house mice).[16,57] Also, exogenous melatonin enhances cell-mediated immune function in male deer mice independent of gonadal steroid hormones.[58] Taken together, these results suggest, but do not establish, a direct effect of melatonin on immune function.

IN VITRO STUDIES SUGGEST A DIRECT ROLE OF MELATONIN ON IMMUNE FUNCTION

In vitro studies are valuable because they remove the confounding influence of concurrent circulating hormones. However, the results of many *in vitro* studies are contradictory; *in vitro* melatonin has been reported to enhance,[57,59,60] inhibit,[61,62] or have no effect[63,64] on immune function.

We have conducted a series of studies designed to tease apart the direct and indirect effects of melatonin on one aspect of immune function by examining the influence of *in vitro* melatonin on splenocyte proliferation in female prairie voles held in long (LD 16:8) or short (LD 8:16) days.[65] Splenocytes were removed under sterile conditions, and splenocyte proliferation was evoked by the T-cell mitogen concanavalin A. Addition of melatonin *in vitro* enhanced splenocyte proliferation in comparison to splenocyte cultures receiving no melatonin (see FIGURE 2). These results support the hypothesis that melatonin exerts a direct effect on splenocyte proliferation, potentially via high-affinity melatonin receptors localized on splenocytes.

Using the techniques described by Pang and colleagues,[66] we have established the existence of iodo-melatonin binding in *Microtus* spleens (G. Bentley, D.L. Drazen, G.E. Demas, and R.J. Nelson, unpublished data). In a follow-up study, splenocyte proliferation was examined in mice that were treated with luzindole, a melatonin receptor antagonist, 30 minutes before removal of the spleens. Melatonin enhancement of splenocyte proliferation was attenuated among luzindole-treated mice (D.L. Drazen, D. Bilu, and R.J. Nelson, unpublished data) (see FIGURE 3). Studies with Mel1a knockout mice are currently underway to specify which melatonin receptor is mediating the enhancing effects of melatonin on splenocyte proliferation.

SUMMARY

Taken together, the results of recent studies in our lab demonstrate that *in vitro* melatonin treatment enhances cell-mediated immunity in rodents. In addition, these findings support the hypothesis that melatonin exerts a direct effect on splenocyte proliferation, possibly via high-affinity melatonin receptors localized on splenocytes. The effects of prior steroid hormone or prolactin concentrations on *in vitro* splenocyte proliferation require further testing because these hormone concentrations vary greatly in different photoperiodic conditions or with melatonin treatment. Also, splenocyte proliferation after specific melatonin receptor antagonists should

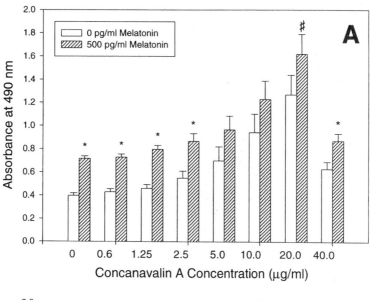

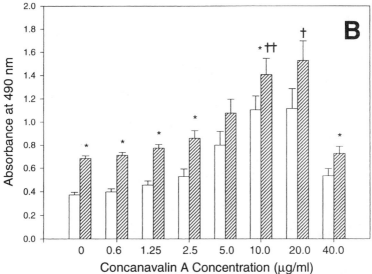

FIGURE 2. Mean (± SEM) proliferation values (represented as absorbance units) from (**A**) short- (LD 8:16) and (**B**) long-day (LD 16:8) housed female prairie voles in response to stimulation with concanavalin A (ConA), and with or without 500 pg/mL melatonin added to each assay well. **A:** #, Significantly different from all other groups, excluding 0 pg/mL MEL at ConA 20 ($p < 0.001$); *, significantly different from paired control ($p < 0.001$). **B:** †, Significantly different from all other groups, excluding 500 pg/mL MEL at ConA 10 and 0 pg/mL MEL at ConA 20 (p < 0.001); ††, significantly different from all other groups, excluding 500 pg/mL MEL at ConA 20 ($p < 0.001$); * significantly different from paired control ($p < 0.001$).

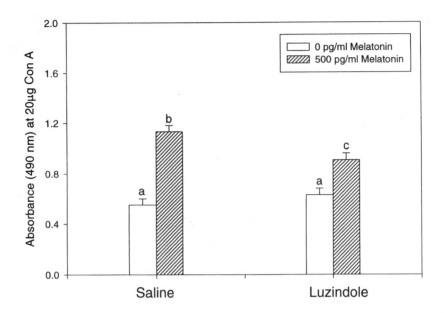

FIGURE 3. Mean (± SEM) proliferation values (represented as absorbance units) from male C57BL/6 house mice in response to optimal stimulation with ConA, either with or without the addition of 500 pg/mL melatonin added to each assay well, and after luzindole or saline injection. Bars that share letters are *not* significantly different from one another ($p < 0.001$).

reveal the receptor subtype involved in melatonin enhancement of splenocyte proliferation. Finally, the use of mice with specific melatonin receptor knockouts should aid in dissecting the role of each melatonin receptor subtype.

ACKNOWLEDGMENTS

We thank Brian Spar, Lance Kriegsfeld, Donna Bilu, Greg Demas, George Bentley, and Staci Bilbo for assistance and allowing us to report unpublished data in this paper. Preparation of this review and for the unpublished data herein were supported by USPHS Grant MH5735 and NSF Grant IBN 97-23420.

REFERENCES

1. ARENDT, J. 1998. Complex effects of melatonin. Therapie **53:** 479–488.
2. GOLDMAN, B.D. & R.J. NELSON. 1993. Melatonin and seasonality in mammals. *In* Melatonin: Biosynthesis, Physiological Effects and Clinical Applications. H.S. Yu & R.J. Reiter, Eds.: 225–252. CRC Press. New York.
3. HELDMAIER, G. & T. RUF. 1992. Body temperature and metabolic rate during natural hypothermia in endotherms. J. Comp. Physiol. B **162:** 696–706.
4. SAARELA, S. & R.J. REITER. 1994. Function of melatonin in thermoregulatory processes. Life Sci. **54:** 295–311.

5. BARTNESS, T.J., J. BRADLEY, M.H. HASTINGS, E.L. BITTMAN & B.D. GOLDMAN. 1993. The timed infusion paradigm for melatonin delivery: What has it taught us about the melatonin signal, its reception, and the photoperiodic control of seasonal responses? J. Pineal Res. **15:** 161–190.

6. LYNCH, G.R., H.W. HEATH & C.M. JOHNSTON. 1981. Effect of geographical origin on the photoperiodic control of reproduction in the white-footed mouse, *Peromyscus leucopus*. Biol. Reprod. **25:** 475–484.

7. PUCHALSKI, W. & G.R. LYNCH. 1994. Photoperiod time measurement in Djungarian hamsters evaluated from T-cycle studies. Am. J. Physiol. **267:** R191–R201.

8. BRONSON, F.H. & P.D. HEIDEMAN. 1994. Seasonal regulation of reproduction in mammals. *In* The Physiology of Reproduction vol. 2, 2nd edit. E. Knobil & J.D. Neill, Eds.: 541–584. Raven Press. New York.

9. NELSON, R.J. 1987. Photoperiod-nonresponsive morphs: a possible variable in microtine population density fluctuations. Am. Nat. **130:** 350–369.

10. PRENDERGAST, B.J. & D.A. FREEMAN. 1999. Pineal-independent regulation of photo-nonresponsiveness in the Siberian hamster (*Phodopus sungorus*). J. Biol. Rhythms **14:** 62–71.

11. HELDMAIER, G. & G.R. LYNCH. 1986. Pineal involvement in thermoregulation and acclimitization. Pineal Res. Rev. **4:** 97–139.

12. REITER, R.J. 1991. Melatonin: The chemical expression of darkness. Mol. Cell. Endocrinol. **79:** C153–158.

13. NELSON, R.J. & G.E. DEMAS. 1996. Seasonal changes in immune function. Q. Rev. Biol. **71:** 511–548.

14. NELSON, R.J., G.E. DEMAS & S.L. KLEIN. 1998. Photoperiodic mediation of seasonal breeding and immune function in rodents: a multi-factorial approach. Am. Zool. **38:** 226–237.

15. YELLON, S.M., O.R. FAGOAGA & S.L. NEHLSEN-CANNARELLA. 1999. Influence of photoperiod on immune cell functions in the male hamster. Am. J. Physiol. **45:** R97–R102.

16. MAESTRONI, G.J. 1993. The immunoneuroendocrine role of melatonin. J. Pineal Res. **14:** 1–10.

17. SPURLOCK, M.E. 1997. Regulation of metabolism and growth during immune challenge: an overview of cytokine function. J. Anim. Sci. **75:** 1773–1783.

18. JOHNSON, R.W. 1997. Inhibition of growth by pro-inflammatory cytokines: an integrated view. J. Anim. Sci. **75:** 1244–1255.

19. KRAMER, T.R., R.J. MOORE, R.L. SHIPPEE, K.E. FRIEDL, L. MARTINEZ-LOPEZ, M.M. CHAN & E.W. ASKEW. 1997. Effects of food restriction in military training on T-lymphocyte responses. Int. J. Sports Med. **18**(Suppl 1): S84–90.

20. LIN, J.X. & W.J. LEONARD. 1997. Signaling from the IL-2 receptor to the nucleus. Cytokine Growth Factor Rev. **8:** 313–332.

21. DEMAS, G.E., V. CHEFER, M.C. TALAN & R.J. NELSON. 1997. Metabolic costs of an antigen-stimulated immune response in adult and aged C57BL/6J mice. Am. J. Physiol. **273:** R1631–R1637.

22. DIXON, F., H. JACOT-GUILLARMOD & P.J. MCCONAHEY. 1966. The antibody responses of rabbits and rats to hemocyanin. J. Immunol. **97:** 350–355.

23. DEMAS, G.E., A.C. DEVRIES & R.J. NELSON. 1997. Effects of photoperiod and 2-deoxy-D-glucose-induced metabolic stress on immune function in female deer mice. Am. J. Physiol. **272:** R1762–R1767.

24. MONJAN, A.A. 1981. Stress and immunologic competence: Studies in animals. *In* Psychoneuroimmunology. R. ADER, Ed.: 185–228. Academic Press. New York.

25. DEMAS, G.E. & R.J. NELSON. 1998. Photoperiod, ambient temperature, and food availability interact to affect reproductive and immune function in adult deer mice (*Peromyscus maniculatus*). J. Biol. Rhythms **13:** 253–262.

26. MASORO, E.J. & S.N. AUSTAD. 1996. The evolution of the antiaging action of dietary restriction: a hypothesis. J. Gerontol. S. Biol. Sci. Med. Sci. **51:** B387–B391.

27. MUNCK, A. & P.M. GUYRE. 1991. Glucocorticoids and immune function. *In* Psychoneuroimmunology. R. ADER, D.L. FELTEN & N. COHEN, Eds.: 447–474. Academic Press. New York.

28. BERCZI, I. 1986. The influence of the pituitary-adrenal axis on the immune system. *In* Pituitary Function and Immunity. I. BERCZI, Ed.: 49–133. CRC Press. Boca Raton..
29. MCEWEN, B.S., C.A. BIRON, K.W. BRUNSON, K. BULLOCH, W.H. CHANBERS, F.S. DHABHAR, R.H. GOLDFARB, R.P. KITSON, A.H. MILLER, R.L. SPENCER & J.M. WEISS. 1997. The role of adrenocorticoids as modulators of immune function in health and disease: neural, endocrine and immune interactions. Brain Res. Rev. **23:** 79–133.
30. DEMAS, G.E. & R.J. NELSON. 1996. Photoperiod and temperature interact to affect immune parameters in adult male deer mice (*Peromyscus maniculatus*). J. Biol. Rhythms **11:** 94–102.
31. CAROLEO, M.C., A.D. FRASCA, G. NISTICO & G. DORIA. 1992. Melatonin as immuno-modulator in immunodeficient mice. Immunopharmacology **23:** 81–89.
32. PIOLI, C., C. CARLEO, G. NISTICO & G. DORIA. 1993. Melatonin increases antigen presentation and amplifies specific and nonspecific signals for T-cell proliferation. Int. J. Immunopharmacol. **15:** 463–468.
33. JANKOVIC, B.D., K. ISAKOVIC & S. PETROVIC. 1970. Effect of pinealectomy on immune reactions in the rat. Immunology **18:** 1–6.
34. VERMEULEN, M., M. PALERMO & M. GIORDANO. 1993. Neonatal pinealectomy impairs murine antibody-dependent cellular cytotoxicity. J. Neuroimmunol. **43:** 97–101.
35. HANSSON, I., R. HOLMDAHL & R. MATTSSON. 1993. Pinealectomy ameliorates collagen II–induced arthritis in mice. Clin. Exp. Immunol. **92:** 432–436.
36. KUCI, S., J. BECKER, G. VEIT, G.R. HANDGRETINGER, A. ATTANASIO, G. BRUCHETT, J. TREUNER, D. NIETHAMMER & D. GUPTA. 1988. Circadian variations in the immunomodulatory role of the pineal gland. Neuroendocrinol. Lett. **10:** 65–80.
37. DEL GOBBO, V., V. LIBRI, N. VILLANI, R. CALIO & G. NISTICO. 1989. Pinealectomy inhibits interleukin-2 production and natural killer cell activity in mice. Int. J. Immunopharmacol. **11:** 567–573.
38. LOPEZ-GONZALES, M.A., J.R. CALVO, C. OSUNA & J.M. GUERRERO. 1992. Interaction of melatonin with human lymphocytes: evidence for binding sites coupled to potentiation of cyclic AMP stimulated vasoactive intestinal peptide and activation of cyclic GMP. J. Pineal Res. **12:** 97–104.
39. CARDINALI, D.P., L.I. BRUSCO, R.A. CUTRERA, P. CASTRILLON & A.I. ESQUIFINO. 1999. Melatonin as a time-meaningful signal in circadian organization of immune response. Biol. Signals. Recept. **8:** 41–48.
40. BOUCEK, R.J. & T.R. ALVAREZ. 1970. 5-Hydroxytryptamine: a cytospecific growth stimulator of cultured fibroblasts. Science **167:** 898–899.
41. POFFENBARGER, M. & G.M. FULLER. 1976. Is melatonin a microtubule inhibitor? Exp. Cell Res. **103:** 135–141.
42. WINSTON, M., E. JOHNSON, J.K. KELLEHER, S. BANERJEE & L. MARGULIS. 1974. Melatonin: cellular effects on live stentors correlated with the inhibition of colchicine-binding to microtubule protein. Cytobios **9:** 237–243.
43. PIERPAOLI, W., J. BALAKRISHNAN, E. SACHE, J. CHOAY & G.J.M. MAESTRONI. 1987. Neuroendocrine and bone marrow factors for control of marrow transplantation and tissue regeneration. Ann. N.Y. Acad. Sci. **496:** 27–38.
44. MAESTRONI, G.J.M., A. CONTI & W. PIERPOLI. 1986. Role of the pineal gland in immunity. Circadian synthesis and release of melatonin modulates the antibody response and antagonizes the immunosuppressive effect of corticosterone. J. Neuroimmunol. **13:** 19–39.
45. BECKER, J., G. VEIT, R. HANDGRETINGER, A. ATANASIO, G. BRUCHETT, I. REUNER, D. NIETHAMMER & T.K. DAS GUPTA. 1988. Circadian variations in the immunomodulatory role of the pineal gland. Neuroendocrinol. Lett. **10:** 65–72.
46. CHAMPNEY, T.H., G.C. ALLEN, M. ZANNELLI & L.A. BEAUSANG. 1998. Time-dependent effects of melatonin on immune measurements in male Syrian hamsters. J. Pineal Res. **25:** 142–146.
47. GROSSMAN, C.J. 1985. Interactions between the gonadal steroids and the immune function. Science **227:** 257–261.
48. SCHUURS, A.H. & H.A. VERHEUL. 1990. Effects of gender and sex steroids on the immune response. J. Steroid Biochem. **35:** 157–172.

49. WINGFIELD, J.C., J. JACOBS & N. HILLGARTH. 1997. Ecological constraints and the evolution of hormone-behavior interrelationships. Ann. N.Y. Acad. Sci. **807:** 22–41.

50. BLOM, J.M., J.M. GERBER & R.J. NELSON. 1994. Day length affects immune cell numbers in deer mice: interactions with age, sex, and prenatal photoperiod. Am. J. Physiol. **267:** R596–R601.

51. NELSON, R.J. & J.M BLOM. 1994. Photoperiodic effects on tumor development and immune function. J. Biol. Rhythms **9:** 233–249.

52. DEMAS, G.E. & R.J. NELSON. 1998. Short-day enhancement of immune function is independent of steroid hormones in deer mice (*Peromyscus maniculatus*). J. Comp. Physiol. B **168:** 419–426.

53. BRAINARD, G.C., M. WATSON-WHITMEYER, R.L. KNOBLER & F.D. LUBIN. 1988. Neuroendocrine regulation of immune parameters: photoperiod control of the spleen in Syrian hamsters. Ann. N.Y. Acad. Sci. **540:** 704–706.

54. CHAMPNEY, T.H. & D.N. MCMURRAY. 1991. Spleen morphology and lymphoproliferative activity in short photoperiod exposed hamsters. *In* Role of Melatonin and Pineal Peptides in Neuroimmunomodulation. F. Franschini & R.J. Reiter, Eds.: 219–223. Plenum Press. New York.

55. CALVO, J.R., M. RAFIL-EL-IDRISSI, D. POZO & J.M. GUERRERO. 1995. Immunomodulatory role of melatonin: specific binding sites in human and rodent lymphoid cells. J. Pineal Res. **18:** 119–126.

56. RAFIL-EL-IDRISSI, M., J.R. CALVO, D. POZO, A. HARMOUCH & J.M. GUERRERO. 1995. Specific binding of 2-[^{125}I]iodomelatonin by rat splenocytes: characterization and its role on regulation of cyclic AMP production. J. Neuroimmunol. **57:** 171–178.

57. GUERERO, J.M. & R.J. REITER. 1992. A brief survey of pineal gland–immune system interrelationships. Endocr. Res. **18:** 91–113.

58. DEMAS, G.E. & R.J. NELSON. 1998. Exogenous melatonin enhances cell-mediated, but not humoral, immune function in adult male deer mice (*Peromyscus maniculatus*). J. Biol. Rhythms **13:** 245–252.

59. FRASCHINI, F., F. SCAGLIONE, G. DEMARTINI, V. LUCINI & P. SACERDOTE. 1990. Melatonin action on immune responses. *In* Advances in Pineal Research 4. R.J. Reiter & A. Lukaszyk, Eds.: 225–233. John Libbey. London.

60. ATRE, D. & E.J. BLUMENTHAL. 1998. Melatonin: immune modulation of spleen cells in young, middle-aged, and senescent mice. Mech. Ageing Dev. **103:** 255–268.

61. PERSENGIEV, S.P. & S. KYURKCHIEV. 1993. Selective effect of melatonin on the proliferation of lymphoid cells. Int. J. Biochem. **25:** 441–444.

62. DI STEFANO, A. & L. PAULESU. 1994. Inhibitory effect of melatonin on production of IFN gamma or TNF alpha in peripheral blood mononuclear cells of some blood donors. J. Pineal Res. **17:** 164–169.

63. MAESTRONI, G.J., A. CONTI & W. PIERPAOLI. 1987. Role of the pineal gland in immunity. II. Melatonin enhances the antibody response via an opiatergic mechanism. Clin. Exp. Immunol. **68:** 384–391.

64. ROGERS, N., C. VAN DEN HEUVEL & D. DAWSON. 1997. Effect of melatonin and corticosteroid on *in vitro* cellular immune function in humans. J. Pineal Res. **22:** 75–80.

65. DRAZEN, D.L., S.L. KLEIN, S.M. YELLON & R.J. NELSON. 2000. *In vitro* melatonin treatment enhances splenocyte proliferation in prairie voles. J. Pineal Res. **28:** 34–40.

66. POON, A.M. & S.F. PANG. 1992. 2-[^{125}I]Iodomelatonin binding sites in spleens of guinea pigs. Life Sci. **50:** 1719–1726.

Effects of Preprotachykinin-I Peptides on Hematopoietic Homeostasis

A Role for Bone Marrow Endopeptidases

P. GASCÓN,[a] J. QIAN, D.D. JOSHI, T. TELI, A. HAIDER, AND P. RAMESHWAR

Department of Medicine-Hematology, UMDNJ-New Jersey Medical School, Newark, New Jersey 07103, USA

ABSTRACT: Hematopoiesis is maintained by "fine-tuned" regulation among cytokines, neuropeptides, neurotransmitters, and neurotrophic factors. Neurotransmitters, derived from PPT-I exert immune and hematopoietic regulation. PPT-I is also expressed locally in bone marrow (BM) stromal cells. PPT-I peptides induce the production of cytokines in BM cells, resulting in regulation of both committed progenitors (CFU-GM) and primitive hematopoietic progenitors (CAFC). Both types of progenitors are regulated differently by the two major PPT-I peptides, SP and NK-A. Endopeptidases, present in BM cells, can digest SP to produce SP(1-4) and SP(4-11). In this study, we investigated the hematopoietic effects of these fragments on CFU-GM and CAFC. Similar to the two major intact PPT-I peptides (SP and NK-A), we observed different hematopoietic effects by SP(1-4) and SP(4-11). Whereas SP(1-4) exerted inhibitory effects on CFU-GM and CAFC, SP(4-11) mediated stimulatory effects. Similar to NK-A, the inhibitory effects of SP(1-4) can be partly explained by the induction of suppressive cytokines (TGF-β, TNF-α, and INF-γ). Use of antagonists and screening of a dodecapeptide expression library determined that the effects of SP(1-4) were mediated by NK-1. These results show that PPT-I peptides and their endopeptidase-derived fragments may add to the fine-tuned regulation on hematopoiesis. Furthermore, PPT-I may be exerting autoregulation to protect hematopoietic stem cells. These studies have relevance to stem cell protection and BM transplant.

INTRODUCTION

Hematopoiesis in the adult occurs mainly in the bone marrow (BM), a primary lymphoid organ. Innervation of the primary and secondary lymphoid organs provides the anatomical link in the neuro-endocrine-immune-hematopoietic axis.[1–6] Communication among the different systems of this axis is mediated by soluble factors, such as cytokines, neuropeptides, neurotransmitters, and neurotrophic factors.[7–9] BM stromal cells are important components of the BM microenvironment and constitute a major source of soluble factors that contribute to the "crosstalk" among the different tissues of the axis.[10–12] Our laboratory has been studying the

[a]Address for correspondence: Pedro Gascón, MD, PhD., UMDNJ-New Jersey Medical School, 185 South Orange Ave, MSB Room E-579, Newark, NJ 07103. Voice: 973-972-0625 or 973-972-4913.

rameshwa@umdnj.edu

role of the PPT-I peptides (tachykinins), in particular SP and NK-A, in the regulation of hematopoiesis.[13–15] These are very conserved peptides with pleiotropic functions, among those, neurotransmission and regulation of immune and hematopoietic functions.[9] BM has two potential sources of PPT-I peptides: a neural source from the fibers that innervate the BM cavity and a nonneural source from BM resident cells such as stromal cells that also express the cognate receptors for PPT-I peptides.[16,17] SP, the most studied tachykinin, and the major PPT-I peptides, interact with three neurokinin receptors, NK-1, NK-2, and NK-3, with binding preference for NK-1.[16,17] NK-A shows high affinity for NK-2.[18]

In vitro studies indicate that SP and NK-A exert stimulatory and inhibitory hematopoietic effects, respectively.[13,19] These effects correlate with the induction of cytokines in BM stromal cells that exert positive and negative hematopoieitc effects.[13,19] An important question in stem cell biology is the need for the stem cell to remain quiescent. We asked whether the stimulatory effect of SP on BM progenitors, secondary to the induction of multiple growth factors by the BM stromal cells,

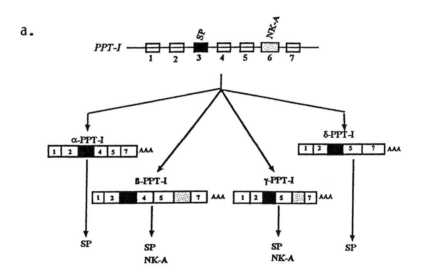

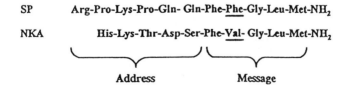

FIGURE 1. a: Schematic representation of PPT-I, its spliced variants, and its major peptides, SP and NK-A. **b:** Amino acid sequence of SP and NK-A. The sequences of the address and message portions are indicated in the bracket.

could induce the proliferation of stem cells and compromise this important homeo-static mechanism. It is clear that the system requires a negative feedback to maintain homeostasis. One mechanism could be the negative hematopoietic effects of NK-A.[13] This would indicate a feedback by a peptide from the same gene (see FIGURE 1). Even if this occurs, the question is How does the stimulatory hematopoietic effect of SP get blunted? Because endopeptidases are ubiquitous and can use SP as their substrates,[20] we studied the hematopoietic effects of SP(1-4), a fragment of the endopeptidase digest.

We studied the roles of two SP fragments, SP (1-4) and SP(4-11), on myeloid hematopoietic progenitors (CFU-GM) and on primitive hematopoietic cells, using the cobblestone-forming cells assay (CAFC). We also used specific antagonists to determine which neurokinin receptor is involved in the effects of the different SP fragments. We found negative hematopoietic effects on committed and primitive hematopoietic progenitors. To better understand these effects of SP(1-4), we deter-mined the induction of three negative hematopoietic regulators, TGF-β, TNF-α, and IFNγ. Indeed the results indicate that SP(1-4) induces each of these cytokines in BM mononuclear cells.

MATERIALS AND METHODS

Peptides and Antagonists

SP(1-4) and SP(4-11) were purchased from Sigma (St. Louis, MO), and CP-96, 345-1 and SR 48968 were purchased from Pfizer Inc. (Groton, CT) and SANOFI Recherche (Montpellier Cedex, France), respectively. Peptides and antagonists were dissolved and stored as described.[21]

Preparation of BM Stroma

BM aspirate was obtained from the posterior iliac crest of a normal healthy vol-unteer into heparin. Informed consent was obtained from each donor according to the guidelines of the Institutional Review Board, UMDNJ-New Jersey Medical School, Newark, NJ. Confluent stromal cells were prepared in 25 cm^2 flasks from BM aspirates as described.[21]

Clonogenic Assays

BM mononuclear cells (BMNC) were isolated from BM aspirate by Ficoll-Hypaque (Sigma) density gradient and then cultured for CFU-GM in methylcellu-lose, as described.[21] Each culture was done in duplicate with 10^5 cells/mL and con-tained three units recombinant human GM-CSF and various concentrations of either SP(1-4) or SP(4-11). The Immunology Department of Genetics Institute (Cam-bridge, MA) provided the GM-CSF. Peptides were omitted in control cultures. All day 10 colonies with greater than 20 cells were enumerated. Cultures with antago-nists contained 10^{-9} M of either SP(1-4) or SP(4-11) and various concentrations of NK-1 antagonist (CD-96,345-1) and/or NK-2 antagonist (SR 48968).

Isolation of CD34+ Cells

CD34+ cells were positively selected from BMNC with an isolation kit (Dynabeads M-450 CD34) purchased from Dynal Inc. (Lake Success, NY). Two sequential isolation procedures were performed and follow manufacturers' instructions. The percentages of CD34+ cells were determined by flow cytometry. Cells were double labeled with PE-conjugated murine anti-CD34 (Becton Dickinson Immunocytometry Systems, San José, CA) and Tri-color-conjugated murine anti-CD45 (Caltag Laboratories, Burlingame, CA). Cells stained dim for CD45, and >90% were positive for CD34. Less than 1% was positive for von Willebrand Factor.

Cobblestone-Forming Assay

BM stroma were detached from flasks with collagenase (Sigma), and $10^4/0.1$ mL were transferred to 96-well tissue culture plates. Culture media (CAFC media) contained a-MEM (Life Technologies). Plates were incubated until confluent and then subjected to 150 Gy, delivered by a cesium source. The following day, nonadherent cells were removed and 200 CD34+ cells added in 0.2 mL CAFC media with various concentrations of SP(1-4). Each peptide concentration was assayed in 12 wells. Control wells contained only CAFC media. After three wells, cobblestone areas with greater then 20 cells were enumerated.

Stimulation of Bone Marrow Mononuclear Cells

BM aspirate was obtained from the posterior iliac crest of normal healthy volunteers after obtaining informed consent. A mononuclear fraction was isolated by Ficoll-Hypaque density gradient (Sigma, St Louis, MO). Bone marrow mononuclear cells (BMNC) (10^6/mL) were resuspended in RPMI 1640 (Sigma) containing 10% FCS (Hyclone Laboratories, Logan, Utah). Cells, 1 mL/well in 24-well plates, were stimulated with various concentrations of SP (1-4) (Sigma). Controls included cells cultured in media alone. At day 3, cell-free supernatants were collected, aliquotted, and stored at $-70°C$ until ready to be assayed for cytokine levels.

Quantitation of TGF-β

Growth inhibition of CCL 64 cells forms the basis of the bioassay used to quantitate active TGF-β. Each sample was tested in triplicate with 50 μL of unknown sample. The quantity of TGF-β was determined by a standard curve established with standard TGF-β versus cell growth. TGF-β concentrations in the standard curve ranged from 0.001 to 10 ng/mL. Samples with TGF-β levels greater than 20 ng/mL were verified by repeating the assay in the presence or absence of neutralizing rabbit polyclonal anti-hTGF-β. TGF-β and the antibody were purchased from R & D Systems (Minneapolis, MN).

Quantitation of IFN-γ

Wish cells, 5×10^3 were added to 96-well plates. Duplicate IFN-γ standard (NIH reference standard Gg23-901-53) was serially diluted beginning at 10 RU/mL to twelve dilutions. Standards (50 mL) or equivalent volumes of unknown samples were added to wells. Unknown samples were added in triplicate as either undiluted or serially diluted, depending of the quantity of IFN-γ. Controls include eight wells per plate with cells in media. Except for four wells with media alone (zero cytopathic effect, CPE), on day 2, 5×10^3 vesicular stomatitis virus (VSV) was added to all other wells. The four wells with cells and media alone represent total or 4 CPE. After 48 h, wells were scored for CPE by a blinded observer. One unit is equivalent to a CPE of 2. For samples with low concentrations of IFN-γ, twice the concentration of undiluted samples (100 mL) was tested. The sensitivity of the assay was 4 U/mL. The results are presented as the units neutralized by horse anti-IFN-γ, Boehringer Mannheim (Indianapolis, IN).

Quantitation of Tumor Necrosis Factor-α

The assay uses the ability of tumor necrosis factor-α (TNF-α) to exert cytotoxic effects on L929 cells. The principle of readout is similar to IFN-γ. L929, 5×10^4, were added to 96-well plates, and at day 2, standard TNF-α (R & D Systems) and an unknown quantity were added for IFN-γ. Actinomycin D (1 mg/mL) was added to each well. On day 3, a blinded observer scored for cytotoxicity. The results represent cytotoxicity neutralized by anti-human TNF-α (R & D Systems).

RESULTS

Effects of SP(1-4) on CFU-GM and CAFC

SP has an stimulatory effect on CFU-GM proliferation and induces stimulatory cytokines (see TABLE 1) that can mediate stem cell proliferation. There are two potential SP sources in the BM: a neural and a nonneural, mostly represented by the BM stroma.[15] Inasmuch as cytokines produced by stromal cells can induce PPT-I expression by autocrine and paracrine mechanisms, it is possible that there are times when the BM microenvironment could contain SP at high concentrations. If this occurs, SP could turn the biological system in the BM into a continuous stimulation. Because the hematopoietic system has to be in homeostasis, there has to be a logical feedback. We have shown that NK-A is a hematopoietic inhibitor (TABLE 1). Furthermore, both SP and NK-A are derived from the same gene (FIG. 1). However, because there are four transcripts of SP and only two can produce NK-A, it would not appear that NK-A is the only and natural feedback of SP.

Endopeptidases are ubiquitous and can be produced by cells such as fibroblasts and endothelial cells.[20] Endopeptidases can digest SP into smaller fragments, sug-

TABLE 1. Relative effects of PPT-1 peptides on hemotopoiesis

Peptides	CAFC	BFU-E	CFU-GM	HR
NK-A	—	↑	↓↓	MIP-1α, TGF-β[13]
SP(1-4)	—	↓	↓↓	see TABLE 2
SP(4-11)	↑↑	↑↑	↑↑	IL-3, IL-6, GM-CSF, SCF[24]
SP	↑↑	↑↑	↑↑	IL-3, IL-6, GM-CSF, SCF[14,19,22]

TABLE 2. Induction of IFN-γ, TNF-α, and TGF-β by SP(1-4)

SP(1-4) (nM)	IFN-γ (U/mL)	TNF-α (U/mL)	TGF-β (pg/mL)
media	<0.5	<4	<5
10	320 ± 25	80 ± 10	60 ± 10
1.0	320 ± 18	60 ± 10	120 ± 15
0.1	160 ± 30	40 ± 5	80 ± 5
0.01	70 ± 15	20 ± 4	40 ± 8
0.001	70 ± 12	8 ± 2	20 ± 4
0.0001	20 ± 8	<4	18 ± 4

gesting that SP could be its own natural regulator. To this end, we studied the effects of the SP (1-4) on CFU-GM.

SP(1-4) at 1 nM shows comparable suppression on CFU-GM as NK-A, whereas the carboxy terminus, SP(4-11), shows similar stimulation as SP (TABLE 1). Interestingly, there was no effect on CAFC (TABLE 1), suggesting that SP(1-4) may be protecting the primitive hematopoietic stem cell similar to NK-A. SP(4-11) and SP shows comparable effects on CAFC (TABLE 1).

Induction of TNF-α, TGF-β, and IFN-γ by SP(1-4)

The summary shown in TABLE 1 indicates that the hematopoietic effects of NK-A, SP, and SP(4-11) correlate with the cytokine profile. We next determined if SP(4-11) can induce cytokines, associated with negative hematopoiesis. Indeed, the results show that the amino terminus fragment of SP(1-4) induces IFN-γ, TNF-α, and TGF-β (see TABLE 2). Unlike a bell-shaped pattern reported for SP,[19,22] the fragment (1-4) shows a dose-response for each cytokine studied. Preliminary studies using a peptide library screening and molecular modeling suggest that the NK-1 type receptor may be involved. However, the mechanism may be different, inasmuch as NK-1 has been reported to exhibit a desensitization effect in the presence of high concentrations of ligand.[23]

CONCLUSION

The results of this study support our basic hypothesis of a bidirectional communication between the hematopoietic and nervous systems (see FIGURE 2). We showed that the first four amino acids of neurotransmitter, SP, stimulate the production of negative hematopoietic regulators that affect stem cell proliferation and differentiation. Furthermore this fragment appears to protect the stem cell. Taken together, the results fulfill every step of the model (FIG. 2).

Considering that SP(1-4) is a fragment of a molecule with potent stimulatory effects at both the primitive and matured progenitor levels (TABLE 1), the data suggest that in addition to PPT-I providing its own feedback (FIG. 1, TABLE 1), SP itself could be providing its own regulation.

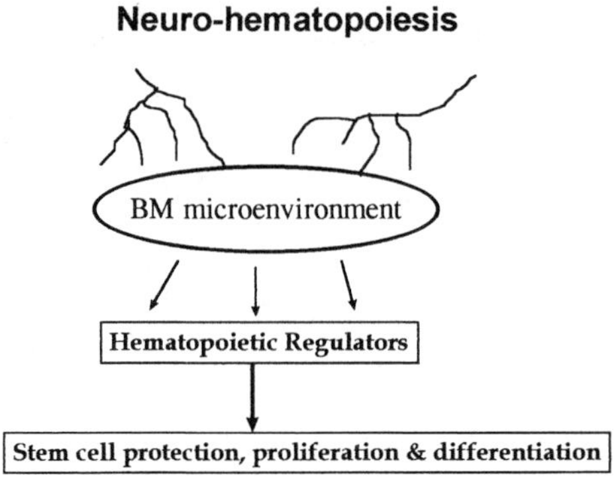

Neuro-hematopoiesis

FIGURE 2. Diagrammatic representation of the working hypothesis of a bidirectional communication between the hematopoietic and nervous systems.

SP(1-4) is included in the address portion of the SP molecule, yet it exerts an effect analogous to a message (FIG. 1b). This leaves the intriguing question of whether this fragment of SP shares the same interacting site as the intact molecule. Another interesting finding that adds to the question of interacting sites on NK-1 is the dose-response effect (TABLE 2) compared to the bell-shaped curve[19,22] observed for SP. These questions will be answered by ongoing research in our laboratory. We are currently combining molecular modeling and screening of a random dodecapeptide library for the SP(1-4) binding site to understand the interactions between SP(1-4) and NK-1. This study is our continued effort to unravel the complex mechanism of hematopoietic regulation by a family of neurotransmitters, the tachykinins.

ACKNOWLEDGMENTS

This work was supported by Grants HL-54973 and HL-57675, both from the National Institutes of Health, and awards from the UMDNJ Foundation and Ruth Estrin Goldberg Memorial for Cancer Research.

REFERENCES

1. WEIHE, E., D. NOHR, S. MICHEL, S. MÜLLER, H.J. ZENTEL, T. FINK & J. KREKEL. 1991. Molecular anatomy of the neuro-immune connection. Int. J. Neurosci. **59:** 1–23.
2. YAMAZAKI, K. & T.D. ALLEN. 1990. Ultrastructural morphometric study of efferent nerve terminals on murine bone marrow stromal cells, and the recognition of a novel anatomical unit: The "Neuro-Reticular Complex." Am. J. Anat. **187:** 261–276.
3. ZBIGNIEW, T., K. GIBSON-BERRY & S.Y. FELTEN. 1996. Noradrenergic and peptidergic innervation of the mouse femur bone marrow. Acta Histochem. **98:** 453–457.

4. HUKKANEN, M., Y.T. KOTTINEN, R.G. REES, S.J. GIBSON, S. SANTAVIRTA & J.M. POLAK. 1992. Innervation of bone from healthy and arthritric rats by substance P and calcitonin gene related peptide containing sensory fibers. J. Rheumatol. **19:** 1252–1259.

5. BJURHOLM, A., A. KREICBERGS, E. BRODIN & M. SCHULTZBERG. 1998. Substance P- and CGRP-immunoreactive nerves in bone. Peptides **9:** 165–171.

6. DE LEEUW, F.W., G.H. JANSEN, E. BATANERO, D.F. VAN WICHEN, J. HUBER & H.J. SCHUURMAN. 1992. The neural and neuro-endocrine component of the human thymus. Brain Behav. Immunol. **6:** 234–248.

7. GOCHLER, L.E., R.P.A. GAYKEMA, K.T. NGUYEN, J.E. LEE, F.J.H. TILDERS, S.F. MAIER & L.R. WATKINS. 1999. Interleukin-1β in immune cells of the abdominal vagus nerve: a link between the immune and nervous systems? J. Neurosci. **19:** 2799–2806.

8. MULLINS, M.W., J. CIALLELLA, V. RANGNEKAR & J.P. MCGILLIS. 1993. Characterization of a calcitonin gene-related peptide (CGRP) receptor on mouse bone marrow cells. Regul. Pept. **49:** 65–72.

9. RAMESHWAR, P. 1997. Substance P: a regulatory neuropeptide for hematopoiesis and immune functions. Molecule of the Month Section. Clin. Immunol. Immunopathol. **85:** 120–133.

10. DORSHKIND, K. 1990. Regulation of hemopoiesis by bone marrow stromal cells and their products. Annu. Rev. Immunol. **8:** 111–137.

11. COOMBE, D.R. 1996. The role of stromal cell heparan sulphate in regulating haemopoiesis. Leuk. & Lymphoma **21:** 399–406.

12. PENN, P.E., D. JIANG, R. FEI, E. SITNICKA & N.S. WOLF. 1993. Dissecting the hematopoietic microenvironment. IX. Further characterization of murine bone marrow stromal cells. Blood **81:** 1205–1213.

13. RAMESHWAR, P. & P. GASCÓN. 1996. Induction of negative hematopoietic regulators by neurokinin-A in bone marrow stroma. Blood **88:** 98–106.

14. RAMESHWAR, P. & P. GASCÓN. 1995. Substance P(SP) mediates production of stem cell factor and interleukin-1 in bone marrow stroma: potential autoregulatory role for these cytokines in SP receptor expression and induction. Blood **86:** 482–490.

15. RAMESHWAR, P. & P. GASCÓN. 1997. Hematopoietic modulation by the tachykinins. Acta Haematol. **98:** 59–64.

16. RAMESHWAR, P., A. PODDAR & P. GASCÓN. 1997. Hematopoietic regulation mediated by interactions among the neurokinins and cytokines. Leuk. & Lymphoma **28:** 1–10.

17. MAGGI, C.A. 1997. The effects of tachykinins on inflammatory and immune cells. Regul. Pept. **70:** 75–90.

18. REGOLI, D., Q.T. NGUYEN & D. JUKIC. 1994. Neurokinin receptor subtypes characterized by biological assays. Life Sci. **54:** 2035–2045.

19. RAMESHWAR, P., D. GANEA & P. GASCÓN. 1993. *In vitro* stimulatory effect of substance P on hematopoiesis. Blood **81:** 391–398.

20. LAOUAR, A. & B. BAUVOIS. 1992. Characterization and modulation of cell surface proteases on human myeloblastic (HL-60) cells and comparison to normal myeloid cells. Immunol. Lett. **34:** 257–266.

21. RAMESHWAR, P., A. PODDAR, G. ZHU & P. GASCÓN. 1997. Receptor induction regulates the synergistic effects of substance P with IL-1 and PDGF on the proliferation of bone marrow fibroblasts. J. Immunol. **158:** 3417–3424.

22. RAMESHWAR, P. & P. GASCÓN. 1994. Induction of IL-3 and GM-CSF by substance P on bone marrow cells is partially mediated through the release of IL-1 and IL-6. J. Immunol. **152:** 4044–4054.

23. GRADY, E.F., A.M. GARLAND, P.D. GAMP, M. LOVETT, D.G. PAYAN & N.M. BUNNETT. 1995. Delineation of the endocytic pathway of substance P and its seven-transmembrane domain NK1 receptor. Mol. Biol. Cell **6:** 509–524.

24. QIAN, J., A. HAIDER, T. TELI, T. TUAN, P. GASCÓN & P. RAMESHWAR. 1999. Effects of SP(1-4) on cobblestone-forming cells. Implications for endopeptidases as hematopoietic regulators. *In* International Congress of Immunology. G.P. Talwar, I. Nath, N.K. Ganguly & K.V.S. Rao, Eds.: 575–581. Monduzzi Editori. Bologna.

Neuropeptide Control of Bone Marrow Neutrophil Production

A Key Axis for Neuroimmunomodulation

CAROLINE S. BROOME AND JALEEL A. MIYAN[a]

Neuroscience and Cell Biology Research Group,
Department of Biomolecular Sciences,
University of Manchester Institute of Science and Technology,
P.O. Box 88, Manchester M60 1QD, United Kingdom

ABSTRACT: Nerve fibers project into the bone marrow and terminate in association with stromal cells. Nerve terminals are also associated with antigen-processing and -presenting cells throughout the body and have been shown to be important in leukocyte trafficking and wound healing as well as hemopoiesis. Here we show that neuropeptide input to the bone marrow is vital to normal granulopoiesis and that deletion of the neuropeptides, substance P, and calcitonin gene-related peptide (CGRP), with the neurotoxin, capsaicin, abrogates normal blood cell production. Norepinephrine, neurokinins *a* and 2, and vasoactive intestinal peptide all have inhibitory effects on *in vitro* CFU-GM colony formation. Substance P, neurokinin 1, nerve growth factor, and CGRP have stimulatory effects on CFU-GM. Furthermore, *in vitro* experiments show that, apart from CGRP, all the neuroactive substances we tested operate through effects on accessory cells, stimulating the release of regulatory molecules that have a direct effect on purified CFU-GM.

INTRODUCTION

Blood cells must be constantly replaced throughout life to maintain circulating cell numbers. Host challenges must also be met with an appropriate increase in output of the specific cell types required, and these must be removed when the response is no longer required. Currently accepted models involve proinflammatory cytokines that stimulate the release and redistribution of neutrophils and monocytes/macrophages from the marrow and circulation to sites of injury in the periphery, activate them functionally, and stimulate production of new granulocytes from marrow.[1–3] The activity of multipotent stem and progenitor cells is further regulated by intimate association with bone marrow stromal cells, which "present" growth factors and adhesion molecules.[4–6] Recent research implicates both the neuroendocrine system of humoral factors[7] as well as direct nerve fiber projections into the marrow and other lymphoid organs.[8–10]

[a]Address for correspondence: Dr. Jaleel Miyan, Department of Biomolecular Sciences, University of Manchester Institute of Science & Technology, P.O.Box 88 Sackville Street, Manchester M60 1QD, UK. Voice: 0161-200 4205; fax: 0161-236 0409.
J.A.Miyan@umist.ac.uk

Nerve terminals associate with particular compartments and specific cell types. In the skin, gut, and mucosa, neuropeptide-containing nerve fibers are associated with epidermal Langerhans' cells, dendritic cells, mast cells, and macrophages.[11-15] These interactions have been implicated in local inflammation, hypersensitivity reactions, and skin disorders (psoriasis and dermatitis), as well as wound healing.[11-13,16] Indeed, deletion of neuropeptide-containing nerves has been correlated with a loss of immune function.[17-20] In the bone marrow, nerve terminals synapse on perivascular stromal cells[21] and are implicated in the control of blood cell production and release from the marrow into the peripheral blood circulation as well as being involved in the retention of progenitor cells.[22,23] Furthermore, spinal cord and brain injuries have been associated with immune dysfunction.[24] There are clear pathways for bidirectional information exchange between the neural and immune-hemopoietic systems.[25,26] Thus, although there is some controversy over certain aspects,[27,28] there is good evidence supporting a direct role for neural input in host defence. In this paper we investigate the role of some of the neurotransmitters identified in nerve fibers in the bone marrow.

MATERIALS AND METHODS

All procedures were performed on 6- to 12-week-old CD1 male mice purchased from Charles River, UK. Mice were kept in a 12:12 light:dark cycle, switching at 8.00 am and 8.00 pm, respectively, and treatments were performed between 9.00 and 13.00 hours.

Intraperitoneal injections of the neurotoxin capsaicin (Sigma, UK) were given under general anesthesia (halothane) at a dosage of 50 mg per kilogram body weight daily for three days. Control animals were injected with the carrier solution in each group. At the appropriate times, bone marrow was taken for analysis by flushing out previously cleaned femurs with sterile PBS or culture medium. Blood samples were taken by cardiac puncture from anesthetized animals.

In vitro effects of neuroactive agents were tested on colony-forming assays of unfractionated normal bone marrow and on highly enriched CFU-GM. Marrow was collected in Iscove's modified medium (Gibco, UK); 10^5 cells were plated into 1 mL methylcellulose culture medium containing fetal calf serum (FCS), bovine serum albumin (BSA) (Stem Cell Technologies, Vancouver), and recombinant IL-3 (Pharmingen, San Diego) to give optimal colony-forming activity. Blood samples were assayed for colony-forming activity by plating 100 μL of untreated blood into 1 mL of methylcellulose containing FCS, BSA, and IL-3. Cultures were incubated in a fully humidified atmosphere of 5% CO_2 in air for seven days when colonies were counted. Enriched (95%) CFU-GM were obtained by counterflow centrifugal elutriation.[29]

Five × 10^6 cells/mL were cultured for 10 minutes, and 24, and 48 hours in the presence of SP, NK-1, CGRP, and norepinephrine to test collected supernatants (SNs) for the presence of active growth factors/cytokines. This was determined by the ability of the SNs to support the growth of CFU-GM.

RESULTS

In Vivo *Effects of Neuropeptide Deletion*

Capsaicin acts with exceptional selectivity on peptide-containing nonmyelinated, nocioceptive nerve fibers involved with pain perception.[30–33] With appropriate controls, effects of both excitation and long-term damage of these fibers can be studied, because capsaicin evokes peptide release from nerve terminals prior to loss of nerve activity.[34] Immediately after capsaicin injection there is a brief decrease in marrow cellularity followed by a rise (see FIGURE 1), presumably reflecting stimulation of release (drop) and hemopoietic activity followed by the rise due to retention of cells, as neuropeptide stimulation is lost by the capsaicin effect. Opposite effects are observed in the blood reflecting release of cells into the blood and subsequent loss of cells from the circulation (see FIGURE 2). Colonies from capsaicin-treated mice were much larger than the colonies formed from the vehicle control–injected mice, reflecting an upregulation of proliferation. No increase in peripheral blood colony-forming activity was observed even in splenectomized animals, suggesting a specific, local effect of neuropeptide deletion to the target bone marrow.

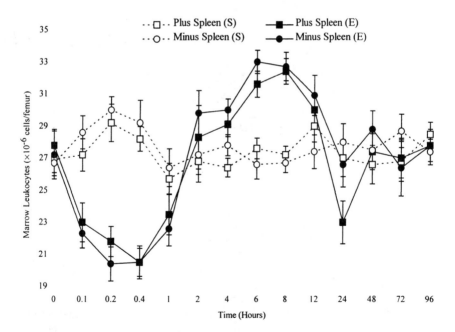

FIGURE 1. Immediate and long-term marrow response to a single capsaicin injection. The sudden drop in cellularity probably reflects immediate release of cells in response to acute release of neuropeptides. The overshoot in recovery may follow the stimulation of hemopoietic output by endogenous peptide release. The number of nucleated cells in one femur (mean ± SEM, $n = 12$) for both experimental (E, *solid lines*) and control injected (S, *dotted lines*) procedures is shown.

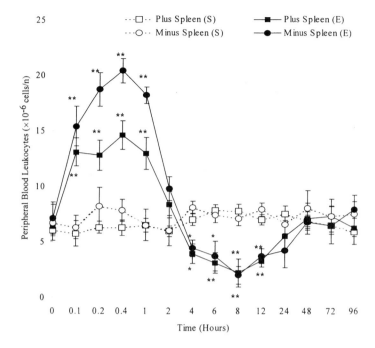

FIGURE 2. Immediate and long-term response in peripheral blood cellularity to a single capsaicin injection. The rise in peripheral blood leukocytes reflects the release of cells from the marrow and probably also a component due to release of cells from marginated sites in the circulatory system itself. The undershoot in recovery probably reflects retention of cells in the marrow as neuropeptide stimulation is lost.

A marked decrease in both marrow and blood cellularity follows further capsaicin treatment together with a fall in marrow CFU-GM activity to 58% of control values ($14{,}220 \pm 1269$, n = 5) (see FIGURE 3a). The colonies that do grow in culture from treated animals contain fewer cells ($p < 0.001$) than those from control mice. In cytospin preparations of colonies grown from marrow three days after treatment, it is clear that they are largely made up of macrophages with very few neutrophils compared to normal CFU-GM colonies (FIG. 3b and c).

In Vitro *Effects of Transmitters*

The action of SP, NK-1, NK-A, NK-2, NGF, CGRP, and norepinephrine on CFU-GM colony formation from unfractionated normal BMMNCs or from enriched CFU-GM was determined using *in vitro* cultures. The numbers of colonies formed were markedly *decreased* in cultures containing norepinephrine (see FIGURE 4), NK-A, and NK-2, whereas colonies were markedly *increased* in cultures containing SP, NK-1, NGF, and CGRP (see FIGURE 5). Only CGRP showed a direct effect on CFU-GM that was very similar to its effect on whole marrow. All the other substances tested had no direct effect on purified CFU-GM. However, these substances did elicit soluble factors from whole marrow that could act directly on CFU-GM. Stimulating whole marrow

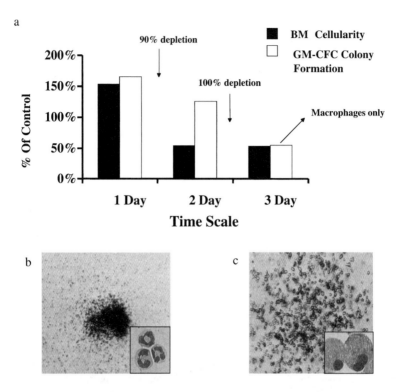

FIGURE 3. Effects of sequential capsaicin injection on bone marrow leukocyte and CFU-GM counts. With the reduction in marrow cellularity and CFU-GM activity, there is also a shift in CFU-GM commitment from granulocyte-macrophage (**b,** ×40) to macrophage alone (**c,** ×40). Few neutrophils are observed in cytospin preparations of colonies grown from animals receiving the complete capsaicin treatment. The insets of **b** and **c** show micrographs (×1000) of cytospin preparations from the colonies illustrating the neutrophil (**b**) and macrophage (**c**) morphologies of the majority cells from the colonies.

cultures with neurotransmitter and then testing the conditioned media in enriched CFU-GM cultures exposed the release of soluble factors (see FIGURE 6).

Our controls included no addition of conditioned supernatant and addition of IL-3 alone. The ten-minute conditioned media could also be viewed as effective controls for the presence of residual neurotransmitter in the supernatant. Comparison between the effects of media conditioned for ten minutes and those conditioned for longer demonstrates the presence of factors released by neurotransmitter treatment.

DISCUSSION

Nerve fibers entering the bone marrow present a neural source for molecules that have physiological effects on bone marrow hemopoietic activity.[8–10,22,26] The fact

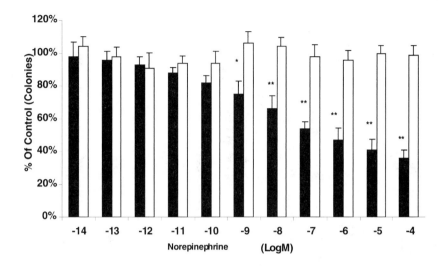

FIGURE 4. Dose-response curve for the effect of norepinephrine on whole marrow (*solid bars*) and purified CFU-GM (*hatched bars*). There is no direct inhibitory effect of norepinephrine on purified CFU-GM. The inhibitory effect of norepinephrine on whole marrow is abolished in the presence of 10^{-6} M prazosin, suggesting an action through alpha-adrenergic pathways. Similar data sets are obtained when testing vasoactive intestinal peptide, neurokinin-A, and neurokinin-2. None of these factors had a direct effect on CFU-GM. KEY: ■, whole bone marrow; □, purified CFU-GM.

that interference with nerve fiber also has an effect suggests that these neurotransmitters do indeed have a role in modulating the activity and output of the marrow.[22] In addition, our experiments demonstrate that these substances operate through accessory cells, inasmuch as none, except CGRP, have a direct effect on progenitor cells. This fits with anatomical evidence that nerve terminals are associated with perivascular and probably other stromal cells in the marrow.[21] Because stromal cells are critical to normal marrow function as well as to mobility and trafficking of cells, it seems likely that neural input modulates these functions. In the rest of the immune-hemopoietic system, CGRP and SP-immunoreactive fibers have been identified in many locations throughout the body and have been shown to have close associations with specific host defence cell types, including macrophages, antigen-processing cells, mast cells, and immune cells.[10,11,26] In addition to the data presented here, capsaicin treatment has also been reported to inhibit immune function,[17–20] suggesting that the neuropeptide system may mediate CNS modulation of both immune and myeloid responses. A subset of peptidergic nerve fibers in the skin are specifically associated with epidermal Langerhans' cells,[12,13] and CGRP has been shown to downregulate antigen presentation by these cells.[12] Together, these findings suggest the existence of a neuroimmune network monitoring host status and coordinating appropriate output of the host defence system.[35]

A feature of the data we have collected is that the observed effects of stimulating and/or deleting neuropeptide input on marrow CFU-GM are independent of effects

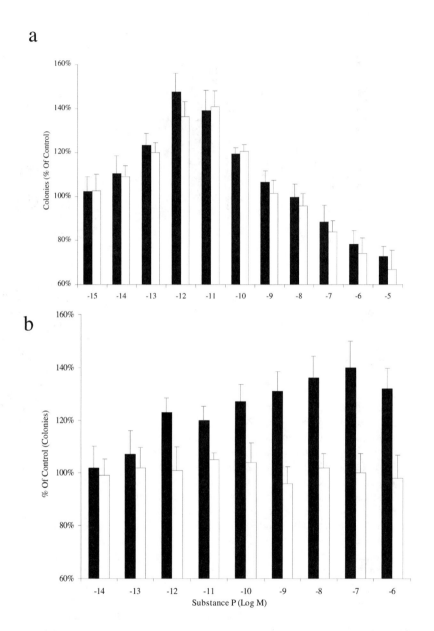

FIGURE 5. Dose-response curve for the effect of CGRP (**a**) and substance P (**b**) on whole marrow (*black*) and purified CFU-GM (*clear*) colony-forming activity. CGRP was the only neuroactive substance tested that had the same effect on whole marrow as on purified progenitors, suggesting a direct effect on CFU-GM progenitors. Neurokinin-A, neurokinin-2, and NGF had very similar stimulatory effects as substance P on whole marrow.

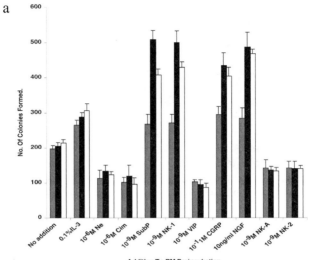

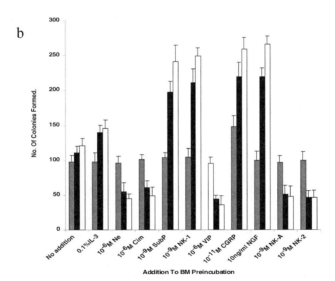

FIGURE 6. Stimulation of colony formation in whole marrow (**a**) and CFU-GM (**b**) by neurotransmitter-conditioned media. Whole marrow was incubated for 10 minutes, and 24 and 48 hours in the presence of the different neurotransmitters or growth factors. The 10-minute time point acts as a control for the residual presence of neuroactive substance. This is important for CGRP alone that has a direct effect on CFU-GM, and a small effect is observed. The 24- and 48-hour incubated media show significant stimulatory or inhibitory effects on colony formation by purified CFU-GM, similar to their effects on whole marrow. This suggests the presence of factors released by the accessory cells stimulated by the neuroactive substances. KEY: ▨, 10 minutes; ■, 24 hours; ☐, 48 hours.

on peripheral blood CFU-GM.[36] These observations support the model we propose of direct, that is to say, hardwired, neural control of bone marrow hemopoiesis, because there is no systemic effect that should have been reflected in changes in blood CFU-GM. We have already shown that mobilization and/or retention of cells is under neural control,[22] but the data from the current experiments suggest that the neuropeptides are not involved in the release of CFU-GM into the periphery. Rather, they appear to be involved in the stimulation of proliferation and differentiation to neutrophils. Furthermore, neuropeptides apparently do not stimulate the release of substances that might have access to circulating CFU-GM, inasmuch as no effect is observed on this population. The localized effect suggests the modulation of cell surface factors such as adhesion molecules.

The key cell type interfacing with the neural system is the modified macrphage, variously known as a Langerhans' cell, dendritic cell, or stroma cell. The macrophage is recognized as an "immune mobile brain"[37] because it can produce the entire sequence of molecules associated with the HPA stress response as well as a range of biogenic amines to control local inflammatory activity. Clearly these cells require further study with regard to their association with nerve terminals and to the neural regulation of host defence activity.

ACKNOWLEDGMENT

This work was supported by the BBSRC.

REFERENCES

1. WATKINS, L.R., S.F. MAIER & L.E. GOEHLER. 1995. Immune activation: the role of pro-inflammatory cytokines in inflammation, illness responses and pathological pain states. Pain 63(3): 289–302.
2. BERCZI, I., I.M. CHALMERS, E. NAGY & R.J. WARRINGTON. 1996. The immune effects of neuropeptides. Bailliere's Clin. Rheumatology 10(2): 227–257.
3. DINARELLO, C.A. 1997. Role of pro- and anti-inflammatory cytokines during inflammation: experimental and clinical findings. J. Biol. Regul. Homeostatic Agents 11(3): 91–103.
4. DEXTER, T.M., L.H. COUTINHO, E. SPOONCER, C.M. HEYWORTH, C.P. DANIEL, R. SCIRO, J. CHANG & T.D. ALLEN. 1990. Stromal cells in haemopoiesis. Ciba Found. Symp. 148: 76–86.
5. CLARK, B.R., J.T. GALLAGHER & T.M. DEXTER. 1992. Cell adhesion in the stromal regulation of haemopoiesis. Bailliere's Clin. Haematology 5(3): 619–652.
6. MAYANI, H., L.J. GUILBERT & A. JANOWSKA-WIECZOREK. 1992. Biology of the hemopoietic microenvironment. Eur. J. Haematol. 49(5): 225–233.
7. MCEWEN, B.S., C.A. BIRON, K.W.BRUNSON, K. BULLOCH, W.H. CHAMBERS, F.S. DHABHAR, R.H. GOLDFARB, R.P. KITSON, A.H. MILLER, R.L. SPENCER & J.M. WEISS. 1997. The role of adrenocorticoids as modulators of immune function in health and disease: neural, endocrine and immune interactions. Brain Res. Rev. 23: 79–133.
8. CALVO, W. 1968. The innervation of the bone marrow in laboratory animals. Am. J. Anat. 123(2): 315–328.
9. TABAROWSKI, Z., K. GIBSON-BERRY & S.Y. FELTEN. 1996. Noradrenergic and peptidergic innervation of the mouse femur bone marrow. Acta Histochem. 98(4): 453–457.

10. STEVENS-FELTEN, S.Y. & D.L. BELLINGER. 1997. Noradrenergic and peptidergic innervation of lymphoid organs. Chem. Immunol. **69:** 99–131.
11. MCKAY, D.M. & J. BIENENSTOCK. 1994. The interaction between mast cells and nerves in the gastrointestinal tract. Immunol. Today **15**(11): 533–538.
12. HOSOI, J., G.F. MURPHY, C.L. EGAN, E.A. LERNER, S. GRABBE, A. ASAHINA & R.D. GRANSTEIN. 1993. Regulation of Langerhans' cell function by nerves containing calcitonin gene-related peptide. Nature **363**(6425): 159–163.
13. MÜLLER, T. 1996. The different morphological types of dendritic cells and their innervation in stratified squamous epithelia of the rat as revealed by methylene blue staining. Biomed. Res. **7**(2): 149–157.
14. FELTEN, D.L., N. COHEN, R. ADER, S.Y. FELTEN, S.L. CARLSON & T.L. ROSZMAN. 1991. Neurochemical links between the nervous and immune systems. *In* Psychoneuroimmunology, Second Edition. R. Ader, D.L. Felten & N. Cohen, Eds. Academic Press. New York.
15. STRAUB, R.H., J. WESTERMANN, J. SCHOLMERICH & W. FALK. 1998. Dialogue between the CNS and immune system in lymphoid organs. Immunol. Today **19:** 409–413.
16. RICHARDS, A.M. & J. MITSOU. 1997. Neural innervation and healing. Lancet **350:** 339–340.
17. HELME, R.D., A. EGLEZOS, G.W. DANDIE, P.V. ANDREWS & R.L. BOYD. 1987. The effect of substance P on the regional lymph node antibody response to antigenic stimulation in capsaicin-pretreated rats. J. Immunol. **139**(10): 3470–3473.
18. NILSSON, G., K. ALVING & S. AHLSTEDT. 1991. Effects on immune responses in rats after neuromanipulation with capsaicin. Int. J. Immunopharmacol. **13**(1): 21–26.
19. SANTONI, G., M. PERFUMI, A.M. BRESSAN & M. PICCOLI. 1996. Capsaicin-induced inhibition of mitogen and interleukin-2-stimulated T cell proliferation: its reversal by *in vivo* substance P administration. J. Neuroimmunol. **68**(1-2): 131–138.
20. KRADIN, R., J. MACLEAN, S. DUCKETT, E.E. SCHNEEBERGER, C. WAEBER & C. PINTO. 1997. Pulmonary response to inhaled antigen: neuroimmune interactions promote the recruitment of dendritic cells to the lung and the cellular immune response to inhaled antigen. Am. J. Pathol. **150**(5): 1735–1743.
21. YAMAZAKI, K. & T.D. ALLEN. 1990. Ultrastructural morphometric study of efferent nerve terminals on murine bone marrow stromal cells, and the recognition of a novel anatomical unit: the "neuro-reticular complex." Am. J. Anat. **187**(3): 261–276.
22. AFAN, A.M., C.S. BROOME, A.D. WHETTON, S.E. NICHOLLS & J.A. MIYAN. 1997. Bone marrow innervation regulates cellular retention in the murine haemopoietic system. Br. J. Haematol. **98:** 569–577.
23. MIYAN, J.A., C.S. BROOME & A.M. AFAN. 1998. Coordinated host defense through an integration of the neural, immune and haemopoietic systems. Domest. Anim. Endocrinol. **15:** 297–304.
24. CRUSE, J.M., R.E. LEWIS, G.R. BISHOP, W.F. KLIESCH & E. GAITAN. 1992. Neuroendocrine-immune interactions associated with loss and restoration of immune system function in spinal cord injury and stroke patients. Immunol. Res. **11:** 104–116.
25. BLALOCK, J.E. 1994. Shared ligands and receptors as a molecular mechanism for communication between the immune and neuroendocrine systems. Ann. N.Y. Acad. Sci. **741:** 292–298.
26. WEIHE, E., D. NOHR, S. MICHEL, S. MULLER, H.J. ZENTEL, T. FINK & J. KREKEL. 1991. Molecular anatomy of the neuro-immune connection. Int. J. Neurosci. **59**(1-3): 1–23.
27. BENESTAD, H.B., I. STROM-GUNDERSEN, P.O. IVERSON, E. HAUG & A. NJA. 1998. No neuronal regulation of murine bone marrow function. Blood **91**(4): 1280–1287.
28. MIYAN, J.A., C.S. BROOME & A.D. WHETTON. 1998 Neural regulation of haemopoiesis. Blood **92:** 2971–2972.
29. WILLIAMS, D.E., J.E. STRANEVA, R.N. SHEN & H.E. BROXMEYER. 1987. Purification of murine bone-marrow-derived granulocyte-macrophage colony forming cells. Exp. Hematol. **15:** 243.
30. JANCSO, G. 1981. Intracisternal capsaicin: selective degeneration of chemosensitive primary sensory afferents in the adult rat. Neurosci. Lett. **27**(1): 41–45.

31. BEVAN, S. & J. SZOLCSANYI. 1990. Sensory neuron-specific actions of capsaicin: mechanisms and applications. Trends Pharmacol. Sci. **11**(8): 330–333.
32. DRAY, A. 1992. Neuropharmacological mechanisms of capsaicin and related substances. Biochem. Pharmacol. **44**(4): 611–615.
33. HOLZER, P. 1991. Capsaicin: cellular targets, mechanisms of action, and selectivity for thin sensory neurons. Pharmacol. Rev. **43**(2): 143–201.
34. MOUSSEAU, D.D., X. SUN & A.A. LARSCH. 1994. An antinociceptive effect of capsaicin in the adult mouse mediated by the NH2-terminus of substance P. J. Pharmacol. Exp. Ther. **268**(2): 785–790.
35. DOWNING, J.E.G. & J.A. MIYAN. 2000. Neural immunoregulation: emerging roles for nerves in immune homeostasis and disease. Immunol. Today **21**(6): 281–289.
36. BROOME, C.S., A.D. WHETTON & J.A. MIYAN. 2000. Neuropeptide control of bone marrow neutrophil production is mediated by both direct and indirect effects on CFU-GM. Br. J. Haematol. **108**(1):140–150.
37. OTTAVIANI, E. & C. FRANCESCHI. 1997. The invertebrate phagocytic immunocyte: clues to a common evolution of immune and neuroendocrine systems. Immunol. Today **18**: 169–174.

Light and Immunomodulation

JOAN E. ROBERTS[a]

Department of Natural Sciences, Fordham University,
113 West 60th Street, New York, New York 10023, USA

ABSTRACT: The immune system is susceptible to a variety of stresses. Recent work in neuroimmunology has begun to define how mood alteration, stress, the seasons, and daily rhythms can have a profound effect on immune response through hormonal modifications. Central to these factors may be light through an eye-brain hormonal modulation. In adult primates, only visible light (400–700 nm) is received by the retina. This photic energy is then transduced and delivered to the visual cortex and, by an alternative pathway, to the suprachiasmatic nucleus (SCN), the hypothalamic region that directs circadian rhythm. Visible light exposure also modulates the pituitary and pineal glands, leading to neuroendocrine changes. Melatonin, norepinephrine, and acetylcholine decrease with light activation, whereas cortisol, serotonin, GABA, and dopamine levels increase. The synthesis of vasoactive intestinal polypeptide (VIP), gastrin releasing peptide (GRP), and neuropeptide Y (NPY) in rat SCN has been shown to be modified by light. These induced neuroendocrine changes can lead to alterations in mood and circadian rhythm as well as immune modulation. An alternative pathway for immune modulation by light is through the skin. Visible light (400–700 nm) can penetrate epidermal and dermal layers of the skin and may directly interact with circulating lymphocytes to modulate immune function. In contrast to visible light, *in vivo* exposure to UV-B (280–320 nm) and UV-A (320–400 nm) radiation can alter normal human immune function only by a skin-mediated response. It is therefore important, when reporting neuroendocrine immune findings, to control the intensity, timing and wavelength of ambient light.

IMMUNOLOGY

The Immune Response

In very simple terms, the immune system involves a variety of white blood cells that work in concert to rid the body of the presence of a foreign pathogen (antigen). The primary cell types involved in an immune response are the macrophages, the T helper/inducer cells CD4$^+$ (T4), natural killer (NK) cells, B cells, and the T suppresser/cytotoxic cells CD8$^+$ (T8). The function of the macrophages is to first recognize and interact with antigen. The original antigen can also be recognized by other antigen-presenting cells such as dendritic cells or B lymphocytes. The T4 helper cells, NK cells, and B cells attack and destroy the antigen. The T8 suppresser cells turn off (anergize) the immune response.

[a]Address for correspondence: Professor Joan E. Roberts, Department of Natural Sciences, Fordham University, 113 West 60th Street, New York, NY 10023. Voice: 212-636-6323; fax: 212-636-7217.
JRoberts@fordham.edu

435

When the macrophage recognizes a pathogen as foreign (antigenicity), this antigen is ingested and fragmented into antigenic peptides. Pieces of these peptides are bound to major histocompatibility complex (MHC) molecules and are displayed on the surface of the macrophage. The binding of different macrophage-antigen-peptide MHC complexes to receptors on the T cells[1] now activates the resting helper T4 cells to release chemical signals known as lymphokines or cytokines (see FIGURE 1). These substances are biologically active factors (peptides) that regulate proliferation, differentiation, and maturation of various types of lymphoid and accessory cells.

Cytokine Control of the Immune Response

A diverse group of cytokines/lymphokines modulate the immune response. Among them are the interleukins 1 through 13 (IL-1–13), growth factors (GM-CSF), interferons (IFN-γ), and tumor necrosis factor (TNF). This has been reviewed elsewhere.[2] They function by stimulating or suppressing the activities of the specific immune cells as seen in FIGURE 1.

One of the original signals to activate the immune response is the release of IL-1 by macrophages. IL-1 activates T4 cells and stimulates the hypothalamus. The activated T4 cells release IL-2 and γ interferon (IFN-g), which induces proliferation of NK cells and macrophages, induces the B cells to produce antibodies, and anergizes

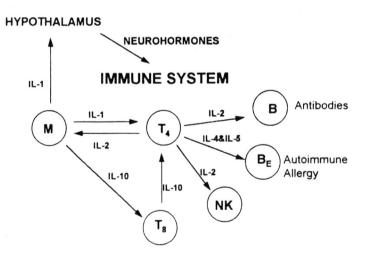

FIGURE 1. The cytokine/lymphokine control of the immune response. Macrophages (M) release IL-1, which activates T4 cells and stimulates the hypothalamus to release neurohormones. Activated T4 cells release IL-2 and other factors that stimulate the proliferation and differentiation of M and natural killer (NK) cells. IL-2 also directs the B cells to make specific antibodies against the antigen present. There can be a single switch with IL-4 and IL-5, which now direct the B cells to make immunoglobin E and other factors that lead to an allergic or autoimmune response. IL-10 released from the M and T8 cells shuts down (anergizes) the immune response.

the T8 cells. When a bacterial or viral infection is arrested, the immune response is shut down through the macrophage release of cytokine IL-10, which stimulates the suppresser T8 cells and suppresses the functioning of the T helper cells, B cells, and NK cells.

Although B cells can be stimulated by IL-2 and IFN-γ to make specific antibodies against antigens, the presence of IL-4 and IL-5 (synergy) induces B cells to synthesize immunoglobin E (IgE) instead of antibodies. IgE is involved in allergic and autoimmune responses. The IL-4 stimulation of synthesis of IgE can be blocked (antagonism) by the presence of IFN-γ.

Among its many properties,[3] IL-6 is important in T cell and NK proliferation and stimulates B cell immunoglobin production.

PHOTOIMMUNOLOGY

All wavelengths of light have the potential to modify the immune response. This includes the change of seasons (cirannual) and daily (circadian) light.[4] The timing, intensity, and *wavelength* of light contribute to immune modulation. Ionizing and nonionizing ultraviolet (UV) radiation (below 400 nm) have been found to suppress immune function.[5,6] This is a skin-mediated response. Visible radiation may affect the immune system through both skin-mediated and eye-brain–mediated mechanisms (see FIGURE 2). Wavelengths above 400 nm can penetrate epidermal and dermal layers of the skin and directly interact with circulating lymphocytes which modulate immune function. There is also a possible indirect mechanism, which would involve light above 400 nm transmitted through the retina to the brain. There, specific areas such as the pituitary, hypothalamus, and the pineal glands are stimulated to produce neurochemicals[7] that could direct changes in immune function.[8–11] Either or both pathways may be involved.

Skin-Mediated Response

The wavelengths of light transmitted through different layers of skin do not vary dramatically from lower mammals to primates. The longer the wavelength of light, the deeper the penetration in skin. The shortest wavelengths of UV light elicit the strongest immune response,[12–15] whereas the skin-mediated visible light response is weak but detectable.[16]

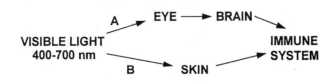

FIGURE 2. Visible light can affect the immune response through an eye-brain– or skin–mediated response.

Ultraviolet Radiation (200–400 nm)

Ultraviolet radiation (UR) may be divided into three components: UV-C (200–290 nm), UV-B (290–315 nmn), and UV-A (315–400 nm). *In vivo* exposure to UV radiation alters normal immune function by a skin-mediated response. Each UV subgroup (A, B, C) induces an immunosuppressive response, but by differing mechanisms. In general the effects that have been observed in humans are: inhibition of allergic contact dermatitis, inhibition of delayed hypersensitivity to an injected antigen, prolongation of skin-graft survival, and induction of a tumor-susceptible state.[5,6] This induced cutaneous anergy apparently proceeds via suppressor cells and serum factors. UV radiation can alter the normal antigen presenting function of nsepidermal Langerhans cells (LC), blocking their ability to activate T4 helper cells while allowing the activation of T8 suppressor cells. UV radiation can also upregulate and, in some cases, induce the secretion by keratinocytes of immunosuppressive factors.[14] Hersey[17] found that UV radiation reduces the number of T helper lymphocytes (13%), increases the number of T suppressor lymphocytes (29%), and reduces the ratio of T helper/T suppressor lymphocytes (32%). T cell proliferation requires IFN-γ and IL-2, and these are downregulated after UV irradiation.[1,18]

Visible Light (400–700 nm)

As has been reported to date, visible light has little direct skin-mediated suppression of the immune response. Even in the presence of phototoxic agents such as eosin and rose bengal, visible light does not produce suppression of contact hypersensitivity with T8 suppressor cells.[16] Light directly applied to the skin has been shown to alter circadian rhythm[19] and may alter the immune response through a hormone- and/or cytokine-mediated response.[4]

PHOTONEUROIMMUNOLOGY

Eye-brain mechanisms are both species specific and age dependent and are determined by the wavelengths of light transmitted through the eye and reaching the retina that can then be transmitted to the brain.

Species Specificity

The wavelengths of light that might induce an eye-brain–mediated immune response depend upon the transmission properties of the eye of the particular species (see FIGURE 3). In lower animals, UV-B, UV-A, and visible light may be transmitted to the retina because these wavelengths are not filtered by their cornea or lens. Therefore, both UV and visible light might induce an eye-brain–mediated response. In adult primates, including humans, the cornea cuts out all light below 295 nm, while the lens filters out light between 295 and 400nm, so that only visible light (400–700 nm) reaches the primate retina. This photic energy is transduced in the retina and sent to the visual cortex for vision and through alternative pathways to the hypothalamic, pineal, and limbic structures.[20, 21]

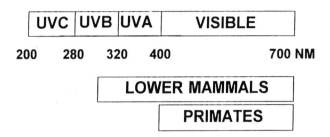

FIGURE 3. The light transmitted to the retina and transduced to the brain differs with species. In lower animals UV-B, UV-A, and visible light are transmitted to the retina. In adult primates the lens filters UV-B and UV-A, so only visible light reaches the retina.

Age

Age is also a factor involved in the transmission of specific wavelengths of light to the brain of primates, because the filtering characteristics of the lens change throughout life.[22]

The young human lens transmits light in the range of 320 nm to the retina (see FIGURE 4). The physiological function of this UV light in the development of the brain has yet to be determined. This UV light is completely filtered by the human lens by puberty. The elderly lens prevents much of the blue light (400–450 nm) from reaching the retina. This presumably protects the elderly from light-induced retinal damage[23] at a time when their quenchers (glutathione) and antioxidant enzyme systems have decreased production and/or effectiveness. Aphakia (removal of the lens) and certain forms of blindness may also change the wavelength characteristics of light impinging on the retina and transmitted to the brain.[24]

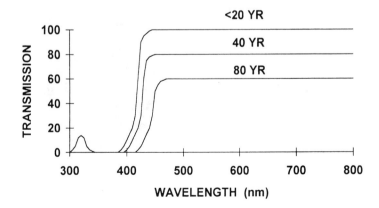

FIGURE 4. Changes in the transmission characteristics of the human lens with age. The young human lens transmits UV-B (320 nm), the adult human lens transmits only visible light (above 400 nm), and the elderly humans filters much of the blue light (400–450).

Retinal Light Transmitted to the Brain

Neural Chemical Control

Photons reaching the photoreceptor layer of the retina are transduced. This process is mediated by the release of retinal serotonin and dopamine and the suppression of melatonin.[25] *N*-acetyltransferase, which converts serotonin to melatonin, is specifically blocked by light. This enhances the production of serotonin and decreases the production of melatonin. Dopamine production is enhanced by light-induced activation of the enzymes tyrosine hydroxylase and phenylalanine decarboxylase.

Retina-Hypothalamus

Although most of the light energy received by the retina is relayed to the visual cortex for vision, an alternative pathway (see FIGURE 5) from the retina relays a small part to the suprachiasmatic nucleus (SCN), which is part of the hypothalamic region in the brain.[21,26] The SCN is thought to direct circadian rhythm and therefore controls a variety of events in the body such as temperature, reproductive cycles, appetite, and mood.[27] The pituitary and pineal gland are also involved in visible light–induced neuroendocrine changes. The neuroendocrine hormones that are particularly sensitive to modification of circadian rhythm are growth hormone, thyroid-stimulating hormone, thyroid hormones, prolactin, plasma cortisol, and melatonin.[4,7] Circadian rhythm is phase shifted by visible light.

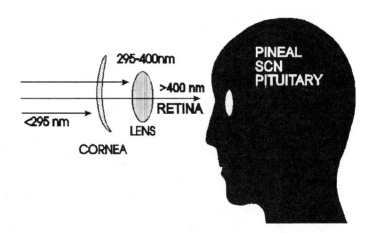

FIGURE 5. In primates UV light is filtered by the lens and cornea, and only visible light is transmitted to the retina. This light is transduced and sent to the visual cortex and, through an alternative pathway, to the SCN in the hypothalamus. There are further neural pathways that directly connect the hypothalamus with the pineal and pituitary glands. Irradiation of the eye leads to induction of the production of neurotransmitters and neuropeptide hormones from the SCN, pituitary, and pineal gland.

TABLE 1. **Neurotransmitters/hormones with immunomodulatory properties**[a]

Hormone/Neurotransmitter	Effect
Immune enhancers	
Prolactin	Activates macrophages Proliferates NK cells Produces IL-2
Growth hormone	Activates antibody synthesis Activates macrophages Produces IL-2
Somatostatin	Proliferates T, NK, and B cells and macrophages
Vasointestinal protein	Proliferates T and NK cells and macrophages
Substance P	Proliferates T and NK cells and macrophages
α-Melanin stimulating hormone	Proliferates NK cells Downregulates IL-1 and TNF-α Upregulates IL-10
Thyroxine	Activates T cells
β-Endorphin	Activates T cells and macrophages Suppresses B cells
Acetylcholine	Stimulates T and NK cells Increases IFN-γ
Melatonin	Activates T, NK, and B cells Upregulates IL-2
Serotonin	Proliferates T cells
Dopamine	Stimulates T and NK cells through stimulation of acetylcholine
Estrogen	Promotes IFN-γ Activates autoimmune response
Immune suppressors	
ACTH/CRH/cortisol	Impairs T and NK cell and macrophages Blocks antibody production Inhibits IL-4, Ig-E
Serotonin	Deactivates immune response through ACTH/CRH/cortisol modulation
Epinephrine/norepinephrine	Blocks IL-1, IL-2
Testosterone	impairs immune function through enhanced cortisol production

[a]See Refs. 34–36.

VISIBLE LIGHT EFFECTS IN HUMANS

All of the neurohormones shown in TABLES 1–3 that are modulated by light have been shown to affect immune response. Therefore, there may be one or more fundamental photoneuroendocrine–mediated mechanisms that control part of the immune system. This has been demonstrated in a few human studies.

We[28] and others[29,30] have found a small but significant enhancement in the number of peripheral lymphocytes induced by visible light through the eye. The proliferation of T4 and T8 cells in response to visible light was also reflected in seasonal changes.

In those studies, most subjects' response to visible light was a small but significant increase in the number of T lymphocytes. This result contrasts with what has been seen for UV irradiation in humans. Ultraviolet light (200–400 nm) reduces the number of T4 lymphocytes (13%), increases the number of T8 lymphocytes (29%), and reduces the ratio of T4/T8 lymphocytes (32%).[17] T cell proliferation requires IFN-γ and IL-2, and these are downregulated after UV irradiation.[18]

TABLE 2. Neurotransmitters modified by visible light[a]

Modification	Neurotransmitter
Increased by light	Serotonin
	Dopamine
	GABA
Decreased by light	Melatonin
	Norepinephrine
	Acetylcholine

[a]See Ref. 37.

TABLE 3. Effects of light on neuropeptides

Wavelength of light	Effect	Neuropeptide
UVA	Induces	α-Melanocyte-stimulating hormone (MSH)
		Adrenocorticotropic hormone (ACTH)
Visible light	Upregulates	Gastrin-releasing peptide (GRP)
		Corticotropin-releasing hormone (CRH)
		Neuropeptide Y
		Follicle-stimulating hormone (FSH)
	Downregulates	Vasoactive intestinal peptide (VIP)

CIRCADIAN IMMUNE RESPONSE

Circadian (daily) rhythm has a profound effect on immune responsiveness in humans. This has been reviewed by Levi[31] and Maestroni.[32] Briefly, the immune response to antigen presentation differs both quantitatively and qualitatively, depending upon the time of exposure. Also, the proliferation and circulation of T, B, or NK lymphocytes in the peripheral blood differs throughout the day. T lymphocyte response to antigen and proliferation of those cells is most efficient in the morning. On the other hand B cells have maximum antigen response, proliferation, and circulation in the evening. The enhanced expression of IL-2 receptors and proliferation of NK cells appear in the early afternoon. The mRNA synthesis for T cells peaks at 1 A.M., for B cells at 10 A.M., and for NK cells at 7 A.M.

Cirannual (seasonal) rhythms in immune response have been documented in many species.[33] T cell immunity was found to be depressed in most species in the winter even when natural light sources (photoperiod) are kept constant. On the other hand we have found a direct correlation between changes in immune response during visible light treatment and the seasons in humans.[4]

CONCLUSION

In conclusion, light modulates the immune system through both eye-brain and skin responses. The longer the wavelength, the greater the penetration of light through ocular and dermal tissues. The potential to suppress or activate the immune response depends on the wavelength. Light also induces specific changes in the production of neuroendocrine hormones, which in turn can indirectly modulate the immune response. Since light affects neuroendocrine processes, the wavelength, intensity, and timing of ambient light must be taken into consideration in designing and interpreting immunological experiments.

REFERENCES

1. SCHWARZ, T. & T.A. LUGER. 1989. Effect of uv irradiation on epidermal cell cytokine production. J. Photochem. Photobiol. **4:** 1–13.
2. THOMSON, A. 1994. The Cytokine Handbook, 2nd edit. Academic Press. New York.
3. AKINA, S., T. TAGA & T. KISHIMOTO. 1993. Interleukin-6 in biology and medicine. Advances Immunol. **54:** 1–60.
4. ROBERTS, J.E. 1995. Visible light induced changes in the immune response through an eye-brain mechanism (Photoneuroimmunology). J. Photochem. Photobiol. B: Biology **29:** 3–15.
5. PARRISH, J.A., M.L. KRIPKE & W.L. MORRISON. 1983. Photoimmunology. Plenum Press. New York.
6. PAMPHILON, D.H., A.A. ALNAQDY & T.B. WALLINGTON. 1991. Immunomodulation by ultraviolet light: clinical studies and biological effects. Immunol. Today **12:** 119–123.
7. BRAINARD, G.C. 1991. Photic parameters that regulate the neuroendocrine system and influence behavior in humans and animals. Photodermatol. Photoimmunol. Photomed. **8:** 34–39.
8. HAOUR, F., C. MARQUETTE, E. BAN, M. CRUMEYROLLE-ARIA, W. ROSTENE, H. TSIANG & G. FILLION. 1995. Receptors for interleukin-1 in the central nervous and neuroendocrine systems: role in infection and stress. Ann. Endocrinol. **56:** 173–179.

9. SPECTOR, N.H., Ed. 1988. Neuroimmunomodulation. Gordon and Breach Science Publishers. New York.
10. CARLSON, S.L. & D. FELTEN. 1989. Involvement of hypothalamic and limbic structures in neural-immune communication. *In* Neuroimmune Network: Physiology and Diseases. 219–226. Alan Liss. New York.
11. KHANSARI, D.N., A.J. MURGO & R.E. FAITH. 1990. Effects of stress on the imune system. Immunology Today 2: 170–175.
12. KRIPKE, M.L. 1988. Immunoregulation of carcinogenesis: past, present and future. J. Natl. Cancer Inst. 80: 722–727.
13. MORISON, W.L. 1989. Effects of ultraviolet radiation on the immune system in humans. Photochem. Photobiol. 50: 515–524.
14. CRUZ, P.D. 1991. Effects of UV radiation on induction of cutaneous immune responses. Photodermatol. Photoimmunol. Photomed. 8: 44.
15. NOONAN, F.P. & E.C. DeFABO. 1992. Immunosuppression by ultraviolet B radiation: initiation by urocanic acid. Immunol. Today. 13(7): 250–254.
16. MORISON, W.L. & M. KRIPKE. 1987. Photoimmunology and skin cancer. Photochem. Photobiophys. Suppl. 467–474.
17. HERSEY, P., M. BRADLEY, E. HASIC & G. HARAN. 1983. Immunological effects of solarium exposure. Lancet 1(8324): 545–548.
18. ARANEO, B.A., T. DOWELL, H.B. MOON & R.A. DAYNES. 1989. Regulation of murine lymphokine production in vivo. J. Immunol. 143: 1737–1744.
19. CZEISLER, C.A., M.P. JOHNSON, J.F. DUFFY, E.N. BROWN, E.N. BROWN, J.M. RONDA & R.E. KRONAUER. 1990. Exposure to bright light and darkness to treat physiologic maladaptation to night work, N. Engl. J. Med. 322: 1253–1259.
20. SADUN, A.A., J.D. SCHAECHTER & L.E.A SMITH. 1984. Retinalhypothalamic pathway in man: light mediation of circadian rhythms. Brain Res. 302: 371–377.
21. REME, C.E., A. WIRZ-JUSTICE & M. TERMAN. 1991. The visual input stage of the mammalian circadian pacemaking system: I. Is there a clock in the mammalian eye? J. Biol. Rhythms 6: 5–29.
22. DILLON, J. 1991. Photophysics and photobiology of the eye. J. Photochem. Photobiol. B. Biol 10: 23–40.
23. MAINSTER, M.A. 1987. Light and macular degeneration: a biophysical and clinical perspective. Eye 1: 304–310.
24. ZUCLIC, J.A. 1984. Ultraviolet induced damage in the primate cornea and retina. Curr. Eye Res. 3: 27–34.
25. DENIS, P., J.P. NORDMANN, P.P. ELENA & M. DUSSAILANT. 1993. Physiological roles of dopamine and neuropeptides in the retina. Fundam. Clin. Pharmacol. 7(6): 193–304.
26. TAKAHASHI, J.S., P.J. DeCOURSEY, L. BAUMAN & M. MENAKER. 1984. Spectral sensitivity of a novel photoreceptive system mediating entrainment of mammalian circadian rhythms. Nature 308: 186–188.
27. TERMAN, M., Ed. 1988–1990. Soc. Light Treatment Biol. Rhythms Abstr. 1988–1990.
28. ROBERTS, J.E., R. WHITT, DeS. LAWLESS, J.S. TERMAN, M. TERMAN & J. DILLON. 1992. Immune response to visible light treatment of SAD patients. *In* Biological Effects of Light. M.F. Holick & A.M. Kligman, Eds.: 125–129. Walter de Gruyter. New York.
29. ROSENTHAL, N.E., C. BROWN, D.A. OREN, G. GALLETTO & P. SCHWARTZ. 1991. Effects of light on mood and T-cell values in HIV infected individuals with and without winter-SAD. Soc. Light Treatment Biol. Rhythms Abstr. 3: 16.
30. KASPER, S., N.E. ROSENTHAL, S. BARBERI, A. WILLIAMS, L. TAMERKIN, S.L.B. ROGERS & S.R. PILLEMER. 1991. Immunological correlates of seasonal fluctuations in mood and behavior and their relationship to phototherapy. Psychiatry Res. 35: 253–264.
31. LEVI, F., C. CANON, M. DIPALMA, I. FLORENTIN & J-L. MISSET. 1991. When should the immune clock be reset? Ann. N.Y. Acad. Sci. 618: 312–339.
32. MAESTRONI, G.J.M. & A. CONTI. 1996. Melatonin and the immune-hematopoietic system. Therapeutic and adverse pharmacological correlates. Neuroimmunomodulation 3: 325–332.

33. ZAPATA, A.G., A. VARAS & M. TORROBA. 1992. Seasonal variations in the immune system of lower vertebrates. Immunol. Today **13:** 167–173.
34. SATOH, R.S., T. NAKAMURA, T. TAGA, T. MATSUDA, T. HIRANO, T. KISHIMOTO & Y. KAZIRO. 1988. Induction of neuronal differentiation in PC 12 cells by B-cell stimulatory factor 2/interleukin 6. Mol. Cell. Biol. **8:** 3546–3549.
35. SIRIANNI, M.C., S. FAES, B. ANNIBALE, S. DELUCA, M. BOIRIVANT, G. DELLEFAVE & F. PALLONE. 1991. Gut neuropeptides and the immune system. Adv. Neuroimmunol. **1:** 173–179.
36. VANDENBERG, P., J. ROZING & L. NAGELKERKEN. 1991. Opioid peptides as cytokine in T cell activation. Adv. Neuroimmunol. **1:** 189–203.
37. BRAINARD, G., J. FRENCH, P. HANNON, M. ROLLAG, J. HANIFIN & W. STORM. 1991. Effects of bright illumination on melatonin, prolactin and cortisol rhythms in subjects during sustained wakefulness. Soc. Light Treatment Bio. Rhythms Abstr. **3:** 16.
38. INOUYE,S.-I.T., K. SHINOHARA, K. TOMINAGA, Y. OTORI, C. FUKUHARA & J. YANG. 1990. A circadian pacemaker in the suprachiasmatic nucleus and its interaction with light. *In* Frontiers of Photobiology. A. Shima, M. Ichahashi, Y. Fujiwara & H. Takebe, Eds.: 257–262. Elsevier. Amsterdam.

Complex Coping Patterns and Their Role in Adaptation and Neuroimmunomodulation

Theory, Methodology, and Research

LYDIA R. TEMOSHOK[a]

Institute of Human Virology, University of Maryland, Baltimore, Maryland 21201, USA

ABSTRACT: This paper describes the evolution of a model of adaptative coping, as well as an example of the converse, a maladaptive coping pattern, *type C*. It was hypothesized that the more closely a coping process resembles the inverted U-shaped function that characterizes homeostasis for most biological systems, the more likely it is to be adaptive, and to be associated with more positive health outcomes. Maladaptive learned coping patterns, such as type C coping, represent deviations from homeostasis in that they fail to recognize, respond appropriately to, and/or resolve stressors, thus keeping the physiological stress response chronically engaged, with subsequent long-term damage to implicated biological systems. This interpretation of how maladaptive coping patterns such as type C can influence health outcomes is consistent with findings from the author's 20-year program of research on the type C pattern, its assessment, and its association with poorer health indicators and outcomes in cancer (malignant melanoma) and HIV/AIDS.

THEORY AND RESEARCH

Although animal research related to neuroimmunomodulation (NIM) has produced generally consistent results showing the negative effects of stress on tumor growth and other biological outcomes (see, e.g., Refs. 1–3), studies of psycho-neuroimmunologic (PNI) factors in humans have produced inconsistent, and often apparently contradictory, results.[4] It is likely that the failure of NIM animal research on the immunosuppressive effects of stressors to be reproduced consistently in humans is attributable to the more complex and varied ways in which the more advanced human cortex has evolved to deal with stressors. Previously, I attempted to explain these seeming discrepancies in the psychosocial oncology literature (through the mid-eighties) by positing a dynamic model of how a maladaptive coping pattern, type C, might operate across the trajectory of cancer etiology and progression.[5]

The burgeoning research literature on PNI and HIV/AIDS suggests that similarly inconsistent results on the health outcomes of psychosocial factors are accumulat-

[a]Address for correspondence: Dr. L.R. Temoshok, Institute of Human Virology, University of Maryland, 725 West Lombard St., Baltimore, MD 21201. Voice: 410-706-2621; fax: 410-706-3243.

temoshok@umbi.umd.edu

ing, particularly when, as in the psychosocial oncology literature,[6] insufficient attention is focused on coping patterns and other contextual factors. Such factors are highlighted in several studies, which, when considered together, suggest that a "simple" stressor-immunosuppression model is inadequate, and that prediction of actual health outcomes (versus hypothesized mediating mechanisms) is most accurate when complex coping patterns and contexts are taken into account.

For example, individuals with AIDS who scored higher on Kobasa's conceptually complex *hardiness* scale—which assesses commitment, control, and the ability to see adversity as a challenge—were more likely to be alive at follow-up than those scoring lower on these coping dimensions.[7] HIV-infected individuals with higher levels of type C coping[8] were more likely to progress to defined AIDS diagnosis at 6- and 12-month follow-up than those with other patterns of coping.[9] Depression, which has been inconsistently associated with HIV outcomes across several studies, was shown to be unrelated to HIV progression when it was the result of bereavement, in which depression might be interpreted as an adaptive working through of loss.[10] Bereaved individuals who were able to find meaning in their loss situations had slower CD4 cell decline and lower mortality over a two- to three-year follow-up than those who were not able to do so.[11] Another study by the same group of investigators showed, however, that when bereavement was combined with negative expectancies, AIDS-related symptoms developed more rapidly among initially asymptomatic HIV-infected men.[12] Far from being inconsistent, these studies combine to support an articulated understanding of how various coping responses work and whether they are adaptive or maladaptive can modify the health outcomes of bereavement stress.

A MODEL OF ADAPTIVE COPING APPLICABLE TO STUDIES OF CANCER AND HIV/AIDS

My previous model of type C coping was based on the recognition that adaptation is a dynamic process. What is adaptive at one point in time (e.g., when seeking information and second medical opinions concerning a possible cancer diagnosis) may be less adaptive at another (e.g., when postsurgery recovery favors rest and tranquility). Moreover, what may be adaptive for one context may not be adaptive for another. For example, I have hypothesized that while the type C pattern of focusing on pleasing others and not expressing anger in order to present a pleasant façade may help lubricate social relationships, when chronically engaged, this type of coping may have negative implications for physiological and immunological functioning.[5]

This model was elaborated in two subsequent iterations, in which I emphasized that the goal of coping is to maintain psychological-physiological homeostasis,[13] and that the more closely a coping process resembles the inverted U-shaped function that characterizes homeostasis for most biological processes, the more likely it is to be adaptive and to be associated with positive health outcomes.[14] Deviations from this normal physiological pattern are likely to be maladpative. If such maladaptive coping occurs chronically in response to stressors, the cumulative effect will be dysfunction and disease. The physiological adaptiveness hypothesis (see FIGURE 1) depicts the adaptive inverted U-shaped function, in contrast to three hypothetically maladaptive patterns of response to a stimulus.

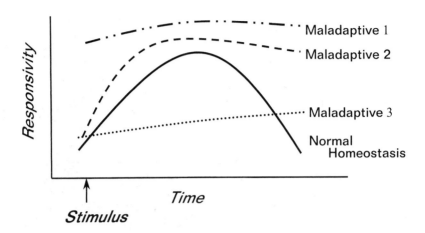

FIGURE 1. Physiological adaptiveness hypotheses.

Pattern 1 is maladaptive because the organism is already so hyperaroused that the ceiling effect comes into play, such that the stimulus generates very little response. An example of this would be a person so overwhelmed by loss of a loved one that he or she is unable to respond to any other environmental demands, such as the need to pay one's monthly mortgage bills (with devastating consequences if this pattern is sustained over time). Although the stressor is responded to quite strongly in maladaptive pattern 2, the arousal continues long after the adaptive pattern has returned to a resting or baseline level of arousal. This pattern is typical of some persons with obsessive compulsive disorder, in which certain thoughts continue to generate anxiety and sometimes compulsive repetitive behaviors that are ineffective, of course, in dealing with the initial trigger of the anxiety. In maladaptive pattern 3, there is minimal response to the stimulus, probably not enough to deal with the stimulus if it constitutes a problem demanding a solution or response. This pattern describes the immunological picture of someone with AIDS, whose depleted and dysfunctional immune system is unable to mount an effective response against opportunistic infections and pathogens that would cause no problem for someone with a normally functioning immune system.

To elaborate on this hypothesis, coping with stressors is most effective when all systems are working together in a coordinated and synchronous manner, and when the system best able to address and resolve the problem posed by the stressor takes the lead, as it were. For example, a psychosocial stressor—let us say a demand by one's boss to work late to finish a project—is best dealt with by the central nervous system (CNS), focusing attention and mental effort on completing the project as well and as quickly as possible. To the extent that other bodily systems are involved—for example, if anger and resentment about working late increase blood pressure, cause muscle tension, headaches, and so forth—these responses are not adaptive, may detract from the CNS's ability to do its job effectively, and may have more permanent negative effects on systems and organs affected by these responses.

Findings from a pilot study of psychological and physiological factors predicting longer survival in men with AIDS[15] support this notion that persons who respond to stressors with a more adaptive inverted U-shaped function will have better health outcomes. The best predictor of longer survival (controlling for initial CD4+ cell count, or months since diagnosis and nature of AIDS-defining diagnosis) was having a large difference between heart rate peak in response to experimental instructions to "relive" five emotionally stressful events that occurred in the past week *combined with* a low resting baseline between each of the five emotion-evoking episodes.[16] This physiological response maps as the adaptive pattern in FIGURE 1, in contrast to maladaptive patterns 1–3, which were all associated with significantly shorter survival times.

Interestingly, when the trajectory of HIV disease is plotted on the X axis and immune responsiveness on the Y axis, a U-shaped function (*not* inverted, as in the adaptive homeostatic model) describes the overall immune response to stressors across a number of studies in the HIV PNI literature.[16] This interpretation is consistent with the view of HIV as a potent system dysregulator of normal homeostasis, such that early in HIV disease, the immune system is inappropriately activated[17] and does not show the expected decline in lymphocytic proliferative responses to stressors,[18] whereas the relatively decimated immune systems of persons with AIDS may be able only to downregulate (maladaptively) in the face of stressors or the challenge of opportunistic infections and other pathogens.

MECHANISMS UNDERLYING LINKS BETWEEN COPING PATTERNS AND DISEASE OUTCOMES

My research on the type C behavior pattern suggests that the chronic suppression of anger and other dysphoric emotions, along with the presentation of a strong and pleasant façade in the face of a stressful situation may contribute to progression of malignant melanoma.[8] There are two hypothetical pathways or sets of mechanisms by which this may occur, the psychosocial and the psychoneuroimmunologic,[19] although it is likely that these pathways interact with and synergize each other. Following the psychosocial pathway, by not expressing emotion and by appearing stoically in control, the type C individual does not elicit social support from friends and relatives, and may not even get his or her medical needs met if symptoms or side effects are not communicated. Thus, the type C pattern is maladaptive from a strictly behavioral perspective because it does not address or resolve the problem of getting the best treatment for one's cancer and gaining the social support needed for recovery.

The type C pattern is characterized by a dysynchrony between a psychological response of suppression and nonexpression combined with an inappropriate physiological stress response.[8] In a study comparing the responses of melanoma patients, cardiovascular disease patients, and normal controls, Kneier and I found that melanoma patients were significantly more likely to rate themselves as "not upset" by a potentially stressful statement presented on a slide, at the same time that their skin conductance response to that slide indicated a stress response.[20] In other words, when the type C pattern was engaged, potential stressors were not dealt with appropriately by psychological means, but instead an inappropriate physiological stress response occurred. Considerable PNI and NIM research has shown that the hormonal alterations induced by stress alter the synthesis and release of cytokines by leukocytes[21] and have a generally immunosuppressive effect on natural killer cell activity (NKCA),[22] which has a key role in controlling metastases.[23] To the extent that an individual responds repeatedly and chronically to stressful situations—of which the stress of a cancer diagnosis and its treatment is among the most challenging—with an exaggerated physiological stress response that results in decreased NKCA, this individual will have an increased risk of metastases. Thus, the individual who chronically engages a type C coping pattern in response to stress will have a significantly poorer cancer prognosis than someone who addresses these same stressors with a more appropriately expressive and active coping pattern that reduces the physiological stress response.

METHODOLOGY AND RESEARCH: ASSESSING THE TYPE C BEHAVIOR PATTERN

The ways in which I have attempted to assess the type C coping pattern evolved over the years, as the pattern became more discernible to me, and my understanding of how such a coping pattern could affect immune functioning and cancer outcome became simultaneously clearer and more articulated. The first assessment of type C was adapted from Rosenman and Friedman's well-known assessment of the type A or "coronary-prone" behavior pattern.[24] I had observed in interviewing patients with malignant melanoma that not only did they show no evidence of the type A behavior pattern, but they were not type B either, which Rosenman and Friedman had described as the absence of type A. In fact, the dominant behavior pattern of my melanoma patients seemed to be the *polar opposite* of type A in nearly all respects. Thus, because I was formulating the hypothesis that the behavior pattern of these cancer patients was somehow involved in the progression and possibly the etiology of their cancer, I decided to call this the type C or "cancer-prone" behavior pattern.

My first study with colleagues at the University of California San Francisco found that delay in seeking medical attention for suspicious lesions (this inattention to one's own needs, bodily sensations, or symptoms that anything might be wrong was conceived as part of the type C constellation of behaviors) contributed the most variance in multiple regression analyses to tumor thickness, the best prognostic indicator for malignant melanoma.[25] Emotional as well as behavioral aspects of the type C pattern were also assessed by raters of videotaped patient interviews, using 17 semantic differential scales that contrasted typical type A emotions and behaviors (e.g., active, impatient, hostile) versus what we hypothesized to be type C characteristics (e.g., passive, bland, appeasing). Separate from delay behavior, the semantic differential ratings of type C vs. type A emotions and behaviors were significantly correlated with tumor thickness, most strongly for patients under age 55.[25]

In my next study, with A. Kneier[20] (which was actually published before the one just described), we tried to capture the "repressive" or "suppressive" aspect of type C, which appeared to contribute to the behavior of delay in seeking medical attention for suspicious lesions in our first study. When we asked patients why they delayed seeing a doctor, they all seemed to recognize that their growing and/or discolored lesion could represent a medical problem, even possibly cancer, but they put this in the back of their minds and focused their attention on the needs of others in their family and environment.[8] In thinking about how to assess this repressive or suppressive pattern, we first considered using the method described by Weinberger, Schwartz, and Davidson,[26] which contrasted responses to *two* scales, the Taylor Manifest Anxiety Scale (MAS)—a trait measure based on reported anxiety symptoms—and the Marlowe-Crowne (M-C) Social Desirability Scale, which was designed to assess tendencies to respond to questionnaires in a socially desirable direction. By using subjects' responses on these two measures, Weinberger *et al.* categorized them as either truly high anxious (high MAS, low M-C), truly low anxious (low MAS, low M-C), repressors (low MAS, high M-C), and defensive high anxious (high MAS, high M-C).

The problem with using this two-scale method for our melanoma patients was that we were conducting our assessments at the point when the subjects were coming in for their biopsy results and were likely to be overtly anxious about this; thus, this method would not be able to capture their tendency to respond to potentially (rather than actually) stressful stimuli in a repressive manner. Another drawback to this method was that it did not seem capable of furthering our understanding of just *how* the repressive aspects of the type C pattern might influence physiological processes. Therefore, we devised a method that contrasted the type C tendency to underreport negative or socially undesirable symptoms (such as anxiety or a suspicious lesion) with a physiologically reactive response indicative of stress. We hypothesized that individuals who coped with potential stressors by deploying a type C pattern would exhibit a dysynchrony between their psychological and their physiological responses, defined in this study as the sum of all responses to potentially disturbing statements presented on slides in which the person's skin conductance response (SCR) was *above* the mean SCR across all statements for that individual, *in conjunction with* a self-report of perturbation *below* that individual's mean self-report score. As hypothesized, melanoma patients had significantly more coping reactions that were dysynchronous in the direction of repression or suppression, in contrast to cardiovascular disease patients, who displayed the opposite pattern (higher reports of psychological perturbation vs. SCR reactivity, and controls, who had a more synchronous pattern (psychological and physiological reactivity correlated).[20]

I was still dissatisfied with this method, however, because the physiological process measured by skin conductance is not a mediating mechanism for cancer progression, although it may reflect more complex biological processes that may be more directly implicated (i.e., stressor-induced activation of the sympathetic nervous system and the sympathetic-adrenal medullary and hypothalamic-pituitary adrenal axes,[27] which, in turn, influence activity of the immune system). Thus, my next study focused on an immune measure that is directly related to disease outcome in malignant melanoma: the number of lymphocytes at the base of the deepest invasion of the tumor, according to a pathologist's rating of paraffin-embedded sections of the primary lesions using the light microscope. Patients' emotional expressiveness, rated across five highly inter-correlated dimensions from specific videotaped interview segments about how they felt when they were first told they might have melanoma, was strongly and significantly correlated with having more lymphocytes at the base of the tumor.[28] This study was also important in that it identified the inappropriately dampened expression or *nonexpression* of emotion as the pathogenic core of the type C pattern, similar to the convergence of studies on hostility (an emotional expression variable) as the key aspect of type A that influences cardiovascular disease.[29]

NEEDED: A USER-FRIENDLY METHOD TO ASSESS TYPE C THAT HAS PREDICTIVE VALIDITY

The problem with the methods of assessing aspects of the type C coping pattern described above is that they all involved a great deal of equipment (computerized physiological monitoring apparatus or videotape cameras), space, and personnel. There was also a fair amount of demand on study participants. All these factors limited the number of participants in any one study, with consequent limits on statistical power. I tried using various scales that measured components and aspects of the type C pattern, but these failed to predict potential immune mechanisms, biological prognostic indicators, or intermediate health outcomes. Moreover, study participants did not like filling out pages of self-report scales and often scribbled notes in the margins to indicate that their real thoughts or feelings were not represented or were distorted by a given item. Clearly, another method was needed.

In the early 1980s, I had worked with Rex Green, a psychologist who had developed a computerized multidimensional scaling program for describing a person according to a series of similarity ratings along a number of dimensions.[30] While piloting these multidimensional similarity ratings, I soon became aware that (a) people liked doing the task, (b) they felt the resulting description was remarkably accurate, and (c) "objective" observers also perceived the accuracy of the resulting descriptions when they were compared to a picture of the person derived from an hour-long psychological interview.

I was also struck with how much descriptions of actual (but disguised) patients in my book on the type C pattern[8] elicited strong feelings of recognition by people with cancer and their friends and relatives. Thus, I decided to combine these two "techniques" and compose a paragraph or vignette about a person emoting, behaving, and thinking in type C ways in response to a situation of having to face possible diagnosis with a serious disease. For contrast, I also composed vignettes describing someone coping in a more adaptive manner (i.e., seeking information, asking questions of one's physician, seeking the support of family and friends, expressing feelings and needs), and then someone responding in a very maladaptive "helpless/hopeless" way (i.e., feeling overwhelmed, avoiding friends and family, not being able to act effectively in any way).[8] The task for the respondent was simply to rate on a 1-to-5 or 1-to-10 point scale, "How similar do you think your reactions are to the reactions of (name of person in vignette)?" I found it was helpful to match the gender of the person in the vignette to that of the respondent.

Because the vignettes are about other people, being asked to rate similarity to the emotions and behaviors of *someone else*, rather than rating one's own emotions and behaviors on a series of scale items, appears to minimize defensiveness about reporting socially less desirable states and behaviors. Thus, the method is particularly useful for assessing the type C coping pattern, of which a key characteristic is the desire to please others and present the self in socially desirable ways.

The vignette method is also very flexible: by altering the details of the situation, but not the general ways in which people are described as thinking, feeling, and behaving, it is possible to vary the stories such that they could be presented as repeated measures, while retaining vivid relevance to the person's changing challenges or stressors. This has been done in an Italian study of HIV progression, in which the vignettes were adapted to the general stage of disease of participants at the beginning of the study, and then at 6- and 12-month follow-ups.[9] Another adaptation was for a study of HIV patients in San Francisco and Los Angeles who had recently experienced a traumatic event (an earthquake).[31] The vignette-similarity rating method was also applied to assessing the complex concept of forgiveness across different levels or contexts (i.e., self, interpersonal, health care, community, and spiritual), for persons living with HIV/AIDS in India.[32] The general experience of researchers using the vignette method has been that it is well accepted and even liked by study participants (good face validity) and is a strong and significant predictor of health outcomes (high predictive validity).[33]

CONCLUDING COMMENTS

In this paper, I have described the evolution of an integrative model of adaptive coping over the course of two decades of NIM and PNI studies on cancer and HIV/AIDS. In this model, the more closely a coping process resembles an inverted U-shaped function, the more likely it is to be adaptive and to be associated with more positive health outcomes. Maladaptive learned patterns, such as type C coping, represent deviations from homeostasis, including dysynchronies in responding to stressful stimuli across systems. It was hypothesized that HIV wreaks its havoc by dysregulating the immune system, as well as central nervous system and autonomic functioning, and inducing maladaptive, U-shaped response processes to stressful psychological and biological stimuli. This interpretation of how maladaptive coping or responding to stressors can influence health outcomes in cancer and HIV/AIDS, and findings discussed here that support these connections suggest that interventions that bring at least one system back into a regulated, adaptive coping pattern may have beneficial health effects. One of the main challenges in conducting such research is to devise methods to assess adaptive or maladaptive coping that have high predictive validity. In describing how my assessment methods have also evolved over the years to better "capture" or approximate the complex reality subsumed by these complex coping patterns, I hope to stimulate further research on these critical questions.

REFERENCES

1. ADER, R., D.L. FELTEN & N. COHEN. 1991. Psychoneuroimmunology, 2d edit. Wiley. New York.
2. TEMOSHOK, L., H.V.S. PEEKE, C.W. MEHARD *et al.* 1987. Stress-behavior interactions in hamster tumor growth. Ann. N.Y. Acad. Sci. **496:** 501–509.
3. GIRALDI, T. 2000. Stress and chemotherapy: combined effects on immunity and disease progression in animal models. The 4th International Congress of the International Society for Neuroimmunomodulation. Ann. N.Y. Acad. Sci. **917:** this volume.

4. CONTI, A. 2000. Oncology in NIM: past, present and future. The 4th International Congress of the International Society for Neuroimmunomodulation. Ann. N.Y. Acad. Sci. **917:** this volume.

5. TEMOSHOK, L. 1987. Personality, coping style, emotion, and cancer: toward an integrative model. Cancer Surv. **6:** 837–857.

6. GREER, S. 2000. What's in a name: neuroimmunolomodulation or psychoneuroimmunology? The 4th International Congress of the International Society for Neuroimmunomodulation. Ann. N.Y. Acad. Sci. **917:** this volume.

7. SOLOMON, G.F., L. TEMOSHOK, A. O'LEARY & J. ZICH. 1987. An intensive psychoimmunologic study of long-surviving persons with AIDS: pilot work, background studies, hypotheses, and methods. Ann. N.Y. Acad. Sci. **496:** 647–655.

8. TEMOSHOK, L. & H. DREHER. 1992. The Type C Connection: The Behavioral Links to Cancer and Your Health. Random House. New York.

9. SOLANO, L., M. COSTA, S. SALVATI et al. 1993. Psychosocial factors and clinical evolution in HIV-1 infection: a longitudinal study. J. Psychosom. Res. **37:** 39–51.

10. KEMENY, M.E., H. WEINER, S.E. TAYLOR et al. 1994. Repeated bereavement, depressed mood, and immune parameters in HIV seropositive and seronegative gay men. Health Psychol. **13:** 14–24.

11. BOWER, J.E., M.E. KEMENY, S.E. TAYLOR et al. 1998. Cognitive processing, discovery of meaning, CD4 decline, and AIDS-related mortality among bereaved HIV-seropositive men. J. Consult. Clin. Psychol. **66:** 979–986.

12. REED, G.M., M.E. KEMENY, S.E. TAYLOR et al. 1999. Negative HIV-specific expectancies and AIDS-related bereavement as predictors of symptom onset in asymptomatic HIV-positive gay men. Health Psychol. **18:** 354–363.

13. TEMOSHOK, L.R. 1990. On attempting to articulate the biopsychosocial model: psychological-psychophysiological homeostasis. In Personality and Disease. H. Friedman, Ed.: 203–225. Wiley. New York.

14. TEMOSHOK, L.R. 1997. The complexity of cause: linking emotional dynamics to health outcomes. In The (Non)expression of Emotions in Health and Disease. A. Vingerhoets, F. van Bussel & S.J. Boelhouwer, Eds.: 15–24. Tilburg University Press. Tilburg, The Netherlands.

15. O'LEARY, A., L. TEMOSHOK, S.R. JENKINS et al. 1989. Autonomic reactivity and immune function in men with AIDS. Psychophysiology **26:** S47.

16. TEMOSHOK, L. 1993. HIV/AIDS, psychoneuroimmunology and beyond: a commentary and review. Adv. Neuroimmunol. **3:** 141–149.

17. ASCHER, M.S. & H.W. SHEPPARD. 1988. AIDS as immune system activation: a model for pathogenesis. Clin. Exp. Immun. **73:** 165–167.

18. IRONSON, G., A. LAPERRIERE, M. ANTONI et al. 1990. Changes in immune and psychological measures as a function of anticipation and reaction to news of HIV-1 antibody status. Psychosom. Med. **52:** 247–270.

19. TEMOSHOK, L.R. 1995. On biobehavioral models of cancer stress and disease course. Am. Psychol. **50:** 1104–1105.

20. KNEIER, A.W. & L. TEMOSHOK. 1984. Repressive coping reactions in patients with malignant melanoma as compared to cardiovascular disease patients. J. Psychosom. Res. **29:** 139–153.

21. GLASER, R., B. RABIN, M. CHESNEY et al. 1999. Stress-induced immunomodulation: implications for infectious diseases? J. Am. Med. Assoc. **281:** 2268–2270.

22. HERBERT, T.B. & S. COHEN. 1993. Stress and immunity in humans: a meta-analytic review. Psychosom. Med. **55:** 364–379.

23. HERBERMAN, R.B. 1991. Principles of tumor immunology. In American Cancer Society Textbook of Clinical Oncology. A.I. Holleb, D.J. Fink & G.P. Murphy, Eds.: 69–79. American Cancer Society. Atlanta, GA.

24. ROSENMAN, R.H., M. FRIEDMAN, R. STRAUS et al. 1964. A predictive study of coronary heart disease. JAMA **189:** 15–26.

25. TEMOSHOK, L.R., B.W. HELLER, R.W. SAGEBIEL et al. 1985. The relationship of psychosocial factors to prognostic indicators in cutaneous malignant melanoma. J. Psychosom. Res. **29:** 139–153.

26. WEINBERGER, D.A., G.E. SCHWARTZ & R.J. DAVIDSON. 1979. Low-anxious, high-anxious, and repressive coping styles: psychometric patterns and behavioral and physiological responses to stress. J. Abnorm. Psychol. **88:** 369–380.
27. RABIN, B.S. 1999. Stress, immune function, and health: the connection. Wiley-Liss & Sons, Inc. New York.
28. TEMOSHOK, L. 1985. Biopsychosocial studies on cutaneous malignant melanoma: psychological factors associated with prognostic indicators, progression, psychophysiology, and tumor-host response. Soc. Sci. Med. **20:** 833–840.
29. DEMBROSKI, T.M., J.M. MACDOUGALL, R.S. ELIOT et al. 1983. Stress, emotions, behavior, and cardiovascular disease. In Emotions in Health and Illness: Theoretical and Research Foundations. L. Temoshok, C. Van Dyke & L.S. Zegans, Eds.: 61–72. Grune & Stratton. New York.
30. TEMOSHOK, L. & R.S. GREEN. 1984. PRAT: A real time multidimensional scaling assessment of object relations for psychotherapy. In Proceedings, Second Annual Conference of the American Association for Medical Systems and Informatics (AAMSI). B.T. Williams, Ed.: 85–96. AAMSI. New York.
31. TEMOSHOK, L. & J.M. MOULTON. 1991. Dimensions of biopsychosocial research on HIV disease: perspectives from the UCSF Biopsychosocial AIDS Project. In Stress, Coping and Disease. P.M. McCabe, N. Schneiderman, T. Field & J. Skyler, Eds.: 211–236. Erlbaum. Englewood Cliffs, NJ.
32. TEMOSHOK, L.R. & P.S. CHANDRA. 1999. The meaning of forgiveness in a specific situational and cultural context: persons living with HIV/AIDS in India. In Forgiveness: Theory, Research, and Practice. M. McCullough, K. Pargament & C. Thoresen, Eds.: 41–64. Guilford Publications. New York.
33. MESSICK, S. 1995. Validity of psychological assessment: validation of inferences from persons' responses and performances as scientific inquiry into score meaning. Am. Psychol. **50:** 741–749.

The Immune System and Schizophrenia

An Integrative View

NORBERT MÜLLER,[a] MICHAEL RIEDEL, RUDOLF GRUBER,
MANFRED ACKENHEIL, AND MARKUS J. SCHWARZ

Psychiatric Hospital, Ludwig-Maximilian University, Munich, Germany

ABSTRACT: Immune alterations in schizophrenia have been described for decades. Modern immunological methods and new insights into the highly developed and functionally differentiated immune system allow an integrative view of both the older and the recent findings of immunological abnormalities in schizophrenia. Both the unspecific and the specific arms of the immune system seem to be involved in the dysfunction of the immune system in schizophrenia. The unspecific, "innate" immune system shows signs of overactivation in unmedicated schizophrenic patients, as indicated by increased monocytes and γδ-cells. Increased levels of interleukin-6 (IL-6) and the activation of the IL-6 system in schizophrenia might be the result of the activation of monocytes/macrophages, too. On the other hand, several parameters of the specific cellular immune system are blunted, such as, for example, the decreased T helper-1 (TH-1)–related immune parameters in schizophrenic patients both *in vitro* and *in vivo*. It seems that a TH-1–TH-2 imbalance with a shift to the TH-2 system is associated with schizophrenia. During antipsychotic therapy with neuroleptics, the specific TH-1–related immune answer becomes activated, but in addition the B cell system and antibody production increase.

INTRODUCTION

Immunological alterations in schizophrenia have been described in the international literature since the beginning of the last century.[1–3] However, for several reasons, the focus of interest moved away from the immune system. One reason was the introduction of neuroleptics into the therapy of schizophrenia, leading to the dopamine hypothesis as the center of research activities. Another reason was that the components and functions of the immune system were not well understood during those times.

Schizophrenia is a heterogenous disorder in its clinical symptomatology, the acuity of its symptoms, its course, its treatment response and probably also its etiology. Besides causing methodological pitfalls, this heterogeneity might contribute to the heterogeneity of the results of biological investigations, which can be found in several fields of biological research in schizophrenia. Widespread heterogeneity can

[a]Address for correspondence: Prof. Dr. med. Dipl.-Psych. Norbert Müller, Psychiatrische Klinik der Ludwig-Maximilians-Universität, Nußbaumstr. 7, 80336 München, Germany. Voice: 089-5160-3397; fax: 089-5160-4548.
nmueller@psy.med.uni-muenchen.de

also be observed in the results of immunological studies in schizophrenia (overview in Ref. 4).

RELATIONSHIP BETWEEN CLINICAL CHARACTERISTICS AND IMMUNE ALTERATIONS

Signs of an inflammatory disease process in schizophrenia have been observed in a subgroup of schizophrenic patients.[5] Clinical features of this subgroup showing signs of immunological or inflammatory disease have been studied by several groups of researchers. It was observed that the symptomatolgy—for instance, paranoid symptoms or negative symptoms,[6,7] the acuity,[8-10] and the drug treatment[11-18] influence the immunological parameters. Also, the clinical response to treatment with neuroleptics seems to be related to immune parameters.[19]

The discussion of this relationship between the clinical characteristics of schizophrenia and parameters of the immune system may help to define subgroups characterized by disturbances of the immune system. Moreover, a critical review has to take into consideration these results in order to classify the immune alterations with regard to clinical features of schizophrenia on the one hand and to the function of the immune system on the other. Therefore, a short description of the immune system is necessary for further understanding its dysfunction in schizophrenia.

THE CONCEPT OF INNATE AND ADAPTIVE IMMUNITY IN HUMANS

The immune system developed over millions of years of evolution. In order to defend against a variety of invading life-threatening microorganisms, such as bacteria and viruses, a highly differentiated system consisting of different lines of defense was established. A widespread heterogeneity was the consequence: two functionally different immune systems both representing different types of barriers and each consisting of cellular and humoral immune components. The "innate" immune system is the phylogenetically elder, "primitive" one. Its cellular arm is represented by monocytes/macrophages, granulocytes, and natural killer (NK) cells. The humoral arm consists of acute-phase proteins and the complement system. This "unspecific" immune system represents the first line of defense.

The specific part of the immune system of higher organisms including humans is the "adaptive" immune system, consisting of the cellular arm of the T and B cells and the humoral arm of specific antibodies. This system includes higher functions, such as memory, and can be conditioned. In case of reexposure to a specific antigen, this system can recognize the enemy and initiate a specific immune response (see TABLE 1).

The innate and adaptive immune systems are functionally balanced. Within the adaptive immune system is another balance involving the activation of the cellular and humoral immune systems. The cellular arm of the adaptive immune system is mainly activated by the T helper–1 (TH-1) system—helper cells that produce the activating "immunotransmitter" interleukin-2 (IL-2), interferon-γ (IFN-γ), and tumor necrosis factor–α (TNF-α). The humoral arm of the adaptive immune system

TABLE 1. Components of the unspecific "innate" and the more specific cellular "adaptive" immune systems in humans

Components	Innate	Adaptive
Cellular	Monocytes macrophages granulocytes γ/δ-cells	T and B cells
Humoral	Complement, APP, mannose–binding lectin (MBL)	Antibodies

is activated mainly via the TH-2 system—helper cells that produce mainly IL-4, IL-10, and IL-6.

ACTIVATION OF THE INNATE UNSPECIFIC IMMUNE SYSTEM IN SCHIZOPHRENIA

Although systematic investigations of the innate immune system in schizophrenia are lacking, there are several hints that this part of the immune system may be more activated in schizophrenic patients than in controls. There is a report that monocytes are increased in schizophrenic patients compared to controls,[10] and our own investigations of unmedicated schizophrenic patients also showed increased amounts of monocytes in schizophrenia compared to controls (unpublished results). An increase in the number of cells of the "first immune barrier" was also found in $\gamma\delta^+CD8^+$ cells in unmedicated schizophrenics.[20]

One of the key cytokines that initiates the immune response and especially activates the B cell system is interleukin-6 (IL-6). Activated monocytes and macrophages are the major sources of the production and release of IL-6. Vice versa, increased levels of IL-6, as mentioned in the next paragraph, may be the result of the activation of the monocyte/macrophage system leading to an overproduction of IL-6 by the innate immune system.

IL-6 IN THE CENTRAL NERVOUS SYSTEM

IL-6 is a pleiotropic cytokine that is released from various cell types in the blood (macrophages, monocytes, T and B cells). One function of IL-6 is to activate B cells to synthesize antibodies.[21] However, as with several other cytokines, IL-6 is not only synthesized and released in immune cells of the peripheral blood; it is also produced by activated astrocytes and microglia cells in the central nervous system (CNS). Several findings suggest that IL-6 may mediate the exacerbation of autoimmune disorders in the CNS;[22] for example, IL-6 supports the differentiation of B cells, local IgG synthesis in the CNS, and blood-brain barrier disturbance.[23,24] In the hypothalamus,

IL-6 can induce the release of growth hormone–releasing hormone and TSH, and it stimulates *in vitro* the secretion of prolactin and growth hormone from pituitary cells.[25]

A strong relationship between IL-6 and neurotransmitter production has been reported by various studies. IL-6 can stimulate neurons *in vitro* to secrete dopamine and probably other catecholamines as well.[26] The peripheral application of IL-6 in animal experiments enhanced the dopaminergic and serotonergic turnover in the hippocampus and frontal cortex, without affecting noradrenaline.[27] Conversly, noradrenaline can stimulate astrocytes to release IL-6.[22] Both observations point to a direct influence of activating cytokines, especially IL-6, on the catecholaminergic neurotransmitter system.

IL-6 AND SCHIZOPHRENIA

Several reports have shown increased IL-6 levels in schizophrenia.[13,28–30] Several authors have described a relationship between increased IL-6 levels and clinical features of schizophrenia: high IL-6 levels were related to the duration of the disorder[28] and to treatment resistance.[30] These findings suggest that IL-6 serum levels may be especially high in patients with an unfavorable course of the disease. However, methodological concerns must be considered.

However, investigations of sIL-6R (soluble IL-6 receptor) levels in the CSF showed that high levels of sIL-6R can be found in schizophrenic patients, especially those with a more marked paranoid-hallucinatory syndrome.[31] These investigations also point to a more altered IL-6 system in patients with an unfavorable course of the disease: longer duration of illness, greater treatment resistance, or more marked paranoid-hallucinatory symptomatology.

Another study found reduced levels of sgp130 in the CSF of schizophrenic patients compared to depressed patients and psychiatrically healthy controls.[32] This result supports the view of a disturbance in the IL-6 system in schizophrenia, because gp130 is part of the IL-6 system. The soluble protein spg130 acts as an antagonist to the gp130 receptor and mediates the inhibition of the IL-6 system.[33] Functionally, decreased sgp130 levels in the CSF point to a decrease in the inhibition of the IL-6 system and an increase in its activation.

ANTIPSYCHOTIC THERAPY AND THE IL-6 SYSTEM

There are several observations that antipsychotic therapy with neuroleptics is accompanied by a functional decrease of the IL-6 system. A significant decrease of IL-6 during therapy with neuroleptics was described by Maes and coworkers.[13] Two studies found a significant decrease of sIL-6R levels during antipsychotic therapy with neuroleptics.[13,16] Studies from human CNS cell cultures also showed an inhibitory effect of various neuroleptics on the production of IL-6 after stimulation with lipopolysacharides, more marked with phenothiazines than with butyrophenones (unpublished results). Similar observations have been described by other authors, too.[30]

T HELPER–2 CELL ACTIVATION IN SCHIZOPHRENIA

IL-6 is a product not only of macrophage/monocyte activation, but also of the activation of the TH-2 system. Therefore it cannot be known whether a functional increase of the IL-6 system is a product of TH-2 activation or of the monocyte/macrophage line. However, other results point to activation of the TH-2 system in schizophrenia.

IL-10 is a cytokine that is produced by TH-2 cells. An increase of IL-10 in schizophrenic patients compared to healthy controls has been reported.[6] Another study observed a strong relationship between IL-10 levels and schizophrenic negative symptoms in the cerebrospinal fluid of 62 unmedicated schizophrenics.[34] In schizophrenics treated with haloperidol, a significant relationship between CSF IL-10 levels and the severity of schizophrenic psychosis, measured by the Bunney-Hamburg psychosis rating scale,[35] was found.[34] These findings suggest that IL-10 levels in the CSF are related to the severity of the psychosis, especially to the negative symptoms.

Another characteristic cytokine that is produced by TH-2 cells is IL-4. An increase of IL-4 levels in the CSF of juvenile schizophrenic patients has recently been reported.[36] The production of IgE is also a sign of the activation of the TH-2 immune response. Increased levels of IgE in schizophrenic patients compared to controls have been observed.[37] The latter findings suggest that the probable increase of the TH-2 system in schizophrenia not only is a phenomenon of the peripheral immune system, it also seems to play a role in the CNS immune system.

Earlier descriptions of elevated CD3+ and CD4+ cells in unmedicated schizophrenics are consistent with the hypothesis of a shift to the TH-2 system with diminished TH-1 immune response in schizophrenia.[15,38]

As shown in FIGURE 1, there is a functional balance between the TH-1 and TH-2 systems. It would be expected that overactivation of the TH-2 system would be asso-

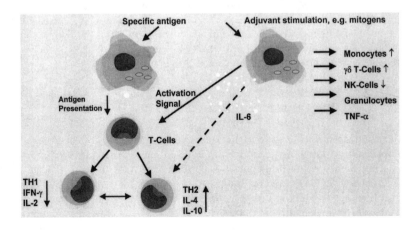

FIGURE 1. Model of the immune response in schizophrenia: increase of the unspecific "innate" immune response, impaired cellular TH-1 activation, and shift to a TH-2 response.

ciated with underactivation of the TH-1 system. Many different findings over decades of years point to decreased activation of the TH-1 system in schizophrenia.

THE T HELPER–1 SYSTEM AND SCHIZOPHRENIA

The key characteristics of the TH-1 system are the production of interferon-γ and IL-2. One of the often-replicated findings in schizophrenia is the decreased *in vitro* production of IL-2.[6,39–42] This phenomenon has often been interpreted as the consequence of an exhaustion of the lymphocytes after overproduction of IL-2, but it may reflect as well the reduced capacity of lymphocytes to produce IL-2. The observation of decreased production of IL-2 fits well with another finding: decreased production of interferon-γ.[10,43] Both findings indicate decreased production of TH-1–related cytokines and underactivation of the TH-1 system in schizophrenia. Lack of activation of the TH-1–related cellular immune system has also been postulated by other researchers.[38] Our findings of decreased production of lymphocytes after stimulation with different specific antigens may also reflect reduced capacity for a TH-1–mediated immune response in schizophrenia. Especially after stimulation with tuberculin, which provokes a TH-1–mediated immune answer, the reaction was blunted.[15]

sICAM-1: MARKER FOR TH-1 ACTIVATION

Recently, decreased levels of soluble intercellular adhesion molecule–1 (sICAM-1) in the serum of schizophrenic patients have been described (Wieselmann, personal communication; Ref. 44). ICAM-1 is a molecule that mediates the adhesion of lymphocytes to other lymphocytes, to endothelial cells, and to parenchymal cells; but it also mediates the signal for the activation of the cellular immune system. ICAM-1 is part of the TH-1 immune response.[45,46] Therefore, decreased levels of the soluble form of ICAM-1, which is shedded from lymphocytes, seem to represent the state of activation of the TH-1 system. However, reduced sICAM-1 levels have recently been found in not only the serum, but also the CSF of schizophrenic patients (Schwarz *et al.*, manuscript in preparation). The latter finding suggests that the decreased activation of the TH-1 system may not be restricted to the peripheral immune system, because CSF parameters reflect more directly the immune pathology of the CNS.

One of the classic epidemiological findings in schizophrenia research is the negative association between schizophrenia and rheumatoid arthritis.[47] This negative association can be interpreted as two sides of the TH-1/TH-2-balance—represented by increased sICAM-1 levels in rheumatoid arthritis and decreased sICAM-1 levels in schizophrenia. Because sICAM-1 is also a key molecule that mediates the inflammatory reaction in rheumatoid arthritis, increased sICAM-1 levels are regularly found in rheumatoid arthritis.[48] Rheumatoid arthritis is a disorder that is primarily mediated by the cellular TH-1–related immune system.

BLUNTED REACTION OF THE CUTANEOUS CELLULAR
IMMUNE RESPONSE IN SCHIZOPHRENIA

Also, the blunted cutaneus reaction to antigens of the Multitest Mérieux that can be observed in schizophrenic patients (Müller *et al.*, manuscript in preparation) points to a blunted response of cell-mediated immunity in schizophrenia. A very early description of this phenomenon, from long before the era of neuroleptics, is that by Molholm of the hyposensitivity of schizophrenic patients, compared to a control group, to intracutaneously injected guinea pig serum.[49] Not only was such a blunted reaction of a cell-mediated (TH-1) immune response observed in the cutaneus reaction to antigens, but also decreased antibody production after vaccination with salmonella was found in unmedicated schizophrenic patients.[11] Descriptions of immune reactions before the era of neuroleptics exclude the possibilty that the observed phenomena may be artefacts of the effects of neuroleptics. Antipsychotic therapy is associated with various effects on the immune system, but these effects may counterregulate the immune effects of the disease. Neuroleptics mainly activate the TH-1 system.

THE TH-1 SYSTEM AND ANTIPSYCHOTIC THERAPY

Recent findings indicate that neuroleptics may have TH-1–stimulating effects. *In vitro* studies show that the decreased interferon-g production becomes normalized after therapy with neuroleptics.10 The increase of soluble IL-2 receptors has been described by several groups.[16,18,50] Since sIL-2R are shedded from activated T cells, the increase may reflect an increase of activated IL-2–bearing T cells.

The increase of CD4+CD45RO+ cells during therapy with neuroleptics was observed by two groups.[6,51] CD4+CD45RO+ cells are one of the primary sources of interferon-g production. The increase of this subpopulation during therapy may contribute to an increase in interferon-γ production. The reduced sICAM-1 levels in the serum of schizophrenics do not normalize during short-term neuroleptic therapy, but a statistically nonsignificant tendency to increase sICAM-1 could be observed.[44] On the other hand, the leucocyte function antigen–1 (LFA-1) molecule on CD4+ cells shows increased expression during antipsychotic therapy.[17] LFA-1 is the counter-molecule to ICAM-1. Moreover, the blunted reaction to vaccination with salmonella was not observed in patients who were treated with neuroleptics.[11] These studies indicate that the TH-1–mediated immune response increases during antipsychotic therapy. The B cell–mediated immune response also increases during antipsychotic treatment.

B CELLS AND ANTIPSYCHOTIC TREATMENT

Activated B cells are antibody-producing cells. Several observations in the literature point out that B cells are activated during antipsychotic treatment and antibody production may increase. Already during the 1970s *in vitro* studies showed an increase of antibody production after stimulation with phenothiazines.[52,53]

Many studies described increased antibody production in schizophrenic patients, and those observations led to discussion of a possible autoimmune origin of schizophrenia.[54] Nevertheless, the role of antipsychotic treatment was not considered in several of these studies. Although findings have repeatedly shown that about 20–35% of schizophrenic patients show features of an autoimmune process, the role of actual or former therapy with neuroleptics may not have been adequately taken into consideration.

An increase of IgG—antibodies are mainly IgG-antibodies—in the CSF has been described, especially in patients with predominantly negative symptoms.[7] Increased antibodies against heat shock protein 60 in schizophrenia is an interesting recent finding, because it may reflect a mechanism of loss of neuronal protection.[55–57] However, antibodies against heat shock protein 60 are found especially in patients during neuroleptic therapy.

An increased number of patients with activated B cells ($CD5^+CD19^+$ cells) compared to healthy controls has been described in neuroleptic-treated schizophrenic patients. Our own study shows an increase in the number of activated B cells during antipsychotic therapy.[51] It seems that not only the TH-1 cell system is activated during neuroleptic therapy, but also the antibody production by activated B cells.

During antipsychotic therapy, both arms of the specific adaptive immune system seem to become activated: the specific cellular immunity of the TH-1 system and also the B cell system with its humoral arm, which produces antibody. Activation of the unspecific innate immune system can be found mainly in unmedicated schizophrenic patients, which suggests that it may reflect the disease process rather than the antipsychotic treatment.

OUTLOOK

A number of immunological methods and various clinical features of schizophrenic patients—acuity or chronicity, subtype, course, state of medication—have to be taken into account in the discussion of the heterogenous results of immunological studies. Moreover, it must be borne in mind that schizophrenia is not a disease entity but a syndrome. Therefore, results have to be interpreted cautiously.

However, alterations of the immune system in schizophrenia have been observed for a long time. In the context of both modern, sophisticated immunological methods and the growing body of knowledge of the multiple functions of immune cells, cytokines, soluble factors, and so on, more precise suggestions and explanations regarding the interrelationships between the immune functions are possible. Especially the functional differentiation between the innate and the adaptive immune systems and the conceptualization of T helper-1 and T helper-2 cells allow one to understand more precisely the functional deficits in schizophrenia. This will lead to a more consistent theory of the immune disturbances in schizophrenia and the role of antipsychotic therapy, and will have implications for an immune therapy in schizophrenia.

REFERENCES

1. BRUCE, L.C. & A.M.S. PEEBLES. 1903. Clinical and experimental observations on catatonia. J. Mental Sci. **49:** 614–628.
2. DAMESHEK, W. 1930. White blood cells in dementia praecox and dementia paralytica. Arch. Neurol. Psychiatry **24:** 855.
3. LEHMANN-FACIUS, H. 1939. Serologisch-analytische Versuche mit Liquores und Seren von Schizophrenen. Allg. Z. Psychiatrie **110:** 232–243.
4. MÜLLER, N. & M. ACKENHEIL. 1998. Psychoneuroimmunology, the cytokine network in the CNS, and the implications for psychiatric disorders. Progr. Neuro-Psychopharmacol. Biol. Psychiatry **22:** 1–31.
5. KÖRSCHENHAUSEN, D., H. HAMPEL. M. ACKENHEIL, R. PENNING & N. MÜLLER. 1996. Fibrin degradation products in post mortem brain tissue of schizophrenics: a possible marker for underlying inflammatory processes. Schizophr. Res. **19:** 103–109.
6. CAZZULLO, C.L., S. SCARONE, B. GRASSI, C. VISMARA, D. TRABATTONI & M. CLERICI. 1998. Cytokines production in chronic schizophrenia patients with or without paranoid behavior. Prog. Neuro-Psychopharmacol. Biol. Psychiatry **22:** 947–957.
7. MÜLLER, N. & M. ACKENHEIL. 1995. Immunoglobulin and albumin contents of cerebrospinal fluid in schizophrenic patients: the relationship to negative symptomatology. Schizophrenia Res. **14:** 223–228.
8. KORTE, S., V. AROLT, M. PETERS, CH. WEITZSCH, D. ECKHOFF, M. ROTHERMUND & H. KIRCHNER. 1998. Increased serum neopterin levels in acutely ill and recovered schizophrenic patients. Schizophrenia Res. **32:** 63–67.
9. SPERNER-UNTERWEGER, B., CH. BARNAS, D. FUCHS, G. KEMMLER, H. WACHTER, H. HINTERHUBER & W.W. FLEISCHHACKER. 1992. Neopterin production in acute schizophrenic patients: an indicator of alterations of cell-mediated immunity. Psychiatry Res. **42:** 121–128.
10. WILKE, I., V. AROLT, M. ROTHERMUNDT, CH. WEITZSCH, M. HORNBERG & H. KIRCHNER. 1996. Investigations of cytokine production in whole blood cultures of paranoid and residual schizophrenic patients. Eur. Arch. Psychiatry Clin. Neurosci. **246:** 279–284.
11. ÖZEK, M., K. TÖRECI, I. AKKÖK & Z. GÜVENER. 1971. The influence of treatment with neuroleptics upon the antibody-formation. Psychopharmacologia **21:** 401–412.
12. SAUNDERS, J.C. & E. MUCHMORE. 1964. Phenothiazine effect on human antibody synthesis. Br. J. Psychiatry **110:** 84–89.
13. MAES, M., E. BOSMANS, J. CALABRESE, R. SMITH & H.Y. MELTZER. 1995. Interleukin-2 and Interleukin-6 in schizophrenia and mania: effects of neuroleptics and mood-stabilizers. J. Psychiatr. Res. **29:** 141–152.
14. MASSERINI. C., A. VITA, R. BASILE, R. MORSELLI, P. BOATO, C. PERUZZI, L. PUGNETTI, P. FERRANTE & C.L. CAZZULLO. 1990. Lymphocyte subsets in schizophrenic disorders. Relationship with clinical, neuromorphological and treatment variables. Schizophrenia Res. **3:** 269–275.
15. MÜLLER, N., M. ACKENHEIL, E. HOFSCHUSTER, W. MEMPEL & R. ECKSTEIN. 1991. Cellular immunity in schizophrenic patients before and during neuroleptic therapy. Psychiatry Res. **37:** 147–160.
16. MÜLLER, N., M. EMPEL, M. RIEDEL, M.J. SCHWARZ & M. ACKENHEIL. 1997. Neuroleptic treatment increases soluble IL-2 receptors and decreases soluble IL-6 receptors in schizophrenia. Eur. Arch.. Psychiatry Clin Neurosci. **247:** 308–313.
17. MÜLLER, N., M. HADJAMU, M. RIEDEL, J. PRIMBS, M. ACKENHEIL & R. GRUBER. 1999. The adhesion-molecule receptor expression on T helper cells increases during treatment with neuroleptics and is related to the blood-brain barrier permeability in schizophrenia. Am. J. Psychiatry **156:** 634–636.
18. POLLMÄCHER, T., D. HINZE-SELCH, J. MULLINGTON & F. HOLSBOER. 1995. Clozapine-induced increase in plasma levels of soluble Interleukin-2 receptors. Arch. Gen. Psychiatry **52:** 877–878.
19. MÜLLER, N., M. ACKENHEIL, E. HOFSCHUSTER, W. MEMPEL & R. ECKSTEIN. 1993. T-cells and psychopathology in schizophrenia: relationship to the outcome of neuroleptic therapy. Acta Psychiatr. Scand. **87:** 66–71.

20. MÜLLER, N., B.C. SCHLESINGER, M. HADJAMU, M. RIEDEL, M. SCHWARZ, J. PRIMBS, M. ACKENHEIL, R. WANK & R. GRUBER. 1998. Cytotoxic gamma/delta cells (γ/δ^+CD8^+) are elevated in unmedicated schizophrenic patients and related to the blood-brain barrier and the HLA allele DPA 02011. Schizophrenia Res. **12:** 69–71.

21. PLATA-SALAMAN, C.R. 1991. Immunoregulators in the nervous system. Neurosci. Behav. Rev. **15:** 185–215.

22. DUNN, A.J. 1992. Endotoxin-induced activation of cerebral catecholamine and serotonin metabolism: comparison with interleukin-1. J. Pharmacol. Exp. Ther. **261:** 964–969.

23. FREI, K., U.V. MALIPIERO, T.P. LEIST, R. M. ZINKERNAGEL, M.E. SCHWAB & A. FONTANA. 1989. On the cellular source and function of interleukin 6 produced in the central nervous system in viral diseases. Eur. J. Immunol. **19:** 689–694.

24. MURAGUCHI, A., T. HIRANO, B. TANG, T. MATSUDA, Y. HORII, K. NAKAJIMA & T. KISHIMOTO. 1988. The essential role of B-cell stimulating factor 2 (BSF-2/IL-6) for the terminal differentiation of B cells. J. Exp. Med. **167:** 332–344.

25. SPANGELO, B.L., A.M. JUDD, P.C. ISAKSON & R.M. MACLEOD. 1989. Interleukin-6 stimulates anterior pituitary hormone release in vitro. Endocrinology **125:** 575–577.

26. HAMA, T., Y. KUSHIMA, M. MIYAMOTO, M. KUBOTA, N. TAKEI & H. HATANAKA. 1991. Interleukin-6 improves the survival of mesencephalic catecholaminergic and septal cholinergic neurons from postnatal, two-week-old rats in cultures. Neuroscience **40:** 445–452.

27. ZALCMAN, S., J.M. GREEN-JOHNSON, L. MURRAY, D.M. NANCE, D. DYCK, H. ANISMAN & A.H. GREENBERG. 1994. Cytokine-specific central monoamine alterations induced by interleukin-1, -2 and -6. Brain Res. **643:** 40–49.

28. GANGULI, R., Z. YANG, G. SHURIN, R. CHENGAPPA, J.S. BRAR, A.V. GUBBI & B.S. RABIN. 1994. Serum interleukin-6 concentration in schizophrenia: elevation associated with duration of illness. Psychiatry Res. **51:** 1–10.

29. FROMMBERGER, U.H., J. BAUER, P. HASELBAUER, A. FRAULIN, D. RIEMANN & M. BERGER. 1997. Interleukin-6 (IL-6) plasma levels in depression and schizophrenia: comparison between the acute state and after remission. Eur. Arch. Psychiatry Clin. Neurosci. **247:** 228–232.

30. LIN, A., G. KENIS, S. BIGNOTTI, G.J.B. TURA, R. DE JONG, E. BOSMANS, R. PIOLI, C. ALTAMURA, S. SCHARPÉ & M. MAES. 1998. The inflammatory response system in treatment-resistant schizophrenia: increased serum interleukin-6. Schizophrenia Res. **32:** 9–15.

31. MÜLLER, N., P. DOBMEIER, M. EMPEL, M. RIEDEL, M. SCHWARZ & M. ACKENHEIL. 1997. Soluble IL-6 receptors in the serum and cerebrospinal fluid of paranoid schizophrenic patients. Eur. Psychiatry **12:** 294–299.

32. SCHWARZ, M.J., N. MÜLLER, M. RIEDEL, H. TRAPMAN & M. ACKENHEIL. 1999. Altered regulation of Interleukin-6 in CSF of schizophrenic patients. Submitted.

33. NARAZAKI, M., K. YASUKAWA, T. SAITO *et al.* 1993. Soluble forms of the interleukin-6-signal transducing receptor component of gp 130 in human serum possessing a potential to inhibit signals through membrane anchored gp 130. Blood **82:** 1120–1126.

34. VAN KAMMEN, D.P., C.G. MCALLISTER-SISTILLI & M.E. KELLEY. 1997. Relationship between immune and behavioral measures in schizophrenia. *In* Current Update in Psychoimmunology. G. Wieselmann, Ed.: 51–55. Springer Verlag. New York.

35. BUNNEY, W.E., JR. & D.A. HAMBURG. 1963. Methods for reliable longitudinal observation of behavior. Arch. Gen. Psychiatry **9:** 280–294.

36. MITTLEMAN, B.B., F.X. CASTELLANOS, L.K. JACOBSON, J.L. RAPOPORT, S.E. SWEDO & G.M. SHEARER. 1997. Cerebrospinal fluid cytokines in pediatric neuropsychiatric disease. J. Immunol. **159:** 2994–2999.

37. RAMCHAND, R., J. WEI, C.N. RAMCHAND & G.P. HEMMINGS. 1994. Increased serum IgE in schizophrenic patients who responded poorly to neuroleptic treatment. Life Sci. **54:** 1579–1584.

38. SPERNER-UNTERWEGER, B., C. MILLER, B. HOLZNER, B. WIDNER, W.W. FLEISCHHACKER & D. FUCHS. 1999. Measurement of neopterin, kynurenine and tryptophan in sera of schizophrenic patients. *In* Psychiatry, Psychimmunology, and Viruses. N. Müller, Ed.: 115–119. Springer. New York.

39. VILLEMAIN, F., L. CHATENOUD, A. GALINOWSKI, F. HOMO-DELARCHE, D. GENESTET, H. LOO, E. ZARIFARAIN & J.F. BACH. 1989. Aberrant T-cell–mediated immunity in untreated schizophrenic patients: deficient interleukin-2 production. Am. J. Psychiatry **146**: 609–616.

40. GANGULI, R., J.S. BRAR, K.R. CHENGAPPA, M. DELEO, Z.W. YANG, G. SHURIN & B. RABIN. 1995. Mitogen-stimulated interleukin 2 production in never-medicated, first episode schizophrenics—the influence of age of onset and negative symptoms. Arch. Gen. Psychiatry **52**: 878.

41. HORNBERG, M., V. AROLT, I. WILKE, A. KRUSE & H. KIRCHNER. 1995. Production of interferons and lymphokines in leukocyte cultures of patients with schizophrenia. Schizophrenia Res. **15**: 237–242.

42. BESSLER, H., Z. LEVENTAL, L. KARP, I. MODAI, M. DJALDETTI & A. WEIZMAN. 1995. Cytokine production in drug-free and neuroleptic-treated schizophrenic patients. Biol. Psychiatry **38**: 297–302.

43. ROTHERMUND, M., V. AROLT, CH. WEITZSCH, D. ECKHOFF & H. KIRCHNER. 1996. Production of cytokines in acute schizophrenic psychosis. Biol. Psychiatry **39**: 1294–1297.

44. SCHWARZ, M.J., M. RIEDEL, M. ACKENHEIL & N. MÜLLER. 2000. Deceased levels of soluble intercellular adhesion molecule–1 (sICAM-1) in unmedicated and medicated schizophrenic patients. Biol. Psychiatry. **47**: 29–33.

45. VAN SEVENTER, G.A., Y. SHIMIZU, K.J. HORGAN & S. SHAW. 1990. The LFA-1 ligand ICAM-1 provides an important costimulatory signal for T-cell receptor mediated activation of resting T-cells. J. Immunol. **144**: 4579–4586.

46. KUHLMAN, P., V.T. MOY, B.A. LOLLO & A.A. BRIAN. 1991. The accessory function of murine intercellular adhesion molecule–1 in T-lymphocyte activation: contribution of adhesion and co-activation. J. Immunol. **146**: 1773–1782.

47. VINOGRADOV, S., I.I. GOTTESMAN, H.W. MOISES & S. NICOL. 1991. Negative association between schizophrenia and rheumatoid arthritis. Schizophr. Bull. **17**: 669–678.

48. NEIDHART, M., F. PATAKI & K. FEHR. 1995. Increased soluble endothelial adhesion molecules in rheumatoid arthritis correlate with circulating cytokines and depletion of CD45R0+ T-lymphocytes from blood stream. Schweiz. Med.Wochenschr. **125**: 424–428.

49. MOLHOLM, H.B. 1942. Hyposensitivity to foreign protein in schizophrenic patients. Psychiatr. Q. (NY) **16**: 565–571.

50. MAES, M., H.Y. MELTZER & E. BOSMANS. 1994. Immune-inflammatory markers in schizophrenia: comparison to normal controls and effects of clozapine. Acta Psychiatr. Scand. **89**: 346–351.

51. MÜLLER, N., M. RIEDEL, M. SCHWARZ, R. GRUBER & M. ACKENHEIL. 1997. Immunomodulatory effects of neuroleptics to the cytokine system and the cellular immune system in schizophrenia. *In* Current Update in Psychoimmunology. G. Wieselmann, Ed.: 57–67. Springer Verlag. New York.

52. GALLIEN, M., J.P. SCHNETZLER & J. MORIN. 1977. Antinuclear antibodies and lupus cells in 600 hospitalized phenothiazine treated patients. Ann. Med. Psychol. Med. **1**: 237–248.

53. ZARRABI, M.H., S. ZUCKER, F. MILLER, R.M. DERMAN, G.S. ROMENO, J.A. HARTNETT & A.O. VARMA. 1979. Immunologic and coagulation disorders in chlorpromazine-treated patients. Ann. Intern. Med. **91**: 194–199.

54. GANGULI, R., R.S. RABIN, R.H. KELLY, M. LYTE & U. RAGU. 1987. Clinical and laboratory evidence of autoimmunity in acute schizophrenia. Ann. N.Y.. Acad Sci. **496**: 676–685.

55. SCHWARZ, M.J., M. RIEDEL, R. GRUBER, N. MÜLLER & M. ACKENHEIL. 1998. Autoantibodies against 60-kDa heat shock protein in schizophrenia. Eur. Arch. Psychiatry Clin. Neurosci. **248**: 282–288.

56. SCHWARZ, M.J., M. RIEDEL, R. GRUBER, M. ACKENHEIL & N. MÜLLER. 1999. Antibodies to heat-shock proteins in schizophrenic patients—implications for disease mechanism. Am. J. Psychiatry **156:** 1103–1104.
57. KILIDIREAS, K., N. LATOV, D.H. STRAUSS, D.G. AVIVA, G.A. HASHIM, J.M. GORMAN & S.A. SADIQ. 1992. Antibodies to human 60-kD heat-shock protein in patients with schizophrenia. Lancet **340:** 569–572.

Prenatal Influences on Neuroimmune Set Points in Infancy

CHRISTOPHER L. COE[a] AND GABRIELE R. LUBACH

Harlow Center for Biological Psychology, University of Wisconsin-Madison, Madison, Wisconsin 53706, USA

ABSTRACT: Many factors during fetal life and early infancy have been found to affect the development of immune responses in animals. This study investigated whether acute exposure of the fetal monkey to high levels of corticosteroids would also have a lingering effect on the expression of immune responses still manifest postpartum in yearling juveniles. One month prior to parturition, pregnant rhesus monkeys were administered dexamethasone for two days. Lymphocyte proliferative responses to mitogen were then examined in their offspring when they were between 1.0–1.5 years of age. In addition, cell sensitivity to corticosteroid feedback was assessed by testing the ability of a gradation of cortisol doses to inhibit proliferation. Monkeys generated from dexamethasone-treated pregnancies tended to have lower responses to concanavalin A. Further, their cells were less sensitive to *in vitro* incubation with cortisol, suggesting that elevated adrenal activity *in vivo* had downregulated hormone receptors on their cells. These findings concur with the view that steroidal hormones *in utero* can influence the fetal immune system, resulting in prolonged effects on immune responses after birth. The similarity of the dexamethasone condition to the clinical treatment used in obstetrical practice raises a potential concern about the widespread antenatal exposure of premature infants to steroidal drugs.

Over the last two decades it has become increasingly clear that many nonimmune processes, including stress, trauma, and poor nutrition, can influence immune competence and vulnerability to disease. While these relationships can be demonstrated at any point in the life span, it has been the guiding hypothesis of our research that these effects are particularly important during infancy and old age. A greater sensitivity of the immune system to extrinsic influence in immature and elderly individuals may be due in part to the developmental changes occurring at both stages: maturation in the infant and the onset of immune senescence in the aged. Our prior research with nonhuman primates has focused particularly on the vulnerability of the young infant, especially the ways in which prenatal conditions may set the stage for different immune set points after birth, creating a developmental bias for health or an increased risk for disease.

It is of historical interest that observations of immune alterations in young animals and children were important for validating the initial belief that environmental

[a]Address for correspondence: Christopher L. Coe, Ph.D., Department of Psychology, University of Wisconsin, 1202 West Johnson Street, Madison, WI 53706. Voice: 608-263-3550; fax: 608-262-6020.
ccoe@facstaff.wisc.edu

and psychological processes could alter immune competence.[1–3] In nonhuman primates, we and others showed that there is a transient inhibition of many cellular and humoral responses following separation of the young monkey from the mother.[4,5] While these findings were extremely informative about how stressful life events can affect immune changes, the alterations were typically transient, lasting only 1–2 weeks. This recovery suggested that certain homeostatic set points had been established even earlier in development. In keeping with this conclusion, studies in rodents have indicated that processes accounting for the number and ratios of lymphocyte subsets are preset early in fetal development. As a consequence, following acute depletion of circulating cells with drugs such as hydroxyurea, cell numbers in adult rats rebound right back to the original level seen prior to treatment.[6]

By manipulating infant monkeys immediately at birth, we obtained confirmatory evidence for the hypothesis that longer-lasting effects occur more readily when the perturbations are experienced by a very immature host. For example, if an infant monkey is reared from birth by humans, rather than by its biological mother, there are changes in cell subsets and lymphocyte proliferative and cytolytic activity that persist through at least two years of age.[7,8] Our ongoing research has extended this type of evaluation back into fetal life, and has shown that a number of pregnancy manipulations can also alter the development and expression of immune responses in the infant postpartum. In previous studies we have found that periods of maternal arousal, endocrine activation, and social stressors can affect the behavioral and immune status of the infant at birth.[9,10] When the endocrine physiology of the gravid female was altered for two weeks by stimulation with the adrenocorticotrophic hormone (ACTH), significant immune differences were still evident in the offspring as yearlings.[11] As juveniles, these offspring were administered the cytokine interleukin-1; they mounted a smaller fever response and released lower amounts of interleukin-6 in both blood and cerebrospinal fluid, suggesting that critical aspects of the proinflammatory cascade had been altered by the *in utero* treatment. The following study extends this research by examining the influence of another prenatal condition involving corticosteroid hormones.

The gravid female was administered dexamethasone (dex) for two days in a manner comparable to that used in obstetrical practice to accelerate maturation of the premature infant's lung function.[12] While studies in animals and a few in humans have periodically raised some concern about potential side effects of dexamethasone on infant development, the remarkable respiratory and vascular benefits have outweighed these reservations.[13] Steroidal effects have been observed on lymphocyte responses in human neonates, but it is generally believed that in time the immune effects subside.[14–16] If so, humans would differ from rodents, sheep, and monkeys, in which more lasting effects have been observed.[17–20] The current study also indicates that traces of the prenatal steroid treatments are still evident on lymphocyte responses in the yearling monkey.

METHODS

Subjects

Mother and infant rhesus monkeys (*Macaca mulatta*) from a 550+ breeding colony at the Harlow Primate Laboratory were tested in this study. Twenty-one juvenile monkeys, between 11–18 months of age, were the specific focus. Ten had been exposed *in utero* to a two-day dexamethasone condition; five were exposed to dexamethasone after undisturbed pregnancies; and an additional five gravid females received dexamethasone after a 5.5-week period of psychological disturbance. For control values, blood samples were collected from 11 animals: eight from infants from undisturbed pregancies, and three from dams that had been administered saline injections for two days in the same manner as the dex-treated ones. None of the offspring experienced any invasive treatments postnatally. Their physical growth and behavioral development were monitored, and blood samples were collected periodically across the first year of life.

Housing

Their mothers were multiparous females born and reared in our laboratory from defined pedigrees with known experimental histories. Date of conception was determined by mating each female during a four-day period at the time of ovulation. Once conception was verified, the gravid female was transferred to another room in the animal quarters, where she remained undisturbed until the experimental manipulation was initiated. Thereafter, the female's pregnancy continued normally until parturition and the postnatal evaluation of her infant. Housing conditions of the mother-infant pairs were also standardized. Each dyad was housed in a stainless steel cage ($0.9 \times 0.9 \times 0.9$ m) within visual and auditory contact of other monkeys. At six months of age, the infant was rehoused into small social groups of 4–8 weanlings, each housed in a wire mesh pen ($1.9 \times 1.9 \times 2.0$ m). These groups were left undisturbed, and the housing conditions remained stable, until the current blood samples were collected. Commercial monkey chow (Purina) was provided daily, supplemented with fruit, and water was available ad libitum. The light:dark schedule was 16:8, with lights on at 0600; samples were collected between 0900 and 1000. Ambient room temperature was maintained at 21°C.

Prenatal Manipulations

The two-day dexamethasone treatment began on day 145 postconception after either an undisturbed pregnancy (Dex, $n = 5$) or 5.5 weeks of a daily stress condition (Dex-and-Stress, $n = 5$). The latter condition was included because dexamethasone treatments of premature human infants often occur in the context of problematic pregnancies. To create this type of pregnancy, the female was disturbed acutely by being relocated to a darkened room down the hallway from the main housing area for 10 min between 1430 and 1600 daily between days 105 and 145 postconception. While located there in a small transfer cage, a computer programmed the one-second sounding of an alarm horn, which elicited a startle response three times randomly during the 10-min period.

Dexamethasone was administered intramuscularly at 12-h intervals for two days (0.125 mg/kg body weight, comparable to the human dose used in the United States). Three control females were injected with four equivalent volumes of saline IM to mimic the handling involved in the dexamethasone treatments. Blood samples were collected from the gravid female on the day before and the morning after the last injections to assess the efficacy of the dexamethasone dose, as determined by the transient suppression of her endogenous cortisol release. After the dexamethasone treatments, the females remained undisturbed in their home cages until the natural birth of their infants. In addition to saline controls, eight more control infants were generated from undisturbed pregnancies.

Lymphocyte Proliferation

Mononuclear cells (MNC, monocytes and lymphocytes) were isolated from the juvenile monkey's blood by centrifugation. The plasma was removed, and the remaining cells were diluted 1:2 in Dulbecco's phosphate-buffered saline (DPBS) and layered over Histopaque 1077 (Sigma, St. Louis, MO). The MNC were washed twice in DPBS and suspended in Iscove's modified Dulbecco's media supplemented with 5% fetal bovine serum, 1% GMS-X, 1% MEM nonessential amino acids, and 1% antibiotic/antimycotic solution (IMDM-C) (Gibco, Grand Island, NY). Then, 10^5 of the infant's cells were stimulated with concanavalin A (Con A, Sigma) in quadruplicate wells of a 96-well U-bottom tissue culture plate. The plates were incubated for two days, at which point 1 μC_i (3H) thymidine was added to each well. Twenty-four hours later, the cells were harvested onto glass fiber filters with a PHD (Cambridge Technology) cell harvester and thymidine incorporation determined by counting the filters in 3 mL Ecoscint (National Diagnostics, Manville, NJ) on an Isocap 300 LSC. In addition to stimulating the cells with two concentrations of Con A (1.25 and 5 μg/mL), the cultures were exposed to a gradation of four cortisol doses (10^{-8} to 10^{-5} molar, Sigma) concurrent with Con A. The capacity of cortisol to inhibit the proliferative responses to mitogen was determined, both as a "percent of untreated control wells," and by generating a regression line from the four proliferative values and determining the quantity of cortisol needed to cause a 50% inhibition.

Statistical Analyses

The data were analyzed with one- and two-way analyses of variance, with prenatal condition and infant gender as between-factors. The two dexamethasone conditions (Dex, Dex-and-Stress) were combined in most ANOVAs, but also considered separately. Proliferative activity to the two concentrations of Con A, and the effect of the four doses of cortisol were analyzed as repeated measures; thus the Greenhouser-Geiser correction was applied for the *p* values.

RESULTS

Maternal Treatment

An effective dose of dexamethasone was administered to the pregnant females, as evidenced by a suppression of endogenous adrenal activity. On the morning after the two-day treatment, plasma cortisol levels averaged only 2.6 µg/dL, significantly below both the pretreatment morning level (33.7 µg/dL) and the values seen after two days of saline injections in the control females (31.3 µg/dL). Pregnant monkeys in the Dex-and-Stress condition underwent a comparable decrease in cortisol after the dexamethasone treatment.

Gestation Length and Birth Weight

Neither gestation length nor infant birth weight were significantly affected by the dexamethasone treatment as compared to the saline controls or normative values obtained previously on larger samples of undisturbed monkeys. Gestation length in the dex-treated pregnancies averaged 170.5 days (±2.5 days), as compared to a norm of 169 days. Birthweight averaged 521 g (±17 g), as compared to a norm of 510 g (±18 g).

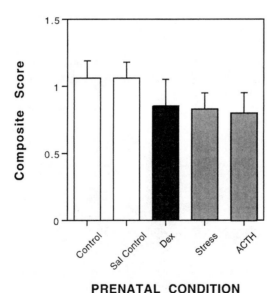

PRENATAL CONDITION

FIGURE 1. Neuromotor measures from the Infant Behavioral Assessment Scale (IBAS), showing the effect of prenatal manipulations on neuromotor maturation at two weeks postpartum. Data on Dex-treated infants are presented with respect to values determined from other prenatal conditions. They appeared similar to infants from other disturbed pregnancies (six-week prenatal Stress [$n = 18$] and two-week ACTH treatment [$n = 12$]), and less mature in their coordination and muscle tone than ones from saline and undisturbed control pregnancies ($n = 13$ and 15, respectively). (Adapted from Refs. 21 and 24.)

Neuromotor Maturation

Infants from dex-treated pregnancies appeared physically healthy at birth and were not overtly abnormal on behavioral test measures. When their neuromotor and attentional processes were evaluated at two weeks of age with a standardized test battery, they did not differ significantly from the current control infants. However, when their neuromotor development was considered in the context of prior data on a larger sample of control and perturbed infants, their reflexes did seem slightly immature, in the range of infants from other prenatally disturbed pregnancies (see FIGURE 1).[21]

Proliferative Activity

Infants from dex-treated pregnancies had lower proliferative responses to both doses of Con A than did the control infants (F[1,19] = 3.71, p = 0.069) (TABLE 1). It was of interest that this effect of prenatal dexamethasone treatment was more consistent in the offspring from undisturbed pregnancies, rather than in those from pregnancies also involving a prior 5.5-week period of maternal disturbance. In addition, the lower proliferative activity was associated with a differential response of the cells to *in vitro* incubation with cortisol (see FIGURE 2). At the high dose of cortisol (10^{-5} M) all animals showed a marked inhibition of the response to mitogen, and this suppressive effect of the steroid was more evident with the lower concentration of Con A. However, when compared to those of control animals, the cells of the dex-treated animals proved to be less sensitive to this cortisol feedback. The insensitivity was demonstrated by higher cortisol levels needed to inhibit proliferative responses. Especially with the lower proliferation induced by the 1.5-μg/mL concentration of Con A, there was a clear difference in cellular reactivity to cortisol based on prenatal condition ($F[2,18]$ = 4.66, p = 0.023). Here it is again noteworthy that this cellular insensitivity to cortisol was most evident in the monkeys from pregnancies involving only Dex treatment, more so than for those generated from the Dex-and-Stress

TABLE 1. Mean (SE) proliferative responses to Con A in juvenile monkeys from the three prenatal conditions, and the molar concentration of cortisol required to induce a 50% inhibition of the reponse to mitogen

Experimental condition	Con A Alone[a]		50% Inhibition[b]	
	5.0	1.25	5.0	1.25
Control (n = 11)	29308 (8914)	6978 (3929)	6.6 (0.1)	7.6 (0.3)
Dexamethasone (n = 5)	15994 (7224)	1548 (433)	6.3 (0.7)	6.7 (0.4)
Stress-and-Dex (n = 5)	5710 (1540)	4251 (2763)	6.0 (0.6)	7.6 (0.2)

[a]Proliferative responses in wells stimulated with only Con A. Infants from dex-treated and dex-and-stress pregnancies lower at p = 0.069.

[b]Molar concentration of cortisol required to induce a 50% decline based on regression line from four hormone-treated wells (10^{-8}–10^{-5} M). Smaller numbers in the exponent (10^x) indicate that more cortisol was required to induce the inhibitory effect. For 1.25 Con A stimulation, the five infants from dex-treated pregnancies differed from controls at p = 0.023.

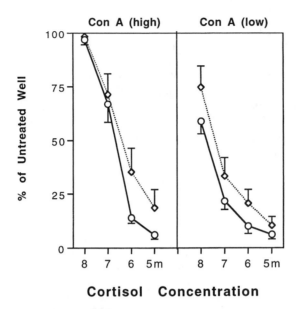

Cortisol   Concentration

FIGURE 2. Percent inhibition of lymphocyte proliferation to Con A (5 and 1.25 μg/mL) induced by incubation with cortisol *in vitro* at doses of 10^{-8} to 10^{-5} M. MNC of infants generated from Dex-treated pregnancies tended to be less sensitive to the inhibitory actions of cortisol, especially at the lower concentration of mitogen. This insensitivity to cortisol *in vitro* occurred in conjunction with a lower proliferative response to Con A, with and without cortisol. Key: ——○—— , control; ······◇······ , dex-treated.

pregnancies. The latter juveniles appeared to have been impacted at an intermediate level, and the pattern of cell inhibition induced by cortisol was more similar to the control profile.

DISCUSSION

This study supports the view that certain drugs and stressful events experienced by the pregnant female monkey can influence fetal development, concurring with considerable research on other animals and humans.[22,23] It also extends our previous findings showing that psychological stressors and endocrine activation in the gravid female can affect the infant monkey postpartum, in both its behavioral reactivity and its immune responses. Our prior immune studies had focused on the neonate or evaluated infants across the first six months of life.[9,10] While we had evidence that behavioral alterations, in the juvenile monkey's emotionality and social behavior,[24] were more long lasting, we had previously reported only one immune alteration lasting into the second year of life.[11] That immune effect involved an alteration in the proinflammatory responses seen in juveniles following challenge with IL-1. Now we have additional evidence for a developmental impact on other immune responses that also extends into the second year of life. Further, the current findings are unique in that the prenatal manipulation was brief—only two days of dexamethasone as compared to a 14-day treatment of the dam with ACTH—and the alteration in lymphocyte proliferation was evident without any further experimental provocation of the juvenile monkey.

Like mice and rats, the rhesus monkey seems to be particularly sensitive to prenatal corticosteroid treatment, possibly more so than humans. In studies where the administered dose was fivefold higher (5 mg per monkey), a two-day dexamethasone treatment induced a significant reduction in the size of the hippocampal region of the infant's brain postnatally.[25] Doses of dexamethasone in this range and higher have also been found to slow fetal growth, and to decrease the size of thymus and spleen in the monkey,[26] although we did not observe an effect on birth weight with our lower dose of 0.125 mg/kg (approximately 1 mg per monkey). While the persistent effects on proliferative responses could reflect a teratogenic effect of steroids on fetal organs,[27] we believe that the more parsimonious explanation is that there was a subtle shift in physiological set points. In this case, it is likely that higher levels of endogenous adrenal activity in the monkeys from dex-treated pregnancies may account for both the lower lymphocyte proliferative responses and the decreased sensitivity of the cells to *in vitro* exposure to cortisol. This type of insensitivity is usually interpreted to mean that there has been a downregulation of hormone receptors, either fewer receptors or ones of lower affinitiy. Uno *et al.* have previously reported a greater stress reactivity in monkeys that had been exposed to dexamethasone prenatally, and their hippocampal damage may alter the ability of this critical brain area to exert regulatory control over the hypothalamic-pituitary-adrenal axis. These findings in the monkey differ from conclusions about the benign side effects of antenatal steroid treatment in human infants, where the actions are generally believed to be more transient, even though lymphocytes of human newborns have been found to be quite hormone sensitive.[14] More concern about the implications of these monkey data for children may be warranted now that some obstetricians are employing protracted treatments with multiple doses of steroid treatment.[29]

In summary, a two-day dexamethasone treatment during the latter month of pregnancy impacted the young monkey such that its MNC proliferated less in response to mitogenic stimulation. Further, these cells evinced a blunted reaction to incubation with cortisol *in vitro,* which is typically intepreted to mean that the cells had fewer or downregulated receptors. A reasonable explanation for these observations would be the sustained maintenance of higher circulating levels of pituitary-adrenal hormones in offspring from dex-treated pregnancies. While this report is restricted to the effects of prenatal dexamethasone treatment, it should be mentioned that we have preliminary data indicating that the proliferative and cytokine reponses of juvenile monkeys from psychologically stressed pregnancies also deviate from the norms found for monkeys from undisturbed pregnancies.[30] Thus, in a larger context, it suggests that many pregnancy conditions may be capable of altering the trajectory of postnatal immune development. One enigmatic finding that needs to be explored further was the smaller influence of dexamethasone on infants from stressed mothers, as compared to mothers from previously undisturbed pregnancies, possibly suggesting a different mode of drug action on a compromised than on a healthy fetus.

ACKNOWLEDGMENT

This research was supported by NIMH grant MH41659 to C.L.C. Acknowledgments are due to H. Crispen and A. Slukvina for technical assistance.

REFERENCES

1. ADER, R. & S.B. FREIDMAN. 1965. Differential experiences and suceptibility to transplanted tumor in the rat. J. Comp. Physiol. Psych. **59:** 361–364.
2. MEYER, R.J. & R.J. HAGGERTY. 1962. Streptococcal infections in families. Factors altering individual susceptibility. Pediatrics **29:** 539–549.
3. SOLOMON, G.F., S. LEVINE & J.K. KRAFT. 1968. Early experience and immunity. Nature **220:** 821–822.
4. COE, C.L. 1993. Psychosocial factors and immunity in nonhuman primates. A review. Psychosomat. Med. **55:** 298–398.
5. LAUDENSLAGER M.L. & M.R. REITE. 1984. Loss and separations: immunological consequences and health implications. *In* Review of Personality and Social Psychology: 285–311. Sage. Beverly Hills, CA.
6. FRIETAS, A.A. & B.B. ROCHA. 1993. Lymphocyte lifespans: homeostasis, selection, and competition. Immunol. Today **14**(1): 25–34.
7. LUBACH, G.R., C.L. COE & W.B. ERSHLER. 1995. Effects of early rearing environment on immune responses of infant rhesus monkeys. Brain Behav. Immun. **9:** 31–46.
8. COE, C.L., G.R. LUBACH, M.L. SCHNEIDER, D.J. DIERSCHKE & W.B. ERSHLER. 1992. Early rearing conditions alter immune responses in the developing infant primate. Pediatrics **90**(3): 505–509.
9. COE, C.L., G.R. LUBACH, J.W. KARASZEWSKI & W.B. ERSHLER. 1996. Prenatal endocrine activation alters postnatal cellular immunity in infant monkeys. Brain Behav. Immun. **10:** 221–234.
10. COE, C.L., G.R. LUBACH & J. KARASZEWSKI. 1999. Prenatal stress and immune recognition of self and nonself in the primate neonate. Biol. Neonate. **76**(5): 301–310.
11. REYES, T.R. & C.L. COE. 1997. Prenatal manipulations reduce the proinflammatory response to a cytokine challenge in juvenile monkeys. Brain Res. **769:** 29–35.
12. HALLIDAY, H.L. 1999. Clinical trials of postnatal corticosteroids. Inhaled and systemic. Biol. Neonate **77**(Suppl. 1): 29–40.
13. DERKS, J.B., E.J.H. MULDER & G.H.A. VISSER. 1995. The effects of maternal betamethasone administration on the fetus. Brit. J. Obstet. Gynecol. **102:** 40–46.
14. KAVELAARS, A., B. CATS, G.H.A. VISSER, B.J.M. ZEGERS, J.M. BAKKER, E.P. VAN REES & C.J. HEIJNEN. 1996. Ontogeny of the response to human peripheral blood T cells to glucocorticoids. Brain Behav. Immun. **10:** 288–297.
15. KAUPPILA, A., A.L. HARTIKAINEN-SORRI, M. KOIVISTO & P. RYHANEN. 1983. Cell-mediated immunocompetence of children exposed in utero to short- or long-term action of glucocorticoids. Gynecol. Obstet. Invest. **15:** 41–48.
16. SMOLDERS-DE HAAS, H., J. NEUVEL, B. SCHMAND, P.E. TERFFES, J.G. KOPPE & J. HOEKS. 1990. Physical development and medical history of children who were treated antenatally with corticosteroids to prevent respiratory distress syndrome. 10–12 year follow-up. Pediatrics **86:** 65–70.
17. EISHI, Y., K. HIROKAWA & S. HATAKEYAMA. 1983. Long-lasting impairment of immune and endocrine systems of offspring induced by injection of dexamethasone into pregnant mice. Clin. Immunol. Pathol. **26:** 334–349.
18. BAKKER, J.M., E. DONNE-SMIDT, A. KAVELAARS, C.J. HEIJEN, F.J.H. TILDERS & E.P. VAN REES. 1995. Effects of short-term dexamethasone treatment during pregnancy on the development of the immune system and the hypothalamo-pituitary adrenal axis in the rat. J. Neuroimmunol. **63:** 183–192.
19. JOBE, A.H., H. WAD, L.M. BERRY, M. IKEGAMI & M.G. ERVIN. 1998. Single and repetitive maternal glucocorticoid exposures reduce fetal growth in sheep. Gen. Obstet. Gynecol. **178:** 880–885.

20. MURPHY, K.K. & F.R. MOYA. 1994. Effect of betamethasone on maternal, fetal, and neonatal rat cellular immunity. Early Human Devel. **36:** 1–11.
21. SCHNEIDER, M.L, C.L. COE & G.R. LUBACH. 1992. Endocrine activation mimics the adverse effects of prenatal stress on the neuromotor development of the infant primate. Devel. Psychobiol. **25:** 427–439.
22. WADHWA, P.D. 1998. Prenatal stress and life-span development. Encyc. Mental Health **3:** 265–280.
23. KAY, G., N. TARCIC, T. POLYREVT & M. WEINSTOCK. 1998. Prenatal stress depresses immune function in rats. Physiol. Behav. **63**(3): 397–402.
24. COE, C. L., G.R. LUBACH & M.L. SCHNEIDER. 1999. Neuromotor and socio-emotional behavior in the young monkey are presaged by prenatal conditions. *In* Stress and Soothing. M. Lewis & D. Ramsay, Eds.: 19–38. Lawrence Erlbaum. Mahwah, NJ.
25. UNO, H., L. LOHMILLER, C. THIEME, J.W. KEMNITZ, M.J. ENGLE, E.B. ROECKER & P.M. FARRELL. 1990. Brain damage induced by prenatal exposure to dexamethasone in fetal rhesus macaques. I. Hippocampus. Dev. Brain Res. **53:** 157–167.
26. JOHNSON, J.W.C., W. MITZNER, W.T. LONDON, A.E. PALMER & R. SCOTT. 1979. Betamethasone and the rhesus fetus: multisystemic effects. Am. J. Obstet. Gynecol. **133:** 677–684.
27. SAWYER, R., A. HENDRICKX, B. OSBURN & T. TERRELL. 1977. Abnormal morphology of the fetal monkey (*Macaca mulatta*) thymus exposed to a corticosteroid. J. Med. Primatol. **6:** 145–150.
28. UNO, H., S. EISELE, A. SAKAI, S. SHELTON, E. BAKER, O.J. DEJESUS & J. HOLDEN. 1994. Neurotoxicity of glucocorticoids in the primate brain. Horm. Behav. **28:** 236–248.
29. BANKS , B.A., A. CNAAN, M.A. MORGAN, J.T. PARER, J.D. MERRILL, P.L. BALLARD & R.A. BALLARD. 1999. Multiple courses of antenatal corticosteroids and outcome of premature neonates. Am. J. Obstet. Gynecol. **181:** 709–717.
30. KRAMER, M., C.L. COE, C. KIRSCHBAUM, P. NETTER & E. FUCHS. 2001. Prenatal stress diminishes cytokine production after an endotoxin challenge and induces glucococticoid resistance in juvenile rhesus monkeys. J. Clin. Endocr. Metab. In press.

Illness, Cytokines, and Depression

R. YIRMIYA,[a,b] Y. POLLAK,[a] M. MORAG,[a] A. REICHENBERG,[a] O. BARAK,[a]
R. AVITSUR,[a] Y. SHAVIT,[a] H. OVADIA,[c] J. WEIDENFELD,[c] A. MORAG,[d]
M.E. NEWMAN,[e] AND T. POLLMÄCHER[f]

*Departments of [a]Psychology, [c]Neurology, [d]Clinical Virology, and [e]Psychiatry,
The Hebrew University and Hadassah Hospital, Jerusalem, Israel*

[f]Max Planck Institute for Psychiatry, Munich, Germany

ABSTRACT: Various medical conditions that involve activation of the immune
system are associated with psychological and neuroendocrine changes that
resemble the characteristics of depression. In this review we present our recent
studies, designed to investigate the relationship between the behavioral effects
of immune activation and depressive symptomatology. In the first set of experiments, we used a double-blind prospective design to investigate the psychological consequences of illness in two models: (1) vaccination of teenage girls with
live attenuated rubella virus, and (2) lipopolysaccharide (LPS) administration
in healthy male volunteers. In the rubella study, we demonstrated that, compared to control group subjects and to their own baseline, a subgroup of vulnerable individuals (girls from low socioeconomic status) showed a significant
virus-induced increase in depressed mood up to 10 weeks after vaccination. In
an ongoing study on the effects of LPS, we demonstrated significant LPS-
induced elevation in the levels of depression and anxiety as well as memory
deficits. These psychological effects were highly correlated with the levels of
LPS-induced cytokine secretion. In parallel experiments, we demonstrated
in rodents that immune activation with various acute and chronic immune
challenges induces a depressive-like syndrome, characterized by anhedonia,
anorexia, body weight loss, and reduced locomotor, exploratory, and social
behavior. Chronic treatment with antidepressants (imipramine or fluoxetine)
attenuated many of the behavioral effects of LPS, as well as LPS-induced
changes in body temperature, adrenocortical activation, hypothalamic serotonin release, and the expression of splenic TNF-α mRNA. Taken together, these
findings suggest that cytokines are involved in the etiology and symptomatology
of illness-associated depression.

INTRODUCTION

Depression is a common, disturbing concomitant of medical conditions. The
reported prevalence of major depression episodes in physically ill patients varies
from 5% to more than 40%. However, because depression is often unrecognized and
undertreated in sick patients, the prevalence reported in most studies is probably
underestimated.[1] The high prevalence of depression in various medical conditions is

[b]Address for correspondence: Professor Raz Yirmiya, Department of Psychology, The
Hebrew University of Jerusalem, Mount Scopus, Jerusalem 91905, Israel. Voice: 972-2-
5883695; fax: 972-2-5881159.
msrazy@mscc.huji.ac.il

reflected by the special psychiatric diagnostic entity "depression due to a general medical condition."[2] To make a diagnosis of this condition "the clinician should establish the presence of a general medical condition, and determine that the depression is etiologically related to the general medical condition through a physiological mechanism" (see Ref. 2, p. 367). Several lines of evidence suggest that this physiological mechanism involves the immune system—that is, the depression associated with various medical conditions is not merely a reaction to the incapacitation, pain, and losses that accompany the physical disease process, but may be directly caused by activation of the immune system.[3]

The physiological and psychological effects of immune activation (collectively termed *sickness behavior*) are mediated by cytokines derived from activated immune and other cells.[4–6] Most immune challenges produce their initial effects in the periphery, but information regarding their presence is almost immediately transmitted to the brain, in a sensory-like process. Within the brain, this immune-related information activates several areas, and induces glia cells and neurons to release cytokines, such as interleukin (IL)-1 and tumor necrosis factor-alpha (TNF-α), which serve as neurotransmitters and neuroregulators.[4,5] The aim of the present review is to present the current knowledge on the role of cytokines in mediating the depressive-like symptoms that accompany various medical conditions in humans and experimental models of these conditions in animals.

DEPRESSION ASSOCIATED WITH INFECTIOUS AND NONINFECTIOUS DISEASES IN HUMANS

Infectious illnesses are often associated with a range of depressive symptoms, including fatigue, psychomotor retardation, anorexia, somnolence, lethargy, muscle aches, cognitive disturbances, and depressed mood.[7] The evidence for these alterations is mainly anecdotal, and only few studies examined these symptoms systematically. Experimentally induced viral infections (e.g., common cold, influenza),[8,9] as well as natural occurrence of upper respiratory tract illness or influenza,[10–12] produce depressed mood and other depressive symptoms, as well as various neuropsychological impairments. Similar disturbances have also been reported following chronic infections with herpesvirus, cytomegalovirus, Epstein-Barr virus, gastroenteritis, Borna disease virus and HIV.

Many noninfectious conditions, such as autoimmune diseases, stroke, trauma, Alzheimer's disease and other neurodegenerative diseases, are also associated with chronic activation of the immune system and secretion of cytokines. High incidence of depression has been demonstrated in patients afflicted with many of these conditions, including multiple sclerosis, rheumatoid arthritis, systemic lupus erythematosus, allergy, stroke, and Alzheimer's disease.[3,6] When studied, immune dysregulation was found to precede the development of depression, suggesting that rather than being a psychological reaction to the medical condition per se, illness-associated depression is causally related to immune activation.

We have recently used a double-blind prospective design to investigate the immediate and prolonged psychological and physiological effects of a specific viral infection in humans.[13] Subjects were teenage girls who were vaccinated with live

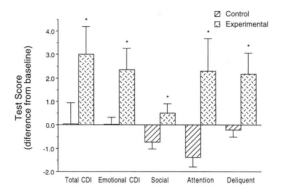

FIGURE 1. Effects of vaccination with live attenuated Rubella virus on psychological parameters measured in 12-year-old girls with low socioeconomic status before, and 10 weeks after, the vaccination. Compared to their own baseline and to the levels in girls who were already immune to Rubella before vaccination (control group), subjects who seroconverted following vaccination (experimental group) showed significantly increased levels of total and emotional depression, measured by the Children Depression Inventory, and significantly higher incidence of social and attention problems and delinquent behavior, assessed by the Achenbach Child Behavior Checklist. (Adapted from Morag et al.[13])

attenuated rubella virus. Based on analysis of levels of antibodies to rubella, subjects were divided into two groups: an experimental group, consisting of subjects who were initially seronegative and were infected following vaccination; and a control group, consisting of subjects who were already immune to rubella before vaccination. Compared to control subjects and to their own baseline, subjects from low, but not middle or high, socioeconomic status (SES) within the experimental group exhibited more severe depressed mood, as well as more social and attention problems and delinquent behavior (see FIGURE 1).[13] The particular vulnerability to immunization-induced depression may be associated with several characteristics of low SES, including higher incidence of stressful life events and fewer sources of social support, which modulate the responsiveness to immune challenges. Thus, even a mild viral infection can produce a prolonged increase in depressive symptomatology in vulnerable individuals.

ADMINISTRATION OF CYTOKINES AND LPS IN HUMANS PRODUCES DEPRESSIVE SYMPTOMS

Administration of cytokines in humans produces marked behavioral and neuroendocrine symptoms that are similar to those induced by viral infection. Administration of alpha interferon (IFN-α), IL-2, or TNF-α was found to cause flu-like symptoms as well as depressive symptoms, including depressed mood, dysphoria, anhedonia, helplessness, mild-to-severe fatigue, anorexia and weight loss, hypersomnia, psychomotor retardation, decreased concentration, and confusion.[14] The fact that these symptoms appear almost immediately after cytokine administration and usually disappear shortly after termination of the cytokine treatment, strongly suggests a causal role for cytokines in producing the depressive symptoms.

To further examine the role of cytokines in the psychologcial alterations that accompany infection and inflammation, we have recently conducted a study on the effects of LPS on affective and cognitive variables in healthy volunteers. A within-subjects cross-over design was used, in which each subject completed a battery of psychological and neuropsychological tests at various time points following LPS injection on one day, and following saline injection on another day. Neither the experimenter nor the subject knew the group assignment (i.e., a double-blind design). LPS produced a marked increase in the levels of circulating cytokines and cortisol, as well as mild fever and anorexia, but no other flu-like symptoms. The levels of anxiety and depression were significantly elevated in LPS-injected subjects. LPS produced no alterations in attention and executive functions, but it did produce a marked impairment in both verbal and nonverbal memory functions. The levels of anxiety, depression, and memory impairments were significantly and positively correlated with the levels of blood cytokines, demonstrating the important role of cytokines in mediating the emotional and cognitive responses to illness.

BEHAVIORAL EFFECTS OF INFECTIOUS AND AUTOIMMUNE DISEASES IN ANIMALS: MEDIATION BY PERIPHERAL AND BRAIN CYTOKINES

In animals, systemic protozoan, bacterial or viral infections are associated with anorexia and body weight loss, hypersomnia, psychomotor retardation, fatigue, and impaired cognitive abilities, exploration and social behavior.[4–6] Similar symptoms, as well as increased anxiety behavior, were also reported using mouse models of autoimmune disease,[15,16] indicating that behavioral changes can also accompany non-infectious conditions.

The behavioral effects of disease processes are mediated by cytokines, as evidenced by infection-like sickness behavior symptoms following exogenous administration of cytokines (particularly IL-1β and TNF-α), which act centrally and synergistically to induce sickness behavior. Moreover, the behavioral effects of immune challenges can be attenuated by pretreatment with cytokine synthesis blockers and cytokine antagonists, as well as by manipulations in cytokine genes, such as transgenic overexpresion or gene knockout.[4–6,17]

One particularly important aspect of depression that has recently been modeled in animals is anhedonia—that is, the diminished capacity to experience pleasure. Suppression of intracranial self-stimulation (ICSS) is a very useful animal model to study anhedonia. LPS-induced suppression of ICSS has been demonstrated more than three decades ago.[18] This report was recently corroborated by the findings that exogenous administration of IL-2 produce a specific and long-lasting decrease in ICSS.[17,19] Administration of LPS,[20] IL-1β,[19] or antigenic challenge with sheep red blood cells[21] was also associated with suppression of ICSS.

The consumption of and preference for sweet solutions can also serve as a model for hedonic processes. Studies in our laboratory, as well as others, demonstrated that various immune challenges attenuate the consumption of and preference for sweet solutions, while having minimal effects on water drinking (see FIGURE 2A).[3,17,22] Autoimmune diseases in animals are also associated with anhedonia. Thus, mice that spontaneously develop systemic autoimmune lupus-like disease also show blunted sensitivity to sucrose, which can be reversed by an immunosuppressive treatment.[23] Moreover, we have recently demonstrated that induction of experimental autoimmune encephalomyelitis (EAE) in SJL/J female mice by adoptive transfer of lymph node cells is associated with sickness behavior symptoms, including anorexia, loss of body weight, reduced social exploration, and decreased intake of and preference for sucrose solution (FIG. 2B).[16] Interestingly, the onset and recovery of the behavioral symptoms preceded the onset and recovery of the neurological signs, respectively. Since EAE is considered as an established animal model for multiple sclerosis (MS) in humans, it is suggested that EAE-induced behavioral changes may serve as a model for the depressive symptomatology that characterizes most MS patients.

Finally, we have found that various immune challenges produce a dramatic decrease in libido and sexual performance of female rats.[24,25] Such a reduction in sexual interest or desire and difficulties in sexual functioning are features commonly associated with depression, and they are also viewed as manifestations of the general loss of interest and pleasure in activities that were previously considered pleasurable.[2] In conclusion, various immune challenges induce anhedonia and many behavioral alterations that resemble the core symptoms of depression. These findings suggest that immune activation produces a depression-like syndrome in animals.

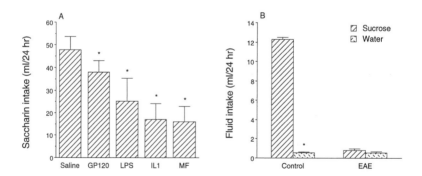

FIGURE 2. Effects of various immune challenges on the consumption of sweet solutions. **A.** For each immune challenge, animals were presented with two graduated tubes containing a 10-mM saccharin solution or water. Data represents the mean (±SEM) saccharin solution consumption over a 24-h period in nondeprived rats, following administration of saline, HIV-1 gp120, LPS, interleukin-1β (IL-1), or *Mycoplasma fermentans* (MF). The intake of saccharin solution following saline was computed by averaging the intake in all the individual experiments from which this graph was derived. **B.** Effects of EAE on the intake of sucrose solution and water. Consumption was measured in female SJL mice presented with a dilute sucrose solution and water over a period of six hours (average of two sessions). *Significantly different from saline/control group.

ANTIDEPRESSANTS ATTENUATE THE DEPRESSIVE-LIKE
SYMPTOMS INDUCED BY IMMUNE ACTIVATION IN ANIMALS

Antidepressants have been used successfully in treating depressive symptoms associated with various medical conditions[1] and depression induced by IFN administration in humans.[26] To further elucidate the relationship between immune activation and depression and explore the mechanisms underlying the therapeutic action of antidepressants, we employed an experimental animal model. Specifically, we examined the effects of antidepressants on LPS-induced behavioral and neuroendocrine alterations in rats. We demonstrated that chronic, but not acute, administration of the tricyclic antidepressant (TCA) imipramine (daily injection for 3–5 weeks) attenuated or completely abolished the behavioral effects of LPS, including decreased saccharine preference, anorexia, body weight loss, reduced social activity, and suppression of locomotor and exploratory behavior in the open field test (see FIGURE 3).[22] The dissociation between the effects of acute and chronic imipramine treatment is important, because in clinical settings imipramine is also effective in alleviating depression only following chronic, but not acute, administration.

In subsequent experiments we showed that chronic administration of fluoxetine, a serotonin reuptake inhibitor (SSRI), also significantly attenuated LPS-induced reduction in food consumption and body weight, although it did not affect LPS-induced decrease in social interaction and activity in the open field test. Chronic fluoxetine treatment also had marked effects on changes in body temperature: in control mice LPS induced a biphasic response, characterized by initial hypothermia followed by prolonged hyperthermia; in contrast, fluoxetine-treated mice showed no hypothermic response, beginning the hyperthermic response earlier than controls. Finally, chronic treatment with fluoxetine significantly attenuated LPS-induced secretion of corticosterone.

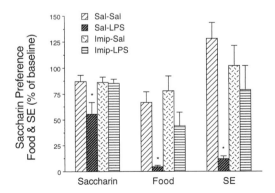

FIGURE 3. Effects of chronic imipramine treatment on LPS-induced behavioral suppression. Saccharin preference, food consumption, and social exploration (SE) were measured following an acute injection with LPS in rats that were treated chronically with either saline or imipramine (daily injections of 10 mg/kg for 3–5 weeks). *Significantly different from all other groups. (Adapted from Yirmiya.[22])

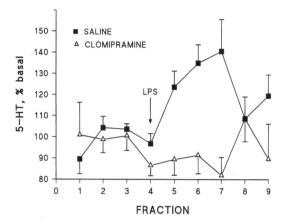

FIGURE 4. Effects of chronic clomipramine treatment on LPS-induced changes in se-rotonin (5-HT) concentration within the hypothalamus. Following chronic treatment (five weeks of daily injections) with either saline ($n = 11$) or clomipramine ($n = 7$), the concen-tration of 5-HT within the anterior hypothalamus was measured by an *in vivo* microdialysis system. Measurements (fractions) were taken every 30 min, four times before and five times after an i.p. injection with LPS (100 µg/kg).

Several mechanisms may underlie the effects of antidepressants on LPS-induced behavioral suppression. One possibility is that antidepressants attenuate LPS-induced cytokine secretion. Indeed, several recent reports have demonstrated that TCAs and SSRIs can attenuate the *in vitro* secretion of cytokines by cells taken from either rodents or humans.[27,28] To further explore these effects, we recently measured LPS-induced expression of TNF-α and IL-1β mRNA in splenocytes of rats and mice treated chronically with antidepressants. In collaboration with Professor E. Weihe and Dr. M. Bette from the Department of Anatomy and Cell Biology, University of Marburg, Germany, we demonstrated, using *in situ* hybridization, that chronic treat-ment with fluoxetine, but not imipramine, produced a small attenuation of LPS-induced increase in TNF-α mRNA expression. Neither fluoxetine nor imipramine produced any attenuation in LPS-induced increase in IL-1β mRNA levels. Similar results were obtained in our laboratory using PCR analysis.[6] These findings suggest that suppression of cytokine production is not a general mechanism by which anti-depressants modulate the responses to LPS.

To begin to explore the possibility that antidepressants attenuate the effects of immune challenges on neurochemical systems within the brain, we recently exam-ined the effects of chronic treatment with the TCA clomipramine on LPS-induced secretion of brain serotonin (5-HT). On the last day of antidepressant treatment, rats were implanted with a dialysis probe into the hypothalamus, and the effect of LPS on 5-HT concentrations was assessed 24 h later in freely moving rats. In rats that were chronically treated with saline, LPS produced a significant elevation in hypo-thalamic 5-HT concentration. This effect was completely abolished by chronic clo-mipramine treatment, suggesting that antidepressants can attenuate the serotonergic activation induced by an immune challenge (see FIGURE 4).

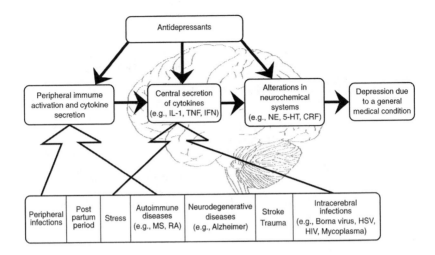

FIGURE 5. Immune activation and depression due to a general medical condition: possible mechanisms for modulation by antidepressants.

CONCLUSIONS

Accumulating evidence indicates that immune activation during various medical conditions is associated with a depressive syndrome in both humans and experimental animals. Taken together with the reports that brain cytokines influence the neurochemical systems involved in depression, these findings support the hypothesis that immune activation, via the release of peripheral and brain cytokines, may be involved in the etiology and symptomatology of "depression due to a general medical condition" (see FIGURE 5). This hypothesis has direct implications for antidepressant therapy. Future research should examine the effects of antidepressant drugs on immune functions and cytokine secretion, as well as the effects of cytokine synthesis blockers and antagonists on depressive disorders associated with medical conditions.

ACKNOWLEDGMENTS

This work was supported by a grant from the German Israeli Foundation for Research and Development and by Grant 97-204 from the United States–Israel Binational Science Foundation.

REFERENCES

1. KATON, W., & M.D. SULLIVAN. 1990. Depression and chronic medical illness. J. Clin. Psychiatry **51:** 3–11.
2. 1994. DSM-IV, Diagnostic and Statistical Manual of Mental Disorders, 4th edit. American Psychiatric Association. Washington, DC.

3. YIRMIYA, R. 1997. Behavioral and psychological effects of immune activation: implications for "depression due to a general medical condition." Curr. Opinion Psychiatry 10: 470–476.

4. MAIER, S.F. & L.R. WATKINS. 1998. Cytokines for psychologists: implications of bidirectional immune-to-brain communication for understanding behavior, mood, and cognition. Psychol. Rev. 105: 83–107.

5. DANTZER, R., A. AUBERT et al. 1999. Mechanisms of the effects of cytokines. In Cytokines, Stress and Depression. R. Dantzer, E.E. Wollman & R. Yirmiya, Eds.: 83–106. Kluwer Academic/Plenum Publishers. New York.

6. YIRMIYA, R., J. WEIDENFELD et al. 1999. Cytokines, "depression due to a general medical condition," and antidepressant drugs. In Cytokines, Stress and Depression. R. Dantzer, E.E. Wollman & R. Yirmiya, Eds.: 283–316. Kluwer Academic/Plenum Publishers. New York.

7. HICKIE, I. & A. LLOYD. 1995. Are cytokines associated with neuropsychiatric syndromes in humans? Int. J. Immunopharmacol. 17: 677–683.

8. SMITH, A.P., D.A.J. TYRRELL et al. 1988. The effects of experimentally induced respiratory virus infections on performance. Psychiatr. Med. 18: 65–71.

9. SMITH, A.P., D.A.J. TYRRELL et al. 1992. Mood and experimentally induced respiratory virus infections and illness. Psychol. Health 6: 205–212.

10. HALL, S. & A.P. SMITH. 1996. Investigating the effects and aftereffects of naturally occurring upper respiratory tract illnesses on mood and performance. Physiol. Behav. 59: 569–577.

11. CAPURON, L. D. LAMARAQUE et al. 1999. Attentional and mnemonic deficit associated with infectious disease in humans. Psychol. Med. 29: 291–297.

12. MEIJER, A., Z. ZAKAY-RONES & A. MORAG. 1988. Post-influenzal psychiatric disorder in adolescents. Acta Psychiatr. Scand. 78: 176–181.

13. MORAG, M., R. YIRMIYA et al. 1998. Influence of socioeconomic status on behavioral, emotional, and cognitive effects of rubella vaccination: a prospective, double blind study. Psychoneuroendocrinology 23: 337–351.

14. MEYERS, C.A. 1999. Mood and cognitive disorders in cancer patients receiving cytokine therapy. In Cytokines, Stress and Depression. R. Dantzer, E.E. Wollman & R. Yirmiya, Eds.: 75–82. Kluwer Academic/Plenum Publishers. New York.

15. SCHROTT, L.M. & L.S. CRNIC. 1996. Anxiety behavior, exploratory behavior, and activity in NZB X NZW F1 hybrid mice: role of genotype and autoimmune disease progression. Brain Behav. Immun. 10: 260–274.

16. POLLAK, Y., H. OVADIA et al. 2000. Behavioral aspects of experimental autoimmune encephalomyelitis (EAE). J. Neuroimmunol. 104: 31–36.

17. ANISMAN, H. & Z. MERALI. 1999. Anhedonic and anxiogenic effects of cytokine exposure. In Cytokines, Stress and Depression. R. Dantzer, E.E. Wollman & R. Yirmiya, Eds.: 199–233. Kluwer Academic/Plenum Publishers. New York.

18. MILLER, N.E. 1964. Some psychophysiological studies of motivation and of the behavioral effects of illness. Bull. Br. Psychiatr. Soc. 17: 1–20.

19. ANISMAN, H., L. KOKKINIDIS et al. 1998. Differential effects of interleukin (IL)–1, IL-2, and IL-6 on responding for rewarding lateral hypothalamic stimulation. Brain Res. 779: 177–187.

20. BOROWSKI, T., L. KOKKINIDIS et al. 1998. Lipopolysaccharide, central in vivo biogenic amine variations, and anhedonia. NeuroReport 9: 3797–3802.

21. ZACHARKO, R.M., S. ZALCMAN et al. 1997. Differential effects of immunologic challenge on self-stimulation from the nucleus accumbens and the substantia nigra. Pharmacol. Biochem. Behav. 58: 881–886.

22. YIRMIYA, R. 1996. Endotoxin produces a depressive-like syndrome in rats. Brain Res. 711: 163–174.

23. SAKIC, B., J.A. DENBURG et al. 1996. Blunted sensitivity to sucrose in autoimmune MRL-lpr mice: a curve shift study. Brain Res. Bull. 41: 305–311.

24. YIRMIYA, R., R. AVITSUR et al. 1995. Interleukin-1 inhibits sexual behavior in female but not in male rats. Brain Behav. Immun. 9: 220–33.

25. AVITSUR, R. & R. YIRMIYA. 1999. The immunobiology of sexual behavior: gender differences in the suppression of sexual activity during illness. Pharmacol. Biochem. Behav. **64:** 787–796.
26. LEVENSON, J.L. & H.J. FALLON. 1993. Fluoxetine treatment of depression caused by interferon-alpha. Am. J. Gastroenterol. **88:** 760–761.
27. XIA, Z., J.W. DEPIERRE & L. NASSBERGER. 1996. Tricyclic antidepressants inhibit IL-6, IL-1β and TNF-α release in human blood monocytes and IL-2 and interferon-γ in T-cells. Immunobiology **34:** 27–37.
28. MAES, M., C. SONG *et al.* 1999. Negative immunoregulatory effects of antidepressants: inhibition of interferon-gamma and stimulation of interleukin-10 secretion. Neuropsychopharmacology **20:** 370–379.

Experimental Immunomodulation, Sleep, and Sleepiness in Humans

THOMAS POLLMÄCHER,[a,b] ANDREAS SCHULD,[b] THOMAS KRAUS,[b]
MONIKA HAACK,[b] DUNJA HINZE-SELCH,[c] AND JANET MULLINGTON[d]

[b]Max Planck Institute of Psychiatry, Munich, Germany

[c]The Stanley Division of Developmental Neurovirology, Johns Hopkins University,
Baltimore, Maryland, USA

[d]Department of Neurology, Beth Israel Deaconess Medical Center and
Harvard Medical School, Boston, Massachusetts, USA

ABSTRACT: Infection, inflammation, and autoimmune processes are accompanied by serious disturbances of well-being, psychosocial functioning, cognitive performance, and behavior. Here we review those studies that have investigated the effects of experimental immunomodulation on sleep and sleepiness in humans. In most of these studies bacterial endotoxin was injected intravenously to model numerous aspects of infection including the release of inflammatory cytokines. These studies show that human sleep-wake behavior is very sensitive to host defense activation. Small amounts of endotoxin, which affect neither body temperature nor neuroendocrine systems but slightly stimulate the secretion of inflammatory cytokines, promote non–rapid-eye-movement sleep amount and intensity. Febrile host responses, in contrast, go along with prominent sleep disturbances. According to present knowledge tumor necrosis factor-α (TNF-α) is most probably a key mediator of these effects, although it is likely that disturbed sleep during febrile host responses involves endocrine systems as well. There is preliminary evidence from human studies suggesting that inflammatory cytokines such as TNF-α not only mediate altered sleep-wake behavior during infections, but in addition are involved in physiological sleep regulation and in hypnotic effects of established sedating drugs.

INTRODUCTION

Infection, inflammation, and autoimmune processes are accompanied by serious disturbances of well-being, psychosocial functioning, cognitive performance, and behavior. In particular, sleep and subjective alertness are very sensitive to ongoing host defense processes. For example, subjective sleep duration changes already prior to the occurrence of overt symptomatology during experimental influenza or rhinovirus infections in humans[1] and hypersomnia may persist for years after the acute symptomatic phase of Epstein Barr Virus (EBV) infection.[2]

[a]Address for correspondence: Thomas Pollmächer, M.D., Max Planck Institute of Psychiatry, Kraepelinstrasse 10, 80804 Munich, Germany. Voice: +49-89-30622-572; fax: +49-89-30622-562.

topo@mpipsykl.mpg.de

Although sleepiness was already recognized by Aristotle[3] as a symptom of febrile diseases, we still know little about immune-mediated alterations in sleep-wake behavior and about the underlying mechanisms in humans. Earlier we reviewed in detail the scanty knowledge on sleep and sleepiness during human infectious diseases, mainly viral infections.[4] To summarize these findings, infections consistently induce some degree of subjective sleepiness. The amount of sleep, however, may be increased (for example, EBV infection[2]), decreased (for example, symptomatic HIV infection[5]), or unchanged, but differently distributed across the nychthemeron (for example, African sleeping sickness[6]). Hence, clinical data suggest that ongoing host defense processes have a complex and variable influence on human sleep-wake behavior.

To understand the underlying mechanisms, experimental studies using defined immunological challenges and a standardized assessment of sleep and wakefulness are needed. Animal studies started in the 1980s. By now there is abundant evidence that in rats and rabbits bacterial, viral, and fungal infections go along with an increased amount of non–rapid-eye-movement (nonREM) sleep, whereas the amount of REM sleep is slightly reduced or unaffected.[7] Moreover, these studies showed that in animals infections increase the amount of EEG delta waves during nonREM sleep, as assessed by EEG spectral analysis or equivalent measures. Therefore, it has been generally concluded that infections increase the amount and intensity of nonREM sleep in animals. Further studies revealed that the key mediators of infection-induced alterations in sleep-wake behavior are cytokines,[8] which are well known for the induction of other adaptive changes in CNS functions such as fever[9] and activation of the hypothalamic-pituitary-adrenal (HPA) system.[10] In particular the proinflammatory cytokines interleukin-1 (IL-1) and tumor necrosis factor–α (TNF-α) both increase nonREM sleep amount and intensity, and these effects can be blocked by specific antibodies or by endogenous antagonists of cytokine actions such as IL-1 receptor antagonist[11] or soluble TNF receptor [sTNF-R] p55.[12]

The present paper summarizes the studies that have investigated the effects of immunomodulation on sleep and sleepiness in humans. Most of these studies[13–19] have used bacterial endotoxin, well known for its stimulating effect on cytokine secretion.[20] So far, only two studies have investigated the effects of cytokines on human sleep. In one study IL-6 was used,[21] and in the other study, granulocyte colony-stimulating factor.[22] Although the studies reviewed here support the pivotal role of cytokines as immunomodulators of sleep and wakefulness, they point to important differences between animals and humans. In particular, increase of non-REM sleep amount and intensity is much less consistently seen in humans than in animals and occurs only when host defense activation is subtle and not accompanied by fever. In contrast, human febrile host responses to endotoxin go along with prominent sleep disruption. The reasons for these species differences and the clinical and physiological implication of these experimental findings will be discussed.

EFFECTS OF EXPERIMENTAL IMMUNOMODULATION
ON SLEEP IN HUMANS

Effects of Bacterial Endotoxin

Endotoxins are the major cell wall components of gram-negative bacteria. They are lipopolysaccharides (LPS) and account for about 80% of the cell wall mass of the respective microorganisms.[23] Research during the past 100 years has firmly established that endotoxins are the key molecules that activate the unspecific immune system during early gram-negative bacterial infection.[24,25] Bound to LPS-binding protein, they activate immunocompetent cells, mainly macrophages, through the CD14 receptor and induce the release and *de novo* synthesis of a plethora of mediators including pro- and anti-inflammatory cytokines.

Human host responses to endotoxins have been characterized in many studies.[20] At present there are two purified preparations available for use in humans: one from *Escherichia coli* is used mainly in the U.S. and one from *Salmonella abortus equi* preferred in Europe. Salmonella-derived endotoxin is relatively more potent, but the effects in humans do not differ qualitatively between the two preparations. Both have been administered intravenously in the great majority of studies and induce a dose-dependent, self-limited host response that lasts between 8 and 12 hours. The host response includes an increase in rectal temperature, an initial drop in leukocyte counts followed by an increase, and increases in the circulating amounts of ACTH, cortisol, and numerous cytokines and soluble cytokine receptors (TNF-α, sTNF-R p55 and p75, IL-6, IL-10, IL-1 receptor antagonist [IL-1Ra], G-CSF, and others). As we have discussed in detail earlier[14,26] there is no consistent evidence that endotoxin increases circulating IL-1ß levels in humans. Similar to the other host responses endotoxin-induced physical sickness symptoms are dose dependent. These symptoms are flu-like and include headache, muscle aches, short-lasting chills and nausea. FIGURE 1 shows schematically the temporal pattern of host responses to endotoxin. Already during the first hour following the injection of endotoxin a prominent increase in the levels of TNF-α and sTNF-Rs occurs. The occurrence of sickness symptoms is closely related to this steep increase in TNF-α levels. Activation of the TNF system is followed by increases in IL-6 and cortisol levels that parallel the increase in rectal temperature. As shown in FIGURE 1, all these responses to endotoxin are monophasic, and baseline levels are reached 12 hours following injection or even earlier.

Human host responses to endotoxin depend on the time of day. Temperature and cortisol responses are much less pronounced in the morning at 0900 hours compared to the evening at 1900 hours, despite similar amounts of IL-6 and TNF-α released into circulation.[27] Hence, it is likely that the biological activity of inflammatory cytokines varies across the day in humans as it has been shown for TNF-α–induced lethality in mice.[28]

TABLE 1 summarizes methodological details of those studies in which endotoxin was administered to humans in the afternoon or evening and subsequent night sleep was monitored. These studies differ with respect to the endotoxin preparation used, the amount and time of injection, and the strength of the ensuing host response. The latter fact is illustrated by the variation in the maximum febrile response that ranged

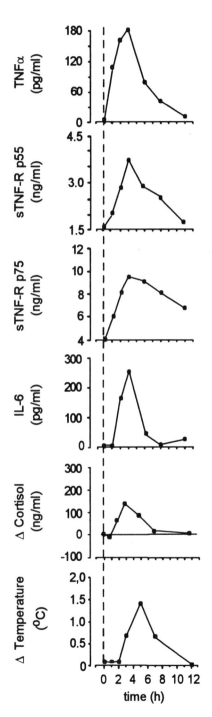

FIGURE 1. Schematic representation of host responses to bacterial endotoxin in healthy volunteers, based on data from various studies using *Salmonella abortus equi* endotoxin. The time courses of rectal temperature and cortisol levels are depicted as difference data (relative changes compared to placebo control) because the variables show prominent circadian variations. For more details see text.

TABLE 1. Studies that have investigated the effects of bacterial endotoxin on human night sleep

	Number of subjects[a]	Amount of endotoxin (ng/kg) injected[b]	Mean maximum rectal temperature (°C)
Mullington *et al.*, 2000	5	0.8	38.9
Karacan *et al.*, 1968	4	2[c]	38.7
Bauer *et al.*, 1995	7[d]	Unknown[e]	38.7
Trachsel *et al.*, 1994	9/8[f]	0.4/0.8	37.8
Pollmächer *et al.*, 1993	15	0.4	37.6
Mullington *et al.*, 2000	5	0.4	37.5
Mullington *et al.*, 2000	7	0.2	No significant increase

NOTE: The studies are listed according to their effects on rectal temperature.
[a]If not specified otherwise, the subjects were healthy volunteers.
[b]If not specified otherwise the *Salmonella abortus equi* endotoxin preparation described in detail by Pollmächer *et al.*, 1993, was used.
[c]In this study a different *Salmonella abortus equi* endotoxin preparation was used, which is not described in detail in the paper.
[d]These subjects were patients suffering from major depression.
[e]In this study an autolysate of gram-negative and gram-positive bacteria was used. The preparation contained amounts of endotoxin that were not standardized.
[f]The nine subjects included in this study who received 0.4 ng/kg are a subgroup of the 15 subjects reported on by Pollmächer *et al.*, 1993.

from 38.9°C to no significant increase in rectal temperature. Rectal temperature is the only physiological parameter that allows one to compare the extent of host defense activation by endotoxin between all the different studies, because in older studies cytokines could not be measured, and in more recent studies methodological differences impair quantitative comparisons of cytokine levels. However, the studies that have been carried out by our group clearly show that there are strong positive correlations between the endotoxin-induced increase in rectal temperature and the release of cytokines and cortisol.[14] Hence, rectal temperature is a valid measure of the overall response strength, which is of pivotal importance for the effects of endotoxin on sleep.

In all studies reporting febrile responses (rectal temperature exceeding 38.0°C) endotoxin disrupted night sleep. Sleep continuity was disturbed, and the amount of wakefulness or at least the number of nocturnal awakenings were increased. The amount of nonREM sleep was reduced particularly prior to and around the peak of the host response, although the total amount across the entire night was not reduced in two studies.[16,19] The total amount of nonREM sleep during the night was reduced in one study only.[13] Amounts of endotoxin that induced subpyrogenic host responses (rectal temperature below 38.0°C) had either no effect on nonREM sleep and wakefulness[19] or yielded an increase in nonREM sleep[14,15,19] that occurred either with a concomitant decrease in wakefulness[14,19] or without.[15]

The effects of subpyrogenic doses of endotoxin on nonREM sleep need more detailed consideration. Endotoxin administered at 1900 hours[14,15] raised rectal temperature to near 38.0°C and induced an increase in light (stage 2) nonREM sleep; whereas deep nonREM sleep—that is, stages 3 and 4 (slow wave sleep, SWS)—was not affected. In accordance with these effects on visually scored sleep stages, sleep intensity, quantified by EEG spectral delta power, was unchanged. The lowest dose of endotoxin (0.2 ng/kg) that has ever been administered to humans did not affect rectal temperature or cortisol levels at all, but consistently stimulated IL-6 and TNF-α secretion.[19] This small dose of endotoxin increased the amount of deep non-REM sleep (stages 3 and 4, SWS), and did promote sleep intensity—that is, EEG spectral delta power.

The effects of endotoxin on human REM sleep are less complex than those on nonREM sleep. In all published studies (see TABLE 1) REM sleep was found to be suppressed, and this effect increased with the degree of host defense activation.

Two studies investigated the effects of endotoxin on daytime sleep in humans.[17,18] In both experiments a paradigm of six scheduled daytime naps with controlled wakefulness in between was used. This paradigm was adopted from the Multiple Sleep Latency Test, a standardized tool to assess excessive daytime sleepiness.[29] In the first study[17] 0.8 ng/kg endotoxin injected at 0900 hours increased rectal temperature to about 37.4°C and stimulated TNF-α, IL-6, and cortisol secretion but had very little effect on sleep. Only during the first scheduled nap, one hour following the administration of endotoxin, did a significant reduction in REM sleep amount occur. The amount of nonREM sleep was not affected but correlated negatively with the peak IL-6 concentration, suggesting that more prominent host defense activation would suppress nonREM sleep. This idea was confirmed by the second study.[18] In this study a more prominent host response (mean maximal rectal temperature 37.8 °C) was achieved by pretreatment with granulocyte colony-stimulating factor (G-CSF), which is known to enhance endotoxin-induced host responses.[26] In parallel, nonREM sleep amount was decreased and the amount of wakefulness was increased during the first nap following the injection of endotoxin. In this study REM sleep was not found to be suppressed, which might be explained by the very low amount of REM sleep that occurred already at baseline.

Effects of Cytokines on Sleep

To date there are only two studies in humans that have investigated the effects of cytokines on polygraphically recorded sleep. In one study IL-6 (0.5 μg/kg body weight, subcutaneously) was administered to 16 healthy volunteers at 1900 hours, and sleep was recorded starting at 2300 hours.[21] IL-6 induced prominent increases in its own plasma levels and in those of cortisol. Sublingual temperature rose continuously to about 37.5°C at 2300 hours, when temperature measurement was stopped. IL-6 suppressed REM sleep, but wakefulness and nonREM sleep were not affected when the entire night was considered. Spectral EEG delta power was not assessed. Hence, IL-6 induced a subpyrogenic host response and had effects on night sleep similar to the effects of subpyrogenic amounts of endotoxin.

The second study assessed the effects of G-CSF on night sleep in 10 healthy volunteers.[22] G-CSF is a hematopoietic cytokine[30] known primarily for its prominent effects on the circulating number and the function of granulocytes. In addition,

G-CSF is supposed to have anti-inflammatory properties[31] and induces subtle increases in the circulating amounts of TNF-α, sTNF-R p55, sTNF-R p75, and IL-1Ra, but has no effect on IL-1β, IL-6, cortisol, and human growth hormone (hGH) levels, and rectal temperature.[22,26] After injection at 2100 hours G-CSF (300 μg, subcutaneously) induced increases in the circulating amounts of sTNF-R p55, sTNF-R p75, and IL-Ra that occurred rapidly and were consistent when sleep recordings started at 2300 hours. In contrast, the plasma TNF-α levels were not significantly increased until the early morning hours. During the first hours of sleep, when only the levels of cytokine antagonists were increased, deep nonREM sleep amount and spectral EEG delta power were reduced. Hence, the effects of G-CSF on night sleep are opposite to those of the lowest dose of endotoxin investigated so far.[19]

EFFECTS OF IMMUNOMODULATION ON SLEEPINESS

Sleepiness is a very common symptom of infectious diseases, and clinical experience suggests that therapeutic use of cytokines in patients with cancer, multiple sclerosis, and other conditions may induce sleepiness. However, the available experimental database is extremely small.

Only four studies published so far have investigated the effects of experimental immunomodulation on subjective sleepiness in humans. In all these studies visual analogue scales were used to assess sleepiness. Two studies were carried out in the evening. We found that injection of endotoxin at 1900 hours had no effect on sleepiness measured hourly until the onset of sleep around 2300 hours, but subjects were less sleepy the following morning.[14] In contrast,[21] it was reported that IL-6, injected at 1900 hours, induced an increase in subjective sleepiness until 2200 hours, whereas these researchers did not find any effect the next morning. Endotoxin administered at 0900 hours in the morning had no effect on the time course of sleepiness across the day in one of our studies.[17] However, in the second study,[18] where the host response was more pronounced due to priming with G-CSF, we found a transient increase in subjective sleepiness. This increase showed a remarkable time course: it started two hours following endotoxin injection, peaked at three hours, and then rapidly declined. Notably, this increase in sleepiness followed the first scheduled nap after endotoxin administration, which was characterized by disturbed sleep. Moreover, the increase in subjective sleepiness was not followed by an increased amount of sleep in the subsequent naps. Hence, in this study, endotoxin increased subjective sleepiness after it had induced disturbed sleep, but increased sleepiness did not lead to more sleep subsequently.

MECHANISMS UNDERLYING THE EFFECTS OF IMMUNOMODULATION ON SLEEP AND SLEEPINESS IN HUMANS

Before discussing the underlying mechanisms, we will briefly summarize the results of the studies reviewed above. The effects of immunomodulation on human sleep crucially depend on the degree of host defense activation. With respect to REM sleep this relationship is quite simple, because the more the primary host defense is activated, the more REM sleep is suppressed. However, the influence of immuno-modulation on wakefulness and nonREM sleep is more complex. FIGURE 2 integrates the respective results into a model of the relationship between the degree of host defense activation and changes in wakefulness, nonREM sleep, and spectral EEG delta power. Subtle host defense activation that is reflected only in an increase in the production of inflammatory cytokines, but does not go along with HPA system activation and increased body temperature, enhances nonREM sleep amount and EEG spectral delta power, and reduces the amount of wakefulness. With increasing host defense activation, including mild HPA system activation and subpyrogenic rectal temperatures, this sleep-promoting effect diminishes up to a "neutral" point where nonREM sleep, wakefulness, and spectral EEG power are not affected at all. Finally, even more prominent host defense activation in the typical febrile range results in reduced nonREM sleep and increased wakefulness—that is, in disturbed sleep.

As already mentioned and reviewed in detail earlier,[8] there is convincing evidence in animals that inflammatory cytokines, in particular IL-1β and TNF-α, are the most important mediators of the increased amount and intensity of nonREM sleep during infections. A major role of these immune mediators in human sleep responses to infection is very probable, too, although the mechanisms are likely to be not identical. There is some data suggesting that the roles of individual cytokines differ between species. For example, IL-6 has a suppressive effect on REM sleep in humans,[21] but does not affect sleep in rabbits.[32] Moreover, in contrast to animals, a major role of IL-1β in the effects of endotoxin on human sleep is less likely, because endotoxin does not induce measurable increases in the circulating amounts of IL-1β (albeit increased IL-1ß synthesis within the CNS cannot be excluded). Animal and human studies congruently suggest an important role of TNF-α in promoting nonREM sleep. The firm evidence in animals is supported in humans by at least two independent results: (1) by the finding that in the subpyrogenic range of host defense nonREM sleep amount correlates positively to TNF-α peak levels;[14] and (2) the find-

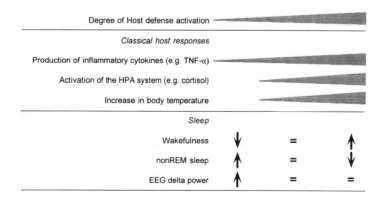

FIGURE 2. Schematic representation of the relationship between the degree of host defense activation during an infection and the respective alteration in sleep. For details see text.

ing that the increase in soluble TNF receptors induced by G-CSF goes along with nonREM sleep and EEG spectral delta power suppression.[22]

The mechanisms underlying the prominent disruption of sleep during febrile host responses in humans cannot be easily deduced from the preclinical data. For unknown reasons rats and rabbits typically do not show reductions in nonREM sleep amount and increased wakefulness during infections or comparable experimental conditions that induce fever.[7,8] The increase in rectal temperature by itself cannot explain nonREM sleep suppression in humans, because passive body heating has opposite effects.[33,34] In our view, the most probable explanation at present is that HPA system activation, which becomes very prominent only in the febrile host response range, causes disturbed sleep through central CRH release, well known to suppress nonREM sleep.[35]

As reviewed above, the available data on the effects of experimental immuno-modulation on subjective sleepiness are extremely scanty, rendering any discussion of the underlying mechanisms difficult. It is tempting to speculate that, similar to their important role in modulating sleep during infections, cytokines are causally involved in effects on subjective sleepiness. Preclinical studies have often assumed that increased nonREM sleep during infections in animals is an equivalent of increased sleepiness in humans. However, this is not necessarily the case, as is well illustrated by the effects of endotoxin on sleepiness in volunteers,[18] who did not sleep more despite being more sleepy. However, sleepiness was preceded by a reduction in sleep amount. Other studies yielded equivocal results regarding the effects of experimental immunomodulation on sleepiness (see above). Therefore, the mechanisms underlying the effects of immunmodulation on subjective sleepiness are definitely unknown at present, and they may differ considerably from the mechanisms underlying the effects on sleep.

CLINICAL AND PHYSIOLOGICAL SIGNIFICANCE OF THE EFFECTS OF IMMUNOMODULATION ON SLEEP AND SLEEPINESS IN HUMANS

As outlined in the introduction and reviewed in detail earlier,[4] infectious diseases in humans go along with a variable degree of sleep alterations, ranging from severe hypersomnia to prominent sleep disruption. The studies reviewed herein suggest that one major reason for this variability is the variability in host defense activation. Based on experimental data one would predict that subtle host defense activation, as occurs, for example, in the very early presymptomatic phase or in the post-acute chronic phase of viral infections, would result in hypersomnia, whereas the symptomatic peak of an acute febrile illness would coincide with considerably disturbed sleep. These alterations in sleep-wake behavior are probably mediated by inflammatory cytokines, in particular TNF-α. Notably, sleep is very sensitive to both subtle increases in the circulating amounts of TNF-α (promoting nonREM sleep and intensity) and increases in the levels of sTNF-Rs (suppressing nonREM sleep amount and intensity). In clinical practice postviral fatigue syndromes—for instance, following EBV infection, can be resistant to various kinds of stimulant drugs.[2] Therefore, the clinical efficacy of endogenous antagonists of cytokine activity—for example, of sTNF-R p55—should be tested in such conditions. Moreover, cytokines and cytokine antagonists may be of interest for sleep medicine in general, for conditions ranging from psychophysiological insomnia to narcolepsy. Finally, very recent studies suggest that some sedating drugs exert their effects on sleep-wake behavior through immunomodulation. For example, benzodiazepines[36] and thalidomide[37,38] increase systemic TNF-α levels in humans. The same holds true for the sedating antipsychotic clozapine,[39] which has effects on sleep strikingly similar to those of subpyrogenic doses of endotoxin.[40]

Although little doubt remains that infections induce cytokine-mediated alterations in sleep-wake behavior, two related questions remain to be discussed: whether altered sleep during infections has an adaptive value and whether cytokines are also involved in sleep regulation under physiological conditions.

It is a widespread belief that sleep helps us to overcome infections, and due to the prominent nonREM sleep–promoting effects of host defense activation in animals, it is tempting to speculate that indeed nonREM sleep supports host defense. Then, however, sleep deprivation should compromise host defense. Despite considerable efforts, this could not be demonstrated unequivocally.[41] Therefore, an immunosupportive function of sleep, and of nonREM sleep in particular, remains to be defined. The studies reviewed in the present paper do not contribute much to this controversy. However, they suggest that if nonREM sleep supports the host defense against acute infections in humans, this happens in the early phases of the process, because nonREM sleep is promoted only by subtle host defense activation.

Since the discovery that during sleep deprivation muramyl peptides accumulate in urine,[42] the idea has been pursued that the immune system is involved in physiological sleep regulation. Recent studies in healthy animals showed that nonREM sleep and spectral EEG power are suppressed when the biological activity of IL-1β[43] or TNF-α[12] is antagonized. Moreover, transgenic mice lacking the TNF p55 receptor show a reduced amount of spontaneous nonREM sleep, further supporting the idea that under baseline conditions inflammatory cytokines are involved in nonREM sleep regulation.[44] The nonREM sleep–suppressive effect of G-CSF in healthy volunteers[22] that probably occurs through enhanced shedding of soluble TNF receptors yields the first indirect evidence that cytokines are also involved in human nonREM sleep regulation. To establish this role definitively, however, more studies are needed that directly investigate the effects of cytokines and cytokine antagonists on human sleep.

ACKNOWLEDGMENTS

This work was supported by grants from the Volkswagenstiftung, Hannover, Germany (I/71979) and from the German Israel Foundation (I-0495-135.02/96)

REFERENCES

1. SMITH, A. 1992. Sleep, colds, and performance. *In* Sleep, Arousal, and Performance. R.J. Broughton & R.D. Ogilvie, Eds.: 233–242. Birkhäuser. Boston.
2. GUILLEMINAULT, C. & S. MONDINI. 1986. Mononucleosis and chronic day time sleepiness: a long-term follow-up study. Arch. Intern. Med. **146:** 1333–1335.

3. ARISTOTLE. On the Soul. Parva Naturalia. On Breath. *In* Aristotle in Twenty-three Volumes, Vol. 8. W.S. Hett, Trans.: 316–345. Harvard University Press. Cambridge, MA.

4. POLLMÄCHER, T., J. MULLINGTON, C. KORTH & D. HINZE-SELCH. 1995. Influence of host defense activation on sleep in humans. Adv. Neuroimmunol. **5:** 155–169.

5. POLLMÄCHER, T. & F. HOLSBOER. 1996. Sleep-wake disturbances in HIV-infected patients—a potential model of the interactions between sleep and the immune system. Sleep Res. Soc. Bull. **2:** 37–42.

6. BUGUET, A., J. BERT, P. TAPIE, F. TABARAUD, F. DOUA, J. LONSDORFER, P. BOGUI & M. DUMAS. 1993. Sleep-wake cycle in human African trypanosomiasis. J. Clin. Neurophysiol. **10:** 190–196.

7. TOTH, L.A. 1995. Sleep, sleep deprivation and infectious disease: studies in animals. Adv. Neuroimmunol. **5:** 79–92.

8. KRUEGER, J.M., S. TAKAHASHI, L. KAPÁS, S. BREDOW, R. ROKY, J. FANG, R. FLOYD, K.B. RENEGAR, N. GUHA-THAKURTA, S. NOVITSKY & F. OBÁL. 1995. Cytokines in sleep regulation. Adv. Neuroimmunol. **5:** 171–188.

9. KLUGER, M.J. 1991. Fever: role of pyrogens and cryogens. Physiol. Rev. **71:** 93–117.

10. TURNBULL, A.V. & C. RIVIER. 1995. Regulation of the HPA axis by cytokines. Brain Behav. Immun. **9:** 253–275.

11. IMERI, L., M.R. OPP & J.M. KRUEGER. 1993. An IL-1 receptor and an IL-1 receptor antagonist attenuate muramyl dipeptide- and IL-1–induced sleep and fever. Am. J. Physiol. **265:** R907–913.

12. TAKAHASHI, S., D.D. TOOLEY, L. KAPAS, J.D. FANG, J.M. SEYER & J.M. KRUEGER. 1995. Inhibition of tumor necrosis factor in the brain suppresses rabbit sleep. Eur. J. Physiol. **431:** 155–160.

13. KARACAN, I., S.M. WOLFF, R.L. WILLIAMS, C.J. HURSCH & W.B. WEBB. 1968. The effects of fever on sleep and dream patterns. Psychosomatics **9:** 331–339.

14. POLLMÄCHER, T., W. SCHREIBER, S. GUDEWILL, H. VEDDER, K. FASSBENDER, K. WIEDEMANN, L. TRACHSEL, C. GALANOS & F. HOLSBOER. 1993. Influence of endotoxin on nocturnal sleep in humans. Am. J. Physiol. **264:** R1077–R1083.

15. TRACHSEL, L., W. SCHREIBER, F. HOLSBOER & T. POLLMÄCHER. 1994. Endotoxin enhances EEG alpha and beta power in human sleep. Sleep **17:** 132–139.

16. BAUER, J., F. HOHAGEN, E. GIMMEL, F. BRUNS, S. LIS, S. KRIEGER, W. AMBACH, A. GUTHMANN, H. GRUNZE, R. FRITSCH-MONTERO, A. WEISSBACH, U. GANTER, U. FROMMBERGER, D. RIEMANN & M. BERGER. 1995. Induction of cytokine synthesis and fever suppresses REM sleep and improves mood in patients with major depression. Biol. Psychiatry **38:** 611–621.

17. KORTH, C., J. MULLINGTON, W. SCHREIBER & T. POLLMÄCHER. 1996. Influence of endotoxin on daytime sleep in humans. Infect. Immun. **64:** 1110–1115.

18. HERMANN, D., J. MULLINGTON, D. HINZE-SELCH, W. SCHREIBER, C. GALANOS & T. POLLMÄCHER. 1998. Endotoxin-induced changes in sleep and sleepiness during the day. Psychoneuroendocrinol. **23**(2): 427–437.

19. MULLINGTON, J., C. KORTH, D. HERMANN, A. ORTH, C. GALANOS, F. HOLSBOER & T. POLLMÄCHER. 2000. Dose-dependent effects of endotoxin on human sleep. Am. J. Physiol. **278:** R947–955.

20. BURRELL, R. 1994. Human responses to bacterial endotoxin. Circ. Shock **43:** 137–153.

21. SPÄTH-SCHWALBE, E., K. HANSEN, F. SCHMIDT, H. SCHREZENMEIER, L. MARSHALL, K. BURGER, H. FEHM & J. BORN. 1998. Acute effects of recombinant human interleukin-6 on endocrine and central nervous sleep functions in healthy men. J. Clin. Endocrinol. Metab. **83:** 1573–1578.

22. SCHULD, A., J. MULLINGTON, D. HERMANN, D. HINZE-SELCH, T. FENZEL, F. HOLSBOER & T. POLLMÄCHER. 1999. Effects of granulocyte colony-stimulating factor on night sleep in humans. Am. J. Physiol. **276:** R1149–R1155.

23. RIETSCHEL, E.T., T. KIRIKAE, F.U. SCHADE, U. MAMAT, G. SCHMIDT, H. LOPPNOW, A.J. ULMER, U. ZÄHRINGER, U. SEYDEL, F. DI PADOVA, M. SCHREIBER & H. BRADE. 1994. Bacterial endotoxin: molecular relationships of structure to activity and function. FASEB J. **8:** 217–225.

24. WESTPHAL, O., U. WESTPHAL & T. SOMMER. 1978. The history of pyrogen research. *In* Microbiology—1977. D. Schlesinger, Ed.: 221–238. American Society for Microbiology. Washington, DC.
25. PARRILLO, J.P. 1993. Pathogenetic mechanisms of septic shock. N. Engl. J. Med. **328:** 1471–1477.
26. POLLMÄCHER, T., C. KORTH, J. MULLINGTON, W. SCHREIBER, J. SAUER, H. VEDDER, C. GALANOS & F. HOLSBOER. 1996. Effects of granulocyte colony-stimulating factor on plasma cytokine and cytokine receptor levels and on the *in vivo* host response to endotoxin in healthy men. Blood **87:** 900–905.
27. POLLMÄCHER, T., J. MULLINGTON, C. KORTH, W. SCHREIBER, D. HERMANN, A. ORTH, C. GALANOS & F. HOLSBOER. 1996. Diurnal variations in the human host response to endotoxin. J. Infect. Dis. **174:** 1040–1045.
28. HRUSHESKY, W.J.M., T. LANGEVIN, Y.J. KIM & P.A. WOOD. 1994. Circadian dynamics of tumor necrosis factor alpha (cachetin) lethality. J. Exp. Med. **180:** 1059–1065.
29. CARSKADON, M.A., W.C. DEMENT, M.M. MITLER, T. ROTH, P.R. WESTBROOK & S. KEENAN. 1986. Guideliness for the multiple sleep latency test (MLST): a standard measure of sleepiness. Sleep **9:** 519–524.
30. STEWARD, W.P. 1993. Granulocyte and granulocyte-macrophage colony-stimulating factors. Lancet **342:** 153–157.
31. HARTUNG, T. 1999. Immunomodulation by colony-stimulating factors. Rev. Physiol. Biochem. Pharmacol. **136:** 1–164.
32. OPP, M.R., J.R.F. OBAL, A.B. CADY, L. JOHANNSEN & J.M. KRUEGER. 1989. Interleukin-6 is pyrogenic but not somnogenic. Physiol. Behav. **45:** 1069–1072.
33. HORNE, J.A. & L.H.E. STAFF. 1983. Exercise and sleep: body heating effects. Sleep **6:** 36–46.
34. BUNNELL, D.E. & S.M. HORVATH. 1985. Effects of body heating during sleep interruption. Sleep **8:** 274–282.
35. FRIESS, E., K. WIEDEMANN, A. STEIGER & F. HOLSBOER. 1995. The hypothalamic-pituitary-adrenocortical system and sleep in man. Adv. Neuroimmunol. **5:** 111–125.
36. HAACK, M., D. HINZE-SELCH, T. FENZEL, T. KRAUS, M. KÜHN, A. SCHULD & T. POLLMÄCHER. 1999. Plasma levels of cytokines and soluble cytokine receptors in psychiatric patients upon hospital admission: effects of confounding factors and diagnosis. J. Psychiatr. Res. **33:** 407–418
37. JACOBSON, J.M., J.S. GREENSPAN, J. SPRITZLER, N. KETTER, J.L. FAHEY, J.B. JACKSON, L. FOX, M. CHERNOFF, A.W. WU, L.A. McPHAIL, G.J. VASQUEZ & D.A. WOHL. 1997. Thalidomide for the treatment of oral aphtous ulcers in patients with human immunodeficiency virus infection. N. Engl. J. Med. 336: 1487–1493.
38. WOLKENSTEIN, P.J., J. LATARJET, J.-C. ROUJEAU, C. DUGUET, S. BOUDEAU, L. VAILLANT, M. MAIGNAN, M.-H. SCHUHMACHER, B. MILPIED, A. PILORGET & H. BOCQUET. 1998. Randomised comparison of thalidomide versus placebo in toxic epidermal necrolysis. Lancet 352: 1586–1589.
39. POLLMÄCHER, T., D. HINZE-SELCH & J. MULLINGTON. 1996. Effects of clozapine on plasma cytokine and soluble cytokine receptor levels. J. Clin. Psychopharmacol. **16:** 403–409.
40. HINZE-SELCH, D., J. MULLINGTON, A. ORTH, C.J. LAUER & T. POLLMÄCHER. 1997. Effects of clozapine on sleep: a longitudinal study. Biol. Psychiatry **42:** 260–266.
41. BENCA, R.M. & J. QUINTANS. 1997. Sleep and host defenses—a review. Sleep **20:** 1027–1037.
42. PAPPENHEIMER, J.R. , G. KOSKI, V. FENCL, M.L. KARNOVSKY & J. KRUEGER. 1975. Extraction of sleep-promoting factor S from cerebrospinal fluid and from brains of sleep-deprived animals. J. Neurophysiol. **38:** 1299–1311.
43. OPP, M.R. & J.M. KRUEGER. 1994. Anti interleukin-1β reduces sleep and sleep rebound after sleep deprivation in rats. Am. J. Physiol. **266:** R688–R695.
44. FANG, J., Y. WANG & J.M. KRUEGER. 1997. Mice lacking the TNF 55 kDa receptor fail to sleep more after TNF-α treatment. J. Neurosci. **17:** 5949–5955.

Psychoneuroimmunology and HIV/AIDS

GEORGE F. SOLOMON,[a,b] GAIL H. IRONSON,[c] AND ELIZABETH G. BALBIN[d]

[b]*Department of Psychiatry and Biobehavioral Sciences, University of California, Los Angeles, Los Angeles, California, USA*

[c]*Department of Psychology and Psychiatry, University of Miami, Miami, Florida, USA*

[d]*Behavioral Medicine Research Program, University of Miami, Miami, Florida, USA*

PSYCHOSOCIAL PREDICTORS OF DISEASE PROGRESSION IN HIV/AIDS

Several psychosocial factors have been explored as possible predictors of disease progression in HIV infection beyond the biological factors known to affect progression such as genetics and age of host and viral strain. These psychosocial variables include: *stressors, depression and distress, coping, social support and loss, disclosure and emotional expression,* and *cognitive mindset.*

It is beyond the scope of this brief presentation to describe the considerable but sometimes conflicting evidence that these psychosocial variables have considerable relevance to rates of progression of HIV infection and to morbidity and mortality with AIDS. There are, of course, also important *behavioral variables* that may contribute to the course of HIV infection including: selecting an AIDS-competent physician, adherence to medical regimens, and avoidance of reinfection by more virulent strains by practicing safer sex or not sharing needles (probably), as well as (possibly) exercise and vitamin supplements.

PSYCHOLOGY OF HEALTH AND LONG SURVIVAL WITH HIV/AIDS

Our current research concerns an intensive investigation of two unique groups of HIV-positive individuals. The first are long-term survivors (LTS) of AIDS. These individuals have survived twice as long as expected after having had an opportunistic infection or neoplasm. In 1996, when the study started, the length of time to define long-term survivor status was four years. (With the widespread availability of protease inhibitors, this time has increased, but our subjects had to meet the four-year criterion before starting on protease inhibitors.) The second group is a "rare" group of HIV-positive people with very low CD4$^+$ cell counts (less than 50/mm^3) who have had a period of at least nine months with no AIDS-related symptoms. This group is quite rare because most people with CD4 counts of less than 50 are seriously symptomatic.[1] As was true for the LTS group, individuals in this "healthy low-CD4 group" (HLC) had to meet the inclusion criteria before starting on protease inhibitors. A third group of HIV-positive individuals has been used as a comparison

[a]Address for correspondence: George F. Solomon, M.D., 10724 Wilshire Blvd. #602, Los Angeles, CA 90024.

gfsolomon@pol.net

(COMP) group. This comparison group initially had CD4 counts of between 150 and 400/mm[3]; they are being followed longitudinally for three years. Over the past two years, we have begun reporting results contrasting the LTS ($n = 60$) versus COMP ($n = 120$) group and the HLC ($n = 60$) versus COMP ($n = 120$) groups on major psychological variables. The psychological variables examined in the comparisons involve four factors, which we hypothesized might be related to long survival: health care, connectedness, maintaining perspective, and life involvement.[2] So far, we have found some evidence for each of the factors. Long-term survivors were significantly higher than the comparison group in having a collaborative relationship with doctor,[3] being partnered, having high life involvement[4] and emotional expression;[5] and were significantly lower on hopelessness.[3] The healthy low-CD4 group, interestingly, had relatively preserved natural killer cell cytotoxicity (NKCC) and NK cell numbers, suggesting that NKCC may be a factor protecting the health of these people and compensating in some way for the loss in CD4 (helper T) cells.[6] Since NKCC is one of the immune variables for which there is strong evidence of a stress-immune connection,[7] we looked for psychological variables that might relate to this relative preservation. The HLC group had both lower perceived stress and lower depression than the COMP group.[8] Finally, the two unusual groups (LTS and HLC) were combined and compared across three subscales (compliance, defiance, collaboration) assessing their relationships with treating physicians. The "unusual" groups were significantly higher on the collaborative relationship with doctor scales.[3] Comparisons on other psychological characteristics revealed that the LTS+HLC group scored significantly higher on life involvement and on a composite of adaptive minus maladaptive coping scales. Both our study and other studies on long survivorship[2] lend support to the four factors noted above (health care, connectedness, maintaining perspective, and life involvement) and to the notion that psychosocial factors make important contributions to the maintenance of health and long survival with HIV/AIDS.

PSYCHONEUROIMMUNE PATHWAYS IN HIV

We have mentioned studies illustrating a prospective relationship between psychosocial factors and disease progression in HIV/AIDS and cited studies relating psychosocial factors to health and long survival. Let us now consider the immune pathways by which stress, distress, and poor coping might contribute to progression of HIV infection. There is ample literature, too great to review herein, showing there is an impact of stressors on the immune system in healthy people.[7,9]

PNI Studies in HIV Populations

The immune measures most affected by stress[7] that are particularly relevant to HIV infection include, but are not limited to, helper and cytotoxic T cells, T cell activity, NK cell activity, and herpes virus antibody titers. As noted, both stressors and distress have been related prospectively to CD4 decline. There are only a few studies relating psychological variables directly to other immune measures in HIV populations. Lower T cell proliferation to PHA was predicted by an increase in denial surrounding notification of HIV serostatus, and both lower proliferation to

PHA and denial increase predicted subsequent faster disease progression.[10] NK cell cytotoxicity has also been shown to be stress responsive in an HIV population; individuals receiving notification of HIV seropositivity had a significant drop in NKCC.[11] Furthermore, a stress management intervention using massage produced a significant increase in NKCC, as well as a significant increase in cytotoxic CD8 lymphocytes, providing more evidence of a stress-immune link in an HIV-positive population.[12] Finally, several studies have been done relevant to latent viruses in HIV. In a cross- sectional study of HIV-infected individuals, Robertson et al. found that distress was related to higher antibody titers (and, thus, poorer control of latent virus) for HSV but not EBV or CMV.[13] A stress management intervention with HIV-positive gay men had a favorable impact on EBV, HSV-2, and HHV-6 titers.[14,15] Thus, there are a number of immune measures for which there is a psychoimmune link in HIV populations, but more needs to be done to discern transduction of psychological influence into HIV-relevant immunological processes. As of yet, there is not adequate research in persons with HIV linking psychological stress to viral load, cytokine production, CD8 number and cytotoxicity, and percentage of "naïve" T cells.

Endocrine Linkages

Distress-related endocrine changes may also contribute to HIV progression either directly or through impacting the immune system. NK cell activity is synergistically inhibited by cortisol and HIV envelope peptide.[16] Corticosteroids impair many aspects of cellular immunity including NK cell activity, responsiveness to mitogens, cytokine production, and T cell populations.[17] Another stress hormone, norepinephrine, accelerates HIV replication via suppression of cytokine production.[18] Recently, there has been interest in the possible role of dehydroepiandrosterone (DHEA) in HIV.[19] DHEA has been shown to have inhibitory effects on HIV replication *in vitro,* and serum levels of DHEA may be an independent predictor of HIV progression. It is interesting to note that stress management interventions have been shown to have a significant impact in reducing cortisol[12,20] and in buffering a decrease in the DHEA/cortisol ratio seen in a nonintervention HIV-positive control group.[21]

CONCLUSION

Psychosocially influenced neuroendocrine-immune relationships appear to be quite relevant to the clinical course, morbidity, and mortality of HIV/AIDS. It is likely that sensitivity to psychosocial influences on health and longevity with HIV/AIDS will remain important even in the new era of highly active antiretroviral treatment.

ACKNOWLEDGMENT

We wish to thank the National Institute of Health for funding the research reported in the section on Psychology of Health and Long Survival with HIV/AIDS (RO1MH53791).

REFERENCES

1. MOSS, A.O., P. BACCHETTI & D. OSMOND. 1988. Seropositivity for HIV and development of AIDS or AIDS-related condition: three-year follow-up of the San Francisco General Hospital cohort. Br. Med. J. **296:** 745–752.
2. IRONSON, G., G. SOLOMON, D. CRUESS, J. BARROSO & M. STIVERS. 1995. Psychosocial factors related to long-term survival with HIV/AIDS. Clin. Psychol. Psychother. **2:** 249–266.
3. IRONSON, G., G. SOLOMON, E. BALBIN, C. O'CLEIRIGH, M. STIVERS, J. PAVONE, H. OHATA, N. SCHNEIDERMAN, N. KLIMAS & M.A. FLETCHER. 1998. Characteristics of long term survivors of AIDS. Presented at the annual meeting of the American Psychosomatic Society, Clearwater, FL, March 1998.
4. BALBIN, E, G. IRONSON, C. O'CLEIRIGH, J. PAVONE, M. STIVERS, J. OHATA, K. BAUM, N. SCHNEIDERMAN, M.A. FLETCHER & G. SOLOMON. 1998. Life involvement is associated with long term survival of patients with AIDS. Paper presented at the annual meeting of the Society of Behavioral Medicine, March, New Orleans, LA.
5. O'CLEIRIGH, C.M., G.H. IRONSON, E.G. BALBIN, J. OHATA, N. SCHNEIDERMAN, M.A. FLETCHER & G. SOLOMON. 1999. Emotional expression is associated with long-term survival of patients with AIDS. Poster presented at the annual meeting of the Society of Behavioral Medicine, San Diego, CA, April 1999.
6. IRONSON, G., E. BALBIN, M.A. FLETCHER, G. SOLOMON, P. GUEVARA & N. SCHNEIDERMAN. 1999. Relative preservation of natural killer cell cytotoxicity in healthy AIDS patients with low CD4 counts. Neuroimmunomodulation **6:** 226.
7. HERBERT, T.B. & S. COHEN. 1993. Stress and immunity in humans: a meta-analytic review. Psychosom. Med. **55:** 364–379.
8. BALBIN, E., G. IRONSON, G. SOLOMON, R. WILLIAMS & N. SCHNEIDERMAN. 1999. Low perceived stress and depression as protective factors in asymptomatic HIV+ people with CD4 counts under 50. Neuroimmunomodulation **6:** 204.
9. RABIN, B.S. 1999. Stress Immune Function and Health: The Connection. Wiley-Liss. Pittsburgh, PA.
10. IRONSON, G., A. FRIEDMAN, N. KLIMAS, M. ANTONI, M.A. FLETCHER, A. LaPERRIERE, J. SIMONEAU & N. SCHNEIDERMAN. 1994. Distress, denial, and low adherence to behavioral interventions predict faster disease progression in gay men infected with human immunodeficiency virus. Int. J. Behav. Med. **1:** 90–105.
11. IRONSON, G., A. LasPERRIERE, M. ANTONI, P. O'HEARN, N. SCHNEIDERMAN, N. KLIMAS & M.A. FLETCHER. 1990. Changes in immune and psychological measures as a function of anticipation and reaction to news of HIV antibody status. Psychosom. Med. **52:** 247–270.
12. IRONSON, G., T. FIELD, F. SCAFIDI, M. HASHIMOTO, M. KUMAR, A. KUMAR, A. PRICE, A. GONCALVES, I. BURMAN, C. TETENMAN, R. PATARCA & M.A. FLETCHER. 1996. Massage therapy is associated with enhancement of the immune system's cytotoxic capacity. Int. J. Neurosci. **84:** 205–217.
13. ROBERTSON, K.R., J.W. WILKINS, J. HANDY, C. VAN DER HORST, W.T. ROBERTSON, J.G. FRYER, D. EVANS & C.D. HALL. 1993. Psychoimmunology and AIDS: psychological distress and herpes simplex virus in human immunodeficiency virus–infected individuals. Psychol. Health **8:** 317–327.
14. LEVY, J.A., C.E. MACKEWICZ & E. BARKER. 1996. Controlling HIV pathogenesis: the role of the noncytotoxic anti-HIV response of CD8+ T cells. Immunol. Today **17**(50): 217–224.
15. LUTGENDORF, S.K., M.H. ANTONI, G. IRONSON, N. KLIMAS, M. KUMAR, K. STAN & P. McCABE. 1997. Cognitive-behavioral stress management decreases, dysphoric mood and herpes simplex virus-type 2 antibody titers in symptomatic HIV-seropositive gay men. J. Consult. Clin. Psychol. **35:** 31–43.
16. NAIR, M.P.N. & S.A. SCHWARTZ. 1995. Synergistic effect of cortisol and HIV-1 envelope peptide on the NK activity of normal lymphocytes. Brain Behav. Immun. **9:** 20–30.
17. CUPPS, T. & A. FAUCI. 1982. Corticosteroid-mediated immunoregulation in man. Immunol. Rev. **65:** 133–155.

18. COLE, S.W., Y.D. KORIN, J.L. FAHEY & J.A. ZACK. 1998. Norepinephrine accelerates HIV replication via protein kinase A–dependent effects on cytokine production. J. Immunol. **161:** 610–616.
19. RABKIN, J.G. & S.J. FERRANDO. 1997. DHEA and HIV illness. Aids Reader **7:** 28–36.
20. GOODKIN, K., D.J. FEASTER, D. ASTHANA, N.T. BLANEY, M. KUMAR, T. BALDEWICZ, R.S. TUTTLE, K.J. MAHER, M.K. BAUM, P. SHAPSHAK & M.A. FLETCHER. 1998. A bereavement support group intervention is longitudinally associated with salutary effects on the CD4 cell count and number of physician visits. Clin. Diagn. Lab. Immunol. **5:** 392–391.
21. CRUESS, D.G., M.H. ANTONI, M. KUMAR, G.H. IRONSON, P. MCCABE, J.B. FERNANDEZ, M.A. FLETCHER & N. SCHNEIDERMAN. 1999. Cognitive behavioral stress management buffers decreases in dehdroepiandrosterone sulfate (DHEA-S) and increases in the cortisol/DHEA-S ration and reduces mood disturbance and perceived stress among HIV-seropositive men. Psychoneuroendocrinology **24:** 537–549.

Cooperation of Pituitary Hormone Prolactin with Interleukin-2 and Interleukin-12 on Production of Interferon-γ by Natural Killer and T Cells

LINA MATERA[a] AND MARCELLA MORI

Department of Internal Medicine, University of Turin, Turin, Italy

ABSTRACT: The pituitary hormone prolactin (PRL) is also produced by cells of the immune system and participates in early and late T cell activating events. We have previously shown a modulatory role of PRL during maturation of dendritic cells (DC). Production of IL-12 by T cell receptor (TCR)–activated DC is necessary for T cells to acquire the Th1 cytokine (i.e., IFN-γ secreting) profile, which is associated with activation of cellular response. In a separate work, PRL has been shown to increase IFN-γ synthesis by natural killer (NK) cells. We have extended that study by exploring the ability of PRL to induce IFN-γ production by T and NK cells in the presence of the specific stimuli IL-12 and IL-2. The individual effect of PRL, IL-12, and IL-2 was specific for NK cells, and IL-2 and IL-12 were much more efficient than PRL. Cooperation of IL-2 and PRL was observed on NK cells. IL-2–induced synthesis of IFN-γ was increased by physiological concentrations of PRL but was unaffected or inhibited by high concentrations. By contrast, optimal enhancement of IL-12–induced IFN-γ release was observed with T cells but not with NK cells. Unexpectedly, interaction between PRL and IL-12 occurred only at high concentrations of PRL. These data indicate a complex role of PRL in the cytokine network and point to a revaluation of the proposed immunosuppression by stress-related hyperprolactinemia.

INTRODUCTION

Prolactin (PRL), a pituitary peptide hormone, has been shown to influence the development and function of immune cells. Hypophysectomized rats present abnormalities of the immune system, including increased thymic atrophy and lymphopenia, which can be restored after graft of syngeneic pituitary.[1] Severe anemia, immunological anergy, and death are observed when hypophysectomy is combined with anti-PRL antibody treatment, indicating the involvement of extra-pituitary PRL in maintenance of hemopoiesis and immunocompetence. PRL receptors (R) belong to the superfamily of receptors for the hemopoietin/cytokines and are expressed, although at low density, on B and T lymphocytes[2] and NK[3] cells and on hemopoietic

[a]Address for correspondence: Lina Matera, Department of Internal Medicine, University of Turin, Corso A.M. Dogliotti, 14, 10126 Turin, Italy. Voice: +39-011-696-1816; fax: +39-011- 663-4751

matera@molinette.unito.it

progenitors.[4] PRL has been shown to interact with hemopoietin and cytokines. The GM-CSF–induced development of erythroid cells *in vitro*[4] is increased by PRL through upmodulation of the EPO-R, and PRL has been shown to support the differentiation of erythroid progenitors in the absence of a functional erythropoietin (EPO) receptor.[5]

PRL acts in the immune system as a growth and differentiating factor for NK cells, either alone or in combination with IL-2, with which it shares target transcription factors. One of these, IRF-1, is the transcription factor for the perforin gene, which is activated by IFN-γ and IL-2 in NK cells.[6] IRF-1 is one of the first genes activated by PRL.[7] We have also shown that PRL induces the synthesis and release of IFN-γ by NK cells,[8] an activity that has been assigned to IL-2.[9–11] Redundancy is a common feature of cytokines, and in the case of PRL it may perhaps explain the failure to detect any disturbance in the immune system development and function of PRLR-deficient mice.[12] On the other hand, the existence of dose-specific interaction of PRL with other cytokines indicates that their coordinate action may be necessary in adult life to achieve a given function. An accurate study of the functional links of PRL with other cytokines will therefore shed light on the role of this hormone in the immune system. IL-12 shares many functions with IL-2,[13–15] including functional activation of and IFN-γ release by NK cells[16] and maturation of the Th1 cytokine profile.[17,18] Unpublished data from our laboratory have shown that PRL can induce maturation of Th1 (IFN-γ)– but not Th2 (IL-4)–secreting cells from blood cord lymphocytes. In addition to stimulating antitumor cytotoxixc cells, PRL may also act as a pro-inflammatory cytokine, through IL-2/IL-12-dependent/independent upmodulation of IFN-γ. Conceivably, enhancing versus suppressing effects of PRL depend on the concentration of the hormone in the circulation. Here we have shown the cooperative action of PRL and IL-2/IL-12 on the production of IFN-γ by mature NK and T cells from adult blood.

MATERIALS AND METHODS

Factors

Recombinant IL-2 was kindly provided by CHIRON (Chiron Italia S.r.l.), recombinant IL12 from NIBSC (National Institute for Biological Standars and Control, UK); extractive pituitary PRL was a gift from Genzyme Corporation (Framingham, MA).

Purification of NK and T cells

NK and T cells have been purified by heparinized blood of blood bank normal donors as previously described.[19] Briefly, PBL were isolated as a nonadherent population after a 2-h incubation of PBMC on plastic flasks. B cells were depleted by passage on a nylon wool column. The nonbinding cells were depleted of high-affinity E rosette-forming cells by Ficoll centrifugation (E_{HA}) and were used as the NK-enriched cell populations consisting of more than 70% CD16+CD56+, less than 2% CD3+ cells.[19] Purified (greater than 95% CD3+) T cells were obteined from the E_{HA} after osmotic lysis of contaminant sheep red blood cells.

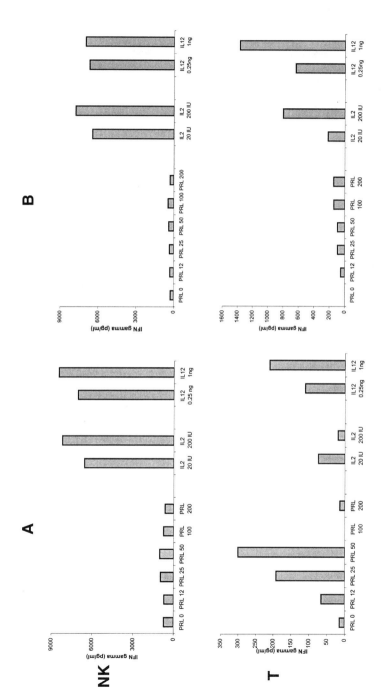

FIGURE 1. Individual effect of hPRL, rIL-2 and rIL-12 on the IFN-γ release by NK and T cells from two donors (A and B). NK and T cells were isolated and cultured in the presence or absence of PRL, rIL-2 (20 and 200 IU/mL) or IL-12 (0.25 and 1 ng/mL). After three days the supernatants were collected and tested for cytokine production by ELISA.

IFN-γ Release

IFN-γ release was detected in 100-mL culture supernatant freshly collected or kept at −20°C. IFN-γ was assessed by ELISA kits (Duoset, R&D, Minneapolis, MN).

RESULTS

Individual Effect of PRL, IL-2, and IL-12 on IFN-γ Release by NK and T Cells

The effect of the three cytokines alone on release of IFN-γ by NK and T cells was studied in two different donors. As shown in FIGURE 1, IL-2 and IL-12 were much more effective than PRL at stimulating the IFN-γ secretory activity of NK cells from both donors. By contrast, the effect of the three cytokines on T cells was donor dependent. A much higher IFN-γ release was in fact induced by PRL compared to IL-2 and IL-12 in T cells of donor B.

Comparative Effect of PRL on IFN-γ Release by NK and T Cells

PRL triggering of the signaling machinery requires dimerization by a single hormone molecule. This occurs at physiological concentrations, whereas in excess conditions every receptor becomes engaged and cross-linking cannot occur.[20] This is

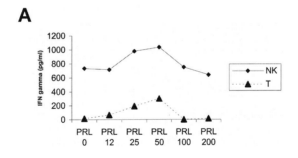

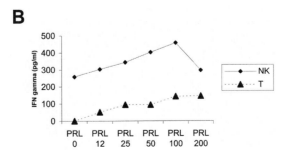

FIGURE 2. Pattern of IFN-γ release by NK and T cells upon hPRL stimulation in two different donors. NK and T cells were obteined as described in MATERIALS AND METHODS.

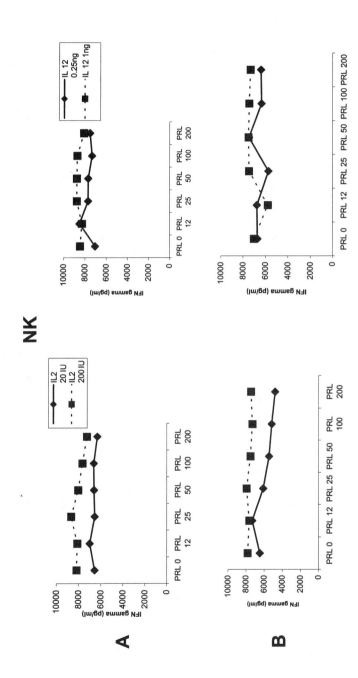

FIGURE 3. Combined effect of hPRL and rIL–2 (20 and 200 IU/mL) or rIL–12 (0.25 and 1 ng/mL) on IFN-γ release by NK cells.

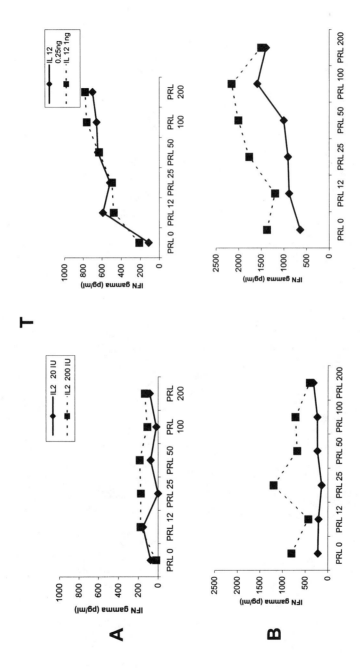

FIGURE 4. Combined effect of hPRL and rIL-2 (20 and 200 IU/mL) or rIL-12 (0.25 and 1 ng/mL) on IFN-γ release by T cells.

exemplified in FIGURE 2, which shows the pattern seen in two donors. Optimal IFN-γ release by NK cells peaked at 50 ng/ml (donor A) and 100 ng/ml (donor B), and baseline values were observed with the highest concentration of PRL. NK and T cells of donor A were activated by the same concentrations of PRL, whereas T cells of donor B were activated by 200 ng/ml in a dose-dependent fashion. The requirement for different concentrations of PRL may reflect a different number of PRL-R. In agreement with our previous data,[21] NK cells of both donors were far more responsive than T cells.

Combined Effect of PRL and IL-2

In both donors, physiological concentrations of PRL increased the IFN-γ release induced on NK cells by low concentrations of IL-2. A general trend of no effect to inhibition (FIGURE 3; donor B, IL-2 20 IU) was observed with the highest concentrations of PRL. No clear effect of PRL could be observed on T cells.

Combined Effect of PRL and IL-12

In contrast with the effect observed with IL-2, the effect of IL-12 was more evident on T cells. Only in donor A was the expected stimulation by physiological concentrations of PRL observed in NK cells cultured with low-dose IL-12. T cells of donor B were better stimulated by IL-12 than by IL-2, and the stimulatory activity of IL-12 was further increased by PRL, with an anusual peak at 100 ng/ml, FIGURE 4. In contrast with that observed with IL-2 (present data and Ref. 21) and with IL-12 on NK cells of donor B, the enhancing effect of PRL was observed with optimal concentrations of IL-12. Similar levels of IFN-γ release were induced by IL-2 and IL-12 on T cells of donor A, but these values were strongly increased (sixfold) by PRL only in IL-12 cultures. Again, this enhancing effect was seen at high PRL concentrations and was observed with either low or optimal concentrations of IL-12, FIGURE 4.

DISCUSSION AND PERSPECTIVES

The activity of cytokines in the immune system is characterized by pleiotropism and cooperation. One cytokine can act on the native as well as on the adaptive arms of the immune system, and a given action can be carried out by two or even more cytokines acting in concert. Sometimes this picture is quite complex. Upon antigen capture or microbial infection, DCs produce various cytokines, such as IL-12, that induce maturation of T lymphocytes towards the Th1 cytokine profile.[22] Th1 cytokines (mainly IFN-γ and IL-2) then induce the maturation of the effector cytotoxic T and NK cells. IL-12 itself can directly activate NK and T cells, either alone or in combination with IL-2.[21,23] Activation of cytotoxic cells by IL-2 and IL-12 is secondary to synthesis of IFN-γ, which, in turn, increases the cytotoxic function of NK and T cells by upmodulating the gene for perforin,[6] a key molecule in the lytic machinery.

Consistent evidence for a functional role of PRL in the immune system is its synergistic effect on the IL-2–induced activation of NK cells (LAK cells).[24] This PRL-induced NK enhancement can be neutralized by an anti–IFN-γ antibody, and new

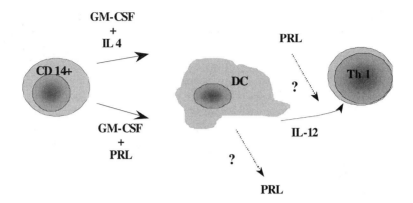

FIGURE 5. Model of the possible steps involving PRL action/release in the T cell activation pathway.

synthesis of IFN-γ has been demonstrated in NK cells after PRL activation.[8] Here we show that the synergistic effect of PRL can, at least in part, rest on upmodulation of IFN-γ secretion. However, the major finding with IFN-γ release is absence of enhancement or even inhibition of the IL-2 effect by high concentrations of PRL.

IL-2 and IL-12 are known to exert combined actions on NK and T cells.[15] It was of interest, therefore, to explore the possibile interaction between PRL and IL-12. Results show that while the individual effect of IL-2 and IL-12 is specifically and unequivocally directed to NK cells, cooperation of PRL with IL-2 and IL-12 can be differentiated on the basis of the cell population. Interaction with IL-2 was observed with NK cells, wherease interaction of PRL with IL-12 was observed with T cells, and this pattern was mutually exclusive. An indication of the cell specificity of the IL-12–PRL interaction was the absence of inhibition by high concentrations of PRL on the IL-12–induced IFN-γ production by NK cells. This was instead observed with T cells. Another distinguishing feature of the PRL effect on T cells was the enhancing effect of high concentrations of the hormone on IL-12 action. The selective cooperation of PRL and IL-2 on T cells is in line with our unpublished observation that PRL can interact with IL-12 during long-term maturation of Th1 cells. The stimulatory effects of high concentrations of PRL with IL-12, a DC cytokine, are reminiscent of the effect seen with maturation of DC from blood monocytes (in press). Together, these data confirm that PRL is minimally effective on the immune response when used alone and that its major individual effect is modulation of an ongoing response. The interactions of PRL with IL-2 and IL12 underlie different signaling mechanisms and different target cell populations and may offer a model to better define the biology of these two cytokines. Finally, the fact that high concentrations of PRL can depress NK IFN-γ while increasing T cell IFN-γ suggest a fine tuning of the immune response by PRL. A model of the possible steps involving PRL action/release in the T cell activation pathway is proposed in FIGURE 5. Further studies in this direction are needed to better define the role of PRL in the complex cytokine network and hence the immune consequences of transient (stress-related) or chronic hyperprolactinemia.

REFERENCES

1. NAGY, E. *et al.* 1991. Hypophysectomized rats depend on residual prolactin for survival. Endocrinology **128:** 2776–2784.
2. RUSSEL, D.H. *et al.* 1985. Prolactin receptors on human T and B lymphocytes: antagonism of prolactin binding by cyclosporin. J. Immunol. **134:** 3027–3031.
3. MATERA, L. *et al.* 1988. Prolactin receptors on large granular lymphocytes: dual regulation by cyclosporin A. Brain Behav. Immun. **2:** 1–10.
4. BELLONE, G. *et al.* 1995. Regulatory action of prolactin on the *in vitro* growth of CD34+ve human hemopoietic progenitor cells. J. Cell. Physiol. **163:** 221–231.
5. SOCOLOVSKY, M. *et al.* 1998. The prolactin receptor rescues EpoR-/-erythroid progenitors and replaces EpoR in a synergistic interaction with c-kit. Blood **92:** 1491–1496.
6. DUNCAN, G.S. *et al.* 1996. The transcription factor interferon regulatory factor–1 is essential for natural killer cell function *in vivo*. J. Exp. Med. **184:** 2043–2048.
7. YU-LEE, L.Y. 1997. Molecular actions of prolactin in the immune system. Proc. Soc. Exp. Biol. Med. **215:** 35–52.
8. MATERA, L. *et al.* 2000. Up-modulation of interferon-γ mediates the enhancement of spontanous cytotoxicity in prolactin-activated natural killer cells. Immunology. **98:** 386–392.
9. BIRON, C.A. *et al.* 1999. Natural killer cells in antiviral defense: function and regulation by innate cytokines. Annu. Rev. Immunol. **17:** 189–220.
10. FEHNIGER, T.A. *et al.* 1999. Costimulation of human natural killer cells is required for interferon gamma production [review]. Transplant. Proc. **31:** 1476–1478.
11. TUO, W. *et al.* 1999. Comparative effects of interleukin-12 and interleukin-4 on cytokine responses by antigen-stimulated memory CD4+ T cells of cattle: IL-12 enhances IFN-gamma production, whereas IL-4 has marginal effects on cytokine expression. J. Interferon Cytokine Res. **19:** 741–749.
12. BOUCHARD, B. *et al.* 1999. Immune system development and function in prolactin receptor–deficient mice. J. Immunol. **163:** 576–582.
13. TRINCHIERI, G. 1998. Immunobiology of interleukin-12 [review]. Immunol. Res. **17:** 269–278.
14. GATELY, M.K. *et al.* 1998. The interleukin-12/interleukin-12–receptor system: role in normal and pathologic immune responses. Annu. Rev. Immunol. **16:** 495–521.
15. HENNEMANN, B. *et al.* 1999. Expression of SCM-1alpha/lymphotactin and SCM-1beta in natural killer cells is upregulated by IL-2 and IL-12. DNA Cell. Biol. **18:** 565–571.
16. BILLIAU, A. *et al.* 1998. Immunomodulatory properties of interferon-gamma. An update [review]. Ann. N.Y. Acad. Sci. **856:** 22–32.
17. ROMAGNANI, S. 1991.Type 1 T helper and type 2 T helper cells: functions, regulation and role in protection and disease [review]. Int. J. Clin. Lab. Res. **21:** 152–158.
18. DEL PRETE, G. 1998. The concept of type-1 and type-2 helper T cells and their cytokines in humans [review]. Int. Rev. Immunol. **16:** 427–455.
19. MATERA, L. 1996. Role of prolactin in the *in vitro* development of interleukin-2–driven antitumoral lymphokine-activated killer cells. Immunology **89:** 619–626.
20. ELBERG, G. *et al.* 1990. Mitogenic and binding properties of monoclonal antibodies to the prolactin receptor in Nb2 rat lymphoma cells. J. Biol. Chem. **265:** 14770–14776.
21. CESANO, A. *et al.* 1994. Independent and synergistic effect of interleukin-2 and prolactin on development of T- and NK-derived LAK effectors. Immunopharmacology **28:** 67–75.
22. BANCHEREAU, J. & R.M. STEINMAN. 1998. Dendritic cells and the control of immunity. Nature **392:** 245–252.
23. MATERA, L. *et al.* 1992. Modulatory effect of prolactin on the resting and mitogen-induced activity of T, B and NK lymphocytes. Brain Behav. Immun. **6:** 409–417.
24. GAIDANO, G. *et al.* 1996. AIDS-related Burkitt's-type lymphomas are a target for lymphokine-activated killers induced by interleukin-2 and prolactin. Proc. Soc. Exp. Biol. Med. **213:** 196–205.

Role of Cyclophilins in Somatolactogenic Action

MICHAEL A. RYCYZYN[a] AND CHARLES V. CLEVENGER

Department of Pathology and Laboratory Medicine, University of Pennsylvania Medical Center, Philadelphia, Pennsylvania 19104, USA

ABSTRACT: Prolactin (PRL) and growth hormone (GH) are members of the somatolactogenic hormone family, the pleiotropic actions of which are necessary for vertebrate growth and mammary differentiation. The basis for the specific function of these hormones has remained uncertain; however, their action is associated with internalization and translocation into the nucleus. A yeast two-hybrid screen identified an interaction between PRL and cyclophilin B (CypB), a peptidyl prolyl isomerase (PPI) found in the endoplasmic reticulum (ER), extracellular space, and nucleus. The interaction between CypB and PRL/GH was confirmed *in vitro* and *in vivo* through the use of recombinant proteins and coimmunoprecipitation studies. The exogenous addition of CypB potentiated the proliferation of PRL- and GH-dependent cell lines 18- and 40-fold, respectively. The potentiation of PRL action by CypB was accompanied by a dramatic increase in the nuclear retrotranslocation of PRL. Immunogold electron microscopy has revealed this retrotransport to occur via a vesicular pathway. A CypB mutant, termed CypB-NT, was generated that lacked the putative wild-type N-terminal nuclear localization sequence. Although CypB-NT demonstrated levels of PRL binding and PPI activity equivalent to wild-type CypB, it was incapable of mediating the nuclear retrotranslocation of PRL or enhancing PRL-driven proliferation. These studies reveal CypB as an important chaperone facilitating the nuclear retrotransport and action of the somatolactogenic hormone family.

INTRODUCTION

The neuroendocrine hormone prolactin (PRL) was initially identified as being of pituitary origin;[1,2] however, synthesis of PRL is not limited to the pituitary, as expression has been detected in the decidua, breast, and T lymphocytes.[3–9] Initially, PRL was thought to function solely within the breast; however, the functional pleiotropism of PRL with regards to reproductive functions, osmoregulation, behavior, and immunoregulation was subsequently recognized.[10] Structural analysis of PRL has revealed it to be related to members of the cytokine/hematopoietin family such as growth hormone (GH), erythropoietin, granulocyte-macrophage colony stimulating factor (GM-CSF), and interleukins 2–7.[11]

[a]Address for correspondence: Michael A. Rycyzyn, Ph.D., Department of Pathology and Laboratory Medicine, University of Pennsylvania Medical Center, 510 Stellar-Chance Laboratories, 422 Curie Boulevard, Philadelphia, PA 19104. Voice: 215-898-0776; fax: 215-573-8944.

mrycyzyn@mail.med.upenn.edu

The effects of PRL are mediated through its receptor (prolactin receptor, PRLr), a member of the class I cytokine receptor family, which is present on numerous cell types including mammary epithelia, T and B lymphocytes, and macrophages.[12,13] The initial event in PRL signaling is the dimerization of the receptor,[14,15] which mediates the juxtaposition of the intracytoplasmic domains containing a region of membrane-proximal homology to other cytokine receptors—that is, box 1/variable box/box2 and X box. The box 1 and 2 motifs have been implicated in Jak2 binding and consist of hydrophobic/proline and hydrophobic/acidic residues, respectively. The box 1 motif is essential for PRLr function as its deletion abrogates PRLr function,[16] while tyrosine residues present with the C terminus of the rat PRLr may also contribute to the engagement of STAT5 and the activation of Jak2.[17] PRLr dimerization results in the rapid phosphorylation of the PRLr signaling domains[18] along with the activation of PRLr-associated kinases such as Jak2,[19,20] Fyn,[21] Shc-Grb2-Sos,[22] Vav,[23] and Bag-1/Bcl-2.[24] These activation events induce several signaling cascades resulting in the transactivation of the PRL-responsive gene loci involved in the proliferation and differentiation of mammary tissue.[21,26,27] These data indicate that PRL acts at the endocrine, paracrine, and autocrine levels in regulating T-lymphocyte proliferation and survival[28–31] and the terminal maturation of mammary tissues.[32,33]

PRL is internalized within 30 minutes of its addition to cells expressing PRLr. The internalization of both ligand and receptor into an endosomal/multivesicular body/lysosomal pathway is thought to be mediated by di-leucine motifs within the intracellular domain of the PRLr.[8,34,35] An appreciable amount of the internalized hormone can be stored by T cells for up to one week. Alone, PRL is weakly mitogenic to breast cancer cell cultures and nonmitogenic to cultures of murine T lymphocytes;[8,26] however, it does act as a potent comitogen with both interleukin (IL)–2 (on T cells) and epidermal growth factor (EGF, on human breast cancer cells). When both IL-2–stimulated T cells and EGF-stimulated breast cancer cells are cultured in media containing PRL, appreciable amounts of PRL (up to 10–20% of total intracellular PRL) can be detected within the cell nucleus by biochemical, immunofluorescent, and immunogold electron microscopy approaches.[8,35,36]

How could an extracellular hormone, such as PRL, undergo translocation into the cell nucleus? The internalization of proteins from the extracellular medium through a *trans*-Golgi/ER (endoplasmic reticulum) pathway into the cytosol or nucleus has been previously observed with several bacterial toxins and viral proteins, and is a process known as retrotranslocation.[37–40] The model most extensively studied regarding retrotranslocation is Shiga toxin. Studies have addressed this issue by generating Shiga toxin that contains known tyrosine sulfation and N-glycosylation sites.[39] Shiga toxin is known to enter cells by clathrin-coated pit-mediated endocytosis. When HeLa cells were cultured in defined medium containing ^{35}S-sulfate, retrotransport of the Shiga toxin from endosomes to the *trans*-Golgi network (TGN) was confirmed by the radiolabeling of the tyrosine sulfation site by the TGN-localized enzyme sulfotransferase. The retrotransport between the TGN and ER has been well characterized for resident proteins that carry retrieval signals—that is, KDEL. Shiga toxin has no such retrieval signal, but the retrotransport of Shiga toxin from the TGN to the ER was confirmed by N-glycosylation of the toxin. When a KDEL peptide was introduced into Shiga toxin, it had no effect on the kinetics of retrotransport; yet it did trap the toxin in the ER, while non–KDEL-containing toxin was free to pass through the ER. This indicates that known ER targeting signals are not necessarily needed in order for protein transport to the ER to take place. Lacking a KDEL sequence, colloidal gold-labeled PRL can be clearly visualized within the ER/Golgi apparatus within two hours after its internalization via a vesicular pathway, suggesting that its internalization may follow pathways parallel to Shiga toxin.

Previous work in our laboratory has shown that nuclear prolactin contributes to IL-2–stimulated proliferation by providing a necessary, but not sufficient, function within the cell.[41] In the absence of comitogenic stimulation (such as IL-2 or EGF), the nuclear retrotranslocation does not occur—an observation noted by other labs.[42] Retrotranslocation of PRL to the nucleus has been observed in several PRL-responsive tissues including the breast, T lymphocytes, liver,[43] ovary,[44] and adrenal.[45] Numerous other peptide hormones such as EGF, NGF, and PDGF,[46] insulin,[47] FGF,[48] and IL-5[49] have also been observed with the nucleus after their introduction into the extracellular medium. This would indicate that the nuclear retrotranslocation of peptide hormones is a widespread phenomenon that could regulate numerous physiologic processes.

IDENTIFICATION OF A PRL BINDING PROTEIN

Since PRL has neither an intrinsic enzymatic activity nor a recognizable nuclear localization signal sequence (NLS), we reasoned that the nuclear retrotranslocation and function of PRL must be mediated by the interaction of PRL with other proteins. To identify such proteins, a molecular screening approach using yeast two-hybrid analysis[50] was employed. When a human PRL "bait" construct was used to screen a cDNA library from Jurkat cells using standard approaches, fully 10% of the sequences obtained were full-length cyclophilin B (CypB). CypB is a 22-kDa member of the greater immunophilin family consisting of CypA-D, Cyp40, FK506 binding protein, and Tor.[51] The immunophilins are a family of peptidyl-prolyl isomerases (PPI) that serve as protein chaperones and mediate the effects of cyclosporin A (CsA), FK506, and rapamycin. Cyclophilin B is localized to the ER, nucleus, and extracellular space, where it can be found in breast milk and serum at concentrations of 150 ng/ml.[52] This interaction between PRL and CypB was specific, as reporter transactivation was not observed in single transfectants expressing either PRL or CypB, or with irrelevant baits (such as bicoid) cotransfected with CypB. This *in vivo*

TABLE 1. Functional characterization of the interaction between PRL and CypB

	Nb2 proliferation	Nuclear translocation	% Nuclear (+)	Nb2 growth	Jak2 Act.	K_D PRL-PRLr
PRL alone	+	+	10–20	+	+	1.46 nM
PRL + CypB[a]	++++	++++	95–100	++	+	1.2 nM
PRL + CypB-NT	+	±	<10	N.D.	N.D.	N.D.
CypB alone	−	−	0	−	−	N.D.

[a]CypB enhanced hGH-driven proliferation 40-fold.

interaction between CypB and PRL is novel and was subsequently confirmed *in vitro* using purified recombinant proteins (all data summarized in TABLE 1).

FUNCTIONAL CHARACTERIZATION OF THE PRL/CYPB INTERACTION

The interaction between PRL and CypB *in vitro* was examined using a typical "pull-down" assay. CypB does bind PRL *in vitro*; this interaction is increased approximately eightfold by the inclusion of Ca^{2+}, reducing reagent, or CsA. Pull-down experiments between CypA and PRL were also tested and failed to demonstrate any detectable binding of PRL and CypA. In parallel studies, the ability of GH, another somatolactogenic hormone, to directly interact with CypB was tested; like PRL, GH was found to interact directly with CypB. The exogenous addition of CypB at physiological concentrations into the defined medium of responsive cell lines potentiated PRL- and hGH-driven proliferation 18- and 40-fold, respectively. In the absence of ligand, CypB at any concentration was neither mitogenic for, nor toxic to the Nb2 cells, whereas the addition of varying concentrations of CypB had no effect on IL-2– or IL-3–driven proliferation. Therefore, it appears that somatolactogenic action is significantly potentiated by physiologic concentrations of CypB. Scatchard analysis revealed CypB did not alter the affinity of binding between PRL and its receptor, nor does CypB alter the activation of receptor-associated Jak2. This indicates that the potentiation of PRL signaling is not occurring due to an alteration of the receptor complex.

CypB MEDIATES THE NUCLEAR TRANSLOCATION OF PRL

Given the previous data from our laboratory and others indicating that a nuclear retrotranslocation of PRL occurred during the IL-2–driven proliferation of T cells and the EGF-driven proliferation of breast cancer cells, the effects of CypB and PRL on internalization were tested. The addition of exogenous PRL into the defined medium of T47D cells resulted in a primarily cytosolic internalization of ligand; however, 10–20% of the nuclei also demonstrated PRL accumulation. When costimulated with CypB, PRL internalization appeared to be quantitatively increased, with approximately 100% of the cell nuclei demonstrating intense anti-PRL indirect immunofluorescence. Confocal microscopic analysis confirmed PRL staining within the nuclear plane. An examination of the amino terminus of CypB revealed a putative nuclear localization sequence (NLS). A CypB mutant, termed CypB-NT, was generated that lacked this NLS, and its function was tested in both T47D and Nb2 cells. While this mutant exhibited the same PRL binding properties and enzymatic activity as wild-type CypB, the inclusion of CypB-NT into the culture medium resulted in the absence of detectable anti-PRL immunofluorescence in any nucleus with a corresponding loss of enhanced PRL-driven growth. This confirmed a role for the N terminus of CypB in the nuclear retrotransport of PRL and the growth-enhancing properties of nuclear PRL.

SUMMARY

PRL is a necessary hormone regulating the growth and differentiation of human breast epithelium and lymphocytes, with its effects being mediated through its receptor expressed throughout the body. PRL is also retrotranslocated into the cell nucleus of several PRL-responsive tissues as a function of comitogenic stimulation. The findings described above demonstrate that CypB significantly enhances cell proliferation driven by the PRL/PRLr complex at physiological concentrations and facilitates the internalization and nuclear retrotranslocation of PRL. Precedent data indicate that after internalization into endosomal compartments, this complex can retrotransport through the *trans*-Golgi network and into the ER. We speculate that the ER transporter complex Sec61 may assist in the translocation of the CypB/PRL complex into the cytosol. Indeed, a 22-kDa protein that exhibits PPI activity (CypB) has been shown to associate with the Sec61 complex along with nascent pre-PRL.[53] Such a pathway would allow PRL to move directly into the nucleus via the nuclear localization sequence within CypB. Although the specific function of the intranuclear PRL/CypB complex is unknown, previous data have indicated that cyclophilins can bind to and modulate the activity of transcription factors.[54] It is possible that intranuclear PRL may serve as a protein scaffold linking the PPI activity of CypB to transcription factors; yet we can not rule out the possibility that PRL may also be involved in modulating transcription factor activity directly. With the important physiologic and pathologic functions of PRL and GH, the modulation of the function of such intranuclear CypB-ligand complexes via CypB mutants or peptide analogs could be of appreciable therapeutic value. Thus, ongoing studies into the basis for ligand retrotranslocation should provide novel insights into the mechanisms and actions of the PRL/PRLr complex as well the larger cytokine/cytokine receptor superfamily to which it belongs.

ACKNOWLEDGMENTS

This work was supported by NIH Grants CA69294 and DK50771 (to C.V.C.), and F32 DK10043 (to M.A.R.).

REFERENCES

1. RIDDLE, O. & P.F. BRAUCHER. 1931. Studies on the physiology of reproduction in birds. XXX. Control of the special secretion of the crop-gland in pigeons by an anterior pituitary hormone. Am. J. Physiol. **97:** 617–625.
2. RIDDLE, O., R.W. BATES & S.W. DYKSHORN. 1933. The preparation, identification and assay of prolactin—a hormone of the anterior pituitary. Am. J. Physiol. **105:** 191–216.
3. CLEVENGER, C.V. & T.L. PLANK. 1997. Prolactin as an autocrine/paracrine growth factor in breast tissue. J. Mammary Gland Biol. Neoplasia **2:** 59–68. d
4. MERSHON, J., W. SALL, N. MITCHNER & N. BEN-JONATHON. 1995. Prolactin is a local growth factor in rat mammary tumors. Endocrinology **136:** 3619–3623.
5. DIMATTIA, G.E., B. GELLERSEN, H.G. BOHNET, & H.G. FRIESEN. 1986. A human B-lymphoblastoid cell line produces prolactin. Endocrinology **122:** 2508–2517.

6. GINSBURG, E. & B.K. VONDERHAAR. 1995. Prolactin synthesis and secretion by human breast cancer cells. Cancer Res. **55:** 2591–2595.

7. GELLERSEN, B., R. KEMPF, R. TELGMANN & G.E. DIMATTIA. 1994. Nonpituitary human prolactin gene transcription is independent of pit-1 and differentially controlled in lymphocytes and in endometrial stroma. Mol. Endocrinol. **8:** 356–373.

8. CLEVENGER, C.V., D.H. RUSSELL, P.M. APPASAMY & M.B. PRYSTOWSKY. 1990. Regulation of IL2-driven T-lymphocyte proliferation by prolactin. Proc. Natl. Acad. Sci. USA **87:** 6460–6464.

9. MONTGOMERY, D.W., C.F. ZUKOSKI, G.N. SHAH, A.R. BUCKLEY, T. PACHOLCZYK & D.H. RUSSELL. 1987. Concanavalin A–stimulated murine splenocytes produce a factor with prolactin-like bioactivity and immunoreactivity. Biochem. Biophys. Res. Commun. **145:** 692–698.

10. NICOLL, C.S. 1974. Physiological actions of prolactin. *In* Handbook of Physiology, Section 7: Endocrinology. R.O. Greep & E.B. Astwood, Eds.: 253–292. American Physiological Society. Washington, DC.

11. BAZAN, J.F. 1990. Haematopoietic receptors and helical cytokines. Immunol. Today **11:** 350–354.

12. DARDENNE, M., M.C.L. DEMORALES, P.A. KELLY & M.-C. GAGNERAULT. 1994. Prolactin receptor expression in human hematopoietic tissues analyzed by flow cytofluorometry. Endocrinology **134:** 2108–2114.

13. PELLEGRINI, I., J.-J. LEBRUN, S. ALI & P.A. KELLY. 1992. Expression of prolactin and its receptor in human lymphoid cells. Mol. Endocrinol. **6:** 1023–1031.

14. GERTLER, A., J. GROSCLAUDE, C.J. STRASBURGER, S. NIR & J. DJIANE. 1996. Real-time measurements of the interactions between lactogenic hormones and prolactin-receptor extracellular domains from several species support the model hormone-induced transient receptor dimerization. J. Biol. Chem. **271:** 24482–24491.

15. SOMMERS, W., M. ULTSCH, A.M. DEVOS & A.A. KOSSIAKOFF. 1994. The X-ray structure of a growth hormone-prolactin receptor complex. Nature **372:** 478–481.

16. LEBRUN, J.-J., S. ALI, A. ULLRICH & P.A. KELLY. 1995. Proline-rich sequence-mediated Jak2 association to the prolactin receptor is required but not sufficient for signal transduction. J. Biol. Chem. **270:** 10664–10670.

17. LEBRUN, J.-J., S. ALI, V. GOFFIN, A. ULLRICH, & P.A. KELLY. 1995. A single phosphotyrosine residue of the prolactin receptor is responsible for activation of gene transcription. Proc. Natl. Acad. Sci. USA **92:** 4031–4035.

18. CHANG, W.-P., Y. YE, & C.V. CLEVENGER. 1998. Stoichiometric structure/function analysis of the prolactin receptor signaling domains by receptor chimeras. Mol. Cell. Biol. **18:** 896–905.

19. CAMPBELL, G.S., L.S. ARGETSINGER, J.N. IHLE, P.A. KELLY, J.A. RILLEMA & C. CARTER-SU, 1994. Activation of JAK2 tyrosine kinase by prolactin receptors in Nb2 cells and mouse mammary gland explants. Proc. Natl. Acad. Sci. USA **91:** 5232–5236.

20. RUI, H., J.-J. LEBRUN, R.A. KIRKEN, P.A. KELLY & W.L. FARRAR. 1994. Jak2 activation and cell proliferation induced by antibody-mediated prolactin receptor dimerization. Endocrinology **135:** 1299–1306.

21. CLEVENGER, C.V. & M.V. MEDAGLIA. 1994. The protein tyrosine kinase p59^{fyn} is associated with prolactin receptor and is activated by prolactin stimulation of T-lymphocytes. Mol. Endocrinol. **8:** 674–681.

22. CLEVENGER, C.V., T. TORIGOE & J.C. REED. 1994. Prolactin induces rapid phosphorylation and activation of prolactin receptor associated Raf-1 kinase in a T-cell line. J. Biol. Chem. **269:** 5559–5565.

23. ERWIN, R.A., R.A. KIRKEN, M.G. MALBARA, W.L. FARRAR & H. RUI. 1995. Prolactin activates Ras via signaling proteins SHC, growth factor receptor bound 2, and son of sevenless. Endocrinology **136:** 3512–3518.

24. CLEVENGER, C.V., W. NGO, S.M. LUGER & A.M. GEWIRTZ. 1995. Vav is necessary for prolactin-stimulated proliferation and is translocated into the nucleus of a T-cell line. J. Biol. Chem. **270:** 13246–13253.

25. CLEVENGER, C.V., K. THICKMAN, W. NGO, W.-P. CHANG, S. TAKAYAMA & J.C. REED. 1997. Role of Bag-1 in the survival and proliferation of the cytokine-dependent lymphocyte line Ba/F3 and Nb2. Mol. Endocrinol. **11:** 608–618.

26. CLEVENGER, C.V., A.L. SILLMAN, J. HANLEY-HYDE & M.B. PRYSTOWSKY. 1992. Requirement for prolactin during cell cycle regulated gene expression in cloned T-lymphocytes. Endocrinology **130:** 3216–3222.

27. YU-LEE, L.Y. 1990. Prolactin stimulates transcription of growth-related genes in Nb2 T lymphoma cells. Mol. Cell. Endocrinol. **68:** 21–28.

28. GALA, R.R. 1991. Prolactin and growth hormone in the regulation of the immune system. Proc. Soc. Exp. Biol. Med. **198:** 513–527.

29. YU-LEE, L.Y. 1997. Molecular actions of prolactin in the immune system. Proc. Soc. Exp. Biol. Med. **215:** 35–52.

30. KOOIJMAN, R., E.L. HOOGHE-PETERS & R. HOOGHE. 1996. Prolactin, growth hormone, and insulin-like growth factor–1 in the immune system. Adv. Immunol. **63:** 377–454.

31. PRYSTOWSKY, M.B. & C.V. CLEVENGER. 1994. Prolactin as a second messenger for interleukin 2. Immunomethods **5:** 49–55.

32. KELLY, P.A., S. ALI, M. ROZAKIS, L. GOUJON, M. NAGANO, I. PELLEGRINI, D. GOULD, J. DJIANE, M. EDERY, J. FINIDORI & M.C. POSTEL-VINAY. 1993. The growth hormone/prolactin receptor family. Rec. Prog. Horm. Res. **48:** 123–164.

33. SHIU, R.P.C., L.C. MURPHY, D. TSUYUKI, Y. MYAL, M. LEE-WING & B. IWASIOW. 1987. Biological actions of prolactin in breast carcinoma. Rec. Prog. Horm. Res. **43:** 277–299.

34. VINCENT, V., V. GOFFIN, M. ROZAKIS-ADCOCK, J.-P. MORNON & P.A. KELLY. 1997. Identification of cytoplasmic motifs required for short prolactin receptor internalization. J. Biol. Chem. **272:** 7062–7068.

35. CLEVENGER, C.V., A.L. SILLMAN & M.B. PRYSTOWSKY. 1990. Interleukin-2 driven nuclear translocation of prolactin in cloned T-lymphocytes. Endocrinology **127:** 3151–3159.

36. RAO, Y.-P., D.J. BUCKLEY, M.D. OLSON & A.R. BUCKLEY. 1995. Nuclear translocation of prolactin: collaboration of tyrosine kinase and protein kinase C activation in rat Nb2 node lymphoma cells. J. Cell. Physiol. **163:** 266–276.

37. DE VIRIGLIO, M., H. WENINGER, & N.I. IVESSAR. 1998. Ubiquitination is required for the retrotranslocation of a short-lived luminal endoplasmic reticulum glycoprotein to the cytosol for degradation by the proteasome. J. Biol. Chem. **273:** 9734–9743.

38. HAZES, B. & R.J. READ. 1997. Accumulating evidence suggests that several AB toxins subvert the endoplasmic reticulum–associated protein degradation pathway to enter target cells. Biochemistry **36:** 11051–11054.

39. JOHANNES, L. & B. GOUD. 1998. Surfing on a retrograde wave: how does Shiga toxin reach the endoplasmic reticulum? Trends Cell Biol. **8:** 158–162.

40. WIERTZ, E.J.H.J., D. TORTORELLA, M. BOGYO, J. YU, , W. MOTHES, T.R. JONES, T.A. RAPAPORT & H.L. PLOEGH. 1997. Sec61-mediated transfer of a membrane protein from the endoplasmic reticulum to the proteasome for destruction. Nature **384:** 432–438.

41. CLEVENGER, C.V., S.W. ALTMANN & M.B. PRYSTOWSKY. 1991. Requirement of nuclear prolactin for interleukin-2–stimulated proliferation of T lymphocytes. Science **253:** 77–79.

42. PERROT-APPLANAT, M., O. GUALILLO, H. BUTEAU, M. EDERY & P.A. KELLY. 1997. Internalization of prolactin receptor and prolactin in transfected cells does not involve nuclear translocation. J Cell Sci. **110:** 1123–1132.

43. BUCKLEY, A.R., P.D. CROWE & D.H. RUSSELL. 1988. Rapid activation of protein kinase C in isolated rat liver nuclei by prolactin, a known hepatic mitogen. Proc. Natl. Acad. Sci. USA **85:** 8649–8653.

44. NOLIN, J.M. 1978. Intracellular prolactin in rat corpus luteum and adrenal cortex. Endocrinology **102:** 402–406.

45. NOLIN, J.M. 1980. Incorporation of regulatory peptide hormones by individual cells of the adrenal cortex: prolactin adrenocorticotropin differences. Peptides **1:** 249–255.

46. RAKOWICZ-SZULCZYNSKA, E.M., U. RODECK, M. HERLYN & H. KOPROWSKI. 1986. Chromatin binding of epidermal growth factor, nerve growth factor, and platelet-derived growth factor in cells bearing the appropriate surface receptors. Proc. Natl. Acad. Sci. USA **83:** 3728–3732.

47. SMITH, R.M. & L. JARETT. 1987. Ultrastructural evidence for the accumulation of insulin in nuclei of intact 3T3-L1 adipocytes by an insulin-receptor mediated process. Proc. Natl. Acad. Sci. USA **84:** 459–463.

48. BALDIN, V., A.M. ROMAN, I. BOSC-BIERNE, F. AMALRIC & G. BOUCHE. 1990. Translocation of bFGF to the nucleus is G1 phase cell cycle specific in bovine aortic endothelial cells. EMBO J. **9:** 1511–1517.

49. JANS, D.A., L.J. BRIGGS, S.E. GUSTIN, P. JANS, S. FORD & I.G. YOUNG. 1997. The cytokine interleukin-5 (IL-5) effects cotransport of its receptor subunits to the nucleus *in vitro*. FEBS Lett. **410:** 368–372.

50. FIELDS, S. & O.-K. SONG. 1989. A novel genetic system to detect protein-protein interactions. Nature **340:** 245–246.

51. SCHREIBER, S.L. 1991. Chemistry and biology of the immunophilins and their immunosuppressive ligands. Science **251:** 283–287.

52. ALLAIN, F., C. BOUTILLON, C. MARILLER & G. SPIK. 1995. Selective assay for CyPA and CyPB in human blood using highly specific anti-peptide antibodies. J. Immunol. Methods **178:** 113–120.

53. KLAPPA, R., R.B. FREEDMAN & R. ZIMMERMAN. 1995. Protein disulphide isomerase and a lumenal cyclophilin-type peptidyl-prolyl *cis-trans* isomerase are in transient contact with secretory proteins during late stages of translocation. Eur. J. Biochem. **232:** 755–764.

54. LEVERSON, J.D. & S.A. NESS. 1998. Point mutations in v-Myb disrupt a cyclophilin-catalyzed negative regulatory mechanism. Mol. Cell **1:** 203–211.

Prolactin Regulation of Apoptosis-Associated Gene Expression in T Cells

ARTHUR R. BUCKLEY[a,b,c] AND DONNA J. BUCKLEY[b]

[b]College of Pharmacy and [c]Department of Molecular and Cellular Physiology, College of Medicine, University of Cincinnati Medical Center, Cincinnati, Ohio 45267-0004, USA

ABSTRACT: Evidence accumulated over the last two decades indicates important actions for prolactin (PRL) in regulation of several functions of the immune system. That PRL can serve to facilitate immune cell proliferation is well established. In addition, PRL appears to play a salient role in the genesis and/or potentiation of certain autoimmune diseases. Recent evidence from several laboratories has extended the spectrum of PRL actions in immunological systems to include regulation of lymphocyte pool size through the process of apoptosis. Experimental results obtained using lactogen-dependent rat pre-T cell lines, the Nb2 lymphoma, have demonstrated that PRL suppresses cell death mechanisms activated by cytokine/hormone deprivation and cytotoxic drugs such as glucocorticoids. In this paper, we review results from studies conducted to investigate the mechanism(s) underlying PRL-regulated apoptosis suppression. Effects of the hormone on expression of apoptosis-associated genes of the Bcl-2 family as well as the protooncogene *pim-1* in proliferating Nb2 sublines and in cells exposed to apoptotic stimuli are presented. It is concluded that PRL-mediated apoptosis suppression in immune cells reflects a complex interaction among several gene products.

It is now well established that prolactin (PRL) plays a pivotal role in regulating the immune response.[1] Its administration to hypophysectomized rats restores immunocompetence,[2–4] and in combination with interleukin-2 (IL-2), phytohemagglutinin, and *Staphylococcus aurieus cowan,* it enhances mitogenesis in natural killer and T and B lymphocytes.[5,6] Rodent and human lymphocytes synthesize and secrete PRL[7–11] and express cell surface PRL receptors.[12,13] Moreover, PRL is directly mitogenic in the rat pre-T Nb2 lymphoma cell line,[14] a system in which IL-2 also stimulates proliferation.[15] Due to the robust proliferative response stimulated by PRL in this lactogen-dependent lymphoma, it has become a widely employed paradigm for the investigation of molecular mechanisms coupled to PRL receptor stimulation in T-lineage lymphocytes. The PRL receptor expressed in Nb2 cells has been cloned[16] and, together with its counterparts in other cells and tissues, has been found to be a member of the cytokine/hormone receptor superfamily that also includes the receptor for IL-2 and growth hormone.[17,18]

[a]Address for correspondence: Arthur R. Buckley, Ph.D., College of Pharmacy and Department of Molecular and Cellular Physiology, University of Cincinnati Medical Center, 3223 Eden Avenue, P.O. Box 670004, Cincinnati, OH 45267-0004. Voice: 513-558-2575; fax: 513-558-0978.

Arthur.Buckley@uc.edu

In addition to a role as a facilitator of immune cell proliferation, PRL may also represent a central determinant of lymphocyte pool size through its capacity to regulate apoptosis. Recent results obtained in our laboratory, as well as in those of others, indicate that PRL suppresses the cell death program activated by cytokine/ growth factor deprivation as well as that induced by cytotoxic drugs. Witorsch and coworkers[19,20] were the first to demonstrate that, just as with thymocytes, treatment of lactogen-starved Nb2 lymphoma cells with glucocorticoids, such as dexamethasone (DEX), produced cell death. These researchers subsequently demonstrated that the addition of PRL to the DEX-treated cultures blocked apoptosis. Since Nb2 lymphoma cells have been previously characterized as a pre-T lymphocyte at an intermediate stage of differentiation, these observations suggested that PRL may subserve the maintenance of certain T cell populations by suppressing apoptosis.

Apoptosis, a form of cellular self-destruction that is distinct from necrosis, is characterized by a number of specific morphological and biochemical changes. These include nuclear condensation and fragmentation, formation of apoptotic bodies, activation of specific proteases (caspases), and cleavage of genomic DNA.[21–23] Hydrolysis of DNA at polylinker regions yielding multiples of approximately 200-bp fragments is mediated by endogenous endonucleases presumably activated by apoptotic stimuli–induced cysteine proteases (caspases).[24] The process of apoptosis plays a central role in regulating the magnitude of specific cell populations under normal conditions such as during development of multicellular organisms. It may also be activated in cells during inflammatory and other physiological or pathological responses including cancer.[25,26] In the immune system, apoptosis underlies thymic selection of T lymphocytes. Therefore, the observation of a selective survival advantage afforded by PRL in the Nb2 paradigm suggested that in addition to regulation of growth- and differentiation-associated gene expression, it may also regulate transcription of genes that positively or negatively mediate apoptosis. In this paper, we discuss genes and gene families related to apoptosis regulation that appear to be controlled by PRL in Nb2 T cells.

PRL REGULATION OF bcl-2 FAMILY MEMBERS

The protein product of the founding member of the *bcl-2* gene family of apoptosis regulators is a 26-kDa membrane-associated protein that can complex with itself or dimerize with other homologous family members through an interaction involving several BH domains.[27–30] Originally identified as a protooncogene expressed in lymphoid neoplasia, Bcl-2 represents a well-characterized suppressor of apoptosis.[31,32] Unlike many other protooncogenes, its overexpression in tumors promotes cell survival but not proliferation. The accumulated evidence to date indicates that the relative levels of Bcl-2 and a second family member, Bax, are key determinants of whether cells succumb to apoptotic stimuli or survive. Thus, when Bax is expressed at elevated levels compared to Bcl-2, apoptosis is favored; if Bcl-2 predominates, cells are afforded a survival advantage.[27]

Prolactin deprivation for a period of 18–24 h induces growth arrest in the early G1 phase of the cell cycle in lactogen-dependent Nb2-11 cells. Stimulation with nanogram quantities of PRL reinitiates cell cycle progression in a partially synchronous manner. This characteristic has resulted in the wide use of this model to investigate signaling mechanisms and gene expression triggered as a consequence of PRL-stimulated proliferation. Notably, prolonged culture of Nb2 cells in the absence of hormone activates apoptosis coupled to cell cycle arrest.[19,33] To determine whether *bcl-2* or *bax* were expressed in such quiescent cells and to assess whether PRL altered the expression of either apoptosis-associated gene, stationary Nb2-11 cells were employed in initial experiments.

Three *bcl-2* transcripts (9.4, 7.3, and 4.2 kb) were observed by Northern blot analysis to be expressed in the Nb2-11 cell line.[34] Each was present at nearly undetectable levels in quiescent cells. However, the addition of PRL to the cultures stimulated a time- and concentration-dependent accumulation of the *bcl-2* mRNAs.[34] Maximally increased *bcl-2* expression was observed within 2–4 h subsequent to hormone addition, with maximal protein expression occurring by six hours. Prolactin-induced *bcl-2* expression appeared to be a direct effect of the hormone and not due to increased stability of its mRNA.[34]

A 1.0-kb *bax* transcript was also detected in stationary Nb2-11 cells. Its expression increased slowly with time subsequent to PRL treatment, with maximal levels observed at 8–12 hours. In contrast, the Bax protein, although apparent in quiescent cells, decreased to undetectable levels 4–6 h following PRL treatment but was again detectable two hours later.[34]

In quiescent cells, a condition that favors a modest induction of apoptosis, Bcl-2 was depressed while Bax was expressed at higher levels. In contrast, PRL treatment, which stimulates a growth response in addition to cellular survival, rapidly augmented the Bcl-2:Bax ratio. Thus, these observations suggested that the mechanism by which PRL inhibits apoptosis provoked by growth factor/cytokine deprivation involved its direct signaling to the *bcl-2* gene to increase its transcription together with the simultaneous attenuation of Bax.

Glucocorticoids also activate cell death in Nb2 cells, and this effect can be antagonized by PRL. Treatment of stationary Nb2-11 cells with the potent glucocorticoid DEX causes time- and concentration-dependent fragmentation of DNA. Addition of PRL at concentrations that only minimally stimulate proliferation (0.1 ng/mL), significantly abrogated the cytolytic effects of DEX.[33] Upon further evaluation, PRL was found to be required during the initial six hours subsequent to the addition of the glucocorticoid to be effective, suggesting that its suppression of apoptosis most likely reflected rapid accumulation of suppressor or a decreased expression of facilitory proteins. While a modest, twofold increase in *bax* mRNA was observed 6–12 h following the addition of PRL to DEX-treated Nb2-11 cultures, its protein level remained unchanged. However, PRL enhanced *bcl-2* transcripts to a level sixfold above those observed in cultures treated with DEX alone within six hours. Importantly, the observed increase in its mRNA resulted in significant accumulation of the Bcl-2 protein with similar kinetics.[33] Therefore, the requirement for PRL during the initial six hours following exposure of the cells to DEX, together with the observation that just as with cells cultured with PRL only, hormone addition to DEX-treated cultures increased Bcl-2 levels relative to those of Bax, strongly suggested that cell survival afforded by PRL may reflect an important contribution by this oncoprotein.

The expression of other Bcl-2 family members was also assessed including *mcl-1, bad,* and *bcl-x_L,* in the Nb2 paradigm.[35] Expression of *mcl-1* transcripts was detected;

it was constitutive and did not appear to be significantly altered by PRL. Moreover, *bad* mRNA was undetectable by Northern blot analysis. Of the Bcl-2 family members evaluated, only $bcl-x_L$ was found to be responsive to hormone treatment.

Similar to the antiapoptotic actions of *bcl-2*, $bcl-x_L$ is a suppressor of this process that interacts with BH domains present within other family members.[36] $Bcl-x_L$ also has been reported to suppress redistribution of cytochrome c, a proapoptotic event,[37–39] and may interfere with the activation of certain caspases.[40] In exponentially proliferating Nb2-11 cells, its mRNA was readily detected but was absent in stationary cultures. However, treatment with PRL provoked a 20-fold increase in the level of its transcript within four hours, which was similar to results obtained with respect to *bcl-2*.[34,35] Moreover, its protein product accumulated to levels sixfold above those observed in stationary cultures by six hours subsequent to addition of PRL. However, in contrast to Bcl-2, this effect of PRL appeared to be indirect, since cycloheximide-mediated inhibition of protein synthesis reduced the level of the $Bcl-x_L$ protein by more than 50 percent.[35] Notably, neither the stimulatory effect of PRL on $bcl-x_L$ mRNA expression nor its protein product was altered by DEX. Therefore, at least two protein members of the *bcl-2* family—Bcl-2 and Bcl-x$_L$—may participate by suppressing apoptosis activated in Nb2-11 cells under the conditions of lactogen deprivation or following exposure to DEX.

PROLACTIN REGULATION OF *pim-1* EXPRESSION

The protooncogene *pim-1* encodes a conserved cytosolic serine-threonine kinase that is expressed in myeloid and lymphoid tissues and is thought to be required for lymphocyte activation.[41,42] Its expression is induced by cytokines including interleukins and colony-stimulating factors, as well as by erythropoietin.[43,44] Originally identified in malignant lymphomas,[45] *pim-1* has been linked to proliferation[43,44] as well as to apoptosis in hematopoietic cells.[46] Since its expression had been previously linked to activation of cytokine/hormone family receptors in lymphoid cells, we sought to determine whether PRL similarly affected *pim-1* in Nb2 cell lines.[47]

Expression of *pim-1* mRNA and protein in early G1-arrested Nb2-11 cells was nearly undetectable. However, the addition of PRL to these quiescent cultures rapidly stimulated its accumulation. Increased *pim-1* mRNA was observed as early as 15 min following PRL and reached levels nearly 60-fold above that found in control cultures within 4 hours. Interestingly, PRL induced a biphasic response with respect to gene activation; its initial peak preceded a second rise in the level of its mRNA at 12–18 hours. Results from [^{3}H]-thymidine pulse-labeling experiments revealed that the early PRL-stimulated mRNA peak corresponded with early–mid–G1 cell cycle progression, while the later, second increase occurred during the G1/S phase transition. Treatment of quiescent cells with IL-2, which also elicits a proliferative response in these cells,[15] similarly induced the initial peak in *pim-1* expression, although the subsequent rise in its level was less apparent. Results from other experiments revealed that PRL-induced *pim-1* expression was a concentration-dependent, direct effect of the hormone and not due to increased stability of its mRNA. These results suggested that, similar to interferon factor-1 and *c-myc*,[48,49] *pim-1* represented a PRL-regulated immediate–early gene.

Pim-1 expression was also studied in Nb2-11 cells exposed to the apoptotic stimulator DEX.[33] Here, PRL markedly increased its expression 15-fold again within four hours, followed by a second peak in the level of its transcript at 12 hours. In addition, significantly elevated levels of the Pim-1 protein accumulated in parallel to the observed alterations in its mRNA in cells treated with DEX in combination with PRL.

Expression of *pim-1* was also investigated in the PRL-independent Nb2-SFJCD1 subline. This cell line, produced by prolonged lactogen starvation of a PRL-dependent line and cloning of surviving cells,[50] proliferates in the complete absence of added mitogen and is resistant to glucocorticoid-induced apoptosis.[20,51,52] Karyotypic analysis showed that the Nb2-11 and Nb2-SFJCD1 cell lines exhibit many chromosomal alterations identical to those of the parental, PRL-dependent cell line plus several additional changes indicating that they arose from the latter line via clonal evolution.[50] In control Nb2-SFJCD1 cultures, *pim-1* expression was found to be constitutive; it was augmented by the addition of PRL in a biphasic manner with kinetics similar to those observed in its PRL-dependent counterpart.[47]

Previously, Gout[51] demonstrated that culturing autonomous Nb2-SFJCD1 cells in the presence of butyrate (BT), a naturally occurring four-carbon fatty acid produced endogenously by bacterial fermentation of dietary fiber, arrested growth and induced transient reversion of this line to a PRL-dependent phenotype. Just as with the effect of lactogen withdrawal in Nb2-11 cells, exposure of Nb2-SFJCD1 cultures to BT arrested their growth early in the G1 phase of cell cycle;[53] introduction of PRL to such cultures reinitiated cell cycle progression.[51,53] Presumably as a consequence of cell cycle arrest, BT also profoundly reduced the expression of *pim-1* as well as of *c-myc* at the mRNA and protein levels. Similarly to the effect of PRL on proliferation in BT-pretreated cultures, hormone stimulation produced a rapid rise in the level of expression of each protooncogene.[53]

In other studies, the effect of BT was determined on the sensitivity of Nb2-SFJCD1 cells to apoptotic stimuli.[52] It was found that exposure to BT, in addition to causing cell cycle arrest, increased the basal level of apoptotic cells in the cultures by nearly sixfold. Thus, in a small but significant population of cells, the death program was activated by the fatty acid. More importantly, however, it was observed that DEX profoundly activated apoptosis in a concentration-dependent manner in the previously resistant cells. Moreover, the addition of PRL abrogated this effect of the glucocorticoid. The results from time-course experiments indicated that, similar to its demonstrated effect in PRL-dependent Nb2-11 cells, the presence of hormone was required within the first six hours following the addition of DEX to suppress its activation of apoptosis. These results suggested that PRL-coupled apoptosis gene expression was most likely occurring within this early temporal window similar to its requirement in lactogen-dependent cells.

The expression of the Bcl-2 family genes, *bcl-2* and *bax,* as well as *pim-1* were studied to determine whether the alterations in their expression subsequent to the addition of PRL to DEX-treated Nb2-11 cultures were also apparent in BT-pretreated Nb2-SFJCD1 cells under similar conditions.[52] The expression of *bax* at both the mRNA and protein levels was found to be unaltered by the addition of DEX-alone or it in combination with PRL. A 50% reduction in *bcl-2* mRNA was observed in DEX-treated cultures; nevertheless, it did not appear to produce any deviation in the level of its protein product. The addition of PRL also failed to increase Bcl-2 protein. Thus, in BT-pretreated Nb2-SFJCD1 cells treated with DEX alone or with DEX+PRL the Bcl-2:Bax ratio remained unchanged compared to control cultures. These results lead us to conclude that these two apoptosis-regulatory proteins most likely did not contribute to the anti-apoptotic effect afforded by PRL in these BT-pretreated cells.

Compared to the expression of the Bcl-2 family members, *pim-1* was markedly altered by PRL in autonomous cells previously treated with BT, then challenged with DEX. Increased *pim-1* mRNA was apparent within 1 h and reached significantly elevated levels (fivefold) within 4 h following the addition of DEX+PRL. More importantly, the presence of PRL in the DEX-treated cultures triggered a marked increase in Pim-1 protein synthesis within the same time period. Thus, PRL provoked increased transcription/translation of *pim-1* in the presence of a potent apoptotic stimulus, suggesting an important role for this kinase as a mediator of lactogen-provoked suppression of the death program.

PRL SIGNALING TO APOPTOSIS SUPPRESSION

In numerous previous studies, lactogen-stimulated Nb2 cells have been utilized to investigate PRLR activation of signal transduction pathways linked to regulation of specific gene transcription. To date, PRL has been reported to activate several tyrosine kinases (Jak2,[54–56] FYN,[57] and ZAP-70[58,59]) serine-threonine kinases (MAPK,[60] protein kinase C,[61] S6 kinase,[62] and phosphatidylinositol 3-kinase[63]) and guanine nucleotide proteins (Ras[64,65] and Vav[66]). Of the pathways investigated, activation of Jak2 tyrosine kinase and its subsequent phosphorylation of signal transducers and activators of transcription (Stat)-family member transcription factors have been most commonly implicated in the expression of PRL-responsive genes.[67] Moreover, in several hematopoietic cell systems, *pim-1* has been reported to be regulated by this signaling mechanism.[68,69] Since the 5'-promoter region of the *pim-1* gene contains several γ-interferon activation sequences (GAS) that specifically bind Stat factors to stimulate transcription, it appeared likely that its PRL-induced expression most likely reflected activation of Jak/Stat.

To test this hypothesis, promoter/reporter experiments employing a 1268-bp segment upstream of the transcription initiation site of the *5'-pim-1* promoter were conducted using a premyeloid cell line (FDC/Nb2) that stably expresses the Nb2 form of the PRL receptor. A series of deletion mutants of the promoter were transiently transfected into the cells, and the effect of PRL addition was determined on reporter gene expression. The results indicated that two elements [distal (DE), −427 to −336 bp and proximal (PE), −104 to −1], but not several GAS or GAS-like sequences, were required for promoter activation by PRL.[70] In other experiments, the effect of PRL to stimulate transcription factors present within Nb2-11 cells to bind to the DE and PE was evaluated by gel mobility shift analysis. The results indicated that factors within PRL-treated Nb2 cells rapidly and specifically bound to these promoter sequences; however, no binding was observed to GAS-like sequences present within the promoter. Finally, results from DNAse I protection experiments revealed a nuclear factor–1 (NF-1)–like motif within the promoter that appeared to repress *pim-1* expression in unstimulated Nb2 cells. Treatment with PRL produced a time-dependent reduction in protein binding to the *pim-1* NF-1–like segment. From these results we concluded that the PRLR induces *pim-1* expression by a mechanism that involves activation of specific transcription factors that stimulate the DE and PE and derepress the NF-1–containing element. Therefore, it appears that mechanisms independent of the Jak2/Stat signaling pathway are most likely responsible for PRL-induced transcription of *pim-1*.

SUMMARY

The accumulated evidence to date suggests a role for at least three gene products—*bcl-2, bcl-xL,* and *pim-1*—in PRL-mediated suppression of apoptosis in T-lineage lymphocytes. Each of these was rapidly induced by PRL in quiescent Nb2 T cells within the six hour time period demonstrated to be critical for hormone-mediated cytoprotection. Moreover, the expression of each was induced by lactogen treatment in Nb2-11 cells under conditions in which apoptosis was activated. However, while increased levels of *bcl-2* mRNA were observed following addition of PRL to DEX-treated Nb2-SFJCD1 cells previously exposed to BT, the level of its protein remained unchanged, resulting in a static Bcl-2:Bax ratio. This observation suggests that this protooncogene may not represent a key intermediate in apoptosis suppression in this system. Notably, quite different results were obtained when expression of $bcl-x_L$ was determined under similar conditions. Prolactin increased its mRNA and protein levels as an early consequence of hormone exposure in DEX-treated cells, indicating that this Bcl-2 family member may participate in lactogen-mediated apoptosis suppression.

The demonstrated effects of PRL on Bcl-2 family member apoptosis suppressors notwithstanding, the results obtained also strongly suggest that the protein product of the *pim-1* protooncogene is a key mediator of apoptosis suppression in the Nb2 paradigm. First, its expression was rapidly stimulated by PRL in lactogen-deprived and DEX-treated Nb2-11 cells, conditions that favor apoptosis. Second, Pim-1 was constitutively expressed at relatively high levels in apoptosis-resistant Nb2-SFJCD1 subline. Third, marked attenuation in expression of Pim-1 accompanied BT-treatment of this line, causing the cells to revert to an apoptosis-sensitive phenotype. Fourth, addition of PRL to BT-pretreated Nb2-SFJCD1 cells exposed to glucocorticoid was rapidly followed by marked expression of *pim-1* at the mRNA and protein levels. Finally, PRLR signaling to *pim-1* transcription reflected a union of positive and negative transcription factor influences that appear to be distinct from the Jak/Stat pathway. Thus, it can be concluded from these observations that PRL directly signals to activate *pim-1* transcription, and the resulting increase in its protein product mediates apoptosis suppression by phosphorylating key, yet to be defined, cellular proteins that are critical to progression of the apoptotic program.

Recent evidence provided by Clevenger and coworkers[71] suggested that yet another protein—Bag-1, a Bcl-2–associated protein that has also been linked to signaling by the serine kinase Raf-1—may participate in growth and survival functions of PRL in Nb2 cells. Its level of expression was reported to be diminished in lactogen-dependent cells upon withdrawal of PRL or the addition of DEX. In glucocorticoid-resistant Nb2-SFJCD1 cells, neither condition affected its level of expression. Taken together, PRL appears to regulate a spectrum of apoptosis-associated intermediates to facilitate survival in cells in which the death program has been activated. These range from direct mediators of the apoptotic process itself ($Bcl-x_L$) to associated proteins (Bag-1) and those responsible for modulation of signaling mechanisms (Pim-1, Bag-1). Future studies will likely focus upon determining the relationships among these proteins and others in mediating PRL-regulated apoptosis suppression.

ACKNOWLEDGMENT

This work was supported in part by NIH Grant DK53452 and a grant from the Ohio Cancer Research Associates.

REFERENCES

1. YU-LEE, L-Y. 1997. Molecular actions of prolactin in the immune system. Proc. Soc. Exp. Biol. Med. **215:** 35–52.
2. BERCZI, I., E. NAGY, K. KOVACS & E.HORVATH. 1981. Regulation of humoral immunity in rats by pituitary hormones. Acta Endocrinol. **98:** 506–513.
3. NAGY, E. & I. BERCZI. 1981. Prolactin and contact sensitivity. Allergy **36:** 429–432.
4. BERCZI, I., E.NAGY, S.L. ASA & K. KOVACS. 1984. The influence of pituitary hormones on adjuvant arthritis. Rheumatology **27:** 682–688.
5. MATERA, L., A. CASANO, G. ELLONE & E. OOBERHOLTZER. 1992. Modulatory effect of prolactin on the resting and mitogen-induced activity of T, B, and NK lymphocytes. Brain Behav. Immun. **6:** 409–417.
6. ATHREYA, B.H., J. PLETCHER, F. ZULIAN, D.B. WEINER & W.V. WILLIAMS. 1993. Subset-specific effects of sex hormones and pituitary gonadotropins on human lymphocyte proliferation *in vitro*. Clin. Immunol. Immunopathol. **66:** 201–211.
7. MONTGOMERY, D.W., C.F. ZUKOSKI, G.N. SHAH, A.R. BUCKLEY, T. PACHOLECYZK & D.H. RUSSEL. 1987. Concanavalin A stimulated murine splenocytes produce a factor with prolactin-like bioactivity and immunoreactivity. Biochem. Biophys. Res. Commun. **145:** 692–698.
8. O'NEAL, K.D., D.W. MONTGOMERY, T.M. TRUONG & L-Y. YU-LEE. 1992. Prolactin gene expression in human thymocytes. Mol. Cell. Endocrinol. **87:** R19–R23.
9. MONTGOMERY, D.W., G.K. SHEN, E.D. ULRICH, L.L. STEINER, P.R. PARISH & C.F. ZUKOSKI. 1992. Human thymocytes express a prolactin-like messenger ribonucleic acid and synthesize bioactive prolactin-like proteins. Endocrinology **131:** 3019–3026.
10. SABHARWAL, P., R.GLASER, W. LAFUSE, S. VARMA, Q. LIA, S. ARKINS, R. KOOIJMAN, L. KUTZ, K.W. KELLEY & W.B. MALARKEY. 1992. Prolactin synthesized and secreted by human peripheral blood mononuclear cells: an autocrine growth factor for lymphoproliferation. Proc. Natl. Acad. Sci. USA **89:** 7713–7716.
11. PELLEGRINI, I., J.J. LABRUN, S. ALI & P.A. KELLY. 1993. Expression of prolactin and its receptor in human lymphoid cells. Mol. Endocrinol. **6:** 1023–1031.
12. RUSSELL, D.H., R. KIBLER, L. MATRISIAN, D.F. LARSON, B. POULOS & B.E. MAGUN. 1985. Prolactin receptors on human T and B lymphocytes: antagonism of prolactin binding by cyclosporine. J. Immunol. **134:** 3027–3031.
13. GAGNERAULT, M-C., P. TOURINE, W. SAVINO, P.A. KELLY & M. DARDENNE. 1993. Expression of prolactin receptors in murine lymphoid cells in normal and autoimmune situations. J. Immunol. **150:** 5673–5681.
14. GOUT, P.W., C.T.BEER & R.L. NOBEL. 1980. Prolactin-stimulated growth of cell cultures established from malignant Nb2 rat lymphomas. Cancer Res. **40:** 2433–2436.

15. CROZE, F., A. WALKER & H.G. FRIESEN. 1988. Stimulation of growth of Nb2 lymphoma cells by interleukin-2 in serum-free and serum-containing media. Mol. Cell. Endocrinol. **55:** 253–259.
16. ALI, S., I. PELLEGRINI & P.A. KELLY. 1991. A prolactin-dependent immune cell line (Nb2) expresses a mutant form of prolactin receptor. J. Biol. Chem. **266:** 20110–20117.
17. KELLY, P.A., J. DJIANE, D. BANVILLE, S. ALI, M. EDERY & M. ROZAKIS. 1991. The growth hormone/prolactin receptor gene family. Endocr. Rev. **12:** 235–251.
18. PAUL, W.E. & R.A. SEDER. 1994. Lymphocyte responses and cytokines. Cell **76:** 241–251.
19. FLETCHER-CHIAPPINI, S.E., M.M. COMPTON, H.A. LA VOIE, E.B. DAY & R.J. WITORSCH. 1993. Glucocorticoid-prolactin interactions in Nb2 lymphoma cells: antiproliferative versus anticytolytic effects. Proc. Soc. Exp. Biol. Med. **202:** 345–352.
20. WITORSCH, R.J., E.B. DAY, H.A. LA VOIE, N. HASHEMI & J.K. TAYLOR. 1993. Comparison of glucocorticoid-induced effects in prolactin-dependent and autonomous rat Nb2 lymphoma cells. Proc. Soc. Exp. Biol. Med. **203:** 454–460.
21. KERR, J.F., A.H. WYLLIE & A.R. CURRIE. 1972. Apoptosis: a basic biological phenomenon with wide-ranging implications in tissue kinetics. Br. J. Cancer **26:** 239–257.
22. RAFF, M.C. 1992. Social controls on cell survival and cell death. Nature **356:** 397–400.
23. PEITSCH, M.C., C. MULLER & J. TSCHOPP. 1993. DNA fragmentation during apoptosis is caused by frequent single-strand cuts. Nucleic Acids Res. **21:** 4206–4209.
24. ENARI, M., H. SAKAHIRA, H. YOKOYAMA, K. OKAWA, A. IWAMATSU & S. NAGATA. 1998. A caspase-activated DNase that degrades DNA during apoptosis, and its inhibitor ICAD. Nature **391:** 43–50.
25. KERR, J.F., C.M. WINTERFORD & B.V. HARMON. 1994. Apoptosis. Its significance in cancer and cancer therapy. Cancer **73:** 2013–2026.
26. THOMPSON, C.B. 1995. Apoptosis in the pathogenesis and treatment of disease. Science **267:** 1456–1462.
27. OLTVAI, Z.N., C.L. MILLIMAN & S.J. KORSMEYER. 1993. Bcl-2 heterodimerizes *in vivo* with a conserved homolog, Bax, that accelerates programmed cell death. Cell **74:** 609–619.
28. OHTA, K., K. IWAI, Y. KASAHARA, N. TANIGUCHI, S. KRAJEESKI, J.C. REED & T. MIYAWAKI. 1995. Immunoblot analysis of cellular expression of Bcl-2 family proteins, Bcl-2, Bax, Bcl-X and Mcl-1, in human peripheral blood and lymphoid tissues. Int. Immunol. **7:** 1817–1825.
29. YIN, X.M., Z.N. OLTVAI & S.J. KORSMEYER. 1994. BH1 and BH2 domains of Bcl-2 are required for inhibition of apoptosis and heterodimerization with Bax. Nature **369:** 321–323.
30. ZHA, H., C. AIME-SEMPE, T. SATO & J.C. REED. 1996. Proapoptotic protein Bax heterodimerizes with Bcl-2 and homodimerizes with Bax via a novel domain (BH3) distinct from BH1 and BH2. J. Biol. Chem. **271:** 7440–7444.
31. BAKHSHI, A., J.P. JENSEN, P. GOLDMAN, J.J. WRIGHT, O.W. MCBRIDE, A.L. EPSTEIN & S.J. KORSMEYER. 1985. Cloning the chromosomal breakpoint of t(14;18) human lymphomas: clustering around JH on chromosome 14 and near a transcriptional unit on 18. Cell **41:** 899–906.
32. CLEARY, M.L. & J. SKLAR. 1985. Nucleotide sequence of a t(14;18) chromosomal breakpoint in follicular lymphoma and demonstration of a breakpoint-cluster region near a transcriptionally active locus on chromosome 18. Proc. Natl. Acad. Sci. USA **82:** 7439–7443.
33. KRUMENACKER, J.S., D.J. BUCKLEY, M.A. LEFF, J.T. MCCORMACK, G. DE JONG, P.W. GOUT, J.C. REED, T. MIYASHITA, N.S. MAGNUSON & A.R. BUCKLEY. 1998. Prolactin-regulated apoptosis of Nb2 lymphoma cells: pim-1, bcl-2, and bax expression. Endocrine **9:** 163–170.
34. LEFF, M.A., D.J. BUCKLEY, J.S. KRUMENACKER, J.C. REED, T. MIYASHITA & A.R. BUCKLEY. 1996. Rapid modulation of the apoptosis regulatory genes bcl-2 and bax by prolactin in rat Nb2 lymphoma cells. Endocrinology **137:** 5456–5462.

35. KOCHENDOERFER, S., D.J. BUCKLEY & A.R. BUCKLEY. 2000. Role of bcl-xL in prolactin-mediated apoptosis suppression in Nb2 lymphoma cells. Submitted.

36. YANG, E., J. ZHA, J. JOCKEL, L.H. BOISE, C.B. THOMPSON & SJ. KORSMEYER. 1995. Bad, a heterodimeric partner for Bcl-XL and Bcl-2, displaces Bax and promotes cell death. Cell **80:** 285–291.

37. MINN, A.J., P. VELEZ, S.L. SCHENDEL, H. LIANG, S.W. MUCHMORE, S.W. FESLK, M. FILL & C.B. THOMPSON. 1997. Bcl-x(L) forms an ion channel in synthetic lipid membranes. Nature **385:** 353–357.

38. VANDERHEIDEN, M.G., N.S. CHANDEL, E.K. WILLIAMSON, P.T. SCHUMACKER & C.B. THOMPSON. 1997. Bcl-xL regulates the membrane potential and volume homeostasis of mitochondria. Cell **91:** 627–637.

39. LI, F., A. SRINIVASAN, Y. WANG, R.C. ARMSTRONG, K.J. TOMASELLI & L.C. FRITZ. 1997. Cell-specific induction of apoptosis by microinjection of cytochrome c. Bcl-xL has activity independent of cytochrome c release. J. Biol. Chem. **272:** 30299–30305.

40. CHINNAIYAN, A.M., K. O'ROURKE, B.R. LANE & V.M. DIXIT. 1997. Interaction of CED-4 with CED-3 and CED-9: a molecular framework for cell death. Science **275:** 1122–1126.

41. HOOVER, D., M. FRIEDMAN, R. REEVES & N.S. MAGNUSON. 1991. Recombinant human human pim-1 protein exhibits serine/threonin kinase activity. J. Biol. Chem. **266:** 14018–14022.

42. FRIEDMAN, M., M.S. NISSEN, D.S. HOOVER, R. REEVES & N.S. MAGNUSON. 1992. Characterization of the proto-oncogene pim-1 kinase activity and substrate recognition sequence. Arch. Biochem. Biophys. **298:** 594–601.

43. DAUTRY, F., D. WEIL, J. YU & A. DAUTRY-VERSAT. 1988. Regulation of pim and myb mRNA accumulation by interleukin-2 and interleukin-3 in murine hematopoietic cell lines. J. Biol. Chem. **263:** 17615–17620.

44. LILLY, M., T. LE, P. HOLLAND & S.L. HENDRICKSON. 1992. Sustained expression of the pim-1 kinase is specifically induced in myeloid cells by cytokines whose receptors are structurally related. Oncogene **7:** 727–732.

45. BERNS, A., H.T. CUYPERS, G. SELTON & J. DOMEN. 1987. Pim-1 activation in T-cell lymphomas. *In* Viral Carcinogenesis. N.O. Kjeldgaard & J. Forchhamer, Eds.: 211. Alfred Benzen Symposium.

46. LILLY, M. & A. KRAFT. 1997. Enforced expression of the Mr 33,000 Pim-1 kinase enhances factor-independent survival and inhibits apoptosis in murine myeloid cells. Cancer Res. **57:** 5348–5355.

47. BUCKLEY, A.R., D.J. BUCKLEY, M.A. LEFF, D.S. HOOVER & N.S. MAGNUSON. 1995. Rapid induction of pim-1 expression by prolactin and interleukin-2 in rat Nb2 lymphoma cells. Endocrinology **136:** 5252–5259.

48. YU-LEE, L-Y., J.A. HRACHOVY, A.M. STEVENS & L.A. SCHWARZ. 1990. Interferon-regulatory factor 1 is an immediate–early gene under transcriptional regulation by prolactin in Nb2 T cells. Mol. Cell. Biol. **10:** 3087–3084.

49. MURPHY, P.R., G.E. DIMATTIA & H.G. FREISEN. 1988. Role of calcium in prolactin-stimulated c-myc gene expression and mitogenesis in Nb2 lymphoma cells. Endocrinology **122:** 2476–2485.

50. HORSMAN, D.E., S. MASUI & P.W. GOUT. 1991. Karyotypic changes associated with loss of prolactin dependency of rat Nb2 node lymphoma cell cultures. Cancer Res. **51:** 282–287.

51. GOUT, P.W. 1987. Transient requirement for prolactin as a growth initiator following treatment of autonomous Nb2 node rat lymphoma cell cultures with butyrate. Cancer Res. **47:** 1751–1755.

52. BUCKLEY, A.R., J.S. KRUMENACKER, D.J. BUCKLEY, M.A. LEFF, N.S. MAGNUSON, J.C. REED, T.MIYASHITA, G. DE JONG & P.W. GOUT. 1997. Butyrate-induced reversal of dexamethasone resistance in autonomous rat Nb2 lymphoma cells. Apoptosis **2:** 518–528.

53. BUCKLEY, A.R., M.A. LEFF, D.J. BUCKLEY, N.S. MAGNUSON, G. DE JONG & P.W. GOUT. 1996. Alterations in pim-1 and c-myc expression associated with sodium butyrate–induced growth factor dependency in autonomous rat Nb2 lymphoma cells. Cell Growth Differ. **7:** 1713–1721.

54. CAMPBELL, G.S., L.S. ARGETSINGER, J.N. IHLE, P.A. KELLY, J.A. RILLEMA & C. CARTER-SU. 1994. Activation of JAK2 tyrosine kinase by prolactin receptors in Nb2 cells and mouse mammary gland explants. Proc. Natl. Acad. Sci. USA **91:** 5232–5236.

55. RUI, H., R.A. KIRKEN & W.L. FARRAR. 1994. Activation of receptor-associated tyrosine kinase JAK2 by prolactin. J. Biol. Chem. **269:** 5364–5368.

56. KIRKEN, R.A., H. RUI, O.M.Z. HOWARD & W.L. FARRAR. 1994. Involvement of JAK-family tyrosine kinases in hematopoietin receptor signal transduction. Prog. Growth Fac. Res. **5:** 195–211.

57. CLEVENGER, C.V. & M.V. MEDAGLIA. 1994. The protein tyrosine kinase P59fyn is associated with prolactin (PRL) receptor and is activated by PRL stimulation of T-lymphocytes. Mol. Endocrinol. **8:** 674–681.

58. MONTGOMERY, D.W., J.S. KRUMANCKER & A.R. BUCKLEY. 1998. Prolactin stimulates phosphorylation of the human T-cell antigen receptor complex and ZAP-70 tyrosine kinase: a potential mechanism for its immunomodulation. Endocrinology **139:** 811–814.

59. KRUMENACKER, J.S., D.W. MONTGOMERY, D.J. BUCKLEY, P.W. GOUT & A.R. BUCKLEY. 1998. Prolactin receptor signaling: shared components with the T-cell antigen receptor in Nb2 lymphoma cells. Endocrine **9:** 313–320.

60. BUCKLEY, A.R., Y-P. RAO, D.J. BUCKLEY, P.W. GOUT. 1994. Prolactin-induced phosphorylation and nuclear translocation of MAP kinase in Nb2 lymphoma cells. Biochem. Biophys. Res. Commun. **204:** 1158–1164.

61. BUCKLEY, A.R., D.W. MONTGOMERY, R. KIBLER, C.W. PUTNAM, C.F. ZUKOSKI, P.W. GOUT, C.T. BEER & D.H. RUSSELL. 1986. Prolactin stimulation of ornithine decarboxylase and mitogenesis in Nb2 node lymphoma cells: the role of protein kinase C and calcium mobilization. Immunopharmacology **12:** 37–51.

62. CAREY, G.B. & J.P. LIBERTI. 1995. Stimulation of receptor-associated kinase, tyrosine kinase, and MAP kinase is required for prolactin-mediated macromolecular biosynthesis and mitogenesis in Nb2 lymphoma. Arch. Biochem. Biophys. **316:** 179–189.

63. AL-SAKKAF, K.A., P.R.M. DOBSON & B.L. BROWN. 1996. Activation of phosphatidylinositol 3-kinase by prolactin in Nb2 cells. Biochem. Biophys. Res. Comm. **221:** 779–784.

64. ERWIN, R.A,. R.A. KIRKEN, M.G. MALABARBA, W.L. FARRAR & H. RUI. 1995. Prolactin activates Ras via signaling proteins SHC, growth factor receptor bound 2, and son of sevenless. Endocrinology **136:** 3512–3518.

65. RAO, Y-P., D.J. BUCKLEY & A.R. BUCKLEY. 1995. Rapid activation of mitogen-activated protein kinase and p21ras by prolactin and interleukin 2 in rat Nb2 node lymphoma cells. Cell Growth Differ. **6:** 1235–1244.

66. CLEVENGER, C.V., W. NGO, D.L. SOKOL, S.M. LUGER & A.M. GEWIRTZ. 1995. Vav is necessary for prolactin-stimulated proliferation and is translocated into the nucleus of a T-cell line. J. Biol. Chem. **270:** 13246–13253.

67. WANG, Y-F. & L-Y. YU-LEE. 1996. Multiple Stat complexes interact at the IRF-1 GAS in prolactin-stimulated Nb2 T cells. Mol. Cell. Endocrinol. **121:** 19–28.

68. YIP-SCHNEIDER, M.T., M. HORIE & H.E. BROXMEYER. 1995. Transcriptional induction of pim-1 protein kinase gene expression by interferon g and posttranscriptional effects on costimulation with steel factor. Blood **85:** 3494–3502.

69. MUI, A.L., H. WAKAO, A.M. O'FARRELL, N. HARADA & A. MIYAJIMA. 1995. Interleukin-3, granulocyte-macrophage colony-stimulating factor, and interleukin-5 transduce signals through two STAT5 homologs. J. Leukocyte Biol. **57:** 799–803.

70. BORG, K.E., M. ZHANG, D. HEGGE, R.L. STEPHEN, D.J. BUCKLEY, N.S. MAGNUSON & A.R. BUCKLEY. 1999. Prolactin regulation of pim-1 expression: positive and negative promoter elements. Endocrinology **140:** 5659–5668.

71. CLEVENGER, C.V., K. THICKMAN, W. NGO, W-P. CHANG, S. TAKAYAMA & J.C. REED. 1997. Role of Bag-1 in the survival and proliferation of the cytokine-dependent lymphocyte line Ba/F3 and Nb2. Mol. Endocrinol. **11:** 608–618.

Growth Hormone and Prolactin Expression in the Immune System

RON KOOIJMAN,[a] SARAH GERLO, ASTRID COPPENS, AND
ELISABETH L. HOOGHE-PETERS

Department of Pharmacology, Medical School,
Free University of Brussels (V.U.B.), Belgium

ABSTRACT: Prolactin (PRL) and growth hormone (GH) are pituitary hormones that play pivotal roles in lactation and body growth, respectively. In addition, both hormones have been implicated as modulators of immune responses. Since the expression of GH and PRL by leukocytes points to autocrine or paracrine roles during immune responses, our study is aimed at PRL- and GH-production in leukocytes. We show that human peripheral blood granulocytes, which express GH and PRL mRNA, contain high molecular-weight immunoreactive variants of GH and PRL (37 and 43 kDa, respectively), but not the pituitary-sized hormones. Secretion of these variants, or biologically active material as assessed by the Nb2 bioassay, was not detected. On the other hand, certain leukemic myeloid cells secrete 23-kDa, pituitary-sized, PRL, which is biologically active.

INTRODUCTION

Prolactin (PRL) and growth hormone (GH) are mainly produced by the anterior pituitary, where their expression is regulated by the pituitary transcription factor Pit-1. Their best recognized functions are lactation and stimulation of body growth, respectively. In rodents and man, many leukocytes bear receptors for PRL and GH, which both belong to the cytokine-receptor superfamily. Furthermore, both hormones are produced by leukocytes, and they also have been shown to modulate the immune system.[1] The presence of both hormones and their receptors in the same lymphoid tissues leads to the hypothesis that PRL and GH act in an autocrine or paracrine way. Our study is aimed at the understanding of the mechanism of PRL and GH production in leukocytes and their relevance to the immune response.

THE ROLE OF PIT-1 IN GH REGULATION
IN THE IMMUNE SYSTEM

The role for PRL in the immune system has recently been explored using PRL- and PRL-receptor knockout mice.[2,3] Both studies demonstrate that PRL is not a

[a]Address for correspondence: Ron Kooijman, Department of Pharmacology, Medical School, Free University of Brussels, Laarbeeklaan 103, B-1090 Brussels, Belgium. Voice: +32-24774461; fax: +32-24774464.
rkooi@farc.vub.ac.be

necessary factor for the immune system. However, many groups showed that PRL exhibit immunomodulatory functions.[1] For prolactin, an alternative regulation mechanism via a far-upstream alternative promoter, independent of the pituitary transcription factor Pit-1, has been found in the myometrium, the decidualized endometrium, and the immune system.[4,5] To evaluate the role of GH in the immune system, many groups have studied the relation between hormone levels in serum and immune responses. Immunological parameters have been studied in hypophysecto-mized rats, hypopituitary dwarf mice, and GH-deficient patients. However, autocrine and paracrine functions for GH have been suggested by several investigators observing GH expression by leukocytes.

The presence of an alternative GH regulation mechanism in the immune system would imply that animals and humans with a GH deficiency are not necessarily deficient in extrapituitary GH. Therefore, local effects of leukocyte-derived GH should be taken into account when studying the roles of GH in the immune system. In earlier studies we addressed a possible alternative regulation mechanism for GH in the immune system as compared to that in the pituitary by studying GH expression in bone-marrow-derived leukocytes from normal and hypopituitary Snell dwarf mice. These mice have a mutated gene for Pit-1 that is deficient in DNA binding.[6] By immunocytochemistry, we showed that $65 \pm 24\%$ of the bone-marrow-derived granulocytes from normal mice contained immunoreactive GH, while $5.8 \pm 1.5\%$ of the granulocytes expressed detectable amounts of GH mRNA as assessed by *in situ* hybridization. In dwarf mice, we found that $57 \pm 31\%$ of the bone marrow granulocytes were stained with GH antiserum, and that $8.8 \pm 3.7\%$ of bone marrow cells expressed GH transcripts. The presence of GH mRNA in dwarf mice was confirmed by reversed transcription (RT)-PCR.[7] Our observation that GH expression in bone marrow granulocytes from dwarf mice is similar to that in normal mice, points to a Pit-1-independent expression of GH in murine leukocytes. The idea that Pit-1 is not involved in GH expression in murine leukocytes is also supported by the finding of Weigent *et al.*,[8] who showed that GH expression in subpopulations of cultured thymic and splenic lymphocytes from DW/J GH-deficient dwarf mice is normal.

In man, gene duplication gave rise to two GH genes. GH-N (normal) is expressed in the pituitary under the control of Pit-1, and GH-V (variant) is expressed in the placenta. Melen *et al.*[9] showed that GH-V is expressed in peripheral blood mononuclear cells (PBMC) from a woman with a Pit-1 deficiency, whereas the GH-N gene transcripts were absent. Pit-1 is expressed in human lymphoid and myeloid cell lines[10] and PBMC, and could regulate GH expression. FIGURE 1A shows Pit-1 transcripts in the human pituitary and freshly isolated PBMC by RT-PCR followed by Southern blotting. Pit-1 protein was detected by Western blotting using a polyclonal antiserum (FIG. 1B). Pit-1 exists as two forms (31 and 33 kDa) due to the use of alternative translation start sites. Our control experiments show that anti-Pit-1 indeed recognizes two proteins in a PRL-secreting pituitary adenoma. The 31-kDa protein is also recognized in extracts from normal human pituitary and PBMC. Furthermore, the T-cell mitogen phytohemagglutinin (PHA) upregulated Pit-1 expression during a three-day culture period. This effect might be involved in the enhancing effect of PHA on GH secretion by PBMC.[11,12] Further investigations are necessary to assess the exact role of Pit-1 in GH regulation.

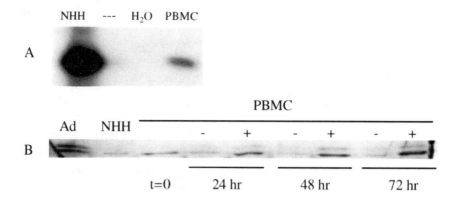

FIGURE 1. Expression Pit-1 in human PBMC. (A) Evidence of Pit-1 gene expression in human PBMC by RT-PCR and Southern blotting. (B) Effects of the T-cell mitogen PHA on Pit-1 protein expression in human PBMC. Cells were cultured in RPMI/10% FCS for different periods of time in the absence (−) or presence (+) of 10 mg/mL PHA. Whole cells were solubilized in Laemmli sample buffer containing 2-mercaptoethanol. Proteins from the normal human hypophysis (NHH) and the pituitary adenoma (Ad) were obtained by sonication of minced tissues. Subsequently, proteins were subjected to Western blotting using an antiserum against human Pit-1.

EXPRESSION OF GH AND PRL
IN GRANULOCYTES AND BONE MARROW

To further address the possible autocrine or paracrine role for GH in the human immune system, we focused on GH expression in granulocytes and bone marrow. Since GH affects the development of hematopoietic cells[13] and several granulocyte functions,[14] we investigated GH expression in peripheral blood granulocytes, synovial granulocytes from patients with rheumatoid arthritis, bone-marrow-derived leukocytes, and *in vitro* cultured stromal cells from bone marrow.

Granulocytes express GH mRNA and immunoreactive GH.[15] To characterize immunoreactive GH and to address GH secretion, we performed Western blot analysis on whole cell extracts and Nb2 bioassays on culture medium. Using three different polyclonal antisera and three different monoclonal antibodies, we could not detect 22 kDa GH in freshly isolated granulocytes from peripheral blood, but several immunoreactive proteins with different molecular weights were detected (see FIGURE 2A). The 37-kDa protein was the only band that was recognized by different antibodies. It was detected by two out of three polyclonal antisera and by one out of three monoclonal antibodies. The 37-kDa band completely disappeared when the GH binding antibodies in the two antisera were adsorbed by recombinant human GH. A similar control experiment could not be performed for the monoclonal antibody, because it is directed toward an internal epitope (Dr. L. Retegui, personal communication). This immunoreactive 37-kDa GH was also detected in PBMC and bone-marrow-derived leukocytes (FIG. 2B). Other tissues tested, such as muscle, heart, and liver, did not contain the 37-kDa band (data not shown).

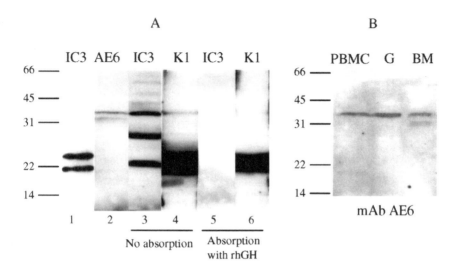

FIGURE 2. Western blot analysis of immunoreactive GH in leukocytes. Human granulocytes (better than 99% pure) and PBMC (better than 97% pure) were isolated from peripheral blood. Bone marrow cells from the sternum were obtained from patients undergoing cardiac surgery. Recombinant human GH (22 kDa), purified 20-kDa GH, and whole cells were solubilized in Laemmli sample buffer containing 2-mercaptoethanol. Subsequently, proteins were resolved by SDS-polyacrylamide gel electrophoresis and subjected to immunoblotting. (**A**) Detection of immunoreactive GH in granulocytes by two polyclonal antisera [IC3 (NIADDK) and K1] and a monoclonal antibody (AE6). *Lane 1* contains recombinant 22-kDa GH and purified 20-kDa GH, and *lanes 2–6* contain granulocyte lysates. Detection of immunoreactive bands with the polyclonal antisera disappeared by absorption with rhGH (*lanes 5* and *6*). (**B**) Expression of 37-kDa immunoreactive GH in PBMC, granulocytes (G), and bone-marrow cells (BM), as detected by mAb AE6.

Similar results were found for PRL. Granulocytes expressed PRL transcripts (see FIGURE 3A) and contained a high molecular-weight immunoreactive PRL-like protein of 43 kDa (FIG. 3B). This protein was recognized by two antisera. However, neither of these antisera detected 23-kDa PRL.

To study the secretion of bioactive GH and PRL, we cultured different cell types in a serum-free medium for 3 to 48 h and assayed for lactogenic activity using rat Nb2 lymphoma cells. These cells express PRL receptors and are completely dependent on lactogenic hormones (PRL, GH, placental lactogens) for proliferation. In contrast to PBMC,[11,12] granulocytes and bone-marrow-derived leukocytes never secreted detectable levels of bioactive GH or PRL (below 1 pg/mL and below 3 pg/mL, respectively). On the other hand, stromal bone marrow cells, the human leukemia cell line EoL-1, and freshly isolated peripheral blood leukocytes (50% blasts) from a patient with AML secreted significant amounts of lactogenic material. Using inhibitory antisera, we showed that this lactogenic material in all cases completely consisted of PRL (see FIGURE 4). Interestingly, all cell types that secreted biologically active PRL also secreted 23-kDa PRL as assessed by Western blotting.

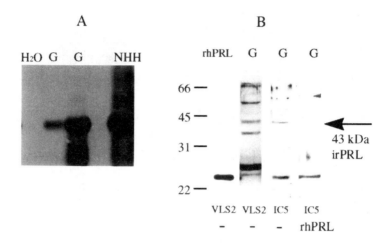

FIGURE 3. (**A**) Expression of PRL transcripts by peripheral blood granulocytes. Granulocytes (G) were isolated to a purity of more than 99% and assayed for PRL mRNA by RT-PCR followed by Southern blotting. Normal human hypophysis (NHH) and H_2O were used as positive and negative controls, respectively. (**B**) Immunoreactive PRL in cellular extracts from peripheral blood granulocytes (G) as detected by immunoblotting using two different antisera (VLS2 and IC5). Binding to the 43-kDa band was blocked by adsorption to rhPRL.

CONCLUDING REMARKS

An alternative, Pit-1 independent, regulation mechanism exists for GH in the murine immune system, and for GH-V in the human immune system. This result implies that a pituitary GH deficiency does not necessarily concur with an impaired GH production in the immune system.

Since several groups already established GH and PRL production by PBMC, we investigated expression and secretion of these hormones in granulocytes. Although human granulocytes contain both immunoreactive GH and PRL in addition to GH and PRL transcripts, we never detected secretion of lactogenic activity as assessed with the Nb2 bioassay. Several immunoreactive, high molecular-weight variants of both GH and PRL were found to be secreted, but we never detected secretion of 22-kDa GH or 23-kDa PRL. The secretion of biologically active PRL in other cell types always concurred with the secretion of 23-kDa PRL. Taken together, we have no indications that the immunoreactive hormones with a high molecular weight are functional autocrine of paracrine factors, nor that they are products of either GH or PRL genes.

The lack of secretion of 23-kDa GH and biologically active GH in bone-marrow-derived leukocytes and stromal cells does not support the idea that local production of GH in bone marrow is important for hematopoiesis and immune function, but further investigations are necessary to address GH expression in minor subpopulations. On the other hand, our study confirms earlier results of Bellone *et al.*[16] that bone-marrow-derived stromal cells synthesize and secrete 23-kDa PRL. Since PRL from

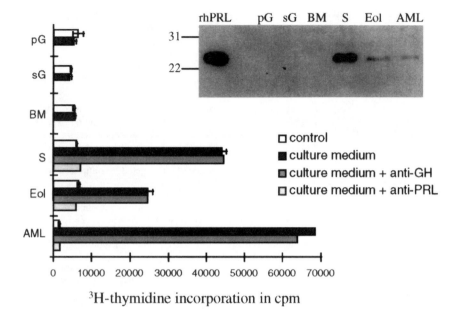

^{3}H-thymidine incorporation in cpm

FIGURE 4. Secretion of immunoreactive PRL and lactogenic activity by different types of leukocytes. Cells were cultured in serum-free medium for 18 h: peripheral blood granulocytes (pG), synovial granulocytes from patients with rheumatoid arthritis (sG), bone marrow cells (BM), *in vitro* cultured stromal bone marrow cells (S), EoL-1 human leukemia cell line (Eol), and peripheral blood leukocytes from a patient with an acute myeloblastic leukemia (AML). Immunoreactive PRL in the culture medium was detected by Western blotting (*insert*), whereas lactogenic activity was measured using the Nb2 bioassay in the presence of normal rabbit serum, anti-GH, or anti-PRL. Culture medium without cells was used as a control.

stromal bone marrow cells enhanced erythropoiesis *in vitro,* a paracrine role for PRL in hematopoiesis is conceivable.[16]

The secretion of biologically active PRL by leukemic cells[17,18] (see FIGURE 4) prompted us to further investigate PRL secretion by primary leukemic cells. So far, we have found *in vitro* secretion of biologically active PRL by leukemic cells from two out of three patients with AML. Using similar culture conditions, we never found secretion of PRL by PBMC from healthy donors. Additional studies are required to assess whether synthesis and secretion of biologically active PRL is a property of certain types of leukemia.

ACKNOWLEDGMENTS

This research was funded by the Flemish Government (GOAs), the Fund for Scientific Research-Flanders, Belgium (F.W.O.) and institutional grants from the V.U.B. Ron Kooijman is a research associate of the Fund for Scientific Research-Flanders,

Belgium (F.W.O.). We are very grateful to Dr. L.A. Retegui (University of Buenos Aires, Argentina) for supplying her monoclonal antibodies against human growth hormone, and Dr. Y.N. Sinha for providing his PRL antiserum VLS-2.

REFERENCES

1. KOOIJMAN, R., E.L. HOOGHE-PETERS & R. HOOGHE. 1996. Prolactin, growth hormone and insulin-like growth factor-I in the immune system. Adv. Immunol. **63:** 377–453.
2. BOUCHARD, B., C.J. ORMANDY, J.P. DI SANTO et al. 1999. Immune system development and function in prolactin receptor-deficient mice. J. Immunol. **163:** 576–582.
3. HORSEMAN, N.D., W. ZHAO, E. MONTECINO-RODRIGUEZ et al. 1997. Defective mammopoiesis, but normal hematopoiesis, in mice with a targeted disruption of the prolactin gene. EMBO J. **16:** 6926–6935.
4. GELLERSEN, B., R. KEMPF, R. TELGMANN et al. 1994. Nonpituitary human prolactin gene transcription is independent of Pit-1 and differentially controlled in lymphocytes and in endometrial stroma. Mol. Endocrinol. **8:** 356–373.
5. BERWAER, M., J.A. MARTIAL & J.R.E. DAVIS. 1994. Characterization of an up-stream promoter directing extrapituitary expression of the human prolactin gene. Mol. Endocrinol. **8:** 635–642.
6. LI, S., E.B. CRENSHAW III, E.J. RAWSON et al. 1990. Dwarf locus mutants lacking three pituitary cell type results from mutations in the POU-domain gene pit-1. Nature **347:** 528–533.
7. KOOIJMAN, R., A. MALUR, S.C. VAN BUUL-OFFERS et al. 1997. Growth hormone expression in murine bone marrow leukocytes is independent of the pituitary transcription factor Pit-1. Endocrinology **138:** 3949–3955.
8. WEIGENT, D.A. & J.E. BLALOCK. 1994. Effect of the administration of growth-hormone-producing lymphocytes on weight gain and immune function in dwarf mice. Neuroimmunomodulation **1:** 50–58.
9. MELEN, L., G. HENNEN, R.P. DULLAART et al. 1997. Both pituitary and placental growth hormone transcripts are expressed in human peripheral blood mononuclear cells (PBMC). Clin. Exp. Immunol. **110:** 336–340.
10. DELHASE, M., P. VERGANI, A. MALUR et al. 1993. The transcription factor Pit-1/ GHF-1 is expressed in hematopoietic and lymphoid tissues. Eur. J. Immunol. **23:** 951–955.
11. VARMA, S., P. SABHARWAL, J.F. SHERIDAN et al. 1993. Growth hormone secretion by human peripheral blood mononuclear cells detected by an enzyme-linked immunoplaque assay. J. Clin. Endocrinol. Metab. **76:** 49–53.
12. HATTORI, N., A. SHIMATSU, M. SUGITA et al. 1990. Immunoreactive growth hormone (GH) secretion by human lymphocytes: augmented release by exogenous GH. Biochem. Biophys. Res. Commun. **168:** 396–401.
13. MERCHAV, S. 1998. The haematopoietic effects of growth hormone and insulin-like growth factor-I. J. Pediatr. Endocrinol. Metab. **11:** 677–685.
14. FU, Y.K., S. ARKINS, G. FUH et al. 1992. Growth hormone augments superoxide anion secretion of human neutrophils by binding to the prolactin receptor. J. Clin. Invest. **89:** 451–457.
15. KOOIJMAN, R., D. BERUS, A. MALUR et al. 1997. Human neutrophils express GH-N gene transcripts and the pituitary transcription factor Pit-1b. Endocrinology **138:** 4481–4484.
16. BELLONE, G., P. ASTARITA, E. ARTUSIO et al. 1997. Bone marrow stroma-derived prolactin is involved in basal and platelet-activating factor-stimulated in vitro erythropoiesis. Blood **90:** 21–27.
17. MATERA, L., M. CUTUFIA, M. GEUNA et al. 1997. Prolactin is an autocrine growth factor for the Jurkat human T-leukemic cell line. J. Neuroimmunol. **79:** 12–21.
18. HATFILL, S.J., R. KIRBY, M. HANLEY et al. 1990. Hyperprolactinemia in acute myeloid leukemia and indication of ectopic expression of human prolactin in blast cells of a patient of subtype M4. Leuk. Res. **14:** 57–62.

The Role of Bim, a Proapoptotic BH3-Only Member of the Bcl-2 Family, in Cell-Death Control

ANDREAS STRASSER,[a] HAMSA PUTHALAKATH, PHILIPPE BOUILLET, DAVID C.S. HUANG, LIAM O'CONNOR, LORRAINE A. O'REILLY, LEONIE CULLEN, SUZANNE CORY, AND JERRY M. ADAMS

The Walter and Eliza Hall Institute, Post Office Royal Melbourne Hospital, Melbourne, Australia

ABSTRACT: Apoptosis is an evolutionarily conserved process for killing unwanted cells. Genetic and biochemical experiments have indicated that three groups of proteins are necessary for activation of the cell-death effector machinery: cysteine proteases, their adaptors, and proapoptotic Bcl-2 family members. Antiapoptotic Bcl-2 family members are needed for cell survival. We have cloned Bim, a proapoptotic Bcl-2 family member that shares with the family only a 9–16 aa region of homology [Bcl-3 homology region(BH3)], but is otherwise unique. Bim requires its BH3 region for binding to Bcl-2 and activation of apoptosis. Analysis of Bim-deficient mice has shown that Bim is essential for the execution of some but not all apoptotic stimuli that can be antagonized by Bcl-2. Bim-deficient mice have increased numbers of lymphocytes, plasma cells, and myeloid cells, and most develop fatal autoimmune glomerulonephritis. In healthy cells, Bim is bound to the microtubule-associated dynein motor complex, and is thereby sequestered from Bcl-2. Certain apoptotic signals unleash Bim and allow it to translocate to intracellular membranes, where it interacts with Bcl-2 or its homologues. These results indicate that BH3-only proteins are essential inducers of apoptosis that can be unleashed by certain death signals. Unleashed BH3-only proteins neutralize the prosurvival function of Bcl-2-like molecules, and this is thought to liberate Apaf-l-like adapters to activate caspase zymogens, which then initiate cell degradation.

THE ROLE OF APOPTOSIS
IN NORMAL DEVELOPMENT AND IN DISEASE

Apoptosis is a physiological process for killing unwanted cells.[1] Alongside cell immigration, cell division, and cell export, apoptosis is a critical determination of overall cell production.[2] Apoptosis is used in multicellular organisms for sculpting tissues during embryogenesis, as a regulator of cellular homeostasis, and as a defense mechanism against infectious microorganisms.[3,4] Abnormalities in cell-death control have been implicated as an initiating event or contributing factor in the

[a]Address for correspondence: Andreas Strasser, The Walter and Eliza Hall Institute, Post Office Royal Melbourne Hospital, 3050 Vic, Melbourne, Australia. Voice: + 61-3-9345-2624; fax: + 61-3-9347-0852.
strasser@wehi.edu.au

development of several diseases. Inappropriate survival of cells that are normally doomed can lead to cancer,[5] particularly in combination with mutations that deregulate cell cycle control,[6] and can cause autoimmune disease.[7,8] Conversely, premature death of cells that are normally long-lived has been postulated—but not yet proven—to be a cause of neurodegenerative disorders and muscular atrophy.[9]

THE MOLECULAR CONTROL OF APOPTOSIS

Genetic and biochemical experiments have identified a framework of the molecular control of apoptosis.[4] Three groups of proteins have been shown to be essential for activating the effector phase of apoptosis: cysteine proteases,[10] their adapters,[11] and proapoptotic members of the Bcl-2 family.[12] Antiapoptotic members of the Bcl-2 family are needed for cell survival.[12] Cysteine proteases have a cysteine in their catalytic site and cleave protein substrates at aspartate residues (the so-called P1 position), and are therefore called caspases.[10] Caspases must recognize an exposed stretch of four amino acids (P1–P4 positions) within a substrate to proteolyze it. Caspases can be subdivided according to their preferences for different amino acids in the P2 to P4 positions, which endows them with different substrate specificities.[10] They can also be classified according to the presence or absence of long N-terminal prodomains that have regulatory function (see below). One subclass of caspases, including caspases-1 and -11, has long prodomains, and their preferred substrate recognition sequence is YVAD. They play critical roles in intracellular processing of cytokines, such as IL-1β and IL-18, and appear to be dispensable for apoptosis.[13] Caspases are present in cells as zymogens that have very little yet functionally significant enzymatic activity. They must themselves be cleaved at aspartic acid residues by caspases to produce fragments of approximately 20-kDa and 10-kDa size and facilitate assembly of the fully active tetrameric ($p20_2p10_2$) enzyme.[10] So-called initiator caspases have long regulatory prodomains that can undergo homotypic interaction with specific adapter proteins. The caspase recruitment domain (CARD) region in procaspase-9 binds to the CARD in Apaf-1,[14] and one of the two death effector domains (DED) in procaspase-8 binds to the DED domain in FADD (also called MORT1).[15,16] Biochemical studies have indicated that adapter proteins mediate aggregation of procaspases, and thereby promote their autocatalytic activation.[14,17,18] Initiator caspases can activate their own precursors and so-called effector caspases (e.g., caspase-3), and thereby initiate a proteolytic avalanche that culminates in cellular collapse.[10] Effector caspases induce late apoptotic events, such as membrane blebbing, chromatin condensation, internucleosomal DNA cleavage, by cleaving vital structural components of the cell (e.g., lamin, gelsolin), and by proteolytic activation of latent enzymes (e.g., PAK2, Acinus, caspase-activated DNAse).[19–21]

THE BCL-2 FAMILY

Members of the Bcl-2 protein family are major regulators of apoptosis.[12] Bcl-2, the prototypic member of this family, and its closest homologs (Bcl-x_L, Bcl-w, A1,

Mcl-1, Boo) share three or four regions of homology (Bcl-2 homology or BH1–BH4 regions), and all inhibit apoptosis.[12,22] Other members of the family promote apoptosis. They can be further subdivided into two groups. Bax, Bak, Bok/Mtd, and Bcl-x$_S$ (a splice form of the *bcl*-x gene) have two or three BH regions, whereas Bad, Bik/Nbk, Blk, Bid, Hrk/DP5, and Bim/Bod only possess a short (9–16 aa) BH3 domain, but are otherwise unique.[12] Several of the pro- and antiapoptotic members of the Bcl-2 family also have a membrane-spanning domain at the C-terminus. This region is (at least in part) responsible for the localization of these proteins at the cytosolic aspect of the nuclear envelope, endoplasmic reticulum (ER), and the outer mitochondrial membrane.[23] Members of the Bcl-2 family can undergo homotypic and heterotypic interaction. Antiapoptotic members can bind to each other and to proapoptotic members, and certain proapoptotic members have been reported to interact with each other.[12] The BH3-only proteins require only their BH3 domain for binding to and neutralizing the activity of antiapoptotic Bcl-2 family members, and it appears that this is the only mechanism by which they induce cell death.[12] Structural analysis has shown that the BH3 region forms an amphipathic α-helix that binds via hydrophobic and electrostatic interactions into a cleft on the surface of Bcl-x$_L$.[24] It is less clear how Bax, Bak, Bok/Mtd, and Bcl-x$_S$ induce apoptosis. Some studies have indicated that they also function by inactivating Bcl-2-like molecules,[12] but others provided evidence that they kill cells by forming pores in mitochondria,[25] either directly or by interacting with certain channel proteins.[26,27] Although Bcl-2 was the first mammalian apoptosis regulator identified,[22] its biochemical function remains controversial.[12] Genetic evidence and some biochemical studies have shown that Bcl-2 and its functional homologs keep Apaf-1-like adapter proteins at bay and thereby prevent activation of initiator caspases. Other biochemical experiments have indicated that Bcl-2-like proteins form channels in mitochondria or prevent release of cytochrome *c*, which then activates Apaf-1.[12] The latter models do not explain why Bcl-2-like proteins that are not localized on mitochondria (e.g., adenovirus E1B19kD protein or certain mutants of Bcl-2) can inhibit apoptosis as potently as wild-type Bcl-2.[28,29] We believe that Bcl-2-like proteins inhibit the function of Apaf-1-like adapter proteins by a mechanism that remains to be discovered, and that release of cytochrome *c* from mitochondria constitutes a mechanism for amplifying caspase activation.[12,30]

APOPTOSIS SIGNALING

Apoptosis can be induced by multiple independent signaling pathways that all converge upon activation of effector caspases.[4] Experiments with mutant mice lacking individual caspases or their adapters and those overexpressing Bcl-2-like proteins have identified two major signaling pathways. Apoptosis induced by ligation of CD95 (also called Fas or APO-1) or related death receptors requires caspase-8[31,32] and its adapter FADD,[33–35] and cannot be blocked by Bcl-2 or its functional homologues, at least in lymphocytes.[36] In contrast, apoptosis induced by glucocorticoids, DNA damage, and other intracellular signals requires caspase-9[37,38] and its adapter Apaf-1,[39,40] and can be inhibited by antiapoptotic Bcl-2 family members.[41,42] Different intracelleular stimuli trigger Apaf-1-mediated activation of caspase-9 by distinct signaling routes. For example, the tumor suppressor p53 is required for DNA damage-induced apoptosis in quiescent (but interestingly not cycling) lymphocytes, while the glucocorticoid receptor is needed for glucocorticoid-induced cell death.[43–45]

ISOLATION AND CHARACTERIZATION OF BIM, A BH3-ONLY MEMBER OF THE BCL-2 FAMILY

We have screened a λ-phage cDNA expression library (from a p53-/- T lymphoma line[45]) with Bcl-2 as a bait to find interactive partners and thereby investigate its biochemical function. This led to the identification of Bim, a BH3-only member of the Bcl-2 family that also has a transmembrane region.[46] There are three splice forms of Bim: Bim_S, Bim_L, and Bim_{EL}. They all have a BH3 domain, but vary in a region toward the N-terminus. Transient transfection with Bim expression constructs rapidly induced apoptosis, and none of the Bim isoforms could be stably expressed in mammalian cell lines, unless Bcl-2 or a homolog was coexpressed. Bim-induced apoptosis could also be inhibited by baculovirus protein p35, a broad-spectrum caspase inhibitor, but not by the cowpox virus serpin CrmA, which blocks caspases-1 and -8. This indicated that caspase-9 or other initiator caspases, but not caspase-8, are needed for Bim-induced apoptosis. Bim_S was a much more potent inducer of apoptosis than Bim_L or Bim_{EL}, indicating that the extra region present in Bim_L and Bim_{EL} attenuates proapoptotic activity (see below).[46] Experiments with mutated forms of Bim (all isoforms) demonstrated that the BH3 region and the transmembrane region are both required for cell killing.[46] Northern blot analysis and immunohistochemical staining with specific monoclonal antibodies showed that Bim_L and Bim_{EL} are expressed in lymphoid tissues, myeloid cells, neurons, and epithelial cells.[46,47,51] Thus far, we have not detected Bim_S in any cell type.

BIM IS ESSENTIAL FOR HEMOPOIETIC CELL HOMEOSTASIS AND SOME APOPTOTIC PATHWAYS

Gene targeting in ES cells was performed to investigate the essential role of Bim. The BH3 domain encoding exon was replaced by a *neo* cassette. By Western blotting we found only very little truncated Bim protein in cells from *bim*–/– mice (probably due to instability of the truncated Bim), demonstrating that we had created a true null allele.[48] Intercrosses of *bim*+/– mice yielded only about a third of the expected number of *bim*–/– offspring, demonstrating that Bim plays a critical role in embryogenesis. Interestingly, the yield of *bim*+/– heterozygotes was also significantly below the expected frequency, indicating that there is a gene dosage effect. Embryonic lethality occurred prior to E9.5 (due to a currently unknown reason), and was observed on a mixed as well as the inbred C57BL/6 and 129 genetic backgrounds.[48]

The *bim*–/– mice that were born appeared normal and had no obvious abnormalities other than a 3- to 5-fold increase in mature B and T cells, macrophages, and granulocytes.[48] Numbers of erythroid cells and megakaryocytes were normal, but platelet numbers were reduced by 50% compared to control mice. This may indicate that platelet shedding is an apoptosis-like process that involves Bim. These results demonstrated that Bim is a critical regulator of hemopoietic cell homeostasis.

In tissue culture *bim–/–* lymphocytes (pre-T cells, pre-B cells, mature resting, and activated B and T cells) were resistant to certain apoptotic stimuli that are inhibitable by Bcl-2 (e.g., cytokine withdrawal, calcium flux). Survival of cells from *bim+/–* heterozygotes was intermediate between that of wt and *bim–/–* cells, demonstrating that the dose of Bim is critical. Bim-deficient lymphocytes, however, had nearly normal sensitivity to other apoptotic stimuli that can be blocked by Bcl-2 (e.g., DNA damage, glucocorticoids, PKC activation).[48] It therefore appears that different death stimuli require different BH3-only proteins for apoptosis induction.

BIM PRECLUDES SYSTEMIC AUTOIMMUNE DISEASE

When *bim–/–* mice grew older (around 4–8 months), they accumulated a 50- to 200-fold increase in immunoglobulin (Ig)-secreting plasma cells (mostly IgG) and a corresponding increase in serum Ig levels. Within a year approximately 60% of the *bim–/–* mice developed fatal autoimmune glomerulonephritis, characterized by immune-complex deposits in the kidney and high titers of IgG autoantibodies to nuclear antigens (e.g., dsDNA, histones). This systemic lupus erythematosus (SLE)-like disease was very similar to the autoimmunity observed in (C57BL/6xSJL)F2 mice expressing a *bcl-2* transgene in B lymphocytes.[7] Interestingly, a significant portion (about 30%) of *bim+/–* heterozygotes also developed fatal immune-complex glomerulonephritis, reinforcing the notion that there is a gene-dosage effect.

POSTTRANSLATIONAL REGULATION OF THE PROAPOPTOTIC ACTIVITY OF BIM

Initial Northern blot analysis showed that *bim* mRNA levels are not increased in lymphocytes by death stimuli that require Bim for induction of apoptosis.[46] We therefore used the yeast 2-hybrid system to examine how the proapoptotic activity of Bim is regulated at the posttranslational level. We found that Bim_L and Bim_{EL}, but not Bim_S, bound to LC8 dynein light chain both in yeast and mammalian cells.[49] Single amino acid substitutions in Bim_L that disrupt its interaction with LC8 increased its killing potency to that of Bim_S,[49] proving that interaction with LC8 is a physiological regulator of Bim proapoptotic activity. In healthy cells, most endogenous Bim_L and Bim_{EL} molecules were bound via LC8 to the microtubule-associated dynein motor complex, and thereby sequestered from Bcl-2 and its homologs. Certain apoptotic stimuli, such as growth-factor withdrawal, disrupted the interaction between LC8 and the dynein motor complex.[49] This freed Bim to translocate together with LC8 to Bcl-2 and neutralize its antiapoptotic activity. This process did not require caspase activity, and therefore constitutes an initiating event in apoptosis signaling.

CONCLUSIONS AND PERSPECTIVES

These results demonstrate that BH3-only members of the Bcl-2 family play a critical role in apoptosis of mammalian cells, similar to the BH3-only protein Egl-1, which is essential for programmed cell death in *C. elegans*.[50] It appears that in mammals different BH3-only proteins are activated by distinct posttranslational mechanisms,[49] and are needed for the execution of different death stimuli.[48] It is also possible that different cells can use distinct BH3-only proteins for the execution of a given death stimulus. Our analysis of *bim–/–* mice has also shown that abnormalities in BH3-only proteins can cause diseases, such as autoimmunity and perhaps also cancer.[48] To further investigate the role of BH3-only proteins in cell-death control, animal development, and disease we will generate mice lacking members of this family that have not yet been studied. Intercrosses of such animals will unravel the combined activities of these proteins.

ACKNOWLEDGMENTS

Our laboratories are supported by the NHMRC (Reg. Key 973002), the U.S. NCI (CA43540 and CA80188), the Anti-Cancer Council of Victoria (Melbourne), the Dr. Josef Steiner Cancer Research Foundation (Bern), the Leukemia Society of America, and the Cancer Research Institute (New York). We are grateful to all of our past and present colleagues at the Walter and Eliza Hall Institute, particularly Drs. A. Harris, D. Vaux, D. Metcalf, F. Koentgen, D. Tarlinton, S. Bath, L. Harrison, T. Kay, and G. Hausmann, for help with experiments and insightful discussions. We thank L. Barnett, S. Novakovic, and J. Beaumont for technical assistance, and J. Birtles for editorial help.

REFERENCES

1. KERR, J.F.R. *et al.* 1972. Apoptosis: a basic biological phenomenon with wide-ranging implications in tissue kinetics. Br. J. Cancer **26:** 239–257.
2. RAFF, M.C. 1996. Size control: the regulation of cell numbers in animal development. Cell **86:** 173–175.
3. VAUX, D.L. *et al.* 1994. An evolutionary perspective on apoptosis. Cell **76:** 777–779.
4. VAUX, D.L. *et al.* 1996. The molecular biology of apoptosis. Proc. Natl. Acad. Sci. U.S.A. **93:** 2239–2244.
5. STRASSER, A. *et al.* 1997. The role of the *bcl-2/ced-9* gene family in cancer and general implications of defects in cell death control for tumourigenesis and resistance to chemotherapy. Biochim. Biophys. Acta **1333:** F151–F178.
6. STRASSER, A. *et al.* 1990. Novel primitive lymphoid tumours induced in transgenic mice by cooperation between *myc* and *bcl-2*. Nature **348:** 331–333.
7. STRASSER, A. *et al.* 1991. Enforced *BCL2* expression in B-lymphoid cells prolongs antibody responses and elicits autoimmune disease. Proc. Natl. Acad. Sci. U.S.A. **88:** 8661–8665.
8. WATANABE-FUKUNAGA, R. *et al.* 1992. Lymphoproliferation disorder in mice explained by defects in Fas antigen that mediates apoptosis. Nature **356:** 314–317.
9. BARR, P.J. *et al.* 1994. Apoptosis and its role in human disease. Biotechnology **12:** 487–493.
10. THORNBERRY, N.A. *et al.* 1998. Caspases: enemies within. Science **281:** 1312–1316.
11. VAUX, D.L. 1997. CED-4—The third horseman of apoptosis. Cell **90:** 389–390.

12. STRASSER, A. *et al.* 2000. Apoptosis signaling. Ann. Rev. Biochem. **69:** 217–245.

13. LI, P. *et al.* 1995. Mice deficient in IL-1b-converting enzyme are defective in production of mature IL-1b and resistant to endotoxic shock. Cell **80:** 401–411.

14. SRINIVASULA, S.M. *et al.* 1998. Autoactivation of procaspase-9 by Apaf-1-mediated oligomerization. Mol. Cell **1:** 949–957.

15. BOLDIN, M.P. *et al.* 1996. Involvement of MACH, a novel MORT1/FADD-interacting protease, in Fas/APO-1- and TNF receptor-induced cell death. Cell **85:** 803–815.

16. MUZIO, M. *et al.* 1996. FLICE, a novel FADD homologous ICE/CED-3-like protease, is recruited to the CD95 (Fas/Apo-1) death-inducing signaling complex. Cell **85:** 817–827.

17. MUZIO, M. *et al.* 1998. An induced proximity model for caspase-8 activation. J. Biol. Chem. **273:** 2926–2930.

18. MARTIN, D.A. *et al.* 1998. Membrane oligomerization and cleavage activates the caspase-8 (FLICE/MACHa1) death signal. J. Biol. Chem. **273:** 4345–4349.

19. RUDEL, T. *et al.* 1997. Membrane and morphological changes in apoptotic cells regulated by caspase-mediated activation of PAK2. Science **276:** 1571–1574.

20. SAHARA, S. *et al.* 1999. Acinus is a caspase-3-activated protein required for apoptotic chromatin condensation. Nature **401:** 168–173.

21. SAKAHIRA, H. *et al.* 1998. Cleavage of CAD inhibitor in CAD activation and DNA degradation during apoptosis. Nature **391:** 96–99.

22. VAUX, D.L. *et al.* 1988. *Bcl-2* gene promotes haemopoietic cell survival and cooperates with *c-myc* to immortalize *pre-B* cells. Nature **335:** 440–442.

23. LITHGOW, T. *et al.* 1994. The protein product of the oncogene *bcl-2* is a component of the nuclear envelope, the endoplasmic reticulum and the outer mitochondrial membrane. Cell Growth Differ. **5:** 411–417.

24. SATTLER, M. *et al.* 1997. Structure of Bcl-x_L-Bak peptide complex: recognition between regulators of apoptosis. Science **275:** 983–986.

25. ANTONSSON, B. *et al.* 1997. Inhibition of Bax channel-forming activity by Bcl-2. Science **277:** 370–372.

26. MARZO, I. *et al.* 1998. Bax and adenine nucleotide translocator cooperate in the mitochondrial control of apoptosis. Science **281:** 2027–2031.

27. SHIMIZU, S. *et al.* 1999. Bcl-2 family proteins regulate the release of apoptogenic cytochrome *c* by the mitochondrial channel VDAC. Nature **399:** 483–487.

28. ZHU, W. *et al.* 1996. Bcl-2 mutants with restricted subcellular location reveal spatially distinct pathways for apoptosis in different cell types. EMBO J. **15:** 4130–4141.

29. HUANG, D.C.S. *et al.* 1997. Bcl-2, Bcl-X_L and adenovirus protein E1B19kD are functionally equivalent in their ability to inhibit cell death. Oncogene **14:** 405–414.

30. HENGARTNER, M.O. 1998. Death cycle and Swiss army knives. Nature **391:** 441–442.

31. SMITH, K.G.C. *et al.* 1996. CrmA expression in T lymphocytes of transgenic mice inhibits CD95 (Fas/APO-1)-transduced apoptosis, but does not cause lymphadenopathy or autoimmune disease. EMBO J. **15:** 5167–5176.

32. VARFOLOMEEV, E.E. *et al.* 1998. Targeted disruption of the mouse *Caspase 8* gene ablates cell death induction by the TNF receptors, Fas/Apo1, and DR3 and is lethal prenatally. Immunity **9:** 267–276.

33. NEWTON, K.A. *et al.* 1998. A dominant interfering mutant of FADD/Mort1 enhances deletion of autoreactive thymocytes and inhibits proliferation of mature T lymphocytes. EMBO J. **17:** 706–718.

34. YEH, W.C. *et al.* 1998. FADD: essential for embryo development and signaling from some, but not all, inducers of apoptosis. Science **279:** 1954–1958.

35. ZHANG, J. *et al.* 1998. Fas-mediated apoptosis and activation-induced T-cell proliferation are defective in mice lacking FADD/Mort1. Nature **392:** 296–300.

36. STRASSER, A. *et al.* 1995. Bcl-2 and Fas/APO-1 regulate distinct pathways to lymphocyte apoptosis. EMBO J. **14:** 6136–6147.

37. KUIDA, K. *et al.* 1998. Reduced apoptosis and cytochrome c-mediated caspase activation in mice lacking caspase 9. Cell **94:** 325–337.

38. HAKEM, R. *et al.* 1998. Differential requirement for caspase 9 in apoptotic pathways in vivo. Cell **94:** 339–352.

39. CECCONI, F. *et al.* 1998. Apaf-1 (CED-4 homologue) regulates programmed cell death in mammalian development. Cell **94:** 727–737.
40. YOSHIDA, H. *et al.* 1998. Apaf1 is required for mitochondrial pathways of apoptosis and brain development. Cell **94:** 739–750.
41. SENTMAN, C.L. *et al.* 1991. *bcl-2* inhibits multiple forms of apoptosis but not negative selection in thymocytes. Cell **67:** 879–888.
42. STRASSER, A. *et al.* 1991. *Bcl-2* transgene inhibits T cell death and perturbs thymic self-censorship. Cell **67:** 889–899.
43. LOWE, S.W. *et al.* 1993. p53 is required for radiation-induced apoptosis in mouse thymocytes. Nature **362:** 847–849.
44. CLARKE, A.R. *et al.* 1993. Thymocyte apoptosis induced by p53-dependent and independent pathways. Nature **362:** 849–852.
45. STRASSER, A. *et al.* 1994. DNA damage can induce apoptosis in proliferating lymphoid cells via p53-independent mechanisms inhibitable by Bcl-2. Cell **79:** 329–339.
46. O'CONNOR, L. *et al.* 1998. Bim—A novel member of the Bcl-2 family that promotes apoptosis. EMBO J. **17:** 384–395.
47. O'REILLY, L.A. *et al.* 1998. Rapid hybridoma screening method for the identification of monoclonal antibodies to low abundance cytoplasmic proteins. BioTechniques **25:** 824–830.
48. BOUILLET, P. *et al.* 1999. Bcl-2 family member Bim required for some apoptotic pathways and to preclude autoimmunity. Science **286:** 1735–1738.
49. PUTHALAKATH, H. *et al.* 1999. The pro-apoptotic activity of the Bcl-2 family member Bim is regulated by interaction with the dynein motor complex. Mol. Cell **3:** 287–296.
50. CONRADT, B. *et al.* 1998. The *C. elegans* protein EGL-1 is required for programmed cell death and interacts with the Bcl-2-like protein CED-9. Cell **93:** 519–529.
51. O'REILLY, L.A. *et al.* 2000. The pro-apoptotic BH3-only protein Bim is expressed in hemopoietic, epithelial, neuronal and germ cells. Am. J. Pathol. **157:** 449–461.

Stress and Chemotherapy

Combined Effects on Tumor Progression and Immunity in Animal Models

TULLIO GIRALDI,[a,c] SONIA ZORZET,[a] LAURA PERISSIN,[b] AND VALENTINA RAPOZZI[b]

[a]Department of Biomedical Sciences, University of Trieste, Trieste, Italy

[b]Department of Biomedical Sciences and Technologies, University of Udine, I-33100 Udine, Italy

ABSTRACT: In mice bearing Lewis lung carcinoma, rotational and restraint stress specifically increases the formation of lung metastasis, and restraint stress markedly attenuates the antitumor effects of cyclophosphamide. The aim of this investigation was therefore to examine the effects of restraint stress on tumor metastasis in mice bearing MCa mammary carcinoma, and on the effectiveness of CCNU and DTIC. Restraint stress increases MCa mammary carcinoma metastasis, causes a marked reduction in cyclophosphamide activity, and a minor attenuation of the effects of CCNU and DTIC. The possible occurrence of seasonal factors, observed for the increase by rotational stress of Lewis lung carcinoma metastasis, was also determined for cyclophosphamide effectiveness. The survival time of control mice is longer in February than in June, and is not appreciably modified by rotational stress. The effects of cyclophosphamide are similar in both seasonal periods, and are similarly attenuated by rotational stress. The seasonal effects of rotational stress, and the reduction of the effects of cyclophosphamide caused by rotational stress, are accompanied by corresponding variations in the number of CD3+ and CD4+ splenic T-lymphocyte subsets and in the CD4+/CD8+ ratio, respectively. The reported effects of stress on tumor progression and on the effectiveness of cyclophosphamide thus appear to occur via modulation of immune responses of the host directed against the tumor. These data appear of interest for their experimental implications, and suggest the opportunity to consider the role that the stress during treatment may play in determining the effectiveness of clinical antitumor chemotherapy.

INTRODUCTION

Clinical oncologists are giving increased attention to the quality of life of their cancer patients, and investigations focused on the role that psychosocial factors may play in the progression of clinical cancers by means of neuroendocrine modulation of immune functions of the host continues to be carried on with encouraging results.[1,2] In this connection, model systems consisting of laboratory animals bearing

[c]Author for correspondence: Tullio Giraldi, Department of Biomedical Sciences, University of Trieste, I-34100 Triesete, Italy. Voice: +39 (0)40 6763537; fax +39 (0)40 577435.
giraldi @ univ.trieste.it

transplanted tumors and subjected to stress paradigms offered a valuable experimental tool and provided useful results.[3] Studies are available showing that the exposure to stress causes specific effects on the immune system of the host and concomitantly influences tumor growth.[4] Yet, the specific effects of stress on malignant metastatic dissemination in experimental systems received limited attention, in spite of the clinical relevance of tumor metastatic spread.[5] Moreover, although immune responses of the host may participate in determining the efficacy of antitumor drugs,[6] little attention appears to have been given to the neuroimmunomodulation induced by stress on the outcome of antineoplastic chemotherapy. Indeed, the latter aspect may deserve investigation, since low dosages of cyclophosphamide and melphalan were equally or more effective in causing cures in mice bearing MOPC-315 plasmacytoma[7–9] than higher dose levels of the same drugs. Mice cured with the low-dosage treatment schedules showed a strong acquired immune resistance to further tumor challenges that did not occur using high dosages of both antitumor drugs,[7,8,10,11] and that was shown to depend on the appearance of Lyt 2+ T cells.[10,12] Findings consistent with a dosage-dependent immunoregulatory action of melphalan and cyclophosphamide, crucial in curing MOPC-315 plasmocytoma in mice, also were obtained in rats bearing KMT-17 fibrosarcoma upon treatment with bleomycin.[13]

As far as metastasis is concerned, several paradigms, including rotational and restraint stress, have been shown to specifically increase the metastatic spread of Lewis lung carcinoma in syngeneic mice, in a way that is independent of the effects of the stressor on the growth of the primary tumor.[14,15] The increase in metastasis formation caused by rotational stress was shown to vary in magnitude with a highly significant circannual rhythm, with the acrophase coinciding with the summer solstice; the magnitude of the increase in metastasis formation negatively correlated with the number of splenic CD3+ and CD4+ T-lymphocyte subsets.[16] On the other hand, in mice bearing Lewis lung carcinoma, the application of restraint stress caused the attenuation of the cytotoxic effects of cyclophosphamide, reducing the increase in life span and the number of long-term survivors caused by the drug. Physical restraint and cyclophosphamide concomitantly reduced the CD4+/CD8+ ratio in an additive way.[17]

On the basis of these findings and considerations, the aim of the present investigation has been to examine the effects of restraint and rotational stress on the effectiveness of cyclophosphamide, CCNU, and DTIC in mice bearing MCa mammary carcinoma, and to relate them to the numerosity of CD3+, CD4+, CD8+ splenic T-lymphocyte subpopulations and NK cells. The results obtained are reported below.

MATERIALS AND METHODS

Animals and Tumor Transplantation

For the experiments with Lewis lung carcinoma, the animals used are female C57BL/6 and C57BL/6 X DBA/2F$_1$ (BD2F1) mice weighing 18–20 g, purchased from Charles River, Calco, Como, Italy. Lewis lung carcinoma, originally provided by the National Cancer Institute, Bethesda, Maryland, is maintained in C57BL/6 mice by subcutaneous injection in the axillary region of 50 mm^3 of minced tumor tissue aseptically prepared from donors similarly inoculated two weeks before. For experimental purposes, the tumor is propagated in BD2F1 mice by intramuscolar injection of a tumor cell suspension containing 10^6 viable tumor cells.[14]

For the experiments with MCa mammary carcinoma, the animals used are female CBA/Lac mice weighing 18–20 g, obtained from a locally established breeding colony, grown according to the standard procedure for inbred strains. MCa mammary carcinoma, originally obtained from the Department of Experimental Biology and Medicine of the Rudjer Boskovic Institute (Zagreb, Croatia) is maintained and propagated, for experimental purposes, in CBA/Lac mice by intramuscular injection of a tumor cell suspension containing 10^6 viable tumor cells.[18]

Measurement of Tumor Growth and Metastasis Formation

Primary tumor volume was determined 14 days after tumor inoculation by caliper measurements of its short and long axis. The number and volume of metastases were determined at necroscopy after sacrifice on day 21 from tumor inoculation by examining the surface of the lungs with a low-power stereo microscope. The details of the procedures used have been reported in detail elsewhere.[14]

Experimental Stress Paradigms

In order to reduce the variable stress resulting from shipment and housing,[19–21] the animals were kept in a protected environment for 2 weeks preceding each experiment and throughout the duration of the experiment. The protected environment consisted of cabinets containing the animal cages with laminar air flow, minimizing acoustic, olfactory, and visual communication among the cages. The cabinets were placed in a room remote from the animals' rooms, where staff entered only once every 5 days to check the animals for water and flood supplies, which were available *ad libitum.* The light–dark cycle in the room was 12–12 h, with an intensity in the cages of approximately 5 lux. Temperature and relative humidity were constant at 20°C and 60%, respectively. The animals were kept 5 per cage in order to avoid the effects of overcrowding or isolation on tumor progression.[19,20] Restraint stress consisted of tying the animals' legs with string fixed to small plastic boards; daily sessions lasting 1 h were repeated on days 1–6 from tumor inoculation. Rotational stress was applied to the animals in the low-stress environment by spinning the cages at 45 rpm for 10 min every hour from the time of tumor inoculation until sacrifice on day 21.

Drug Treatment

Cyclophosphamide (CYCLO, CY) was kindly provided by Schering, while CCNU and DTIC were obtained from Rhone-Poulenc and Roner, respectively. To avoid the stress of repeated handling and intraperitoneal injections,[4,22] the drug was administered orally admixed in powdered food on days 1–6 from tumor implantation. Drug concentration was selected to provide the daily dosage indicated in the tables, on the basis of a measured average daily food consumption of 5.0 ± 0.1 g per mouse. The dosage used for each drug is the optimal one for the treatment schedule employed, as previously determined in separate experiments.

Measurement of Splenic T-Lymphocyte Subpopulations and NK Cells

Spleens were removed immediately following sacrifice by cervical dislocation. They were disaggregated and then passed through a double layer of gauze to obtain single-cell suspensions. The cells were washed and lymphocytes were separated from red blood cells by Ficoll-Hypaque centrifugation (Sigma, St. Louis, MO).[23] The final suspension of splenic lymphocytes was labeled with antimouse mono- clonal antibodies using a PBS staining medium, pH 7.4, containing 0.5% BSA and 0.1% NaN_3. Aliquots of 10^6 viable cells in 0.5 mL of staining medium, counted by the trypan-blue exclusion test, were incubated in the dark for 30 min at 4°C with 50 µL of rat antimouse monoclonal antibodies to CD3 (0.5 µg), CD4 (1 µg), CD8 (1 µg), or NK 1.1 (1 µg) (Pharmingen, San Diego, CA). Stained cells were examined using an EPICS flow cytometer (Coulter, Miami, FL); each analysis consisted of 10,000 events counted.[24] Results for single-color analysis are expressed as total number of positive cells collected from the spleen of each animal.

Statistical Analysis

Data were subjected to the appropriate factorial ANOVAs assessing significance against an alpha-level $p < 0.05$; the significance of the effects of individual experi- mental variables and of their interaction(s) is indicated in the tables. Survival was analyzed using Kaplan-Meyer and Cox proportional hazard methods, and the results

TABLE 1. Effects of Cyclophosphamide and rotational stress on the survival time of mice bearing Lewis lung carcinoma

CYCLO	Rotational stress	Seasonal period	Mean survival time (days)	Long-term survivors
–	–	June	26.8	0/10
–	+		25.8	0/10
+	–		34.4	4/10[a]
+	+		27.8	0/10
–	–	February	47.8	0/10
–	+		42.9	0/10
+	–		56.3	6/10[a]
+	+		38.2	0/10
HR = 0.206 $(0.066–0.064)^b$	HR = 8.24 $(2.51–27.8)^b$	HR = 0.083 $(0.026–0.265)^b$		

NOTE: Groups of 10 mice were implanted s.c. with Lewis lung carcinoma on day 0. The ani- mals received cyclophosphamide (240 mg/kg/day orally) on days 1–6, and were subjected to rotational stress on days 1–21, as indicated. The survival time was recorded and analyzed using the Kaplan-Meier method. Values are reported as mean survival time and as the fraction of mice with a survival time > 90 days.
[a]Different from the other experimental groups, Pearson chi-square $p < 0.05$.
[b]Multivariate Cox proportional hazard analysis, $p < 0.0001$ (95% CI).

are indicated in TABLE 1. Standard procedures, implemented in the Systat package (SYSTAT Inc., Evanston, IL), were used.

RESULTS

The first series of experiments examined the effects of the treatments in terms of primary tumor volume measured 2 weeks after implantation, and of lung metastasis volume 1 week later at necroscopy after sacrifice. Data reported in TABLE 2 illustrate the results obtained in mice bearing MCa mammary carcinoma. ANOVA indicates that in drug-untreated controls, restraint stress causes a significant increase in lung metastasis formation, although its effects on the primary tumor are insignificant. The effects of cyclophosphamide are significant and similarly pronounced on primary tumor and metastasis volume; the reduction in metastasis volume and in the number of mice with metastasis is significantly attenuated upon the combination of restraint stress with drug treatment. CCNU and DTIC do not cause any significant effect on the primary tumor; CCNU significantly decreases metastasis incidence and volume, whereas DTIC reduces metastasis incidence only. The number of mice with metastasis after treatment with CCNU and DTIC is increased by restraint stress to values that do not differ significantly from those of drug-untreated controls.

In mice bearing Lewis lung carcinoma, cyclophosphamide is highly effective on primary tumor and metastasis; the further application of rotational stress significantly attenuates the effectiveness of cyclophosphamide. The effects of rotational stress on the growth of the primary tumor and on the formation of lung metastasis in drug-untreated controls significantly depend on the seasonal period, and consist of an increase in summer and a decrease in winter. After treatment with cyclophosphamide, the fraction of mice without primary tumor or metastasis is markedly reduced, and the effectiveness of cyclophosphamide is significantly attenuated by rotational stress; these effects do not significantly depend on the seasonal period (see TABLE 3).

Further experiments were performed in mice bearing Lewis lung carcinoma, in order to determine the effects of cyclophosphamide and its combination with rotational stress on the survival time of the animals. Kaplan-Meier analysis and log-rank test indicate a significant effect of the treatments on survival when the data are stratified on the eight experimental groups (Mantel chi-square = 51.18, $p < 0.0001$). Univariate Cox proportional hazard estimation confirms a significant effect ($p < 0.008$) for cyclophosphamide treatment (HR = 0.232, 95% C.I. 0.077–0.697), for rotational stress (HR = 6.84, 95% C.I. 2.16–21.6), and for the seasonal period (HR = 0.160, 95% C.I. 0.053–0.479). Multivariate Cox proportional hazard analysis also significantly confirms ($p < 0.0001$) that cyclophosphamide treatment is a negative risk factor (HR = 0.206, 95% C.I. 0.066–0.640), that rotational stress is a significant positive risk factor (HR = 8.24, 95% C.I. 2.51–27.8), and that the seasonal period has a significant relevance for survival (HR = 0.083, 95% C.I. 0.026–0.265). The mean survival time of the untreated animals appears to be greater in winter than in summer, and to be prolonged by cyclophosphamide; rotational stress lacks effects by itself, but attenuates the increase in survival caused by cyclophosphamide. The significant fraction of long-term survivors in the cyclophosphamide group (4/10 in June and 6/10 in February, Pearson chi-square $p < 0.05$) is reduced to 0/10 in both

TABLE 2. Effects of restraint stress, and cyclophosphamide, CCNU, and DTIC on primary-tumor growth and metastasis formation in mice bearing MCa mammary carcinoma

Drug	Drug treatment	Restraint stress	Primary tumor volume (cm³)	Number of mice with tumor/total number	Metastasis volume (mm³)	Number of mice with metastasis/total number
CYCLO	−	−	0.51 ± 0.21	9/9	49.8 ± 30.6	9/9
	−	+	0.85 ± 0.72	9/9	116.3 ± 39.4	9/9
	+	−	0.04 ± 0.02	6/9[a]	14.0 ± 0.0	2/9[a,b]
	+	+	0.24 ± 0.19	9/9	26.6 ± 10.3	8/9
ANOVA			CY		Stress, CY, stress*CY	
CCNU	−	−	1.70 ± 0.45	9/9	37.8 ± 21.4	9/9
	−	+	1.86 ± 0.28	9/9	90.4 ± 55.1	9/9
	+	−	1.54 ± 0.36	9/9	4.5 ± 0.7	2/9[a]
	+	+	1.60 ± 0.36	9/9	9.2 ± 6.4	5/9
ANOVA					CCNU	
DTIC	−	−	1.69 ± 0.45	9/9	37.7 ± 21.4	9/9
	−	+	1.86 ± 0.28	9/9	90.4 ± 55.1	9/9
	+	−	1.61 ± 0.32	2/9	37.7 ± 37.6	3/9[a]
	+	+	1.56 ± 0.37	5/9	24.3 ± 23.8	6/9
ANOVA					DTIC, stress*DTIC	

NOTE: Each value is the mean ± SD obtained using groups of 9 mice that were implanted i.m. with MCa mammary carcinoma on day 0. The animals received orally cyclophosphamide (240 mg/kg/day on days 1–6, CYCLO), CCNU (9.5 mg/kg/day on days 1–14), or DTIC (60 mg/kg/day on days 1–14), and were subjected to restraint stress on days 1–6, as indicated.
[a]Different from drug untreated controls, Pearson chi-square $p < 0.05$.
[b]CYCLO different from CYCLO + stress, Pearson chi-square $p < 0.05$.

TABLE 3. Effects of Cyclophosphamide and rotational stress on primary-tumor growth and lung metastasis formation in mice bearing Lewis lung carcinoma

CYCLO	Rotationl stress	Seasonal period	Primary tumor volume (cm^3)	Number of mice with tumor/total number	Metastasis volume (mm^3)	Number of mice with metastasis/total number
–	–	June	2.03 ± 0.20	10/10	27.5 ± 8.42	10/10
–	+		2.43 ± 1.29	10/10	82.5 ± 25.7	10/10
+	–		0	0/10[a]	0	0/10[a]
+	+		0.69 ± 0.24	10/10	14.7 ± 4.55	10/10
–	–	February	2.28 ± 0.49	10/10	32.4 ± 19.6	10/10
–	+		1.68 ± 0.45	10/10	10.5 ± 5.46	10/10
+	–		0.34 ± 0.26	4/10[a]	0	0/10[a]
+	+		0.81 ± 0.45	10/10	1.47 ± 0.15	6/10
ANOVA			Stress, CY, seas.*stress, seas.*CY, seas*CY*stress		Seas., CY, Stress, Seas.*stress, Seas.*CY, Seas.*CY*stress	

NOTE: Each value is the mean ± SD obtained using groups of 10 mice that were implanted s.c. with Lewis lung carcinoma on day 0. The animals received cyclophosphamide (240 mg/kg/day orally, CYCLO) on days 1–6, and were subjected to rotational stress (RS) on days 1–21, as indicated.
[a]Different from the other groups, Pearson chi-square $p < 0.05$.

TABLE 4. Effects of Cyclophosphamide and rotational stress on splenic T-lymphocyte subpopulations and NK cells

Rotational stress	CYCLO	Seasonal period	CD3+	CD4+	CD8+	CD4+/CD8+ ratio	NK
–	–	June	23.5 ± 3.14	13.6 ± 1.81	10.7 ± 1.63	1.27 ± 0.08	2.66 ± 0.73
+	–		13.9 ± 1.27	7.32 ± 1.11	5.92 ± 0.74	1.26 ± 0.29	2.30 ± 1.01
–	+		10.6 ± 2.12	6.61 ± 1.09	4.11 ± 1.13	1.68 ± 0.43	1.41 ± 0.32
+	+		6.99 ± 1.30	4.08 ± 0.40	2.65 ± 0.71	1.61 ± 0.34	1.04 ± 0.22
–	–	February	21.0 ± 3.45	15.7 ± 3.42	9.12 ± 0.90	1.71 ± 0.24	3.32 ± 1.80
+	–		31.0 ± 6.67	23.1 ± 2.77	7.50 ± 2.15	3.25 ± 0.81	4.25 ± 2.02
–	+		13.1 ± 2.47	10.0 ± 0.99	3.38 ± 1.30	3.37 ± 1.44	2.01 ± 1.49
+	+		10.2 ± 1.10	7.40 ± 0.85	1.59 ± 0.32	4.84 ± 1.39	1.91 ± 0.41
ANOVA			Seas.,CY Seas.*stress Seas.*CY Seas.*stress*CY	Seas.,CY Seas.*stress Seas.*CY Stress*CY Seas.*stress*CY	Stress,Cy Seas.*stress*CY	Seas.,stress,CY Seas.*stress Seas.*CY	Seas., CY

NOTE: Each value is the mean ± SD ($\times 10^6$) obtained using groups of five mice that were subjected to rotational stress (RS) and were treated with cyclophosphamide (CYCLO), as indicated.

seasonal periods. The pronounced effects of cyclophosphamide in terms of survival thus appear to be sharply reduced by rotational stress, and not to depend on the seasonal period (TABLE 1).

Finally, data in TABLE 4 illustrate the effects of the treatments on splenic T-lymphocyte subsets and on NK cells in normal mice. ANOVA indicates a significant interaction of rotational stress, cyclophosphamide, and seasonal period on CD3+ and CD4+ subsets. A reduction in these subsets is caused by rotational stress in June, whereas an increase is observed in February. In both seasonal periods cyclophosphamide causes a decrease in these subsets, which are further reduced by the combination of drug treatment with rotational stress.

DISCUSSION

The application of stress paradigms, such as rotational and restraint stress, has been previously shown in the authors' laboratory to specifically increase the formation of spontaneous lung metastasis in mice bearing Lewis lung carcinoma.[14,15] Restraint stress also has been shown in the same animal-tumor system to markedly attenuate the antitumor effects of cyclophosphamide, both in terms of tumor and metastasis size at sacrifice, and also more meaningfully of the animals' survival.[17] The aim of the present investigation therefore has been to examine the effects of restraint and rotational stress on tumor metastasis in mice bearing a different tumor, and on the effectiveness of the treatment with different antitumor drugs.

Indeed, when tumor and metastasis size are determined at the end of treatment in mice bearing MCa mammary carcinoma, rotational stress increases metastasis formation and markedly attenuates the pronounced antitumor effects of cyclophosphamide, as observed in mice bearing Lewis lung carcinoma. In these experimental conditions, CCNU displays a similarly effective antitumor action, whereas the effects of DTIC are less pronounced; for the latter drugs, the application of rotational stress causes a tendency toward the reduction of their effects, which does not reach statistical significance.

Rotational stress has been shown to increase metastasis formation in mice bearing Lewis lung carcinoma, displaying a circannual rhythm; metastasis was increased in summer and decreased in winter.[16] The data currently reported confirm this finding, and further indicate that the effects of cyclophosphamide on tumor and metastasis size are similarly attenuated by rotational stress in both seasonal periods. The examination of the survival time of the animals provides additional information, which is particularly relevant in a therapeutic perspective. Multivariate Cox proportional hazard analysis indicates a significant effect for the seasonal period and rotational stress, as well as for cyclophosphamide treatment. The survival time of control mice is approximately twice as long in February as compared with June, and is not appreciably modified by rotational stress. On the other hand, cyclophosphamide causes an increase in survival time that is substantially equivalent in both seasonal periods; the combined application of cyclophosphamide and rotational stress reduces the mean survival time of the animals by a similar extent. A similar proportion of cures caused by cyclophosphamide (4/10 and 6/10 long-term survivors in June and February, respectively), is reduced to 0/10 upon application of rotational stress in both seasonal periods.

The seasonal effects of rotational stress in mice bearing Lewis lung carcinoma, and the reduction of the effects of cyclophosphamide caused by rotational stress in mice bearing the same tumor, were accompanied by corresponding variations in the number of CD3+ and CD4+ splenic T-lymphocyte subsets[16] and in the CD4+/CD8+ ratio,[17] respectively. The data presented reveal a significant effect of rotational stress and cyclophosphamide on the number of CD3+ and CD4+ subsets, which is additive when the treatments are combined. These results support the view that the reported effects of the stress paradigms on tumor metastasis and on the effectiveness of the tested antitumor drugs are caused via modulation of immune responses of the host directed against the tumor.

In conclusion, these data appear of interest for their experimental implications, showing that tumor metastasis in laboratory mice can be influenced by stress paradigms in a way that may also display significant seasonal factors. Moreover, stress may also influence the effectiveness of antitumor drugs, although seasonal factors appear of little relevance for these effects. The effects of stress on tumor progression and response to chemotherapy appear to occur via modulation of T-lymphocyte immune functions of the host. In a clinical perspective, psychosocial factors have been shown to significantly influence tumor progression in cancer patients.[1,2,25,26] However, these investigations concerned patients who had already completed their treatment, including chemotherapy. The data presented suggest the opportunity to also consider in future investigations the role that the stress during the period of acute treatment, deriving from life events as well as from the treatments themselves, may play in determining the effectiveness of clinical antitumor chemotherapy.

REFERENCES

1. ANDERSEN, B.L., W.B. FARRAR, D. GOLDENKREUTZ, L.A. KUTZ, R. MACCALLUM, M.E. COURTNEY & R. GLASER. 1998. Stress and immune responses after surgical treatment for regional breast cancer. JNCI **90:** 30–36.
2. CROYLE, R.T. 1998. Depression as a risk factor for cancer: renewing a debate on the psychobiology of disease, stress and cancer. JNCI **90:** 1856–1857.
3. JUSTICE, A. 1985. Review of the effects of stress on cancer in laboratory animals: importance of time of stress application and type of tumor. Psychol. Bull. **98:** 108–138.
4. MOYNIHAN, J.A., G.J. BRENNER, R. COCKE, J.D. KARP, S.M. BRENEMAN, J.M. DOPP, R. ADER, N. COHEN, L.J. GROTA & Y. FELTEN. 1994. Stress-induced modulation of immune function in mice. *In* Handbook of Human Stress and Immunity. R. Glaser & J. Kiecolt-Glaser, Eds.: 1–22. Academic Press. San Diego.
5. BAMMER, K. 1981. Stress, spread and cancer. *In* Stress and Cancer. K. Bammer & B.H. Newberry, Eds.: 137–163. Hogrefe. Toronto.
6. DEVITA, V.T., S. HELLMAN & S.A. ROSENBERG. 1991. Biologic Therapy of Cancer. Lippincott. Philadelphia-New York.
7. BEN-EFRAIM, S., R.C. BOCIAN, M.B. MOKYR & S. DRAY. 1983. Increase in the effectiveness of melphalan therapy with progression of MOP-315 plasmacytoma tumor growth. Cancer Immunol. Immunother. **15:** 101–107.
8. MOKYR, M.B. & S. DRAY. 1983. Some adavntages of curing mice bearing a large subcutaneous MOPC-315 tumor with a low dose rather than a high dose of cyclophosphamide. Cancer Res. **43:** 3112–3119.
9. BERKO, R., K. SEISSMAN, M. COLVIN, R.C. BOCIAN, S. BEN-EFRAIM & S. DRAY. 1988. Tumoricidal and immunomodulatory activities of drugs and implications for therapy of mice bearing a late stage MOPC-315 plasmacytoma. Int. J. Immunopharmacol. **10:** 825–834.

10. MOKYR, M.B., R.B. BRUNDETT, M. COLVIN & S. DRAY. 1986. Ability of cyclophosphamide in the absence of cross-linking activity to exert the immunomodulatory effect required for the cure of mice bearing a large MOPC-315 tumor. Cancer Res. **46:** 3313–3320.

11. HENGST, J.C., M.B. MOKYR & S. DRAY. 1981. Cooperation between cyclophosphamide tumoricidal activity and host antitumor immunity in the cure of mice bearing large MOPC-315 tumors. Cancer Res. **41:** 2163–2167.

12. MOKYR, M.B., E. BAKER, L.M. WEISKIRCH, B.Y. TAKESUE & J.M. PYLE. 1989. Importance of Lyt 2^+ T-cells in the curative effectiveness of a low dose of melphalan for mice bearing a large MOPC-315 tumor. Cancer Res. **49:** 4597–4606.

13. MORIKAWA, K., M. HOSOKAWA, J. HAMADA, M. SUGAWARA & H. KOBAYASHI. 1985. Host-mediated therapeutics effects produced by appropriately timed administration of bleomycin on a rat fibrosarcoma. Cancer Res. **45:** 1502–1506.

14. GIRALDI, T., L. PERISSIN, S. ZORZET, P. PICCINI & V. RAPOZZI. 1989. Effects of stress on tumor growth and metastasis in mice bearing Lewis lung carcinoma. Eur. J. Cancer Clin. Oncol. **25:** 1583–1588.

15. GIRALDI, T., L. PERISSIN, S. ZORZET, V. RAPOZZI & M.G. RODANI. 1994. Metastasis and neuroendocrine system in stressed mice. Int. J. Neurosci. **74:** 265–278.

16. PERISSIN, L., S. ZORZET, V. RAPOZZI, R. CARIGNOLA, A. ANGELI & T. GIRALDI. 1998. Seasonal effects of rotational stress on Lewis lung carcinoma metastasis and T-lymphocyte subsets in mice. Life Sci. **63:** 711–719.

17. ZORZET, S., L. PERISSIN, V. RAPOZZI & T. GIRALDI. 1998. Restraint stress reduces the antitumor efficacy of cyclophosphamide in tumor-bearing mice. Brain Behav. Immun. **12:** 23–33.

18. GIRALDI, T., G. SAVA, L. PERISSIN & S. ZORZET. 1985. Proteinases and proteinase inhibition by cytotoxic and antimetastatic drugs in transplantable solid metastasizing tumors in mice. Anticancer Res. **5:** 355–360.

19. RILEY, V., M.A. FITZMAURICE & D.H. SPACKMAN. 1981. Psychoneuroimmunologic factors in neoplasia: studies in animals. *In* Psychoneuroimmunology. R. Ader, Ed.: 31–102. Academic Press. New York.

20. LABARBA, R.C. 1970. Experimental and environmental factors in cancer. Psychosom. Med. **32:** 258–276.

21. RILEY, V., M.A. FITZMAURICE & D.H. SPACKMAN. 1981. Animals models in biobehavioral research: effects of anxiety stress on immunocompetence and neoplasia. *In* Perspective on Behavioral Medicine. S.M. Weiss, J.A. Herd & B.H. Fox, Eds.: 371–400. Academic Press. New York.

22. PERISSIN, L., S. ZORZET, P. PICCINI, V. RAPOZZI & T. GIRALDI. 1991. Effects of rotational stress on the effectiveness of cyclophosphamide and razoxane in mice bearing Lewis lung carcinoma. Clin. Exp. Metastasis **9:** 541–549.

23. HUNT, S.U. 1987. Preparation of lymphocytes and accessory cells. *In* Lymphocytes: A Pratical Approach. C.G.B. Klaus, Ed.: 1–34. IRL Press. Oxford.

24. DASIC, G., S. PACOR, A. BERGAMO, G. SALERNO, B. VRANESIC, R. JUKIC, J. TOMASIC & G. SAVA. 1994. Effects of L-(adamant-2-yl)glycyl-L-alanyl-D-isoglutamine on the antitumor action of cyclophosphamide, 5-FU, cisplatin and dacarbazine on advanced carcinomas of the mouse. Int. J. Oncol. **5:** 275–284.

25. FAWZY, F.I., N.W. FAWZY & C.S. HYUN. 1994. Short-term psychiatric intervention for patients with malignant melanoma: effects on psychological state, coping, and the immune system. *In* The Psychoimmunology of Cancer: Mind and Body in the Fight for Survival? C.E. Lewis, C. O'sullivan & J. Barraclough, Eds.: 291–319. Oxford Univ. Press. Oxford.

26. SPIEGEL, D. 1996. Psychological distress and disease and disease course for women with breast cancer: one answer, many questions. JNCI **88:** 629–631.

Modulation of Anticancer Cytokines IL-2 and IL-12 by Melatonin and the Other Pineal Indoles 5-Methoxytryptamine and 5-Methoxytryptophol in the Treatment of Human Neoplasms

PAOLO LISSONI[a]

Division of Radiation Oncology, San Gerardo Hospital, Monza, Milan, Italy

INTRODUCTION

It is known that lymphocytes, namely T lymphocytes and NK cells, play a fundamental role in mediating the destruction of cancer cells[1] through complex interactions with macrophages and dendritic cells (DC).[2] Interleukin-2 (IL-2), mainly produced by T-helper-1 (TH1) lymphocytes, is the main growth factor for T lymphocytes and the main molecule responsible for the evolution of NK into LAK cells.[3] The increase in lymphocyte number represents the main prognostic factor, which can predict the efficacy of cancer immunotherapy with IL-2.[4] In contrast, the evidence of inflammatory response activation prior to immunotherapy has been proven to correlate with clinical resistance to IL-2 therapy of cancer.

In addition, the recent advances in the psychoneuroimmunology have demonstrated that lymphocyte response to cytokine administration does not depend only on the sensitivity of cytokine receptors expressed by immune cells, but also on a physiological neuroendocrine regulation of the immune system.[5] Opioid peptides and pineal hormones seem to constitute the main neuroactive substances involved in the neuroimmunomodulation (NIM). The opioid substances would have a major immunosuppressive effect on the anticancer immunity.[6] Ot the other hand, the pineal gland has been proven to exert a fundamental immunostimulatory action on the immune responses, including the anticancer immune reaction.[7] More to the point, the pineal hormone melatonin (MLT) may have several evident immunomodulating effects by acting on specific melatoninergic receptors,[8] through various mechanisms, including stimulation of IL-2 production by TH1-lymphocytes, inhibition of macrophage-mediated suppressive events, and possible activation of the DC system.[9,10] In particular, MLT has been proven to enhance lymphocyte proliferation and activation in response to IL-2,[11] by acting on specific MLT receptors mainly expressed by TH1-lymphocytes,[8] whereas their expression by TH2-lymphocytes is still controversial.[8,9] However, it has to be taken into consideration that the immunomodulating and the oncostatic properties of the pineal gland would not depend only on MLT itself, but also on other indole and peptidergic substances. Within the indole group, at least two other pineal indoles have been proven *in vitro* to exert oncostatic activity,

[a]Address for correspondence: Dr. Paolo Lissoni, Divisione di Radioterapia Oncologica, Ospedale S. Gerardo, Via Donizetti 106, Monza (Milan), Italy. Voice: ++/39/039/233.3681; fax ++/039/233.3414.

consisting of 5-methoxytryptamine (5-MTT) and 5-methoxytryptophol (5-MTP).[12] *In vitro*, 5-MTT has appeared to exert a direct antiproliferative effect on cancer cell lines superior to that of MLT itself.[12] In contrast, very few data are available on the possible immunomodulatory effects of pineal indoles other than MLT.[13]

After more than 30 years of experimental investigation showing several important biological activities of MLT, including antiproliferative, immunomodulating, antioxidant, myelotrophic, and neurotrophic effects,[14] the clinicians now seem to start adequate clinical trials with MLT and other immunomodulating agents in the treatment of human diseases. In particular, several clinical studies have suggested important therapeutic applications of MLT and its absolute lack of toxicity.[14] In contrast, at present there are only very preliminary studies in human data concerning the other pineal indoles, 5-MTT and 5-MTP, showing an apparent lack of toxicity and potential anti-inflammatory immunomodulating effects.[13] In any case, the lack of toxicity and the potential oncostatic activity would justify further clinical studies with 5-MTT and 5-MTP in the treatment of human neoplasms. Finally, the advances in tumor immunobiology have recently demonstrated the evident anticancer activity of another cytokine, interleukin-12 (IL-12), mainly produced by DC after antigen activation.[2] Unfortunately, the clinical application of IL-12 in the treatment of human neoplasms is still in its infancy, whereas in experimental conditions the association of IL-2 plus IL-12 has been proven to constitute the most effective cytokine combination in inducing objective tumor regression.[15]

The present investigations have been performed in an attempt to evaluate the immunomodulatory effects of MLT and other pineal indoles on IL-2 and IL-12 immunobiological effects in metastatic cancer patients.

MATERIALS AND METHODS

In a biological clinical study, we have evaluated the influence of MLT on a low-dose IL-2-induced lymphocyte increase with respect to the results obtained with low-dose IL-2 combined with MLT plus the two other pineal indoles, 5-MTT and 5-MTP. The study was performed on 30 consecutive patients with untreatable metastatic solid tumors that did not respond to earlier conventional chemotherapies and for which no other effective standard therapy was available.

Tumor histotypes were as follows: eleven non-small-cell lung cancer (NSCLC); eight colorectal cancer; six gastric cancer; five pancreatic cancer. Dominant metastasis sites were, as follows: fourteen lung; nine liver; four liver + lung; three bone. After being rated according to tumor histotype and disease site, patients were randomized to receive subcutaneous (s.c.) low-dose IL-2 alone (3 million IU/day s.c. in the evening, for 6 days/week for 4 consecutive weeks, corresponding to one complete cycle), IL-2 plus MLT alone (20 mg/day orally in the evening every day), or IL-2 plus MLT plus 5-MTT (10 mg/day orally in the afternoon every day) plus 5-MTP (5 mg/day orally at noon every day).

The doses of pineal indoles were established according to the results observed in a large number of earlier studies for MLT[7,11] and in preliminary clinical studies for 5-MTTT and 5-MTP.[13] Moreover, MLT and 5-MTP were given during the dark part of the day and during the period of maximum light, respectively, to reproduce the timing of their physiological maximum increase in the blood.[16] Finally, 5-MTT was also given during the daylight to avoid its possible transformation into MLT itself by N-acetyl-transferease, which is activated by the darkness.[16] The immunobiological response to IL-2 alone or IL-2 plus pineal indoles was evaluated according to the increase in lymphocyte and eosinophil numbers,[4] by collecting venous blood samples prior to immunotherapy, and at weekly intervals until the end of the immunotherapeutic cycle.

In a second study, we have evaluated the influence of MLT on IL-2 –IL-12 interactions, by comparing the results observed in seven groups of metastatic renal cell cancer patients treated with MLT alone (20 mg/day orally every day in the evening), s.c. low-dose IL-2 alone (3 million IU/day in the evening for 6 days/week), s.c. low-dose IL-12 alone (0.5 μg/kg b.w. in the morning once/week), IL-2 plus MLT, IL-12 plus MLT, IL-2 plus IL-12 (by injecting IL-12 three days prior to IL-2) or IL-2 plus IL-12 plus MLT. Each group consisted of six courses of treatment, and each course consisted of two weeks of therapy. Because of their fundamental prognostic significance during cancer immunotherapy with cytokines, the biological response was evaluated by analyzing changes in the number of lymphocytes in venous blood samples collected before the onset of treatments and after two weeks of administration.

The experimental protocols were explained to each patient and written consent obtained. Data were reported as mean ± SE, and statistically analyzed by Student's *t*-test, the chi-square test, and the analysis of variance, as appropriate.

RESULTS

FIGURES 1 and 2 illustrate the mean number of lymphocytes and eosinophils, respectively, obseved in metastatic cancer patients before treatment and at the time of

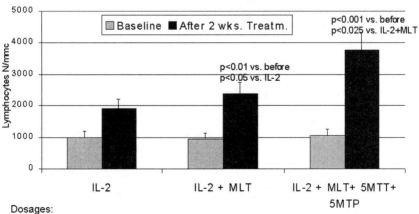

FIGURE 1. Lymphocyte mean number observed in metastatic cancer patients before and after low-dose IL-2 alone, IL-2 plus MLT, or IL-2 plus MLT plus 5-MTT and 5-MTP.

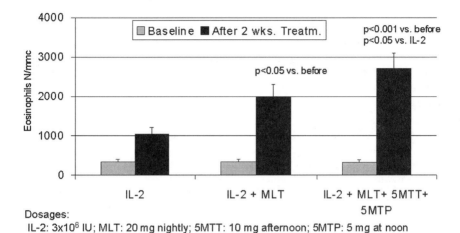

FIGURE 2. Eosinophil mean number observed in metastatic cancer patients before and after low-dose IL-2 alone, IL-2 plus MLT, or IL-2 plus MLT plus 5-MTT and 5-MTP.

their maximum increase during administration of low-dose IL-2 alone or IL-2 plus pineal indoles. The mean number of lymphocytes and eosinophils increased in response to low-dose IL-2 alone, but the only eosinophil increase reached statistical significance with respect to the values found before ($p < 0.05$). The concomitant administration of MLT induces an increase in the mean number of lymphocytes, which

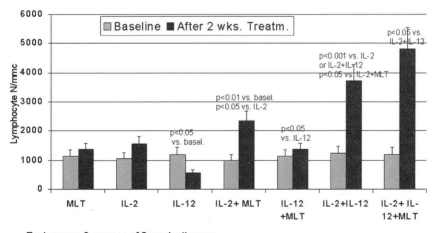

FIGURE 3. Lymphocyte mean number observed in metastatic cancer patients before and after low-dose IL-2 alone, MLT alone, IL-12 alone, IL-2 plus MLT, IL-12 plus MLT, IL-2 plus IL-12, and IL-2 plus IL-12 plus MLT.

was statistically significant with respect to that obseved after IL-2 alone ($p < 0.05$). In addition, the further association with 5-MTT and 5-Mtp induced a signifi canly higher increase in the mean number of lymphocytes with respect to that found with IL-2 plus MLT ($p < 0.025$). The increase in the mean number of eosinophils was also significantly higher after IL-2 plus MLT than after IL-2 alone ($p < 0.05$), whereas no significant difference was found in the mean number of eosinophils obseved after IL-2 plus MLT alone and IL-2 plus the 3 pineal indoles.

Changes in the mean number of lymphocytes obseved in metastatic renal cell cancer patients after MLT, IL-2, IL-12, or their combinations are illustrated in FIGURE 3. MLT alone induced no significant changes in the mean number of lymphocytes. IL-2 alone increased the of mean number lymphocytes, without, however, statistical significance with respect to the values observed before the two weeks of treatment. IL-12 alone induced a statistically significant decrease in the mean number of lymphocytes ($p < 0.05$ vs. before), which was significantly abrogated by the concomitant administration of MLT ($p < 0.05$ vs. IL-12 alone). The concomitant injection of low-dose IL-2 and IL-12 induced a very pronounced lymphocytosis, which was statistically significant with respect to each of the other combinations ($p < 0.001$ vs. IL-2 alone and IL-12 alone, $p < 0.01$ vs. IL-2 plus MLT). Finally, the concomitant administration of MLT induced a further significant increase in the mean number of lymphocytes with respect to IL-2 plus IL-12 ($p < 0.05$). The mean number of platelets decreased after both IL-2 and IL-12 alone, without, however, significant differences with respect to the counts seen before. In contrast, the combination of IL-2 plus IL-12 induced a significant decline in the mean number of platelets (96 ± 12 vs. $179 \pm 15 \times 10^3/mm^3$, $p < 0.05$). Cytokine-induced thrombocytopenia was nullified by the concomitant administration of MLT, and the mean number of platelets observed after IL-2 plus IL-12 plus MLT was significantly higher than that found after IL-2 plus IL-12 alone (153 ± 9 vs. $96 \pm 12 \times 10^3/mm^3$, $p < 0.05$).

MLT induced sleepiness and sedation, while neither 5-MTT nor 5-MTP induced sleepiness. In contrast, most patients reported an enhanced capacity for mental concentration after being given 5-MTP, and the symptomatology was already improved by the joint administration of 5-MTT and 5-MTP. In particular, asthenia occurred significantly less frequently in patients treated with IL-2 plus the three pineal indoles than in those receiving IL-2 alone or IL-2 plus MLT alone (1/12 vs. 9/28, $p < 0.05$).

DISCUSSION

According to our previous clinical investigations,[17] this study shows that MLT, which is the most investigated pineal immunomodulating hormone, may amplify the lymphocytosis induced by low-dose IL-2. Moreover, this study shows that the concomitant administration of other less investigated pineal indoles, such as 5-MTT and 5-MTP, may further amplify MLT-induced increase in the lymphocyte mean number in response to low-dose IL-2. The therapeutic implications of this finding in the cancer immunotherapy of human neoplasms need to be established by successive clinical studies. However, because of the fundamental importance of lymphocytosis in mediating the efficacy of IL-2 cancer immunotherapy,[1–4] it is possible to suggest that the impressive lymphocyte increase in response to IL-2 plus the three known pineal indoles with respect to IL-2 plus MLT may further improve the already clinically relevant clinical efficacy of this neuroimmune combination in the treatment of metastatic solid-tumor patients, who failed to respond to the standard anticancer therapies.[17] At present, however, it is still obscure whether 5-MTT and 5-MTP may further enhance MLT-induced amplification of IL-2 activity by acting on specific receptors expressed by immune cells, or whether by interacting with those for MLT. Moreover, at present it is still unknown whether the greater biological activity obtained with the three pineal indoles rather than with MLT alone may depend or not on a possible simultaneous replacement therapy of more pineal endocrine deficiencies. Cancer progression has been proven to be associated with a progressive decline in MLT nocturnal secretion.[18] In experimental conditions, MLT deficiency has appeared to reduce Il-2 secretion and activity.[19] Therefore, the exogenous administration of MLT could also represent an endocrine replacement therapy in advanced cancer patients. In contrast, at present there are no data about 5-MTT and 5-MTP blood concentrations in cancer patients in relation to the clinical history of their neoplastic disease. However, preliminary experimental studies would suggest that a deficiency of MLT tends to be associated with that involving other pineal indoles.[20] If successive studies will confirm a concomitant diminished production of 5-MTT and 5-MTP with the neoplastic progression, we could affirm that a total pineal indole replacement therapy can enhance the IL-2-dependent anticancer immunity with respect to the exogenous administration of the only MLT in advanced cancer patients. Moreover, the total pineal endocrine replacement therapy would reduce IL-2 toxicity further than does MLT alone.

In addition, this study shows that the pineal indole MLT may enhance the immunobiological activity not only of IL-2 but also that of the other fundamental anticancer cytokine in humans, IL-12. According to the preliminary results of this study, MLT would manipulate IL-12 activity by abrogating IL-12-induced lymphocytopenia with the following potential increase in the *in vivo* immunobiological action of IL-12 alone or IL-2 plus IL-12, which would constitute the most effective cytokine combination to induce lymphocytosis described up to now in cancer patients. Moreover, MLT would be effective in reducing the toxicity of the IL-2–IL-12 combination, particularly asthenia and thrombocytopenia.

Therefore, by taking into consideration the fundamental role of lymphocytosis to achieve *in vivo* an immune-system-mediated control of the neoplastic disease, the following conclusions from the present study seem to be justified:

1. The stimulatory effect of the pineal hormone MLT on IL-2-induced lymphocytosis can be further amplified by a total endocrine pineal replacement therapy, which can be reached by the simultaneous administration of the three main pineal indoles (MLT, 5-MTT, and 5-MTP).

2. IL-2-induced lymphocytosis may be extremely amplified by IL-12, which in contrast induces lymphocytopenia when it is injected alone, and the concomitant administration of MLT may further enhance the lymphocytosis induced by the IL-2–IL-12 combination and reduce its toxicity, namely thrombocytopenia.

Thus, this study may suggest the psychoneuroimmune bases for the future immunobiotherapies in the treatment of metastatic human neoplasms.

SUMMARY

Lymphocyte number still remains one of the most important immune parameters predicting the prognosis of advanced cancer patients. IL-2 and IL-12 are the main antitumor cytokines in humans, and their effect is modulated by the neuroendocrine system, mainly by the pineal gland through the circadian release of melatonin (MLT) and perhaps that of other indole hormones, such as 5-methoxytryptamine (5-MTT), and 5-methoxytryptophol (5-MTP). MLT has been proven to exert important antitumor immunomodulating effects, whereas the possible immunomodulatory properties of the other pineal indoles are still controversial. In an attempt to better define the pineal neuroendocrine regulation of the anticancer cytokine network, we have evaluated in metastatic solid-tumor patients the effects on lymphocyte number induced by different neuroimmune regimens, consisting of MLT alone (20 mg/day orally in the evening), subcutaneous (s.c.) low-dose IL-2 alone (3 MIU/day in the evening for 6 days/week), s.c. low-dose IL-12 alone (0.5 mcg/kg once/week in the morning), IL-12 plus MLT, IL-2 plus MLT, and IL-2 plus MLT plus 5-MTT (10 mg/day orally in the afternoon) plus 5-MTP (5 mg/day orally at noon). The results showed the following evidence: (1) MLT alone is unable to induce lymphocytosis; (2) MLT significantly enhances IL-2-induced lymphocytosis; (3) IL-12 alone determines lymphocytopenia, which can be reversed by MLT; (4) IL-2 plus IL-12 induces a very pronounced lymphocytosis, which can be further amplified by MLT; (5) a total pineal endocrine replacement therapy with MLT, 5-MTT, and 5-MTP further increases IL-2-induced lymphocytosis with respect to MLT plus IL-2 alone. Therefore, this study confirms that IL-2- and IL-12-dependent anticancer immunity is under a pineal modulation.

REFERENCES

1. ATZPODIEN, J. & H. KIRCHNER. 1990. Cancer, cytokines and cytotoxic cells: interleukin-2 in the immunotherapy of human neoplasms. Klin. Wochenschr. **68:** 1–11.
2. DI NICOLA, M., A. ANICHINI, R. MORTARINI, M. BREGNI, G. PARMIANI & A.M. GIANNI. 1998. Human dendritic cells: natural adjuvants in antitumor immunotherapy. Cytok. Cell. Molec. Ther. **4:** 265–273.
3. GRIMM, E.A., A. MAZUMDER, H.Z. ZHANG & S.A. ROSENBERG. 1982. Lymphokine-activated killer cell phenomenon. J. Exp. Med. **155:** 1823–1841.
4. LISSONI, P. 1996. Prognostic markers in interleukin-2 therapy. Cancer Biother. Radiopharm. **11:** 285–287.
5. JANKOVIC, B.D. 1994. Neuroimmunomodulation. From phenomenology to molecular evidence. Ann. N.Y. Acad. Sci. **741:** 1–38.
6. MANFREDI, B., P. SACERDOTE & M. BIANCHI. 1993. Evidence for an opioid inhibitory tone on T-cell proliferation. J. Neuroimmun. **44:** 43–47.
7. MAESTRONI, G.J.M. 1993. The immunoneuroendocrine role of melatonin. J. Pineal Res. **14:** 1–10.
8. GARCIA-MAURINO, S., M.G. GONZALES-HABA, J.R. CALVO, M. RAFII-EL-IDRISSI, V. SANCHEZ-MARGALET, R. GOBERNA & J.M. GUERRERO. 1997. Melatonin enhances IL-2, IL-6 and IFN-gamma production by human circulating CD4+ cells: a possible nuclear receptor-mediated mechanisms involving T helper type 1 lymphocytes and monocytes. J. Immunol. **159:** 574–581.
9. MAESTRONI, G.J.M. 1995. T-helper-2 lymphocytes as a peripheral target of melatonin. J. Pineal Res. **18:** 84–89.

10. LOTZE, M.T., B. HELLERSTEDT, L. STOLINSKI, T. TUETING, C. WILSON, D. KINZLER, H. VU, J.T. RUBIN, W. STORKUS, H. TAHARA, E. ELDER & T. WHITESIDE. 1997. The role of interleukin-2, interleukin-12, and dendritic cells in cancer therapy. Cancer J. Sci. Am. **3:** S109–S114.
11. LISSONI, P., S. BARNI, G. TANCINI, A. ARDIZZOIA, G. RICCI, R. ALDEGHI, F. BRIVIO, E. TISI, F. ROVELLI, R. RESCALDANI, G. QUADRO & G.J.H. MAESTRONI. 1994. A randomised study with subcutaneous low-dose interleukin-2 alone vs. interleukin-2 plus the pineal neurohormone melatonin in advanced solid neoplasms other than renal cancer and melanoma. Br. J. Cancer **69:** 196–199.
12. SZE, S.F., T.B. NG & W.K. LIU. 1993. Antiproliferative effect of pineal indoles on cultured tumor cell lines. J. Pineal Res. **14:** 27–33.
13. LISSONI, P., S. PITTALIS, F. ROVELLI, S. ZECCHINI, M. CASATI, M. TREMOLADA & F. PELIZZONI. 1996. Immunomodulatory properties of a pineal indole hormone other than melatonin, the 5-methoxytryptophol. J. Biol. Regul. Homeostatic Agents **10:** 27–30.
14. BRZEZINNSKI, A. 1997. Melatonin in humans. N. Engl. J. Med. **336:** 186–195.
15. WIGGINTON, J.M., K.L. KOMSCHLIES, T.C. BACK, J.L. FRANCO, M.J. BRUNDA & R.H. WILTROUT. 1996. Administration of interleukin 12 with pulse interleukin 2 and the rapid and complete eradication of murine renal carcinoma. J. Natl. Cancer Inst. **88:** 38–43.
16. MCISAAC, W.M., G. FARRELL, R.G. TABORSKY & A.N. TAYLOR. 1965. Indole compounds: isolation from bovine pineal tissue. Science **148:** 102–109.
17. LISSONI, P., M. LAUDON, S. BARNI, F. BRIVIO, E. TISI, F. ROVELLI, V. CHATIKHINE, L. FUMAGALLI, G.J.M. MAESTRONI, A. CONTI & G. TANCINI. 1998. Long-term results of cancer immunotherapy with subcutaneous low-dose interleukin-2 plus melatonin. Int. J. Immunother. **XIV:** 169–174.
18. BARTSCH, C., H. BARTSCH & T.H. LIPPERT. 1992. The pineal gland and cancer: facts, hypotheses and perspectives. Cancer J. **5:** 194–199.
19. DEL GOBBO, V., V. LIBRI, N. VILLANI, R. CALLO & G. NISTICÒ. 1989. Pinealectomy inhibits interleukin-2 production and natural killer activity in mice. Int. J. Immunopharmacol. **11:** 567–571.
20. SKENE, D.J., T. SMITH & J. ARENDT. 1986. Radioimmunoassay of pineal 5-methoxytryptophol in different species: comparison with pineal melatonin content. J. Endocrinol. **110:** 177–184.

What's in a Name?

Neuroimmunomodulation or Psychoneuroimmunology?

STEVEN GREER[a]

St. Raphael's Hospice, London Road, North Cheam, Surrey, United Kingdom

ABSTRACT: Compelling evidence is presented to support the hypothesis that psychological processes affect immune function. Consequently, it is argued that psychological processes should be included in human immunological studies and that neuroimmunomodulation could accurately by called psychoneuroimmunology.

INTRODUCTION

To suggest to the International Society for Neuroimmunomodulation that it should consider changing its name to Psychoneuroimmunology may well be regarded as hubris. Be that as it may, the issue is an important one that goes to the heart of a long-standing problem in medicine, namely the split between mind and body. Although perceptive clinicians have always recognized that mind and body are inextricably interwoven, Cartesian dualism remains deeply entrenched in medicine. All too often in medical research, psychological processes are ignored as a confounding nuisance.

The central question addressed here is whether psychological processes affect immune functions. Opinion is sharply divided. One observer,[1] in somewhat caustic language, describes psychoneuroimmunology (PNI) as a "still-born discipline"; "it is as though the whole conglomerate error of scientific thought over the last centuries . . . had infected this fetal pseudoscience." More restrained voices have argued that the evidence for direct links between the central nervous system (CNS) and immune system is unconvincing and that even if such links exist, they do not necessarily include psychological processes.[2,3] In striking contrast, other researchers claim that there is overwhelming evidence for communication each way between the CNS and immune system,[4,5] and that the influence of psychological processes on immune competence is reasonably well established.[5,6] Which of these views is correct? A detailed review of the literature is beyond the scope of the present paper, but arguably this question can be answered by focusing on some salient studies in this field.

The earliest published evidence suggesting a psychological influence on immune function was a study in 1963 by Black *et al.*, who reported that direct suggestion under hypnosis inhibited immediate-type hypersensitivity response[7] as well as the Mantoux reaction.[8] In the following year, Solomon and Moos published a seminal paper[9] that gave impetus to psychoimmunological research. The various psychological processes,

[a]Address for correspondence: Steven Greer, M.D., F.R.C. Psych., Consultant Psychiatrist, St. Raphael's Hospice, London Road, North Cheam, Surrey SM3 9DX, United Kingdom. Voice: 44-020-8335-4575; fax: 44-020-8335-4569.

the effect of which on immune function has been studied, can be grouped under the following headings:

1. *Bereavement.* In a controlled study of bereaved spouses, Bartrop *et al.*[10] first reported a significant reduction in mitogen-induced lymphocyte proliferation following bereavement. Similar findings were obtained in a study of bereaved men by Schleifer *et al.*,[11] but Monjan *et al.*'s study of bereaved men found no difference from matched controls in lymphocyte proliferation.[12] In another study, involving homosexual men whose partners had died of AIDS, immunological measurements were carried out before bereavement and up to one year later in these subjects as well as in a control group of nonbereaved homosexual men matched for age and HIV serostatus. In HIV-positive men, bereavement was significantly associated with decreased mitogen-induced lymphocyte proliferation, an effect that was not explained by the use of alcohol, tobacco, or other "recreational" drugs, or treatment with AZT.[13]

Natural killer (NK) cell activity has also been assayed in bereaved subjects, but results have been conflicting.[14,15] The most recent bereavement study represents an advance on previous studies in two respects: (i) assessments were made of how subjects coped with bereavement, and (ii) disease outcome was ascertained.[15]

In this study, homosexual HIV-positive men whose partners had died of AIDS were followed up for several years. Repeated measurements of CD4 lymphocyte levels were made, and coping responses to bereavement assessed. The important results of this study were that men who made deliberate efforts to find meaning in their lives following bereavement showed significantly less rapid decreases in CD4 levels and lower AIDS-related mortality rates. These results were independent of health status at baseline, health behaviors, and other confounding variables.

2. *Coping Style.* The relationship between coping style and immune function reported in the previous study[16] was also examined in another series of homosexual HIV-positive men by Goodkin *et al.*[17] Using a different measure of coping, they found, after controlling for alcohol and other drug use and nutritional status, that an active coping style was positively associated with NK cell activity.

3. *Psychological Stress.* In a series of investigations, Kiecolt-Glaser and her colleagues demonstrated that various psychologically stressful situations, such as medical students' final exams, marital strife, and the experience of looking after a spouse with dementia, resulted in decreased immune functions including higher levels of herpes virus antibody, mitogen-induced lymphocyte proliferation percentage of NK cells, and NK cell activity.[18–20]

Although most studies report that stressors lead to decreased immune function, this is not always the case. Increases in some immune functions in response to stressors have also been reported.[21] The authors of a critical review[22] point out that what is needed is to establish which immune functions are influenced by stressors, in which direction and under which circumstances, and that the timing of measurement could crucially affect the result.

A landmark study by Cohen *et al.*[23] revealed that psychological stress predicted the probability of developing upper respiratory tract infection, a result that was confirmed independently by Stone *et al.*[24] It seems likely that the observed association between psychological stress and subsequent respiratory infection is due to lowered immunity, but direct evidence for this is lacking.

A major study of psychological stress among women with regional breast cancer has been conducted by Andersen *et al.*[25] Stress levels and immune responses following surgery were measured before adjuvant therapy. After ruling out potentially confounding variables, the results revealed that stress levels significantly predicted: (i) lower NK cell activity; (ii) diminished response of NK cells to recombinant interferon-gamma; and (iii) decreased lymphocyte proliferation to plant lectins and to a monoclonal antibody directed against the T-cell receptor. The authors concluded that these results show that the physiologic effects of stress inhibit cellular immune responses that are relevant to cancer prognosis, including NK cell activity and T-cell responses. That conclusion is supported by two studies that have reported that lowered mitogen-induced lymphocyte proliferation in women with breast cancer is associated with a poor prognosis.[26,27]

4. *Depression.* Depression is associated with impaired cellular immunity. Patients with depressive illness show a reduction in mitogen-induced lymphocyte response, in a number of lymphocytes, and in NK cell activity.[28–31] These findings have been confirmed in a meta-analysis of 40 studies.[32] Humoral immunity is also affected by clinical depression, with reported increases in IgA, IgM, and IgE having been observed.[33]

5. *Emotional Support.* Perceived emotional support (often called "social support" in the literature) appears to enhance immune activity.[34]

A series of elderly men and women who reported that they had confiding relationships showed greater mitogen-induced lymphocyte proliferation than matched controls.[35] In another study, cancer patients' spouses who experienced emotional support also showed increased proliferative response as well as increased NK cell activity compared to spouses without emotional support.[36] However, Perry *et al.*[37] were unable to confirm the relationship between emotional support and immune function in their study of HIV-positive men.

6. *Psychological Interventions.* Perhaps the most compelling and clinically relevant evidence for a psychological effect on immune functions comes from recent studies of psychological intervention among patients with cancer and with HIV. Fawzy and his colleagues conducted a randomized trial of psychiatric intervention in patients with malignant melanoma.[38,39] Psychiatric intervention resulted in enhanced immune function, as shown by increases in CD8 cells, NK cells, and NK cell activity; these changes extended beyond the time of intervention and were observed six months later. At 5–6 years follow-up, the mortality among patients who received psychiatric intervention was significantly lower than among the control group. A randomized study of women with nonmetastatic breast cancer by Walker *et al.*[40] demonstrated that relaxation therapy and guided imagery were associated with greater lymphokine-activated killer-cell activity. Another randomized study, this time of women with regional and metastatic breast cancer, reported that psychotherapy was associated with lower plasma cortisol and prolactin levels and, in contrast to other studies, lower percentages of CD8 cells, NK cells, and CD4 cells, as well as lower mitogen-induced lymphocyte proliferation.[41] Last, a cognitive-behavioral stress-management program has been evaluated in a randomized study of symptomatic HIV-

positive homosexual men[42]; psychological intervention was found to be associated with reduced anxiety and reduced herpes simplex virus-type 2 immunoglobulin G antibody titers.

PROBLEMS IN PNI RESEARCH

Research in PNI is beset by formidable problems, both in methodology and in the interpretation of results.

Methodology

Measurement of immune function can be affected by age, sex, alcohol, tobacco, and other drugs, nutrition, and sleep[34,43]; moreover, immune assays are highly variable.[44] To require that all these factors should be controlled for is, perhaps, a counsel of perfection. Certainly few researchers have met these rigorous requirements fully.[34] As far as psychological measurements are concerned, a conspicuous drawback has been the failure to assess coping when studying the effect of stressors. Without measures of coping, it is unclear whether the stressors actually resulted in distress. To measure the effect of stressors in isolation would seem to be akin to listening to the sound of one hand clapping.[45]

Interpretation of Results

The interpretation of observed changes in immune function is problematic: (1) there is disagreement about the concept of global immunocompetence; (2) lymphoid cells in the peripheral blood constitute only about 5% of the total pool of immuno-cytes[22]; (3) the clinical relevance of the reported statistically significant changes in immune function remains largely unknown.

In a young, complex interdisciplinary field of research, such difficult problems are to be expected, and the fact that there are some inconsistent findings comes as no surprise. None of these shortcomings, however, invalidate the weight of evidence indicating a psychological influence on immune function.

SUMMARY AND CONCLUSIONS

1. There is compelling evidence that psychological processes can influence immune function.
2. Most PNI research has focused on cellular immunity; more data about humoral immunity are required.
3. Psychological processes that have been shown to affect immune function include various stressors, clinical depression, hypnosis, and certain kinds of psychological intervention.
4. In PNI studies of the effects of stressors, attention needs to be paid to the measurement of coping.
5. Whether and to what extent psychologically induced changes in immune function are clinically relevant remains to be established. There are some

early indications that psychological interventions may induce changes in immune function that have prognostic significance in certain cancers. This challenging work needs to be replicated.

6. Finally, the growing evidence documenting significant associations between psychological processes and the immune system demands the inclusion of psychological variables in immunological studies. PNI can make an important contribution to our understanding of the complexities of mind–body interactions and thereby to the practice of whole-person medicine.

REFERENCES

1. BIERMAN, S.F. 1996. Mind matters. Advances **12:** 51–60.
2. HALL, J.G. 1985. Emotion and immunity. Lancet **i:** 326–327.
3. LANGMAN, R. & M. COHN. 1993. No data yet show that the nervous system can contribute to the self-non-self discrimination by the immune system. Advances **9:** 39–50.
4. BLALOCK, J.E. 1994. The syntax of immune-neuroendocrine communication. Immunol. Today **15:** 504–511.
5. HALL, N.R.S., M. O'GRADY & D. CALANDRA. 1994. Transformation of personality and the immune system. Advances **10:** 7–15.
6. URSIN, H. 1994. Stress, distress and immunity. Ann. N.Y. Acad. Sci. **741:** 204–211.
7. BLACK, S. 1963. Inhibition of immediate-type hypersensitivity response by direct suggestion under hypnosis. Br. Med. J. **1:** 925–929.
8. BLACK, S., J.H. HUMPHREY & J.S.F. NIVEN. 1963. Inhibition of Mantoux reaction by direct suggestion under hypnosis. Br. Med. J. **1:** 1649–1652.
9. SOLOMON, G.F. & R.H. MOOS. 1964. Emotions, immunity and disease: a speculative theoretical integration. Arch. Gen. Psychiatry **11:** 657–674.
10. BARTROP, R.W., E. LUCKHURST, L. LAZARUS, L.G. KILOH & R. PENNY. 1977. Depressed lymphocyte function after bereavement. Lancet **i:** 834–836.
11. SCHLEIFER, S.J., S.E. KELLER, M. CAMERINO, J.C. THORNTON & M. STEIN. 1983. Suppression of lymphocyte stimulation following bereavement. JAMA **250:** 374–377.
12. MONJAN, A.A. 1984. Effects of acute and chronic stress upon lymphocyte blastogenesis in mice and humans. *In* Stress, Immunity and Ageing. C.L. Cooper, Ed.: 81–108. Dekker. New York.
13. KEMENY, M.E., H. WEINER, R. DURAN, S.E. TAYLOR, B. VISSCHER & F.L. FAHEY. 1995. Immune system changes after the death of a partner in HIV-positive gay men. Psychosom. Med. **57:** 547–554.
14. IRWIN, M., M. DANIELS, T.L. SMITH, E. BLOOM & H. WEINER. 1987. Impaired natural killer cell activity during bereavement. Brain Behav. Immun. **1:** 98–104.
15. IRWIN, M., M. DANIELS, E. BLOOM, T.L. SMITH & H. WEINER. 1987. Life events, depressive symptoms and immune function. Am. J. Psychiatry **144:** 437–441.
16. BOWER, J.E., M.E. KEMENY, S.E. TAYLOR & J.L. FAHEY. 1998. Cognitive processing, discovery of meaning, CD4 decline and AIDS-related mortality among bereaved HIV-seropositive men. J. Consult. Clin. Psychol. **66:** 979–986.
17. GOODKIN, K., N.T. BLANEY, D. FEASTER, M.A. FLETCHER, M.K. BAUM, E. MANTERO-ATIENZA, N.G. KLIMAS, C. MILLON, J. SZAPOCZNIK & C. EISDORFER. 1992. Active coping style is associated with natural killer cell cytotoxicity in asymptomatic HIV-1 seropositive homosexual men. J. Psychosom. Res. **36:** 635–650.
18. KIECOLT-GLASER, J.K., W. GARNER, C. SPEICHER, G.M. PENN, J. HOLLIDAY & R. GLASER. 1984. Psychosocial modifiers of immunocompetence in medical students. Pschosom. Med. **46:** 7–14.
19. KIECOLT-GLASER, J.K., L.D. FISHER, P. OGROCKI, H.J.C. STOUT, C.E. SPEICHER & R. GLASER. 1987. Marital quality, marital disruption, and immune function. Psychosom. Med. **49:** 13–34.

20. KIECOLT-GLASER, J.K., J.R. DURA, C.E. SPEICHER, O.J. TRASK & R. GLASER. 1991. Spousal caregivers of dementia victims: longitudinal changes in immunity and health. Psychosom. Med. **53:** 345–362.

21. FITTSCHEN, B., K.-H. SCHULZ, H. SCHULZ, A. RAEDLER & M. KEREKJARTO. 1990. Changes of immunological parameters in health subjects under examination stress. Int. J. Neurosci. **51:** 3–4.

22. SCHULZ, K.-H. & H. SCHULZ. 1992. Overview of psychoneuroimmunological stress— and intervention studies in humans with emphasis on the uses of immunological parameters. Psycho-Oncol. **1:** 51–70.

23. COHEN, S., D.A.J. TYRRELL & A.P. SMITH. 1991. Psychological stress and susceptibility to the common cold. New Engl. J. Med. **325:** 606–612.

24. STONE, A., G.D. BOVBJERG, J. NEALE, A. NAPOLI, H. VALDIMARSDOTTIR, D. COX, F. HAYDEN & J. GWALTNEY. 1992. Development of common cold symptoms following experimental rhino-virus infection as related to prior stressful life events. Behav. Med. **18:** 115–120.

25. ANDERSEN, B.L., W.B. FARRAR, D. GOLDEN-KREUTZ, L.A. KUTZ, R. MACCALLUM, M.E. COURTNEY & R. GLASER. 1998. Stress and immune responses after surgical treatment for regional breast cancer. J. Nat. Cancer Inst. **90:** 30–36.

26. MANDEVILLE, R., G. LAMOUREUX, S. LEGAULT-POISSON & R. SOISSON. 1982. Biological markers and breast cancer: a multiparametric study. Cancer **50:** 1280–1288.

27. BURFORD-MASON, A., G.M.L. GYTE & S.M. WATKINS. 1989. Phytohaemagglutinin responsiveness of peripheral lymphocytes and survival in patients with primary breast cancer. Breast Cancer Res. Treat. **13:** 243–250.

28. KRONFOL, Z., J.D. HOUSE & J. SILVA, JR. 1986. Depression, urinary free cortisol excretion and lymphocyte function. Br. J. Psychiat. **148:** 70–73.

29. DARKO, D. & J.C. GILLIN. 1989. Peripheral white blood cells and HPA axis neurohormones in major depression. Intern. J. Neurosci. **45:** 153–159.

30. IRWIN, M., U. LACHER & C. CALDWELL. 1992. Depression and reduced natural killer cytotoxicity: a longitudinal study of depressed patients and control subjects. Psychol. Med. **22:** 1045–1050.

31. SCHLEIFER, S.J., S.E. KELLER, J.A. BARTLET, H.M. ECKHOLDT & B.R. DELANEY. 1996. Immunity in young adults with major depressive disorder. Am. J. Psychiat. **153:** 477–482.

32. HERBERT, T.B. & S. COHEN. 1993. Depression and immunity: a meta-analytic review. Psychol. Bull. **113:** 472–486.

33. SONG, C., T. DINAN & B.E. LEONARD. 1994. Changes in immunoglobulin, complement and acute phase protein levels in depressed patients and normal controls. J. Affect. Dis. **30:** 283–288.

34. COHEN, S. & T.B. HERBERT. 1996. Health psychology: psychological factors and physical disease from the perspective of human psychoneuroimmunology. Annu. Rev. Psychol. **47:** 113–142.

35. THOMAS, P.D., J.M. GOODWIN & J.S. GOODWIN. 1985. Effect of social support on stress-related changes in cholesterol level, uric acid level, and immune function in an elderly sample. Am. J. Psychiat. **142:** 735–737.

36. BARON, R.S., S.E. CUTRONA, D. HICKLIN, D.W. RUSSELL & D.M. LUBAROFF. 1990. Social support and immune function among spouses of cancer patients. J. Pers. Soc. Psychol. **59:** 344–352.

37. PERRY, S., B. FISHMAN, L. JACOBSBERG & L. FRANCES. 1992. Relationships over 1 year between lymphocyte subsets and psychosocial variables among adults with infection by human immunodeficiency virus. Arch. Gen. Psychiat. **49:** 396–401.

38. FAWZY, F.I., M.E. KEMENY, N.W. FAWZY, R. ELASHOFF, D. MORTON, N. COUSINS & J.L. FAHEY. 1990. A structured psychiatric intervention for cancer patients. II. Changes over time in immunological measures. Arch. Gen. Psychiat. **47:** 729–735.

39. FAWZY, F., N.W. FAWZY, C.S. HYUN, R. ELASHOFF, D. GUTHRIE, J.L. FAHEY & D.L. MORTON. 1993. Malignant melanoma: effects of an early structured psychiatric intervention, coping and affective state on recurrence and survival 6 years later. Arch. Gen. Psychiat. **50:** 681–689.

40. WALKER, L.G., M.B. WALKER, E. SIMPSON, K. FIELDEN, A. OGSTON, A. SEGAR, S.D. HEYS, A.K. AH-SEE, A.W. HUTCHEON & O. EREMIN. 1997. Guided imagery and relaxation therapy can modify host defences in women receiving treatment for locally advanced breast cancer. Br. J. Surg. **84**(Suppl. 1): 31.

41. VAN DER POMPE, G., H.J. DUIVENVOORDEN, M.H. ANTONI, A. VISSER & C.J. HEIJNEN. 1997. Effectiveness of a short-term group psychotherapy program on endocrine and immune function in breast cancer patients: an exploratory study. J. Psychosom. Res. **42**: 453–466.

42. LUTGENDORF, S.K., M.H. ANTONI, G. IRONSON, N. KLIMAS, M. KUMAR, K. STARR, P. MCCABE, K. CLEVEN, M.A. FLETCHER & N. SCHNEIDERMAN. 1997. Cognitive-behavioural stress management decreases dysphoric mood and herpes's simplex Virus-type 2 antibody titres in symptomatic HIV-seropositive gay men. J. Consult. Clin. Psychol. **65**: 31–43.

43. IRWIN, M., A. MASCOVICH, J.C. GILLIN, R. WILLOUGHBY, J. PIKE & T.L. SMITH. 1994. Partial sleep deprivation reduces natural killer cell activity in humans. Psychosom. Med. **56**: 493–498.

44. SCHLEIFER, S.J., H.M. ECKHOLDT, J. COHEN & S.E. KELLER. 1993. Analysis of partial variance as a statistical approach to control day to day variation in immune assays. Brain Behav. Immun. **7**: 243–252.

45. WATSON, M. & S. GREER. 1998. Personality and coping. *In* Psychooncology. J.C. Holland, Ed.: 91–98. Oxford Univ. Press. New York.

Sympathetic Innervation Affects Superantigen-Induced Decrease in CD4Vβ8 Cells in the Spleen

ADRIANA DEL REY,[a] ALEXA KABIERSCH, SIGRID PETZOLDT, ANKE RANDOLF, AND HUGO O. BESEDOVSKY

Division of Immunophysiology, Institute of Physiology, Philipps-University, Marburg, Germany

ABSTRACT: The stimulation by superantigens of T cells expressing an appropriate Vβ chain results in a strong proliferative response that is followed by a state of energy specific for the antigen used. This model was used to continue our studies on immunoregulatory host neuroendocrine responses. We have recently found that four days after administration of the superantigen staphylococcal enterotoxin B (SEB) into mice, that is, at an early stage of the anergic phase, the decrease in the percentage of splenic CD4Vβ8 was accompanied by a decrease in the splenic concentration of the sympathetic neurotransmitter noradrenaline (NA) as compared to vehicle-injected mice. No comparable changes were detected in the kidney. At this point, blood levels of NA, adrenaline, and corticosterone were comparable in SEB- and vehicle-injected mice. We have also found that the decrease in splenic CD4Vβ8 cells was not observed in animals that had been chemically sympathectomized prior to the administration of the superantigen. These results indicate that the sympathetic response induced by SEB may have immunoregulatory implications.

INTRODUCTION

We have previously shown that the immune response to sheep red blood cells is paralleled by a decrease in noradrenaline (NA) concentration and turnover rate in the spleen, and that the decrease in splenic NA concentration is more sustained in immunologically high-responder animals.[1,2] Furthermore, we and others have reported that sympathetic innervation in the spleen can affect the immune response to conventional antigens like sheep red blood cells, trinitrophenyl-*N*-(2-aminoethyl) car-banylethyl dextran, and phosporylcholine containing a polysaccharide extract.[1,3] However, *in vivo* antigenic challenge does not necessarily culminate in specific immune effector functions, but may induce clonal unresponsiveness (for review, see Refs. 4 and 5). For example, injection of superantigens into adult animals initially leads to a strong proliferation of T cells expressing appropriate Vβ elements. This expansion phase is followed by a decline in the number of these cells by an

[a]Address for correspondence: Adriana del Rey, Institute of Physiology, Philipps-University, Deutschhausstrasse 2, 35037 Marburg, Germany. Voice: +49-6421-2862175; fax: +49-6421-2868925.

besedovs@mailer.uni-marburg.de

apoptosis-mediated mechanism, and the remaining cells are unresponsive to restimulation by the superantigen *in vitro* (T-cell anergy). The aim of our studies was to determine whether this type of immune response also affects neurotransmitter concentration in lymphoid organs, and if so, whether such a neural response has immunoregulatory consequences. The results reported here represent a first attempt at clarifying these questions. The experiments were performed at an early stage of the anergic phase of the response to staphylococcal enterotoxin B (SEB), a superantigen derived from gram-positive bacteria.

MATERIAL AND METHODS

Animals

Balb/c male mice (nine weeks old) were obtained from Harlan-Winkelmann, Germany. Animals were housed individually for one week before experiments were started and kept single-caged throughout in temperature- and light (12-h cycles)-controlled rooms. Animals were fed *ad libitum.*

Reagents

SEB from *Staphylococcus aureus* and 6-hydroxydopamine hydrochloride (6-OH-DA) were obtained from Sigma-Aldrich Chemie GmbH, Steinheim, Germany. Tricolor-labeled rat monoclonal antibody to mouse CD4 (clone CT-CD4) and FITC-labeled rat monoclonal antibody to mouse CD8 (clone CD8a) were obtained from Caltag-Medac GmbH, Hamburg, Germany, and PE-labeled antimouse Vβ8.1, 8.2 (clone MR5-2) from Pharmingen, Hamburg, Germany.

Experimental Procedure

SEB (10 μg/mouse) or physiological saline (0.9% NaCl) was injected i.p. into mice. Animals were killed by cervical dislocation four days later and blood was collected in EDTA-coated tubes. The spleen was weighed and divided into two portions; one was used for the determination of cell composition, and the other portion and the kidney were immediately frozen until NA determinations were performed.

Chemical Denervation

Mice received either 6-OH-DA (150 mg/kg in 0.01% ascorbic acid) or ascorbic acid injected i.p. (two injections, 24 h apart). SEB was injected 12 days later, as described previously.

Catecholamine Determinations

Noradrenaline concentration in tissues and plasma was determined by HPLC, as previously described.[6]

Flow Cytometry Analysis

Immediately after collection, cell suspensions from one half of the spleen of each individual mouse were prepared, and aliquots were used for flow cytometry analysis using standard techniques. Cells were double stained with TC-labeled anti-CD4 or FITC-labeled anti-CD8 and PE-labeled anti-Vβ8.

Statistical Analysis

Results are expressed as mean ± SE. Data were analyzed using one-way analysis of variance (ANOVA) followed by the Fisher test for multiple comparisons. Differences were considered significant at $p < 0.05$.

RESULTS AND DISCUSSION

The best *in vivo* characterized effect of SEB during the anergic phase of this immune response is the change in the percentage of cells expressing Vβ8 chains (for review, see Refs. 4 and 5). This is one of the major T-cell subpopulations that specifically recognizes the superantigen SEB. As shown in TABLE 1, four days after administration of SEB into mice, the percentage of CD4Vβ8 cells was decreased, and that of CD8Vβ8 was increased. The dose of SEB used did not affect the body weight. We have simultaneously determined that the splenic NA concentration in the SEB-injected mice was decreased when compared to that of saline-injected mice

TABLE 1. CD4Vβ8 and CD8Vβ8 cell subpopulations and noradrenaline levels 4 days after SEB administration

	Control	SEB
% CD4 cells among nucleated cells	25.6 ± 0.6	20.8 ± 0.8[a]
% Vβ8 cells among CD4 cells	24.7 ± 0.4	21.8 ± 0.4[a]
% CD8 cells among nucleated cells	11.1 ± 0.4	12.3 ± 0.5
% Vβ8 cells among CD8 cells	27.5 ± 0.3	31.4 ± 0.2[a]
Spleen weight (mg)	91.8 ± 3.9	137.5 ± 5.2[a]
NA (ng/g spleen)	641 ± 63	433 ± 51[a]
NA (ng/spleen)	58.2 ± 4.2	58.9 ± 4.9
Kidney weight (mg)	199.1 ± 2.2	189.8 ± 3.7
NA (ng/g kidney)	379 ± 24	332 ± 19
NA (ng/kidney)	75.4 ± 4.6	63.0 ± 3.8
NA (ng/mL plasma)	7.35 ± 1.49	7.49 ± 2.04

NOTE: Animals received physiological saline (control) or SEB and were killed 4 days later. The parameters included in the table were evaluated as described in Material and Methods.
[a]$p < 0.05$, as compared to control.

(TABLE 1). The spleen of SEB-injected mice was enlarged at this time, and this resulted in no differences in NA content in the whole organ between control and SEB-treated mice. No significant changes in NA concentration or content were detected in the kidney or in NA concentration in plasma. At this point, the blood levels of adrenaline and corticosterone were also comparable in both groups of mice (data not shown).

Increased cell number and a decreased sympathetic activity leading to blood retention are the main causes that could account for spleen enlargement. In any case, according to the results obtained, the immune response to SEB is expected to develop in the spleen in a microenvironment where NA concentration is reduced. We have therefore studied whether a further reduction in splenic NA content and concentration, as induced by chemical sympathectomy, could affect the SEB-induced change in the percentage of CD4Vβ8 and CD8Vβ8 cells in the spleen. Groups of mice were chemically denervated or received the vehicle alone (control). Twelve days later, both groups received SEB, and mice were killed after four days. As shown in FIGURE 1A, NA concentration in the spleen of SEB-, vehicle-injected mice was comparable to that shown in TABLE 1 for SEB-treated animals. As expected from the 6-OH-DA treatment, the concentration and content of NA in the spleen of SEB-injected, denervated mice was much more markedly reduced. In these animals, the percentage of CD4Vβ8 cells was significantly increased as compared to that of SEB-injected control mice (FIG. 1B). Interestingly, CD8Vβ8 cells seem not to have been affected by the denervation, since the percentage of this cell subtype was comparable in both groups of mice. For comparison, the ratio CD4Vβ8/CD8Vβ8 cells in the spleen of normal animals, and of vehicle- or denervated mice that received SEB 4 days before, is shown in FIGURE 2.

The observation that the SEB-induced diminution in the percentage of CD4Vβ8 cells is not detected in denervated mice suggests that splenic sympathetic innervation may play a functional role. In our view, two main, not mutually exclusive, mechanisms may explain this finding. One mechanism could involve the proapoptotic effects of NA. Apoptosis of the stimulated cells has been proposed as the main cause of the specific decrease in cell number after SEB inoculation,[7,8] and we have recently found that NA can trigger apoptosis in T cells via β-adrenergic receptors (manuscript in preparation). For example, in vitro exposure of splenic cells to 10^{-5} M NA for four hours results in about an 80% increase in the percentage of apoptotic cells among Thy 1.2 cells, and in about an 85% increase in apoptotic cells among CD4 cells. The percentage of apoptotic cells was evaluated by assessing exposure of phosphatidylserine using FITC-labeled Annexin V, and decrease of mitochondrial potential using 3,3′-dihexyloxacarbocyanine iodide. Using propidium iodide fluorescence as indicator, other authors have also reported that NA can induce apoptosis in splenic lymphocytes.[9] It is therefore conceivable that a marked decrease in NA concentration in the spleen, such as that obtained in chemically denervated mice, might impede the contribution of the neurotransmitter to apoptosis of CD4 cells. Preliminary results indicate that these cells are more sensitive than CD8 to NA-induced apoptosis. The decrease in NA concentration in the spleen of intact, SEB-injected animals could represent a means to restrict NA-induced apoptosis. The second mechanism involved could be related to effects of the neurotransmitter on cell traffic.

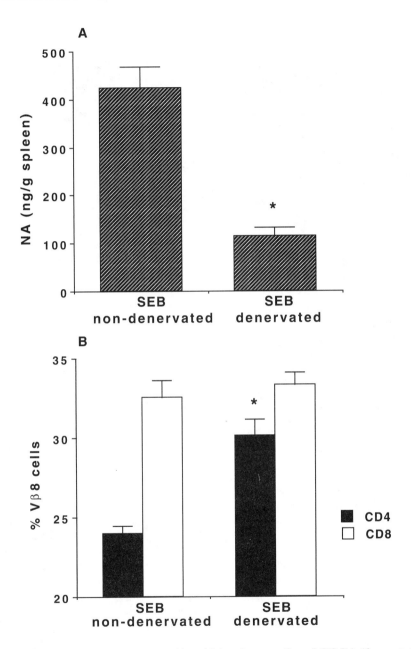

FIGURE 1. Mice received ascorbic acid (nondenervated) or 6-OH-DA (denervated). SEB was injected 12 days later, and NA concentration in the spleen (**A**) and the percentage of CD4Vβ8 among CD4 cells and of CD8Vβ8 among CD8 cells in the spleen (**B**) were determined after 4 days. Each column represents the mean ± SE of the results obtained from 6–7 animals/group. *$p < 0.05$ as compared to the corresponding parameter of the nondenervated mice.

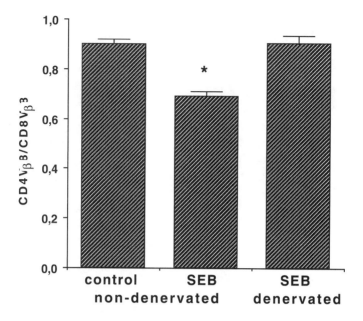

FIGURE 2. The ratio CD4Vβ8/CD8Vβ8 cells in the spleen of normal animals (control; $n = 4$), and of vehicle (nondenervated; $n = 7$), or denervated mice ($n = 6$) that received SEB four days before, is shown. Each column represents the mean ± SE. *$p < 0.05$, as compared to control and denervated mice.

We have recently reported that, under certain conditions, NA can increase lymphoid cell mobilization from the spleen by a smooth-muscle-independent, β-adrenergic mediated mechanism.[10] It has been shown that stimulated T cells express more β-adrenergic receptors than resting cells. For example, after stimulation of quiescent T lymphocytes by IL-2, there is an increase in β-adrenergic receptor activity.[11] It is intriguing that the percentage of CD8Vβ8 cells seems not to be affected by sympathectomy, but the results obtained would be in agreement with the finding that CD8 lymphocytes express fewer β-adrenergic receptors than CD4 cells.[12] The evidence mentioned earlier allows us to postulate that an intact innervation would favor the migration of stimulated CD4Vβ8 cells from the spleen, thus resulting in a proportional decrease in their number. This mechanism would be absent in denervated animals. We are at present performing experiments to determine whether one or both of these potential mechanisms play a role in the phenomenon described, and whether those CD4Vβ8 cells found in the spleen of denervated, SEB-injected mice are functional or anergic.

ACKNOWLEDGMENT

This work was supported by the Deutsche Forschungsgemeinschaft (SFB 297).

REFERENCES

1. ESEDOVSKY, H.O., A. DEL REY, E. SORKIN, M. DA PRADA & H.A. KELLER. 1979. Immunoregulation mediated by the sympathetic nervous system. Cell. Immunol. **48:** 346–355.
2. DEL REY, A., H.O. BESEDOVSKY, E. SORKIN, M. DA PRADA & P. BONDIOLOTTI. 1982. Sympathetic immunoregulation: difference between high- and low-responder animals. Am. J. Physiol. **242:** R30–R33.
3. MILES, L., J. QUINTANS, E. CHELMICKA-SCHORR & E.G.W. ARNASON. 1981. The sympathetic nervous system modulates antibody response to thymus-independent antigens. J. Neuroimmunol. **1:** 101–105.
4. HERMAN, A., J.W. KAPPLER, P. MARRACK & A.M. PULLEN. 1991. Superantigens: mechanism of T-cell stimulation and role in immune responses. Annu. Rev. Immunol. **9:** 745–772.
5. FLEISCHER, B. & H.O. SJÖGREN. 1991. Superantigens. Springer Verlag. Heidelberg.
6. KABIERSCH, A., A. DEL REY, C.G. HONEGGER & H.O. BESEDOVSKY. 1988. Interleukin-1 induces changes in norepinephrine metabolism in the rat brain. Brain Behav. Immun. **2:** 267–274.
7. WAHL, C., T. MIETHKE, K. HEEG & H. WAGNER. 1993. Clonal deletion as direct consequence of an *in vivo* T cell response to bacterial superantigen. Eur. J. Immunol. **23:** 1197–1200.
8. D'ADAMIO, L., K.M. AWAD & E. REINHERZ. 1993. Thymic and peripheral apoptosis of antigen-specific T cells might cooperate in establishing self tolerance. Eur. J. Immunol. **23:** 747–753.
9. JOSEFSSON, E., J. BERGQUIST, R. EKMAN & A. TARKOWSKI. 1996. Catecholamines are synthesized by mouse lymphocytes and regulate function of these cells by induction of apoptosis. Immunology **88:** 140–146.
10. ROGAUSCH, H., A. DEL REY, J. OERTEL & H.O. BESEDOVSKY. 1999. Norepinephrine stimulates lymphoid cell mobilization from the perfused rat spleen via β-adrenergic receptors. Am. J. Physiol. **276:** R724–R730.
11. DAILEY, M.O., J. SCHREURS & H. SCHULMAN. 1988. Hormone receptors on cloned T lymphocytes. Increased responsiveness to histamine, prostaglandins and β-adrenergic agents as a late stage in T cell activation. J. Immunol. **140:** 2931–2936.
12. LANDMANN, R.M.A., H. BITTIGER & F.R. BÜHLER. 1981. High affinity beta-2-adrenergic receptors in mononuclear leucocytes: similar density in young and old normal subjects. Life Sci. **29:** 1761–1771.

Variability of Interactions Between Neuroendocrine and Immunological Functions in Physiological Aging and Dementia of the Alzheimer's Type

E. FERRARI,[a] M. FIORAVANTI, F. MAGRI, AND S.B. SOLERTE

Department of Internal Medicine, University of Pavia,
Piazza Borromeo 2, 27100 Pavia, Italy

ABSTRACT: A link between neuroendocrine and immunological changes has been suggested in the pathophysiology of dementia of the Alzheimer's type (DAT). Healthy young and old subjects and patients with DAT were recruited to evaluate the chrononeuroendocrine organization of cortisol, GH, and melatonin (MLT) secretions. The study was carried out together with the evaluation of natural killer (NK) cell function: cytotoxic activity (NKCC) and TNF-α and IFN-γ release after exposure to IL-2 (100 U/mL). Moreover, a cerebral morphometric analysis of hippocampus and temporal lobe (MRI) was performed. The activation of hypothalamo–pituitary–adrenal (HPA) axis and the decrease of GH, and MLT nocturnal peaks were associated with normal NKCC and TNF-α/IFN-γ in healthy elderly subjects, whereas in DAT patients the same neuroendocrine changes occurred together with abnormal NKCC (spontaneous and IL-2/IFN-β-modulated) and with alterations of TNF-α/INF-γ generation from NK. Moreover significant correlations among the increase of NKCC and TNF-α and the decrease of cognitive function were found in the DAT group. These correlations were associated with the impairment of nocturnal GH and MLT levels and with the relatively higher serum cortisol concentrations. Moreover, the impairment of cortisol suppression after dexamethasone (1 mg orally at 23:00) was significantly correlated with the increase of spontaneous release of TNF-α and with IL-2-modulated NKCC. Finally the imunoneuroendocrine alterations found in DAT were associated with the reduction of cerebral volume in hippocampus and temporal lobes. Taken together these data indicate that the immmunoneuroendocrine balance is maintained in physiological aging, whereas NK immune dysregulation in DAT could contribute to altering the neuroendocrine functions and to extend the progression of neurodegeneration and dementia.

INTRODUCTION

Multiple interactions among immunoneuroendocrine factors could contribute to physiologic aging brain and to develop the Alzheimer's disease (AD) neuropathology.

[a]Address for correspondence: Dr. E. Ferrari, Department of Internal Medicine, Geriatrics and Gerontology Clinic, Post-graduate School of Geriatrics and Endocrinology, University of Pavia, Piazza Borromeo 2, 27100 Pavia, Italy. Voice: 0039-382-27769; fax: 0039-382-28827.
ferrari@unipv.it

Within this context, neuroendocrine changes related to hypothalamo–pituitary–adrenal axis (HPA) and to GH and melatonin (MLT) secretion have been reported in normal aging and dementia.[1–8] Furthermore, a dysregulation of the immune system has been linked either with neuroimmune disorders associated with dementia of the Alzheimer's type (DAT),[9–16] or with functional changes of endocrine and neuroendocrine patterns.[17–24]

Concerning the pathophysiology of DAT, no conclusive data related to immunoneuroendocrine interactions with the mechanism of neurodegeneration are reported in the literature. However, experimental and clinical evidences would seem to suggest that immune factors could negatively influence the neuroendocrine control of GH, MLT and cortisol secretions. In particular, the immune cell activity and the immunomodulated cytokine release could affect the neuroendocrine regulation of cortisol, GH and MLT secretion.[17–24] All these changes might contribute to the development of neurodegeneration in brain areas involved in the physiologic regulation of learning and memory (hippopcampus and frontotemporal cortex), thereby inducing cognitive impairment and dementia. Indeed, glucocorticoids can potentially increase the neurodegenerative risk at the hippocampal level, and hence influence the cognitive functions in normal and pathological aging.[25–29] On the other hand, the atrophy of hippocampus may fourthly sustain the activation of HPA axis and its impaired sensitivity toward the steroid negative feedback.[7,30,31]

These evidences raised the question of the importance of having new insights on the modulatory effect of the immune system on the neuroendocrine system in order to analyze, in a selected group of patients with DAT, the complex mechanism suggested in the development of brain neuropathology.

SUBJECTS AND METHODS

Healthy subjects and old patients with DAT were included in the study. The recruitment concerned 22 healthy young subjects, age range 19–43 yr (mean age 26.8 ± 1.1 SEM), 52 healthy old subjects, age range 66–90 yr (mean age 80.3 ± 0.84 SEM), and 20 old patients with DAT, age range 69–90 yr (mean age 81.1 ± 1.41 SEM). Healthy old subjects were carefully selected on the basis of the SENIEUR protocol, in order to exclude clinical and immunological alterations.[32] The diagnosis of probable or possible DAT was performed according to the criteria of the DSM III-R,[33] and confirmed with the diagnostic standards of NINCDS-ADRDA criteria.[34] All patients with DAT had a Hachinsky ischemic score of less than 4.[35] Diagnosis of DAT was also supported by clinical and neurological examination and by brain imaging (MRI or CT scan). The severity of dementia and the degree of cognitive impairment were assessed by using the Clinical Dementia Rating (CDR) and the Mini Mental State Examination (MMSE) score.[36] Finally, patients with DAT were free of any medication and of diseases known to affect immune function. The study was conducted in accordance with the declaration of Helsinki and was approved by the Ethical Committee of the Department of Internal Medicine of the School of Medicine of the University of Pavia. Written informed consent was also obtained from all subjects or, where appropriate, from their caregivers.

Healthy subjects and old patients with DAT were studied at least seven days after the hospital admission, in order to allow their synchronization to the hospital-life schedule (meals at 8 A.M., 12:00 noon, and 6 P.M.; sleep in darkness from 7 P.M. to 6 A.M.), and all the subjects were studied on a normocaloric diet. The circadian rhythm of serum cortisol (at baseline and after suppression with dexamethasone: 1 mg orally at 11 P.M.), GH and melatonin (MLT) were simultaneously evaluated in every healthy subjects and DAT patients by samplings every four hours during the day (from 8 A.M. to 8 P.M.) and every two hours during the night (from 8 P.M. to 4 A.M.). The statistical significance of the hormonal fluctuations throughout the 24-h cycle was validated by the single and mean cosinor methods;[38] comparison of the rhythm parameters among the three groups was carried out by the mesor test and the amplitude-acrophase Hotelling's test.[39]

In order to avoid the venipuncture stress, blood samples were obtained throughout an indwelling catheter inserted into an antecubital vein before the study. Blood samples were immediately centrifuged and extracted serum was stored at $-20°C$ until the immunometric assay. Cortisol and GH measurements were performed by time-resolved fluoroimmunoassay (DELFIA-WALLAC Turke, Finland) and the results were expressed as µg/dL and ng/mL, respectively; the intra- and interassay coefficients of variation were always below 7%, and the minimal detectable concentration was 0.54 µg/dL for cortisol and 0.05 ng/mL for GH. Plasma melatonin (MLT) was determined by radioimmunoassay (Nichols Institute BV, Wychen, NL) with diethyl-ether extraction of 500-mL volume of anticoagulated plasma, and the results were expressed as pg/mL; the intra- and interassay coefficients of variation were below 10% and the low detection limit was 3 pg/mL.

In the three groups of subjects a cerebral morphometric analysis of the hippocampus and temporal cortex was performed in agreement with previous studies[8,37]; the MRI analysis was conducted with a Toshiba MRT-35 system operating at 0.35 T. The sequence analysis, protocol of employement, and calibration procedures were described elsewhere.[8]

The separation of NK cells (immunological procedure) was obtained in a completely sterile manner, as previously described.[13-15] In summary, peripheral blood mononuclear cells (PBMC) were isolated by Ficoll-Hypaque density gradient. The enriched fraction of PBMC containing T/NK cells was used for the magnetic cell separation procedure (MACS, Miltenyi Biotech GmbH, Bergisch, Gladbach, Germany), in which the negative unlabeled fraction represents the enriched nonmagnetic NK cell fraction (CD 16+, CD 56+, CD 3− cells). The efficency of separation was measured with flow cytometry (FACScan Becton Dickinson, Mountain View, CA); the purity of NK cells exceeded 97% and viability was above 95%. After magnetic separation, NK cells were resuspended in complete RPMI 1640 medium and concentrated to a final measured density of 7.75×10^6 cells/mL of complete medium. These cells were incubated for 20 h without modulators (spontaneous conditions), with IL-2 (100 U/mL/ cells of Proleukin, Chiron Corporation, Emeryville) and IFN-β (650 U/mL/cells of Betantrone, Italfarmaco, Milano, Italy) in order to measure spontaneous and cytokine-modulated NK cell cytotoxicity (NKCC) against tumoral targets K562.[40,41] TNF-α and IFN-γ concentrations in the supernatant fluids of NK cells were measured, in spontaneous conditions and after exposure with IL-2 (100 U/mL) and cortisol

(10^{-6} M/mL) by a standard ELISA procedure (Bender MedSystems Diagnostics GmbH, Wien, Austria).

Because of the skewed distribution of cortisol, GH, and MLT values, a nonparametric statistical analysis was performed: data were analyzed by the Friedman ANOVA and Kendall coefficient of concordance test and the Kruskal-Wallis ANOVA, and were compared using the Mann-Whitney U-test. The correlations between hormonal secretions and clinical data were calculated by the Spearman's Rank Order correlation coefficient. ANOVA F-test, paired Student's *t*-test, and linear regression analysis were used for immunological data. The threshold level of significance was $p < 0.05$ (two-tailed).

RESULTS

FIGURE 1 and TABLE 1 summarize the circadian pattern and the population mean cosinor summary, respectively, of serum cortisol (baseline and after DXM administration), GH, and plasma melatonin of healthy subjects(of young and old age) and of DAT patients. The cortisol circadian profile was clearly flattened in elderly subjects, both demented and not, when compared to healthy young subjects. The most relevant differences among the three groups of subjects occured at the evening and nighttime. Indeed the serum cortisol nadir values were significantly higher in old than in young subjects, and even more in DAT patients. The nocturnal increase of serum cortisol (namely, the difference between the values recorded at 8 A.M. and at midnight) was significantly impaired in old subjects, and particularly in DAT patients, by comparison to healthy young subjects (9.26 ± 0.88, 8.02 ± 1.83, and 16.10 ± 1.39, respectively; $p < 0.001$). The reduction of the nocturnal increase of serum cortisol was significantly related to the subjects' age ($r = -0.40$, $p < 0.001$).

The circadian rhythm of serum cortisol reached statistical significance in the three groups of subjects. By comparison to healthy young subjects, the cortisol circadian mesor was significantly higher in aged subjects, and in particular in the demented ones. Besides, a reduction in the amplitude of cortisol rhythm occurred in healthy elderly subjects, in particular when demented. Both the increase of the nadir values and the reduction of the amplitude of the circadian fluctuations were significantly related to the subjects' age ($r = 0.29$, $p < 0.01$ and $r = -0.27$, $p < 0.05$, respectively); on the contrary, the effects of the age on the increase of the cortisol mean levels reached statistical significance only in the DAT group ($r = 0.59$, $p < 0.001$). The mean serum cortisol levels, recorded after DXM administration, were significantly higher in DAT patients than in healthy old and young subjects. The circadian rhythm of serum cortisol after DXM did not reach statistical significance in DAT patients. Furthermore, the percent decrease of the cortisol circadian mesor related to DXM administration was significantly lower in healthy old subjects, and especially in DAT patients, than in healthy young subjects (63.2%, 52.7%, and 79.8%, respectively).

A selective impairment of MLT nocturnal peak occurred in healthy elderly subjects, demented or not, by comparison to young controls. Thus, the circadian profile of plasma melatonin was clearly flattened in aged people.

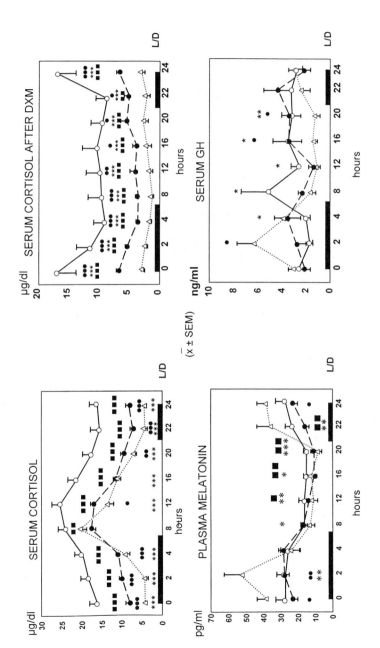

FIGURE 1. Circadian profile of serum cortisol (before and after DXM), GH, and plasma melatonin in healthy young (*open triangles*) and elderly (*closed circles*) subjects , and in patients with DAT (*open circles*). L/D = light/dark. $\bullet$ $p < 0.05$, $\bullet\bullet$ $p < 0.01$, $\bullet\bullet\bullet$ $p < 0.001$, young versus elderly subjects; * $p < 0.05$, ** $p < 0.01$, *** $p < 0.001$, young subjects versus DAT patients; $\blacksquare$ $p < 0.05$, $\blacksquare\blacksquare$ $p < 0.01$, $\blacksquare\blacksquare\blacksquare$ $p < 0.001$, healthy elderly subjects versus DAT patients.

TABLE 1. Population mean cosinor summary of the circadian rhythms evaluated

	p	Mesor (Mean ± SEM)	Amplitude (Mean ± SEM)	Acrophase (hours) (95% CI)
Serum cortisol (μg/dL)				
Young subjects	0.0001	10.76 ± 0.79	6.58 ± 0.66	10:06 (09:18 to 10:52)
Old subjects	0.0001	12.37 ± 0.56	4.97 ± 0.35	10:12 (09:35 to 10:47)
DAT patients	0.0001	20.48 ± 1.82	4.66 ± 0.60	10:39 (09:02 to 12:31)
Cortisol after DXM (μg/dL)				
Young subjects	0.0036	2.06 ± 0.46	0.85 ± 0.28	21:11 (18:03 to 01:10)
Old subjects	0.0007	4.34 ± 0.52	1.12 ± 0.32	22:24 (19:20 to 02:10)
DAT patients	0.2675	10.4 ± 2.21	1.32 ± 0.70	00:21
Plasma melatonin (pg/mL)				
Young subjects	0.0002	21.12 ± 3.23	17.16 ± 2.91	01:30 (00:16 to 03:08)
Old subjects	0.0001	17.39 ± 1.66	9.26 ± 1.28	03:45 (02:53 to 04:49)
DAT patients	0.1003	20.12 ± 2.63	6.55 ± 2.71	02:00
Serum GH (ng/mL)				
Young subjects	0.0007	2.31 ± 0.31	1.89 ± 0.35	02:42 (00:13 to 04:07)
Old subjects	0.0178	2.80 ± 0.34	0.76 ± 0.35	21:27 (02:52 to 17:03)
DAT patients	0.1993	1.20 ± 0.25	0.25 ± 0.19	12:35

NOTE: Mesor test: **, $p < 0.01$; ***, $p < 0.001$; Hotelling's test: ■, $p < 0.05$; ■■, $p < 0.01$; ■■■, $p < 0.001$.

The circadian rhythm of plasma MLT reached statistical significance in healthy young and old subjects, but not in DAT patients. The amplitude of the plasma MLT circadian fluctuations was clearly dampened in healthy old subjects, and especially in DAT patients, by comparison to healthy young subjects.

Significant inverse correlations were found among the subjects' age and the nocturnal peak, the index, and the circadian amplitude of plasma MLT ($r = -0.44$, $p < 0.001$; $r = -0.43$, $p < 0.001$, and $r = -0.44$, $p < 0.001$, respectively).

By comparison to healthy young subjects, the circadian profile of GH of healthy elderly subjects and of DAT patients showed the absence of the physiological sleep-related nocturnal peak, while abnormal diurnal peaks were found. A statistically significant circadian rhythm of GH was detectable in healthy young and old subjects, but not in DAT patients.

FIGURE 2 shows the cerebral morphometric analysis concerning the hippocampus and temporal lobe volumes. The volumes of right and left hippocampus and of temporal lobes were significantly lower in healthy old subjects, and particularly in the demented ones, when compared to healthy young subjects ($p < 0.001$). These volumetric reductions were significantly related to both the subjects' age and the impairment of cortisol nocturnal increase.

FIGURE 3 shows the mean variations of NKCC (percent increase after IL-2 and IFN-β) in healthy subjects (of young and old age) and in patients with DAT. Significantly higher NKCC was demonstrated in the DAT group than in healthy subjects ($p < 0.001$), whereas no differences were found between healthy young and old subjects.

FIGURE 4 reports the mean variations of spontaneous TNF-α and IFN-γ release from NK in healthy subjects (of young and old age) and in patients with DAT. Elevated TNF-α and IFN-γ release from NK was demonstrated in DAT patients compared to healthy subjects ($p < 0.001$), without differences between healthy groups.

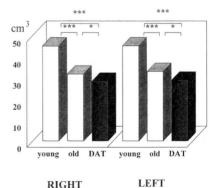

FIGURE 2. Cerebral morphometric analysis of hippocampus and temporal lobes in healthy young and elderly subjects (*open bars*) and in patients with DAT (*closed bars*). *$p < 0.05$, **$p < 0.01$, ***$p < 0.001$.

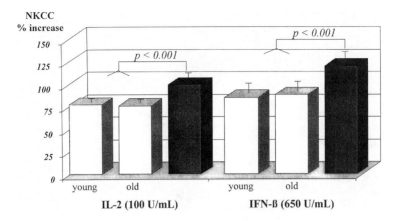

FIGURE 3. Mean variations of NK cell cytotoxicity (NKCC) after IL-2 and IFN-β exposure in healthy young and elderly subjects (*open bars*) and in patients with DAT (*closed bars*).

The percent decrease of TNF-α and IFN-γ release from NK after cortisol exposure was significantly reduced in DAT patients (22% and 42%, respectively) in comparison to healthy subjects (46% and 58%, respectively; $p < 0.001$).

FIGURE 5 shows the correlations and linear regression analysis among cortisol mesor, NKCC (percent increase after IL-2), and TNF-α (spontaneous release) in patients with DAT. Significant positive correlations were found among the increase of NKCC and TNF-α levels and cortisol mesor (expressed as mcg/dL).

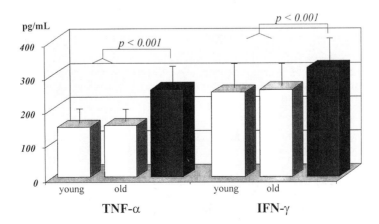

FIGURE 4. Mean variations of spontaneous release of TNF-α and IFN-γ from NK cells in healthy young and elderly subjects (*open bars*) and in patients with DAT (*closed bars*).

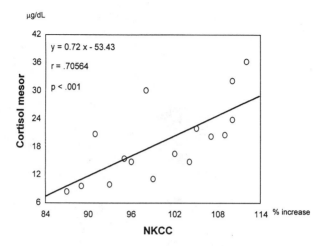

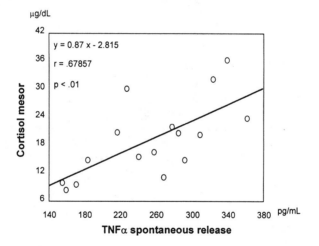

FIGURE 5. Correlations and linear regression analysis among cortisol mesor, NKCC (percentage increase after IL-2), and TNF-α (spontaneous release) in patients with DAT.

FIGURE 6 reports the correlations and linear regression analysis among cortisol mesor after DXM (expressed as percent decrease of the cortisol mesor before DXM), cortisol levels at 8 A.M. after DXM (expressed as percent decrease of cortisol at 8 A.M. before DXM), NKCC (after IL-2), and TNF-α (spontaneous release) in patients with DAT. Significant correlations were demonstrated among the increase of NKCC and TNF-α levels and the reduction of cortisol response after DXM (circadian mesor and 8 A.M. values).

Finally, no significant correlations were found among immunological parameters, GH, and MLT.

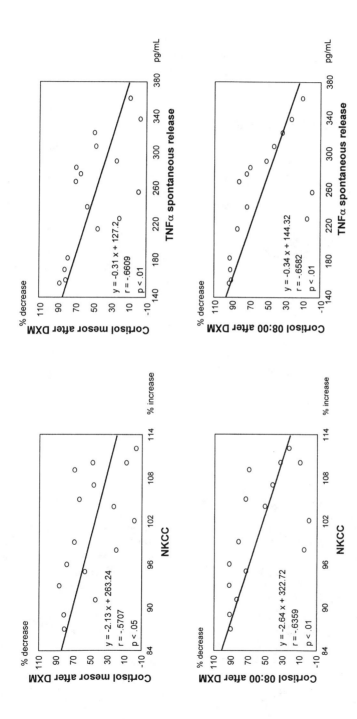

FIGURE 6. Correlations and linear regression analysis among cortisol mesor after DXM (expressed as percent decrease in comparison with cortisol mesor before DXM), cortisol levels at 8 A.M. after DXM (expressed as percent decrease in comparison with cortisol at 8 A.M. before DXM), NKCC (percentage increase after IL–2), and TNF-α (spontaneous release) in patients with DAT.

DISCUSSION

Cells of the immune, neuroendocrine, and central nervous systems can have reciprocal effects on paracrine, autocrine, and endocrine control of release of cytokines, hormones, and growth factors, which in turn regulate the complex multidirectional communications among these systems. Therefore, functional cell biology can offer useful supports in order to understand the events related to aging brain either in physiological conditions or during DAT neurodegeneration.

Growing evidence suggests that immunoneuroendocrine cell-to-cell interactions can be involved in the neurodegenerative mechanism of DAT. The activation of HPA axis and the impairment of GH-IGF-I secretory patterns could be dependent on abnormal signals arising from immune cells, and in particular on cytokine generation and release from circulating mononuclear cells (i.e., monocytes, natural killer, and T lymphocytes).

The main suggestion linked to the association between immune and neuroendocrine systems in DAT may concern the proved neurotoxic effects of adrenal glucocorticoids and cytokines (i.e., IFN-γ, TNF-α, IL-1, IL-6, IL-8) against cholinergic neurons of the hippocampus and of the frontotemporal cortex, while the adverse effects of cytokines on GH-IGF-I secretions can reduce the availability of neurotrophic and pleiotrophic hormones that rescue and protect neural cells from neurotoxic damage.[42,43] Synergy of action between immune and neuroendocrine factors could therefore enhance the risk of amyloidogenesis and of neurodegenerative processes into the brain parenchyma, leading to cognitive loss and DAT. Within this context, our study clearly demonstrated disturbances of immune and neuroendocrine functions in patients with DAT and first reported important correlations between NK functional and secretory activity and neuroendocrine parameters of DAT patients with mild to moderate dementia.

The main features demonstrated in our study concerned the abnormal NKCC and NK secretory pattern, the activation of HPA axis, and the impairment of GH and MLT regulation in DAT patients, whereas no immune changes were reported in healthy elderly subjects.

With respect to HPA activation, we suggest that the immune inputs arising from TNF-α and IFN-γ released by NK cells could enhance, as well as demonstrated for the cytokines IL-1 and IL-6, the non-ACTH-mediated synthesis of glucocorticoids from the adrenal cortex.[44,45] Furthermore, TNF-α and IFN-γ could have a direct immunoendocrine role on HPA activation by stimulating the CRH and ACTH release from the hypothalamo–pituitary axis.[45–47] Finally, both these cytokines can induce a depletion of glucocorticoid receptors, and consequently impair the HPA sensitivity to the feedback mechanism toward glucocorticoids.[48,49] Within this context, our study demonstrated that the overproduction of TNF-α from NK of DAT patients correlated with the decreased response of cortisol to DXM suppression. TNF-α could therefore represent an immunoendocrine mediator of the altered response of HPA system to feedback regulation, thus contributing to induce a vicious-cycle maintaining elevated serum cortisol levels throughout the 24 hours. The impaired sensitivity to glucocorticoids might involve NK secretory activity. In fact, our study demonstrated a lack of suppressive effects by glucocorticoids (cortisol 10^{-6} M) on TNF-α

and IFN-γ release from NK in DAT patients. Our previous studies also demonstrated the same effects on NKCC.[15,50]

Another important point concerns the impairment of GH circadian rhythm in DAT patients. Like that found for the HPA axis, TNF-α and IFN-γ produced by activated NK cells could help antagonize GH secretion and release by means of a direct mechanism on the pituitary gland,[51,52] or by the effects mediated by hypothalamic GHRH[53] and somatostatin.[54] Moreover, these cytokines could decrease the synthesis and the expression of IGFs,[48] independently of GH levels.

In conclusion, immune alterations related to NK functional activity and cytokine release can affect the neuroendocrine regulation of HPA, GH, and MLT in patients with DAT. Like other immune effectors, NK cells could act on endocrine cells by means of the immunoendocrine or paracrine mechanisms. The immunoneuroendocrine link among the NK-derived cytokines, TNF-α and IFN-γ, and the cortisol, GH and MLT secretions, can condition the development of neurotoxic/apoptotic processes in cholinergic neurons of the hippocampus and the frontotemporal cortex, and this damage can also be added to the loss of neuroprotective factors (i.e., IGF-I). All these changes can delineate an immunoneuroendocrine basis of DAT, suggesting new aspects and strategies in the treatment of dementia.

ACKNOWLEDGMENTS

The work was fully supported by a grant from the University of Pavia (F.A.R. 1999/2000, Comitato 6). We thank Drs. L. Cravello and S. Severgnini for technical assistance with the immunological and statistical procedures.

REFERENCES

1. SAPOLSKY, R.M., L.C. KREY & B.S. MCEWEN. 1986. The neuroendocrinology of stress and aging: the glucocorticoid cascade hypothesis. Endocrine Rev. **7:** 284–301.
2. JACOBSON, L. & R. SAPOLSKY. 1991. The role of the hippocampus in feedback regulation of the hypothalamic-pituitary-adrenocortical axis. Endocrine Rev. **12:** 118–134.
3. TOITOU, Y. 1995. Effects of aging on endocrine and neuroendocrine rhythms in humans. Horm. Res. **43:** 12–19.
4. FERRARI, E., F. MAGRI, D. DORI, G. MIGLIORATI, T. NESCIS, G. MOLLA, M. FIORAVANTI & S.B. SOLERTE. 1995. Neuroendocrine correlates of the aging brain in humans. Neuroendocrinology **61:** 464–470.
5. MAGRI, F., M. LOCATELLI, G. BALZA, G. MOLLA, G. CUZZONI, M. FIORAVANTI, S.B. SOLERTE & E. FERRARI. 1997. Changes in endocrine circadian rhythms as markers of physiological and pathological brain aging. Chronobiol. Int. **14:** 385–396.
6. ROSEN, C.J. & C. CONOVER. 1997. Growth hormone/insulin-like growth factor-I axis in aging: a summary of a National Institutes of Aging-sponsored symposium. J. Clin. Endocrinol. Metab. **82:** 3919–3922.
7. YEN, S.S.C. & G.A. LAUGHLIN. 1998. Aging and the adrenal cortex. Exp. Gerontol. **33:** 897–910.
8. MAGRI, F., F. TERENZI, T. RICCIARDI, M. FIORAVANTI, S.B. SOLERTE, M. STABILE, G. BALZA, C. GANDINI, M. VILLA & E. FERRARI. 2000. Association between changes in adrenal secretion and cerebral morphometric correlates in normal aging and senile dementia. Dement. Geriatr. Cogn. Disord. **11:** 90–99.
9. AISEN, P.S. & K.L. DAVIS. 1994. Inflammatory mechanism in Alzheimer's disease: implications for therapy. Am. J. Psychiatry **151:** 1105–1113.

10. HUBERMAN, M., F. SHALIT, I. ROTH-DERI, B. GUTMAN, C. BRODIE, H.E. KO & B. SREDINI. 1994. Correlation of cytokine secretion by mononuclear cells of Alzheimer patients and their disease stage. J. Neuroimmunol. **52:** 147–152.

11. MCGEER, P.L., J. ROGERS & E.G. MCGEER. 1994. Neuroimmune mechanism in Alzheimer's disease pathogenesis. Alzheimer Dis. Assoc. Disord. **8:** 149–158.

12. SINGH, V.K. 1997. Neuroautoimmunity: pathogenetic implications for Alzheimer's disease. Gerontology **43:** 79–94.

13. SOLERTE, S.B., M. FIORAVANTI, S. SEVERGNINI, M. LOCATELLI, M. RENZULLO, N. CERUTTI & E. FERRARI. 1996. Enhanced cytotoxic rersponse of natural killer cells to IL-2 in Alzheimer's disease. Dementia **7:** 343–348.

14. SOLERTE, S.B., M. FIORAVANTI, S. SEVERGNINI, N., PEZZA, N. CERUTTI, M. LOCATELLI, F. TERENZI & E. FERRARI. 1997. Excitatory pattern of γ-interferon on natural killer cell activity in senile dementia of the Alzheimer's type. Dement. Geriatr. Cogn. Disord. **8:** 308–313.

15. SOLERTE, S.B., M. FIORAVANTI, A. PASCALE, E. FERRARI, S. GOVONI & F. BATTAINI. 1998. Increased natural killer cell cytotoxicity in Alzheimer's disease may involve protein kinase C dysregulation. Neurobiol. Aging **19:** 191–199.

16. MUNOZ-FERNANDEZ, M.A. & M. FRESNO. 1998. The role of tumor necrosis factor, interleukin 6, interferon-γ and inducible nitric oxide synthase in the development and pathology of the nervous system. Progr. Neurobiol. **56:** 307–340.

17. BLALOCK, J.E. 1989. A molecular basis for bidirectional communication between the immune and neuroendocrine systems. Physiol. Rev. **69:** 1–32.

18. IMURA, H., J. FUKATA & T. MORI. 1991. Cytokines and endocrine function: an interaction between the immune and neuroendocrine systems. Clin. Endocrinol. **35:** 107–115.

19. SMITH, E.M. 1992. Hormonal activities of cytokines. Chem. Immunol. **52:** 154–169.

20. MAESTRONI, G.J.M. 1993. The immunoneuroendocrine role of melatonin. J. Pineal Res. **14:** 1–10.

21. MCCANN, S.M., S. KARANTH, A. KAMAT, W. LES DEES, K. LYSON, M. GIMENO & V. RETTORI. 1994. Induction by cytokines of the pattern of pituitary hormone secretion in infection. Neuroimmunomodulation **1:** 2–13.

22. IMURA, H. & J. FUKATA. 1994. Endocrine-paracrine interaction in communication between the immune and endocrine systems. Activation of the hypothalamic-pituitary-adrenal axis in inflammation. Eur. J. Endocrinol. **130:** 32–37.

23. CHROUSOS, G.P. 1995. The hypothalamic-pituitary-adrenal axis and immune-mediated inflammation. N. Engl. J. Med. **332:** 1354–1362.

24. BESEDOVSKY, H.O. & A. DEL RAY. 1996. Immuno-neuro-endocrine interactions: facts and hypotheses. Endocr. Rev. **17:** 64–102.

25. SAPOLSKY, R.M., L.C. KREY & B.S. MCEWEN. 1985. Prolonged glucocorticoid exposure reduces hippocampal neuron number: implications for aging. J. Neurosci. **5:** 1221–1226.

26. NEWCOMER, J.W., S. CRAFT, T. HERSHEY, K. ASKIN & M.E. BARDGET. 1994. Glucocorticoid-induced impairment in declarative memory performance in adult humans. J. Neurosci. **14:** 2047–2053.

27. SECKL, J.R. & T. OLSSON. 1995. Glucocorticoid hypersecretion and the age-impaired hippocampus: cause or effect? J. Endocrinol. **145:** 201–211.

28. PORTER, N.M. & P.W. LANDFIELD. 1998. Stress hormones and brain aging: adding injury to insult? Nature Neurosci. **1:** 3–4.

29. LUPIEN, S.J., M. DE LEON, S. DE SANTI, A. CONVIT, C. TARSHISH, M.P.V. NAIR, M. THAKUR, B.S. MCEWEN, R.L. HAUGER & M.J. MEANEY. 1998. Cortisol levels during human aging predict hippocampal atrophy and memory deficits. Nature Neurosci. **1:** 69–73.

30. LUPIEN, S.J. & B.S. MCEWEN. 1997. The acute effects of corticosteroids on cognition: integration of animal and human model studies. Brain Res. Rev. **24:** 1–27.

31. HUIZENGA, N.A.T.M., J.W. KOPER, P. DE LANGE, H.A.P. POLS, R.P. STOLK, D.E. GROBBEE, F.H. DE JONG & S.W.J. LAMBERTS. 1998. Interperson variability but intraperson stability of baseline plasma cortisol concentrations, and its relation to feedback sensitivity of the hypothalamo-pituitary-adrenal axis to a low dose of dexamethasone in elderly individuals. J. Clin. Endocrinol. Metab. **83:** 47–54.

32. LIGHTHART, G.J., J.X. CORBERARD, C. FOURNIER, P. GALANAUD, W. HIJMANS, B. KENNES, H.F. MULLER-HERMELINK & G.C. STEINMAN. 1994. Admission criteria for immunogerontological studies in man: the SENIEUR protocol. Mech. Ageing Dev. **28:** 47–55.

33. AMERICAN PSYCHIATRIC ASSOCIATION. 1987. Diagnostic and statistical manual of mental disorders, 3rd edit., rev. American Psychiatric Association. Washington, DC.

34. MCKHANN, G., D. DRACHMAN, M. FOLSTEIN, R. KATZMANN, D. PRICE & E.M. STADLAN. 1984. Clinical diagnosis of Alzheimer's disease: report of the NINCDS-ADRDA workgroup under the auspices of Department of Healthy and Human Services Task Force on Alzheimer's Disease. Neurology **34:** 939–944.

35. HACHINSKI, V.C., N.A. LASSEN & J. MARSHALL. 1974. Multiinfarct dementia: a cause of mental deterioration in the elderly. Lancet **ii:** 207–210.

36. FOLSTEIN, M., S. FOLSTEIN & P.R. MCHUGH. 1975. Mini mental state. A practical method for grading the cognitive state of patients for the clinician. J. Psychiatr. Res. **12:** 189–198.

37. KESSLAK, J.P., O. NALCIOGLU & C.W. COTMAN. 1991. Quantification of magnetic resonance scans for hippocampal and parahippocampal atrophy in Alzheimer's disease. Neurology **41:** 51–54.

38. HALBERG, F. 1969. Chronobiology. Am. Rev. Physiol. **31:** 378–382.

39. BINGHAM, C., B. ARBOGAST, G.C. GUILLAUME, J.K. LEE & F. HALBERG. 1982. Inferential statistical methods for estimating and comparing cosinor parameters. Chronobiology **9:** 387–439.

40. KORZENIEWSKI, C. & D.M. CALLEWAERT. 1983. An enzyme-release assay for natural cytotoxicity. J. Immunol. Methods **64:** 313–320.

41. PROSS, H. & M. BAYNES. 1977. Spontaneous human lymphocyte mediated cytotoxicity against tumor target cells. A short review. Cancer Immunol. Immunother. **3:** 75–85.

42. DORE, S., S. KAR & R. QUIRION. 1997. Rediscovering an old friend, IGF—I: potential use in the treatment of neurodegenerative diseases. Trends Neurosci. **20:** 326–331.

43. DORE, S., S. KAR & R. QUIRION. 1997. Insulin-like growth factor I protects and rescues hippocampal neurons against beta-amyloid and human amylin-induced toxicity. Proc. Natl. Acad. Sci. USA **29:** 4772–4777.

44. DINARELLO, C.A., J.G. CANNON, S.M. WOLFF, H.A. BERNHEIM, A. BEUTLER & A. CERAMI. 1986. Tumor necrosis factor (cachectin) in an endogenous pyrogen and induces production of interleukin 1. J. Exp. Med. **163:** 1433–1450.

45. BORNSTEIN, S.R. & G.P. CHROUSOS. 1999. Adrenocorticotropin (ACTH) and non-ACTH-mediated regulation of the adrenal cortex: neural and immune inputs. J. Clin. Endocrinol. Metab. **84:** 1729–1736.

46. MILENKOVIC, L., V. RETTORI, G.D. SNYDER, B. BEUTLER & S.M. MCCANN. 1989. Cachectin alters anterior pituitary hormone release by direct action *in vitro*. Proc. Natl. Acad. Sci USA **86:**2418–2422.

47. PAULI, S., A.C. LINTHORST & J.M. REUL. 1998. Tumor necrosis factor-alpha and interleukin-2 differentially affect hippocampal serotoninergic neurotransmission, behavioural activity, body temperature and hypothalamic-pituitary-adrenocortial axis activity in the rat. Eur. J. Neurosci. **10:** 868–878.

48. VOUTILAINEN, R. 1998. Adrenocortical cells are the site of secretion and action of insulin-like growth factors and TNF-α. Horm. Metab. Res. **30:** 432–435.

49. FRANCHIMONT, D., H. MARTENS, M.-T. HAGELSTEIN, E. LOUIS, W. DEWE, G.P. CHROUSOS, J. BELAICHE & V. GEENEN. 1999. Tumor necrosis factor α decreases, and interleukin-10 increases, the sensitivity of human monocytes to dexamethasone: potential regulation of the glucocorticoid receptor. Clin. Endocrinol. Metab. **84:** 2834–2839.

50. SOLERTE, S.B., N. CERUTTI, S. SEVERGNINI, M. RONDANELLI, E. FERRARI & M. FIORAVANTI. 1998. Decreased immunosuppressive effect of cortisol on natural killer cytotoxic activity in senile dementia of the Alzheimer's type. Dement. Geriatr. Cogn. Disord. **9:** 149–156.

51. FRY, C., D.R. GUNTER, C.D. MCMAHON, B. STEELE & J.L. SARTIN. 1998. Cytokine mediated groth hormone release from cultured ovine pituitary cells. Neuroendocrinology **68:** 192–200.

52. WALTON, P.E. & M.J. CRONIN. 1990. Tumor necrosis factor-α inhibits growth hormone secretion from cultured anterior pituitary cells. Endocrinology **125:** 505–512.

53. GAILLARD, R.C., D. TURNILL, P. SAPPINO & A.F. MULLER. 1990. Tumor necrosis factor α inhibits the hormonal response of the pituitary gland to hypothalamic releasing factors. Endocrinology **127:** 101–106.

54. GONZALEZ, M.C., M. RIEDEL, V. RETTORI, W.H. YU & S.M. MCCANN. 1990. Effect of recombinant human γ-interferon on the release of anterior pituitary hormones. Prog. Neuroendocrin. Immunol. **3:** 49–54.

Interleukin-1β and Thymic Peptide Regulation of Pituitary and Glial Cell Cytokine Expression and Cellular Proliferation

BRYAN L. SPANGELO,[a] DERALD D. FARRIMOND,
MELISSA POMPILIUS, AND KAY-LYNN BOWMAN

*Department of Chemistry, University of Nevada Las Vegas,
Las Vegas, Nevada 89154, USA*

ABSTRACT: Interleukin-6 (IL-6) is a B-cell differentiating and T-cell activating cytokine that is expressed in T cells, neutrophils, monocytes, macrophages, and mast cells. Because IL-6 is also synthesized and released by anterior pituitary cells and IL-6 stimulates pituitary hormone release, this cytokine may serve a paracrine or autocrine role within the pituitary. Interleukin-1β (IL-1β) stimulates IL-6 release from anterior pituitary cells through a mechanism that involves lysophosphatidylcholine (LPC 18:0) generation and protein kinase C activation. In the rat C6 glioma cell line, IL-1β synergistically stimulates IL-6 release in the presence of increased intracellular cAMP concentrations. The catecholamines and serotonin also synergistically stimulate IL-6 release in the presence of IL-1β. LPC 18:0 synergistically increases IL-6 release in the presence of norepinephrine, and IL-1β transiently increases LPC 18:0 formation in C6 cells. Therefore, IL-1β induction of LPC 18:0 may lead to increases in IL-6 production via activation of a kinase cascade. The bovine thymic preparation, thymosin fraction 5 (TF5), also stimulates IL-6 release from C6 glioma cells in a protein kinase C–dependent manner. Of interest, TF5 inhibits the proliferation of C6 cells, pituitary adenoma MMQ cells, and promyelocytic HL-60 cells. We suggest that a thymic hormone immune surveillance mechanism may suppress neuroendocrine and hematopoietic tumor formation. Thus, IL-1β and certain thymic peptides act to increase IL-6 expression in neuroendocrine cells. The enhanced production of neuroendocrine cytokines may affect hormone secretion, neurotransmission, and the development of certain neurodegenerative disorders (e.g., Alzheimer's disease). The isolation of the active component of TF5 that inhibits neuroendocrine and hematopoietic tumor cell proliferation will provide a potential therapeutic strategy for the treatment of these tumors.

INTRODUCTION

Interleukin proteins are immune regulating factors that are synthesized and released by lymphocytes, macrophages, and monocytes. Several of these proteins are also produced by a wide variety of cell types, allowing for the designation of

[a]Address for correspondence: Department of Chemistry, University of Nevada, Las Vegas, 4505 Maryland Parkway, Las Vegas, NV 89154-4003. Voice: 702-895-3797; fax: 702-895-3171.

spangelb@nevada.edu

cytokine. Interleukin-6 (IL-6) is a 26,000 molecular weight B-cell differentiation cytokine that is synthesized and released within neuroendocrine structures.[1] Thus, glial elements of the anterior and posterior pituitaries as well as glial cells and astrocytes of the CNS release IL-6. Several roles have been advanced for cytokines produced within the neuroendocrine system, including regulation of hormone secretion and cell proliferation. Inflammatory cytokines produced within the brain may also affect the course of neurodegenerative diseases.[2]

In this paper we will review recent research results documenting the presence of cytokines in the brain and pituitary. The presence of IL-6 in the anterior pituitary and posterior pituitary suggests roles for the autocrine or paracrine regulation of hormone and neuropeptide secretion. We are interested in the regulation of IL-6 release from neuroendocrine cells by IL-1β. Thymic peptides also affect cytokine expression in glial cells. Of interest, certain thymic peptides also inhibit neuroendocrine tumor cell proliferation as well as the proliferation of hematopoietic cells. Therefore, products of the immune system (cytokines, thymic hormones) affect neuroendocrine cytokine and hormone production, and the proliferation of certain neuroendocrine cell lines.

PRESENCE OF CYTOKINES IN NEUROENDOCRINE STRUCTURES

Anterior Pituitary, Posterior Pituitary, and Hypothalamus

Hypothalamic control of neuroendocrine peptide secretion is well documented for several anterior pituitary hormones. For example, growth hormone (GH) secretion is dependent upon the relative levels of inhibitory (e.g., somatostatin) and stimulatory factors (e.g., GH releasing hormone). Pituitary tissue–generated autocrine- or paracrine-acting factors may also facilitate or inhibit hormone release from the anterior pituitary. IL-6 stimulates prolactin, GH, and luteinizing hormone (LH) release from anterior pituitary cells *in vitro*.[3] We hypothesized that IL-6 is produced within this tissue because of the low blood concentrations of this cytokine. (TABLE 1 summarizes the presence of cytokines in the hypothalamic-pituitary-adrenal axis.) IL-6 is

TABLE 1. Cytokine localization in endocrine tissues

| Cytokine | Amino acids | | Hypo-thalamus | Anterior pituitary | Posterior pituitary | Adrenal |
	Precursor	Mature				
IL-1α	271	159	+	+	?	+
IL-1β	269	153	+	+	?	+
IL-2	153	133	?	+	?	?
IL-6	212	184	+	+	+	+
TNF-α	233	157	+	+	?	+

NOTE: Numbers of amino acid residues are presented for the human cytokines.
+ = Cytokine present.
? = Cytokine presence not verified.

synthesized[4] and released[5] within cultures of anterior pituitary tissue, and the release of this cytokine is stimulated by a variety of agents, including IL-1α and IL-1β,[6] vasoactive intestinal polypeptide (VIP),[7] pituitary adenylate cyclase-activating peptide (PACAP),[8] calcitonin gene-related peptide (CGRP),[8] and lipopolysaccharide (LPS).[5,6] Interestingly, none of the classic hypothalamic factors affect IL-6 release (e.g., GHRH, LHRH). In addition, both forms of the IL-6 mRNA (i.e., 1.2 and 2.4 kb) are induced within anterior pituitary and neurointermediate pituitary lobe cells.[4,9] Other cytokines detected within the anterior pituitary include IL-2,[10] IL-1,[11,12] and tumor necrosis factor-α (TNFα).[12]

The cell types within the anterior pituitary responsible for cytokine expression are limited to the folliculostellate cells (for IL-6),[13] thyrotrophs (for IL-1),[11] and somatotrophs (for IL-1 receptor antagonist).[14] The probable cell type within neurointermediate pituitary lobe cell cultures responsible for IL-6 production is the pituicyte.[9] Both pituicytes and folliculostellate cells are glial-like elements which are stimulated by IL-1β for increased IL-6 release.[6,9] Oxytocin and vasopressin have no effect on basal IL-6 release, but both neuropeptides inhibit the IL-1β stimulated release of IL-6 from neurointermediate (but not anterior) pituitary lobe cells.[9]

Cytokines have also been localized to specific brain regions. IL-1β is present in hypothalamic and extrahypothalamic brain sites. Immunoreactive IL-1β neuronal processes and terminals are in the hippocampus,[15] and IL-1β is present in the paraventricular (i.e., magnocellular neurons), periventricular, and supraoptic nuclei of the hypothalamus.[15,16] An inducible IL-6 mRNA is present in the hypothalamus, cerebral cortex, thalamus, and hippocampus.[17] In addition, the mRNAs for IL-6 and the IL-6 receptor are colocalized in the limbic and hypothalamic brain regions.[18] The localizations of IL-1β and IL-6 are both neuronal (basal) and glial (induced) in the CNS.[19] Treatment of medial basal hypothalamic explants with LPS increases IL-6 release and both forms of the IL-6 mRNA *in vitro*, whereas 56 mM K^+ has no effect.[4] Intraperitoneal injections of LPS increases IL-1β immunoreactivity and the expression of the IL-1β mRNA in the rat hypothalamus[20]; however, the level of IL-6 transcripts is not affected by peripheral injections of LPS.[21] The central (icv) injection of LPS does increase the expression of both IL-1β and IL-6 mRNAs in the hypothalamus.[22] As noted in FIGURE 1, the expression of IL-6 in the neuroendocrine system may lead to increases in pituitary hormone secretion.

IL-1β Signal Transduction Pathway

The IL-1β induction of IL-6 release from anterior pituitary cells is not accompanied by increases in intracellular cAMP concentrations.[6] However, IL-1β increases arachidonic acid release and the formation of glycerophosphorylcholine (the product of complete deacylation of phosphatidylcholine) in anterior pituitary cells.[23] Because IL-1β-mobilization of arachidonic acid release from phosphatidylcholine must involve transient formation of lysophosphatidylcholine (LPC), we suggested a role for this lysophospholipid species in IL-1β signal transduction. LPC 18:0 increased IL-6 release, but not prolactin release, from anterior pituitary cells; this stimulation was blocked by the protein kinase C inhibitors H7 and chelerythrine.[24]

Because of the heterogeneous nature of anterior pituitary cell cultures, we continued these investigations using the rat C6 glioma cell line. IL-1β stimulated IL-6 release from C6 cells, and in the presence of dibutyryl cAMP this cytokine induced

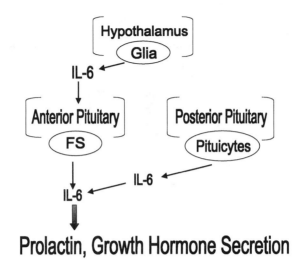

FIGURE 1. Interleukin-6 production within the hypothalamic-pituitary axis may lead to increases in anterior pituitary hormone secretion via a paracrine mechanism. FS, folliculo-stellate cells.

a synergistic release of IL-6.[25] Thus, the combination of these two agents resulted in a release of IL-6 that was much larger than the release attributed to either agent alone (i.e., 30-fold higher). Similarly, IL-1β in the presence of either forskolin or cholera toxin synergistically increased IL-6 release. Each of the catecholamines facilitated the synergistic induction of IL-6 release in the presence of IL-1β. Isoproterenol, a β-receptor agonist, and IL-1β produced a 25-fold synergistic stimulation of IL-6 release. The β-antagonist propranolol completely blocked this synergistic stimulation and the synergistic stimulation caused by norepinephrine and IL-1β. LPC 18:0 also stimulated IL-6 release from C6 cells, and in the presence of norepinephrine, a synergistic enhancement in IL-6 release was measured.[25] Importantly, IL-1β treatment of C6 cells radiolabeled with [³H]choline resulted in an increase in LPC 18:0 and a decrease in the parent phosphatidylcholine lipid species.

We are continuing these experiments with the monoamine serotonin. Pousset *et al.*[26] reported that low concentrations of serotonin (i.e., 10^{-12} to 10^{-10}M) increase IL-6 mRNA expression in rat hippocampal astrocytes. As shown in FIGURE 2, serotonin had no effect on basal IL-6 release from C6 glioma cells; however, in the presence of IL-1β a synergistic induction of IL-6 release was evident. These data indicate that central neurotransmitter levels may affect the production of glial derived cytokines. Specifically, IL-1β and any of the monoamines may stimulate dramatic increases in IL-6 secretion from glial elements. Alternatively, Wu *et al.*[27] demonstrated that perfusion of IL-1β and IL-6 into the anterior hypothalamus increases serotonin release in this region. The co-perfusion of IL-1β and IL-6 synergistically increases hypothalamic serotonin release. Similarly, IL-1β increases the release of norepinephrine and dopamine in the anterior hypothalamus *in vivo*.[28] Thus, increased cytokine expression due to serotonin may act to further increase the release of this

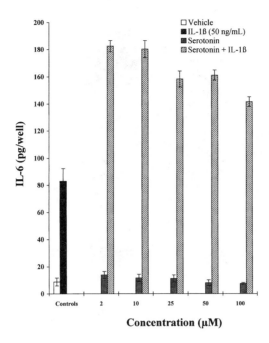

FIGURE 2. Exposure of rat C6 glioma cells to serotonin (5HT) and IL-1β results in the synergistic induction of IL-6 release. Glioma cells (1×10^5 cells/well) were exposed to 50 ng/mL IL-1β in the absence or presence of 5HT (2–100 μM) for 24 hours in serum-free RPMI-1640. IL-6 concentrations were determined with the 7TD1 bioassay.[25]

monoamine. Adding to this cascade is the positive autoregulatory effect of IL-6 on astrocyte IL-6 release.[29] The increased production of this pro-inflammatory cytokine may affect the course of neurodegenerative disorders and CNS infections,[2] and neurotransmission.[30]

The possible IL-1β-mediated signaling events in glial cells are shown in FIGURE 3. The generation of LPC following IL-1 type I receptor activation could activate a kinase cascade (e.g., MAPK). Second messengers from either the catecholamine (e.g., cAMP) or serotonin pathways may converge at the level of kinase activation for the synergistic induction of active transcription factors (e.g., NF-κB). This hypothesis suggests that these trans-acting factors should be activated in the presence of IL-1β, and that this activation should be increased in the presence of IL-1β and any of the catecholamines or serotonin.

Effects on Cell Proliferation

In addition to effects on hormone secretion, cytokines affect the proliferation of neuroendocrine cells. The cytokines IL-1, IL-2, and IL-6 inhibit rat anterior pituitary cell proliferation *in vitro*.[31,32] In contrast, IL-2 and IL-6 actually stimulate the proliferation of pituitary adenomas such as the rat mammosomatotropic cell line GH_3.[32]

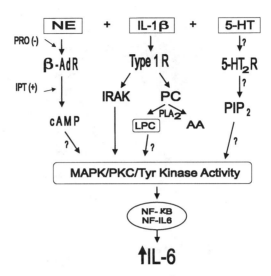

FIGURE 3. IL-1β and the monoamines stimulate the synergistic induction of IL-6 release from C6 glioma cells. AA, arachidonic acid; β-AdR, β-adrenergic receptor; IPT, isoproterenol; IRAK, IL-1 receptor associated kinase; LPC, lysophosphatidylcholine; MAPK, mitogen-activated protein kinase; NE, norepinephrine; NF-IL-6, nuclear factor IL-6; NF-κB, nuclear factor κB; PIP$_2$, phosphatidylinositol-4,5-*bis*phosphate; PC, phosphatidylcholine; PKC, protein kinase C; PLA$_2$, phospholipase A$_2$; PRO,propranolol; 5HT, serotonin.

Approximately one-half of all glioma tumor specimens from human brain tumors coexpress the IL-1 and IL-6 mRNAs,[33] and IL-1β mRNA is detected in 86% of surgically resected gliomas.[34] The dysregulation of cytokine expression may be associated with neoplasia in the brain and pituitary. However, Halfter *et al.*[35] recently reported that the cytokine leukemia inhibitory factor (LIF) was expressed in human glioma cell lines and that LIF suppressed the proliferation of these cells.

EFFECTS OF THYMIC PEPTIDES ON NEUROENDOCRINE FUNCTION

Hormone Release and Cytokine Expression

The thymic peptides belong to another class of immune activating molecules that also affect the functioning of the neuroendocrine system. Thymosin fraction 5 (TF5) is a partially purified preparation of the bovine thymus gland. TF5 contains 30–40 small peptides which are generally acidic and heat-stable. TF5 has numerous biological activities including induction of T-lymphocyte markers, enhanced lymphocyte responses to mitogens, increased antibody production, and increased mixed lymphocyte reactivity.[36] Because TF5 also increases IL-6 production in mitogen-activated splenocyte cultures,[37] this preparation enhances both T-lymphocyte differentiation and cytokine production.

We reported that TF5 stimulates the release of prolactin and GH, but not LH, from rat anterior pituitary cells *in vitro*.[38] Because previously characterized thymosin peptides (e.g., $T\alpha_1$, $T\beta_4$) had no effect on hormone release, a novel thymosin peptide was isolated with hormone-stimulating activities. MB-35 is a highly basic (pI 9.3) peptide of 35 amino acids and a molecular weight of 3756.[39] This peptide stimulates prolactin and GH release without producing any effect on intracellular cAMP concentrations. Interestingly, the amino acid sequence of MB-35 is identical to a section of histone H2A (residues 86-120), a component of nuclear protein A24. Although MB-35 production from A24 has not been demonstrated, it is possible that proteolysis of histone nucleoproteins during the cell cycle may generate peptides (e.g., MB-35) which migrate to the cytoplasm for intracrine actions or are secreted for autocrine, paracrine, or endocrine effects. Several other thymic peptides also influence neuroendocrine function.[36]

As for the cytokine IL-1β noted above, TF5 also increases IL-6 release from rat C6 glioma cells *in vitro*.[40] Circulating thymic peptides may gain access to the CNS across the blood–brain barrier for the enhanced central production of cytokines. Thymic hormones may therefore affect neuronal, neuroendocrine, and inflammatory processes in the brain either directly or indirectly via cytokine production.

Effects on Cell Proliferation

Because cytokines increase hormone release from anterior pituitary cells as well as affect the proliferation of pituitary and pituitary adenoma cells, we hypothesized that TF5 may affect the proliferation of the MMQ cell line. The MMQ cell is a rat pituitary adenoma cell that secretes prolactin and is responsive to dopamine for the inhibition of prolactin release.[41] TF5 suppresses the proliferation of MMQ cells in a cell number and time-dependent manner.[42] This suppression is accompanied with a reduction in cell viability and the increased appearance of the morphological features of apoptosis. The proliferation of the C6 glioma cell was similarly inhibited by TF5, and none of the purified thymosin peptides (i.e., $T\alpha_1$, $T\beta_4$, MB-35) had any effect on either MMQ or C6 cell proliferation. The identity of the active component within TF5 for the inhibition of tumor cell proliferation is unknown. Thus, thymic hormone immune surveillance mechanisms may affect neuroendocrine tumor formation.

We have continued these studies using two non-neuroendocrine cell types, the CRL7686 human melanoma cell line and the human promyelocytic leukemia HL-60 cell line. As shown in FIGURE 4, TF5 effectively inhibits the proliferation of HL-60 cells to 20% of control cultures during a 72-hour incubation period. The TF5 ED_{50} for inhibition of HL-60 cell proliferation is approximately 400 μg/mL. In contrast, CRL7686 melanoma cells are relatively unresponsive to TF5 (60% of control cultures at 1,000 μg/mL TF5). Furthermore, the TF5 ED_{50} for the inhibition of CRL7686 cells is approximately 700 μg/mL. Once again, the purified thymosin peptides (i.e., $T\alpha_1$, $T\beta_4$, MB-35) in concentrations up to 1 μM have no effect on the proliferation of either the HL-60 or CRL7686 cell lines (data not shown). Collectively, these data indicate that the inhibition of HL-60 cells may not be due to a non-specific lethal effect caused by TF5 (i.e., CRL7686 cells were much less responsive). In contrast, prothymosin-α antisense oligonucleotides inhibit proliferation and induce apoptosis in HL-60 cells, indicating the importance of prothymosin α to cell proliferation.[43] However, the

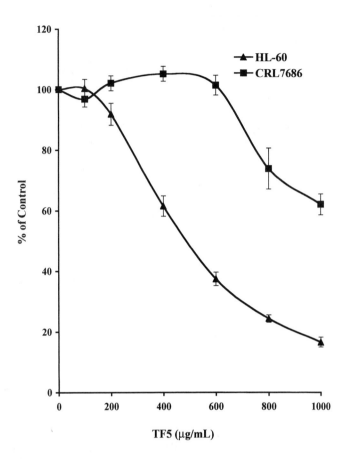

FIGURE 4. Effects of TF5 on the proliferation of human promyelocytic leukemia HL-60 cells and human melanoma CRL7686 cells. HL-60 cells (20,000 cells/well) and CRL7686 cells (25,000 cells/well) were exposed for 72 hours to 100–1,000 µg/mL TF5. Results of the MTT reaction are expressed as a percent of control of either five independent experiments (i.e., HL-60 cells) or two independent experiments (i.e., CRL7686 cells).

isolation of certain thymosin peptides from TF5 may provide a novel treatment strategy for the management of certain types of leukemia.

CONCLUSIONS

Cytokines and thymic peptides affect hormone release from the hypothalamic pituitary axis, as well as the proliferation of pituitary and glial cells. Alterations in circulating hormone levels may subsequently regulate T- and B-lymphocyte activities. Cytokines either enhance or suppress the proliferation of human pituitary adenoma and glioma cells. Our future work will be directed towards the elucidation of

IL-1β signaling events in C6 glioma cells, and the isolation and characterization of the thymic peptide that exerts anti-proliferative effects on HL-60 leukemia cells.

REFERENCES

1. SPANGELO, B.L. & W.C. GOROSPE. 1995. Role of the cytokines in the neuroendocrine-immune system axis. Front. Neuroendocrinol. **16:** 1–22.
2. ENGELBORGHS, S. & P.P. DE DEYN. 1997. The neurochemistry of Alzheimer's disease. Acta Neurol. Belg. **97:** 67–84.
3. SPANGELO, B.L., A.M JUDD, P.C. ISAKSON & R.M. MACLEOD. 1989. Interleukin-6 stimulates anterior pituitary hormone release *in vitro*. Endocrinology **125:** 575–577.
4. SPANGELO, B.L., A.M. JUDD, R.M. MACLEOD, D.W. GOODMAN & P.C. ISAKSON. 1990. Endotoxin-induced release of interleukin-6 from rat medial basal hypothalami. Endocrinology **127:** 1779–1785.
5. SPANGELO, B.L., R.M. MACLEOD & P.C. ISAKSON. 1990. Production of interleukin-6 by anterior pituitary cells *in vitro*. Endocrinology **126:** 582–586.
6. SPANGELO, B.L., A.M. JUDD, P.C. ISAKSON & R.M. MACLEOD. 1991. Interleukin-1 stimulates interleukin-6 release from rat anterior pituitary cells *in vitro*. Endocrinology **128:** 2685–2692.
7. SPANGELO, B.L., P.C. ISAKSON & R.M. MACLEOD. 1990. Production of interleukin-6 by anterior pituitary cells is stimulated by increased intracellular adenosine 3´,5´-monophosphate and vasoactive intestinal peptide. Endocrinology **127:** 403–409.
8. TATSUNO, I., A.SOMOGYVARI-VIGH, K. MIZUNO, P.E. GOTTSCHALL, H. HIDAKA & A. ARIMURA. 1991. Neuropeptide regulation of interleukin-6 production from the pituitary: stimulation by pituitary adenylate cyclase activating polypeptide and calcitonin gene-related peptide. Endocrinology **129:** 1797–1804.
9. SPANGELO, B.L., P.D. deHOLL, L. KALABAY, B.R. BOND & P. ARNAUD. 1994. Neurointermediate pituitary lobe cells synthesize and release interleukin-6 *in vitro*: effects of lipopolysaccharide and interleukin-1β. Endocrinology **135:** 556–563.
10. ARZT, E., G. STELZER, U. RENNER, M. LANGE, O.A. MULLER & G.K. STALLA. 1992. Interleukin-2 and interleukin-2 receptor expression in human corticotrophic adenoma and murine pituitary cell cultures. J. Clin. Invest. **90:** 1944–1951.
11. KOENIG, J.I., K. SNOW, B.D. CLARK, R. TONI, J.G. CANNON, A.R. SHAW, C.A. DINARELLO, S. REICHLIN, S.L. LEE & R.M. LECHAN. 1990. Intrinsic pituitary interleukin-1β is induced by bacterial lipopolysaccharide. Endocrinology **126:** 3053–3058.
12. GATTI, S. & T. BARTFAI. 1993. Induction of tumor necrosis factor-α mRNA in the brain after peripheral endotoxin treatment: comparison with interleukin-1 family and interleukin-6. Brain Res. **624:** 291–294.
13. ALLAERTS, W., P.H.M. JEUCKEN, R. DEBETS, S. HOEFAKKER, E. CLAASSEN & H.A. DREXHAGE. 1997. Heterogeneity of pituitary folliculo-stellate cells: implications for interleukin-6 production and accessory function *in vitro*. J. Neuroendocrinol. **9:** 43–53.
14. SAUER, J., U. RENNER, U. HOPFNER, M.LANGE, A. MULLER, C.J. STRASBURGER, U. PAGOTTO, E. ARZT & G.K. STALLA. 1998. Interleukin-1β enhances interleukin-1 receptor antagonist content in human somatotroph adenoma cell cultures. J. Clin. Endocrinol. Metab. **83:** 2429–2434.
15. LECHAN, R.M., R. TONI, B.D. CLARK, J.G. CANNON, A.R. SHAW, C.A. DINARELLO & S. REICHLIN. 1990. Immunoreactive interleukin-1β localization in the rat forebrain. Brain Res. **514:** 135–140.
16. MOLENAAR, G.J., F. BERKENBOSCH, A.M. VAN DAM & C.M.J.E. LUGARD. 1993. Distribution of interleukin-1β immunoreactivity within the porcine hypothalamus. Brain Res. **608:** 169–174.
17. SCHOBITZ, B., E.R. DE KLOET, W. SUTANTO & F. HOLSBOER. 1993. Cellular localization of interleukin-6 mRNA and interleukin-6 receptor mRNA in rat brain. Eur. J. Neurosci. **5:** 1426–1435.

18. SCHOBITZ, B., D.A.M. VOORHUIS & E.R. DE KLOET. 1992. Localization of interleukin-6 mRNA and interleukin-6 receptor mRNA in rat brain. Neurosci. Lett. **136:** 189–192.

19. LEMKE, R., M. HARTLAGE-RUBSAMEN & R. SCHLIEBS. 1999. Differential injury-dependent glial expression of interleukins-1α, β, and interleukin-6 in rat brain. Glia **27:** 75–87.

20. HILLHOUSE, E.W. & K. MOSLEY. 1993. Peripheral endotoxin induces hypothalamic immunoreactive interleukin-1β in the rat. Br. J. Pharmacol. **109:** 289–290.

21. SCHOBITZ, B., M. VAN DEN DOBBELSTEEN, F. HOLSBOER, W. SUTANTO & E.R. DE KLOET. 1993. Regulation of interleukin-6 gene expression in rat. Endocrinology **132:** 1569–1576.

22. DE SIMONI, M.G., R. DEL BO, A. DE LUIGI, S. SIMARD & G. FORLONI. 1995. Central endotoxin induces different patterns of interleukin (IL)-1β and IL-6 messenger ribonucleic acid expression and IL-6 secretion in the brain and periphery. Endocrinology **136:** 897–902.

23. SPANGELO, B.L., W.D. JARVIS, A.M. JUDD & R.M. MACLEOD. 1991. Induction of interleukin-6 release by interleukin-1 in rat anterior pituitary cells *in vitro*: evidence for an eicosanoid-dependent mechanism. Endocrinology **129:** 2886–2894.

24. SPANGELO, B.L. & W.D. JARVIS. 1996. Lysophosphatidylcholine stimulates interleukin-6 release from rat anterior pituitary cells *in vitro*. Endocrinology **137:** 4419–4426.

25. ZUMWALT, J.W., B.J. THUNSTROM & B.L. SPANGELO. 1999. Interleukin-1β and catecholamines synergistically stimulate interleukin-6 release from rat C6 glioma cells *in vitro*: a potential role for lysophosphatidylcholine. Endocrinology **140:** 888–896.

26. POUSSET, F., J. FOURNIER, P. LEGOUX, P. KEANE, D. SIRE & P. SOUBRIE. 1996. Effect of serotonin on cytokine mRNA expression in rat hippocampal astrocytes. Mol. Brain Res. **38:** 54–62.

27. WU, Y., E.K. SHAGHAGHI, C., JACQUOT, M. PALLARDY & A.M. GARDIER. 1999. Synergism between interleukin-6 and interleukin-1β in hypothalamic serotonin release: a reverse *in vivo* microdialysis study in F344 rats. Eur. Cytokine Netw. **10:** 57–63.

28. SHINTANI, F., S. KANBA, T. NAKAKI, M. NIBUYA, N. KINOSHIT, E. SUZUKI, G. YAGI, R. KATO & M. ASAI. 1993. Interleukin-1β augments release of norepinephrine, dopamine, and serotonin in the rat anterior hypothalamus. J. Neurosci. **13:** 3574–3581.

29. VAN WAGONER, N.J., J. OH, P. REPOVIC & E.N. BENVENISTE. 1999. Interleukin-6 (IL-6) production by astrocytes: autocrine regulation by IL-6 and the soluble IL-6 receptor. J. Neurosci. **19:** 5236–5244.

30. DUNN, A.J., J. WANG & T. ANDO. 1999. Effects of cytokines on cerebral neurotransmission: comparison with the effects of stress. *In* Cytokines, Stress, and Depression. Dantzer *et al.*, Eds.: 117–127. Kluwer Academic/Plenum Publishers. New York.

31. RENNER, U., C.J. NEWTON, U. PAGOTTO, J. SAUER, E. ARZT & G.K. STALLA. 1995. Involvement of interleukin-1 and interleukin-1 receptor antagonist in rat pituitary cell growth regulation. Endocrinology **136:** 3 186–3193.

32. ARZT, E., R. BURIC, G. STELZER, J. STALLA, J. SAUER, U. RENNER & G.K. STALLA. 1993. Interleukin involvement in anterior pituitary cell growth regulation: effects of IL-2 and IL-6. Endocrinology **132:** 459–467.

33. LICHTOR, T. & T.A. LIBERMANN. 1994. Coexpression of interleukin-1β and interleukin-6 in human brain tumors. Neurosurgery **34:** 669–673.

34. SASAKI, A., M. TAMURA, M. HASEGAWA, S. ISHIUCHI, J. HIRATO & Y. NAKAZATO. 1998. Expression of interleukin-1β mRNA and protein in human gliomas assessed by RT-PCR and immunohistochemistry. J. Neuropath. Exp. Neurol. **57:** 653–663.

35. HALFTER, H., J. KREMERSKOTHEN, J. WEBER, U. HACKER-KLOM, A. BARNEKOW, E.B. RINGELSTEIN & F. STOGBAUER. 1998. Growth inhibition of newly established human glioma cell lines by leukemia inhibitory factor. J. Neuro-Oncol. **39:** 1–18.

36. SPANGELO, B.L. & W.C. GOROSPE. 1997. Thymic polypeptides and their role as mediators in neuroendocrine-immune communication. *In* Stress, Stress Hormones and the Immune System. J.C. Buckingham, G.E. Gillies & A.-M. Cowell, Eds.: 357–372. John Wiley & Sons, Ltd.

37. ATTIA, W.Y., M. BADAMCHIAN, A.L. GOLDSTEIN & B.L. SPANGELO. 1993. Thymosin stimulates interleukin-6 production from rat spleen cell *in vitro*. Immunopharmacology **26:** 171–179.
38. SPANGELO, B.L., A.M. JUDD, P.C. ROSS, I.S. LOGIN, W.D. JARVIS, M. BADAMCHIAN, A.L. GOLDSTEIN & R.M. MACLEOD. 1987. Thymosin fraction 5 stimulates prolactin and growth hormone release from anterior pituitary cells *in vitro*. Endocrinology **121:** 2035–2043.
39. BADAMCHIAN, M., B.L. SPANGELO, T. DAMAVANDY, R.M. MACLEOD & A.L. GOLDSTEIN. 1991. Complete amino acid sequence analysis of a peptide isolated from the thymus that enhances release of growth hormone and prolactin. Endocrinology **128:** 1580–1588.
40. TIJERINA, M., W.C. GOROSPE, K. BOWMAN, M. BADAMCHIAN, A.L. GOLDSTEIN & B.L. SPANGELO. 1997. A novel thymosin peptide stimulates interleukin-6 release from rat C6 glioma cells *in vitro*. Neuroimmunomodulation **4:** 163–170.
41. JUDD, A.M., I.S. LOGIN, K. KOVACS, P.C. ROSS, B.L. SPANGELO, W.D. JARVIS & R.M. MACLEOD. 1988. Characterization of the MMQ cell, a prolactin-secreting clonal cell line that is responsive to dopamine. Endocrinology **123:** 2341–2350.
42. SPANGELO, B.L., D.D. FARRIMOND, M. THAPA, C.M. BULATHSINGHALA, K. BOWMAN, A. SAREH, F.M. HUGHES, JR., A.L. GOLDSTEIN & M. BADAMCHIAN. 1998. Thymosin fraction 5 inhibits the proliferation of the rat neuroendocrine MMQ pituitary adenoma and C6 glioma cell lines *in vitro*. Endocrinology **139:** 2155–2162.
43. RODRIGUEZ, P., VINUELA, J.E., ALVAREZ-FERNANDEZ, L. & J. GOMEZ-MARQUEZ. 1999. Prothymosin a antisense oligonucleotides induce apoptosis in HL-60 cells. Cell Death & Differen. **6:** 3–5.

Cytokine Activation of the HPA Axis

ADRIAN J. DUNN[a]

Department of Pharmacology and Therapeutics, Louisiana State University Health Sciences Center, Shreveport, Louisiana 71103, USA

ABSTRACT: The observation that administration of interleukin-1 (IL-1) to animals activates the hypothalamo-pituitary-adrenocortical (HPA) axis stimulated great interest in the significance and mechanism of this response, and in whether other cytokines have similar activities. Interleukin-6 (IL-6) and tumor necrosis factor α (TNFα) share HPA-activating activity, although they are less potent and effective than IL-1, whereas IL-2 and interferon α(IFNα) lack activity. Small increases in body temperature occur in response to IL-1, IL-6 and TNFα, but these changes are prevented by inhibitors of cyclooxygenase (COX) and do not appear to be related to the HPA-activation. The rapid HPA-activating effects of IL-1 are impaired by COX inhibitors, but the more prolonged HPA activation associated with intraperitoneal injections is not affected, indicating multiple mechanisms for IL-1-induced HPA activation. The HPA response to IL-6 is not sensitive to COX inhibitors, but that to TNFα appears to be. The HPA-activating activity of IL-1 is associated with increases in the apparent release of brain noradrenaline (NA) and serotonin (5-HT), but not dopamine, as well as with increased brain tryptophan. The NA changes, but not those in serotonin metabolism and tryptophan, are prevented by COX inhibitors. IL-6 has effects on serotonin and tryptophan like those of IL-1, but no detected effect on NA. TNFα has some effect on NA and tryptophan, but only at relatively high doses. IFNα lacks activity on these neurochemicals. Manipulation of noradrenergic, but not serotonergic systems alters the IL-1–induced HPA activation, suggesting the involvement of NA. However, brain NA does not appear to be essential for HPA activation in mice.

INTRODUCTION

Since the seminal report by Besedovsky that intraperitoneal (i.p.) injection of human interleukin-1β (IL-1β) potently activates the hypothalamo-pituitary-adrenocortical (HPA) axis in rats,[1] the HPA-stimulating effect of IL-1 has been confirmed by many researchers in many species. There seems to be general agreement that this response is a fundamental aspect of immune system communication with the nervous system, and most likely modulates the host's response to infection or tissue damage. Many concur with Besedovsky's original proposal that the systemic elevation of corticosteroids acts as a brake on the immune system, providing negative feedback to limit immune hyperactivity that might result in autoimmune damage, but the physiological significance may extend beyond this.

[a]Address for correspondence: Dr. Adrian J. Dunn, Department of Pharmacology, LSU-HSC, P.O. Box 33932, Shreveport, LA 71130-3932. Voice: 318-675-7850; fax: 318-675-7857.

adunn@lsuhsc.edu

INTERLEUKIN-1 (IL-1)

Although there are very considerable variations in the amino acid sequences of the alpha- and beta-forms of IL-1, as well as among IL-1s from different species, IL-1-induced HPA activation appears to occur with all forms of IL-1 (see TABLE 1).[2] This may be because all known forms of IL-1 interact with the IL-1 type I receptor, the only known active receptor for IL-1. There are, however, significant variations in the binding affinity of the various forms of IL-1 for this receptor.

The characteristics of the HPA response to IL-1 depend on the route of injection. Intravenous (i.v.) injection causes short-lived increases in plasma ACTH and corticosterone in rats and mice. The increases are evident in about 15 minutes, and largely dissipate within one hour.[3] In contrast, the HPA responses to i.p. injection of IL-1 are slower in onset and more prolonged. Elevations of plasma concentrations of ACTH and corticosterone appear within 30 minutes, but the peak responses do not appear until 2 hours.[1,4] The time course of the response of plasma corticosterone to mouse IL-1β is shown in FIGURE 1. Plasma ACTH exhibits a similar time course.

The HPA response to i.v. IL-1 is sensitive to cyclooxygenase (COX) inhibitors, such as indomethacin, in rats[5–7] and mice.[3,8] However, the response to i.p. IL-1 is much less sensitive (see TABLE 2). Only the early phase of the i.p. IL-1β–induced increase in plasma corticosterone in mice was impaired by COX inhibitors,[3] clearly indicating the biphasic nature of the response to IL-1 and suggesting the existence

TABLE 1. HPA responses to cytokine administration in mice

Cytokine	
IL-1α/IL-1β	Potent and prolonged (see FIG. 1)
IL-2	No effect
IL-6	Weak, short-lived response (see FIG. 1)
TNFα	Weak, but slower than IL-6
IFNα	No effect

TABLE 2. Effects of COX inhibitors on HPA activation by cytokines

IL-1β

    Non-selective COX inhibitors, but not lipooxygenase inhibitors, largely prevent the effect of i.v. IL-1

    NS-398 (COX2-selective inhibitor) did not

    COX inhibitors attenuate only the early phase of i.p. IL-1

IL-6

    The responses are not affected

TNFα

    The response is attenuated

of multiple mechanisms for IL-1–induced HPA activation. Indomethacin inhibits both COX and lipoxygenase, but selective inhibitors of lipooxygenase failed to prevent HPA activation by i.v. IL-1β, implicating COX as the important mediator.[3]

The Mechanism of the HPA-activating Effect of IL-1

There is evidence for actions of IL-1 on multiple components of the HPA axis: the brain, the pituitary, and the adrenal, as well as on peripheral nerves. The evidence for direct actions on the pituitary and adrenal derives largely from *in vitro* experiments (and are therefore susceptible to artifact), whereas the *in vivo* evidence strongly favors the need for the pituitary and hypothalamic CRF in normal healthy animals.[9] Hypophysectomy prevents the responses to IL-1 in rats[10,11] and mice.[12] Our results from hypophysectomized mice also indicated no changes in plasma con-

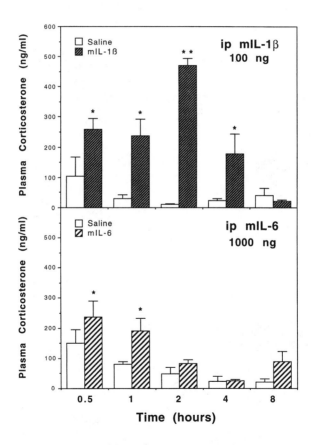

FIGURE 1. Effects of mIL-1β and IL-6 on plasma corticosterone. Mouse IL-1β (100 ng/mouse) (*top*) or mouse IL-6 (1 µg/mouse) (*bottom*) was injected i.p., and samples collected at various subsequent times. Plasma corticosterone was determined by radioimmunoassay. $N = 7$. *Significantly different from the corresponding saline groups (*$p < 0.05$ or **$p < 0.01$, respectively). Data from the bottom figure are from Wang and Dunn.[27]

centrations of ACTH and corticosterone in response to i.p. or i.v. IL-1 lipopolysaccharide (LPS) or Newcastle disease virus (NDV).[12,13] In rats, deafferentation of the hypothalamus[14] and lesions of the hypothalamic paraventricular nucleus (PVN)[15] blocked the plasma ACTH response to IL-1. Neutralizing antibodies to CRF attenuated or blocked the ACTH and corticosterone responses to IL-1 in rats.[16–18] Pretreatment of mice with a neutralizing antibody to CRF prevented the responses in plasma ACTH and corticosterone to i.v. IL-1β, as well as the plasma ACTH response to i.p. IL-1β, but there was a still a small increase in corticosterone.[12] In mice lacking the gene for CRF, the increase in plasma corticosterone in response to i.p. IL-1β was reduced more than 90%, but not completely prevented.[19] These results clearly indicate the necessity for an intact pituitary and CRF for IL-1 to activate the HPA axis, although there may be a very small plasma corticosterone response that is independent of CRF. In adrenalectomized mice IL-1β elicited increases in plasma ACTH (already elevated by adrenalectomy alone), consistent with the observations of Rivier in rats.[5]

It seems most likely that i.v. injected IL-1 acts primarily on a circumventricular organ such as the median eminence or the OVLT. The sensitivity to COX inhibitors could be interpreted to mean that COX in endothelial cells is activated, and that the prostaglandin E_2 (or other COX products) produced travels through the brain to activate CRF secretion. If so, the median eminence is the more attractive site because of its proximity to CRF-containing nerve terminals.[20] On the other hand, i.p. injected IL-1 probably acts by multiple mechanisms, a rapid response like that to i.v. IL-1 from that which rapidly enters the circulation, and slower responses that involve the hypothalamic CRF and perhaps vagal afferents.[21] Moreover, there may be some slower pituitary effects due to IL-6 production, and some small direct effects on the adrenal, perhaps caused by secondary mediators rather than IL-1 itself.

Interleukin-6

Interleukin-6 (IL-6), has long been known to have HPA-activating activity. Human IL-6 increases plasma concentrations of ACTH and corticosterone in rats,[22–25] mice,[26,27] and man,[28,29] and mouse IL-6 is effective in rats[25] and mice.[27] The HPA response to i.p. IL-6 is fast and short-lived compared to that to IL-1 (FIG. 1). The response of plasma ACTH to i.p. mIL-6 was very similar, as were the responses to i.v. mIL-6.[27] The short-lived effects of IL-6 on the HPA axis are consistent with pharmacokinetic studies of IL-6, which indicate a plasma half-life after i.v. injection of around three minutes in rats and seven minutes in mice.[30,31] IL-6 was significantly less potent in activating the HPA axis in mice[27,32] than reported for hIL-6 or mIL-6 in rats.[22–25] IL-6 is significantly less potent than IL-1 (FIG. 1), requiring doses an order of magnitude higher.[24,26,27] Moreover, the maximum response is well below that elicited by IL-1,[27] suggesting that the mechanisms are different. Even doses as high as 2 or 5 µg per mouse failed to induce maximal plasma concentrations of corticosterone.[27] However, in man, plasma cortisol is readily elevated by relatively small doses of IL-6.[28]

The HPA-activating effect of IL-6 in rats has been reported to be sensitive to an antibody to CRF.[22,33] However, IL-6 is known to have a direct stimulatory effect on ACTH secretion from the pituitary[23,25,34] and, in contrast to IL-1, IL-6 stimulates Fos expression in the pituitary gland, but not the PVN.[35,36] These results suggest a pituitary site of action for IL-6 in elevating plasma ACTH and corticosterone, consistent with the rapid time course.

The HPA response to IL-6 is not sensitive to COX inhibitors.[27] The cytokines are "promiscuous" in that administration of one cytokine can stimulate the synthesis and secretion of others. Thus IL-1 administration induces IL-6, so that IL-6 could contribute to the HPA response to IL-1. Pretreatment of mice with a neutralizing monoclonal antibody to mIL-6 indicated that IL-6 contributed to the late phase (2 h but not 4 h) of the plasma ACTH and corticosterone responses to mIL-1β. However, the antibody to IL-6 did not alter the tryptophan or 5-hydroxyindoleacetic acid (5-HIAA) responses.[37]

Tumor Necrosis Factor α

Administration of hTNFα to rats at doses (100–1000 ng i.v.) that failed to affect blood pressure, food consumption, or plasma prolactin concentrations, resulted in significant peak elevations of plasma ACTH within 20 min.[38–41] Most reports found TNFα to be significantly less potent than IL-1 in rats and mice,[40] but Sharp et al. found hTNFα to be almost equipotent with hIL-1β.[38] Our results using mTNFα (i.v. or i.p.) in mice showed a somewhat more prolonged response, but that was less potent than mIL-1β in mice.[32,42]

The activation of the HPA axis by TNFα appears to be mediated at least partially by CRF. The ACTH response was completely blocked, whereas the corticosterone response was partially inhibited by pretreatment with antiserum to CRF.[39] Indomethacin (0.1–1 mg/kg, i.v.) dose-dependently blocked the ACTH response to TNFα (1 mg, i.v.) in rats.[43] The PVN appears to be essential for the ACTH response to TNFα, because lesioning of the PVN abolished the response.[44]

Interferons

Administration of human or mouse interferon α (IFNα) to mice i.p. failed to alter plasma ACTH or corticosterone and the brain concentrations of catecholamines, serotonin, and metabolites at doses (hIFNα: 1,000–10,000 Units/mouse; mIFNα; 400–1,600 Units/mouse) that were behaviorally active 1–2 hours after administration.[45]

ASSOCIATION OF THE NEUROCHEMICAL RESPONSES WITH THE ENDOCRINE RESPONSE

We have been interested in identifying the function(s) of the neurochemical responses. TABLE 3 indicates the antagonists we have tested that failed to attenuate the HPA response to i.p. IL-1β in mice, and TABLE 4 those that have some effects. First we addressed the relationship between the neurochemical responses and the HPA activation. The noradrenergic (NA) response to i.p. injection of IL-1β into mice indicated by increases in the catabolite, 3-methoxy,4-hydroxyphenylethyleneglycol (MHPG), starts early, reaches a peak around two hours, and disappears within eight hours (see FIGURE 2).[4,46] This closely resembles the results reported in rats.[47] The

TABLE 3. Pharmacological treatments that do not affect HPA activation by i.p. IL-1β

α_2-adrenergic antagonist (idazoxan)

β-adrenergic antagonist (propranolol)

Muscarinic antagonists (atropine, scopolamine)

Ganglionic blocker (chlorisondamine)

H_1-receptor antagonist (pyrilamine)

H_2-receptor antagonist (cimetidine)

Lipo-oxygenase inhibitors (BW755C, BWA4C)

NOS Inhibitors (L-NAME, NMA, NIL)

Opiate-receptor antagonist (naloxone)

5-HT_2-receptor antagonist (cinanserin)

Substance P antagonist (BIBP3226)

Y_1-receptor antagonists (L659,877, L703,606, 733,060)

NOTE: Each of the antagonists was tested for its effects on the i.p. IL-1β-induced elevation in plasma corticosterone 2 h after injection.

increases in brain tryptophan and serotonin metabolism (5-HIAA) are significantly slower and do not reach a peak until around four hours (FIG. 2).[4,46]

The time course of the HPA response, indicated by increases in plasma concentrations of ACTH and corticosterone, closely parallels the noradrenergic response.[4,46] Moreover, in individual animals, the correlation between the increases in plasma corticosterone and hypothalamic MHPG is almost perfect. This correlation is indicated even more clearly in a study in which the release of NA from rat hypothalamus was assessed by microdialysis while simultaneously sampling plasma for corticosterone, following i.p. or intravenous injection of IL-1β.[48] The only dissociation of the two responses occurs when mice are treated with COX inhibitors, which prevent the MHPG response to i.p. IL-1β, while the plasma corticosterone response is unimpaired.[3] When the noradrenergic input to the hypothalamus is reduced by injecting the selective NA neurotoxin, 6-hydroxydopamine (6-OHDA) directly into the paraventricular nucleus (PVN) or the ventral ascending noradrener-

TABLE 4. Treatments that affect HPA Activation by i.p. IL-1β

Hypophysectomy

CRF antibodies

Knocking out the CRF gene in mice

Prazosin (α_1-adrenergic antagonist) attenuates

COX inhibitors inhibit the response to i.v., but only the early phase of i.p.

NOTE: Each of the antagonists/treatments was tested for its effects on the i.p. IL-1β-induced elevation in plasma corticosterone 2 h after injection.

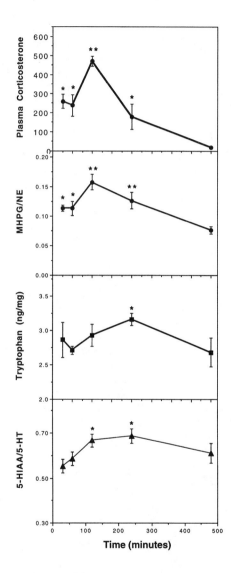

FIGURE 2. Effect of i.p. mIL-1β on hypothalamic catecholamines and indoleamines. Mice were injected with saline or mIL-1β (100 ng i.p.), and plasma and brain samples collected at various subsequent times (the same experiment shown at top of FIG. 1). *Top panel*: Plasma corticosterone (ng/ml); *second panel*: hypothalamic MHPG:NE ratios; *third panel*: hypothalamic tryptophan (ng/mg tissue); *bottom panel*: hypothalamic 5-HIAA:5-HT ratios. $N = 7$. *Significantly different from the corresponding saline groups (not shown, $*p < 0.05$ or $**p < 0.01$).

gic bundle (VNAB) of rats, the plasma corticosterone response to i.p. IL-1 was markedly impaired.[49] However, treatment with α- and β-adrenergic antagonists or the combination did not affect the HPA response to IL-1 in rats.[20,50] Depletions of whole mouse brain NA by 97–99% had little or no effect on the IL-1–induced elevation of plasma corticosterone.[51] In mice, we observed no effects of idazoxan (α_2-adrenoreceptor antagonist), or propranolol (β-adrenoreceptor antagonist), but the α_1-adrenoreceptor antagonist, prazosin, did attenuate the response with a maximal effect of around 50% at 1 mg/kg. Thus, NA does not appear to be essential for the HPA response to IL-1. Most likely the regulation of HPA axis activation involves not only NA, but neuropeptides, such as substance P, neuropeptide Y, or galanin.

As indicated in TABLE 3, serotonergic receptor antagonists did not alter the plasma corticosterone response to IL-1β. Indeed the time course of the tryptophan and 5-HIAA responses to i.p. IL-1β is significantly different from that of plasma ACTH and corticosterone (FIGS. 1 and 2).[46]

As indicated above, COX inhibitors were partially effective in attenuating the plasma ACTH and corticosterone responses to IL-1. The response to i.v. IL-1 was largely effective, but that to i.p. IL-1 less so. Interestingly, the COX2-selective inhibitor NS-398 was ineffective.

ACKNOWLEDGMENTS

The technical assistance of Charles Dempsey is greatly appreciated as is the clerical assistance of Sharon Farrar. This research was supported by grants from the U.S. National Institute of Mental Health (MH46261) and the U.S. National Institute of Neurological Diseases and Stroke (NS25370).

REFERENCES

1. BESEDOVSKY, H.O., A. DEL REY, E. SORKIN & C.A. DINARELLO. 1986. Immunoregulatory feedback between interleukin-1 and glucocorticoid hormones. Science **233:** 652–654.
2. DINARELLO, C.A. 1988. Biology of interleukin 1. FASEB J. **2:** 108–115.
3. DUNN, A.J. & H. CHULUYAN. 1992. The role of cyclo-oxygenase and lipoxygenase in the interleukin-1-induced activation of the HPA axis: dependence on the route of injection. Life Sci. **51:** 219–225.
4. DUNN, A.J. 1988. Systemic interleukin-1 administration stimulates hypothalamic norepinephrine metabolism parallelling the increased plasma corticosterone. Life Sci. **43:** 429–435.
5. RIVIER, C. & W. VALE. 1991. Stimulatory effect of interleukin-1 on adrenocorticotropin secretion in the rat: is it modulated by prostaglandins? Endocrinology **129:** 384–388.
6. MURAKAMI, N. & T. WATANABE. 1989. Activation of ACTH release is mediated by the same molecule as the final mediator, PGE2, of febrile response in rats. Brain Res. **478:** 171–174.
7. MORIMOTO, A., N. MURAKAMI, T. NAKAMORI, Y. SAKATA & T. WATANABE. 1989. Possible involvement of prostaglandin E in development of ACTH response in rats induced by human recombinant interleukin-1. J. Physiol. **411:** 245–256.
8. KRYMSKAYA, L.G., N.Y. GROMYKHINA & V.A. KOZLOV. 1987. Interleukin 1 effect on adrenal gland function in mice. Immunol. Lett. **15:** 307–309.

9. DUNN, A.J. 1990. Interleukin-1 as a stimulator of hormone secretion. Prog. NeuroEndocrinImmunol. **3:** 26–34.
10. GWOSDOW, A.R., M.S.A. KUMAR & H.H. BODE. 1990. Interleukin 1 stimulation of the hypothalamic-pituitary-adrenal axis. Amer. J. Physiol. **258:** E65–70.
11. OLSEN, N.J., W.E. NICHOLSON, C.R. DEBOLD & D.N. ORTH. 1992. Lymphocyte-derived adrenocorticotropin is insufficient to stimulate adrenal steroidogenesis in hypophysectomized rats. Endocrinol. **130:** 2113–2119.
12. DUNN, A.J. 1993. Role of cytokines in infection-induced stress. Ann. N.Y. Acad. Sci. **697:** 189–202.
13. DUNN, A.J. & S.L. VICKERS. 1994. Neurochemical and neuroendocrine responses to Newcastle disease virus administration in mice. Brain Res. **645:** 103–112.
14. OVADIA, H., O. ABRAMSKY, V. BARAK, N. CONFORTI, D. SAPHIER & J. WEIDENFELD. 1989. Effect of interleukin-1 on adrenocortical activity in intact and hypothalamic deafferentated male rats. Exptl. Brain Res. **76:** 246–249.
15. RIVEST, S. & C. RIVIER. 1991. Influence of the paraventricular nucleus of the hypothalamus in the alteration of neuroendocrine functions induced by intermittent footshock or interleukin. Endocrinology **129:** 2049-2057.
16. BERKENBOSCH, F., J. VAN OERS, A. DEL REY, F. TILDERS & H. BESEDOVSKY. 1987. Corticotropin-releasing factor-producing neurons in the rat activated by interleukin-1. Science **238:** 524–526.
17. SAPOLSKY, R., C. RIVIER, G. YAMAMOTO, P. PLOTSKY & W. VALE. 1987. Interleukin-1 stimulates the secretion of hypothalamic corticotropin-releasing factor. Science **238:** 522–524.
18. UEHARA, A., P.E. GOTTSCHALL, R.R. DAHL & A. ARIMURA. 1987. Interleukin-1 stimulates ACTH release by an indirect action which requires endogenous corticotropin releasing factor. Endocrinol. **121:** 1580–1582.
19. DUNN, A.J. & A.H. SWIERGIEL. 1999. Behavioral responses to stress are intact in CRF-deficient mice. Brain Res. **845:** 14–20.
20. RIVIER, C. 1995. Influence of immune signals on the hypothalamic-pituitary axis of the rodent. Front. Neuroendocrinol. **16:** 151–182.
21. WATKINS, L.R., S.F. MAIER & L.E. GOEHLER. 1995. Cytokine-to-brain communication: a review & analysis of alternative mechanisms. Life Sci. **57:** 1011–1026.
22. NAITOH, Y., J. FUKATA, T. TOMINAGA, Y. NAKAI, S. TAMAI, K. MORI & H. IMURA. 1988. Interleukin-6 stimulates the secretion of adrenocorticotropic hormone in conscious, freely-moving rats. Biochem. Biophys. Res. Commun. **155:** 1459–1463.
23. LYSON, K. & S. M. MCCANN. 1991. The effect of interleukin-6 on pituitary hormone release in vivo and in vitro. Neuroendocrinology **54:** 262–266.
24. DEL REY, A. & H.O. BESEDOVSKY. 1992. Metabolic and neuroendocrine effects of pro-inflammatory cytokines. Europ. J. Clin. Invest. 22 Suppl. **1:** 10–15.
25. MATTA, S.G., J. WEATHERBEE & B.M. SHARP. 1992. A central mechanism is involved in the secretion of ACTH in response to IL-6 in rats: comparison to and interaction with IL-1b. Neuroendocrinology **56:** 516–525.
26. PERLSTEIN, R.S., E.H. MOUGEY, W.E. JACKSON & R. NETA. 1991. Interleukin-1 and interleukin-6 act synergistically to stimulate the release of adrenocorticotropic hormone in vivo. Lymph. Cytok. Res. **10:** 141–146.
27. WANG, J.P. & A.J. DUNN. 1998. Mouse interleukin-6 stimulates the HPA axis and increases brain tryptophan and serotonin metabolism. Neurochem. Int. **33:** 143–154.
28. MASTORAKOS, G., G.P. CHROUSOS & J.S. WEBER. 1993. Recombinant interleukin-6 activates the hypothalamic-pituitary-adrenal axis in humans. J. Clin. Endocrinol. Metab. **77:** 1690–1694.
29. STOUTHARD, J.M.L., J.A. ROMIJN, T. VAN DER POLL, E. ENDERT, S. KLEIN, P.J.M. BAKKER, C.H.N. VEENHOF & H.P. SAUERWEIN. 1995. Endocrinologic and metabolic effects of interleukin-6 in humans. Amer. J. Physiol. **268:** E813–819.
30. BOCCI, V. 1991. Interleukins: clinical pharmacokinetics and practical implications. Clin. Pharmacokinet. **21:** 274–284.
31. MULÉ, J.J., J.K. MCINTOSH, D.M. JABLONS & S.A. ROSENBERG. 1990. Antitumor activity of recombinant interleukin 6 in mice. J. Exptl Med. **171:** 629–636.

32. DUNN, A.J. 1992. The role of interleukin-1 and tumor necrosis factor a in the neurochemical and neuroendocrine responses to endotoxin. Brain Res. Bull. **29:** 807–812.

33. ANDO, T., J. RIVIER, H. YANAIHARA & A. ARIMURA. 1998. Peripheral corticotropin-releasing factor mediates the elevation of plasma IL-6 by immobilization stress in rats. Am. J. Physiol. **275:** R1461–R1467.

34. SPANGELO, B.L., A.M. JUDD, P.C. ISAKSON & R.M. MACLEOD. 1991. Interleukin-1 stimulates interleukin-6 release from rat anterior pituitary cells in vitro. Endocrinol. **128:** 2685–2692.

35. CALLAHAN, T.A. & D.T. PIEKUT. 1997. Differential Fos expression induced by IL-1b and IL-6 in rat hypothalamus and pituitary gland. J. Neuroimmunol. **73:** 207–211.

36. TINSLEY, S.L. & A.J. DUNN. Unpublished observations.

37. WANG, J.P. & A.J. DUNN. 1999. The role of interleukin-6 in the activation of the hypothalamo-pituitary-adrenocortical axis induced by endotoxin and interleukin-1b. Brain Res. **815:** 337–348.

38. SHARP, B.M., S.G. MATTA, P.K. PETERSON, R. NEWTON, C. CHAO & K. MCALLEN. 1989. Tumor necrosis factor-a is a potent ACTH secretagogue: comparison to interleukin-1b. Endocrinol. **124:** 3131–3133.

39. BERNARDINI, B., T.C. KAMILARIS, A.E. CALOGERO, E.O. JOHNSON, M.T. GOMEZ, P.W. GOLD & G.P. CHROUSOS. 1990. Interactions between tumor necrosis factor-a, hypothalamic corticotropin-releasing hormone, and adrenocorticotropin secretion in the rat. Endocrinol. **126:** 2876–2881.

40. BESEDOVSKY, H.O., A. DEL REY, I. KLUSMAN, H. FURUKAWA, G. MONGE ARDITI & A. KABIERSCH. 1991. Cytokines as modulators of the hypothalamus-pituitary-adrenal axis. J. Steroid Biochem. Molec. Biol. **40:** 613–618.

41. DARLING, G., D. S. GOLDSTEIN, R. STULL, C. M. GORSCHBOTH & J. A. NORTON. 1989. Tumor necrosis factor: immune endocrine interaction. Surgery **106:** 1155–1160.

42. ANDO, T. & A.J. DUNN. 1999. Mouse tumor necrosis factor-a increases brain tryptophan concentrations and norepinephrine metabolism while activating the HPA axis in mice. Neuroimmunomodulation **6:** 319–329.

43. SHARP, B.M. & S.G. MATTA. 1993. Prostaglandins mediate the adrenocorticotropin response to tumor necrosis factor in rats. Endocrinol. **132:** 269–274.

44. KOVÁCS, K.J., L. TAKÁCS & I.E. ELENKOV. 1993. Involvement of paraventricular corticotropin releasing factor in stimulation of ACTH by different cytokines. Soc. Neurosci. Abstr. **19:** 503.

45. DUNN, A.J., J.-P. WANG & T. ANDO. 1999. Effects of cytokines on central neurotransmission: Comparison with the effects of stress. Adv. Exptl. Med. Biol. **461:** 117–127.

46. DUNN, A.J. 1992. Endotoxin-induced activation of cerebral catecholamine and serotonin metabolism: comparison with interleukin-1. J. Pharmacol. Exptl. Therapeut. **261:** 964–969.

47. KABIERSCH, A., A. DEL REY, C.G. HONEGGER & H.O. BESEDOVSKY. 1988. Interleukin-1 induces changes in norepinephrine metabolism in the rat brain. Brain Behav. Immunol. **2:** 267–274.

48. SMAGIN, G.N., A.H. SWIERGIEL & A.J. DUNN. 1996. Peripheral administration of interleukin-1 increases extracellular concentrations of norepinephrine in rat hypothalamus: comparison with plasma corticosterone. Psychoneuroendocrinol. **21:** 83–93.

49. CHULUYAN, H., D. SAPHIER, W.M. ROHN & A.J. DUNN. 1992. Noradrenergic innervation of the hypothalamus participates in the adrenocortical responses to interleukin-1. Neuroendocrinol. **56:** 106–111.

50. BESEDOVSKY, H. & A. DEL REY. Personal communication.

51. SWIERGIEL, A. H., A. J. DUNN & E. A. STONE. 1996. The role of cerebral noradrenergic systems in the Fos response to interleukin-1. Brain Res. Bull. **41:** 61–64.

In Vivo Immunomodulation by Peripheral Adrenergic and Cholinergic Agonists/Antagonists in Rat and Mouse Models

K. SCHAUENSTEIN,[a] P. FELSNER, I. RINNER,[b] P.M. LIEBMANN, J.R. STEVENSON, J. WESTERMANN,[c] H.S. HAAS, R.L. COHEN,[d] AND D.A. CHAMBERS[d]

Department of General and Experimental Pathology,
University of Graz, A-8010 Graz, Austria

[c]*Department of Anatomy, Medical School Hannover, D-30623 Hannover, Germany*

[d]*Department of Biochemistry and Molecular Biology, College of Medicine,*
University of Illinois, Chicago, Illinois 60612, USA

ABSTRACT: Our work is devoted to defining relationships between the immune system and the adrenergic and cholinergic systems *in vivo*. In the rat model, we have shown that the cells of different immune compartments express the genes of a defined set of adrenergic/cholinergic receptors, and it was shown that lymphocytes are a site of non-neuronal production of norepinephrine and acetylcholine. Furthermore, using implantable slow-release tablets containing adrenergic or cholinergic agonists/antagonists, distinct and partly opposite effects were observed on peripheral immune functions. Concerning sympathetic immunoregulation, our data—in contrast to those of other studies—suggest that an enhanced adrenergic tonus leads to immunosuppression primarily via α_2-receptor-mediated mechanisms. Beta-blockade strongly enhances this effect, most likely by inhibition of pineal melatonin synthesis. In recent experiments on the kinetics it was found that the continuous α-adrenergic treatment entails a strong suppression of cellular responsiveness during the first few hours, which is increasingly followed by a general loss of lymphocytes in blood and lymphoid organs most likely due to enhanced apoptosis. More recently, we have extended our studies to the mouse model. First data obtained with RNAse protection assays suggest a biphasic effect on the gene expression of several cytokines in spleen cells due to adrenergic *in vivo* treatment.

INTRODUCTION

The role of the autonomic nervous system (ANS) in the extrinsic regulation of the immune system is widely accepted.[1–3] Nevertheless, several enigmas still exist precluding a comprehensive view of how changes in the activity of the ANS may actually influence normal or pathogenic immune functions in a given individual, experimental animal, or human being. This concerns, for example, the α/β receptor

[a]Address for correspondence: Professor Konrad Schauenstein, M.D., Department of General and Experimental Pathology, University of Graz, Heinrichstrasse 31A, A-8010 Graz, Austria. Voice: +43 316 380-7660; fax: +43 316 380-9640.
konrad.schauenstein@kfunigraz.ac.at
[b]Died July 29th, 1999.

involvement and effector mechanisms of catecholamine-mediated immunoregulation, the effects of cholinergic signals to the immune system, the modulation of the immune system–brain feedback by autonomic pathways, and the role of non-adrenergic and non-cholinergic neurotransmitters involved in the central control of the ANS. The primary goal of our own studies is to define the *in vivo* relationships between the ANS and the immune system in rodent animal models. Here we will review some of our previous results and present some new preliminary data that address some of the above mentioned puzzles (see FIGURE 1).

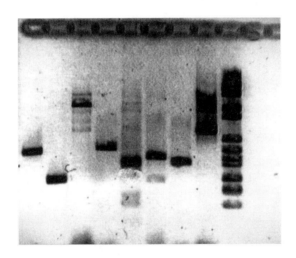

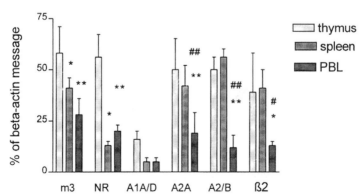

FIGURE 1. (top) Agarose gel electrophoresis of cDNA generated by RT-PCR with mRNA from PBL using specific primers for cholinergic muscarinic m3 (*lane 1*, from left), nicotinic (*lane 2*), and adrenergic α_1A (*lane 3*), α_1D (*lane 4*), α_2A (*lane 5*), α_2B (*lane 6*), β_2 (*lane 7*) receptors, and β-actin (*lane 8*). *Lane 9* = MW marker. **(bottom)** Receptor gene expression in thymus, spleen, and PBLs, *($p < 0.05$), **($p < 0.01$) significantly different from thymus, #($p < 0.05$), ##($p < 0.01$) significantly different from spleen.

ADRENERGIC/CHOLINERGIC RECEPTORS
IN THE IMMUNE SYSTEM OF THE RAT

Adrenergic α-receptors[4] and β-receptors[5–8] and cholinergic muscarinic[9] and nicotinic receptors[10–12] have been detected on the surface of human and rodent lymphocytes of different compartments by specific ligand binding. The reported data show wide quantitative differences and are in some aspects even contradictory, which could be due to species and/or strain differences, different experimental approaches, and to differences in receptor expression and/or function depending on differentiation and/or activation of immunocompetent cells.[6,8,13,14] In recent experiments we investigated the gene expression of cloned adrenergic/cholinergic receptors in rat lymphocytes derived from different immune compartments and at different states of activation. Messenger-RNA was isolated from lymphocytes of thymus, spleen, and peripheral blood (PBL) of male Sprague Dawley rats. PBLs were separated into

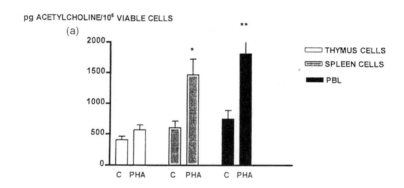

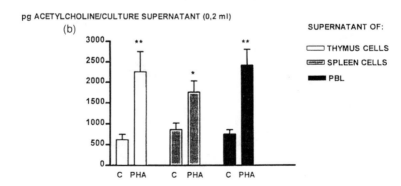

FIGURE 2. Effect of mitogen (PHA) stimulation of thymus, spleen and PBL on cellular content (**a**) and release (**b**) of acetylcholine, as compared to unstimulated controls (C). Acetylcholine was measured by means of a radioimmunoassay. *($p < 0.05$), **($p < 0.01$) significantly different from controls (Reprinted from Rinner et al.[30] by permission of Elsevier Science).

purified T cells, B cells, and CD4$^+$ or CD8$^+$ subsets. Furthermore, PBLs were analyzed before and after *in vitro* stimulation with T-cell (ConA) and B-cell (PWM)
mitogens. The mRNA expression for the following receptors was examined using
specific primers in reverse transcriptase polymerase chain reactions (RT-PCR): cholinergic muscarinic (m3) and nicotinic receptors, and adrenergic α_1A/D, α_2A, α_2B,
α_2C, β_1, and β_2 receptors. The intensities of the electrophoresed PCR products were
quantitatively compared with those of β-actin. The results revealed that (1) lymphocytes from thymus, spleen, and PBL express messages for α_1A/D, α_2A, α_2B, and β_2,
but not α_2C, and β_1 receptors, whereby the mRNA expression is generally lowest in
PBL as compared to thymus and partly (A2A, A2B, β_2) also to spleen (FIG. 1); (2)
in purified B-cells no m3 message could be detected, and the expression of β_2 message was higher as compared to that of T cells; and (3) stimulation of PBL with Con
A decreased the expression of the messages of α_1A/D, α_2A, and β_2 receptors, whereas PWM induced an increase of α_2A mRNA. No differences in the expression of any
receptor genes was noted between CD4$^+$ and CD8$^+$ T cells. Thus, rat lymphocytes
generally transcribe a defined set of adrenergic/cholinergic receptor genes, but their
expression quantitatively differs with tissue origin, phenotype, and activation of the
cells (see FIGURE 2).

CHOLINERGIC SIGNALS TO AND FROM THE IMMUNE SYSTEM

Activation of adrenergic and cholinergic receptors on immune cells has been
shown to affect functional properties of these cells, such as mitogenic stimulation,[15–18] cytokine production,[19–24] and *in vivo* organ distribution.[25,26] As with
receptor expression, the reported data are in many aspects controversial, which may
at least partly be due to differences in receptor gene expression as shown above. The
majority of the existing literature describes catecholamine effects on immune functions, and only few studies are dealing with cholinergic immunomodulation. Concerning the latter, the work of Ingo Rinner in our group should be mentioned. His
results strongly suggested that the cholinergic system importantly takes part in the
brain– immune system dialogue. The main findings were that (1) cholinergic *in vivo*
treatment of rats leads to enhanced lymphocyte functions; (2) the same treatment pri-
or to antigenic challenge interferes with the activation of the HPA axis; and (3) a
peripheral immune response leads to transient changes in the expression of cholinergic receptors in the hippocampus.[18] Furthermore, he showed that acetylcholine
modulates the spontaneous apoptosis of murine thymocytes via a nicotinergic effect
on cortical thymic epithelial cells and may therefore take part in the regulation of
T-cell generation.[27] The sources of this neurotransmitter in the thymus are most likely the developing T cells themselves, as the cholinergic innervation of the thymus is
questionable,[28] and lymphocytes were shown by us to produce[29] and to release acetylcholine depending upon the state of differentiation and activation[30] (FIG. 2). The
impact of these data for our ongoing research activities is two-fold: (1) triggered by
the cholinergic receptor data in the hippocampus, we have recently reviewed the role
of the "limbic system" in neuroimmunomodulation[31]; studies are being initiated to
define the role of excitatory amino acids, as important neurotransmitters in these

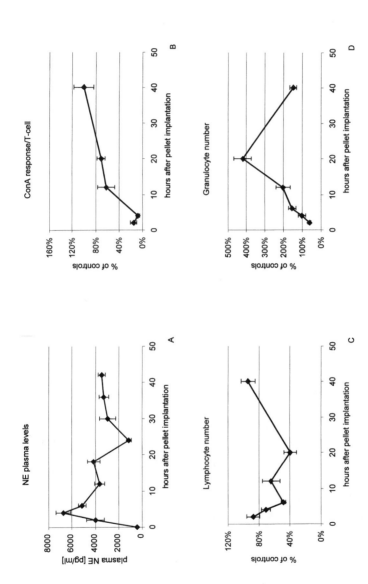

FIGURE 3. Kinetics of α_2-adrenergic *in vivo* effects in the rat. At time 0 two tablets containing norepinephrine (5 mg) and propranolol (20 mg), respectively, were implanted in Sprague Dawley rats. Controls received placebo tablets (= matrix without agents). (**A**) norepinephrine plasma levels; (**B**) ConA response of PBL related to T (CD3$^+$) cells; (**C**) total lymphocyte numbers in peripheral blood as % of controls; (**D**) numbers of granulocytes in peripheral blood as % of controls.

areas, in brain–immune system interactions. (2) The possible immunoregulatory relevance of non-neuronal, lymphocyte-derived acetylcholine and catecholamines[32,33] should be investigated in depth (see FIGURE 3).

ADRENERGIC IMMUNOREGULATION IN THE RAT MODEL

Concerning adrenergic effects, our data in the rat model are in contrast to those of several other studies in showing that increased peripheral catecholamine levels suppress immune functions via α_2-receptor mediated mechanisms and not by activation of β-receptors. This was found both after 20 hours' treatment with subcutaneous implantable pellets containing norepinephrine and as acute effect after intraperitoneal injection of the indirect sympathomimetic agent tyramine.[15,16] The receptor specificity was confirmed by selective agonists and antagonists. Importantly, β-blockade strongly enhanced this immunosuppressive adrenergic effect, even in experiments, where selective α_2-agonists were applied. This latter phenomenon could be effectively counteracted by melatonin,[34] suggesting that this hormone protects lymphocytes from adrenergic stress. The mechanism(s) of such protection is still obscure (TABLE 1).

As a first approach to understanding the mechanism(s) of α_2-mediated immunosuppression, we recently performed kinetic experiments as shown in FIGURE 3. The combined treatment with norepinephrine and β-blocker initially leads to a profound suppression of T-cell responsiveness followed by a significant shift in the differential white blood cell count, that is, an increase in neutrophils and a drop in total lymphocytes. This decrease of lymphocytes was likewise observed in thymus, spleen, and lymph nodes (not shown). Results obtained with the TUNEL technique on tissue sections suggest an increased apoptosis in lymphoid organs due to α-adrenergic treatment (TABLE 1), which may explain this latter phenomenon. Finally, both effects are short-lived and disappear after 40 hours of treatment at the latest, whereby the norepinephrine levels are still markedly elevated (see FIGURE 4).

TABLE 1. **Effect combined norepinephrine and propranolol treatment on the frequency of apoptotic cells**[a]

Apoptotic cells/mm^2	Signficance	Placebo	n	NE + Propr	n
Thymus cortex	$p < 0.05$	164.83 ± 8.9	6	306.60 ± 67.8	5
Thymus medulla	n.s.	68.83 ± 4.4	6	107.50 ± 21.7	6
GC in spleen	$p < 0,05$	677.72 ± 107.8	6	1085.15 ± 102.4	6
GC in LN	$p < 0,05$	648.10 ± 35.2	6	1215.50 ± 221.0	5

[a]Effect of 12 hours combined norepinephrine + propranolol treatment (NE + Propr) on the frequency of apoptotic cells as determined on histologic sections with the TUNEL technique in cortex and medulla of thymus, and in germinal centers (GC) of spleen and lymph nodes (LN) of Sprague Dawley rats. Control rats received tablets without specific agent (placebo).

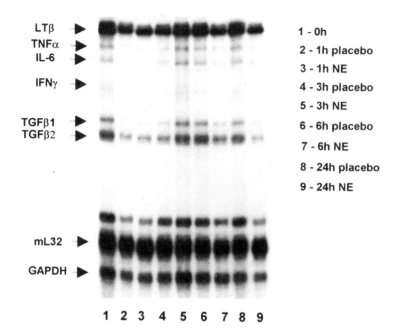

FIGURE 4. Effect of norepinephrine (1.7 mg per tablet) treatment vs. placebo controls on cytokine gene expression of murine spleen. Electrophoresis of products of RNAse protection assays. For details see text.

ADRENERGIC MODULATION IN THE *IN VIVO* MOUSE MODEL

The technique of subcutaneously implanted NE tablets has been used in BALB/c mice to study adrenergic effects *in vivo* on mRNA expression of cytokines in murine spleen cells. Male mice received either an NE tablet or placebo. At various times after implantation spleens were harvested and total RNA was purified and analyzed by RNAse protection assays for TNFα, TGFβ1, TGFβ2, LTβ, and IL-6 mRNA (FIG. 4). At 1 hour of treatment a drop in mRNA expression of all cytokines was seen in both placebo- and NE-treated animals, probably due to the stress of surgical manipulation. After three hours the expression of TNFα, IL-6, TGF-β1, and TGF-β2 showed a 2–3-fold enhancement in NE-treated mice over controls. In contrast, after six hours of NE application, cytokine mRNA was reduced about 2-fold and continued to decrease at 24 hours. No change occurred in mRNA levels of the housekeeping gene L32. In most recent experiments, IL-1 increased in response to NE, whereas MIF showed no change. Thus, *in vivo* cytokine regulation by NE appears selective and specific.

CONCLUSIONS

Our data strongly support the notion that the sympathetic and parasympathetic nervous systems are critically involved in extrinsic immunoregulation. More work is needed to reconcile the existing data from different groups into a coherent and comprehensive view of adrenergic/cholinergic immunomodulation. Besides further studies into the regulation of normal immunity, this goal should also be pursued by analyzing how adrenergic/cholinergic mechanisms influence "abnormal" immune reactions, such as allergy and autoimmunity. Given the fact that adrenergic and cholinergic mediators are to be considered as potent immunomodulators, the final aim of all these studies should be to develop new strategies in the prevention/treatment of pathogenic immune reactions as well as to help to optimally condition the immune defense against exogenous or endogenous pathogens.

ACKNOWLEDGMENTS

This work was supported by the Austrian Science Foundation (Projects 9925, 11130, 10422, 11921, 12579, 12679) and the Jubiläumsfonds der Österreichischen Nationalbank (Projects 5692 and 6730).

REFERENCES

1. MADDEN, K.S., S.Y. FELTEN, D.L. FELTEN, C.A. HARDY & S. LIVNAT. 1994. Sympathetic nervous system modulation of the immune system. II. Induction of lymphocyte proliferation and migration in vivo by chemical sympathectomy. J. Neuroimmunol. **49:** 67–75.

2. FELTEN, D.L., K.D. ACKERMAN, S.J. WIEGAND & S.Y. FELTEN. 1987. Noradrenergic sympathetic innervation of the spleen: I. Nerve fibers associate with lymphocytes and macrophages in specific compartments of the splenic white pulp. J. Neurosci. Res. **18:** 28–21.

3. SHERIDAN, J.F., C. DOBBS, D. BROWN & B. ZWILLING. 1994. Psychoneuroimmunology: stress effects on pathogenesis and immunity during infection. Clin. Microbiol. Rev. **7:** 200–212.

4. RICCI, A., E. BRONZETTI, A. CONTERNO, S. GRECO, P. MULATERO, M. SCHENA, D. SCHIAVONE, S.K. TAYEBATI, F. VEGLIO & F. AMENTA. 1999. alpha 1-adrenergic receptor subtypes in human peripheral blood lymphocytes. Hypertension **33:** 708–712.

5. MAKI, T. 1989. Density and functioning of human lymphocytic beta-adrenergic receptors during prolonged physical exercise. Acta Physiol Scand. **136:** 569–574.

6. MORALE, M.C., F. GALLO, N. BATTICANE & B. MARCHETTI. 1992. The immune response evokes up- and down-modulation of beta 2-adrenergic receptor messenger RNA concentration in the male rat thymus. Mol. Endocrinol. **6:** 1513–1524.

7. MORALE, M.C., Z. FARINELLA & B. MARCHETTI. 1990. Central nervous system (CNS) modulation of immune system development: role of the thymic beta 2-adrenergic receptor. Pharmacol. Res. **22** (Suppl 1): 47–48.

8. MACKENZIE, F.J., J.P. LEONARD & M.L. CUZNER. 1989. Changes in lymphocyte beta-adrenergic receptor density and noradrenaline content of the spleen are early indicators of immune reactivity in acute experimental allergic encephalomyelitis in the Lewis rat. J. Neuroimmunol. **23:** 93–100.

9. BRONZETTI, E., O. ADANI, F. AMENTA, L. FELICI, F. MANNINO & A. RICCI. 1996. Muscarinic cholinergic receptor subtypes in human peripheral blood lymphocytes. Neurosci. Lett. **208:** 211–215.

10. RINNER, I., S. PORTA & K. SCHAUENSTEIN. 1990. Characterization of 3H-N-methylscopolamine binding to intact rat thymocytes. Endocrinol. Exp. **24:** 125–132.

11. BATTAGLIOLI, E., C. GOTTI, S. TERZANO, A. FLORA, F. CLEMENTI & D. FORNASARI. 1998. Expression and transcriptional regulation of the human alpha3 neuronal nicotinic receptor subunit in T lymphocyte cell lines. J. Neurochem. **71:** 1261–1270.

12. TOYABE, S., T. IIAI, M. FUKUDA, T. KAWAMURA, S. SUZUKI, M. UCHIYAMA & T. ABO. 1997. Identification of nicotinic acetylcholine receptors on lymphocytes in the periphery as well as thymus in mice. Immunology **92:** 201–205.

13. PALDI-HARIS, P., J.G. SZELENYI, T.H. NGUYEN & S.R. HOLLAN. 1990. Changes in the expression of the cholinergic structures of human T lymphocytes due to maturation and stimulation. Thymus **16:** 119–122.

14. LOMBARDI, M.S., A. KAVELAARS, M. SCHEDLOWSKI, J.W. BIJLSMA, K.L. OKIHARA, P.M. VAN DE, S. OCHSMANN, C. PAWLAK, R.E. SCHMIDT & C.J. HEIJNEN. 1999. Decreased expression and activity of G-protein-coupled receptor kinases in peripheral blood mononuclear cells of patients with rheumatoid arthritis. FASEB J. **13:** 715–725.

15. FELSNER, P., D. HOFER, I. RINNER, H. MANGGE, M. GRUBER, W. KORSATKO & K. SCHAUENSTEIN. 1992. Continuous in vivo treatment with catecholamines suppresses in vitro reactivity of rat peripheral blood T-lymphocytes via alpha-mediated mechanisms. J. Neuroimmunol. **37:** 47–57.

16. FELSNER, P., D. HOFER, I. RINNER, S. PORTA, W. KORSATKO & K. SCHAUENSTEIN. 1995. Adrenergic suppression of peripheral blood T cell reactivity in the rat is due to activation of peripheral alpha 2-receptors. J. Neuroimmunol. **57:** 27–34.

17. JOHNSON, D.L., R.C. ASHMORE & M.A. GORDON. 1981. Effects of beta-adrenergic agents on the murine lymphocyte response to mitogen stimulation. J. Immunopharmacol. **3:** 205–219.

18. RINNER, I. & K. SCHAUENSTEIN. 1991. The parasympathetic nervous system takes part in the immuno-neuroendocrine dialogue. J. Neuroimmunol. **34:** 165–172.

19. FUJINO, H., Y. KITAMURA, T. YADA, T. UEHARA & Y. NOMURA. 1997. Stimulatory roles of muscarinic acetylcholine receptors on T cell antigen receptor/CD3 complex-mediated interleukin-2 production in human peripheral blood lymphocytes. Mol. Pharmacol. **51:** 1007–1014.

20. STRAUB, R.H., M. HERRMANN, T. FRAUENHOLZ, G. BERKMILLER, B. LANG, J. SCHOLMERICH & W. FALK. 1996. Neuroimmune control of interleukin-6 secretion in the murine spleen. Differential beta-adrenergic effects of electrically released endogenous norepinephrine under various endotoxin conditions. J. Neuroimmunol. **71:** 37–43.

21. RAGHEB, S. & R.P. LISAK. 1998. Secretion of TH-2-type cytokines by acetylcholine receptor (AChR)-stimulated mononuclear cells. Ann. N.Y. Acad. Sci. **841:** 347–350.

22. PETRO, T.M., D.S. PETERSON & Y.K. FUNG. 1992. Nicotine enhances interleukin production of rat splenic T lymphocytes. Immunopharmacol. Immunotoxicol. **14:** 463–475.

23. PRYNC, A.E., E. ARZT, C.S. FERNANDEZ, S. FINKIELMAN & V. NAHMOD. 1992. The inhibitory effect of the muscarinic agonist pilocarpine on lymphocyte activation involves the IL-2 pathway and the increase in suppressor cell function. Int. J. Neurosci. **62:** 277–285.

24. KALINICHENKO, V.V., M.B. MOKYR, L.H. GRAF, JR., R.L. COHEN & D.A. CHAMBERS. 1999. Norepinephrine-mediated inhibition of antitumor cytotoxic T lymphocyte generation involves a beta-adrenergic receptor mechanism and decreased TNF-alpha gene expression . J. Immunol. **163:** 2492–2499.

25. MILLS, P.J., C.C. BERRY, J.E. DIMSDALE, M.G. ZIEGLER, R.A. NELESEN & B.P. KENNEDY. 1995. Lymphocyte subset redistribution in response to acute experimental stress: effects of gender, ethnicity, hypertension, and the sympathetic nervous system. Brain Behav. Immun. **9:** 61–69.

26. LANDMANN, R., M. DURIG, F. GUDAT, M. WESP & F. HARDER. 1985. Beta-adrenergic regulation of the blood lymphocyte phenotype distribution in normal subjects and splenectomized patients. Adv. Exp. Med. Biol. **186:** 1051–1062.

27. RINNER, I., T. KUKULANSKY, P. FELSNER, E. SKREINER, A. GLOBERSON, M. KASAI, K. HIROKAWA, W. KORSATKO & K. SCHAUENSTEIN. 1994. Cholinergic stimulation modulates apoptosis and differentiation of murine thymocytes via a nicotinic effect on thymic epithelium. Biochem. Biophys. Res. Commun. **203:** 1057–1062.

28. NANCE, D.M., D.A. HOPKINS & D. BIEGER. 1987. Re-investigation of the innervation of the thymus gland in mice and rats. Brain Behav. Immun. **1:** 134–147.

29. RINNER, I. & K. SCHAUENSTEIN. 1993. Detection of choline-acetyltransferase activity in lymphocytes. J. Neurosci. Res. **35:** 188–191.

30. RINNER, I., K. KAWASHIMA & K. SCHAUENSTEIN. 1998. Rat lymphocytes produce and secrete acetylcholine in dependence of differentiation and activation. J. Neuroimmunol. **81:** 31–37.

31. HAAS, H.S. & K. SCHAUENSTEIN. 1997. Neuroimmunomodulation via limbic structures—the neuroanatomy of psychoimmunology. Prog. Neurobiol. **51:** 195–222.

32. BERGQUIST, J., A. TARKOWSKI, A. EWING & R. EKMAN. 1998. Catecholaminergic suppression of immunocompetent cells. Immunol. Today **19:** 562–567.

33. RINNER, I., P. FELSNER, P.M. LIEBMANN, D. HOFER, A. WOLFLER, A. GLOBERSON & K. SCHAUENSTEIN. 1998. Adrenergic/cholinergic immunomodulation in the rat model: in vivo veritas? Dev. Immunol. **6:** 245–252.

34. LIEBMANN, P.M., D. HOFER, P. FELSNER, A. WOLFLER & K. SCHAUENSTEIN. 1996. Beta-blockade enhances adrenergic immunosuppression in rats via inhibition of melatonin release. J. Neuroimmunol. **67:** 137–142.

Possible Function of IL-6 and TNF as Intraadrenal Factors in the Regulation of Adrenal Steroid Secretion

ALLAN M. JUDD,[a] GERALD B. CALL, MICHELLE BARNEY, CHRISTOPHER J. McILMOIL, ADAM G. BALLS, ANDREW ADAMS, AND GUSTAVO K. OLIVEIRA

Department of Zoology, Brigham Young University, Provo, Utah 84602, USA

ABSTRACT: Interleukin-6 (IL-6) and tumor necrosis factor α (TNFα) and their mRNAs are present in the human, rat, and bovine adrenal cortex. The release of these cytokines from adrenal cells is regulated by factors that alter adrenal function (e.g., ACTH, angiotensin II, interleukin-1). IL-6 and TNF type 1 receptors are also present on adrenocortical cells. Exposure to IL-6 increases cortisol or corticosterone release from human, bovine, and rat adrenal cells. IL-6 increases basal and ACTH-stimulated aldosterone release, but inhibits angiotensin II-stimulated aldosterone secretion from bovine adrenal cells. IL-6 increases dehydroepiandrosterone (DHEA) release from human cells, but decreases DHEA secretion from bovine cells. TNFα inhibits corticosterone release from normal rat adrenal cells or fragments, but increases corticosterone release from cholestatic rat adrenal slices. TNFα decreases cortisol release from bovine and fetal human adrenal cells, but increases cortisol release from adult human adrenal cells. TNFα inhibits aldosterone secretion from rat and bovine adrenocortical cells. TNFα does not affect DHEA secretion from fetal human adrenocortical cells, but inhibits basal and ACTH-stimulated DHEA release from bovine adrenal cell. Because IL-6 and TNFα are produced in the adrenal gland and modify adrenal steroid secretion, these cytokines may function as intraadrenal factors in the regulation of adrenal steroid secretion.

INTRODUCTION

The production of interleukin-6 (IL-6) and tumor necrosis factor (TNF) in various tissues increases during immunological, inflammatory, and stress responses. These cytokines activate the hypothalamic-pituitary-adrenal axis during inflammatory and immune responses. IL-6 and TNF increase the release of CRH from the hypothalamus, which results in an increase in ACTH release from the anterior pituitary. ACTH in turn augments the release of glucocorticoids from the adrenal cortex.[1,2] However, during chronic stress, there is a poor relationship between ACTH plasma concentrations and the release of glucocorticoids. Therefore, it has been hypothesized that autocrine or paracrine factors may act within the adrenal cortex to regulate glucocorticoid release.[3-6] These intraadrenal factors may also affect the release of aldosterone

[a]Address for correspondence: Allan M. Judd, Department of Zoology, 585 WIDB, Brigham Young University, Provo, Utah 84602. Voice: 801-378-3179; fax: 801-378-7423. Allan_Judd@BYU.EDU

TABLE 1. IL-6 and TNF in the adrenal cortex

Cytokine	Substance measured	Technique utilized	Observations	Ref.
IL-6 (rat)	Activity	Bioassay	LPS, IL-1α, IL-1β, ACTH, AII increase; released primarily from ZG	7–10
	mRNA	Northern blot	Increased by substance listed for IL-6 bioactivity; found in ZG	11
	IL-6	Immunohisto-chemistry	Large amounts in ZG with lesser amounts in ZF, ZR; LPS increases	12
	IL-6	Western blot	LPS increases	7
IL-6 (human)	mRNA	*In situ* hybridization	Band of cells in ZR, also in ZG, ZF	14
IL-6 (bovine)	Activity	Bioassay	LPS, IL-1α, IL-1β, AII, ACTH increase; released from ZG, ZF, ZR	13
TNFα (rat)	Activity	Bioassay	LPS, IL-1α, IL-1β increase; ACTH decreases; primary release from ZG	7,10
	TNFα	Immunohisto-chemistry	Large amounts in ZG with smaller amounts in ZF, ZR	12
	TNFα	Western blot	LPS increases	7
TNFα (human)	mRNA	*In situ* hybridization	Band of cells in ZR, also in ZG, ZF	16
	TNFα	RIA	Found in fetal adrenal; none detected in adult gland	15
TNFα (bovine)	Activity	Bioassay	LPS, IL-1α, IL-1β increase; ACTH decreases; released from ZG, ZF, ZR	13

and dehydroepiandrosterone (DHEA).[3] IL-6 and TNFα may be some of the intraadrenal factors that regulate adrenal function.[1,3,5–7]

ADRENAL IL-6 AND TNF

IL-6 is present in the rat, human, and bovine adrenal gland (TABLE 1). The rat adrenal zona glomerulosa (ZG) and the outer segments of the zona fasciculata (ZF) release IL-6.[1,7–10] Substances involved in inflammation and/or the immune response including lipopolysaccharide (LPS or endotoxin), interleukin-1α (IL-1α), and interleukin-1β (IL-1β) increase the release of IL-6 from rat adrenal cells.[1,7–10] Various regulators of adrenal steroid release including ACTH, angiotensin II (AII), dopamine (through D_2 receptors), serotonin, and adenosine (through A_2 receptors), increase basal IL-6 release from rat adrenocortical cells.[1,7] Interestingly, these secretagogues augment IL-6 release stimulated by LPS, IL-1α, or IL-1β.[7,9] In FIGURE 1, the effects of AII on IL-1α-stimulated IL-6 release from rat adrenal ZG cells are illustrated. AII increased basal IL-6 release and augmented the IL-6 release stimulated by IL-1β. The previously cited studies on IL-6 release were performed utilizing a bioassay for IL-6. Experiments utilizing Western blots have confirmed the presence of IL-6 in the rat adrenal gland and demonstrated that LPS increases adrenal IL-6 content.[15] Immunohistochemical analysis demonstrated that in the rat adrenal gland the cells

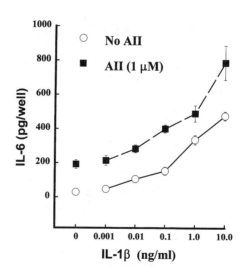

FIGURE 1. The effect of angiotensin II (AII) on IL-1β-stimulated IL-6 release from rat zona glomerulosa cells. The cultured adrenal cells were prepared and the IL-6 measured as explained previously.[9] IL-1β increased ($p < 0.05$ IL-1β concentrations of 0.01 ng/ml and greater vs. medium alone) IL-6 release. AII increased basal IL-6 release ($p < 0.01$ vs. medium alone) and potentiated the IL-6 release stimulated by each concentration of IL-1β ($p < 0.5$ vs. corresponding concentration of IL-1β alone). Incubation interval was 5 h.

of the ZG and outer ZF have high concentrations of IL-6 and a band of cells containing IL-6 is located at the junction of the zona reticularis (ZR) and medulla. Furthermore, the IL-6 content of the adrenal gland is increased by LPS exposure.[16] The rat adrenal gland contains IL-6 mRNA and the cellular content of this mRNA is increased by the secretagogues that increase IL-6 secretion.[7]

Bovine adrenocortical cells also release IL-6, and the release of IL-6 from these cells is regulated by the same factors that regulate rat adrenal IL-6 release. However, unlike the rat, all sections of the bovine adrenal gland release IL-6.[13] Human adrenocortical cells have IL-6 mRNA. The IL-6 mRNA is found in steroid-secreting cells scattered throughout the adrenal cortex, and in a band of cells at the junction of the ZR with the medulla.[14] In the human adrenal, cells that do not secrete steroids also contain IL-6 mRNA.

TNFα is also secreted by rat adrenocortical cells. Similar to IL-6, this cytokine is primarily secreted by ZG cells. LPS, IL-1α, and IL-1β increase TNF release from rat adrenal cells. However, ACTH, dopamine, serotonin, and adenosine decrease basal and secretagogue-stimulated TNF release from rat adrenal cells.[1,8,10] Therefore, IL-6 and TNF release from rat adrenal cells is differentially regulated. TNFα has a similar distribution pattern in the rat adrenal as IL-6. Specifically, TNFα is primarily localized to cells of the ZG and outer ZF and a ring of cells at the ZR and medulla boundary.[12] Western blot analyses of rat adrenal glands confirmed the presence of TNFα and provided evidence that LPS increases the cellular content of this cytokine in adrenal cells.[11]

TNFα is released from bovine adrenal ZG, ZF, and ZR cells. The release of TNFα from bovine adrenocortical cells is regulated in a manner identical to that of TNFα release from rat adrenocortical cells.[13] Jäättelä *et al.* determined that TNFα is present in the human fetal adrenal.[15] *In situ* hybridization has also demonstrated the presence of TNFα mRNA in the adult human adrenal.[16] Cells throughout the adrenal cortex contain the mRNA from this cytokine, but a band of cells at the boundary between the ZR and medulla contain more TNFα mRNA than cells elsewhere in the adrenal cortex. Many of the cells of the adrenal cortex that contain TNFα mRNA are steroid-secreting cells, although cortical cells that do not secrete steroids also contain TNFα mRNA.

IL-6 AND TNFα RECEPTOR IN THE ADRENAL CORTEX

Adrenocortical cells have receptors for IL-6 and TNFα (TABLE 2). Päth *et al.* determined that human adrenocortical cells express IL-6 receptors (IL-6R) with high expression of IL-6R in the ZR and inner ZF, and expression on individual cells in the ZG.[17,18] The human adrenocortical tumor cell line H295R expresses IL-6R ($K_d = 10^{-10}$, 230 receptors/cell) and TNF receptor (TNFR) ($K_d = 10^{-9}$, 110 receptors/cell) as demonstrated by binding of IL-6 or TNFα to these cells.[19] In the rat adrenal gland, IL-6R ($K_d = 10^{-10}$) and TNFR are expressed throughout the adrenal cortex and the TNFR is of the type 1 variety.[19] In the bovine adrenal gland, IL-6 and TNFα binding to adrenocortical cells is present in the ZG, ZF, and ZR (IL-6R $K_d = 10^{-11}$ to 10^{-10}, 100–200 receptors/cell, TNFR $K_d = 10^{-10}$, 200–260 receptors/cell).[19]

TABLE 2. IL-6 and TNF receptors in the adrenal cortex

Receptor and species	Substance measured	Technique utilized	Observation	Ref.
IL-6 (rat)	Receptor	Immunohisto-chemistry	In ZG, ZR, ZF; increased by LPS	19
	Binding	IL-6 binding	$K_d = 10^{-10}$	19
IL-6 (human)	Receptor mRNA	RT-PCR		18
	Receptor	Immunohisto-chemistry	Found in ZG, ZF, and ZR	17,18
	Binding	IL-6 binding	H295R cells; $K_d = 10^{-10}$; 230 receptors/cell	19
IL-6 (bovine)	Binding	IL-6 binding	In ZG, ZF, ZR; $K_d = 10^{-11}$ to 10^{-10}; 100–200 receptors/cell	19
TNFα (rat)	Receptor	Immunohisto-chemistry	TNF type 1 receptor in ZG, ZF, ZR	19
TNFα (human)	Receptor	TNFα binding	H295R cells, $K_d = 10^{-9}$; 110 receptors/cell	19
TNFα (bovine)	Receptor	TNFα binding	In ZG, ZF, ZR. $K_d = 10^{-10}$; 200–260 receptors/cell	19

EFFECTS OF IL-6 AND TNFα ON ADRENAL STEROID SECRETION

IL-6 increases basal and ACTH-stimulated corticosterone release from cultured rat adrenal cells (TABLE 3).[20–22] Similarly, IL-6 increases basal cortisol release from cultured human cells,[17,18,23] and increases basal and ACTH-stimulated cortisol release from bovine adrenocortical cells.[24] In bovine ZG cells, IL-6 increases basal and ACTH-stimulated aldosterone release in concentration-dependent manner, but inhibits AII-stimulated aldosterone release (see FIGURE 2). IL-6 increases aldosterone secretion from human adrenal cells.[17,18] IL-6 also increases DHEA secretion from human adrenocortical cells obtained from patients with renal carcinoma,[17,18] but decreases basal and ACTH-stimulated DHEA from bovine ZR cells.[25] Additional experiments are necessary to determine whether the divergence of IL-6 effects on DHEA secretion represents a difference between species or some environmental factor (e.g., physical and emotional stress related to the renal carcinoma). It is noteworthy that the effects of IL-6 on adrenal steroid secretion is relatively slow and requires 8 to 24 h to become apparent.[17,18,20,21,24,25]

Darling et al.[26] demonstrated that TNFα stimulates cortisol secretion from cultures of adult human adrenocortical cells derived from patients that had a nephrectomy (reason for nephrectomy not stated). However, in fetal human adrenocortical cells,[15,27] and adult bovine ZF cells,[24] TNFα inhibits basal and/or ACTH-stimulated cortisol secretion. Similarly, TNFα inhibits ACTH-stimulated corticosterone release

TABLE 3. The effects of IL-6 and TNFα on steroid release from adrenal cells

Cytokine	Species	Effect on steroid secretion	Ref.
IL-6	Rat	Increased basal and ACTH-stimulated corticosterone	20–22
	Human	Increased cortisol	17,18,23
		Increased DHEA	17,18
		Increased Aldosterone	17,18
	Bovine	Increased cortisol	24
		Decreased basal and ACTH-stimulated DHEA	25
		Increased basal and ACTH-stimulated aldosterone	Current MS
		Deceased AII-stimulated aldosterone	
TNFα	Rat	Decreased corticosterone in normal rats	28
		Increased corticosterone in cholestatic rats	29
		Decreased AII-stimulated aldosterone	30
	Human	Decreased cortisol from fetal adrenal cells	15,27
		Increased cortisol from adult adrenal cells	26
		Modest inhibition of DHEA release from fetal adrenal cells	15,27
		In fetal cells decreases the mRNA for the enzyme DHEA sulftransferase which makes DHEAS.	31
	Bovine	Decreased basal and ACTH-stimulated cortisol	24
		Decreased basal and ACTH-stimulated DHEA.	25
		Decreased basal aldsoterone secretion and aldosterone secretion stimulated by AII and ACTH.	Current MS

from rat adrenocortical cells or adrenal fragments.[28] In contrast, TNFα increases corticosterone secretion from adrenal slices obtained from cholestatic rats.[29] The stimulatory effect of TNFα on glucocorticoid secretion reported by Darling *et al.*[26] in human adrenal cells, and Swain and Maric[29] in rats, may be due to chronic stress (i.e., cholestasis in the rat, chronic disease in the human). In contrast, the difference between the TNFα results may be related to the concentration of TNFα utilized. In the experiments in which TNFα stimulated glucocorticoid release, high concentrations of TNFα were utilized (200 to 500 ng/ml).[26,29] In contrast, low concentrations of TNFα were utilized in experiments in which TNFα inhibited glucocorticoid release (0.1 to 100 ng/ml).[15,24,27,28]

TNFα inhibits aldosterone release stimulated by AII or ACTH in rat adrenocortical cells.[30] In bovine ZG cells, TNFα inhibits basal aldosterone release and the aldosterone release stimulated by AII or ACTH (FIG. 2). In human fetal adrenocortical cells, TNFα has only modest effects on DHEA secretion, but decreases the

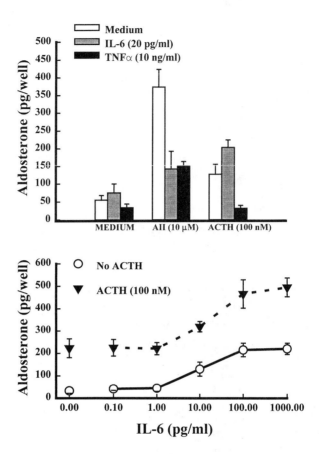

FIGURE 2. The effects of IL-6 and TNFα on aldosterone release from primary cultures of bovine adrenal zona glomerulosa cells. The aldosterone concentration was determined utilizing a kit from ICN Biomedical Inc. (Costa Mesa, CA). **Top**: Angiotensin II (AII) and ACTH increased aldosterone release ($p < 0.01$ vs. medium alone). IL-6 inhibited ($p < 0.01$ vs. AII alone) AII-stimulated aldosterone release and increased ($p < 0.05$ vs. ACTH alone) ACTH-stimulated aldosterone release. TNFα decreased ($p < 0.05$ vs. medium alone) basal aldosterone release and decreased ($p < 0.01$ vs. AII or ACTH alone) aldosterone secretion stimulated by AII or ACTH. **Bottom**: ACTH increased ($p < 0.01$ vs. medium alone) aldosterone secretion. IL-6 at concentrations of 10 ng/ml and greater increased ($p < 0.05$ vs. medium alone or 100 nM ACTH alone) basal and ACTH-stimulated aldosterone release. Incubation interval was 24 h.

mRNAs of the enzymes that synthesize DHEA.[25] The mechanisms through which the mRNAs for the steroidogenic enzymes are inhibited while DHEA is only marginally affected have not been clarified. TNFα decreases basal and ACTH-stimulated DHEA secretion from bovine ZR cells.[25] It is not known whether the divergent effects of TNFα on DHEA secretion in fetal human and bovine ZR cells represents stages in differentiation of the cells (i.e., fetal verus adult adrenocortical cells) or species differences. In human fetal adrenal cells, TNFα decreases the mRNA for dehydroepiandrosterone sulfotransferase, the enzyme that synthesizes dehydroepiandrosterone sulfate (DHEAS) from DHEA.[31]

SUMMARY AND CONCLUSIONS

The adrenal cortex synthesizes and releases IL-6 and TNFα and the release of these cytokines is differentially regulated by various secretagogues. Therefore, it is probable that under various physiological and pathological conditions, the cytokine milieu of the adrenal gland is altered. Since IL-6 and TNFα affect the release of adrenal steroids, this alteration of the adrenal cytokine milieu may modify the release of adrenal hormones. Because the effects of IL-6 on adrenal steroid secretion is slow, the effects of IL-6 on adrenal function are probably most important during chronic conditions. For example, during chronic stress glucocorticoid release remains elevated, but ACTH plasma concentration is near normal.[3-6] We hypothesize that changes in adrenal IL-6 and TNFα secretion during chronic stress may help explain this elevated glucocorticoid secretion.

REFERENCES

1. SPANGELO, B.L., A.M. JUDD, G.B. CALL, J. ZUMWALT & W.C. GOROSPE. 1995. Role of the cytokines in the hypothalamic-pituitary-adrenal and gonadal axes. Neuroimmunomodulation **2:** 299–312.
2. TURNBULL, A.V. & C.L. REVIER. 1999. Regulation of the hypothalamic-pituitary-adrenal axis by cytokines: actions and mechanism of action. Physiol. Rev. **79:** 1–71.
3. EHRHART-BORNSTEIN, M., J.P. HINSON, S.R. BORNSTEIN, W.A. SCHERBAUM & G.P. VINSON. 1998. Intraadrenal interactions in the regulation of adrenocortical steroidogenesis. Endocr. Rev. **19:** 101–143.
4. PIGNATELLI, D., M.M. MAGALHÃES & M.C. MAGALHÃES. 1998. Direct effects of stress on adrenocortical function. Horm. Metab. Res. **30:** 464–474.
5. MARX, C., M. EHRHART-BORNSTEIN, W.A. SCHERBAUM & S.R. BORNSTEIN. 1998. Regulation of adrenocortical function by cytokines: relevance from immun-endocrine interaction. Horm. Metab. Res. **30:** 416–420.
6. BORNSTEIN, S.R. & H. VAUDRY. 1998. Paracrine and neuroendocrine regulation of the adrenal gland-basic and clinical aspects. Horm. Metab. Res. **30:** 292-296.
7. JUDD, A.M. 1998. Cytokine expression in the rat adrenal cortex. Horm. Metab. Res. **30:** 404–410.
8. JUDD, A.M., B.L. SPANGELO & R.M. MACLEOD. 1990. Rat adrenal zona glomerulosa cells produce interleukin-6. Prog. NeuroEndocrinImmunol. **3:** 282–292.
9. JUDD, A.M. & R.M. MACLEOD. 1992. Adrenocorticotropin increases interleukin-6 release from rat adrenal zona glomerulosa cells. Endocrinology **130:** 1245–1254.
10. JUDD, A.M. & R.M. MACLEOD. 1995. Differential release of tumor necrosis factor and IL-6 from adrenal zona glomerulosa cells *in vitro*. Am. J. Physiol. (Endo. Metab.) **268:** E114–E120.
11. RIVIER, C. 1999. Effect of acute alcohol treatment on the release of ACTH, corticosterone, and pro-inflammatory cytokines in response to endotoxin. Alcohol. Clin. Exp. Res. **23:** 673–682.
12. HUSEIN, O.F., M.F. ERICKSON, G.B. CALL, S.D. PAULSEN & A.M. JUDD. 1998. Interleukin-6 and tumor necrosis factor are localized to steroid-secreting cells of the rat adrenal zona glomerulosa. Program and abstracts of the 80th Annual Meeting of The Endocrine Society. No. P2–575.

13. CALL, G.B. & A.M. JUDD. 1996. Bovine adrenal cells release IL-6 and tumor necrosis factor in vitro. Program and abstracts of the 10th International Congress of Endocrinology. No. P1–292.
14. GONZÁLEZ-HERNÁNDEZ, J.A., S.R. BORNSTEIN, M. EHRHART-BORNSTEIN, E. SPÄTH-SCHWALBE, G. JIRIKOWSKI & W.A. SCHERBAUM. 1994. Interleukin-6 messenger ribonucleic acid expression in human adrenal gland in vivo: new clue to a paracrine or autocrine regulation of adrenal function. J. Clin. Endocrinol. Metab. **79:** 1492–1497.
15. JÄÄTTELÄ, M., O. CARPÉN, U.-H. STENMAN & E. SAKSELA. 1990. Regulation of ACTH-induced steroidogenesis in human fetal adrenals by rTNF-α. Mol. Cell. Endocrinol. **68:** R31–R36.
16. GONZÁLEZ-HERNÁNDEZ, J.A., M. EHRHART-BORNSTEIN, E. SPÄTH-SCHWALBE, W.A. SCHERBAUM & S.R. BORNSTEIN. 1996. Human adrenal cells express tumor necrosis factor-alpha messenger ribonucleic acid-evidence for paracrine control of adrenal function. J. Clin. Endocrinol. Metab. **81:** 807–813.
17. PÄTH, G., S.R. BORNSTEIN, E. SPATHSCHWALBE & W.A. SCHERBAUM. 1996. Direct effects of interleukin-6 on human adrenal cells. Endocr. Res. **22:** 867–873.
18. PÄTH, G., S.R. BORNSTEIN, M. EHRHART-BORNSTEIN & W.A. SCHERBAUM. 1997. Interleukin-6 and interleukin-6 receptor in the human adrenal gland: expression and effects on steroidogenesis. J. Clin. Endocrinol. Metab. **82:** 2343–2349.
19. HUSEIN, O., C.J. MCILMOIL & A.M. JUDD. 1999. Rat, human, and bovine adrenocortical cells have receptors for interlukin-6 and tumor necrosis factor. Program and abstracts 81st Annual Meeting of The Endocrine Society. No. P2–179.
20. SALAS, M.A., S.W. EVANS, M.J. LEVELL & J.T. WHICHER. 1989. In vitro effect of rIL 1 and rIL 6 on corticosterone release by isolated rat adrenal gland cells. In Molecular and Cellular Biology of Cytokines. J.J. Oppenhein, M.C. Powanda, M.J. Kluger & C.A. Dinarello, Eds.: 427–432. John Wiley. New York.
21. SALAS, M.A., S.W. EVANS, M.J. LEVELL & J.T. WHICHER. 1990. Interleukin-6 and ACTH act synergistically to stimulate the release of corticosterone from adrenal gland cells. Clin. Exp. Immunol. **79:** 470–473.
22. TOMINAGA, T., J. FUKATA, Y. NAITO, T. USUI, N. MURAKAMI, M. FUKUSHIMA, Y. NAKAI, Y. HIRAI & H. IMURA. 1991. Prostaglandin-dependent in vitro stimulation of adrenocortical steroidogenesis by interleukins. Endocrinology **128:** 526–531.
23. WEBER, M.M., P. MICHL, C.J. AUERNHAMMER, D. ENGELHARDT. 1997. Interleukin-3 and interleukin-6 stimulate cortisol secretion from adult human adrenocortical cells. Endocrinology **138:** 2207–2210.
24. BARNEY, M., G.B. CALL & A.M. JUDD. 1998. Interleukin-6 stimulates and tumor necrosis factor inhibits the release of cortisol from bovine adrenal zona fasciculata cells. Program and abstracts of the Xth International Congress on Hormonal Steroids. No. 120.
25. JUDD, A.M., G.B. CALL, M. BARNEY & O.F. HUSEIN. 1997. Interleukin-6 inhibits basal and ACTH-stimulated dehydroepiandrosterone release from the bovine adrenal zona reticularis. Program and abstracts of the 79th Annual Meeting of The Endocrine Society. No. P2–122.
26. DARLING, G., D.S. GOLDSTEIN, R. STULL, C.M. GORSCHBOTH & J.A. NORTON. 1989. Tumor necrosis factor: immune endocrine interaction. Surgery **106:** 1155–1160.
27. JÄÄTTELÄ, M., V. ILVESMÄKI, R. VOUTILAINEN, U.-H. STENMAN & E. SAKSELA. 1991.Tumor necrosis factor as a potent inhibitor of adrenocorticotropin-induced cortisol production and steroidogenic P450 enzyme gene expression in cultured human fetal adrenal cells. Endocrinology **128:** 623–629.
28. VANDERMEER, M.J.M.M., A.R.M.M. HERMUS, G.J. PESMAN & C.G.J. SWEEP. 1996. Effects of cytokines on pituitary beta-endorphin and adrenal corticosterone release in vitro. Cytokine **8:** 238–247.
29. SWAIN, M.G. & M. MARIC. 1996. Tumor necrosis factor α stimulates adrenal glucocorticoid secretion in cholestatic rats. Am. J. Physiol. (Gastrointest. Liver Physiol. 33) **270:** G987–G991.
30. NATARAJAN, R., S. PLOSZAJ, R. HORTON & J. NADLER. 1989. Tumor necrosis factor and interleukin-1 are potent inhibitors of angiotensin-II-induced aldosterone synthesis. Endocrinology **125:** 3084–3089.

31. PARKER, C.R., A.K. STANKOVIC, O. FAYE-PETERSEN, C.N. FALANY, H. LI & M. JIAN. 1998. Effect of ACTH and cytokines on dehydroepiandrosterone sulfotransferase messenger RNA in human cells. Endocr. Res. **24:** 669–673.

Gaseous Neuromodulators in the Control of Neuroendocrine Stress Axis

P. NAVARRA,[a] C. DELLO RUSSO, C. MANCUSO,
P. PREZIOSI, AND A. GROSSMAN[b]

Institute of Pharmacology, Catholic University Medical School, Rome, Italy

[b]*Department of Endocrinology, St. Bartholomew's Hospital, London, U.K.*

ABSTRACT: The gaseous neuromodulator carbon monoxide has been shown to reduce the stimulated release of stress neuropeptides, such as vasopressin and oxytocin, from the rat hypothalamus *in vitro*, while evidence concerning corticotropin-releasing hormone is controversial. *In vivo* studies have been conducted in the rat, inhibiting heme oxygenase activity—and hence carbon monoxide biosynthesis—in the central nervous system by means of specific heme oxygenase blockers; these studies showed that basal heme oxygenase activity tends to oppose exaggerated increases in vasopressin secretion following immune-inflammatory challenges, whereas it favors the normal rise in circulating ACTH which follows footshock. Another gas normally produced in mammalian brains under basal conditions, hydrogen sulfide, also appears to play a role in the control of the hypothalamo-pituitary-adrenal axis. Indeed, increases in hydrogen sulfide levels within the hypothalamus, either obtained with hydrogen sulfide-enriched media or by the addition of the hydrogen sulfide precursor *S*-adenosyl-methionine, are associated with the inhibition of the stimulated release of corticotropin-releasing hormone from rat hypothalamic explants. Parellel *in vivo* experiments in the rat under resting conditions and after stress-induced adrenocortical activation show that *S*-adenosyl-methionine significantly reduces the rise in serum corticosterone levels caused by 1-h exposure to cold. These results demonstrate the pathophysiological importance of both carbon monoxide and hydrogen sulfide in the regulation of neuroendocrine function.

The concept of intra- and intercellular signaling operated by gaseous messengers is now widely accepted. With regard to nitric oxide, evidence has accumulated over the past few years that endogenous carbon monoxide (CO) plays a role in the control of neuroendocrine adaptive responses to stress. Here we briefly review such evidence, with particular regard to the control of arginine vasopressin (AVP) secretion. Evidence is also presented suggesting that another gas normally produced in mammalian brain, hydrogen sulfide (H_2S), is involved in the control of hypothalamo-pituitary-adrenal (HPA) axis.

[a]Address for correspondence: Institute of Pharmacology, Catholic University Medical School, Largo Francesco Vito 1, 00168 Rome, Italy. Voice: +39 630154367; fax: +39 63050159. pnavarra@rm.unicatt.it

CARBON MONOXIDE

Introduction

Equimolar amounts of CO, iron, and biliverdin are normally generated from the catabolism of the tetrapyrrole ring of hemin (Fe-protoporphyrin-9) by heme oxygenase (HO).[1] Two isoforms of this enzyme have been characterized to date: an inducible isoform, heme oxygenase-1 (HO-1), and a constitutive enzyme, heme oxygenase-2 (HO-2). Apart from the identity between their active centers, HO-1 and -2 differ markedly in amino acid and nucleotide sequence, size, cell and tissue distribution, and regulation.[2] HO-1 can only be detected in macrophages under basal conditions, but is induced in virtually all cell types by a variety of stimuli including hemin itself, oxidative stress, various disease states, and bacterial lipopolysaccharide (LPS), the latter directly or *via* the induction of pro-inflammatory cytokines.[3] Under basal conditions, HO-1 is only found in sparse groups of neurons of the central nervous system (CNS), including those of the paraventricular nuclei (PVN) of the hypothalamus, but its gene expression can be induced, under appropriate stimulation, in cells of the glial lineage as well.[4,5] In spite of such scarce HO-1 expression, the CNS is endowed with very high HO activity under basal conditions, which is mostly accounted for by HO-2.[2] The gene expression and synthesis of HO-2 is regulated by glucocorticoids, which *increase* HO-2 mRNA expression in the brain after long-term *in vivo* treatment.[6] Endogenous CO has been implicated in hippocampal long-term potentiation, non-adrenergic non-cholinergic gastrointestinal relaxation and vasodilatation, and is currently regarded as a neuromodulator in the peripheral and central nervous systems.[7,8]

In Vitro *Studies*

These studies have for the most part been based on a pharmacologic approach reminiscent of that adopted with nitric oxide. The HO substrate hemin and various HO inhibitors have been used to enhance and reduce, respectively, the generation of endogenous CO.

The first reports dealt with the role of HO-CO pathway in the control of corticotropin-releasing hormone (CRH). Parkes and colleagues[9] found that cultured hypothalamic cells exposed to hematin (a hemin isoform also hydrolized by HO) or CO-enriched incubation media increase CRH secretion, whereas a HO inhibitor, zinc-protoporphyrin-9 (ZnPP9) decreased both basal and heme-stimulated CRH release. On the contrary, our group showed that hemin produces a weak, albeit significant, inhibition of KCl-stimulated CRH release from rat hypothalamic explants, this effect being antagonized by ZnPP9.[10] Differences in experimental model, time of exposure, and drug concentration may account for these discrepancies, but the net effect of CO on CRH release *in vitro* remains to be clarified.

Studies on other corticotropin-releasing factors have consistently shown that increased CO generation is associated with the inhibition of K^+-stimulated oxytocin and AVP release from rat hypothalamic explants.[11,12] In the latter, the effect of hemin was counteracted by specific HO inhibitors and mimicked by CO-enriched incubation media, but not by the stable HO end-product biliverdin, suggesting that CO is the sole mediator between the HO pathway and the control of AVP release. A preferential pattern of regulation by CO on AVP release also emerged from another *in vitro* study: bacterial LPS exerted a paradoxical inhibitory action on both CRH and AVP release from rat hypothalamic explants, an effect apparently mediated by inhibitory pathways involving nitric oxide and CO.[13] While the blockade of nitric oxide synthase reverted the minor inhibitory effects of LPS on both CRH and AVP, the HO inhibitors, ZnPP9 and tin-mesoporphyrin-9 (SnMP9), were able to convert the small degree of AVP inhibition into marked stimulation, while having no effect on CRH release.[14]

In Vivo *Studies*

These studies are more recent and relatively few in number, principally because of the apparent inability of most HO inhibitors to cross the blood–brain barrier, as well as by non-specificity and toxicity of hemin when administered *in vivo* to animals.[15]

We have recently conducted a series of experiments *in vivo* in the rat[16] using a well-characterized non-selective HO inhibitor, tin-protoporphyrin-9 (SnPP9). The latter was given by both intraperitoneal (i.p.) and intracerebroventricular (i.c.v.) injection, to clarify the differential effect of systemic *versus* CNS-localized HO inhibition. An immune-inflammatory stimulus, LPS, was used at a dose eliciting significant increases in the circulating levels of stress hormones. The endotoxin was administered either alone or after pretreatment with SnPP9, and serum AVP and corticosterone (Cort) were taken as peripheral markers of the stress response. The hypothalamic content of AVP was also assessed. SnPP9 given i.c.v., but not i.p., significantly influenced the effects of LPS on circulating AVP. In fact, pretreatment with the porphyrin was associated with a marked potentiation of LPS-induced

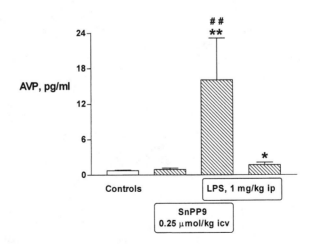

FIGURE 1. Tin-protoporphyrin-9 (SnPP9) significantly potentiates the LPS-induced increase in vasopressin (AVP) circulating levels, but has no effect when given alone. Results are expressed as pg of AVP/ml of serum, the means ± SEM of 8 animals per group. * and **: $p < 0.05$ and $p < 0.01$ vs. controls, respectively. ##: $p < 0.01$ vs. LPS alone.

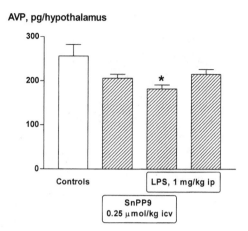

FIGURE 2. The association tin-protoporphyrin-9 (SnPP9) + LPS significantly reduces the hypothalamic content of vasopressin (AVP). Results are expressed as pg of AVP/hypothalamus, the means ± SEM of 8 animals per group. *: $p < 0.05$ vs. controls.

increase in serum AVP levels (see FIGURE 1). On the contrary, SnPP9 did not potentiate in a significant manner the increase in serum Cort induced by LPS (not shown). We also found that the huge increase in circulating AVP observed in the group receiving LPS + SnPP9 was highly correlated with the concomitant depletion of peptide content in the hypothalamus (see FIGURE 2).

While normal HO activity in the CNS appears to blunt the rise in AVP associated with immune-mediated stress, a different phenomenon is observed when stress response is triggered by physicoemotional stimuli such as footshock. In fact, Turnbull and colleagues clearly showed that subcutaneous doses of SnPP9 associated with significant HO inhibition in the CNS are able to *reduce* the ACTH rise following electro-footshock.[17] In previous studies, this group had shown that the inhibition of nitric oxide synthase by nitro-arginine methylester (which blunts the response to footshock[17]) potentiates the effects on the HPA of immune stimuli.[18] Thus, dissociation between the effects of immuno-inflammatory *versus* other types of stress may represent one other biological phenomenon shared by the gases, nitric oxide and CO.

HYDROGEN SULFIDE

Introduction

In contrast to the situation for CO, various enzymatic and nonenzymatic activities appear to be involved in H_2S generation. One pathway is based on cystathionine-β-synthase (CβS),[19] which converts homocysteine to cystathionine. The latter is subsequently transformed to cysteine by cystathionine-γ-lyase (CSE).[20] CβS also hydrolizes cysteine, producing equimolar amounts of serine and H_2S. CβS is markedly activated by S-adenosyl-L-methionine (SAMe).[21] Another enzymatic pathway is based on the ability of CSE to degrade cysteine, yielding pyruvate, NH_3 and H_2S. CSE also transforms cystine into thiocysteine; the latter enters the so-called thiosulfate cycle, which gives rise to H_2S and other inorganic sulfur compounds through nonenzymatic conversion in the presence of glutathione.[22] Finally, H_2S can be generated by enzymatic desulfuration of β-mercaptopyruvate, which derives from cysteine transamination.[23] As a result of these reactions, surprisingly large amounts of H_2S are produced in the CNS under basal conditions: 1.57 and 0.67 µg/g in the whole brain and midbrain of rat and humans are detected by the gas dialysis–ion chromatography technique.[24]

Although the endogenous generation of H_2S has long been known, only recently have Abe and Kimura shown that the gas—at physiological concentrations—facilitates long-term potentiation in the rat hippocampus.[25] H_2S has also been shown to potentiate the relaxing effect of NO in vascular smooth muscle preparations,[26] providing evidence of central and peripheral neuromodulatory activities which are reminiscent of those exerted by CO.

In Vitro *Studies*

To date, the sole evidence in favor of a neuroendocrine effect of H_2S has been on the regulation by the gas of CRH release from hypothalamic explants.[27] Levels of the gas within the hypothalamic tissue can be increased either by incubating tissues in H_2S-enriched media or by adding SAMe to the bath solution. However, no

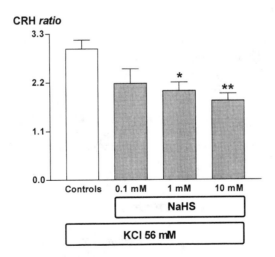

FIGURE 3. NaHS inhibits in a concentration-dependent manner KCl-induced CRH release. Data are expressed as CRH *ratios* (i.e., the *ratios* between the amounts of CRH released in two consecutive 20-min incubation periods, the second in the presence of test substances), the means ± SEM of 8 hypothalami per group. * and **: $p < 0.05$ and $p < 0.01$ vs. controls.

pharmacologic tool is currently available to inhibit H_2S production because of the complexity of enzymatic and nonenzymatic pathways leading to gas production.

The sodium salt of H_2S, NaHS, generates the gas once in solution; NaHS in the range of 0.1–10 mM does not affect basal CRH release (not shown). However, NaHS is able to inhibit, in a concentration-dependent manner, KCl-stimulated CRH release from rat hypothalamic explants, with significant reductions obtained at both 1 mM and 10 mM (see FIGURE 3). According to its role as an indirect H_2S precursor, SAMe should increase endogenous H_2S production. Indeed, the addition of SAMe to the incubation media of rat hypothalami, like NaHS, caused an inhibition of KCl-stimulated CRH release; this was statistically significant at 1 mM (see FIGURE 4).

In Vivo *Studies*

While systemic toxicity prevents NaHS administration *in vivo,*[24] SAMe can be tested in this paradigm; the results of *in vitro* studies suggested to us that SAMe, if given *in vivo,* might possibly inhibit stress-related glucocorticoid increase, while having no effect under resting conditions. Therefore, a series of experiments have been carried out on rats under basal conditions and after a physical stress (i.e., exposure to low temperature). Under resting conditions, repeated SAMe treatments (100 mg/kg i.m. twice daily for a total of five treatments) did not modify serum Cort compared to controls treated with vehicle (not shown). However, such treatment significantly reduced the increase in circulating Cort in rats exposed for 1 h at 4°C with respect to controls (see FIGURE 5).

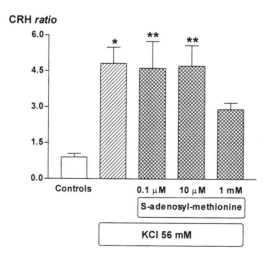

FIGURE 4. *S*-Adenosyl-methionine (SAMe) inhibits KCl-induced CRH release. Data are expressed as CRH *ratios* (i.e., the *ratios* between the amounts of CRH released in two consecutive 20-min incubation periods, the second in the presence of test substances), the means ± SEM of 6 hypothalami per group. * and **: $p < 0.05$ and $p < 0.01$ vs. controls.

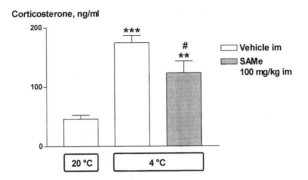

FIGURE 5. *S*-Adenosyl-methionine (SAMe, 100 mg/kg i.m.) significantly reduces the increase in serum corticosterone induced by exposure to low temperature (4°C) for 1 h. Data are expressed as ng corticosterone/ml of serum, the means ± SEM of 8 animals per group. ** and ***: $p < 0.01$ and $p < 0.001$ vs. vehicle at room temperature; #: $p < 0.05$ vs. vehicle at 4°C.

CONCLUSIONS

We have reviewed in this chapter the evidence suggesting that the generation of gases such as CO and H_2S, within the internal *milieu* of the hypothalamus, may influence the neuroendocrine adaptive response to stress, in a manner similar to (but distinct from) that shown earlier by ourselves and others for nitric oxide. The prevailing action seems to be inhibition of exaggerated stress responses, although the net effect may vary with the type of stressor, whether immunological or physico-emotional. While the neuroendocrine actions of nitric oxide and CO may have clear pathophysiological relevance, since bacterial endotoxins can concomitantly activate stress responses and induce the production of the gas, a pathophysiological role for H_2S in the control of stress responses remains to be established.

REFERENCES

1. TENHUNEN, R., H.S. MARVER & R. SCHMIDT. 1969. Microsomal heme oxygenase characterization of the enzyme. J. Biol. Chem. **244:** 6388–6394.
2. MAINES, M.D. 1997. The heme oxygenase system: a regulator of second messenger gases. Ann. Rev. Pharmacol. Toxicol. **37:** 517–554.
3. CANTONI, L., C. ROSSI, M. RIZZARDINI, M. GADINA & P. GHEZZI. 1991. Interleukin-1 and tumor necrosis factor induce hepatic heme oxygenase. Feed-back regulation by glucocorticoids. Biochem. J. **279:** 891–894.
4. EWING, J.F. & M.D. MAINES. 1992. In situ hybridization and immunohistochemical localization of heme oxygenase-2 mRNA and protein in normal rat brain: differential distribution of isozyme 1 and 2. Mol. Cell. Neurosci. **3:** 4559–4570.
5. DWYER, B.E., R.N. NISHIMURA & S.Y. LU. 1995. Differential expression of heme oxygenase-1 in cultured cortical neurons and astrocytes determined by the aid of a new heme oxygenase antibody. Response to oxidative stress. Mol. Brain Res. **30:** 37–47.
6. WEBER, C.M., B.C. EKE & M.D. MAINES. 1994. Corticosterone regulates hemeoxygenase-2 and NO synthase transcription and protein expression in rat brain. J. Neurochem. **63:** 953–962.

7. ZAKHARY, R., S.P. GAINE, J.L. DINERMAN, M. RUAT, N.A. FLAVAHAN & S.H. SNYDER. 1996. Heme oxygenase 2: endothelial and neuronal localization and role in endothelium-dependent relaxation. Proc. Natl. Acad. Sci. USA **93:** 795–798.

8. SNYDER, S.H., S.R. JAFFREY & R. ZAKHARY. 1998. Nitric oxide and carbon monoxide: parallel roles as neural messengers. Brain Res. Rev. **26:** 167–175.

9. PARKES, D., J. KASCKOW & W. VALE. 1993. Carbon monoxide modulates secretion of corticotropin-releasing factor (CRF) from rat hypothalamic cell coltures. Brain Res. **646:** 315–318.

10. POZZOLI, G., C. MANCUSO, A. MIRTELLA, P. PREZIOSI, A.B. GROSSMAN & P. NAVARRA. 1994. Carbon monoxide as a novel neuroendocrine modulator: inhibition of stimulated corticotropin-releasing hormone release from acute rat hypothalamic explants. Endocrinology **135:** 2314–2317.

11. KOSTOGLOU-ATHANASSIOU, I., M.L. FORSLING, P. NAVARRA & A.B. GROSSMAN. 1996. Oxytocin release is inhibited by the generation of carbon monoxide from the rat hypothalamus—further evidence for carbon monoxide as a neuromodulator. Mol. Brain Res. **42:** 301–306.

12. MANCUSO, C., I. KOSTOGLOU-ATHANASSIOU, M.L. FORSLING, A.B. GROSSMAN, P. PREZIOSI, P. NAVARRA & G. MINOTTI. 1997. Activation of heme oxygenase and consequent carbon monoxide formation inhibit the release of arginine vasopressin from rat hypothalamic explants. Molecular linkage between heme catabolism and neuroendocrine function. Mol. Brain Res. **50:** 267–276.

13. NAVARRA, P. 1995. The effects of endotoxin on the neuroendocrine axis. Curr. Opin. Endocrinol. Diabetes **2:** 127–133.

14. KOSTOGLOU-ATHANASSIOU, I., A. COSTA, P. NAVARRA, G. NAPPI, M.L. FORSLING & A.B. GROSSMAN. 1998. Endotoxin stimulates an endogenous pathway regulating corticotropin-releasing hormone and vasopressin release involving the generation of nitric oxide and carbon monoxide. J. Neuroimmunol. **86:** 104–109.

15. MANCUSO, C., P. PREZIOSI, A. GROSSMAN & P. NAVARRA. 1997. The role of carbon monoxide in the regulation of neuroendocrine function. Neuroimmunomodulation **4:** 225–229.

16. MANCUSO, C., E. RAGAZZONI, G. TRINGALI, I. LIBERALE, P. PREZIOSI, A. GROSSMAN & P. NAVARRA. 1999. Inhibition of heme oxygenase in the central nervous system potentiates endotoxin-induced vasopressin release in the rat. J. Neuroimmunol. **99:** 189–194.

17. TURNBULL, A.V., C. KWON SIM, S. LEE & C.L. RIVIER. 1998. Influence of carbon monoxide, and its interaction with nitric oxide, on the adrenocorticotropin hormone response of the normal rat to a physico-emotional stress. J. Neuroendocrinol. **10:** 793–802.

18. RIVIER, C. & G. CHEN. 1994. In the rat, endogenous nitric oxide modulates the response of the hypothalamic-pituitary-adrenal axis to interleukin-1β, vasopressin and oxytocin. J. Neurosci. **14:** 1985–1993.

19. SWAROOP, M., K. BRADLEY, T. OHURA, T. TAHARA, M.D. ROPER, L.E. ROSEMBERG & J.P. KRAUS. 1992. Rat cystathionine β-synthase. J. Biol. Chem. **267:** 11455–11461.

20. ERICKSON, P.F., I.H. MAXWELL, L.-J. SU, M. BAUMANN & L.M. GLODE. 1990. Sequence of cDNA for rat cystathionine γ-lyase and comparison of deduced amino acid sequence with related *Escherichia coli* enzymes. Biochem. J. **269:** 335–340.

21. FINKELSTEIN, J.D., W.E. KYLE, J.J. MARTIN & A.-M. PICK. 1975. Activation of cystathionine synthase by adenosylmethionine and adenosylethionine. Biochem. Biophys. Res. Commun. **66:** 81–87.

22. KOJ, A., J. FRENDO & Z. JANIC. 1967. [^{35}S]Thiosulphate oxidation by rat liver mitochondria in the presence of glutathione. Biochem. J. **103:** 791–795.

23. MEISTER, A., P.E. FRASER & S.V. TICE. 1954. Enzymatic desulfuration of β-mercaptopyruvate to pyruvate. J. Biol. Chem. **206:** 561–575.

24. REIFFENSTEIN, R.J., W.C. HULBERT & S.H. ROTH. 1992. Toxicology of hydrogen sulfide. Ann. Rev. Pharmacol. Toxicol. **32:** 109–134.

25. ABE, K. & H. KIMURA. 1996. The possible role of hydrogen sulfide as an endogenous neuromodulator. J. Neurosci. **16:** 1066–1071.

26. HOSOKI, R., N. MATSUKI & H. KIMURA. 1997. The possible role of hydrogen sulfide as a smooth muscle relaxant in synergy with nitric oxide. Biochem. Biophys. Res. Commun. **237:** 527–531.

27. DELLO RUSSO, C., G. TRINGALI, E. RAGAZZONI, N. MAGGIANO, E. MENINI, M. VAIRANO, P. PREZIOSI & P. NAVARRA. 2000. Evidence that hydrogen sulfide can modulate hypo-thalamo-pituitary-adrenal axis function: *in vitro* and *in vivo* studies in the rat. J. Neuroendocrinol. **12:** 225–233.

Cytokines, Leptin, and the Hypothalamo-Pituitary-Adrenal Axis

R.C. GAILLARD,[a,b] E. SPINEDI,[b,c] T. CHAUTARD,[b] AND F.P. PRALONG[b]

[b]Division of Endocrinology, Diabetology and Metabolism, Department of Medicine, University Hospital (CHUV), CH-1011 Lausanne, Switzerland

[c]Neuroendocrine Unit, IMBICE, La Plata, Argentina

ABSTRACT: The endocrine and immune systems are linked via an elaborated communication system constituted by an array of cytokines and neuropeptides which interact to modulate the integrated response of an organism to infection. Weight loss and anorexia, probably secondary to cytokine release, frequently accompany infection, but leptin could also play a role. Like cytokines, leptin serves as a peripheral messenger to convey signals to the brain. Expression of leptin is stimulated by glucocorticoids, endotoxins, and cytokines; on the other hand, leptin seems to inhibit the activation of the hypothalamo-pituitary-adrenal (HPA) axis. Indeed leptin exerts a direct, dose-dependent inhibition of stimulated cortisol secretion by normal human and rat adrenal cells *in vitro*. These effects are mediated by the long isoform of the leptin receptor, because its transcript is expressed in the adrenal tissue. In addition we investigated the role played by the glucocorticoids in the development of tolerance of the hypothalamo-corticotropic, immune and adipose system responses to repeated endotoxin administration. Unlike that of the corticotropic axis, tolerance of the immune and adipose systems is at least partially glucocorticoid-independent. This crosstalk between the endocrine, immune, and adipose systems may be of prime importance to homeostasis in pathophysiological events occurring during infection.

The endocrine and immune systems are closely linked via an elaborated communication system constituted by an array of cytokines and neuropeptides which interact to modulate the integrated response of an organism to infection.[1,2] It is now quite obvious that in addition to these two systems, the adipose tissue may also be an important partner in this network. Indeed, weight loss and anorexia, probably secondary to cytokine release, frequently accompany infection, but leptin, the product of the *ob* gene, may also play an important role. Like cytokines, leptin serves as a peripheral messenger to convey signals to the brain. Furthermore, the leptin receptor is closely related to the gp-130 family of receptor, a member of the class 1 cytokine receptor group.[3] Thus, the leptin system seems quite likely to be ancestrally related to the cytokines. It is therefore not surprising that endotoxins as well as numerous cytokines can influence leptin levels.[4] Endotoxin and cytokines induce leptin expression even in the face of anorexia, suggesting that this induction of the *ob* gene

[a]Address for correspondence: R.C. Gaillard, M.D., Division of Endocrinology, Diabetology and Metabolism, University Hospital (CHUV), CH-1011 Lausanne, Switzerland. Voice: +41 21 314 05 99; fax: +41 21 314 06 30.

Rolf-Christian.Gaillard@chuv.hospvd.ch

may contribute to the decreased food intake observed during infection.[5] This communication between the immune and adipose systems is bidirectional, since leptin is involved in the regulation of immune responses. Indeed, leptin regulates pro-inflammatory immune responses, by upregulating both phagocytosis and the production of pro-inflammatory cytokines.[6] Leptin induction during inflammation appears to participate in the cytokine cascade activated during infection and injury. The hypothesis that leptin is an important cytokine component of the acute phase response is strongly supported by a very recent study of Faggioni and colleagues that clearly demonstrates that leptin deficiency is accompanied by an increased susceptibility to endotoxin-induced lethality and a decreased induction of anti-inflammatory cytokines.[7] These results led these authors to speculate that disorders characterized by decreased leptin levels, such as cachexia and starvation, might result in an impaired host defense that would increase susceptibility to infection. In addition to its role in the crosstalk between the immune and adipose systems, leptin plays also a key role in the bi-directional communication between the hypothalamo-pituitary-adrenal axis and the adipose system. Overall, the expression of leptin is stimulated by glucocorticoids,[8,9] while leptin seems to inhibit the activation of the HPA axis by lowering ACTH secretion.[10] Thus, the adipose tissue and the HPA axis are probably linked in a classical endocrine feedback loop. It is becoming increasingly obvious that, in addition to regulating food intake, energy expenditure, and immune function, leptin has other physiological roles, among them its action to modulate reproductive physiology and the HPA axis.[10]

The occurrence of a tolerance phenomenon to bacterial endotoxin (LPS) represents a hallmark of chronic endotoxin stimulation. Tolerance can be describe as the hyporesponsiveness of an organism to a repetitive stimulus, such as repeated administration of lipopolysaccharide.[11,12] The mechanism underlying endotoxin tolerance is poorly understood, but it seems that glucocorticoid-dependent and -independent mechanisms may be involved.[13] Among the glucocorticoid-independent mechanism, blockade of the LPS receptors by minimal, inactive LPS structures,[14] blockade of LPS itself by a lipoprotein[15] or blockade of LPS by neutralizing antibodies induced as a consequence of repeated stimulation[16] can be proposed. It is also possible that the effect of cytokines released from LPS-activated macrophages could be blocked by soluble receptors[17] or receptor antagonists.[18] On the other hand, it has been hypothesized that endogenous glucocorticoids may be involved in the LPS-tolerance phenomenon.[13,19]

In this paper, we investigated whether the LPS-tolerance phenomenon also affects LPS-induced leptin secretion, and whether the absence of an appropriate adrenal response, rather than the lack of endogenous glucocorticoids, influences the development of tolerance of the neuroendocrine (corticotropic axis), immune, and adipose tissue responses to repetitive LPS administration. In addition, we studied the interactions between leptin and the HPA axis.

TOLERANCE TO REPEATED LPS ADMINISTRATION

Using Wistar male rats, we first determined the optimal dose of LPS inducing tolerance of the HPA axis and of the immune system when administered intravenously for five consecutive days. Rats were divided into three groups, each group receiving one of the following doses of LPS: 12.5, 25, or 50 µg/kg body weight. Blood samples were drawn on days 1, 3, and 5 (D_1, D_3, and D_5), immediately before as well as 1, 2, 3, and 4 hours after LPS injection. 25 and 50 µg/kg LPS produced the same pattern of responses of ACTH and corticosterone release (HPA axis parameters) as well as of TNFα (immune system parameter): a robust increase on day 1, a slightly less important response on day 3, and no response on day 5. The lower dose of LPS produced an HPA axis response only on day 1 and no effect on days 3 and 5, whereas the TNFα response showed a quite similar pattern to that of the middle LPS dose.

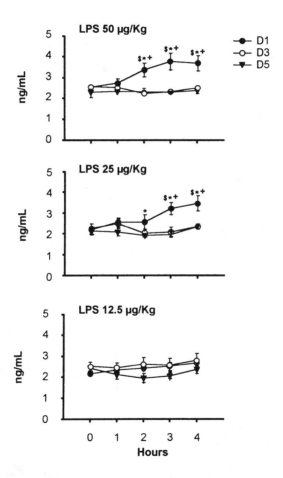

FIGURE 1. Plasma leptin levels (means ± SEM) after intravenous administration at time 0 of 50 (*upper panel*), 25 (*middle panel*), or 12.5 (*lower panel*) µg/kg of bacterial endotoxin (LPS) in intact animals on D_1, D_3, and D_5. \$, $p < 0.05$ or less vs. respective D_3 values (ANOVA, Fischer's test); *, $p < 0.05$ or less vs. respective D_5 values (ANOVA, Fischer's test); +, $p < 0.05$ or less vs. respective time 0 values (paired *t* test). ($n = 5$–6 rats per group). (Adapted from Chautard *et al.*[20] with permission from S. Karger, Basel).

Plasma leptin levels are depicted in FIGURE 1. On day 1, the higher LPS dose induced a significant increase in leptin levels ($p < 0.05$ vs. sample time 0), reaching a plateau at two hours after injection. Full tolerance to LPS was observed on days 3 and 5. The pattern of leptin secretion with the middle dose tested (25 µg/kg) was similar to that described for the higher dose. In contrast, the lowest LPS dose (12.5 µg/kg) failed to induce any change in plasma leptin levels, regardless of the experimental day.

These results demonstrate that, regardless of the mechanism involved, repeated LPS administration can induce tolerance of three different systems implicated in metabolic regulations. At each LPS dose tested, this tolerance resulted in either hyporesponsiveness or nonresponsiveness (at later stage) of the HPA axis, the immune system, and the adipose tissue.[20] These results confirm the existence of an acute effect of LPS on adipocyte function.[4,5] Moreover, and most interestingly, these data provide the first evidence that the adipocyte may also develop tolerance to repeated endotoxemia, as suggested by the finding that such an acute stimulation of leptin secretion was observed only after the first LPS administration. It is therefore possible, in contrast to what has previously been suggested[5] on the basis of acute single LPS administration, that leptin is not constantly elevated during chronic infection.

These results suggest that contrary to what has been hypothesized previously,[5] high circulating levels of leptin are not responsible for the anorexia observed during persistent infection. In contrast, this tolerance phenomenon—decreasing leptin levels—might participate to the body's defense mechanisms against infectious stimuli, maybe by counteracting the anorexigenic effects of TNFα.

ROLE OF GLUCOCORTICOIDS IN THE LPS-TOLERANCE PHENOMENON

To evaluate the role of glucocorticoids in the LPS-tolerance phenomenon, we investigated whether the occurrence of tolerance would be influenced by the absence of an appropriate adrenal response. Tolerance was therefore studied in bilaterally adrenalectomized rats implanted with a subcutaneous pellet containing 75 mg corticosterone (Adx + B) compared to sham-operated rats implanted with a pellet containing placebo. Following the dose–response study discussed before, all experiments were performed with 25 µg LPS/kg body weight for five consecutive days according to the experimental design described above. Of note, body weights were not significantly affected by these experiments. FIGURE 2 displays the corticotropic axis and the TNFα responses to LPS (25 µg/kg) in the sham-operated and Adx + B rats. As expected, the LPS-tolerance phenomenon in sham-operated animals was similar to that observed in intact rats receiving the same LPS dose. In contrast in the Adx + B group, the ACTH responses were more pronounced and sustained on day 1 and 3. Even on day 5, there was still a significant increase in plasma ACTH levels following LPS injections. Therefore, the tolerance of the corticotropic axis to LPS was only partial on day 5, providing evidence that a normal glucocorticoid response to LPS is necessary for the development of full tolerance on the HPA axis. These results also suggest that an inappropriate adrenal response may

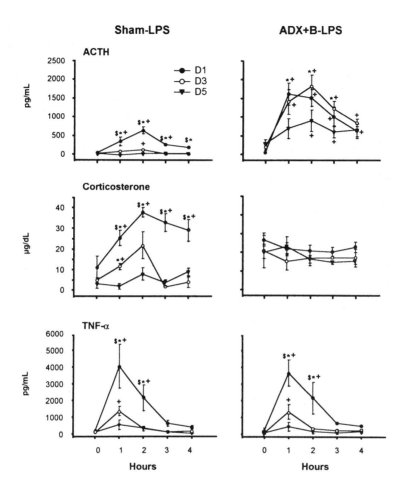

FIGURE 2. LPS (25 µg/kg)-induced ACTH (*upper panel*), corticosterone (*middle panel*), and TNFα (*lower panel*) release in plasma, on three different experimental days (D_1, D_3, and D_5), in sham-operated (*left*) and Adx + B (*right*) animals. Means ± SEM. Statistical significances are as in FIGURE 1. (Adapted from Chautard *et al.*[20] with permission from S. Karger, Basel).

lead to a delay in the appearance of tolerance. The lower panels of FIGURE 2 demonstrate TNFα levels in the sham and Adx + B groups. The pattern of TNFα release in sham-operated animals was similar to that observed in intact rats, demonstrating the occurrence of the tolerance to LPS stimulation. Interestingly the pattern of TNFα secretion in Adx + B animals was comparable to that observed in sham rats on identical days: the tolerance of TNFα secretion to repeated LPS injections was not influenced by the adrenalectomy. This demonstrates that a dynamic adrenal responsiveness to LPS is not mandatory to induce tolerance of the immune system. Moreover, it is possible that the observed tolerance of the corticotropic axis may not only

be related to a glucocorticoid effect, but could also be partly explained by this tolerance of the immune function, as cytokines are potent stimulators of the HPA axis.

FIGURE 3 demonstrates that LPS injection induced in Adx + B rats a pattern of
leptin secretion very similar to that observed in intact and sham-operated rats,
although leptin on day 1 was significantly increased earlier than in intact rats
($p < 0.05$ vs. sample time 0 at 2 h). On days 3 and 5, LPS did not induce any change
in circulating leptin, but values were significantly lower than their respective values
on day 1. The observation that stimulated leptin levels were lower in adrenalectomized rats supplemented with corticosterone than in normal animals suggests that a
normal dynamic response of glucocorticoids participates in LPS-stimulated leptin
secretion. However, our finding of an acute stimulation of leptin secretion by LPS

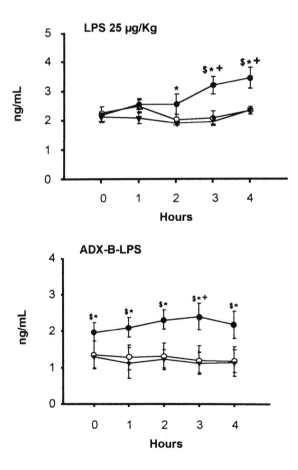

FIGURE 3. LPS (25 µg/kg)-induced leptin release, on three different experimental
days (D_1, D_3, and D_5) in control rats (*top*) and in Adx + B rats. Means ± SEM. Statistical
significances are as in FIGURE 1. (Adapted from Chautard et al.[20] with permission from
S. Karger, Basel).

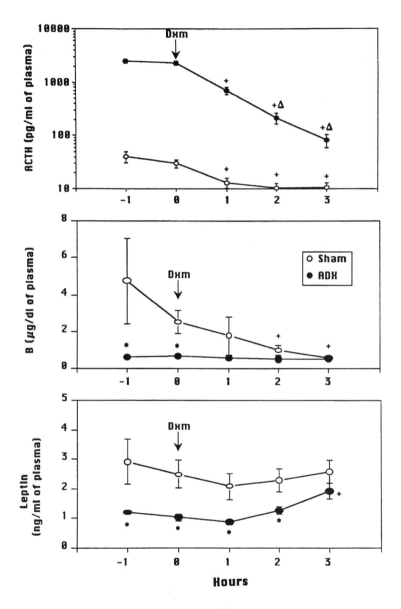

FIGURE 4. Plasma ACTH (*upper*), corticosterone (*middle*), and leptin (*lower*) levels, in sham-operated and adrenalectomized rats (without corticosterone substitution), several times before and after i.v. injection of dexamethasone (30 mg/kg). *, $p < 0.05$ vs. the respective time values in sham-operated rats; +, $p < 0.05$ vs. Adx sample times −1 hour and zero values; Δ, $p < 0.05$ vs. Adx sample time 1 hour values (mean ± SEM, $n = 8$–10 rats per group). (Adapted from Spinedi and Gaillard[21] with permission from the Endocrine Society).

in Adx + B animals demonstrates that this effect of endotoxemia is at least partially glucocorticoid-independent.[20]

The decrease in circulating levels of leptin following Adx is nevetherless consistent with the stimulatory effects of glucocorticoids on leptin secretion. This hypothesis is also supported by other recent data of our laboratory: we observed significantly lower plasma leptin levels in chronically adrenalectomized rats without corticosterone substitution than in sham-operated controls, and corticosterone replacement was found to restore these levels to normal.[21] Moreover, we also found that in addition to glucocorticoid deprivation, high ACTH levels in adrenalectomized rats may contribute to decreased leptin output; this is shown in FIGURE 4. Intravenous dexamethasone was administered in sham-operated and in adrenalectomized rats. This treatment induced a rapid decrease in plasma ACTH levels in sham rats, but had no effect on plasma leptin levels. However, in Adx rats the synthetic glucocorticoid increased plasma leptin concentrations, restoring the levels observed in sham rats. This increase occurred while plasma ACTH levels were decreasing towards basal values in sham animals.

It seems therefore reasonable to suggest that ACTH by itself, at very high circulating levels, could inhibit leptin secretion by the adipose tissue.[21] These results indicate that circulating ACTH and glucocorticoids are able to modulate leptin secretion in plasma. The lack of circulating glucocorticoids and/or increased plasma concentrations of ACTH are responsible for decreasing leptin output, whereas decreased plasma ACTH concentrations allow an increase of leptin secretion.

These data support an important role for circulating ACTH in the regulation of adipose tissue function. Whether ACTH, and possibly any other POMC-derived peptide, could be acting directly at the adipocyte level, and to what degree CRH and catecholamines may participate in this modulation of leptin secretion remain to be determined.

LEPTIN EFFECTS AT THE ADRENAL LEVEL

Since leptin was shown to act directly on peripheral endocrine glands, such as the pancreas[22] and the ovary,[23] we tested the hypothesis that it may also have direct effects in the control of glucocorticoid secretion by the adrenal gland.[24] As shown in FIGURE 5, we have demonstrated that leptin exerts a direct, dose-dependent inhibition of ACTH-stimulated cortisol secretion by normal human and rat adrenal cells *in vitro.* Interestingly, basal cortisol secretion was unaffected by leptin. The inhibition was observed at concentrations of leptin occurring in the human *in vivo,* suggesting its physiological relevance. Moreover, the time course of this effect, with a maximum inhibition occurring after 24 h of exposure to leptin, is consistent with a modulation of adrenal steroidogenesis at the transcriptional level. It appears therefore that leptin is playing a rather long-term regulatory role in the adrenal, in contrast to some of its effects in the CNS, which may be more rapid.

The direct effects of leptin on the adrenal cells are likely mediated by the long isoform of the leptin receptor, OB-Rb, since we were able to demonstrate its expression in human and rat adrenal tissues. Moreover, we observed that leptin had no effect on adrenal cells obtained from *db/db* mice, which completely lack a functional

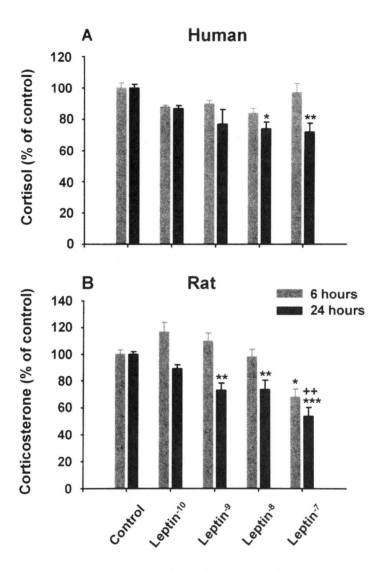

FIGURE 5. (A) Effects of 6-h (*shaded*) or 24-h (*solid*) preincubation with serum-free medium (*control*) or graded concentrations of leptin on ACTH-stimulated cortisol secretion from primary dispersed human adrenal cells. **(B)** Effects of 6-h (*shaded*) or 24-h (*solid*) pre-incubation with serum-free medium (*control*) or graded concentrations of leptin on ACTH-stimulated corticosterone secretion from primary dispersed rat adrenocortical cells. *, $p < 0.05$ vs. control; **, $p < 0.01$ vs. control; ***, $p < 0.001$ vs. control; ++, $p < 0.01$ vs. 10-10 M leptin (leptin 10-10). (Adapted from Pralong *et al.*[24] with permission from the Endocrine Society).

leptin receptor. This latter finding is an indirect demonstration that OB-Rb is functional in normal rat and human adrenal glands, and therefore may be mediating the effect of leptin in this tissue. This loop between adipose tissue and cortisol secretion, via circulating leptin, may represent an important mechanism for modulating glucocorticoid levels in various metabolic states.

CONCLUSION

Taken together these data demonstrate that cytokines, leptin, and glucocorticoids are closely interrelated, allowing a tight communication between the endocrine, immune, and adipose systems. The crosstalk between these three systems implicated in metabolic regulation may be of prime importance to homeostasis in pathophysiological events occurring during infection.

ACKNOWLEDGMENTS

This work was supported by Grant 31-50748.97 from the Swiss National Research Foundation and by a grant from the National and Buenos Aires State Research Council of Argentina.

François P. Pralong is the recipient of a Research Development Career Award from the Professor Dr. Max Cloëtta Foundation.

We are indebted to Marie-Jeanne Voirol and Marco Giacomini for their technical collaboration.

REFERENCES

1. TURNBULL, A.V. & C.L. RIVIER. 1999. Regulation of the hypothalamic-pituitary-adrenal axis by cytokines: actions and mechanisms of action. Physiol. Rev. **79:** 1–71.
2. BESEDOVSKY, H.O. & A. DEL REY. 1996. Immune-neuroendocrine interactions: facts and hypotheses. Endocr. Rev. **17:** 64–102.
3. TARTAGLIA, L.A., M. DEMBSKI, X. WENG, N. DENG, J. CULPEPPER, R. DEVOS, G.J. RICHARDS, L.A. CAMPFIELD, F.T. CLARK & J. DEEDS. 1995. Identification and expression cloning of a leptin receptor, OB-R. Cell **83:** 1263–1271.
4. SARRAF, P., R.C. FREDERICH, E.M. TURNER, G. MA, N.T. JASKOWIAK, D.J. RIVET, J.S. FLIER, B.B. LOWELL, D.L. FRAKER & H.R. ALEXANDER. 1997. Multiple cytokines and acute inflammation raise mouse leptin levels: potential role in inflammatory anorexia. J. Exp. Med. **185:** 171–175.
5. GRUNFELD, C., C. ZHAO, J. FULLER, A. POLLOCK, A. MOSER, J. FRIEDMAN & K.R. FEINGOLD. 1996. Endotoxin and cytokines induce expression of leptin, the ob gene product, in Hamsters. A role for leptin in the anorexia of infection. J. Clin. Invest. **97:** 2152–2157.
6. LOFFREDA, S., S.Q. YANG, H.Z. LIN, C.L. KARP, M.L. BRENGMAN, D.J. WANG, A.S. KLEIN, G.B. BULKLEY, C. BAO, P.W. NOBLE, M.D. LANE & A.M. DIEHL. 1998. Leptin regulates proinflammatory immune responses. FASEB J. **12:** 57–65.
7. FAGGIONI, R., G. FANTUZZI, C. GABAY, A. MOSER, C.A. DINARELLO, K.R. FEINGOLD & C. GRUNFELD. 1999. Leptin deficiency enhances sensitivity to endotoxin-induced lethality. Am. J. Physiol. **276:** R136–R142.

8. DE VOS, P., R. SALADIN, J. AUWERX & B. STAELS. 1995. Induction of ob gene expression by corticosteroids is accompanied by body weight loss and reduced food intake. J. Biol. Chem. **270:** 15958–15961.
9. MURAKAMI, T., M. IIDA & K. SHIMA. 1995. Dexamethasone regulates obese expression inisolated rat adipocytes. Biochem. Biophys. Res. Commun. **214:** 1260–1267.
10. AHIMA, R.S., D. PRABAKARAN, C. MANTZOROS, D. QU, B. LOWELL, E. MARATOS-FLIER & J.S. FLIER. 1996. Role of leptin in the neuroendocrine response to fasting. Nature **382:** 250–252.
11. ZIEGLER-HEITBROCK, H.W. 1995. Molecular mechanism in tolerance to lipopolysaccharide. J. Inflamm. **45:** 13–26.
12. BESSON, P.B. 1967. Tolerance to bacterial pyrogens. I. Factors influencing its development. J. Exp. Med. **86:** 29–44.
13. EVANS, G.F. & S.H. ZUCKERMAN. 1991. Glucocorticoid-dependent and -independent mechanisms involved in lipopolysaccharide tolerance. Eur. J. Immunol. **21:** 1973–1979.
14. WANG, M.H., H.D. FLAD, W. FEIST, H. BRADE, S. KUSUMOTO, E.T. RIETSCHEL & A.J. IMER. 1991. Inhibition of endotoxin-induced interleukin-6 production by synthetic lipid A partial structures in human peripheral blood mononuclear cells. Infect. Immun. **59:** 4655–4664.
15. WARREN, H.S., C.V. KNIGHTS & G.R. SIBER. 1986. Neutralization and lipoprotein binding of lipopolysaccharides in tolerant rabbit serum. J. Infect. Dis. **154:** 784–791.
16. GREISMAN, S.E., E.J. YOUNG & F.A. CARROZZA. 1969. Mechanism of endotoxin tolerance. V. Specificity of the early and late phases of pyrogenic tolerance. J. Immunol. **103:** 1223–1236.
17. SECKINGER, P., J.H. ZHANG, B. HAUPTMANN & J.M. DAYER. 1990. Characterization of a tumor necrosis factor alpha (TNFalpha) inhibitor: evidence of immunological cross-reactivity with TNF receptor. Proc. Natl. Acad. Sci. USA **84:** 5188–5192.
18. HANNUM, C.H., C.J. WICOX, W.P. AREND, F.G. JOSLIN, K.J. DRIPPS, P.L. HEIMDAL, L.G. ARMES, A. SOMMER, A. EISENBERG & R.C. THOMPSON. 1990. Interleukin-1 receptor antagonist activity of a human interleukin-1 inhibitor. Nature **343:** 336–340.
19. SZABO, C., C. THIERMANN, C.C. WU, M. PERRETTI & J.R. VANE. 1994. Attenuation of the induction of nitric oxide synthase by endogenous glucocorticoids accounts for endotoxin tolerance in vivo. Proc. Natl. Acad. Sci. USA **91:** 271–275.
20. CHAUTARD, T., E. SPINEDI, M.J. VOIROL, F.P. PRALONG & R.C. GAILLARD. 1999. Role of glucocorticoids in the response of the hypothalamo-corticotrope, immune and adipose systems to repeated endotoxin administration. Neuroendocrinology **69:** 360–369.
21. SPINEDI, E. & R.C. GAILLARD. 1998. A regulatory loop between the hypothalamo-pituitary-adrenal (HPA) axis and circulating leptin: a physiological role of ACTH. Endocrinology **139:** 4016–4020.
22. EMILSSON, V., Y.L. LIU, M.A. CAWTHORNE, N.M. MORTON & M. DAVENPORT. 1997. Expression of the functional leptin receptor mRNA in pancreatic islets and direct inhibitory action of leptin on insulin secretion. Diabetes **46:** 313–316.
23. SPICER, L.J. & C.C. FRANCISCO. 1997. The adipose obse gene product, leptin: evidence of a direct inhibitory role in ovarian function. Endocrinology **138:** 3374–3379.
24. PRALONG, F.P., R. RODUIT, G. WAEBER, E. CASTILLO, F. MOSIMANN, B. THORENS & R.C. GAILLARD. 1998. Leptin inhibits directly glucocorticoid secretion by normal human and rat adrenal gland. Endocrinology **139:** 4264–4268.

SOCS Proteins: Modulators of Neuroimmunoendocrine Functions

Impact on Corticotroph LIF Signaling

C.J. AUERNHAMMER, C. BOUSQUET, V. CHESNOKOVA, AND S. MELMED[a]

Cedars-Sinai Medical Center, Los Angeles, California 90048, USA

ABSTRACT: Several members of the newly characterized family of suppressor of cytokine signaling (SOCS) proteins–such as SOCS-1, SOCS-3, and CIS–act as negative regulators of the cytokine-induced Jak-STAT signaling cascade. The expression of SOCS proteins is stimulated by a variety of cytokines and hormones in a tissue-specific manner. This article reviews our current understanding of SOCS proteins and their role as modulators of neuroimmunoendocrine functions, for example, in signaling of leptin, growth hormone, and prolactin, specially focusing on the impact of SOCS proteins on corticotroph leukemia inhibitory factor (LIF) signaling. LIF, a member of the gp130 sharing cytokine family, modulates pituitary development, POMC gene expression, and ACTH secretion. Current data on the negative autoregulatory function of the suppressor of cytokine signaling, SOCS-3, in LIF-induced POMC gene expression and ACTH secretion are extensively discussed.

SOCS PROTEINS AND THE JAK-STAT SIGNALING CASCADE

SOCS proteins are a newly characterized family of cytokine-inducible suppressors of cytokine signaling, also named STAT-inducible STAT-inhibitors (SSI), Janus kinase binding protein (JAB), and cytokine-inducible SH2 protein (CIS).[1–6] To date, there are 8 known members of the SOCS protein family, namely CIS and SOCS-1 to SOCS-7.[1–6] All SOCS proteins exhibit a common protein structure, encompassing a variable NH2-terminal region, a central SH2 domain, and a carboxy-terminal SOCS-box motif.[1–6] fSOCS-1 and SOCS-3 demonstrate partially overlapping functions by inhibiting the Jak-STAT signaling cascade of various cytokines[1–28] (TABLE 1). Most studies found no inhibitory activity of SOCS-2 on Jak-STAT signaling,[5,8,13,16,19,26] although this is still controversial.[4,18] Instead, SOCS-2 seems to counteract the inhibitory action of SOCS-1.[18,20] CIS has been identified as a specific inhibitor of STAT5 signaling.[29,30] The functional properties of SOCS-4 to SOCS-7 are yet unknown.

SOCS-1 has been demonstrated to inhibit Jak2 activity. SOCS-1 binds with its SH2 domain and part of its NH2-terminal region to the catalytic JH1 domain of Jak2.[7,8,31] The SOCS-box motif is not required for Jak protein interaction, but seems

[a]Address for correspondence: Shlomo Melmed, M.D., Academic Affairs, Cedars-Sinai Medical Center, 8700 Beverly Blvd., Room 2015, Los Angeles, CA 90048, USA. Voice: 310-423-4691; fax: 310-423-0119.

melmed@csmc.edu

TABLE 1. Suppression of Jak-STAT–mediated cytokine signaling by SOCS-1 and SOCS-3

Cytokine	Suppression of cytokine signaling by	
	SOCS-1	SOCS-3
IL-6	yes[1–3,7–9]	yes[7–9]
LIF	yes[1,3,5,8,9]	yes[4,5,8,9,11]
OSM	yes[1]	yes[1]
IL-11	n.d.	yes[10]
CNTF	n.d.	yes[12]
Leptin	n.d.	yes[13]
GH	yes[16,18]	yes[16,18]
PRL	yes[19,20]	yes[19,20]
EPO	yes[2,5]	yes[5]
TPO	yes[1]	n.d
IFNγ	yes[1,8,21,22]	no[21]/yes[8,22,24]
IFNα/β	yes[21,22]	no[21]/yes[22]
IL-4	yes[25–27]	yes[26]
IL-3	yes[2]	n.d.
IL-2	yes[2]	yes[28]

NOTE: n.d., not determined.

to modulate protein stability.[7,32,33] For SOCS-3, a similar mode of action has been demonstrated.[8,9,34]

SOCS PROTEINS:
MODULATORS OF NEUROIMMUNOENDOCRINE FUNCTIONS

SOCS-3 especially appears as a putative modulator of neuroimmunoendocrine functions. SOCS-3 has been demonstrated to inhibit Jak-STAT signaling of leptin,[13–15] growth hormone,[16–18] and prolactin.[19,20] Acute[13,15] and chronic[14] leptin treatment induces SOCS-3 expression in the hypothalamus[13–15] and peripheral tissues.[14] In contrast, leptin does not induce hypothalamic expression of SOCS-1, SOCS-2, and CIS.[13] Lethal yellow A[y]/a mice, a strain with leptin resistance and hyperleptinemia, exhibit an increased hypothalamic SOCS-3 expression.[13] Thus, SOCS-3 is a potential mediator of leptin resistance. Growth hormone-[16,17] and prolactin-induced[19,20] Jak-STAT signaling can be inhibited by SOCS-1 and SOCS-3, respectively. Northern blot analysis data suggest SOCS-3 to be the main modulator of growth hormone[16] and prolactin[19] signaling, although SOCS-1, SOCS-2, and CIS are also expressed in growth hormone-[16,18] and prolactin-responsive[19] tissues. These data indicate that SOCS-3 is a potential negative feedback regulator of growth hormone signaling, as well as a possible mediator of growth hormone resistance.

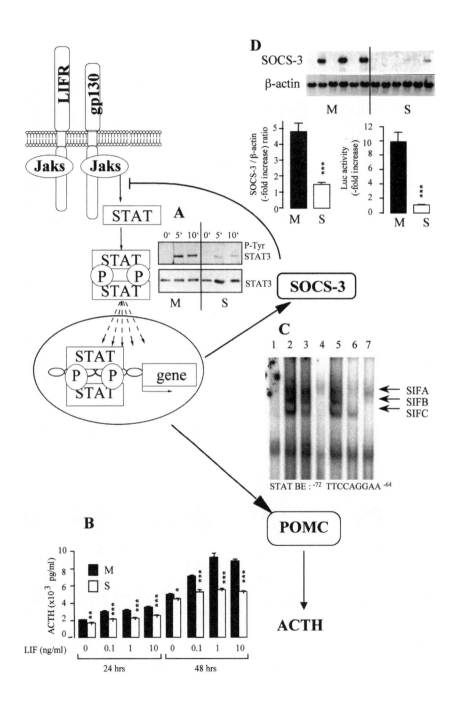

LIF–AUTO/PARACRINE MODULATOR OF
CORTICOTROPH FUNCTION

Cytokines are important neuroimmunoendocrine modulators of HPA axis activity.[35–38] Several cytokines of the gp130-sharing cytokine family (e.g., IL-6, LIF, IL-11) and their respective receptors (e.g., IL-6R, LIFR, IL-11R, gp130) are expressed in the pituitary and act as auto/paracrine stimuli.[10,38,39]

During the past few years, leukemia inhibitory factor (LIF) has been characterized as an important auto/paracrine modulator of corticotroph function and pituitary development.[38–40] Pituitary LIF expression is induced by various inflammatory and stress stimuli. LIF stimulates POMC gene expression and ACTH secretion alone and in synergistic action with CRH. LIF knockout animals show an attenuated HPA axis response to different stimuli. Pituitary-directed overexpression of LIF in mice results in dwarfism, as well as corticotroph hyperplasia and cushingoid features.

LIF signaling involves activation of Jak1 and Jak2, followed by tyrosine phosphorylation of the gp130 receptor subunit, STAT1 and STAT3.[41,42] The essential role of gp130 and STAT3 in corticotroph LIF signaling was demonstrated by gp130 antiserum[42] or overexpression of STAT3 dominant negative mutants,[43] both attenuating LIF-induced POMC gene expression and ACTH secretion.

SOCS PROTEINS: IMPACT ON CORTICOTROPH LIF SIGNALING

As initial studies demonstrated SOCS-1 and SOCS-3 to suppress the Jak-STAT cascade of several gp130-sharing cytokines (e.g., IL-6[1,3,7–9] and LIF[1,3–5]), we exam-

---

FIGURE 1. SOCS-3: suppressor of LIF-induced Jak-STAT signaling in the corticotroph cell. Binding of LIF to its specific LIFR/gp130 receptor complex on the corticotroph cell, stimulates the Jak-STAT signaling cascade. Activation of LIF-induced POMC gene expression and ACTH secretion are STAT3-dependent.[43] SOCS-3 suppresses LIF-induced STAT3 phosphorylation (**A**), thus acting as a negative feedback modulator of corticotroph LIF signaling (**B**). As LIF-induced SOCS-3 gene expression is mediated by an essential STAT1/ STAT3 binding element in the murine SOCS-3 promoter (**C**), SOCS-3 negatively autoregulates its own gene expression (**D**). (Abbreviations: M, mock-transfected AtT-20 cells; S, SOCS-3 overexpressing AtT-20 cells). (**A**) LIF-stimulation of AtT-20M cells results in rapid tyrosine phosphorylation of STAT3. Stable overexpression of SOCS-3 in AtT-20S cells abrogates tyrosine phosphorylation of STAT3.[11] (**B**) LIF-stimulated ACTH secretion was significantly attenuated in SOCS-3, overexpressing AtT-20S cells in comparison to AtT-20M controls[11]. (**C**) Specificity of the putative STAT binding element, located at nt − 72 to −64 in the murine SOCS-3 promoter, was demonstrated by gel shift analysis.[44] Nuclear extracts from AtT-20 cells stimulated with LIF for 15' (*lane* 2) or 30' (*lane* 3) exhibit three distinct bands (SIFA, SIFB, SIFC). These bands are not present in unstimulated control (*lane* 1). Specificity of these bands was proven by specific (*lane* 4) and unspecific (*lane* 5) competition, as well as supershift with STAT3 (*lane* 6) and STAT1 (*lane* 7) antibodies. Thus, the element located at nt −72 to −64 in the murine SOCS-3 promoter is an essential STAT1/STAT3 binding element. (**D**) As demonstrated by luciferase assay and Northern blot analysis, SOCS-3 promoter activity and SOCS-3 gene expression were potently induced by LIF in AtT-20M cells. Overexpression of exogenous SOCS-3 in AtT-20S cells almost completely abolished LIF induction of endogenous SOCS-3 promoter activity and SOCS-3 gene expression.[44] Adapted from Auernhammer and Melmed, Reference 40.

ined the putative role of SOCS proteins in corticotroph LIF signaling. In murine corticotroph AtT-20 cells, LIF,[11,44] IL-11,[10,44] and IL-6[44] potently induced SOCS-3
mRNA expression, peaking early at 30 to 60 min. In contrast, following LIF stimulation, the expression of SOCS-2 was only modestly induced, while the expression
of CIS was unchanged.[11] These data suggested SOCS-3 to be the predominantly regulated SOCS protein in corticotrophs. Also *in vivo* i.p. injection of 5mg LIF in
C57BL/6 mice rapidly induced pituitary SOCS-3 expression ninefold above baseline.[11] Stable overexpression of SOCS-3 in AtT-20 cells caused significant attenuation of LIF[11] or IL-11[10] induced POMC promoter activity, POMC gene expression,
and ACTH secretion. The suppressive effect of SOCS-3 on corticotroph LIF signaling was demonstrated to be due to inhibition of LIF-induced tyrosine phosphorylation of gp130 and STAT3.[11] Specificity of SOCS-3 action on the Jak-STAT signaling
cascade was also demonstrated, as cAMP-induced ACTH secretion was not effected
by overexpression of SOCS-3.[10] These data suggested SOCS-3 to be a negative feedback inhibitor of corticotroph LIF signaling, by inhibiting the Jak-STAT cascade.

Several data suggest a negative autoregulation of SOCS-1[3] and CIS[29] on their
own, respectively, STAT3- and STAT5-dependent gene expression. Negative autoregulation of SOCS protein expression might be an important mechanism to prevent
accumulation of these cytokine-inducible suppressors of cytokine signaling in the
cell. We therefore cloned the promoter region of murine SOCS-3 and characterized
regulation of SOCS-3 expression in the corticotroph.[44] Using a PCR-based genome-
walk technique, approximately 3.8 kb of genomic 5′-region of murine SOCS-3 were
cloned.[44] The full-length clone was sequenced and submitted to Genbank (accession
number AF117732). The major transcription start site was defined by RNAse protection assay and defined as +1. The 5′-genomic region of murine SOCS-3 was sub-
cloned into the pGL3 basic vector in front of the luciferase gene. Reporter gene assay
in transiently transfected AtT-20 cells revealed significant basal, as well as approximately 35-fold higher, LIF-induced SOCS-3 promoter activity.[44] Further characterization of the murine SOCS-3 promoter by deletion and mutation constructs, as well
as gelshift analysis, exhibited an essential STAT1/STAT3 binding element, posi-
tioned at nt −72 to −64.[44] Corticotroph SOCS-3 expression was STAT3- dependent,
as AtT-20 cells overexpressing negative dominant STAT3 mutants showed an attenuated increase of SOCS-3 mRNA following LIF stimulation.[44] Accordingly, overexpression of SOCS-3 blocked its own LIF-induced endogenous gene expression.[44]

In summary, SOCS-3 is a suppressor of LIF-induced Jak-STAT signaling in the
corticotroph cell. LIF and other gp130-sharing cytokines rapidly stimulate pituitary
corticotroph SOCS-3 expression, which is under control of a STAT1/STAT3- responsive promoter element. Our data demonstrate SOCS-3 to be a cytokine-inducible pituitary protein, acting as a suppressor of corticotroph LIF signaling. The negative
autoregulatory feedback of SOCS-3 on its own gene expression prevents accumulation of SOCS-3 in the corticotroph cell. Thus, SOCS-3, in its expression being tightly
controlled, acts as a negative neuroimmunoendocrine modulator of corticotroph LIF
signaling. This regulation provides a mechanism for fast "on" and "off" reactions of
the corticotroph cell to various neuroimmunoendocrine stimuli (SEE FIGURE 1).

REFERENCES

1. STARR, R. *et al.* 1997. A family of cytokine-inducible inhibitors of signaling. Nature **387:** 917–921.

2. ENDO, T.A. *et al.* 1997. A new protein containing an SH2 domain that inhibits JAK kinases. Nature **387:** 921–924.

3. NAKA, T. *et al.* 1997. Structure and function of a new STAT-induced STAT inhibitor. Nature **387:** 924–928.

4. MINAMOTO, S. *et al.* 1997. Cloning and functional analysis of new members of STAT-induced STAT inhibitor (SSI) family: SSI-2 and SSI-3. Biochem. Biophys. Res. Commun. **237:** 79–83.

5. MASUHARA, M. *et al.* 1997. Cloning and characterization of novel CIS family genes. Biochem. Biophys. Res. Commun. **239:** 439–446.

6. HILTON, D.J. *et al.* 1998. Twenty proteins containing a C-terminal SOCS box form five structural classes. Proc. Natl. Acad. Sci. USA. **95:** 114–119.

7. NARAZAKI, M. *et al.* 1998. Three distinct domains of SSI-1/SOCS-1/JAB protein are required for its suppression of interleukin-6 signaling. Proc. Natl. Acad. Sci. USA. **95:** 13130–13134.

8. SUZUKI, R. *et al.* 1998. CIS3 and JAB have different regulatory roles in interleukin-6 mediated differentiation and STAT3 activation in M1 leukemia cells. Oncogene **17:** 2271–2278.

9. NICHOLSON, S.E. *et al.* 1999. Mutational analyses of the SOCS proteins suggest a dual domain requirement but distinct mechanisms for inhibition of LIF and IL-6 signal transduction. EMBO J. **18:** 375–385.

10. AUERNHAMMER, C.J. & MELMED, S. 1999. Interleukin-11 stimulates POMC gene expression and ACTH secretion in corticotroph cells: evidence for a redundant cytokine network in the HPA axis. Endocrinolgy **140:** 1559–1566.

11. AUERNHAMMER, C.J. *et al.* 1998. Pituitary corticotroph SOCS-3: novel intracellular regulation of leukemia-inhibitory factor-mediated proopiomelanocortin gene expression and adrenocorticotropin secretion. Mol. Endocrinol. **12:** 954–961.

12. BJORBAEK, C. *et al.* 1999. Activation of SOCS-3 messenger ribonucleic acid in the hypothalamus by ciliary neurotrophic factor. Endocrinology **140:** 2035–2043.

13. BJORBAEK, C. *et al.* 1998. Identification of SOCS-3 as a potential mediator of central leptin resistance. Mol. Cell. **1:** 619–625.

14. EMILSSON, V. *et al.* 1999. Leptin treatment increases suppressors of cytokine signaling in central and peripheral tissues. FEBS Lett. **455:** 170–174.

15. ELIAS, C.F. *et al.* 1999. Leptin differentially regulates NPY and POMC neurons projecting to the lateral hypothalamic area. Neuron. **23:** 775–786.

16. ADAMS, T.E. *et al.* 1998. Growth hormone preferentially induces the rapid, transient expression of SOCS-3, a novel inhibitor of cytokine receptor signaling. J. Biol. Chem. **273:** 1285–1287.

17. TOLLET-EGNELL, P. *et al.* 1999. Growth hormone regulation of SOCS-2, SOCS-3, and CIS messenger ribonucleic acid expression in the rat. Endocrinology **140:** 3693–3704.

18. FAVRE, H. *et al.* 1999. Dual effects of suppressor of cytokine signaling (SOCS-2) on growth hormone signal transduction. FEBS Lett. **453:** 63–66.

19. HELMAN, D. *et al.* 1998 Cytokine-inducible SH2 protein (CIS3) and JAK2 binding protein (JAB) abolish prolactin receptor-mediated STAT5 signaling. FEBS Lett. **441:** 287–291.

20. PEZET, A. *et al.* 1999. Inhibition and restoration of prolactin signal transduction by suppressors of cytokine signaling. J. Biol. Chem. **274:** 24497–24502.

21. SAKAMOTO, H. *et al.* 1998. A Janus kinase inhibitor, JAB, is an interferon-g-inducible gene and confers resistance to interferons. Blood **92:** 1668–1676.

22. SONG, M.M. *et al.* 1998. The suppressor of cytokine signaling (SOCS) 1 and SOCS3 but not SOCS2 proteins inhibit interferon-mediated antiviral and antiproliferative activities. J. Biol. Chem. **273:** 35056–35062.

23. ITO, S. *et al.* 1999. Interleukin-10 inhibits expression of both interferon alpha- and interferon gamma-induced genes by suppressing tyrosine phosphorylation of STAT1. Blood **93:** 1456–1463.

24. STOIBER, D. *et al.* 1999. Lipopolysaccharide induces in macrophages the synthesis of the suppressor of cytokine signaling 3 and suppresses signal transduction in response to the activating factor IFN-gamma. J. Immunol. **163:** 2640–2647.

25. VENKATARAMAN, C. *et al.* 1999. Repression of IL-4-induced gene expression by IFN-gamma requires Stat1 activation. J. Immunol. **162:** 4053–4061.

26. LOSMAN, J.A. *et al.* Cutting edge: SOCS-1 is a potent inhibitor of IL-4 signal transduction. J. Immunol. **162:** 3770–3774.

27. DICKENSHEETS, H.L. *et al.* 1999. Interferons inhibit activation of STAT6 by interleukin 4 in human monocytes by inducing SOCS-1 gene expression. Proc. Natl. Acad. Sci. USA. **96:** 10800–10805.

28. COHNEY, S.J. *et al.* 1999. SOCS-3 is tyrosine phosphorylated in response to interleukin-2 and suppresses STAT5 phosphorylation and lymphocyte proliferation. Mol. Cell. Biol. **19:** 4980–4988.

29. MATSUMOTO, A. *et al.* 1997. CIS, a cytokine-inducible SH2 protein, is a target of the JAK-STAT5 pathway and modulates STAT5 activation. Blood **89:** 3148–3154.

30. MATSUMOTO, A. *et al.* 1999. Suppression of STAT5 functions in liver, mammary glands, and T cells in cytokine-inducible SH2-containing protein 1 transgenic mice. Mol. Cell. Biol. **19:** 6396–6407.

31. YASUKAWA, H. *et al.* 1999. The Jak-binding protein JAB inhibits Janus tyrosine kinase activity through binding in the activation loop. EMBO J. **18:** 1309–1320.

32. KAMURA, T. *et al.* 1998. The elongin BC complex interacts with the conserved SOCS-box motif present in members of the SOCS, ras, WD-40 repeat, and ankyrin repeat families. Gen. Develop. **12:** 3872–3881.

33. ZHANG, J.G. *et al.* 1999. The conserved SOCS box motif in suppressors of cytokine signaling binds to elongin B and C and may couple bound proteins to proteasomal degradation. Proc. Natl. Acad. Sci. USA **96:** 2071–2076.

34. SASAKI, A. *et al.* Cytokine-inducible SH2 protein-3 (CIS3/SOCS3) inhibits janus tyrosine kinase by binding through the N-terminal kinase inhibitory region as well as SH2 domain. Genes Cells **4:** 339–351.

35. BESEDOVSKY, H.O. & A. DEL REY. 1996. Immune-neuro-endocrine interactions: facts and hypotheses. Endo. Rev. **17:** 64–102.

36. ARZT, E. *et al.* 1999. Pathophysiological role of the cytokine network in the anterior pituitary gland. Front. Neuroendocrinol. **20:** 71–95.

37. TURNBULL, A.V. & C.L. RIVIER. 1999. Regulation of the hypothalamic-pituitary-adrenal axis by cytokines: actions and mechanisms of action. Physiol. Rev. **79:** 1–71.

38. RAY, D. & S. MELMED. 1997. Pituitary cytokine and growth factor expression and action. Endocrin. Rev. **18:** 206–228.

39. MELMED, S. 1997. gp130-related cytokines and their receptors in the pituitary. Trends Endocrinol. Metab. **8:** 391–397.

40. AUERNHAMMER, C.J. & S. MELMED. 2000. Leukemia inhibitory factor–neuroimmune modulator of endocrine function [review]. Endocrine Rev. **21:** 313–345.

41. AUERNHAMMER, C.J. & S. MELMED. 1999. gp130 sharing cytokines. *In* Molecular Regulation. P.M. Conn, Ed. Humana Press. New York. In press.

42. RAY, D.W. *et al.* 1998. Leukemia inhibitory factor regulates proopiomelanocortin transcription. Ann. N.Y. Acad. Sci. **840:** 162–173.

43. BOUSQUET, C. & S. MELMED. 1999. Critical role for STAT3 in murine pituitary adrenocorticotropin hormone leukemia inhibitory factor signaling. J. Biol. Chem. **274:** 10723–10730.

44. AUERNHAMMER, C.J. *et al.* 1999. Autoregulation of pituitary corticotroph SOCS-3 expression: characterization of the murine SOCS-3 promoter. Proc. Natl. Acad. Sci. USA. **96:** 6964–6969.

Macrophage Migration Inhibitory Factor (MIF)

A Critical Neurohumoral Mediator

NIKOLAI PETROVSKY[a] AND RICHARD BUCALA[b,c]

[a]Cytokine and Autoimmunity Research Unit, Department of Endocrinology,
The Canberra Hospital, Yamba Drive, Woden, ACT, Australia 2606

[b]The Picower Institute for Medical Research, 350 Community Drive,
Manhasset, New York 10030,USA

INTRODUCTION

The development and subsequent abatement of an immune response depends upon a complex interplay of humoral and cellular mediators. Cytokines function in this process by recruiting and activating effector cells which fight infection or tissue invasion. Unopposed cytokine action may lead, however, to excess tissue destruction and ultimately prove fatal unless held in check by counterbalancing regulatory forces. The important role of the neuroendocrine system in immune regulation is demonstrated by the increased susceptibility of hypophysectomized or adrenalectomized animals to death from septic shock.[1] Not surprisingly, in view of their close relationship, an increasing number of mediators of neuroendocrine and immune communication have been identified. One of the most significant recently identified factors with both neuroendocrine and immune roles is macrophage migration inhibitory factor (MIF).

MIF was originally described as a factor produced by T lymphoctyes that inhibited the random migration of macrophages.[2] It was not until recently, when MIF was finally cloned and a source of recombinant protein obtained, that some light was finally shed on MIF's role within the wider context of the human neuroendocrine and immune systems.[3–5] The mouse MIF gene maps to the middle region of chromosome 10 and spans approximately 1 kb.[4] Human MIF (115 residues in length) shares a high degree of structural and sequence homology with its murine counterpart.[3] Both mouse and human MIF lack a conventional N-terminal leader sequence indicating its release from cells by a nonclassical protein secretion pathway. MIF shows a weak primary sequence homology (27%) with the enzyme D-dopachrome tautomerase[6] and significant three-dimensional homology with two bacterial enzymes, namely, 4-oxalocrotonate tautomerase and 5-carboxymethyl-2-hydroxymuconate isomerase.[7] X-ray crystallography reveals that MIF forms a homotrimer with six α-helices surrounding three β-sheets that completely wrap around to form a barrel containing a solvent accessible channel.[8–10] Interestingly, given its homology to a number of enzymes, MIF does in fact exhibit enzymatic activity and is capable of catalyzing an isomerization reaction, namely, the conversion of dopachrome to 5,6-dihydroxy-

[c]rbucala@picower.edu

indole-2-carboxylic acid.[11] However, to date there is no evidence that any of the immune effects mediated by MIF relate to its enzymatic properties.

An initial surprise was the finding that MIF, traditionally regarded as a T-cell–derived cytokine, was also a major product of murine anterior pituitary cells.[12] Later work, as described below, has demonstrated that MIF plays a major role in the counterregulation of glucocorticoid-mediated immune suppression as well as having a potential role in the counterregulation of glucocorticoid-mediated changes in glucose homeostasis.

MIF: HORMONE OR CYTOKINE?

By use of a combination of immunocytochemical and immunohistological techniques it was found that pre-formed MIF accounts for about 0.05% of total protein in the anterior pituitary gland.[12] This compares to 0.2% and 0.08%, respectively, for the classical pituitary hormones ACTH and prolactin. Indeed, MIF resides in the same population of secretory granules as ACTH.[13] In keeping with the co-localization of MIF with ACTH, stimulation of cultured pituitary cells with corticotrophin-releasing factor (CRF), the major stimulus for ACTH release, results in the dose-dependent release of MIF.[13] The secretion of MIF was found to occur at lower CRF concentrations than those required to induce ACTH secretion. Anterior pituitary cells, *in vitro,* also secrete large quantities of MIF when stimulated with LPS.[13]

MIF is present in human serum at concentrations ranging from 2–6 ng/ml.[14] The dominant source of human plasma MIF is not currently known, although macrophages, the pituitary, and the liver are all likely to contribute. Although macrophages appear to be the major immune source of MIF, it is also produced by T and B cells. MIF is expressed at high levels in the liver and has been used as a source of purified native MIF.[15] MIF is also expressed in a range of additional cell types including eosinophils,[16] adipocytes,[17] pancreatic islet β cells,[18] the Leydig cells of the testes,[19] and ovarian follicular cell.[20]

Macrophages contain large quantities of stored, pre-formed MIF (estimated to be 2–4 fg/cell) that is released in response to LPS stimulation.[21] The induction of MIF mRNA transcription and secretion of MIF protein are tiggered by 10- to 100-fold lower concentrations of LPS than those required to stimulate TNF-α production. Interestingly, physiological concentrations of glucocorticoids stimulate macrophage secretion of MIF, contrary to the situation with other inflammatory cytokines, which are profoundly inhibited by glucocorticoids.[22] Other stimuli for MIF secretion include gram-positive exotoxins,[23] TNF-α and IFN-γ in monocytes/macrophages,[21] and IL-5 and C5a in eosinophils.[16]

MIF: A PRO-INFLAMMATORY CYTOKINE

Although MIF was originally identified by virtue of its ability to inhibit the random migration of macrophages, it has now been identified as having a wide range of diverse biological activities both within and outside of the immune system. MIF exerts a number of proinflammatory functions. It potentiates septic shock when co-injected with LPS into mice, whereas neutralizing anti-MIF antibodies (anti-MIF) protect mice from an otherwise lethal dose of LPS.[12] Circulating TNF-α levels were reduced by as much as 35% in mice protected from LPS lethality by anti-MIF. Gram-positive exotoxins are extremely potent inducers of MIF secretion.[23] MIF has been shown to be a critical mediator of the activation of immune cells by staphylococcal toxic shock syndrome toxin 1 and streptococcal pyrogenic exotoxin A, the lethal effects of which are significantly reduced by pretreatment with anti-MIF.[23] Anti-MIF has also been shown to inhibit delayed-type hypersensitivity in mice and to inhibit the generation of an antigen-specific T- and B-cell response *in vivo*.[24] Consistent with its role in inflammation, MIF expression is increased in renal allograft rejection,[25] and MIF levels are significantly elevated in the sera of patients with acute uveitis[26] or atopic dermatitis.[27] MIF has also been shown to be present in the alveolar spaces from patients with adult respiratory distress syndrome[28] and in the synovial tissue of rats with adjuvant arthritis[29] as well as patients with rheumatoid arthritis.[30,31] Anti-MIF treatment led to profound, dose-dependent inhibition of adjuvant arthritis in the rat model.[29] Anti-MIF also prevents acute hepatic failure in mice injected with bacillus-Calmette-Guérin and LPS as a model of fulminant hepatitis.[32] The role of MIF in inflammation is further reinforced by the observation that MIF knockout mice(MIF-/-) are resistant to the lethal effects of high-dose LPS, and macrophages from these mice produce less TNF-α than do wild-type mice.[33] Interestingly, MIF-/- mice cleared *Pseudomonas aeruginosa* instilled into the trachea better than did wild-type mice.[33] In an interesting departure from its usual pro-inflammatory role, MIF helps protect the corneal epithelium from NK-mediated lysis by virtue of its ability to inhibit NK cells and, in particular, NK-cell release of perforin.[34]

At least part of the pro-inflammatory effects of MIF may be explained by its ability to induce release of the pro-inflammatory cytokine TNF-α by macrophages. In fact, MIF and TNF-α appear to form a positive feedback loop, as TNF-α is itself able to induce MIF secretion via a tyrosine-kinase-dependent pathway.[21,35] Similarly, the pro-inflammatory cytokine IFN-γ also stimulates MIF secretion.[21]

MIF: A COUNTER-REGULATORY HORMONE

Considered in the context that MIF is released from the same pituitary cells that secrete ACTH, an important anti-inflammatory mediator, the pro-inflammatory effects of recombinant MIF initially appear somewhat paradoxical. Even more surprising is the finding that cortisol, despite being a major anti-inflammatory mediator, itself induces MIF release from macrophages and T cells. Glucocorticoids characteristically downregulate pro-inflammatory cytokine expression by binding to and activating negative regulatory elements in the promoters of cytokine genes and by inducing IκBa, a protein that binds and neutralizes the cytokine transcription factor NF-κB.[36] Cytokines whose mRNAs have been shown to be downregulated by glucocorticoids include IL-1,[37] IL-2 and IFN-γ.[38] IL-3, GM-CSF and TNF-α,[39] IL-6,[40] and IL-8.[41] MIF, therefore, appears to be the only pro-inflammatory mediator whose secretion is induced rather than inhibited by glucocorticoids. The glucocorticoid-initiated secretion of MIF is tightly regulated and follows a bell-shaped dose–response curve with respect to glucocorticoid concentration.[22] At high "anti-inflammatory" glucocorticoid concentrations (at least 10^{-8} M), MIF secretion is shut off.

The observation that glucocorticoids induce the secretion of MIF, a pro-inflammatory factor, suggested that MIF might act as an important counter-regulator to the immunosuppressive effects of glucocorticoids. When added to cultured monocytes, MIF was found to override, in a dose-dependent manner, glucocorticoid-mediated suppression of TNF-α, IL-1β, IL-6, and IL-8 secretion.[22] The ability of MIF to overcome the inhibition of TNF-α secretion varied directly with the concentration of glucocorticoid and decreased with increasing dexamethasone concentration. That MIF has reduced counterregulatory capacity and that its secretion is inhibited at high glucocorticoid concentrations suggests that the major role of MIF is to neutralize the immune effects of low physiological glucocorticoid concentrations; it does this with an escape mechanism operating at high glucocorticoid concentrations, enabling the unopposed immunosuppressive effects of glucocorticoids to protect the host against overwhelming and potentially life-threatening inflammatory reactions.

The concept that MIF plays an important counterregulatory role is supported by the fact that the administration of recombinant MIF to dexamethasone-protected LPS-treated mice completely blocked the protective effects of dexamethasone on LPS lethality.[22] Similarly, recombinant MIF, in a dose-dependent manner, overrides the glucocorticoid-mediated inhibition of T-cell proliferation and IL-2 and IFN-γ production.[24] Interestingly, anti-MIF significantly attenuates the development of antigen-specific T-cell reactivity and primary antibody responses, suggesting that in the absence of MIF the immunosuppressive activity of endogenous glucocorticoids may be markedly increased. Of note, we have recently found that human plasma MIF exhibits significant circadian rhythmicity with a peak at approximately 8 A.M. and with a circadian rhythm that essentially mimics the rhythm of plasma cortisol (N. Petrovsky, unpublished results). This would be consistent with MIF's having a role in counterregulating the immune effects of plasma cortisol within its normal physiological circadian range.

Interestingly, aside from its immune role, MIF is co-secreted with insulin by pancreatic β cells and acts as an autocrine factor to stimulate insulin release.[18] There is also evidence that the intracellular glucose concentration is important in determining MIF expression in adipocytes.[42] Moreover, recent data indicate that MIF can act directly on peripheral muscle, the major site of glucose disposal, to increase glucose transport and glycolytic flux (F. Benigni et al., in preparation). That glucocorticoids are important mediators of insulin resistance suggests that MIF may play an important role in the maintenance of normoglycemia by increasing insulin secretion and promoting glucose disposal, thereby counterregulating glucocorticoid-mediated insulin resistance. The circadian rhythm of plasma MIF may likewise play a role in reducing circadian glucocorticoid-mediated variation in insulin sensitivity.

MIF: THE FUTURE

Despite considerable research progress there are still many unknowns regarding MIF and its biological actions. Whilst it is clear that MIF acts in dual capacities as a hormone and cytokine, it is still not known what tissue is the major source of circulating plasma MIF. It is also not known whether local tissue concentrations (e.g., at the site of inflammation) become more important than circulating plasma levels for determining the biological action of MIF in particular physiological or pathological situations. Furthermore, the way in which MIF exerts its biological activity, the nature of its receptor, and the relevance of MIF's enzymatic activity is still far from completely understood. What does stand out, however, is the consistent evidence that MIF acts as a counterregulator to downmodulate the effects of glucocorticoids on the immune and endocrine systems. MIF thus serves as an excellent model of neuroendocrine immune interaction and provides the opportunity to better understand the role of the neuro-ndocrine system in the regulation of human immune responses.

REFERENCES

1. BERTINI, R., M. BIANCHI & P. GHEZZI. 1988. Adrenalectomy sensitizes mice to the lethal effects of interleukin 1 and tumor necrosis factor. J. Exp. Med. **167:** 1708.
2. GEORGE, M. & J. VAUGHAN. 1962. In vitro cell migration as a model for delayed hypersensitivity. Proc. Soc. Exp. Biol. Med. **111:** 514.
3. WEISER, W.Y., P.A. TEMPLE, J.S. WITEK-GIANNOTTI, H.G. REMOLD, S.C. CLARK & J.R. DAVID. 1989. Molecular cloning of a cDNA encoding a human macrophage migration inhibitory factor. Proc. Natl. Acad. Sci. USA **86:** 7522–7526.
4. MITCHELL, R., M. BACHER, J. BERNHAGEN et al. 1995. Cloning and characterization of the gene for mouse macrophage migration inhibitory factor (MIF). J. Immunol. **154:** 3863.
5. METZ, C.N. & R. BUCALA. 1997. Role of macrophage inhibitory factor in the regulation of the immune response. Adv. Immunol. **66:** 197–223.
6. ROSENGREN, E., P. AMAN, S. THELIN et al. 1997. The macrophage migration inhibitory factor MIF is a phenylpyruvate tautomerase. FEBS Lett. **417:** 85.
7. SUBRAMANYA, H.S., D.I. ROPER, Z. DAUTER et al. 1996. Enzymatic ketonization of 2-hydroxymuconate: specificity and mechanism investigated by the crystal structures of two isomerases. Biochemistry **35:** 792.
8. SUN, H.W., J. BERNHAGEN, R. BUCALA & E. LOLIS. 1996. Crystal structure at 2.6-A resolution of human macrophage migration inhibitory factor. Proc. Natl. Acad. Sci. USA **93:** 5191.
9. SUZUKI, M., H. SUGIMOTO, A. NAKAGAWA et al. 1996. Crystal structure of the macrophage migration inhibitory factor from rat liver. Nature Structural Biology **3:** 259.
10. SUGIMOTO, H., M. SUZUKI, A. NAKAGAWA et al. 1996. Crystal structure of macrophage migration inhibitory factor from human lymphocyte at 2.1 A resolution. FEBS Lett. **389:** 145.
11. ROSENGREN, E., R. BUCALA, P. AMAN et al. 1996. The immunoregulatory mediator macrophage migration inhibitory factor (MIF) catalyzes a tautomerization reaction. Mol. Med. **2:** 143.
12. BERNHAGEN, J., T. CALANDRA, R.A. MITCHELL et al. 1993. MIF is a pituitary-derived cytokine that potentiates lethal endotoxaemia. Nature **365:** 756.
13. NISHINO, T., J. BERNHAGEN, H. SHIIKI et al. 1995. Localization of macrophage migration inhibitory factor (MIF) to secretory granules within the corticotrophic and thyrotrophic cells of the pituitary gland. Mol. Med. **1:** 781.
14. BUCALA, R. 1996. MIF rediscovered: cytokine, pituitary hormone, and glucocorticoid-induced regulator of the immune response. FASEB J. **10:** 1607.
15. BERNHAGEN, J., R.A. MITCHELL, T. CALANDRA et al. 1994. Purification, bioactivity, and secondary structure analysis of mouse and human macrophage migration inhibitory factor (MIF). Biochemistry **33:** 14144.

16. ROSSI, A.G., C. HASLETT, N. HIRANI et al. 1998. Human circulating eosinophils secrete macrophage migration inhibitory factor (MIF). Potential role in asthma. J. Clin. Invest. **101:** 2869.

17. HIROKAWA, J., S. SAKAUE, S. TAGAMI et al. 1997. Identification of macrophage migration inhibitory factor in adipose tissue and its induction by tumor necrosis factor-alpha. Biochem. Biophys. Res. Commun. **235:** 94.

18. WAEBER, G., T. CALANDRA, R. RODUIT et al. 1997. Insulin secretion is regulated by the glucose-dependent production of islet beta cell macrophage migration inhibitory factor. Proc. Natl. Acad. Sci. USA **94:** 4782.

19. MEINHARDT, A., M. BACHER, J.R. MCFARLANE et al. 1996. Macrophage migration inhibitory factor production by Leydig cells: evidence for a role in the regulation of testicular function. Endocrinology **137:** 5090.

20. WADA, S., S. FUJIMOTO, Y. MIZUE & J. NISHIHIRA. 1997. Macrophage migration inhibitory factor in the human ovary: presence in the follicular fluids and production by granulosa cells. Biochem. Mol .Biol. Int. **41:** 805.

21. CALANDRA, T., J. BERNHAGEN, R.A. MITCHELL & R. BUCALA. 1994. The macrophage is an important and previously unrecognized source of macrophage migration inhibitory factor. J. Exp. Med. **179:** 1895.

22. CALANDRA, T., J. BERNHAGEN, C.N. METZ et al. 1995. MIF as a glucocorticoid-induced modulator of cytokine production. Nature **377:** 68.

23. CALANDRA, T., L.A. SPIEGEL, C.N. METZ & R. BUCALA. 1998. Macrophage migration inhibitory factor is a critical mediator of the activation of immune cells by exotoxins of Gram-positive bacteria. Proc Natl Acad Sci USA **95:** 11383.

24. BACHER, M., C.N. METZ, T. CALANDRA et al. 1996. An essential regulatory role for macrophage migration inhibitory factor in T-cell activation. Proc. Natl. Acad. Sci. USA **93:** 7849.

25. LAN, H.Y., N. YANG, F.G. BROWN et al. 1998. Macrophage migration inhibitory factor expression in human renal allograft rejection. Transplantation **66:** 1465.

26. KITAICHI, N., S. KOTAKE, Y. SASAMOTO et al. 1999. Prominent increase of macrophage migration inhibitory factor in the sera of patients with uveitis. Invest. Ophthal. Vis. Sci. **40:** 247.

27. SHIMIZU, T., R. ABE, A. OHKAWARA et al. 1997. Macrophage migration inhibitory factor is an essential immunoregulatory cytokine in atopic dermatitis. Biochem. Biophys. Res. Commun. **240:** 173.

28. DONNELLY, S.C., C. HASLETT, P.T. REID et al. 1997. Regulatory role for macrophage migration inhibitory factor in acute respiratory distress syndrome. Nature Medicine **3:** 320.

29. LEECH, M., C. METZ, L. SANTOS et al. 1998. Involvement of macrophage migration inhibitory factor in the evolution of rat adjuvant arthritis. Arthritis Rheum. **41:** 910.

30. LEECH, M., C. METZ, P. HALL et al. 1999. Macrophage migration inhibitory factor in rheumatoid arthritis: evidence of proinflammatory function and regulation by glucocorticoids. Arthritis Rheum **42:** 1601.

31. ONODERA, S., H. TANJI, K. SUZUKI et al. 1999. High expression of macrophage migration inhibitory factor in the synovial tissues of rheumatoid joints. Cytokine **11:** 163.

32. KOBAYASHI, S., J. NISHIHIRA, S. WATANABE & S. TODO. 1999. Prevention of lethal acute hepatic failure by antimacrophage migration inhibitory factor antibody in mice treated with bacille Calmette-Guerin and lipopolysaccharide. Hepatology **29:** 1752.

33. BOZZA, M., A.R. SATOSKAR, G. LIN et al. 1999. Targeted disruption of migration inhibitory factor gene reveals its critical role in sepsis. J. Exp. Med. **189:** 341.

34. APTE, R. S., D. SINHA, E. MAYHEW et al. 1998. Role of macrophage migration inhibitory factor in inhibiting NK cell activity and preserving immune privilege. J. Immunol. **160:** 5693.

35. HIROKAWA, J., S. SAKAUE, Y. FURUYA et al. 1998. Tumor necrosis factor-alpha regulates the gene expression of macrophage migration inhibitory factor through tyrosine kinase-dependent pathway in 3T3-L1 adipocytes. J. Biochem. **123:** 733.

36. SCHEINMAN, R.I., P.C. COGSWELL, A.K. LOFQUIST & A. BALDWIN, JR. 1995. Role of transcriptional activation of I kappa B alpha in mediation of immunosuppression by glucocorticoids. Science **270:** 283.

37. KERN, J.A., R.J. LAMB, J.C. REED et al. 1988. Dexamethasone inhibition of interleu-kin 1 beta production by human monocytes. Posttranscriptional mechanisms. J. Clin. Invest. **81:** 237.
38. KELSO, A. & A. MUNCK. 1984. Glucocorticoid inhibition of lymphokine secretion by alloreactive T lymphocyte clones. J. Immunol. **133:** 784.
39. HOMO-DELARCHE, F. & M. DARDENNE. 1993. The neuroendocrine-immune axis. Spring Semin. Immunopathol. **14:** 221.
40. RAY, A., K.S. LAFORGE & P.B. SEHGAL. 1990. On the mechanism for efficient repres-sion of the interleukin-6 promoter by glucocorticoids: enhancer, TATA box, and RNA start site (Inr motif) occlusion. Mol. Cell Biol. **10:** 5736.
41. MUKAIDA, N., G.L. GUSSELLA, T. KASAHARA et al. 1992. Molecular analysis of the inhibition of interleukin-8 production by dexamethasone in a human fibrosarcoma cell line. Immunology **75:** 674.
42. SAKAUE, S., J. NISHIHIRA, J. HIROKAWA et al. 1999. Regulation of macrophage migra-tion inhibitory factor (MIF) expression by glucose and insulin in adipocytes in vitro. Mol. Med. **5:** 361.

Functional Cross-talk among Cytokines, T-Cell Receptor, and Glucocorticoid Receptor Transcriptional Activity and Action

E. ARZT,[a,b,d] D. KOVALOVSKY,[b,c] L. MÜLLER IGAZ,[b] M. COSTAS,[b,c] P. PLAZAS,[b,c] D. REFOJO,[b] M. PÁEZ-PEREDA,[d] J.M.H.M. REUL,[d] G. STALLA,[d] AND F. HOLSBOER[d]

[b]Laboratorio de Fisiología y Biología Molecular, University of Buenos Aires, Ciudad Universitaria, 1428 Buenos Aires, Argentina

[c]Members of the Argentine National Research Council (CONICET)

[d]Max-Planck Institute of Psychiatry, Kraepelinstrasse 2–10, 80804 Munich, Germany

ABSTRACT: The main communicators between the neuroendocrine and immune systems are cytokines and hormones. We studied the molecular interaction between immune activators (cytokines and T-cell receptors [TCRs]) and the glucocorticoid receptor (GR) in cells in which glucocorticoids play a key regulatory function: (1) cellular targets of TNF-induced cytotoxicity; (2) the pituitary gland; and (3) thymic cells. Cytokines (TNF-alpha and IL-1) increase glucocorticoid-induced transcriptional activity of the GR via the DNA-glucocorticoid response elements (GREs) in cells transfected with a glucocorticoid-inducible reporter plasmid. As a functional physiological correlate, priming of fibroblastic cells with a low dose of TNF significantly increases the sensitivity to glucocorticoid inhibition of TNF-induced apoptosis (without involving NF-κB). Priming of AtT-20 mouse corticotrophs and Cushing pituitary cells with IL-1 increases the sensitivity to glucocorticoid inhibition of CRH-induced ACTH/POMC expression. In thymocytes, activation of the T-cell receptor counteracts the glucocorticoid-induced thymic apoptosis by downregulating the glucocorticoid action on GRE-driven apoptotic genes. Thus, cytokines and immune mediators prevent their own deleterious effects not only by stimulating glucocorticoid production, but also by modifying the sensitivity of the target cells for the glucocorticoid counter-regulatory action. The functional cross-talk at the molecular level between immune signals and glucocorticoids is essential to determine the biological response to both mediators and constitutes the ultimate level of interaction between the immune and neuroendocrine mediators.

Cytokines activate the hypothalamic-pituitary-adrenal system, causing an elevation of systemic glucocorticoid levels.[1,2] Glucocorticoids inhibit both cytokine gene expression and their pleiotropic actions on target cells.[3–7]

These immunosuppressive and anti-inflammatory actions involve the interaction between the activated glucocorticoid receptor (GR) in the nucleus with different

[a]Address for correspondence: Dr. Eduardo Arzt, Lab. Fisiologia y Biologia Molecular, Dept. Ciencias Biologicas; FCEN—Universidad de Buenos Aires, Ciudad Universitaria, Pabellon II (1428), Buenos Aires, Argentina. Voice: 54-11-4576-3386; fax: 54-11-4576-3321.
earzt@bg.fcen.uba

transcription factors such as AP1 and NF-κB. AP1 proteins include heterodimerization between Jun, Fos and ATF, which transcriptional activity is regulated through interactions with specific protein kinases and a variety of transcriptional coactivators (reviewed in Karin *et al.*).[8] The physical interaction of the GR with the proteins that bind to AP-1 leads to transcriptional interference and inhibition of the expression of AP-1–regulated genes such as IL-2 and IL-6.[9–13] NF-κB proteins are retained in the cytoplasm of unstimulated cells in an inactive form via interactions with one or more of the seven known I-κB proteins (reviewed in Verma *et al.*).[14] In response to a variety of stimuli—including cytokines—I-κB proteins are phosphorylated and degraded, and then free cytoplasmic NF-κB dimers are translocated rapidly to the nucleus, where they regulate κB-dependent gene expression. Cross-coupling of GR with NF-κB was shown to repress inflammatory cytokine (TNF, IL-1) genes[15–17] and actions, since cytokines are not only under the control of, but also induce NF-κB.[18,19] It was also shown that glucocorticoids can inhibit the NF-κB activity, and thus cytokine expression, without physical association, inducing the synthesis of the inhibitor I-κB.[18, 20]

We studied the molecular interaction of immune activators (cytokines and T-cell receptor [TCR]) with the GR in different cellular models in which glucocorticoids exert a key regulatory action: (1) cellular targets of TNF-induced cytotoxicity; (2) the pituitary gland; (3) thymic cells.

INTERACTION OF INFLAMMATORY CYTOKINES WITH GLUCOCORTICOIDS IN CELLULAR TARGETS OF TNF-INDUCED CYTOTOXICITY

Inflammatory cytokines (TNF-α and IL-1) increase the glucocorticoid-induced transcriptional activity of the GR via the DNA-glucocorticoid response elements (GREs) in cells transfected with a glucocorticoid-inducible reporter plasmid. The TNF-α effect is absent in other cell lines that express TNF-α receptors, but not GRs, and is manifest when a GR expression vector is cotransfected, indicating that TNF-α, independent of any effect it may have on GR number, has a direct stimulatory effect on the glucocorticoid-induced transcriptional activity. TNF-α and IL-1 exert the stimulatory action in different types of cells such as glioma, fibroblastic and epithelioid cells, showing that the above described interaction is a general molecular mechanism for TNF/IL-1/GR target cells.[21] This enhancement is very likely the result of a balance between the activation by this cytokine/GRE loop and inhibition through the induction of I-κB synthesis[18,20] and the formation of NFκB/GR complexes.[15–17] Particularly on L929 fibroblastic cells we observe an enhancement of I-κB synthesis by TNF-α or glucocorticoids. However, the anti-apoptotic effect of glucocorticoids in cells transfected with a super-repressor I-κB plasmid is of the same range, indicating that the anti-apoptotic effect of glucocorticoids in these cells does not involve NF-κB but rather GRE target genes. In this context, as a functional physiological correlate of the enhancement of GRE transactivation, priming of fibroblastic cells with a low dose of TNF significantly increases the sensitivity to glucocorticoid inhibition of TNF-induced apoptosis.

INTERACTION OF IL-1 AND GLUCOCORTICOIDS
ON PITUITARY CORTICOTROPHIC CELLS

AtT-20 corticotrophic mouse cells express proopiomelanocortin (POMC) gene and secrete ACTH, both being under glucocorticoid inhibition. In addition, AtT-20 cells express functionally IL-1 receptors,[22] constituting an excellent model for studying IL-1/GR molecular and functional interaction. In these cells, IL-1 stimulates the increased glucocorticoid-induced transcriptional activity of the GR via the GRE. Moreover, the inhibition of ACTH secretion and POMC promoter activity by glucocorticoids is enhanced when the cells are primed with IL-1. This action is also observed in primary cultures of corticotrophs obtained from pituitary adenomas from Cushing patients. These corticotrophs are resistant to glucocorticoid inhibition and become more sensitive to the inhibition when cells are cultured with IL-1, showing a physiological consequence of the molecular interaction that enhances GRE activity.

INTERACTION OF THE T-CELL RECEPTOR AND GLUCOCORTICOIDS
IN THE REGULATION OF THYMIC APOPTOSIS

Activation through T-cell receptor (TCR) with anti-CD3 antibodies (mimicking TCR engagement) and glucocorticoid-induced apoptotic pathways are mutually antagonistic in T-cell hybridomas.[23–24]

T-cell hybridomas transfected with reporter plasmids to assess transcriptional activity levels of factors that bind GRE and κB sites show that anti-CD3 stimulation (which antagonizes GC-mediated apoptosis) decreases GRE-driven activity induced by GC, and that κB-like activity induced by anti-CD3 is modestly changed in the presence of two different inhibitors of anti-CD3-induced apoptosis (glucocorticoids and cAMP). Thus, TCR blockade of glucocorticoid-induced apoptosis involves primarily the inhibition of GRE-regulated genes.

GENERAL CONCLUSIONS

Cross-coupling of distinct pathways in certain situations may repress gene transcription, but in others may activate gene expression. In some physiological situations (cellular targets for inflammatory cytokines), the regulatory loop whereby cytokine transduction signals cross-talk with the GR may result in an enhancement of the transcriptional activity of these nuclear hormone receptors, as occurs in anterior pituitary corticotrophs and targets for TNF action. The above-mentioned interaction between cytokines and glucocorticoids represents a molecular level of their physiological interaction: cytokines enhance GRE on glucocorticoid-responsive genes, making them more susceptible to glucocorticoid regulation and glucocorticoids inhibit cytokine overexpression and biological action. Cytokines modulate the transcriptional activity of glucocorticoid receptors, thus potentiating the counter-regulation by glucocorticoids at the level of their target cells.

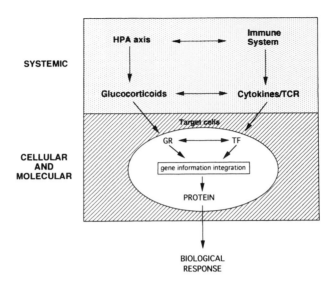

FIGURE 1. Cross-talk of activated GR and transcription factors integrates neuroendocrine-immune information. The interaction between immune mediators (cytokines and T-cell receptor) and glucocorticoids represents a molecular level of their physiological interaction. The functional cross-talk at the molecular level of immune signals and glucocorticoids on many target cells constitutes a general mechanism and is essential to determine the homeostatic biological response.GR, Glucocorticoid receptor; TF, transcription factors.

In another physiological situation, stimulation of the TCR dampens GRE-regulated genes, thus regulating the apoptotic response.

The functional cross-talk at the molecular level of immune signals and glucocorticoids is essential to determine the biological response to both mediators and constitutes the ultimate level of interaction between the immune and neuroendocrine mediators (see FIGURE 1).

ACKNOWLEDGMENTS

This work was supported by grants from the Volkswagen Foundation Germany (I / 74 149), the University of Buenos Aires (UBA), the CONICET, and Agencia Nacional de Promoción Científica y Tecnológica-Argentina.

REFERENCES

1. BESEDOVSKY, H., A. DEL REY, E. SORKIN & C.A. DINARELLO. 1986. Immunoregulatory feedback between interleukin-1 and glucocorticoid hormones. Science **233:** 652–654.
2. SAPOLSKY, R., C. RIVIER, G. YAMAMOTO, P. PLOTSKY & W. VALE. 1987. Interleukin-1 stimulates the secretion of hypothalamic corticotropin-releasing factor. Science **238:** 22–24.

3. SNYDER, D.S. & E.R. UNANUE. 1982. Corticosteroids inhibit murine macrophage Ia expression and interleukin 1 production. J. Immunol. **129:** 1803–1805.

4. GILLIS, S., G.R. CRABTREE & K. SMITH. 1979. Glucocorticoid-induced inhibition of T-cell growth factor production. I. The effect of mitogen-induced lymphocyte proliferation. J. Immunol. **123:** 1624–1631.

5. CUPPS, T.R. & A.S. FAUCI. 1982. Corticosteroid-mediated immunoregulation in man. Immunol. Rev. **65:** 133–155.

6. BEUTLER, B., N. KROCHIN, I.W. MILSARK, C. LUEDKE & A. CERAMI. 1986. Control of cachectin (tumor necrosis factor) synthesis: mechanisms of endotoxin resistance. Science **232:** 977–980.

7. ARZT, E., J. SAUER, T. POLLMÄCHER, M. LABEUR, F. HOLSBOER, J. REUL & G.K. STALLA. 1994. Glucocorticoids suppress interleukin-1 receptor antagonist synthesis following induction by endotoxin. Endocrinology **134:** 672–677.

8. KARIN, M., L. ZHENG-GANG & E. ZANDI. 1997. 1997. AP-1 function and regulation. Curr. Opinion Cell Biol. **9:** 240–246.

9. VACCA, A., M.P. FELLI, A.R. FARINA, S. MARTINOTTI, M. MARODER, I. SCREPANTI, D. MECO, E. PETRANGELI, L. FRATI & A. GULINO. 1992. Glucocorticoid receptor-mediated suppression of the interleukin-2 gene expression through impairment of the cooperativity between nuclear factor of activated T cells and AP-1 enhancer elements. J. Exp. Med. **175:** 637–646.

10. LUCIBELLO, F.C., E.P. SLATER, K.U. JOOSS, M. BEATO & R. MÜLLER. 1990. Mutual transrepression of Fos and the glucocorticoid receptor: involvement of a functional domain in Fos which is absent in FosB. EMBO J. **9:** 2827–2834.

11. DIAMOND, M.I., J.N. MINER, S.K. YOSHINAGA & K.R. YAMAMOTO. 1990. Transcription factor interactions: selectors of positive or negative regulation from a single DNA element. Science **249:** 1266–1272.

12. JONAT, G., H.J. RAHMSDORF, K.-K. PARK, A.C.B. CATO, S. GEBEL, H. PONTA & P. HERRLICH. 1990. Antitumor promotion and anti-inflammation: down-modulation of AP-1 (Fos/Jun) activity by glucocorticoid hormone. Cell **62:** 1189–1204.

13. YANG-YEN, H.F., J.C. CHAMBARD, Y.L. SUN, T. SMEAL, T.J. SCHIMDT, J. DROUIN & M. KARIN. 1990. Transcriptional interference between c-Jun and the glucocorticoid receptor: mutual inhibition of DNA binding due to direct protein-protein interaction. Cell **62:** 1205–1215.

14. VERMA, I.M., J.K. STEVENSON, E.M. SCHWARZ, E.M., VAN ANTWERP & D. MIYAMOTO. 1995. S. Rel/NFκB/IκB family: intimate tales of association and disociation. Gen. Dev. **9:** 2723–2735.

15. RAY, A. & K.E. PREFONTAINE. 1994. Physical association and functional antagonism between the p65 subunit of transcription factor NF-κB and the glucocorticoid receptor. Proc. Natl. Acad. Sci. USA **91:** 752–756.

16. SCHEINMAN, R.I., A. GUALBERTO, C.M. JEWELL, J.A. CIDLOWSKI, & A.S. BALDWIN, JR. 1995. Characterization of mechanisms involved in transrepression of NF-κB by activated glucocorticoid receptors. Mol. Cell. Biol. **15:** 943–953.

17. CALDENHOVEN, E., J. LIDEN, S. WISSINK, A. VAN DE STOLPE, J. RAAIJMAKERS, L. KOENDERMAN, S. OKRET, J.-A. GUSTAFSSON, & P.T. VAN DER SAAG. 1995. Negative cross-talk between RelA and the glucocorticoid receptor: a possible mechanism for the anti-inflammatory action of glucocorticoids. Mol. Endocrinol. **9:** 401–412.

18. SCHEINMAN, R.I., P.C. COGSWELL, A.K. LOFQUIST & A.S. BALDWIN, JR. 1995. Role of transcriptional activation of IκB in mediation of immunosuppression by glucocorticoids. Science **270:** 283–286.

19. BARBARA, J.A.J., W.B. SMITH, J.R. GAMBLE, X. VAN OSTADE, P. VANDENABEELE, J. TAVERNIER, W. FIERS, M.A. VADAS & A.F. LOPEZ. 1994. Dissociation of TNF-α cytotoxic and proinflammatory activities by p55 receptor and p75 receptor-selective TNF-α mutants. EMBO J. **13:** 843–850.

20. AUPHAN, N., J.A. DIDONATO, C. ROSETTE, A. HELMBERG & M. KARIN. 1995. Immunosuppression by glucocorticoids: Inhibition of NFκB activity through induction of IκB synthesis. Science **270:** 286–290.

21. COSTAS, M., T. TRAPP, M. PÁEZ PEREDA, J. SAUER, R. RUPPRECHT, V. NAHMOD, J. REUL, F. HOLSBOER & E. ARZT. 1996. Molecular and functional evidence for in vitro cytokine enhancement of human and murine target cell sensitivity to glucocorticoids: TNF-α priming increases glucocorticoid inhibition of TNF-α-induced cytotoxicity/apoptosis J. Clin. Invest. **98:** 1409–1416.
22. BRISTULF, J., A. SIMONCSITS & T. BARTFAI. 1991. Characterization of a neuronal interleukin 1 receptor and the corresponding mRNA in the mouse anterior pituitary cell line AtT-20. Neurosci Lett. **128:** 173–176.
23. IWATA, M., S. HNAOKA & S. KAZUKI. 1991. Rescue of thymocytes and T cell hybridomas from glucocorticoid-induced apoptosis by stimulation via the T cell receptor/CD3 complex: a possible in vitro model for positive selection of the T cell repertoire. Eur. J. Immunol. **21:** 643–648.
24. ZACHARCHUK, C.M., M. MERCEP, P. CHAKRABORTI, S.S. SIMONS & J.D. ASHWELL. 1990. Programmed T lymphocyte death: cell activation and steroid-induced pathways are mutually antagonistic. J. Immunol. **145:** 4037–4045.

Gender, Neuroendocrine–Immune Interactions and Neuron–Glial Plasticity

Role of Luteinizing Hormone-Releasing Hormone (LHRH)

BIANCA MARCHETTI,[a,b] FRANCESCO GALLO,[b] ZELINDA FARINELLA,[b]
CATALDO TIROLO,[b] NUCCIO TESTA,[b] SALVO CANIGLIA,[b]
AND MARIA C. MORALE[b]

[a]Department of Pharmacology and Gynecology, Medical School,
University of Sassari, 07100 Sassari, Italy

[b]Neuropharmacology, OASI Institute for Research and Care (IRCCS) on
Mental Retardation and Brain Aging, Troina (EN), Italy

ABSTRACT: Signals generated by the hypothalamic–pitutary–gonadal (HPG) axis powerfully modulate immune system function. This article summarizes some aspects of the impact of gender in neuroendocrine immunomodulation. Emphasis is given to the astroglial cell compartment, defined as a key actor in neuroendocrine immune communications. In the brain, the principal hormones of the HPG axis directly interact with astroglial cells. Thus, luteinizing hormone releasing hormone, LHRH, influences hypothalamic astrocyte development and growth, and hypothalamic astrocytes direct LHRH neuron differentiation. Hormonally induced changes in neuron–glial plasticity may dictate major changes in CNS output, and thus actively participate in sex dimorphic immune responses. The impact of gender in neuroimmunomodulation is further underlined by the sex dimorphism in the expression of genes encoding for neuroendocrine hormones and their receptors within the thymus, and by the potent modulation exerted by circulating sex steroids during development and immunization. The central role of glucocorticoids in the interactive communication between neuroendocrine and immune systems, and the impact of gender on hypothalamic–pituitary–adrenocortical (HPA) axis modulation is underscored in transgenic mice expressing a glucocorticoid receptor antisense RNA.

INTRODUCTION

The development and functioning of the nervous, endocrine and immune systems is known to be powerfully influenced by the signals generated by the hypothalamic-pituitary-gonadal (HPG) axis. Indeed, gender-dependent differences of neuroanatomic structures and neurotransmitter and neuropeptidergic innervation and function

[a]Address for correspondance: Bianca Marchetti, Ph.D., Department of Pharmacology, Medical School, University of Sassari, Viale S. Pietro 43/B, 07100 Sassari, Italy. Voice: 01139/0935-936111, ext. 6438; fax: 01139/0935-653-327.

bianca.marchetti@oasi.en.it

are generally responsible for the known sex-dimorphic responses of nervous, endocrine, and immune axes. The biology of reproduction has a major impact on women's lives.The passage from childhood to womanhood is marked by a flow of blood from the uterus. Menstruation is the visible stage of the ovarian cycle, orchestrated primarily by the chief hormone governing reproduction, luteinizing hormone-releasing hormone (LHRH) and by hormones secreted by the pituitary (the gonadotropic hormones, LH and FSH) and ovaries (estrogens and progesterone). A cardinal physiological feature of a living organism resides in its reproductive capacity, essential for species perpetuation, and requires precisely modulated communications between the neuroendocrine and immune systems. Evidence accumulated in the last decades has clearly documented the vital importance of interacting neuroendocrine-immune networks in the regulation of physiological homeostatic mechanisms.[1–13] Within the reproductive system, the early studies of Calzolari[14] almost a century ago, followed by subsequent intuitions of Besedowski[15] and Pierpaoli[16] and more recently others,[17–24] have shown the brain-pituitary-reproductive axis and the brain thymus-lymphoid axis to communicate via an array of internal mechanisms of communication that use similar signals (neurotransmitters, peptides, growth factors, hormones) acting on similar recognition targets (the receptors). Moreover, such communication networks form the basis for the controls of each step and every level of reproductive physiology. The principal conveying signal is LHRH, the key reproductive hormone coordinating the major features of mammalian reproduction (see FIGURE 1). Indeed, from the initiation of a sexually organized response, the detection of sexual odors and the induction of mating behavior, extrahypothalamic and hypothalamic LHRH orchestrates the neuroendocrine modulation of gonadotropin secretion, while its expression within the ovary may directly modulate specific events such as follicular atresia.[25] The presence of LHRH receptors in oocytes[26] may anticipate a potential role of the decapeptide also during the process of fertilization and/or implantation. There are also some specific mechanisms responsible for protecting the mammalian embryo against the potentially hostile immunological maternal environment.[10,27–29] Interestingly, these mechanisms appear to vary according to the different stages of reproduction, from fertilization to implantation and to full development of the fetus. They are also unique since they vary from species to species and result from exceptional genetic and immunological processes.[10,27–29]

Further appreciation of how integrated are the reproductive and immune systems may came from the realization that the "quality" and "intensity" of a coordinated neuroendocrine (NEI) response strictly depends on gender and the integrity of the hypothalamic-pituitary-adrenocortical axis (HPA) axis, in addition to other variables (which may include age, genetic vulnerability, or pathological conditions). Indeed, the neurophysiological and biochemical events that are set into motion when the HPA axis is activated during stressful situations interact remarkably with the specific sex-steroid and immunological backgrounds. A complex interplay between genotype, the circulating gonadal and adrenal hormones, the intrinsic capability to respond to stressful (including inflammatory) stimuli, coupled with a specific immunological setting, may then determine a "major" or "minor" vulnerability to several disease entities, such as psychiatric, neurological or immunological disorders.[7,30–35] In both medicine, and especially in psychiatry, the gender-differentiated predispositions to a number of illnessses are historically exemplified by the sex difference in

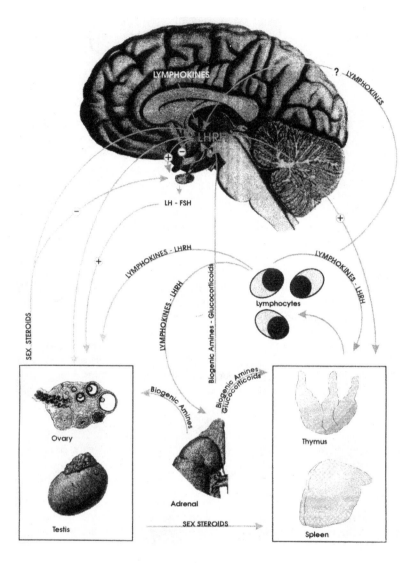

FIGURE 1. Schematic representation of the possible interactions between the hypothalamus-hypophyseal-gonadal axis and the thymus, with LHRH serving as a major channel of communication. Hypothalamic LHRH governs the release of the pituitary gonadotropins LH and FSH, responsible for gonadal production of the sex steroids. The gonadal hormones in turn feed back information to the thymus and hypothalamus. At the thymus level, sex steroids act on specific receptors present on the reticulo-epithelial matrix, and induce both up- and downregulation of target genes involved in the control of T-cell response. On the other hand, the sex steroid background alters the production of thymic peptides (thymosins) and neuropeptides such as LHRH, with autocrine/paracrine regulatory influence within the thymic microenvironment. The direct neural pathways innervating immune and endocrine organs together with the modulatory influence of glucocorticoids and catecholamines are also shown.

the prevalence of depression in women, the vulnerability associated with oral contraceptives, abortion, the premenstrual period, the puerpuerium, and the menopause.[36] By acting on the neuroendocrine and immune systems during the stress response, life events may greatly affect homeostasis and favor the appearance of disease. One of the best example of such psychoimmune-neuroendocrine circuit was revealed by Galen, in approximately 200 A.D., when he observed an increased susceptibility to breast cancer in melancholic women compared to sanguine women. If women are currently thought at higher risk than men to develop certain psychiatric disorders, and the majority of autoimmune disorders, the female sex, however, has a certain number of "biochemical atouts," the potential of which is just starting to be clarified. An abundance of experimental literature has established that the major signals of the HPG axis, the gonadal hormones, are responsible not only for the sexual differentiation of neural circuitry, which mediates a variety of reproductive behaviors and physiological mechanisms, but also for the generation of the sexually driven immunological dimorphisms, as well as the sex-linked differential response of the HPA axis. Interestingly enough, nowdays the female hormones, estrogens, have received increased attention and consideration due to the demonstration of their "beneficial/buffering"—in a word, neuroprotective—effects.[37-40] The precise underlying biochemical and molecular mechanism(s) are, however, far from being completely disclosed, but besides others, their crucial interaction at the neuroendocrine-immune interface may represent a future challenge for this third millennium. In such a scenario, it seems necessary to consider another actor that has been shown to came into play—the brain astrocytic compartment.[43,44] Indeed, astrocytes are elements of the CNS that share with the neuronal, endocrine, and immune cells, similar recognition and transduction capabilities, and that represent key entities during the development of the CNS, in the adult brain as well as during aging and aging-associated diseases such as neurodegenerative disorders.[37-40] It is, thus, not surprising that the HPG axis (and specifically LHRH and estrogens) powerfully and dynamically interact with the astroglial compartment,[41,42] thus realizing a further level of NEI integration.

This paper concentrates on the impact of gender on neuroendocrine-immunomodulation with a major focus on LHRH-driven dimorphisms. The ability of LHRH and estrogens to modulate the activity of neuroendocrine, immune, and glial cells will be reviewed with a major emphasis on hormonally induced neuron-glial plasticity. Different dynamic "*in vitro*" models together with a number of pharmacological tools are proposed to unravel the LHRH–glial relationship at the biochemical and cellular levels. A key regulatory function of astroglia in the differentiation and maturation of the LHRH neuron is suggested on the basis of such experimental paradigms.[41-49] Emphasis will be given to the HPG–HPA interactions in mediating gender differences in immunological responses. Finally, the impact of a dysfunctional HPA system in a transgenic mouse model expressing a glucocorticoid receptor (GR) antisense RNA, for the programming of NEI functions and potential vulnerability to neuromental and autoimmune diseases, are briefly summarized.

GENDER, NEURON–GLIA INTERACTIONS, AND LHRH:
A NEW LEVEL OF NEUROENDOCRINE IMMUNOMODULATION

LHRH-Driven Sexually Dimorphic Responses

The key events underlying gender differences within the HPG axis are dynamically orchestrated by the chief reproductive hormone, LHRH, interacting with specific receptors located in the neuroendocrine-immune-reproductive axis. Indeed, LHRH, a decapeptide manufactured by highly specialized neuroendocrine cells, is the key regulator of the hypothalamic-hypophyseal-gonadal axis and is essential for reproductive competence.[50] This hormone regulates the release of luteinizing hormone (LH) and follicle-stimulating hormone (FSH) from the gonadotropic cells of the anterior pituitary gland.[50,51] Hypothalamic LHRH, released into portal capillaries that perfuse the anterior pituitary, drives the menstrual cycle by stimulation of pituitary LH and FSH. There is a growing recognition that a network of neurons that elaborate three classes of messenger molecules—the classical aminergic neurotransmitters, the amino acids, and the neuropeptides—regulate the secretion of the trigger for the preovulatory surge of pituitary LH secretion on proestrus[51] (see FIGURE 2). The discussion of the intricate interplay between each of these neural components in the control of LHRH release is beyond the scope of this review. However, it is quite apparent that the peptidergic signaling is crucial for the accelerated discharge of LHRH into the hypophyseal portal system in proestrus (FIG. 2). A local hypothalamic network composed of diverse peptidergic signals regulates episodic LHRH secretion and is directly subject to regulation by gonadal steroids.[50] The primary action of steroids is to facilitate the output of peptide signals and to amplify/adjust their postsynaptic responses in a timely fashion. At a central level, sex steroids interact with both aminergic and peptidergic signals, resulting in appropriate and timely coordinated release of pulses of LHRH. The effect of sex steroids and of other modulators such as prolactin and opioids, may also occur at the anterior pituitary level, via an action on the pituitary LHRH receptor system[52–56] (FIG. 2). A further level of control is represented by the ability of the decapeptide to directly modulate its own secretion via an ultra-short feedback mechanism, by exerting both stimulatory and inhibitory actions in LHRH neuronal cells depending on its concentration and duration.[57]

On the other hand, besides the regulation of LHRH secretion at the level of LHRH cell bodies or terminals at the median eminence (ME), LHRH may locally be modulated by dynamic relationships among neuron terminals, glia and basal lamina, as demonstrated for oxytocin and vasopressin.[58] Accordingly, different interplays between products of the astroglial cell compartment (such as growth factors), the neuronal terminals, and the hormonal background may be envisaged, according to the particular reproductive (i.e., specific sex steroid priming) condition (FIG. 2).

Astroglia Is a Key Actor in Neuroendocrine–Immune Communications

Knowledge on neuroglia has rapidly accumulated in the last decades, and an extraordinary body of evidence has now been assembled by different investigators from all fields of neuroscience, supporting a key role role for glia in neuronal physiopathology. Indeed, at nearly a century and a half from the time of development of

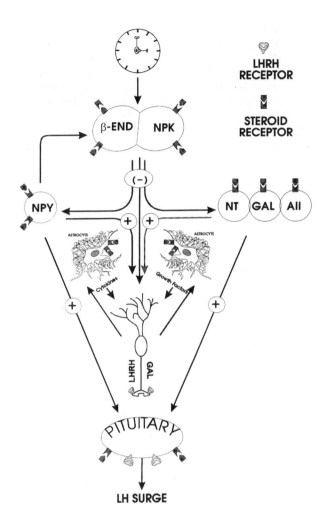

FIGURE 2. Schematic representation of hypothalamic peptidergic and aminergic signals together with integrating environmental factors and hypophyseal-mediated mechanisms in the control of the episodic discharge of LHRH. The possible interference of endogenously produced cytokines is also illustrated. The model includes the LHRH pulse generator, the neural elements (the clock) regulating directly the activity of this generator, and those elements involved in its indirect regulation via the negative feedback action of gonadal steroids, as reviewed by Kalra.[51] Around this unit are also pictured a number of other important factors modulating the phasic LHRH discharge leading to the preovulatory LH surge and ovulation including a number of neuropeptides, such as the opioid peptides, NPY, galanin and neurotensin, with both positive and negative effects. A modulatory influence is represented by the action of sex steroids impinging in this circuitry at both central and peripheral (hypophyseal level) via estrogen receptors, as well as by modifications in the number of pituitary LHRH receptors[53–55] responsible for alterations in the sensitivity of the gonadotropes to LHRH. Besides the classical aminergic and peptidergic reulation at the level of LHRH cell bodies/terminals, the dynamic interactions between LHRH neurons and astroglial cells is also depicted.

knowledge about neuron–glia interactions,[59] the possibility of signals passing from neurons to glial cells, and thus to other neurons, opens up many scenarios for inter-cellular/intracellular cross-talk within single cells of the CNS (see FIGURE 3). The functioning of the nervous system depends upon a continous and sophisticated inter-relationship between neuronal and glial cells. It is not surprising, then, that neuron–glia interactions are involved in the plastic response of the immune system to differ-ent neuroendocrine and/or immune challenges.

There are two broad subgroups of glial cells: the macroglia, which consist of astrocytes, oligodendrocytes, and ependymal cells, and the microglia. In recent years, an array of neurotransmitters, receptors, ion channels, adhesion molecules, and trophic factors have been revealed to be associated with glial cells. An important factor in neuron–astroglial cell interactions is that glia in different brain regions express region-specific properties, including ion channels, neurotransmitter uptake and receptor systems, GF production, and cell-surface adhesion systems.[59] Then, the

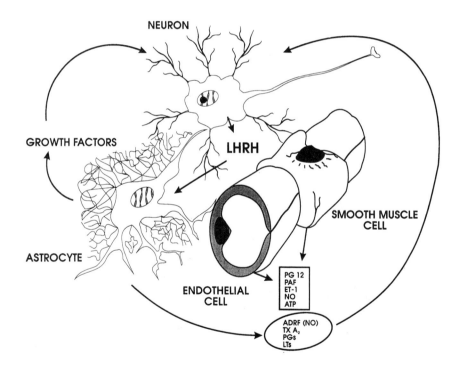

FIGURE 3. Dynamic interaction between the astroglial cell compartment, the endothe-lial cell, and the LHRH neurons. Upon selective stimulation astrocytes may release products able to alter the vascular endothelium. The expression of receptors on astrocytes, their abil-ity to synthesize vasoactive products, and the close spatial relationships of these cells, both with neurons and cell of the vasculature, implicate astroglial cells in bidirectional signaling processes in the CNS. PG, prostaglandin; PAF, platelet activating factor; TXA_2, trombox-ane; NO, nitric oxide; ATP, adenosine triphosphate; ADRF (NO), astrocyte-derived (vaso)-relaxing factor (nitric oxide).

particular nature of the neuronal–glial interaction may depend on the specific neuronal and glial systems involved in a specific brain region. Thus, the dynamics of the cross-talk between neurons and astrocytes appears to be very complex. Neurons and glial cells are likely to be exposed to a number of different extracellular signaling molecules that may vary from moment to moment, and as a function of the particular physiological status (sex, age, stressful situation, immune system activation). Therefore, a sophisticated regulatory network is likely to orchestrate the final appropriate response of both cell types. In the present work we will focus on some of the factors that contribute to the neuron–astroglial signaling, namely steroid hormones and LHRH.

Sex Steroids and Adrenocortical Hormones as Mediators of Neuron–Glia Plasticity: Role of Gender

The role of the sex steroid milieu in the glial microenvironment, has been established, especially by the work of Garcia-Segura *et al.* and other investigators,[60–69] demonstrating that the steroid background is crucial in inducing morphological as well as functional changes of the astroglial cell compartment. In response to estrogens, astrocytes appear to participate in the remodelling of synaptic contacts on hypothalamic neurons that control the release of pituitary secretions in rodents and primates.[63–66] This work is substantiated by findings indicating that the morphology, immunoreactivity, enzymatic activity, and gene expression of astroglia are sexually dimorphic in several brain areas and are modified by different *in vivo/in vitro* experimental manipulations of circulating sex steroids. Glial cells have been shown to harbor receptors for estradiol and progesterone,[63–67] and estradiol is able to induce the appearance of progesterone receptors. In particular, oligodendrocytes, are known to be capable of synthesizing steroids such as pregnenolone and progesterone, and evidences have been presented for the presence of receptors for these hormones on cultured cells.[67,68] Astrocytes were found to possess very few progesterone receptors (PRs); confined to cells derived from female animals.[69] Estradiol has been shown to induce coordinated modifications in the extension of glial and neuronal processes in the arcuate nucleus of the hypothalamus. This hormonal effect results in natural fluctuations in the ensheathing of the arcuate neurons by glial processes and these glial changes are linked to a remodelling of inhibitory GABAergic synapses during the estrous cycle.[61,62]

Studying LHRH neuron–astroglia interactions, we have recently found distinct differences in GFAP- and LHRH-immunopositive fiber tracks during the reproductive cycle, culminating with dramatic changes in LHRH neuron–glia networks in the afternoon of proestrus, in coincidence with the preovulatory LHRH surge. When primary astroglial cell cultures are established, *in vitro,* their sensitivity to 17-beta estradiol varies according to gender, the specific CNS region, the "age" of astroglia (days in culture), and as a function of the specific stimulus/signal (hormones, growth factors) applied.[71] There is abundant evidence that cultured glia possess corticosteroid receptors. Adrenal steroids activate two classes of intracellular receptors, the mineralcorticoid (MR) or type I receptor, and the glucocortioid (GR) or type II receptor.[72] These receptor classes can be distinguished on the basis of the MR's displaying a higher affinity for corticosterone than does the GR, which preferentially binds synthetic glucocorticoids such as dexamethasone.[72] Ligand binding studies have demonstrated the presence of a single population of GRs in both astrocytes and oligodendrocytes.[73,74] Glucocorticoids are known to modulate the expression of a variety of glial proteins, including GFAP, glutamine synthetase (GS), myelin basic protein (MBP), and glycerol phosphate dehydrogenase. Using an *in vitro* model of developing neonatal rat glial cell, we studied developmental expression of GRs as a function of time in culture and showed low levels of GR mRNA expressed at eight days *in vitro* (DIV) with a progressive increase between 12 and 20 DIV and a plateau reaching thereafter, with the mRNA remaining elevated up to 50 DIV.[77] In the intact brain, glial cells have been shown to respond to glucocorticoids.[78] The role of adrenal hormones on GFAP expression has been extensively studied in the last few years, and glucocorticoids appear to powerfully modulate GFAP expression both *in vivo* and *vitro*.[78]

The capability of endogenous sex steroids and glucocorticoid background to powerfully interact with the astroglial cell compartment, may thus be crucial to modulate a sex-dimorphic immune response also via changes in neuron–glial interactions.

THE LHRH NEURON–ASTROGLIA CONNECTION

Astroglia Support LHRH Neuronal Function

In the adult rodent, LHRH is synthesized by diffusely organized forebrain neurons which are scattered over a continuum extending from the septal region anteriorly to the premamillary area (the heaviest concentration being in the anterior hypothalamus, the preoptic area, and the septum), with fibers projecting not only to the median eminence but also through the hypothalamus and midbrain. During this passage, LHRH neurons are known to interact with many types of neurons and glia. Indeed, the architecture of the arcuate nucleus of the hypothalamus is unique in the arrangement of the glial cells within it. Tanycytes, specialized ependymal cells, line the ventricular wall and send their processes in an arching trajectory toward the surface of the brain.[79] Astrocytes of varying morphologies are also located in this region.[80–82] The contribution of glial elements to LHRH axonal targeting was suggested by the early experiments of Kozlowski and Coates,[83] demonstrating the existence of ependymal tunnels and their association with LHRH axons. More recently, relationships of glia to LHRH axonal outgrowth from third ventricular grafts in hypogonadal mice have been described by Silverman and coworkers.[84] Due to the absence of a functional gene for the neuropeptide LHRH, the hypogonadal (hpg) mice have an infantile reproductive tract in adulthood, a condition that can be reversed by the implantation of normal fetal preoptic area tissue that contains LHRH neurons. Interestingly enough LHRH axons were found adjacent to glial elements along their entire traverse from the graft–host interface, and appeared to exit via glial channels.[84] Glial processes seem to provide a permissive substrate for LHRH axonal extension and the presence of chemotropic factors specific for the region of the median eminence underlie the accurate navigation of the growing axon, as has been suggested by Silverman and collaborators.[84] The fact that LHRH axons display a remarkable degree of outgrowth during a time of extensive glial hypertrophy and hyperplasia suggests that the glia may play a facilitatory or permissive role in this particular system.[84] Then, in view of the high requirement for signaling environmental conditions to the LHRH neuronal system, and due to the paucity of synaptic inputs to the LHRH neurons, it seems reasonable to hypothesize that LHRH–astroglial interactions may play a key role in the successful decodification and transduction of appropriate signals from the different regions involved in the control of LHRH release (FIGS. 2 and 3).

Sex Steroids, Growth Factors, LHRH and Neuron–Glial Plasticity

On the basis of electron microscopic results King and Letourneau [85] have noted that LHRH terminals in the median eminence (ME) undergo dramatic changes after gonadal hormone withdrawal, and a possible direct action of "intervening non-neuronal (glial) elements," of the ME has been suggested.[85] Kohama and coworkers[86] have recently demonstrated that glial fibrillary acidic protein (GFAP), the main component of the intermediate filaments in cells of astroglial lineage, increases during proestrus in astrocytes of the hypothalamic arcuate nucleus (ARC). Moreover, these changes were associated with altered astrocyte–neuron contacts and synaptic remodelling during preparation for the preovulatory gonadotropin surge.[86] Interestingly enough, hypothalamic distribution of astrocytes is gender-related.[87] The exquisite interpaly between the circulating gonadal hormones and LHRH–neuron–glial interactions is illustrated by the intricate and interconnected network we have recently shown to occur between GFAP- and LHRH-immunopositive fibers during the estrous cycle, culminating in the afternoon of proestrus.

Finch and coworkers have also recently found evidence that GFAP in the thalamus and hypothalamus increases with reproductive aging,[88] while food restriction delays the age-related increase in GFAP mRNA expression in the hypothalamus.[89] Finally, the development of astrocytes immunoreactive for GFAP in the MBH of hypogonadal mice revealed a marked increase for the glial fibrillary protein.[90] Finally, studies of Ojeda and collaborators[91–94] have documented a key role of astroglia-derived factors in the stimulation of LHRH release and induction of precocious puberty after lesions of the female rat hypothalamus.

Cell–Cell Mechanisms and Soluble Mediators Are Involved in LHRH Neuron–Astroglia Interactions in Vitro

We have used the GT1 cell line[95–97] and primary cultures of astroglial cells and assessed different dynamic models to unravel LHRH–astroglia interactions.[41,42,45–49] From the bulk of our information, LHRH–astroglial cell interactions have been proposed as a prototype for the study of neuroimmune communication within the CNS in the light of (*a*) the commonality of signal molecules (hormones, neurotransmitters, and cytokines) and transduction mechanisms shared by glia, LHRH neuron, and lymphoid cells; (*b*) the central role of glia in the developmental organization and pattern of LHRH neuronal migration during embryogenesis; and (*c*) the strong modulatory role played by sex steroids in mechanisms involved in synaptic and interneuronal organization, as well as in the sexual dimorphisms of neuroendocrine-immune functions.

During their maturation and differentiation *in vitro,* astroglial cells release factors able to accelerate markedly LHRH neuronal phenotypic differentiation as well as the acquisition of mature LHRH secretory potential, with a potency depending on both the "age" and the specific brain localization of the astroglia, as well as the degree of LHRH neuronal differentiation *in vitro*.[41,42,45,48] Different experimental paradigms, such as co-culture and mixed culture models between the immortalized LHRH (GT_{1-1}) neuronal cell line and astroglial cells in primary culture, disclosed the presence of a bidirectional flow of informational molecules regulating both proliferative and secretory capacities of each cell type. Indeed, co-culture with pure LHRH neurons dramatically influenced hypothalamic astrocyte morphology and proliferation,[48] clearly supporting our view of the existence of a bidirectional functional interaction between LHRH neurons and astrocytes. Such regulation disclosed *in vitro* might underlie the plastic changes observed in vivo during the proestrus LHRH surge. Growth factors are key players in LHRH neuron-astroglia cross-talk.[41,42] In particular, basic fibroblast growth factor (bFGF) was identified as a major differentiation factor for the immortalized hypothalamic LHRH neuronal cell line.[41,42,48] A specific synergy/cooperation between bFGF and other growth factors was also revealed at specific stages of LHRH neuron differentiation, indicating that the sequential expression of specific growth factors may participate in the processes of LHRH neuron migration, differentiation and functional regulation.[42] Since bFGF is expressed in GT_{1-1} neurons and glial cells, a possible paracrine/autocrine regulatory loop has been suggested.

Astroglia-Derived Factors Stimulate Leukocyte Proliferation

Astrocytes and microglial cells produce a variety of cytokines, some of which may have a role during maturation and differentiation of the glial cells.[41,42] We then tested a possible immunological nature of glial soluble factors by treating thymic lymphocytes with ACM at different stages of glial differentiation. Thymocytes show a biphasic pattern of response to ACM: 8 and 12 DIV astroglial cell culture medium induced a significant increase in [^{3}H]-thymidine incorporation comparable or even greater than the one observed following a subactive dose of the lectin polyclonal mitogen, concanavalin A (Con-A, 0.3 µg/ml). At later stages of glial maturation (40 DIV) ACM produced a sharp inhibition in T-cell proliferation.

Diffusible Molecules and Cell–Cell Contacts Participate in LHRH–Astroglia Interactions

The ability of astrocytes to synthesize and release a number of prostaglandins (PGE_2, PGF_2) and tromboxane A_2 (TX) in response to arachidonic acid (AA) or calcium ionophore[42] constitutes a major link in LHRH–astroglial interactions, since PGE_2 is an obligatory component in the phasic discharge of LHRH from the mediobasal hypothalamus.[98,99] Another important connection between the LHRH neuron and astroglia is their ability to use and to produce the novel "intercellular" diffusible modulator, NO, and to express NO synthase.[41, 100–103] In the light of the host of receptors present in astrocytes, their ability to synthesize vasoactive products, and close spatial relationship of these cells both with LHRH neurons and cells of the vasculature implicate them in bidirectional signaling processes in the CNS. Signals, in turn, originating from the LHRH neurons could initiate important intracellular changes in astrocytes.[41] The resulting release of prostanoids, and nitrosyl compounds could have profound modulatory effects on the activity of the adjacent (astrocyte/neuronal) cell (FIG. 3).

Plasticity of LHRH Neuron–Astroglia Interactions during Aging: Old Glia Functional Switch under bFGF Treatment Restores Both Neurotrophic and Functional Properties of Astrocytes

Although co-culturing LHRH neurons with young astrocytes (maintained *in vitro* for 8–10 DIV) induced the described neurotrophic and functional effects, the co-culure with "old" glia (maintained in culture for 30 DIV) had significant inhibitory effects both on the growth of LHRH neurons and the release of the decapeptide in the culture medium.[48] Old glia, however, were shown to to display a considerable degree of plasticity, reverting to a growth supporting state when treated with a low dose of bFGF. Moreover, this functional shift led to the release of soluble/diffusible molecules with potent neurotrophic and functional effects on immortalized LHRH neurons.[48]

GENDER, LHRH, AND LHRH-IMMUNE INTERACTIONS

LHRH in the Hypothalamic-Pituitary-Gonadal-Thymic (HPGT) Axis

The fundamental importance of the thymus gland as regulator of reproductive capacity is reflected by the fact that the physiological development of an operative hypothalamic-hypophyseal-gonadal axis (HHGA) necessitates the presence of an intact immune system and normal immune function, since immunosuppressed or incompetent animals show numerous reproductive disorders.[5,9–11,17,20–24] Moreover, inflammatory and infectious diseases often coincide with changes in reproductive functions, including a decline in fertility, an increased incidence of spontaneous abortion, and full-term birth of abnormal progeny.[104] Conversely, hypogonadic patients with the Klinefelter's syndrome appear to have very high rates of lupus erythematosus, and hypogonadic hypogonadotropic patients (with a central deficiency of LHRH), present a number of immune abnormalities (our own unpublished observations).

The primary communication between the immune and the reproductive systems is known to involve the thymus and its peptide secretion,[16,18] and so it seems important to place the LHRH effects within the context of an hypothalamic–pituitary–gonadal–thymic axis (HPGT). Communication between the gonadal axis and the lymphoid organs has been proposed for more than a century, and the studies of Grossman and coworkers[17,23] have even emphasized the existence of such reciprocal relationship between the HHGA and the brain–thymus–lymphoid axis. A schematic representation of the possible interactions between the HHGA and the thymus, with LHRH serving as a primary channel for communication, is given in FIGURE 1 in which a bidirectional network carrying information to both the immune and the neuroendocrine reproductive systems via LHRH is depicted. Direct aminergic and peptidergic innervations of both the gonads and the immune organs[105–107] are also illustrated. While hypophyseal and gonadal hormones feed back information to the thymic cell, providing a modulatory system and regulating thymic cell maturation and thymic peptide production, the thymus and its peptide secretion (thymosin fraction 5 and one of its peptidic constituent, thymosin β4) can exert a modulation of gonadotropin secretion via direct action at the hypothalamic LHRH neuronal level.

LHRH and LHRH Receptors in Immune Organs: Biological Function

Specific LHRH binding sites are present in mouse blood lymphocytes,[19] in rat mast cells,[108] thymocyte and splenocyte[109,110] cultures, as well as in cultured porcine lymphocytes.[111] In addition, LHRH mRNA and/or LHRH-like molecules have been identified in rat thymus, in thymocyte and splenocyte cultures and in human peripheral T lymphocytes.[111–113] Moreover, by synthesizing and sequencing, the rat thymus LHRH thymocyte and hypothalamic LHRH are shown to be identical, with the sequence data obtained 5′ and 3′ to the open reading frame being also identical to hypothalamic LHRH mRNA.[111] Not only is LHRH mRNA expressed in the primary immune organ, but it also appears to be developmentally regulated.[111] Of interest, using the rat immature T-cell line Nb2, Wilson *et al.*[114] have recently reported that the LHRH gene is regulated by PRL at various times during the cell-cycle. Moreover, an alternatively spliced LHRH mRNA exists in Nb2 cells and may produce a new truncated gonadotropin-associated peptide (GAP).[114] Finally, the SH gene, found on the opposite strand of the LHRH gene, is expressed in lymphocytes at the same time and in the same manner as the LHRH gene.[114] Messenger RNA transcripts coding for the LHRH receptor were demonstrated to be present in immunologically competent cells.[112] Using reverse transcription polymerase chain reaction (RT-PCR) and RNA from Nb2 cells, the LHRH-R PCR fragment was sequenced and cloned and the DNA sequence shown to be identical to that previously described.[114] In analogy to what is observed at the anterior pituitary level for the LHRH-R protein,[55] in Nb2 cells the LHRH receptor mRNA was shown to drastically decrease immediately after PRL administration, suggesting possible paracrine regulation between the two hormones within immune cells.[114]

LHRH Coordinates the Hormonal Homeostasis during Pregnancy

The powerful action of LHRH in setting the hormonal homeostasis to high circulating levels of sex steroid hormones during pregnancy, as well as the dynamic alterations in the concentration of prolactin, cortisol, and other hormonal factors, may clearly modify immune responsiveness . The increase in sex steroids that take place in all mammalian species during pregnancy may potentially assist in preventing the maternal–fetal rejection response.[10,27,28] If this rejection response is not depressed, termination of pregnancy may take place before completion of term. However, in most pregnant women, the cell-mediated immune response is markedly depressed and pregnancy is maintained. This can also account for the observation that human skin homografts survive longer on pregnant hosts than on nonpregnant hosts. A number of reports clearly indicate that progesterone participates in the regulation of the immune response during pregnancy. As to the mechanisms of action of sex steroids in modulating immune responsiveness, the presence of receptors for estrogens and testosterone on the reticulo-epithelial matrix of the thymus and peripheral lymphocytes[23] argues in favor of a direct effect of these steroids at the level of the thymus gland.

Gender, Sex Steroids, the Thymus Gland, and the Regulation of Immune Responsiveness

Since steroid hormones mediate profound physiological and developmental effects in higher eukaryotes by interacting with their intracellular receptors in target cells, they provide mechanisms for cellular communication and alterations in phenotypic responses to environmental and internal stimuli.[10] For example, gonadal steroid hormones influence mammalian reproductive function through their action during the perinatal period, and the expression of sex-dimorphic functions in the adult is maintained by adequate levels of circulating hormones, through mechanisms poorly understood. Immunological dimorphism, as reproductive dimorphism, might depend upon two fundamental influences of gonadal steroid hormones: the first one occurring during the perinatal period, when these hormones may permanently alter the developmental pattern of thymocyte selection and turnover, and the establishment of the phenotypic (male vs. female) T-cell repertoire, resulting in permanent effects in a particular subset of T cells.[10] For instance, the development of the medullary epithelium that occurs early in ontogeny may be irreversibly modulated by the sex steroid hormone milieu, giving rise to a population of progenitor cells. The second influence of gonadal hormones may be exerted during adulthood, by maintaining the sex dimorphic immune function, through the production of adequate levels of circulating gonadal hormones.[10] Since the major mechanism of action of most steroids appear to be direct changes in the expression of target genes by altering their rates of transcription, a way to unravel the steroid mechanism of action at a molecular level is to study whether physiological changes in sex steroid levels occurring during the estrous cycle and pregnancy would alter the expression of specific genes for neuroendocrine hormones and their receptors, such as the genes of the LHRH-, β-adrenergic[115] and glucocorticoid[116] receptors (βAR, GR) in the thymus.

LHRH, LHRH Receptors, and LHRH-R mRNA during the Estrous Cycle and Pregnancy

Intrathymic LHRH system activity varies according to the phases of the estrous cycle, but more importantly a sex dimorphic pattern of LHRH synthesis accompanies the sex-dimorphic immune response during ontogeny and cyclicity (see FIGURE 4). Surprisingly enough, LHRH mRNA concentration exhibit clear sex-dependent fluctuation during the rat estrous cycle, which is accompanied by a change in thymocyte sensitivity to LHRH with a maximal response to the natural decapeptide in proestrus (see FIGURE 5). Sealfon *et al.*[117] demonstrated that estradiol and inhibin upregulate LHRH-R mRNA bioactivity in ovine anterior pituitary cell cultures, while progesterone downregulates mRNA bioactivity. Furthermore, Kaiser *et al.*[118] have reported that pulsatile LHRH administration causes a twelve-fold induction in LHRH-R mRNA in superfused primary monolayer cultures of rat pituitary cells. Thus, it is likely that the fluctuation of LHRH mRNA observed in the thymus may reflect the interplay of a number of endocrine influences on thymocytes. The fact that an LHRH-antisense is able to counteract the mitogen-induced lymphocyte proliferation clearly underlines a physiological paracrine/autocrine role of intralymphocytic LHRH in the control of lymphocyte responsiveness. The dramatic decrease in both rodent thymocyte and human peripheral blood lymphocyte response to T-dependent mitogens after ovulation coupled to the diminished lymphocyte response to LHRH in that particular reproductive phase would indicate a possible participation of LHRH in that phenomenon and that sex steroids are capable of modulating that effect. Such a mechanism is then likely to participate in the reduction of immune responsiveness observed during pregnancy.[10] It seems tempting to speculate that sex steroid, altering the expression of target genes within the thymus may modify the responsiveness of the immune cell to different hormones and neurotransmitters. Indeed, the ability of estrogens to directly alter LHRH gene expression has been demonstrated in the placenta.[10]

Gender, β-Adrenergic Receptor Gene Expression and Immunological Dimorphisms

In a previous study, using *in vitro* autoradiography, we demonstrated the presence of β_2-adrenergic receptors (β_2AR) in the rat thymus.[105,106] In the thymus norepinephrine (NE) could therefore act via the β_2AR both as a paracrine hormone available to receptors on thymic cells and as a localized transmitter in nerve terminals that directly contact cortical thymocytes, mast cells, and eosinophils to modulate immune functions. The thymic β_2ARs are preferentially found in the medullar compartment of the gland and show a clear sexual dimorphism in receptor organization during sexual maturation.[105,106] A cyclic variation receptor density accompanies the different phases of the estrous cycle, with a significant increase in receptor density observed during the period of maximal estrogenic stimulation.[105,106] The expression of a

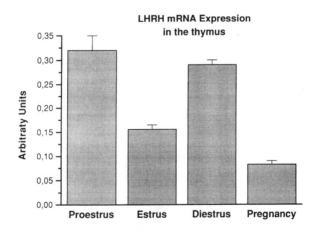

FIGURE 4. Expression of LHRH mRNA within the rat thymus gland as a function of the estrous cycle and pregnancy. Poly(A) mRNAs isolated from female rat thymus gland at the indicated reproductive phases were reverse-transcribed to cDNA and subjected to amplification by the polymerase chain reaction (PCR) after specific primer addition, electrophorized on 2% agarose gel, prepared for transfer and blotted onto nitrocellulose, as described in Ref. 73. After hybridization and washing of the filters underat high-stringency conditions, dry filters were exposed to X-ray film at $-70°C$ with enhancing screens. For quantitative PCR determinations, β-actin was used as internal control. Results represent the mean ± SEM of 2–3 thymic samples, and are expressed in arbitrary optical density units.

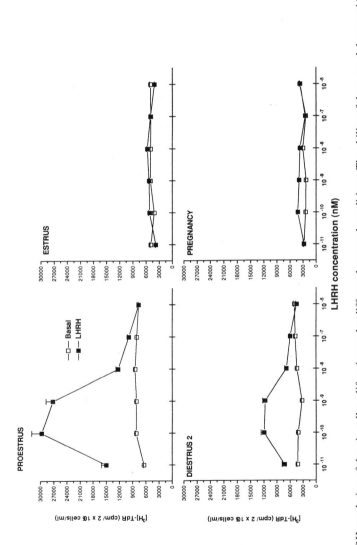

FIGURE 5. LHRH regulation of thymic cell proliferation under different hormonal conditions. The ability of the natural decapeptide LHRH to influence thymocyte proliferation under the different hormonal conditions studied was assessed in thymocyte cell preparations by the incorporation of [³H]-thymidine both in basal and stimulated (Con-A, 2.5 (g/ml) conditions. Thymic cells from the indicated hormonal conditions were prepared as described,[8] and LHRH (10^{-11} to 10^{-5}M) added to the cultures in the absence or in the presence of the T-dependent mitogen, Con-A. Results represent the mean ± SEM of quadruplicate wells, and of three individual determinations. Note the significant increase of proliferative capacity induced by LHRH on proestrus, while a marked drop of proliferative capacity was observed in estrus and pregnant thymic cell preparations.

β_2AR in the rat thymus was further confirmed by the presence in the thymic tissue of a mRNA species of 2.3 Kb which specifically hybridized with a cDNA encoding the full coding sequence of the human β_2AR.[107,115] Interestingly, the β_2AR–stimulated adenylyl cyclase is markedly modulated by the sex steroid hormone background.[115] Indeed, the β_2AR observed in the thymic tissue preparations is functionally coupled to the adenylyl cyclase system, with a sensitivity characteristic of a β_2 subtype receptor. Both a high-affinity state of the receptor for isoproterenol and an isoproterenol-stimulated adenylyl cyclase activity could be detected in the thymus membrane preparations, with the guanine nucleotide converting all of the high-affinity-state receptors into low-affinity-state receptors.[115] Furthermore, an almost 70% loss of the enzyme response to GTP followed castration, suggesting that ovarian steroids may exert potent effects on the β_2AR signalling pathway.[115] In analogy to previous results obtained in other tissues,[104] parallel changes in both β_2AR density and β_2AR mRNA levels followed the hormonal changes associated with the rat estrous cycle, pregnancy, or castration. Such quantitative changes suggest a subtype-specific hormonal regulation of the β_2AR population.[115] The results on the sex steroid-dependent modulation of βAR-stimulated cAMP accumulation and proliferation in rat thymus are consistent with other data obtained in the mammary gland, where the GTP-stimulated adenylate cyclase showed the highest activity during pregnancy.[119] Although the mechanism through which β-adrenergic stimulation alters thymocyte proliferation is unknown, one attractive possibility involves interaction at the level of second messengers. In fact, in T cells, one early transmembrane signal in response to stimulation of the T-cell receptor is the activation of phospholipase C, causing the release of inositol phosphates and calcium mobilization from internal stores and translocation of protein kinase C (PKC).[120] These signals are associated with interleukin 2 (IL-2) receptor α-chain expression and production of cytokines, leading to cell proliferation.[119] Moreover, the membrane translocation and activation of Ca^{2+}-phospholipid-dependent PKC is accompanied by a dramatic decrease in intracellular cAMP.[107] Conversely, stimulation of adenylyl cyclase is known to provide inhibitory signals for T-cell proliferation. In mature T-cells IL-2 is inducible via agonists of the phosphoinositide pathway, resulting in a series of cascading interactions inducing cell proliferation. Because IL-2 has been shown to activate PKC, which in turn inhibits adenylyl cyclase activity, agents affecting either of these biochemical pathways may potentiate or inhibit cell proliferation. For instance, potentiation of proliferation has also been observed with agents that directly inhibit adenylate cyclase activity by activation of G_i, the inhibitory guanine nucleotide regulatory protein, through separate receptors.

Gender, Type II Glucocorticoid (GR) Receptor Gene Expression, and Immunological Dimorphisms

Glucocorticoid hormones are crucial hormones in the control of immunity, being among the most potent anti-inflammatory, anti-allergic and immunosuppressive agents known, and they act in a very complex way, at various steps of the immune system (see FIGURE 6).[30,31,35] The effects of corticosteroids on cells of the immune system, as in other corticosteroid-responsive cells, are mediated through both soluble and nuclear glucocorticoid receptors (GRs). Estrogens and glucocorticoids have been shown to influence GR mRNA concentrations in rat brain and pituitary.[130–132]

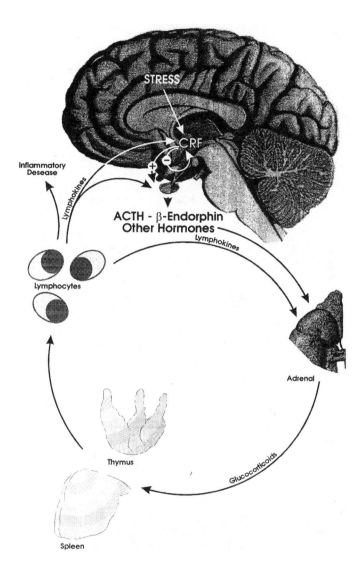

FIGURE 6. The hypothalamo-pituitary-adrenocortical (HPA) axis within the neuroendocrine-immune network. The main regulation of stress-related activity of the HPA axis occurs at the level of the hypothalamus (i.e., the parvocellular components of the paraventricular nuclei) Corticotropin-releasing hormone (CRH) and arginine vasopressin (AVP) are secreted into the hypophyseal portal circulation in a pulsatile fashion and act synergistically to stimulate ACTH secretion by the corticotroph cells, to release the end hormone of the HPA axis, corticosterone or cortisol. Besides the release of ACTH and beta-endorphin from the pituitary, during the stress response, catecholamines are also released from the adrenal glands. Glucocorticoids may act at different (thymus, spleen, lymphoid cells) levels of the immune axis, to countermodulate immune response, while the products of activated immune cells may feed back information at the hypothalamic-pituitary level.

Similar control mechanisms in the thymus could have important implications on the regulatory influence of glucocorticoids on immune functions. One of the major immune compartments where glucocorticoids exert their effects is represented by the thymus gland. Since the observation that glucocorticoids induce atrophy of the cortical area of the thymus there have been many studies on the morphologic changes and cellular events that lead to loss of cell viability. The dramatic alterations of thymus architecture and function accompanying sexual maturation clearly indicate a possible role of sex steroid in the processes of thymic programmed cell death. A way to clarify this issue is to study possible changes in GR gene expression under physiological as well as pharmacological conditions accompanied by marked variations of the sex steroid hormonal milieu, and to correlate such changes with alterations in immune responsiveness. Our results clearly show that thymic GR mRNA concentration is under the control of gonadal and adrenal hormones.[116] We observed an upregulation of GR mRNA content during the luteal (i.e., estrous) phase, and a downmodulation of GR transcript on proestrus, corresponding to the phase of maximal estrogenic stimulation.[116] The hormonal sensitivity of type II GRs in the thymus is further substantiated by the sharp decrease in GR transcript during pregnancy, while the hormonal milieu of lactation lead to a normalization of GR mRNA concentration to levels measured in diestrous rats.[116] Accordingly, castration (OVX) upregulates and estradiol replacement sharply downmodulate GR transcript levels (see FIGURE 7).

It is possible that the hormonal milieu of lactation stimulates GR transcripts within the thymus, and that the estradiol-to-progesterone ratio may be critical in the regulation of type II GR mRNA. In addition, the ability of corticosterone *in vitro* to

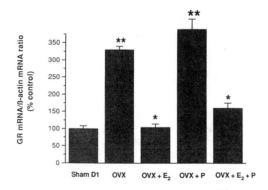

FIGURE 7. Alterations of glucocorticoid receptor (GR) mRNA transcript levels in female thymus after castration and treatment with sex steroids. Total RNA was extracted from thymus of intact female rats on diestrous 1 (D1), three weeks after castration (OVX), and from OVX rats receiving a replacement with 17-β estradiol (E_2), progesterone (P), or the combination of E2 + P for two weeks. Total RNA was hybridized on Northern blots.[8] Results are the mean ± SEM of individual determination in each thymic preparation (six animals/group), expressed as percentages of GR mRNA/β-actin mRNA ratios relative to control values normalized to 100%. ANOVA shows a significant increase of GR transcript levels three weeks after OVX, while E2 treatment completely counteracted the OVX-induced GR transcript rise. *$p < 0.01$ (by Duncan-Kramer test).

influence a cell-mediated immune response in the thymus (i.e., the blastogenic trans-formation of thymocytes) seems to depend upon the sex steroid hormone milieu.[116] Thus, the hormonal conditions accompanied by higher GR transcript levels in the thymus (i.e. OVX, estrus) are characterized by a high degree of corticosterone inhibition of T-cell proliferation. On the other hand, the endogenous adrenal tone is able to influence thymocyte proliferation, and treatment with corticosterone of thy-mocyte cell cultures from adrenalectomized rats produced a sharp inhibition.[116] Of interest, the postnatal development of GR expression within the thymus is sexually dimorphic.[8] The fact that in transgenic mice with impaired GR function the devel-opment of sexually dimorphic response to polyclonal mitogens is inhibited[8] clearly supports a key role for the GR during maturation of T-cell function.[8]

The ability of corticosterone to directly inhibit both GR transcript levels as well as a cell-mediated immune response within the thymus, and the modulation of such inhibitory effect by the sex steroid hormone milieu, may offer an explanation and a molecular mechanism whereby stress may be deleterious for reproduction, also via immunomodulation.[10] On the other hand, hormonally mediated alterations in immunity might also have a pathological implication in sexually related immune diseases.[17] For example, in mouse and humans, lupus erythematosus is more preva-lent in females and estrogen accelerates the disease process, while menstruation is known to exacerbate idiopathic thrombocytopenia purpura.[17] The sex steroid hor-mone milieu, might also have a role in controlling the stress response through immu-nomodulation. Estrogens have been shown to inhibit IL-6 production in IL-1–stimulated cells.[120] Since IL-6 in turn appears to enhance cortisol levels by activat-ing the HPA axis,[121] it would then follow that the estrogenic status might influence the glucocorticoid–lymphokine interactions. It seems therefore highly possible that the degree of susceptibility to, and severity of, inflammatory diseases in response to a given pro-inflammatory trigger may depend on the influence of sex steroids on GR activity. However, it is possible that the sexual dimorphism of immune system activ-ity is related to differential regulation of the HPA axis activity by estrogens since a sexual dimorphism has also been described in HPA axis regulation.[123–133] Indeed, a number of reports gathered in the last decade have clearly demonstrated that the neu-roendocrine response to stress displays profound gender-specific differences, the manifestation of which largely depends on the presence of gonadal steroids.[125–130] Distinct sex differences in the genes encoding CRH in the hypothalamus and GRs in the hippocampus have recently been identified.[37,131] Several previous studies have suggested an influence on the gonadal steroid milieu on CRH and and corticosteroid rceptors. Studies of Patchev and Almeida[37] demonstrate that gonadal setroids exert facilitaing effects on the GC-mediated transcriptional regulation of CRH and GR genes in the rat brain. Interestingly, the absence of a GC feedback mechanism induc-es a persistent increment of ACTH secretion, thus overriding the sexual dimorphism in plasma ACTH concentration.[37]

All together the reports presented suggest, on the one hand, that estrogen may induce an increase in $\beta_2 AR$ and LHRH activities in the thymus, resulting in an increased sensitivity of the thymic cell to locally released and/or circulating cate-cholamines, as well as to endogenous LHRH, not excluding possible intersystems paracrine (i.e., catecholaminergic-LHRH-ergic) paracrine/autocrine/intercrine cross-talk. On the other hand, a sharp decrease of both GR transcripts and thymocyte response to corticosterone follows E_2 treatment/exposure. Such estrogen-induced up- or downregulation of the β_2AR, LHRH, and GR mRNA levels in the thymus may then result in a sophisticated control of lymphocyte sensitivity to endogenous hormones and constitute a molecular mechanism of NEI integration.

LHRH and LHRH-Agonists as Iummunological Response Modifiers

Considerable evidence has been provided that LHRH and its agonists and antagonist analogues are able to markedly influence immune functions. In adult rats, LHRH and its analogues have been shown to increase the absolute and relative thymic weight,[109,110,134–136] and to directly influence thymus morphology and thymocyte proliferative activity of hypophysectomized male rats.[109] More importantly, LHRH agonist (LHRH-A) treatment of aging rats results in a significant increase in thymus weight, and restoration of the morphological appearance of the gland, and to reverse the aging-induced impairment of thymocyte proliferative capacity in response to polyclonal T-dependent mitogens.[109] The biochemical mechanism of action of LHRH after the binding of the neuropeptide to its receptor present in the immune cell appears to be the mobilization of polyphosphoinositide hydrolysis, translocation of the protein kinase C (PKC) and upregulation of the interleukin 2 (IL-2) receptor expression.[120] The physiological significance of the intra LHRH system within the rodent thymus has been also investigated.[24] Treatment of neonatal rats with a very potent LHRH antagonist resulted in irreversible alterations in a series of immune parameters including thymus morphology and cell-mediated and humoral immune responses.[24] Human peripheral T-cell subsets produce LHRH, and its production is increased in T cells activated with phytohemagglutinin (PHA).[113] Such findings coupled with the expression of LHRH mRNA in human lymphocytes further support the idea of LHRH as an important immunomodulator. The fact that changes of intrathymic LHRH mRNA are observed as a function of the stage of the estrous cycle and pregnancy, and the effect of LHRH-antisense on lymphocyte proliferation, clearly underline a physiological role of the hypothalamic decapeptide during the known changes of thymus-dependent immune functions observed in those conditions.

Interestingly enough, Jacobson et al.[138] have recently demonstrated the ability of LHRH-A to modulate the expression of murine lupus in a gonadal steroid-independent fashion, since castrated (SWR X NZB)F1 mice treated with LHRH antagonist displayed decreased total IgG and anti-DNA antibody concentrations, delayed renal disease, and significant prolongation survival,[138] while LHRH increases CD4 T-lymphocyte numbers in an animal model of immunodeficiency.[139] An LHRH agonist might act on the immune system directly by a direct effect on B- or T-lymphocytes. Alternatively the effects might be indirect, through a reduction in gonadotropins or alterations in cytokine production by immune cells. The fact that LHRH analogues are able to modulate murine lupus independently of effects on sex hormone production is of special interest, since they support the possibility that hormones other than gonadal steroids might contribute to the well-known gender differences in expression of autoimmune diseases (see the article by Jacobson in this volume).

Gender, Glucocorticoids, and Autoimmune Diseases of the CNS

The HPG and HPA axes are known to be crucially linked to the development autoimmune diseases, including multiple sclerosis (MS). MS is known to strike women more often than men. Gender differences in experimental autoimmune encephalomyelitis (EAE) parallel those seen in MS. Gonadal hormones are known to influence the clinical disease of the experimental animal model for MS, EAE. Gender differences in EAE have been shown to develop during the induction of the immune response to encephalitogenic peptides, and mechanisms responsible for such gender influences on MS development are actively studied.[140–142] Glucocorticoids are a mainstay in the treatment of autoimmune diseases, and therapeutic effects in inflammatory disorders of the nervous system including MS have been described.[35] Experimental animal studies show that activation of the HPA axis during EAE is crucial for recovery. Indeed, spontaneous recovery from a clinical episode of EAE fully depends on the integrity of the adrenals, while GR antagonists aggravate EAE. Conversely, administration of of GR agonists suppresses neurological signs during EAE.[35] Consistent with these findings, synthetic GCs are still one of the most largely used drugs to treat MS. Strain-related differences in responsiveness of the HPA axis seem to relate to the susceptibility to develop T-cell-mediated autoimmune responses, as seen during experimentally induced autoimmune diseases, such as EAE. Lewis rats have, in fact, a relatively low responsive HPA axis and are highly susceptible to the induction of EAE.[35] Conversely, EAE-resistant rats can be rendered sucseptible to EAE by adrenaletcomy.[35] Clinical studies in patients with MS have shown activation of the HPA axis. Indeed, MS patients have elevated 24-hour cortisol production, a blunted ACTH response to AVP, a reduced cortisol response to CRH and an increased adrenal size, thus supporting a dysfunctional HPA axis in this pathology.[35]

Glucocorticoids are known to have actions during embryogenesis not only on the structural development of organs, but also in the maturation/programming of homeostatic neuroendocrine and immune systems.[143–146] While excess GC exposure in the developing fetus is harmful, reducing birth weight and possibly predisposing to a number of psycho-neuroendocrine and immunological diseases, GCs may have short-term beneficial effects in the brain. The balance between normal and pathological effects of GCs may also depend on a concentration-dependent activation of MRs (activated by low GC levels) versus GRs (activated by high GCs levels). Alterations of the immmnuoendocrine circuit along the HPA axis in various autoimmune diseases, in experimental animals and man, have thus emerged,[30–32] and the potential modulatory role of this feedback regulation in the pathogenesis of autoimmune disease has been suggested.

Through the expression of GC receptor antisense RNA in the brain, Pépin and coworkers have produced transgenic mice with a dysfunctional GR receptor and aberrant HPA axis.[147] This model has supported the hypothesis that disturbed corticoisteroid receptor regulation could be a key factor inducing the CRH and AVP hyperdrive leading to the increased activity of the HPA system and premature escape from the cortisol-suppressant action of dexamethasone seen in affective disorders.[147–151] In previous reports, transgenic (Tg) mice with impaired GR function showed decreased GR mRNA levels in brain, pituitary, and lymphoid organs,[8] reduced thymic and splenic GR binding capacities, and alteration of both trafficking and responsiveness of T-lymphocytes.[8] Moreover, Tg mice display reduced sensitivity to GCs[149] and exaggerated ACTH response to stress and exogenously adminis-trated CRH, but maintained normal early-morning levels of both ACTH and corticosterone in the face of reduced activity of hypothalamic CRH neurons.[147–152] Recently, we studied the intrathymic differentiation during ontogeny in Tg and con-trol mice and revealed a number of alterations.[153] The Tg mice showed a partial blockade of T-cell differentiation and decreased percentages of apoptotic cells dur-ing fetal development, but not in adul life. In contrast, thymic stroma were profound-ly altered from early fetal stages and large epithelium-free areas appeared in the adult thymus.[153] On the other hand, our study revealed a reduction of the splenic TcR alpha beta population accompanied by an increase in the CD4/CD8 ratio. The analysis of different adhesion molecules as well as activation markers demonstrated that most of them were normally expressed in transgenic lymphocytes, whereas CD44 and CD62L expression was altered, indicating the existence of an increased proportion of primed T-cells in these animals.[153] These data suggested a key role for GCs in coordinating the physiological dialogue between the developing thymocytes and their microenvironment.[153] Since the fetal HPA axis is highly sensitive to events occurring early in life, and in the light of the bidirectional communication between the neuroendocrine and immune system, it seemed important to clarify whether a disruption in the thymic developmental response early in fetal life might modulate/modify the neuroendocrine immune response of the adult animal to immunological and endocrinological challenges. We thus studied the susceptibility of the Tg mice to develop an autoimmune disease of the CNS, namely EAE.

For this aim, female B6C3F1 mice intact and Tg received s.c. injections in the flank of myelin olygodendrocyte peptides (MOGs) together with complete Freund's adjuvant and *Mycobacterium tuberculosis*. Clinical signs and body weights were recorded daily for 45 days. The study showed that the neurological signs of EAE developed in 90% of control mice, while only 5% of the Tg animals developed the disease, suggesting that the neuroendocrine immune status of the Tg mice was able to reverse the susceptibility of B6C3F1 into resistance against EAE.

SUMMARY AND CONCLUSION

In the present article we have summarized some aspects of the impact of gender in neuroendocrine-immunomodulation with some potential clinical implications for the susceptibility of developing autoimmune diseases of the CNS. Particular atten-tion was given to one principal system–the LHRH receptor-signaling system–acting as "primum movens" of the cascading actions and interactions concerned with repro-duction. The advances in reproductive immunology have been summarized by fol-lowing the achievements in LHRH-immune studies, from the biochemical to the molecular characterization of a paracrine intralymphocytic LHRH system involved in physiological control immune physiology, and at the same time serving as channel for bidirectional communication with the nervous-reproductive axis. The teleologi-cal assumption that the chief hormone governing the fertility capacity of a living organism "should" directly signal the master gland of the immune system (i.e., the thymus) is now corroborated by a number of biochemical and molecular as well as clinical evidence, all supporting the concept that this neuropeptide may indeed behave as an immunological response modifier. All together, the information presented supports the concept that LHRH participates at both central and peripheral levels in the interaction between the neuroendocrine and immune systems. The reciprocity of the neuroendocrine-immune signaling systems is further supported by the ability of sex steroids to modulate thymus-dependent immune function via direct effects on specific target genes involved in the development of sex dimorphism and sex dimorphic immune responses, including the downregulation of immune response observed during pregnancy. The widespread therapeutic application of LHRH and its potent agonistic and antagonistic analogues in a large number of disorders in pediatric, gynecologic, urologic and oncologic medicine underlines the potential clinical implications of the experimental findings described. Especially, the recently demonstrated direct effect of LHRH-A in murine lupus certainly open a new chapter in the neuroendocrinology of reproduction, the one on the potential immune capabilities of hormones and anti-hormones, which are widely used in a variety of endocrinopathies.

The exquisite functional interplay between the LHRH system and the immune environment is reflected at the CNS level, where a bidirectional functional interaction between the differentiating LHRH neuron and the maturing astroglial cell has been demonstrated for the first time. Glial cells play active roles from embryonic development to adulthood. During development, astroglia direct the migration of neurons to the right targets. From the bulk of the presented information it seems likely that astroglial–LHRH neuronal interactions play a major role in the integration of the multiplicity of brain signals converging on the LHRH neurons, which govern reproduction. Hormonally induced changes in glial plasticity and neuron–glial interactions may lastly dictate some major changes of CNS output, and thus actively participate in sex dimorphic immune responses. The central role of GCs in the interactive communication between the neuroendocrine and immune systems is underscored by the vital role of GCs in autoimmunity. Interaction between gender and the HPA axis is well exemplified by the gender-related differences in the development of an autoimmune disease such as EAE. Interstingly enough transgenic female mice expressing an RNA antisense directed against GR and exhibiting a dysfunctional GR function coupled to aberrant HPA axis are resistant to development of EAE . Such findings may have potential pathophysiological consequences and shape the individual capability to became more or less vulnerable to a number of insults leading to neuropathological states. Characterization of the role of GCs and their underlying mechanisms of action during EAE induction will help us to understand the development of the disease and to generate new ideas for pharmacological targeting with drugs acting at the neuroendocrine–immune interface.

REFERENCES

1. BLALOCK, J.E. 1992. Neuroimmunoendocrinology. J.E. Blalock, Ed. Chem Immunol. 52. S. Karger. Basel.
2. BLALOCK, J.E. 1994. Shared ligands and receptors as a molecular mechanism for communication between the immune and neuroendocrine systems. Ann. N.Y. Acad. Sci. **741:** 292–298.
3. PIERPAOLI,W. & N.H. SPECTOR, Eds. 1994. Neuroimmunomodulation: Interventions in Aging and Cancer. Ann. N.Y. Acad. Sci., Vol. **719.**

4. PIERPAOLI, W. 1990. The pineal gland as ontogenetic scanner of reproduction, immunity, and aging. Ann. N.Y. Acad. Sci. **741:** 46–49.
5. MARCHETTI, B., M.C. MORALE, V. GUARCELLO *et al.* 1990. Crosstalk communication in the neuroendocrine-reproductive axis: age-dependent alterations in the common communication networks. Ann. N.Y. Acad. Sci. **594:** 309–325.
6. MARCHETTI, B., M.C. MORALE, V. GUARCELLO *et al.* 1990. The neuroendocrine-immune connections in the control of reproductive functions. *In* Major Advances in Human Female Reproduction. E.Y. Adashi & S. Mancuso, Eds. Serono Symposia **73:** 279–289.
7. MARCHETTI, B., A. PEIFFER, M.C. MORALE *et al.* 1994. Transgenic animals with impaired type II glucocorticoid receptor expression: a model to study aging of the neuroendocrine immune system. Ann. N.Y. Acad. Sci. **719:** 308–327.
8. MORALE, M.C., N. BATTICANE, F. GALLO *et al.* 1995. Disruption of hypothalamic-pituitary-adrenocortical system in transgenic mice expressing type glucocorticoid receptor antisense ribonucleic acid permanently impairs T-cell functions: effects on T-cell trafficking and T-cell responsiveness during post-natal maturation. Endocrinology **136:** 3949–3960.
9. MARCHETTI, B., F. GALLO, Z. FARINELLA *et al.* 1995. Neuroendocrine immunology (NEI) at the turn of the century: towards a molecular understanding of basic mechanisms and implications for reproductive physiopathology. Endocrine **3:** 845–861.
10. MARCHETTI, B., F. GALLO, Z. FARINELLA & M.C. MORALE. 1996. Unique neuroendocrine-immune (NEI) interactions during pregnancy. *In* The Physiology of Immunity. M. Kendal & J. Marsh, Eds.: 297–328. CRC Press. London.
11. MARCHETTI, B., F. GALLO, C. ROMEO *et al.* 1996. The luteinizing hormone-releasing hormone (LHRH) receptors in the neuroendocrine immune network: biochemical bases and implications for reproductive physiopathology. Ann. N.Y. Acad. Sci. **784:** 209–236.
12. MCCANN, S.M., L. MILENKOVIC, M.C. GONZALEZ *et al.* 1993. Endocrine aspects of neuroimmunomodulation: methods and overview *In* Neurobiology of Cytokines, Part A, Vol. 16: Methods in Neurosciences. E.B. de Souza, Ed.: 187–210. Academic Press. San Diego, CA.
13. MCCANN, S.M., S. KARANTH, A. KAMAT *et al.* 1994. Induction by cytokines of the pattern of pituitary hormone secretion in infection. Neuroimmunomodulation **1:** 2–13.
14. CALZOLARI, A. 1989. Recherches experimentales sur un rapport probable entre la fonction du thymus et celle des testicules. Arch. Ital. Biol. (Tor.) **307:** 71–76.
15. BESEDOWSKI, H.O. & E. SORKIN. 1974. Thymus involvement in sexual maturation. Nature **249:** 356–359.
16. PIERPAOLI, W. & H.O. BESEDOWSKI. 1975. Interdependence of the thymus in programming neuroendocrine functions. Clin. Exp. Immunol. **20:** 323–329.
17. GROSSMAN, C.J. 1984. Regulation of the immune system by sex steroids. Endocr. Rev. **5:** 435.
18. FAROOKHI, R., E. WESOLOWSKI, J.M. TRASLER *et al.* 1988. Modulation by neonatal thymectomy of the reproductive axis in male and female rats during development. Biol. Reprod. **27:** 126.
19. MARCHETTI, B., V. GUARCELLO & U. SCAPAGNINI. 1988. Luteinizing hormone-releasing hormone agonist (LHRH-A) binds to lymphocytes and modulates the immune response. *In* Biology and Biochemistry of Normal and Cancer Cell Growth. L. Castagnetta & I. Nenci, Eds.: 149–152. Harwood Academic Press. London.
20. MARCHETTI, B. 1989. Involvment of the thymus in reproduction. Progr. Neuroendocrin. Immunol. **2:** 64–69.
21. MARCHETTI, B., V. GUARCELLO, G. TRIOLO *et al.* 1989. Luteinizing hormone-releasing hormone (LHRH) as natural messenger in neuro-immune-endocrine communications. *In* Interactions among CNS, Neuroendocrine and Immune Systems. J.W. Hadden, K. Masek & G. Nisticò, Eds.: 127–146. Pythagora Press. Rome-Milan.
22. MARCHETTI, B., V. GUARCELLO, M.C. MORALE *et al.* 1990. A physiological role for the neuropeptide luteinizing hormone-releasing hormone (LHRH) during the maturation of thymus gland function. Intern. J. Neurosci. **51:** 287–289.

23. GROSSMAN, C.J. 1990. Are there underlying immune-neuroendocrine interactions responsible for immunological sexual dimorphism? Progr. Neuroendocrin. Immunol. **3:** 75–80.

24. MORALE, M.C., N. BATTICANE, G. BARTOLONI *et al.* 1991. Blockade of central and peripheral luteinizing hormone-releasing hormone (LHRH) receptors in neonatal rats with a potent LHRH-antagonist inhibits the morphofunctional development of the thymus and maturation of cell-mediated and humoral immune responses. Endocrinology **128:** 1073–1085.

25. BIRNBAUMER, L., N. SHAHABI, J. RIVIER & W. VALE. 1985. Evidence for a physiological role of gonadotropin-releasing hormone (GnRH) or GnRH-like material in the ovary. Endocrinology **116:** 1367.

26. HILLENSJO, T. & W.J. LE MAIRE. 1980 Gonadotropin-releasing hormone agonists stimulates meiotic maturation of follicle-enclosed rat oocytes. Nature **287:** 145–146.

27. HODGEN, G.D. & J. ITSKOVITZ. 1988, 1995. Recognition and maintenance of pregnancy. *In* The Physiology of Reproduction. E. Knobil & J.D. Neill, Eds. Raven Press. New York.

28. SARGENT, I.L. 1993. Maternal and fetal immune responses during pregnancy. Exp. Clin. Immunogenet. **10:** 85.

29. USSA, J.E., A.P. CADAVID & J.G. MALDONADO. 1994. Is the immune system necessary for placental reproduction? A hypothesis on the mechanisms of alloimmunotherapy in recurrent spontaneous abortion. Med. Hypotheses **42:** 193.

30. STERNBERG, E.M. 1989 The role of the hypothalamic-pituitary-adrenal axis in an experimental model of arthritis. Progr. Neuroendocrinimmunol. **2:** 103–108.

31. WICK, G., Y. HU, S. SCHWARZ & G. KROEMER. 1993. Immunoendocrine communication via the hypothalamo-pituitary-adrenal axis in autoimmune diseases. Endocr. Rev. **14:** 539–563.

32. CHROUSOS, G.P. 1995. The hypothalamic-pituitary-adrenal axis and immune-mediated inflammation. N. Engl. J. Med. **332:** 1351–1362

33. HOLSBOER, F., U. BARDELEBE, A. GERKEN *et al.* 1984. Blunted corticotropin releasing factor in depression. N. Engl. J. Med. **311:** 112.

34. MARCHETTI, B., M.V.C. MORALE & J. BROUWER. 1997 Neurochemical, pharmacological and immunological assessments in a transgenic mouse model of neuroendocrine changes in depression. Aging Clin. Exp. Res. **9:** 26–27.

35. MARCHETTI, B., F. GALLO, C. TIROLO *et al.* 1997. Developmental consequences of hypothalamic-pituitary-adrenocortical system disruption: impact on thymus gland maturation and the susceptibility to develop neuroimmune diseases. Dev. Brain Dysfunct. **10:** 503–527.

36. PARRY, B.L. 1995. Mood disorders linked to the reproductive cycle in women. *In* Psychopharmacology: The Fourth Generation of Progress. F.E. Bloom & D.J. Kupfer, Eds.: 1029–1042. Raven Press. New York.

37. PATCHEV, V.K. & O.F.X. ALMEIDA. 1996. Gonadal steroids exert facilitating "buffering" effects on glucocorticoid-mediated transcriptional regulation of corticotropin-releasing hormone and corticosteroid receptor genes in rat brain. J. Neurosci **16:** 7077–7084.

38. BEHL, C., T. SKUTELLA, H. LEZOULAC *et al.* 1997. Neuroprotection against oxidative stress by estrogens: structure-activty relationship. Mol. Pharmacol. **110:** 535–541.

39. SCHNEIDER, L.S. & C.E. FINCH. 1997. Can estrogens prevent neurodegeneration? Drugs & Aging **11:** 87–95.

40. DUBAL, D.B., M.L. KASHON, L.C. PETTIGREW *et al.* 1998. Estradiol protects against ischemic injury. J. Cerbr. Blood Flow Metab. **18:** 1253–1258.

41. MARCHETTI, B. 1996. The LHRH-astroglial network of signals as a model to study neuroimmune interaction: assessment of messenger systems and transduction mechanisms at cellular and molecular levels. Neuroimmunomodulation **3:** 1–27.

42. MARCHETTI, B. 1997. Cross-talk signals in the CNS: role of neurotrophic and hormonal factors, adhesion molecules and intercellular signaling agents in luteinizing hormone-releasing hormone (LHRH)-astroglia interactive network. Trends Biosci. **2:** 1–32.

43. BENVENISTE, E.N. 1995. Cytokine production. *In* Neuroglia. H. Kattenmann & E.R. Ransom, Eds.: 700–716. Oxford University Press. New York and Oxford.

44. GIULIAN, D. 1990. Microglia, cytokines, and cytotoxins: modulators of cellular responses after injury to the central nervous system. J. Immunol. Immunopharmacol. **10:** 15–21.

45. GALLO, F., M.C. MORALE, R. AVOLA & B. MARCHETTI. 1995. Cross-talk between luteinizing hormone-releasing hormone (LHRH) neurons and astroglial cells: developing glia release factors that accelerate neuronal differentiation and stimulate LHRH release from the GT1 cell line and LHRH neurons stimulate astroglia proliferation. Endocr. J. **3:** 863–874.

46. GALLO, F., M.C. MORALE, Z. FARINELLA *et al.* 1996. Growth factors released from astroglial cells in primary culture participate in the crosstalk between luteinizing hormone-releasing hormone (LHRH) neurons and astrocytes: effects on LHRH neuronal proliferation and secretion. Ann. N.Y. Acad. Sci. **784:** 513–516.

47. GALLO, F., R. AVOLA, A. BEAUDET & B. MARCHETTI. 1996. Basic FGF is a major neurotrophic signaling agent during LHRH neuron-astroglia interactions: bFGF priming sensitizes LHRH neurons to growth factor neurotrophic effects [abstr. 624.2]. Vol. 2, 26th Annual Meeting of the Society for Neuroscience.

48. GALLO, F., M.C. MORALE, C. TIROLO *et al.* 2000. Basic fibroblast growth factor acts on both neurons and glia to mediate the neurotrophic effects of astrocytes on LHRH neurons in culture. Synapse: 233–255.

49. MARCHETTI, B., F. GALLO, C. TIROLO *et al.* 1998. Luteinizing hormone-releasing hormone (LHRH) is a primary signaling molecule in the neuroimmune network of signals. Ann. N.Y. Acad. Sci. USA **840:** 205–248.

50. KNOBIL, E. & J. HOTCHKISS. 1988. The menstrual cycle and its neuroendocrine control. *In* The Physiology of Reproduction. E. Knobil & J. Neill, Eds.: 1971–1994. Raven Press. New York.

51. KALRA, S.P. 1993. Mandatory neuropeptide-steroid signaling for the preovulatory luteinizing hormone-releasing hormone discharge. Endocr. Rev. **14:** 507–538.

52. MARCHETTI, B. & F. LABRIE. 1983. Hormonal control luteinizing hormone-releasing hormone activity in the rat anterior pituitary gland. *In* Neuropeptide, Neurotransmitters, and Regulation of Endocrine Processes. E. Endroczi *et al.*, Eds. Akademiai Kiadò, Budapest.

53. MARCHETTI, B., F. LABRIE, G. PELLETIER *et al.* 1983. Hormonal control of pituitary luteinizing hormone-releasing hormone receptors. *In* Recent Advances in Male Reproduction: Molecular Basis and Clinical Implications. R. D'Agata *et al.*, Eds.: 215–226. Raven Press. New York.

54. MARCHETTI, B., J.J. REEVES, G. PELLETIER & F. LABRIE. 1982. Modulation of pituitary luteinizing hormone-releasing hormone receptors by sex steroids and LHRH in the rat. Biol. Reprod. **27:** 133.

55. MARCHETTI, B. & F. LABRIE. 1982. Prolactin inhibits pituitary LHRH receptors in the rat. Endocrinology **111:** 1209.

56. MARCHETTI, B. & U. SCAPAGNINI. 1985. Modulation of opioid influence on pituitary luteinizing hormone-releasing hormone receptors in the female rat. Neuroendocrinol. Lett. **7:** 11–18.

57. KRSMANOVIC, L.Z., S.S. STOJILKOVIC, L.M. MERTZ *et al.* 1993. Expression of gonadotropin-releasing hormone receptors and autocrine regulations of neuropeptide release in immortalized hypothalamic neurons. Proc. Natl. Acad. Sci. USA **90:** 3908–3912 .

58. HATTON, G. I., L. S. PERLMUTTER, A. K SALM, & C.D. TWEEDLE. 1984. Dynamic neuronal-glial interactions in hypothalamus and pituitary: implications for control of hormone synthesis and release, Peptides [Suppl 1] **5:** 121.

59. CAJAL, R.S. 1913. Sobre un nuevo proceder de impregnacion de la neuroglia y sus resultados en los centros nerviosos del hombre y animales. Trab. Lab. Invest. Biol. Univ. Madrid **11:** 219–237.

60. ARENANDER, A. & J. DEVELLIS. 1992. Early response gene induction in astrocytes as a mechanism for encoding and integrating neuronal signals. *In* Neuronal-Astrocytic Interactions. Implications for Normal and Pathological CNS Function. A.C.H.Yu *et al.*, Eds.: 177–188. Elsevier. Amsterdam.

61. GARCIA-SEGURA, L.M., S. LUQUIN, A. PARDUEZ & F. NAFTOLIN. 1994. Gonadal hormone regulation of glial fibrillary acid protein immunoreactivity and glial ultrastructure in the rat neuroendocrine hypothalamus. Glia **10**: 59–69.

62. GARCIA-SEGURA, L.M., J.A. CHOWEN, M. DUENAS *et al.* 1994. Gonadal steroids as promoters of neuro-glial plasticity. Psychoneuroendocrinology **19**: 445–453.

63. GARCIA-SEGURA, L.M., I. TORRES-ALEMAN & F. NAFTOLIN. 1989. Astrocytic shape and fibrillary acidic protein immunoreactivity are modified by estradiol in primary rat hypothalamic cultures. Dev. Brain Res. **47**: 298–302.

64. TORRAN-ALLERAND, C.D., L. ELLIS & K.H. PFENNINGER. 1988. Estrogen and insulin synergisn in neurite growth enhancement in vitro: mediation of steroid effects by interactions with growth factors? Dev. Brain Res. **41**: 87–100.

65. OLMOS, G., F. NAFTOLIN, J. PEREZ *et al.* 1989. Synaptic remodelling in the rat arcuate nucleus during the estrous cycle. Neuroscience **32**: 663–667.

66. LANGUB JR., M.C. & R.E. WATSON JR. 1992. Estrogen receptor-immunoreactive glia, endothelia, and ependima in guinea pig preoptic area and median eminence: electron microscopy. Endocrinology **130**: 364–372.

67. NAFTOLIN, F., C. LERANTH, J. PEREZ & L.M. GARCIA SEGURA. 1993. Estrogen induces synaptic plasticity in adult primate neurons. Neuroendocrinology **57**: 935–939.

68. YUNG-TESTAS, I., Z.Y. HU, E.E. BEAULIEU & P. ROBEL. 1989. Neurosteroids: biosynthesis of pregnenolone and progesterone in primary cultures of rat glial cells. Endocrinology **125**: 2083–2091.

69. YUNG-TESTAS, J.M., J.M. RENOIR, J.H. GASC & E.E. BAULIEU. 1991. Oestrogen-inducible progesterone receptor in primary cultures of rat glial cells. Exp. Cell Res. **193**: 12–19.

70. YUNG-TESTAS, I., J.M. RENOIR, H. BRUGNARD *et al.* 1992. Demonstration of steroid hormone receptor and steroid action in primary cultures of rat glial cells. J. Steroid Biochem. Mol. Biol. **41**: 3–8.

71. MARCHETTI, B., F. GALLO, M.C. MORALE *et al.* 1999 Neuron-glial interaction and estrogens neuroprotective effects om primary mesencephalic cultures. Proceedings of European Congress on Pharmacology, Budapest, July 1999, Abstract, p.136.

72. REUL, J.M.H.M. & E.R. DEKLOET. 1985. Two receptor systems for corticosterone in rat brain: microdistribution and differential occupation. Endocrinology **117**: 2505–2511.

73. KUMAR, S. & J. DEVELLIS. 1988. Glucocorticoid-mediated functions in glial cells. *In* Glial Cell Receptors. H.K. Kimelberg, Ed.: 243–264. Raven Press. New York.

74. CHOU, Y., W.G. LUTTGE & G. SUMNERSA. 1991. Expression of mineralcorticoid type I and glucocorticoid type II receptors in astrocyte glia as a function of time in culture. Dev. Brain Res. **61**: 55–61.

75. PEARCE, B. & G.P. WILKIN. 1995. Eicosanoids, purine, and hormone receptors. *In* Neuroglia. H. Kattenmann & B.R. Ransom, Eds.: 377–386. Oxford University Press. New York and Oxford.

76. ARONSSON, M., K. FUXE, Y. DONG *et al.* 1988. Localization of glucocorticoid receptor mRNA by in situ hybridization. Proc. Natl. Acad. Sci. USA **85**: 9331–9335.

77. AVOLA, R., V. SPINA-PURRELLO, M.C. MORALE *et al.* 1998. Insulin-like growth factor effects on ADP-rybosylation processes and interactions with glucocorticoid during maturation and differentiation of astroglial cells in primary culture. *In* IGFs in the Nervous System, E. Muller, Ed.: 127–134. Springer-Verlag, Berlin.

78. FINCH, C.E. 1997. Stress-mechanisms and the age-related increase of GFAP transcription in brain astrocytes. Dev. Brain Dysfunct. **10**: 350–358.

79. BASCO, I., P.L. WOODHAMS, F. HAJOS & R. BALASZ. 1981. Immunocytochemical demonstration of glial fibrillary acidic protein in mouse tanycytes. Anat. Embryol. **162**: 217–222.

80. CAJAL, R.S. 1913. Sobre un nuevo proceder de impregnacion de la neuroglia y sus resultados en los centros nerviosos del hombre y animales. Trab. Lab. Invest. Biol. Univ. Madrid **11:** 219–237.

81. HORSTMANN, E. 1954. Die faserglial des selachiergehirns. Z. Zellforsch. **39:** 588–617.

82. MILLHOUSE, O.E. 1972. Light and electron microscopic studies of the ventricular wall. Z. Zellforsch. **127:** 149–174.

83. KOZLOWSKI, G.P. & P.W. COATES. 1985. Ependymo-neuronal specializations between LHRH fibers and cells of the cerebroventricular system. Cell Tiss. Res. **242:** 301–311.

84. SILVERMAN, R.C., M.J. GIBSON & A.J. SILVERMAN. 1991. Relationship of glia to GnRH axonal outgrowth from third ventricular grafts in hpg hosts. Exp. Neurol. **114:** 259–274.

85. KING, J.C. & R.J. LETOURNEAU. 1994. Luteinizing hormone-releasing hormone terminals in the median eminence of rats undergo dramatic changes after gonadectomy, as revealed by electron microscopic image analysis. Endocrinology **134:** 1340–1351.

86. KOHAMA, S.G., J.R. GOSS, T.H. MCNEILL & C.E. FINCH. 1995. Glial fibrillary protein increases at proestrus in the arcutae nucleus of mice. Neurosci. Lett. **183:** 164–166.

87. COLLADO, P., C. BEYER, J.B. UTCHISON & S.D. HOLMAN. 1995. Hypothalamic distribution of astrocytes is gender-related in Mongolian gerbils. Neurosci. Lett. **184:** 86–89.

88. KOHAMA, S.G., J.R. GOSS, C.E. FINCH & T.H. MCNEILL. 1995. Increases of glial fibrillary acidic protein in the aging female mouse brain. Neurobiol. Aging **16:** 59–67.

89. NICHOLS, N.R., C.E. FINCH & J.F. NELSON. 1995. Food restriction delays the age-related increase in GFAP mRNA in rat hypothalamus. Neurobiol. Aging **16:** 105–110.

90. MCQUEEN, J.K. & H. WILSON. 1994. The development of astrocytes immunoreactive for glial fibrillary acidic protein in the medio-basal hypothalamus of hypogonadal mice. Mol. Cell Neurosci. **5:** 623–631.

91. OJEDA, S.R. & H.F. URBANSKI. 1994. Puberty in the rat. *In* The Physiology of Reproduction, 2nd edit. E. Knobil & Y.D. Neill, Eds.: 363–409. Raven Press, New York.

92. OJEDA, S.R., H.F. URBANSKI, M.E. COSTA *et al.* 1990. Involvement of transforming growth factor in the release of luteinizing hormone-releasing hormone from the developing female hypothalamus. Proc. Natl. Acad. Sci. USA **87:** 9698–9702.

93. MA, L., M.P. JUNIER, M.E. COSTA & S.R. OJEDA. 1992. Transforming growth factor gene expression in the hypothalamus is developmentally regulated and linked to sexual maturation. Neuron **9:** 657–670.

94. OJEDA, S.R., G.A. DISSEN & M.P. JUNIER. 1993. Neurotrophic factors and female sexual development. Front. Neuroendocrinol. **13:** 120–162.

95. MELLON, P., J. WINDLE, P. GOLDSMITH *et al.* 1990. Immortalization of hypothalamic GnRH neurons by genetically targeted tumorigenesis. Neuron **5:** 1–10.

96. MARTINEZ DE LA ESCALERA, G., F. GALLO, A.L.H. CHOI & R.I. WEINER. 1992. Dopaminergic regulation of the GT1 gonadotropin releasing hormone (GnRH) neuronal cell lines: stimulation of GnRH release via D1-receptors positively coupled to adenylate cyclase. Endocrinology **131:** 2965–2971.

97. MARTINEZ DE LA ESCALERA, G., A.L.H. CHOI & R.I. WEINER. 1992. ß1-Adrenergic regulation of the gt1 GnRH neuronal cell lines: stimulation of the GnRH release via receptors positively coupled to adenylate cyclase. Endocrinology **131:** 1397–1402.

98. NEGRO-VILAR, A., D. CONTE & M. VALENCA. 1986. Transmembrane signals mediating neural peptide secretion: role of protein kinase C activators and arachidonic acid metabolites in luteinizing hormone-releasing hormone. Endocrinology **119:** 2796–2802.

99. OJEDA, S.R., H.F. URBANSKI, K.H. KATZ *et al.* 1986. Activation of two different but complementary biochemical pathways stimulates release of hypothalamic luteinizing hormone-releasing hormone. Proc. Natl. Acad. Sci. USA **83:** 4932–4936.

100. MORETTO, M., F.J. LÓPEZ & A. NEGRO-VILAR. 1993. Nitric oxide regulates luteinizing hormone-releasing hormone secretion. Endocrinology **133**: 2399–2402.
101. BONAVERA, J.J., A. SAHU, P.S. KALRA & S.P. KALRA. 1993. Evidence that nitric oxide may mediate the ovarian steroid-induced luteinizing hormone surge: involvement of excitatory amino acids. Endocrinology **133**: 2481–2487.
102. MURPHY, S., R.L. MINOR, G. WELK & D.G. HARRISON. 1991. CNS astroglial cells release nitrogen oxides with vasorelaxant properties. Cardiovasc. Pharmacol. **17**: S265–S268.
103. MURPHY, S., M.L. SIMMONS, L. AGULLO *et al.* 1993. Synthesis of nitric oxide in CNS glial cells. Trends Neurosci. **16**: 323–328.
104. MARCHETTI, B., M.C. MORALE, N. BATTICANE *et al.* 1991. Aging of the reproductive-neuroimmune axis: a crucial role for the hypothalamic neuropeptide luteinizing hormone-releasing hormone. Ann. N.Y. Acad. Sci. **621**: 159.
105. MARCHETTI, B., M. C. MORALE & G. PELLETIER. 1990. Sympathetic nervous system control of thymus gland maturation: autoradiographic characterization and localization of the β_2-adrenergic receptor in the rat thymus gland and presence of a sexual dimorphism during ontogenic development. Progr. NeuroendocrinImmunol. **3**: 103.
106. MARCHETTI, B., M. C. MORALE & G. PELLETIER. 1990. The thymus gland as a major target for the central nervous system and the neuroendocrine system: neuroendocrine modulation of thymic β_2-adrenergic receptor distribution as revealed by *in vitro* autoradiography. Mol. Cell. Neurosci. **1**: 10.
107. MORALE, M. C., F. GALLO, N. BATTICANE & B. MARCHETTI. 1992. The immune response evokes up- and down-modulation of a β_2-adrenergic receptor messenger RNA concentration in the male rat thymus. Mol. Endocrinol. **6**: 1513.
108. SUNDARAM, K., A. DIDOLKAR, THAU *et al.* 1988. Antagonists of luteinizing hormone releasing hormone bind to rat mast cells and induce histamine release. Agents Actions **25**: 307.
109. MARCHETTI, B., V. GUARCELLO, M.C. MORALE *et al.* 1989. Luteinizing hormone-releasing hormone (LHRH) binding sites in the rat thymus: characteristic and biological function,. Endocrinology **125**: 1025.
110. MARCHETTI, B., V. GUARCELLO, M.C. MORALE *et al.* 1989. Luteinizing hormone-releasing hormone (LHRH) agonist restoration of age-associated decline of thymus weight, thymic LHRH receptors, and thymocyte proliferative capacity. Endocrinology **125**: 1037.
111. MAIER, C.C., B. MARCHETTI, R. DEBOEUF &.J.E. BLALOCK. 1992. Thymocytes express a mRNA that is identical to hypothalamic luteinizing hormone-releasing hormone mRNA. Cell. Mol. Neurobiol. **12**: 447.
112. AZAD, N., N.V. EMANUELE, M.M. HALLORAN *et al.* 1991. Presence of luteinizing hormone-releasing hormone (LHRH) mRNA in rat spleen lymphocytes. Endocrinology **128**: 1679.
113. AZAD, N., N. LA PAGLIA, K. ABEL *et al.* 1993. Immunoactivation enhances the concentration of luteinizing hormone-releasing hormone peptide and its gene expression in human peripheral T-lymphocytes. Endocrinology **133**: 215.
114. WILSON, T.M., L. YU-LEE & M.R. KELLY. 1995. Coordinate gene expression of luteinizing hormone-releasing hormone (LHRH) and the LHRH-receptor following prolactin stimulation in the rat Nb2 T cell line: implications for a role in immunomodulation and cell-cycle gene expression. Mol. Endocrinol. **111**: 171–177
115. MARCHETTI, B., M.C. MORALE, P. PARADIS & M. BOUVIER. 1994. Characterization, expression and hormonal control of a β^2-adrenergic receptor. Am. J. Physiol. (Endocrinol. Metab. 30) **267**: E718-E731.
116. PEIFFER, A., M. C. MORALE, N. BARDEN & B. MARCHETTI. 1994. Modulation of glucocorticoid receptor gene expression in the thymus by the sex steroid hormone milieu and correlation with sexual dimorphism of immune response. Endocr. J. **2**: 181.
117. SEALFON, U.B., D. ZHAO, G.R. CARDONA & W.W. CHIN. 1992 Isolation and characterization of cDNAs encoding the rat pituitary gonadotropin-releasing hormone receptor. Biochem. Biophys. Res Commun. **189**(3): 1645–1652.

118. KAISER, U.B., A. JAKUBOWIAK, A. STEINBERGERGER & W.W. CHIN. 1993. Hormonal regulation of gonadotropin releasing hormnone receptors and messenger RNA activity in ovine pituitary. 75th Annual Meeting of the Endocrinology Society, Las Vegas, Nevada

119. MARCHETTI, B., M. FORTIER, P. POYET et al. 1990. ß2-adrenergic receptor in the rat mammary gland during pregnancy and lactation: characterization, distribution, and coupling to adenylate cyclase, Endocrinology 126: 565.

120. BATTICANE, N., M. C. MORALE, F. GALLO et al. 1991. Luteinizing hormone-releasing hormone signaling at the lymphocyte involves stimulation of interleukin-2 receptor expression. Endocrinology 128: 277–286.

121. TABIBZADEH, S.S., U. SANTHANAM, P.B. SEHGAL & L.T. MAY. 1989. Cytokine-induced production of IFN-beta2/il-6 by freshly explanted human endometrial stromal cells. J. Immunol. 42: 3134.

122. ZANKER, B., G. WAL, K.J. WIEDER & T.B. STROM. 1990. Evidence that glucocorticosteroids block the expression of the human interleukin-6 gene by accessory cells. Transplantation 49: 183.

123. CRITCHLOW, V., R.A. LIEBELT, M. BAR-SELA et al. 1963. Sex differences in resting pituitary adrenal function in the rat. Am. J. Physiol. 205: 807.

124. GALA, R.R. & U. WESTPHAL. 1965. Corticosteroid-binding globulin in the rat: studies on the sex differences, Endocrinology, 77: 841.

125. TURNER, B.B. & D.A. WEAVER. 1985. Sexual dimorphism of glucocorticoid in rat brain. Brain. Res. 343: 16.

126. SPINEDI, E., M.O. SUESCUN, R. HADID et al. 1992 Effects of gonadectomy on the endotoxin-stimulated hypothalamo-pituitary adrenal axis: evidence for a neuroendcorine immunological sexual dimorphism. Endocrinology 131: 2430

127. CHISARI, A., M. CARINO, M. PERONE et al. 1995 Sex and strain variability in the rat hypothalamo-pituitary-adrenal (HPA) axis function. J. Endocrinol. Invest. 18: 25.

128. ATKINSON, H.C. & B.J. WADDEL. 1988. Circadian variations and adrenocoticotropin in the rat: sexual dimorphism and changes across the estrous cycle. Endocrinology 138: 3842.

129. RIVIER, C. 1994 Stimulatory effect of interleukin 1-beta on the hypothalamic-pituitary-adrenal axis of the rat: influence of age, gender and circulating sex steroids. J. Endocrinol. 140: 365

130. CHISARI, A.N., M.J. PERON, A. GIOVANBATTISTA & E. SPINEDI. 1998. Gender-dependent characteristics of the hypothalamo-corticotrope axis function in glucorticoid-replete and glucocorticoid-depleted rats. J. Endocrinol. Invest. 21: 737–743.

131. PEIFFER, A., B. LAPOINTE & N. BARDEN. 1991. Hormonal regulation of type II glucocorticoid receptor messenger ribonucleic acid in rat brain. Endocrinology 129: 2166–2174.

132. PEIFFER, A. & N. BARDEN. 1987. Estrogen-induced decrease of glucocorticoid receptor messenger ribonucleic acid concentration in rat anterior pituitary gland. Mol. Endocrinol. 1: 435–440.

133. PEIFFER, A. & N. BARDEN. 1988. Glucocorticoid receptor gene expression in rat pituitary gland intermediate lobe following ovariectomy. Mol. Cell. Endocrinol. 55: 115–120.

134. GREENSTEIN, B.D., F.T. A. FITZPATRICK, M.D. KENDALL et al. 1987. Regeneration of the thymus in old male rats treated with a stable analogue of LHRH. J. Endocrinol. 112: 345.

135. CHIODI, H. 1977. Thymus hypertrophy induced by castration in old rats and mice. Fed. Proc. 35: 277A.

136. ATAYA, K.M., W. SAKR, C.M. BLACKER et al. 1989. Effect of GnRH agonists on the thymus in female rats. Acta Endocrinol. 121: 833.

137. RAO, L.V., R.P. CLEVELAND & K.M. ATAYA. 1993. Sequential changes in functional lymphocyte subpopulations during long term administration of GnRH agonist in postpubertal female mice. Endocrine J. 1: 451.

138. JACOBSON, J.D., B.C. NISULA & A.D. STEINBERG. 1994. Modulation of the expression of murine lupus by gonadotropin-releasing hormone analogs. Endocrinology 134: 2516.

139. JACOBSON, J.D., M.A. ANSARI, M.E. MANSFIELD *et al.* 1999. Gonadotropin-releasing hormone incerases CD4⁺ T-lyphocytes numbers in an animal model of immunodeficiency. J. Allergy Clin .Immunol. **104:** 653–658.

140. BEBO, B.F. JR., E. ZELINKA-VINCENT, G. ADAMUS *et al.* 1998. Gonadal hormones inflence the immune respons eto PLP 139-151 and the clinical course of relapsing experimental autoimmune encephalomyelitis. J. Neuroimmunol. **84:** 122–130.

141. VOSKHUL, R.R., H. PITCHEKIAN-HALABI, A. McKENZIE-GRAHAM *et al.* 1996. Gender differences in autoimmune demyelination in the mouse: implications for multiple sclerosis. Ann. Neurol. **39:** 724–733.

142. DALAL, M., S. KIM & R.R. VOSKUHL. 1997. Testosterone therapy ameliorates experimental autoimmune encephalomyelitis and induces a T helper 2 bias in autoantigen-specific T lymphocyte response. J. Immunol. **159:** 3–6.

143. McEWEN, B.S. 1998 Protective and damaging effects of stress mediators. N. Engl. J. Med. **238:** 171–179.

144. SAPOLSKY, R. 1992. Stress, the Aging Brain and Mechanisms of Neuron Death. MIT Press. Cambridge, MA.

145. McEWEN, B.S. & R.M. SAPLOSKY. 1995. Stress and cognitive function. Curr. Opin. Neurobiol. **5:** 205–212.

146. SAPOLSKY, R.M. 1996. Stress, glucocorticoids and damage to the nervous system: the current state of confusion. Stress **1:** 1–19.

147. PEPIN, M.C., F. POTHIER & N. BARDEN. 1992. Impaired type II glucocorticoid-receptor function in mice bearing antisense RNA transgene. Nature **355:** 725–728.

148. BARDEN, N. 1995. Do antidepressants stabilize mood through action on the hypothalamic-pituitary-adrenocortical system? Trends Neurosci. **18:** 6–11.

149. HOLBOER, F. & N. BARDEN. 1996. Antidepressant and hypothalamic-pituitary-adrenocortical regulation. Endocr. Rev. **17:** 187–205.

150. STEA, I., N. BARDEN, J.M.H. REUL & F. HOLSBORN. 1994. Dexamethasone nonsuppression in transgenic mice expressing antisense RNA to the glucocorticoid receptor. J. Psychiat. Res. **28:** 1–5.

151. KARANTH, S., A.C.E. LINTHORST, G.K. STALLA *et al.* 1997. Hypothalamic-pituitary adrenocortical axis changes in a transgenic mouse with impaired glucocorticoid receptor function. Endcorinology **138:** 3476–345.

152. DIJKISTRA, I., F.J. TILDERS, G. AGUILERA *et al.* 1998. Reduced activity of hypothalamic corticotropin-releasing hormone neurons in transgenic mice with impaired glucocorticoid receptor function. J. Neurosci. **18:** 3909–3918.

153. SACEDON, R., A.VICENTE, A. VARAS *et al.* 1999. Partial blockade of T-cell differentiation during ontogeneses and marked alterations of the thymic microenvironment in transgenic mice with impaired glucocorticoid receptor function. J. Neuroimmunol. **98:** 157–167.

Thymic Neuroendocrine Self-Antigens

Role in T-Cell Development and Central T-Cell Self-Tolerance

VINCENT GEENEN,[a] HENRI MARTENS, FABIENNE BRILOT,
CHANTAL RENARD, DENIS FRANCHIMONT, AND OUAFAE KECHA

Department of Medicine, Institute of Pathology CHU-B23, Laboratory of Radio-Immunology and Neuroendocrine-Immunology, University of Liège, Belgium

ABSTRACT: The repertoire of thymic neuroendocrine precursors plays a dual role in T-cell differentiation as the source of either cryptocrine accessory signals in T-cell development or neuroendocrine self-antigens presented by the thymic major histocompatibility complex (MHC) machinery. Thymic neuroendocrine self-antigens usually correspond to peptide sequences highly conserved during the evolution of one family. The thymic presentation of some neuroendocrine self-antigens is not restricted by MHC alleles. Oxytocin (OT) is the dominant peptide of the neurohypophysial family. It is expressed by thymic epithelial and nurse cells (TEC/TNCs) of different species. Ontogenetic studies have shown that the thymic expression of the OT gene precedes the hypothalamic one. Both OT and VP stimulate the phosphorylation of p125[FAK] and other focal adhesion-related proteins in murine immature T cells. These early cell activation events could play a role in the promotion of close interactions between thymic stromal cells and developing T cells. It is established that such interactions are fundamental for the progression of thymic T-cell differentiation. Insulin-like growth factor 2 (IGF-2) is the dominant thymic polypeptide of the insulin family. Using fetal thymic organ cultures (FTOCs), the inhibition of thymic IGF-2-mediated signaling was shown to block the early stages of T-cell differentiation. The treatment of FTOCs with an mAb anti-(pro)insulin had no effect on T-cell development. In an animal model of autoimmune type 1 diabetes (BB rat), thymic levels of (pro)insulin and IGF-1 mRNAs were normal both in diabetes-resistant and diabetes-prone BB rats. IGF-2 transcripts were clearly identified in all thymuses from diabetes-resistant adult (5-week) and young (2- and 5-days) BB rats. In marked contrast, the IGF-2 transcripts were absent and the IGF-2 protein was almost undetectable in ±80% of the thymuses from diabetes-prone adult and young BB rats. These data show that a defect of the thymic IGF-2–mediated tolerogenic function might play an important role in the pathophysiology of autoimmune Type 1 diabetes.

[a]Address for correspondence: Pr. Vincent Geenen, M.D., Ph.D., University of Liège, Institute of Pathology CHU-B23, B-4000 Liège 1-Sart Tilman, Belgium. Voice: 32 43 66 25 50; fax: 32 43 66 29 77.
vgeenen@ulg.ac.be

THE DUAL ROLE OF THYMIC NEUROENDOCRINE
SELF-ANTIGENS IN T-CELL DIFFERENTIATION

Before reacting against "non-self" infectious agents, the immune system must be able to tolerate the host molecular structure ("self"). The induction of immune self-tolerance is a multistep process that is initiated inside the thymus during fetal ontogeny (central self-tolerance) and also involves inactivating (anergizing)[1] mechanisms outside the thymus (peripheral self-tolerance).[2] The thymus is the primary lymphoid organ implicated in the development of immunocompetent and self-tolerant T lymphocytes.[3] Our experimental studies since 1985 have established that the thymus also constitutes one privileged meeting point between the two major systems of intercellular signaling, the neuroendocrine and immune systems.[4,5] The thymic parenchyme is the site of synthesis for protein precursors belonging to various neuroendocrine families. Thymic precursors not only provide accessory signals for T-cell growth and development, but they are also the source of neuroendocrine self-antigens which are presented to differentiating T cells. According to the theory of T-cell negative selection,[6–8] the intrathymic presentation of neuroendocrine self-antigens would induce the clonal deletion or developmental arrest of self-reactive T cells. Such self-reactive T cells randomly emerge during the recombination of gene segments coding for the chains of the T-cell receptor of antigen (TCR) and they are bearing one TCR specifically directed toward the complex CMH/self-antigen. The thymus is the major, if not the only one, lymphoid organ wherein permanently occurs a confrontation between the presentation of the self molecular structure and a pure random phenomenon with a potential toxic threat for the host organism. In physiological conditions, this confrontation leads to the deletion or the inactivation of such self-oriented toxicity. Even if other tolerizing mechanisms exist in the periphery, it is now well established that the thymus exerts the dominant tolerogenic control upon the immune system.

According to its nature as the source of either cryptocrine accessory signals or self-antigens, respectively, the thymic repertoire of neuroendocrine precursors recapitulates at the molecular level the dual physiological role of the thymus in T-cell positive and negative selection. The interaction of neuroendocrine self-antigens with their corresponding TCR implies a binding of moderate affinity (from 10^{-6} to 10^{-8} M), but with a high selectivity. On the other hand, cryptocrine signaling between thymic neuroendocrine-related peptides and their cognate neuroendocrine-type receptors expressed by pre-T cells involves a high-affinity binding (from 10^{-10} to 10^{-11} M), albeit with a low specificity.[9] Moreover, a hierarchy of dominance and an economical principle appear in the organization of the polypeptide repertoire expressed in the thymus. This is of high significance since self-tolerance primarily concerns dominant antigenic determinants of self-molecules.[10] This model concurs with the "avidity/affinity hypothesis" that has been proposed as another explanation of the thymic paradox in T-cell life and death.[11] According to this latter hypothesis, T lymphocytes are positively selected if their TCR is barely engaged with self-antigen at low concentrations (10^{-12} M), and are deleted if TCR is strongly engaged with self-peptide at high concentrations (10^{-6} M). However, since the affinity of a TCR for its cognate antigen is rather low (10^{-8} M at the maximum),[12] the intrathymic concentration of self-peptides is of crucial importance for determining positive or negative

T-cell selection. It therefore became a primary objective to define the nature and the amount of peptide/MHC combinations that contribute *in vivo* to positive or negative selection of a particular TCR in a normal thymus.

ONTOGENY OF THYMIC OT AND IGF GENE EXPRESSION

Although the two neurohypophysial genes, OT and vasopressin (VP), are expressed in human and murine thymuses,[13] at the peptide level OT is the dominant member of this family which is synthesized by TEC/TNCs in these species. Using RT-PCR, *in situ* hybridization, and immunocytochemistry (ICC), we recently investigated the ontogeny of neurohypophysial gene expression in the thymus of Balb/c mice. Transcripts of *proOT* and *proVP* are detected without any visible modulation in the thymus already from fetal day (FD) 14 until day 7 after birth. In the murine thymus, neurohypophysial transcripts are located in cells with an epithelial morphology and are absent in the lymphoid compartment.[14] Because of the microscopic size of thymic rudiments before FD 14, it was not possible to analyze earlier the thymic expression of the neurohypophysial genes. Nevertheless, the comparison with previous reports[15] shows that the transcription of neurohypophysial genes in the rodent thymus precedes their expression in the magnocellular neurons of the hypothalamic–neurohypophysial axis. At the peptide level, this difference is more evident since ir-OT is detected in the thymus on FD 15, whereas ICC labels ir-OT in the hypothalamus only on FD 20.[16] Thus, the expression of neurohypophysial genes in the murine thymus coincides with the appearance of T-cell progenitors and slightly precedes their hypothalamic transcription. This observation is highly significant with regard to the physiological role proposed for thymic OT both in T-cell lymphopoiesis and in central tolerance of the hypothalamo-neurohypophysial functions. The early expression of thymic OT is another experimental argument supporting a tolerogenic role of the thymic repertoire of neuroendocrine self-antigen precursors. Indeed, it is logical that the induction of central self-tolerance precedes the appearance of antigenic epitopes in the target organs susceptible to an autoimmune aggression.[17,18] Furthermore, the putative thymic deletion of OT-reactive T-cell clones will allow the immunomodulation by peripheral OT without the risk of inducing an autoimmune hypothalamitis. For example, a non-specific immune activation is usually observed in the postpartum, a period characterized by an increase of lactatory hormones (prolactin and OT) and an enhancement of the estrogen/progesterone ratio.

The components of the IGF axis have also been characterized in the human thymus. Human TEC expresses different members of this axis, with a predominance of IGF-2 and IGF-binding proteins (IGFBP) 2 to 6.[19,20] In the human and rat thymuses, IGF-1 expression is restricted to sparse cells with a macrophage-like morphology and distribution.[20,21] RT-PCR analyses of total RNA from murine fetal and postnatal thymuses revealed that IGF-1, IGF-2, IGF type 1 (IGF-1R) and type 2 (mannose-6-phosphate [M6P]/IGF-2R) receptors are expressed from FD 14 through seven weeks of age. Though RT-PCR conditions are not quantitative, a striking difference appeared between the IGF-2 signals and the others studied. Similar mRNA levels of IGF-1, IGF-1R, and M6P/IGF-2R were detected in all the fetal and postnatal murine thymuses. However, IGF-2 mRNA levels declined after birth, but weak signals were still detected in seven-week old thymuses. By *in situ* hybridization, IGF-2 mRNAs were detected mainly in the epithelial component of the murine thymus. Therefore, the expression of insulin-related genes in the thymus also precedes their peripheral transcription, as in the pancreatic islet cells.

THE ROLE OF THYMIC OT AND IGF IN T-CELL DEVELOPMENT

After their migration from the fetal liver and then from bone marrow, immature T-cell progenitors receive from the thymic parenchyme various types of signals which regulate their differentiation program toward T-cell death or development. These signals are not strictly thymus-specific, but their local action is linked to their expression within a particular microenvironment and at a crucial step of T-cell differentiation. The ability of pre-T cells to respond to thymic OT and IGF-2 was demonstrated by a series of different approaches.

Functional neurohypophysial hormone receptors are expressed by immature T cells and by mature cytotoxic T cells.[22,23] These lymphocyte receptors are different from classic V1a/V2 receptors, and rather appear such as another V1 (V1b or V3?) subtype, as well as the OT type.[23,24] They are able to transduce OT and VP into a phospho-inositide turnover, and to mediate mitogenic effects of neurohypophysial-related peptides on freshly isolated human pre-T cells.[23] Moreover, in a line of pre-T cells derived from a murine thymic lymphoma (RL12-NP), OT and VP quickly stimulate the phosphorylation of p125^{FAK}, a tyrosine-kinase involved in focal adhesion, as well as other proteins implicated in this process like paxillin and a 130-kDa protein (p130^{CAS}?). Neurohypophysial peptide-induced p125^{FAK} phosphorylations are blocked by a V1 antagonist (Manning compound).[25] As demonstrated by others, the role of p125^{FAK} is crucial for T-cell differentiation.[26] The OT-mediated activation of p125^{FAK} in RL12-NP cells suggests that thymic OT intervenes in T-cell selection, either as a promoter of focal adhesion itself, or as an anti-apoptotic inducer of a cryptocrine signaling between TEC and T cells leading to the proliferation and survival of early T-cell precursors.

There is increasing evidence that IGFs are implicated in the development and modulation of the immune response. Thymocytes express both types of IGF receptors (IGF-1R and M6P/IGF-2R).[27,28] Administration of IGF-1 stimulates thymus and spleen growth and T-cell proliferation and development and modulates the regeneration of T cells in a rat model of dexamethasone-induced apoptosis.[29,30] In addition, the thymus of IGF-2 transgenic mice contains high levels of IGF-2 mRNA and displays an increased cellularity, with a higher number of the CD4$^+$ T-cell subset.[31] We also examined the role of IGFs on murine T-cell development by evaluating the effect of anti-IGFs and IGF-receptors neutralizing Abs on the generation of thymocyte subpopulations in fetal thymic organ cultures (FTOCs).[32] Neither anti-IGF-1 nor anti-IGF-2 induced a significant change in the total cell number or the percentage of dead cells as measured by propidium iodide staining. FTOC treatment with anti-IGF-2 mAb, an anti-IGF-1R mAb, or an anti-M6P/IGF-2R polyclonal Ab induced a blockade of T-cell differentiation at the CD4$^-$CD8$^-$ (double negative) T cells, as shown by a significant increase in the percentage of CD4$^-$CD8$^-$ cells and a decrease in the percentage of CD4$^+$CD8$^+$ cells. In addition, the treatment with anti-IGF-1R Ab blocked T-cell differentiation at the CD4+CD8+ stage as shown by a decrease in single positive subsets. Moreover, anti-IGF-2 Ab treatment induced an increase in CD8+ single positive cells, suggesting that thymic IGF-2 has a role in determining differentiation into the CD4 or CD8 lineage. The total percentage of viable cells was not affected by any of the anti-IGF-R Abs tested. However, in FTOCs treated with anti-IGF-2R, there was a 31% decrease in the total cell number. This decrease was more important (81%) with the FTOC treatment by anti-IGF-1R. Although the (pro)insulin gene is slightly expressed in the thymus,[33] FTOCs treated with a specific anti-(pro)insulin mAb were unaffected neither in total cell number, nor in the main steps of T-cell differentiation.[32]

THYMIC PRESENTATION OF NEUROENDOCRINE SELF-ANTIGENS

The synthesis of OT in TEC/TNCs is not coupled to the classic secretion of the non-apeptide and its precursor-associated binding neurophysin in the supernatant of TEC primary cultures. In the murine thymus, ir-OT is not located in secretory granules, but is diffuse in the cytosol, in vesicles of the endoplasmic reticulum, and in close association with cytokeratin filaments.[34] Similar ultrastructural features have also been described for ir-OT and ir-VP synthesized by murine spleen eosinophil-like cells.[35] Those independent observations repeatedly questioned the classic model of neurosecretion which was established for OT and VP in the hypothalamo-neurohypophysial tractus. They further suggested a processing of the OT precursor that differs in the thymus compared to the situation in the hypothalamo-neurohypophysial axons. As discussed above, the thymic function is associated with the presentation of self-antigens to developing T cells. This action was long thought to be mediated by thymic macrophages and dendritic/interdigitating (IDC) cells only, but TEC/TNCs also are actively involved in the induction of central self-tolerance.[36–38] Thus, we hypothesized a processing of thymic proOT that could be related to antigen presentation instead of a classic neurosecretion.

Using affinity-chromatography with a mAb directed against the monomorphic part of human MHC class I molecules,[39] we identified in TEC/TNC plasma membranes a 55-kDa protein that was labelled both by anti-MHC class I mAb and anti-neurophysin antibodies.[40] Since anti-neurophysin Abs do not cross-react with either MHC class I proteins, nor with β2-microglobulin, this 55-kDa membrane protein may represent a hybrid protein including both a neurophysin domain (10 kDa) and an MHC class I heavy chain-related domain (45 kDa). The precise biochemical mechanisms underlying the formation of this hybrid neurohypophysial/MHC class I membrane protein are still to be further deciphered. Some preliminary hypotheses may be advanced, however. The origin of this protein could reside at the posttranscriptional level (such as a *trans*-splicing phenomenon) or at the posttranslational level (such as the ATP-dependent binding of ubiquitin to protein targeted to proteolysis). Following this putative explanation, the MHC class I domain would be implicated in membrane targeting of this hybrid protein, whereas neurophysin binds OT for presentation to pre-T cells. Other authors have shown the translocation of a 45-kDa neurophysin-like material in the cell membranes of cancer cells, and have provided strong arguments supporting the behavior of neurohypophysial-related peptides as candidate tumoral antigens.[41,42] Thus, both in the hypothalamo–neuro-hypophysial axis and in the thymus, the neurophysin part of the OT precursor fulfills the same function: binding of the active nonapeptide OT and tranport to the external limits of neurons or TEC/TNCs. The tyrosine residue in position 2 of OT and VP plays an important role in their binding to neurophysin.[43] Interestingly, the tyrosine residue in the same position plays a crucial role in the binding of antigens to some MHC class I alleles for their presentation.[44] The particular features of thymic OT-mediated T-cell education to the neurohypophysial family can be related to the observation of a dissociation between thymic T-cell education to self and peripheral T-cell recognition of antigens.[45] Selective advantages appear from this model of thy-mic neuroendocrine–self-antigen presentation. A first advantage is the absence of a tight allelic restriction in thymic T-cell education to a neuroendocrine family. Such an allelic restriction of central T-cell tolerance was hardly conceivable and our data indicate that it is not the case in reality. Concerning the presentation of thymic OT, though MHC class I molecules are involved in the process, it is the invariant neuro-physin domain of the hybrid membrane 55-kDa protein that binds OT for presenta-tion to pre-T cells. Another advantage resides in the presentation to pre-T cells of the structure characteristic of the neurohypophysial family.

The antigenic behavior of thymic OT was further demonstrated by another type of experiments. The immunological recognition of OT by specific mAbs at the outer surface of human TEC plasma membrane induced a marked secretion of the cytok-ines interleukin-6 and leukemia inhibitory factor in the supernatant of TEC cultures.[46] Given the nature of the epitopes recognized by anti-OT mAbs, we could conclude that the molecule OT is fully processed at the level of the TEC plasma membrane. The absence of biological effects following the treatment of TEC cul-tures with anti-VP mAbs further confirms that thymic OT behaves as the self-antigen representative of the neurohypophysial hormone family.

Neurotensin (NT) and somatostatin have been extracted from the chicken thymus, especially after hatching, and have been characterized both immunochemically and chromatographically.[47] Ir-NT is expressed at the cell surface of human TEC, and cultured human TECs contain ± 5 ng ir-NT/10^6 cells, of which 5% is associated with plasma cell membranes. HPLC analysis of ir-NT present in human TEC revealed a major peak of ir-NT corresponding to intact NT_{1-13}. Using an affinity column pre-pared with the same anti-MHC class I Ab, NT-related peptides were retained on the column and were eluted together with MHC class I proteins.[48] With regard to the thymic presentation of NT, there is no physical constraint for a non-covalent binding to MHC since this neuropeptide is a linear peptide (in contrast to cyclic OT and IGF-2). In addition, the C-terminal sequence of NT includes tyrosine, isoleucine and leucine residues, which can all be used in the anchorage to most of the MHC class I alleles. Given these characteristics, it is logical to postulate that NT and NT-derived C-terminal fragments could behave as natural ligands for a majority (if not all) of MHC class I alleles. This hypothesis is also in agreement with the high degree of conservation of NT-related C-terminal region throughout evolution.[49]

Neurokinin A (NKA) is the peptide of the tachykinin family encoded in human and rat TEC by the preprotachykinin A (PPT-A) gene.[50] Thymic *PPT-A* expression appears to be glucocorticoid-dependent since adrenalectomy of Sprague-Dawley rats markedly enhances thymic expression of *PPT-A* (and *NPY*) mRNAs (Ericsson and Geenen, unpublished observations). Interestingly, NKA exerts IL-1-like mitogenic effects on murine thymocytes,[51] suggesting that tachykinin receptors are expressed by immature T cells and are implicated as an accessory pathway in T-cell maturation and positive selection. The amino-acid sequence of NKA shares the same C-terminal epitope with other members of the tachykinin family, and the leucine residue in position 9 could be used in the binding to some MHC class I alleles, thus making NKA the self-antigen of the tachykinin family. The other tachykinin encoded by *PPT-A,* substance P (SP), is not detected in TEC, but is present in sensory nerve fibers of the thymus.[52] Thymic-specific receptors for SP are associated with the vasculature in the medulla, where they could control local blood flow and vascular permeability.[53]

For IGFs, the role of binding and transport proteins is ensured by IGFBPs. IGFBPs have co-evolved with IGFs, but are not intrinsic part of IGF precursors, and are encoded by distinct genes. These proteins play a prominent role in regulating the bioavailability and distribution of IGFs.[54,55] Interestingly, some IGFBPs are in close relationship with cell plasma membranes (through binding to integrins or the extracellular matrix), but their relationship with MHC as well as their potential implication in thymic IGF presentation to immature T cells deserves to be further investigated.

A DEFECT OF THYMIC FUNCTION IN
AUTOIMMUNE TYPE 1 DIABETES

The development of an autoimmune disease affecting the neuroendocrine system may be viewed as a failure to develop or to maintain self-tolerance of cellular and molecular components which are constitutively expressed by neuroendocrine cells. Three types of factors are usually thought to be implicated in the pathogeny of autoimmune diseases: (1) The immune effectors are CD4 and CD8 auto-reactive T cells which are specifically oriented against a given target cell or molecule. These auto-reactive T cells are usually thought to result from a spontaneous breakdown of peripheral T-cell tolerance. (2) A series of extra- and intra-MHC genes are related to different autoimmune diseases. Some of these genes intervene in the presentation of target auto-antigens to auto-reactive T lymphocytes, but others certainly not. (3) An environmental factor is involved and establishes a link between the target auto-antigens and auto-reactive T cells. A molecular mimicry between target auto-antigens and microorganisms was shown to intervene at this level.[56] The involvement of microbial superantigens has also been proposed to activate peripheral auto-reactive T cells.[57]

Although the relationship between lymphoepithelial structures and autoimmunity had been suspected by Burnet and Mackay in 1962,[58] the question of a defective central T-cell self-tolerance in the pathophysiology of autoimmune diseases has not been intensively investigated. Also, Burnet repeatedly proposed that the emergence of "forbidden" self-reactive T-cell clones should play a major role in the pathophysiology of autoimmunity. In this perspective, it has been shown that neonatal thymectomy prevents the emergence of diabetes in an animal model of autoimmune type 1 diabetes, the Bio-Breeding (BB) rat.[59] In clinical practice also, thymectomy usually induces a significant improvement in patients suffering from autoimmune myasthenia gravis, especially when a thymoma (hyperplasia of thymic epithelium) is associated.[60] In both cases, the benefit of thymectomy can be explained by the removal of the defective thymic censorship. Such a trouble in central self-tolerance would be responsible for a continuous release and enrichment of the peripheral T-cell pool with intolerant and self-reactive lymphocytes. The development of diabetes is prevented by the transplantation of thymus from diabetes-resistant to diabetes-prone BB rats.[61] The transplantation of the thymus from NOD mice to diabetes-resistant mouse strains was also shown to induce diabetes in the recipients.[62] While bone marrow transplantation is rather ineffective in preventing autoimmune diseases of MRL/+ mice, thymus transplantation is a crucial factor for their prevention. [63] A defective process of thymic T-cell negative selection has been suggested on the basis that the thymus of diabetes-resistant BB rats contains thymocytes predisposed to auto-reactivity.[64] Another argument is the observation that grafts of pure thymic epithelium from NOD mouse embryos to newborn C57BL/6 athymic mice induced CD4 and CD8 T-cell–mediated insulitis and sialitis.[65] At the histological level, a defect in thymic function could be linked to a disorganization of the microenvironment, such as the giant perivascular spaces observed in the NOD mouse thymus,[66] and the epithelial defects of BB rat thymus.[67] Recently, we examined the G75 elution profiles of ir-IGFs in the thymus from Wistar Furth (WF) normal rats and from diabetes-resistant and diabetes-prone BB rats. A peak of ir-IGF-2 above 10 ng/ml was observed in the G75 profile of WF thymus extracts; a peak around 1.5 ng/ml was eluted from diabetes-resistant BB rat thymic extracts, however IGF-2 concentrations were almost undetectable in diabetes-prone BB rats.[68] IGF-2 transcripts were not detected by RT-PCR in the thymus of 11/15 diabetes-prone BB rats, but were clearly identified in the thymus of 15/15 diabetes-resistant BB rats. The defect of thymic IGF-2 expression was evidenced at different ages of the diabetes-prone BB rat. The expression of proinsulin and IGF-1 genes was normal in the thymus of diabetes-prone and diabetes-resistant BB rats. The defect of IGF-2 expression was tissue-specific since IGF-2 transcripts were detected in the brain and liver of diabetes-prone BB rats.[69] Taken together, these observations show a genetically determined defect of *IGF2* expression in the thymus of diabetes-prone BB rats. They also strongly support that a defect in the central T-cell self-tolerance of the insulin family is involved in the pathophysiology of autoimmune type 1 diabetes, at least in this animal model. A recent study has shown that the thymic and pancreatic expression of *IGF2* is not polymorphic enough to explain the human susceptibility to type 1 diabetes, which is associated with *IDDM2*,[70] the genetic locus that includes the contiguous IGF2 and insulin genes. It must be pointed out, however, that the imprinting of *IGF2* could partially explain why the susceptibility to the disease is higher in children from diabetic fathers than those from diabetic mothers.[71,72]

NEUROENDOCRINE SELF VERSUS AUTO-ANTIGENS

In the neurohypophysial family, the bulk of experimental data shows that OT is the self-antigen of the neurohypophysial hormone family. A strong immunological tolerance protects the OT lineage, more than the VP one, from an autoimmune aggression. Indeed, some cases of so-called "idiopathic" central diabetes insipidus result from an autoimmune hypothalamitis oriented toward VP-producing neurons. Given the implication of the OT lineage at different levels of the reproductive process, a stronger tolerance of this lineage is important for the preservation of the species. Thus, in the neurohypophysial family, while OT behaves as the self-antigen, VP is suspected to be the target auto-antigen of the autoimmune process. As discussed previously, this conclusion is also supported by the frequences and the titers of Abs induced by active immunization against neurohypophysial peptides (VP >> OT). An infiltration of the hypothalamo-neurohypophysial tract by inflammatory mononuclear cells can be observed, both after active immunization against VP,[73] and in autoimmune "idiopathic" diabetes insipidus.[17,18]

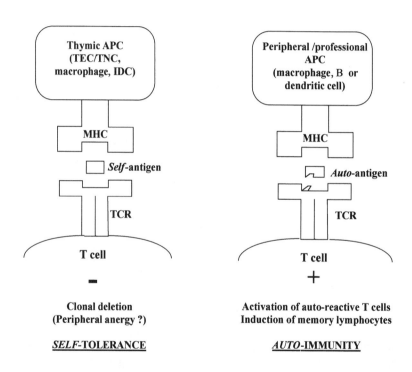

FIGURE 1. The opposite immune responses elicited by the thymic presentation of a self-antigen and the peripheral presentation of an auto-antigen. Thymic antigen-presenting cells (APC) are thymic epithelial and nurse cells (TEC/TNC), macrophages and interdigitating cells (IDC) or denditic cells. Neuroendocrine self-antigens correspond to peptide sequences of a precursor that have been highly conserved during evolution of their corresponding family (i.e., OT for the neurohypophysial peptides, IGF-2 for the insulin family, NKA for the tachykinins). They are very homologous to peripheral related auto-antigens (i.e., VP for the neurohypophysial peptides, insulin for the insulin family), although they are not identical. This biochemical difference between neuroendocrine self- and auto-antigens results in opposite immune responses with a deletion of self-reactive T-cell clones in the thymus (and anergy at the periphery?), and an activation of auto-reactive T cells and induction of memory lymphocytes at the periphery.

Insulin is one important auto-antigen tackled by various auto-reactive components of the immune system both in animal and human type 1 diabetes.[74,75] Moreover insulin is the specific marker of the pancreatic islet endocrine β cells. Oral, intranasal and parenteral administration of insulin or insulin-derived dominant auto-antigens have been shown to inhibit the occurrence of diabetes in animal models of type 1 diabetes.[76,77] However, one cannot exclude the risk of priming or triggering autoimmunity by peripheral administration of an auto-antigen.[78] Reprogramming self-tolerance that has not been installed or that is broken in autoimmune diseases is a very rational strategy for the prevention of devastating diseases such as multiple sclerosis, rheumatoid arthritis or type 1 diabetes. Such reprogramming could be based upon the tolerogenic properties of the thymic epithelium. Instead of the classic immunogenic vaccination (with immune activation and induction of memory/immunocompetent cells), the novel form of tolerogenic vaccination (or negative vaccine, so to use the phrase proposed by Nossal)[79] should provoke the deletion or the anergy of auto-reactive T lymphocytes (FIG. 1). The induction of T-cell tolerance following peptide vaccination has already been obtained with synthetic peptides representing cytotoxic CD8 epitopes of T cells oriented against tumor antigens or viruses.[80] According to Claude Bernard's principles of experimental medicine, the hope appears now that the correction of the defective central self-tolerance could prevent the appearance of autoimmune type 1 diabetes. The tolerogenic vaccination represents a very attractive strategy for preventing autoimmune diseases, the heavy tribute paid by the humans for the efficiency and complexity of their system of immune defenses.

ACKNOWLEDGMENTS

These studies were supported by the Fondation Léon Fredericq and the Special Research Fund of Liège University Medical School, the National Fund of Scientific Research (NFSR), Télévie-NFSR, the Association contre le Cancer (Belgium), the Juvenile Diabetes Foundation International, and the Association Belge du Diabète (Fonds Suzanne et Jean Pirart). Our gratitude is due to Pr. Dale L. Greiner (University of Massachussets, Worcester), who provided us with thymuses and organs from Bio-Breeding rats. We also thank Dr. Magda Desmedt and Pr. Jean Plum (University of Ghent, Belgium), who instructed us on fetal thymic organ culture technology.

V. Geenen is Research Director of the Belgian NFSR and Associate Professor of Liège University Medical School.

REFERENCES

1. NOSSAL, G.J.V. 1983. Cellular mechanisms of immunological tolerance. Annu. Rev. Immunol. **1:** 33–62.

2. GEENEN, V. & G. KROEMER. 1993. The multiple ways to cellular immune tolerance. Immunol. Today **14:** 573–576.

3. SHORTMAN, K. & L. WU. 1996. Early T lymphocyte progenitors. Annu. Rev. Immunol. **14:** 29–45.

4. MARTENS, H., B. GOXE & V. GEENEN. 1996. The thymic repertoire of neuroendocrine self-antigens: Physiological implications in T-cell life and death. Immunol. Today **17:** 312–317.
5. GEENEN, V., M. WIEMANN & H. MARTENS. 1999. Thymus gland: Neuroendocrine-Immunology. *In* Encyclopedia of Neuroscience, 2nd edit. G. Adelman & B. Smith, Eds.: 2039–2042. Elsevier. New York.
6. BURNET, F.M. 1957. A modification of Jerne's theory of antibody production using the concept of clonal selection. Aust. J. Sci. **20:** 67–69.
7. KISIELOW, P., H. BLUTHMANN, U. STAERZ *et al.* 1988. Tolerance in T-cell receptor transgenic mice involves deletion of nonmature CD4$^+$8$^+$ thymocytes. Nature **333:** 742–746.
8. NEMAZEE, D.A. & K. BURKI. 1989. Clonal deletion of B lymphocytes in a transgenic mouse bearing anti-MHC class I antibody genes. Nature **337:** 562–566.
9. GEENEN, V. 1995. La Communication Cryptocrine Intrathymique et la Tolérance Immunitaire Centrale au Soi Neuroendocrine. Professoral thesis, University of Liège.
10. CABANIOLS, J.P., R. CIBOTTI, P. KOURILSKY *et al.* 1994. Dose-dependent T-cell tolerance to an immunodominant self-peptide. Eur. J. Immunol. **24:** 1743–1749.
11. ASHTON-RICKARDT, P.G. & S. TONEGAWA. 1994. A differential-avidity model for T-cell selection. Immunol. Today **15:** 362–366.
12. SYKULEV, Y., A. BRUNMARK, T.J. TSOMIDES *et al.* 1994. High-affinity interactions between antigenic-specific T-cell receptors and peptides associated with allogeneic and syngeneic major histocompatibility complex class I proteins. Proc. Natl. Acad. Sci. USA **91:** 11487–11491.
13. GEENEN, V., O. KECHA & H. MARTENS. 1998. Thymic expression of neuroendocrine self-peptide precursors: role in T-cell survival and self-tolerance. J. Neuroendocrinol. **11:** 811–822.
14. MARTENS, H. 1999. The Dual Role of Thymic Oxytocin in T-lymphocyte Differentiation. Ph.D. Thesis, University of Liège.
15. LAURENT, F.M., C. HINDELANG, M.J. KLEIN *et al.* 1989. Expression of the oxytocin and vasopressin genes in the rat hypothalamus during development: an *in situ* hybridization study. Dev. Brain Res. **46:** 145–154.
16. REPPERT, S.M. & G.R. UHL. 1987. Vasopressin messenger ribonucleic acid in supraoptic and suprachiasmatic nuclei: appearance and circadian regulation during development. Endocrinology **120:** 2483–2487.
17. SCHERBAUM, W.A. & G.R. BOTTAZZO. 1983. Autoantibodies to vasopressin cells in idiopathic diabetes insipidus: evidence for an autoimmune variant. Lancet **1:** 897–901.
18. IMURA, H., K. NAKAO, A. SHIMATSU *et al.* 1993. Lymphocytic infundibuloneurohypophysitis as a cause of central diabetes insipidus. N. Engl. J. Med. **329:** 683–689.
19. GEENEN, V., I. ACHOUR, F. ROBERT *et al.* 1993. Evidence that insulin-like growth factor 2 (IGF-2) is the dominant thymic peptide of the insulin superfamily. Thymus **21:** 115–127.
20. KECHA, O., H. MARTENS, N. FRANCHIMONT *et al.* 1999. Characterization of the insulin-like growth factor axis in the human thymus. J. Neuroendocrinol. **11:** 435–440.
21. ARKINS, S., N. REBEIZ, A. BIRAGYN *et al.* 1993. Murine macrophages express abundant insulin-like growth factor-I class I Ea and Eb transcripts. Endocrinology **133:** 2334–2343.
22. GEENEN, V., F. ROBERT, M. FATEMI *et al.* 1988. Vasopressin and oxytocin: thymic signals and receptors in T-cell ontogeny. *In* Recent Progress in Posterior Pituitary. S. Yoshida & L. Share, Eds.: 303–309. Elsevier, New York.
23. MARTENS, H., F. ROBERT, J.J. LEGROS *et al.* 1992. Expression of functional neurohypophysial peptide receptors by murine immature and cytotoxic T cell lines. Prog. NeuroEndocrinImmunol. **5:** 31–39.
24. ELANDS, J., A. RESINK & E.R. DE KLOET. 1990. Neurohypophysial hormone receptors in the rat thymus, spleen and lymphocytes. Endocrinology **126:** 2703–2710.

25. MARTENS, H., O. KECHA, C. CHARLET-RENARD *et al.* 1997. Neurohypophysial peptides stimulate the phosphorylation of pre-T cell focal adhesion kinases. Neuroendocrinology **67:** 282–289.
26. KANAZAWA, S., D. ILIC, M. HASHIYAMA *et al.* 1996. p59^{FYN}-p125^{FAK} cooperation in development of CD4$^+$CD8$^+$ thymocytes. Blood **87:** 865–870.
27. VERLAND, S. & S. GAMMELTOFT. 1989. Functional receptors for insulin-like growth factors I and II in rat thymocytes and mouse thymoma cells. Mol. Cell. Endocrinol. **67:** 207–216.
28. KOOIJMAN, R., L.E. SCHOLTENS, G.T. RIJKERS & B.J.M. ZEGERS. 1995. Differential expression of type 1 insulin-like growth factor receptors in different stages of human T cells. Eur. J. Immunol. **25:** 931–935.
29. CLARK, R., J. STRASSER, S. MCCABE *et al.* 1993. Insulin-like growth factor I stimulation of lymphopoiesis. J. Clin. Invest. **95:** 540–548.
30. HINTON, P.S., C.A. PETERSON, E.M. DAHLY & D.M. NEY. 1998. IGF-I alters lymphocyte survival in thymus and spleen after dexamethasone treatment. Am. J. Physiol. **274:** R912–R917.
31. KOOIJMAN, R., S.C. VAN BUUL-OFFERS, L.E. SCHOLTENS *et al.* 1995. T-cell development in insulin-like growth factor-II transgenic mice. J. Immunol. **154:** 5736–5745.
32. KECHA, O., F. BRILOT, H. MARTENS *et al.* 2000. Involvement of insulin-like growth factors in early T cell development: a study using fetal thymic organ cultures. Endocrinology **141:** 1209–1217.
33. JOLICŒUR, C., D. HANAHAN & K.M. SMITH. 1994. T-cell tolerance toward a transgenic β-cell antigen and transcription of endogenous pancreatic genes in the thymus. Proc. Natl. Acad. Sci. USA **91:** 6707–6711.
34. WIEMANN, M. & G. EHRET. 1993. Subcellular localization of immunoreactive oxytocin within thymic epithelial cells of the male mouse. Cell Tissue Res. **273:** 79–87.
35. KUMAMOTO, K., T. MATSUURA, T. AMAGAI & M. KAWATA. 1995. Oxytocin-producing and vasopressin-producing eosinophils in the mouse spleen: immunohistochemical, immuno-electron-microscopic and *in situ* hybridization studies. Cell Tissue Res. **281:** 1–10.
36. WEBB, S.R. & J. SPRENT. 1990. Tolerogenicity of thymic epithelium. Eur. J. Immunol. **20:** 2525–2528.
37. LORENZ, R.G. & P.M. ALLEN. 1989. Thymic cortical epithelial cells can present self-antigens *in vivo*. Nature **337:** 560–562.
38. BONOMO, A. & P. MATZINGER. 1993. Thymus epithelium induces tissue-specific tolerance. J. Exp. Med. **177:** 1153–1164.
39. REBAI, S.N. & B. MALISSEN. 1983. Structural and genetic analyses of HLA class I molecules using monoclonal xenoantibodies. Tissue Antigens **22:** 107–117.
40. GEENEN, V., E. VANDERSMISSEN, N. CORMANN-GOFFIN *et al.* 1993. Membrane translocation and relationship with MHC class I of a human thymic neurophysin-like protein. Thymus **22:** 55–66.
41. ROSENBAUM, L.C., E.A. NEUWELT, H.H.M. VAN TOL *et al.* 1990. Expression of neurophysin-related precursor in cell membranes of a small-cell lung carcinoma. Proc. Natl. Acad. Sci. USA **87:** 9928–9932.
42. NORTH, W.G. 2000. Gene regulation of vasopressin and vasopressin receptors in cancer. Exp. Physiol. **85s:** 27s–40s.
43. GRIFFIN, G.H., R. ALAZARD & P. COHEN. 1973. Complex formation between bovine neurophysin-1 and oxytocin, vasopressin and tripeptide analogs of their NH2-terminal region. J. Biol. Chem. **248:** 7975–7978.
44. MARYANSKI, J.L., P. ROMERO, A. VAN PEL *et al.* 1991. The identification of tyrosine as a common key residue in unrelated H-2K^d restricted antigenic peptides. Int. Immunol. **3:** 1035–1042.
45. SIMPSON, E., P.J. ROBINSON, P. CHANDLER *et al.* 1994. Separation of thymic education from antigen presenting functions of major histocompatibility complex class I molecules. Immunology **81:** 132–136.
46. MARTENS, H., B. MALGRANGE, F. ROBERT *et al.* 1996. Cytokine production by human thymic epithelial cells: Control by the immune recognition of the neurohypophysial self-antigen. Regul. Pept. **67:** 39–45.

47. SUNDLER, F., R.E. CARRAWAY, R. HAKANSON *et al.* 1978. Immunoreactive neurotensin and somatostatin in the chicken thymus. A chemical and histochemical study. Cell Tissue Res. **194:** 367–376.
48. VANNESTE, Y., A. NTODOU-THOME, E. VANDERSMISSEN *et al.* 1997. Identification of neurotensin-related peptides in human thymic epithelial cell membranes and relationship with major histocompatibilty complex class I molecules. J. Neuroimmunol. **76:** 161–166.
49. CARRAWAY, R.E., S.E. RUANE & H.R. KIM. 1982. Distribution and immunochemical character of neurotensin-like material in representative vertebrates and invertebrates: Apparent conservation of the COOH-terminal region during evolution. Peptides **3:** 115–123.
50. ERICSSON, A., V. GEENEN, F. ROBERT *et al.* 1990. Expression of preprotachykinin A and neuropeptide-Y messenger RNA in the thymus. Mol. Endocrinol. **4:** 1211–1218.
51. SODER, O. & P.M. HELSTROM. 1989. The tachykinins neurokinin A and physalaemin stimulate murine thymocyte proliferation. Int. Arch. Allergy Appl. Immunol. **90:** 91–96.
52. GEPPETTI, P., E. THEODORSSON-NORHEIM, G. BALLERINI *et al.* 1988. Capsaicin-sensitive tachykinin-like immunoreactivity in the thymus of rats and guinea pigs. J. Neuroimmunol. **19:** 3–9.
53. SHIGEMATSU, K., J.M. SAAVEDRA & M. KURIHARA. 1986. Specific substance P binding sites in rat thymus and spleen: in vitro autoradiographic study. Regul. Pept. **16:** 147–156.
54. CLEMMONS, D.R., W.H. BUSBY, T. ARAI *et al.* 1995. Role of insulin-like grow factor binding proteins in the control of IGF actions. Prog. Growth Factor Res. **6:** 357–366.
55. KELLEY, K.M., Y. OH, S.E. GARGOSKY *et al.* 1996. Insulin-like growth factor-binding proteins (IGFBPs) and their regulatory dynamics. Int. J. Biochem. Cell Biol. **6:** 619–637.
56. ATKINSON, M.A. & N.K. MACLAREN. 1994. The pathogenesis of insulin-dependent diabetes mellitus. N. Engl. J. Med. **331:** 1428–1436.
57. CONRAD, B., E. WEIDMANN, G. TRUCCO *et al.* 1994. Evidence for superantigen involvement in insulin-dependent diabetes mellitus aetiology. Nature **371:** 351–355.
58. BURNET, F.M. & I.R. MACKAY. 1962. Lymphoepithelial structures and autoimmune disease. Lancet **2:** 1030–1033.
59. LIKE, A.A., E. KISLAUKIS, R.M. WILLIAMS & A.A. ROSSINI. 1982. Neonatal thymectomy prevents spontaneous diabetes mellitus in the BB:W rat. Science **216:** 644–646.
60. NEWSOM-DAVIS, J. 1987. Myasthenia gravis. Med. Int. **48:** 1988–1991.
61. GEORGIOU, H.M. & D. BELLGRAU. 1989. Thymus transplantation and disease prevention in the diabetes-prone bio-breeding rat. J. Immunol. **142:** 3400–3405.
62. GEORGIOU, H.M. & T.E. MANDEL. 1995. Induction of insulitis in athymic (nude) mice. The effect of NOD thymus and pancreas transplantation. Diabetes **44:** 49–59.
63. HOSAKA, N., M. NOSE, M. KYOGOKU *et al.* 1996. Thymus transplantation, a critical factor for correction of autoimmune disease in aging MRL/+ mice. Proc. Natl. Acad. Sci. USA **93:** 8558–8562.
64. WHALEN, B.J., A.A. ROSSINI, J.P. MORDES & D.L. GREINER. 1995. DR-BB rat thymus contains thymocyte populations predisposed to autoreactivity. Diabetes **44:** 963–967.
65. THOMAS-VASLIN, V., D. DAMOTTE, M. COLTEY *et al.* 1997. Abnormal T cell selection on nod thymic epithelium is sufficient to induce autoimmune manifestations in C57BL/6 athymic nude mice. Proc. Natl. Acad. Sci. USA **94:** 4598–4603.
66. SAVINO, W., C. CARNAUD, J.J. LUAN *et al.* 1993. Characterization of the extracellular matrix-containing giant perivascular spaces in the NOD mouse thymus. Diabetes **42:** 134–140.
67. DOUKAS, J., J.P. MORDES, C. SWYMER *et al.* 1994. Thymic epithelial defects and predisposition to autoimmune diabetes in BB rats. Am. J. Pathol. **145:** 1517–1525.
68. GEENEN, V., I. ACHOUR, O. KECHA *et al.* 1996. Thymic insulin-like growth factors (IGFs) in man and in an animal model of autoimmune IDDM. Diabetologia **39**(Suppl. 1): A15.

69. KECHA, O., R. WINKLER, H. MARTENS *et al.* 1999. Thymic insulin-related polypeptides in diabetes-prone Bio-Breeding rats. Diabetologia **42**(Suppl. 1): OP16.
70. VAFIADIS, P., R. GRABS, C.G. GOODYER *et al.* 1998. A functional analysis of the role of *IGF2* in *IDDM2*-encoded susceptibility to Type 1 diabetes. Diabetes **47**: 831–836.
71. POLYCHRONAKOS, C., N. GIANNOUKAKIS & C.L. DEAL. 1995. Imprinting of *IGF2*, insulin-dependent diabetes, immune function, and apoptosis: a hypothesis. Dev. Genet. **17**: 253–262.
72. GEENEN, V. 1996. Le Diabète Insulino-Dépendant. Professoral Lecture. Revue Méd. Liège **51**: 684–694.
73. CAU, P. & G. ROUGON-CAPUZZI. 1979. Autoimmune alterations in the neurohypophysis of rabbits immunized against vasopressin. Brain Res. **177**: 265–271.
74. SIMONE, E.A., L. YU, D.R. WEGMANN & G.S. EISENBARTH. 1997. T cell receptor gene polymorphisms associated with anti-insulin, autoimmune T cells in diabetes-prone NOD mice. J. Autoimmun. **10**: 317–321.
75. DANIEL, D., R.G. GILL, N. SCHLOOT & D.R. WEGMANN. 1995. Epitope specificity, cytokine production profile and diabetogenic activity of insulin-specific T cell clones isolated from NOD mice. Eur. J. Immunol. **25**: 1056–1062.
76. ZHANG, Z.J., L. DAVIDSON, G.S. EISENBARTH & H.L. WEINER. 1991. Suppression of diabetes in nonobese diabetic mice by oral administration of porcine insulin. Proc. Natl. Acad. Sci. USA **88**: 10252–10256.
77. DANIEL, D. & D.R. WEGMANN. 1996. Protection of nonobese diabetic mice from diabetes by intranasal or subcutaneous administration of insulin peptide Bv(9–23).Proc. Natl. Acad. Sci. USA **93**: 956–960.
78. BLANAS, E., F.R. CARBONE, J. ALLISON *et al.* 1996. Induction of autoimmune diabetes by oral administration of autoantigen. Science **274**: 1707–1709.
79. NOSSAL, G.J.V. 1998. Four decades of self and non-self: reflections on autoimmunity and tolerance. *In* The Autoimmune Diseases, 3rd edit. N.R. Rose & I.R. Mackay, Eds.: 5–8. Academic Press, San Diego, CA.
80. TOES, R.M., R. OFFRINGA, R.J.J. BLOM *et al.* 1996. Peptide vaccination can lead to enhanced tumor growth through specific T-cell tolerance induction. Proc. Natl. Acad. Sci. USA **93**: 7855–7860.

Human T Lymphopoiesis

In Vitro and *In Vivo* Study Models

J. PLUM,[a] M. DE SMEDT, B. VERHASSELT, T. KERRE, D. VANHECKE,
B. VANDEKERCKHOVE, AND G. LECLERCQ

Department of Clinical Chemistry, Microbiology and Immunology,
University of Ghent, De Pintelaan 185, B-9000 Gent, Belgium

ABSTRACT: Successive steps in T lymphocyte differentiation and T potential of human stem cells (HSC) can be tested in the following models: (a) the infusion of cells in NOD-SCID mice, (b) the injection of cells in rencontituted SCID/hu mice, (c) the differentiation of cells in fetal thymus organ culture (FTOC), and (d) on thymic stromal layers. Using mixed human-murine FTOC, we showed (a) TCRαβ, TCRγδ lymphocytes, NK cells, and dendritic cells complete their differentiation, (b) IL-7Rα signaling and IL-7 are essential, (c) a detailed phenotypic and functional analysis of discrete successive steps of positively selected thymocytes, (d) an efficient transduction of genes in HSC with persistent gene expression throughout the T-lymphocyte differentiation, and (e) adaptation to submerging high oxygen culture increases the test sensitivity to a clonal assay. Other approaches are the *in vivo* SCID/hu reconstitution model. With this method small fragments of human fetal liver and thymus are implanted under the kidney capsule of an adult SCID mouse with result in an impressive human thymus organ, six months after transplantation. We use this model to study thymus T-cell developmental kinetics, development of gene-marked precursor cells and thymic homing of precursor cells.

TOOLS TO STUDY HUMAN T LYMPHOPOIESIS

Basic studies of human T-lymphocyte differentiation are subject to a number of restrictive constraints [ethical constraints, the rarity of pluripotent hematopoietic stem cell (HSC), complexity of genetic background]. However, *in vitro* studies allow analysis of successive steps in differentiation or testing of the T lymphocyte potential of precursor cells. The models used are (a) the infusion of cells in NOD-SCID mice, (b) the injection of cells in rencontituted SCID/hu mice, (c) the growth and differentiation of cells in fetal thymus organ culture (FTOC), and (d) on thymic stromal layers.

The FTOC model was adapted to allow the study of human T-cell differentiation by the use of mice with the SCID mutation.[1] These mice suffer from a severe combined immune deficiency due to natural mutations in gene encoding for repair factors of double-strand breaks. This prevents the completion of V(D)J recombination

[a]Address for correspondence: Dr. J. Plum, Department of Clinical Chemistry, Microbiology and Immunology, University of Ghent, 4BlokA, De Pintelaan 185, B-9000 Gent, Belgium. Voice: 32 9 2403658; fax 32 9 2403659.
  jean.plum@rug.ac.be

reactions necessary to form TCR. This blocks T-cell development at the CD44[+]CD25[+] stage. Therefore, the thymic lobes of the SCID mice have empty spaces, allowing the development of syngeneic or xenogeneic HSC. We and others[2–6] have developed a mixed human-murine FTOC (HM-FTOC) in which human T-cell differentiation takes place. In this novel assay, purified human HSCs are seeded into murine fetal thymic lobes. During the subsequent 5–8 weeks of SCID/hu FTOC of these thymic lobes, all the different human T-cell differentiation stages are obtained, including the most mature T lymphocytes. With this method we have shown that (a) not only T lymphocytes with TCRαβ complete their differentiation, but also TCRγδ lymphocytes, NK cells, and dendritic cells complete their differentiation *in vitro*,[1,7] (b) IL-7Rα signaling and IL-7 are essential, but not sufficient, for human T-lymphocyte development,[8] (c) a detailed phenotypic and functional analysis of discrete successive steps of human T-cell differentiation of positively selected thymocytes can be obtained,[9,10] and (d) an efficient transduction of genes in HSC from cord blood can be achieved with persistent gene expression throughout the T-lymphocyte differentiation process.[11] We have recently adapted our *in vitro* culture method to a submerging high-oxygen culture. This modified technique allows one to address T-cell differentiation with a lower input of cells and points to the possibility of a clonal assay.

Other approaches are the *in vivo* SCID/hu reconstitution model. This model was introduced by McCune *et al.*[12–14] With this method small fragments of human fetal liver and human fetal thymus are implanted under the kidney capsule of an adult SCID mouse. The SCID mutation, as discussed before, leads to an impaired immune system that allows the development of the xenograft. An impressive human thymus organ is seen six months after transplantation. This technique has been used by the Weissman group (Systemix) to delineate HSC. We use this model to study thymus T-cell developmental kinetics[10] (Vanhecke, unpublished data), development of gene-marked precursor cells,[15] and thymic homing of precursor cells (Kerre, unpublished data). Combining our efforts and data from the literature gives us the possibility of clearly relating phenotypical changes with discrete steps of the intrathymic differentiation pathway.

CURRENT STATUS OF FLOW CYTOMETRIC ANALYSIS OF HUMAN T LYMPHOPOIESIS

The Start: The Multipotent Hematopietic Stem Cell

It is now accepted that a single type of cell, the multipotent stem cell, is the precursor to all the major hematopoietic lineages.[16–18] Stem cells divide to replicate themselves (self-renewal), as well as to produce cells that become mature blood cells (multipotency). The search for the hematopietic stem cells began with the use of *in vivo* assays in mice in which lethally irradiated animals were reconstituted with candidate precursor cells and tested for radioprotection and long-term reconstitution.[18] These assays cannot be performed in man. Some of these experiments have been performed in baboons. In this way, it was demonstrated that CD34-bearing cells contain the hematopoietic precursor cells. However, the CD34[+] population is very heterogeneous, and only a minor fraction is considered to contain true stem cells.[19]

Moreover, the current view of CD34 being the marker of the earliest multipotent progenitor cells has been challenged recently, and CD34− cells have been identified with the capacity to form long-term initiating cells or LTC-IC and to differentiate into multiple colonies.[20] It is still not clear whether T- and B-cell development can or must derive from clonogenic lymphoid-restricted stem cells, or from common lymphoid progenitors, or if they derive from multipotent progenitors.

In this respect Galy et al.[21] have shown that the CD10⁺CD34⁺Lin⁻c-kit⁻Thy-1⁻ population in human bone marow gives rise to T, B, NK, and lymphoid dendritic cells, but very few myeloerythroid cells. It is unknown if a single clonogenic cell gives rise to T cells. We have the experience that depending on the sources of stem cells (fetal liver, cord blood, bone marow), some markers differ. CD45RA is virtually absent on the CD34⁺38⁻ stem cells from fetal liver. The recent discovery that IL-7Rα is present on a subset of murine bone marrow cells, and that this Lin⁻IL7Rα⁺Thy-1⁻Sca-1^lo c-kit^lo subpopulation possessed a rapid lymphoid restricted (T, B, NK) reconstitution capacity and lacked myeloid differentiation,[2] has been very stimulating. A counterpart of this population in humans has to be found.

T-Cell Differentiation and Development in the Thymus

The most immature intrathymic precursor cells that are able to develop are phenotypically similar to the extrathymic-derived progenitor cells. These cells express CD34, are negative for lineage markers (CD3, CD4, C8), and a subset of those cells are CD38 dim.

Recently we addressed the phenotypic changes during early T-cell development by introducing CD34⁺CD38⁻ fetal liver cells in FTOC.[7] We showed that the CD34⁺CD38⁻ precursor cells, which are CD4⁻CD7⁻cytoplasmatic(cy)CD3⁻HLA-DR^−/++, differentiate into a CD4⁺ population, which remained CD7⁻cyCD3⁻HLA-DR⁺ and a CD4⁻ population that expressed CD7 and cyCD3. The CD4⁺CD7⁻cyCD3⁻ cells differentiate into phenotypically and functionally mature dendritic cells, but do not differentiate into T or NK cells. The CD4⁻CD7⁺cyCD3⁺ population later differentiates into a CD4⁺CD7⁺ cyCD3⁺HLA-DR⁻ population, which has no potential to differentiate into dendritic cells, but is able to differentiate into NK cells and γδ and αβ T lymphocytes. These findings support the notion that the T/NK split occurs downstream of the NK/dendritic split.

We also addressed the phenotypic changes of the CD34⁺ population in function of time of FOTC. We found that CD38 and CD7 were already expressed on the majority of the CD34⁺, after 4–5 days of culture. After 11 days, CD1 is expressed by half of the CD34⁺ population and one-third expressed CD2. After 18 days, the majority population is CD2 positive. We do not know if these phenotypic changes correlate with a restiction in lymphoid or T potential.

Upon differentiation the human cells upregulate the expression of CD1a At this stage in development TCR gene rearrangement is initiated. The human thymocytes start to express CD4 without CD3 and are generally referred to as CD4 immature single-positive (SP) cells. A minority of these cells express TCRβ protein. When CD8α is coexpressed with CD4, the majority of cells have the pre-TCR complex, TCRβ and pre-T-α together with CD3. This is the first round of selection that allows the survival expanson and further differentiation of the thymocytes with productive TCRβ rearrangements.

The next step is the expression of CDβ and corresponds to the CD4$^+$CD8$^+$ DP stage in development. At that stage the thymocytes rearrange the TCRα locus and are subjected to positive and negative selection.

Mature functional CD4 or CD8 SP thymocytes differentiate from immature CD4$^+$ 8$^+$ DP precursors through a process of positive selection and terminal differentiation. To study CD4/CD8 lineage commitment, human postselection CD69$^+$ thymocytes were separated into distinct subpopulations based on the differential expression of CD27, CD1, and CD45RA/RO. We demonstrate that these CD69$^+$ subpopulations represent transitional stages of a common differentiation pathway during which CD69$^+$ thymocytes that are initially CD27$^-$ CD1$^+$CD45RA$^-$ will sequentially up-regulate CD27, downregulate CD1, and eventually acquire CD45RA upon maturation.

Examination of CD4 and CD8 expression on these CD69$^+$ subsets identified an early postselection CD69$^+$CD27$^-$CD4SP population that gives rise to both CD4SP and CD8SP mature T cells when cultured in mouse thymus organs. In addition, a CD4$^+$ 8$^+$ DP population was identified that is CD69$^+$ and CD27$^+$, which only gives rise to CD8SP progeny upon culture. Although these results suggest that development of CD4SP and CD8SP cells may proceed through distinct intermediates, examination of active biosynthesis of CD4 and CD8 by the various subsets demonstrated that cells that have selectively terminated CD4 synthesis are already present in the CD27$^-$CD4SP and CD27$^+$ DP populations before culture. These data support a model of thymocyte differentiation whereby the decision of thymocytes to differentiate into one or the other lineage occurs concomitantly with, or very soon after, acquisition of CD69 and before the cells acquire CD27, downregulate CD1, or acquire functional properties.[9]

Positive selection of T-cell precursors is an MHC-dependent, multistep process by which functionally mature CD4$^+$8$^-$ helper and CD4$^-$8$^+$ cytotoxic SP T cells are generated from immature CD4$^+$8$^+$ DP thymocytes. We investigated the requirement for TCR/MHC class II interactions during different stages of positive selection of human CD4 SP thymocytes. We show that sorted CD69$^-$ CD48$^+$ DP preselection thymocytes cultured in fetal thymus lobes of normal mice were subject to positive selection and differentiated to CD3(high) CD69$^+$, mature CD8 SP, and CD4 SP cells. When cultured in thymus lobes from MHC class-II-deficient mice, these precursors failed to develop into mature CD4 SP T cells, indicating that in the hybrid cultures, murine MHC class II molecules are required for the development of mature human CD4 SP T cells. We have previously identified CD4 SP intermediate thymocytes that have received at least some of the signals involved in positive selection, since these cells are CD69$^+$, CD3/TCR(high), and CD8β$^-$, but that are still phenotypically and functionally immature. Here we demonstrate that in contrast to preselection thymocytes, these CD4 SP intermediate thymocytes can give rise to phenotypically mature and functionally CD4 SP progeny both in normal and in MHC class-II-deficient thymus lobes. These results suggest that TCR/MHC interactions are required for the initial stages of positive selection, but are not essential during terminal differentiation to functionally mature CD4 SP T cells.[23]

In contrast to thymic differentiation of TCR αβ cells, differentiation stages of TCR γδ cells are largely unknown. This report shows that CD1, a known marker of immature TCR αβ thymocytes, was expressed on some postnatal TCR γδ thymocytes. Only CD1$^+$ TCR γδ thymocytes expressed recombination-activating

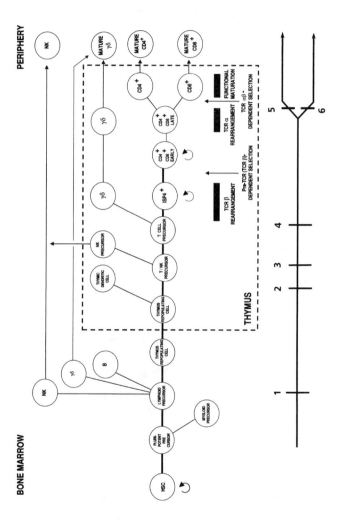

FIGURE 1. Model of lymphoid development in man. Self-renewing HSCs reside in the bone marrow. These stem cells differentiate in precursor cells, some of which can seed the thymus (thymus-repopulating cells). There they generate dendritic cells, NK cells, TCR-γδ T cells, but mainly TCR-αβ T cells. The latter are generated by an immature single positive (ISP4$^+$) that proliferates, rearranges the TCR-β genes, and is subject to pre-TCR selection. Immediate descendants are CD4$^+$CD8$^+$ DP thymocytes that rearrange the TCR-α genes and, when positively selected, differentiate to CD4$^+$ or CD8$^+$ SP, mature thymocytes. These leave the thymus as naive T cells. Normal TCR-αβ development is disturbed in disease (developmental block is indicated on the scheme) like (1) reticular dysgenesis, (2) Di George syndrome, (3) X-linked SCID and Jak3 deficiency SCID, (4) RAG-1 or RAG-2 deficiency SCID, (5) MHC class II deficiency, and (6) ZAP-70 or TAP-2 deficiency.

gene-1 mRNA, and they were shown to differentiate into CD1⁻ TCR γδ thymocytes. Functionally, sorted CD1⁻ TCR γδ thymocytes proliferated in the presence of immobilized anti-CD3 antibodies plus exogenous rIL-2 or rIL-15. Interestingly, in contrast to CD1⁻ TCR αβ cells, CD1⁻ TCR γδ thymocytes also proliferated extensively when cultured with exogenous rIL-2 or rIL-15 alone. FACS analysis as well as reverse-transcription–PCR analysis showed that only CD1⁻ TCR γδ thymocytes expressed IL-2Rβ protein and mRNA. The differential expression of maturation markers, such as CD27, CD45RO, and CD45RA, as a function of expression of CD1 was similar in TCR γδ and TCR αβ thymocytes. An important exception is the expression of CD4 and CD8. Whereas TCR αβ thymocytes are mainly CD4⁻CD8 DP at the immature CD1⁺ stage and CD4 or CD8 SP at the mature CD1⁻ stage, CD1(bright) TCR γδ thymocytes all expressed CD4, but only some of them expressed CD8. Some CD1⁻ TCR γδ thymocytes also expressed CD8, but were negative for CD4. Collectively, our data clearly show that CD1 is a useful marker to distinguish immature human TCR γδ thymocytes from functional mature γδ cells based on recombination-activating gene-1 expression, *in vitro* differentiation, and phenotypic and functional characteristics.[24]

It is clear that phenotypic changes during T lymphopoiesis are correlated with important stages in T-cell development. The confrontation of these phenotypic changes with the expression of RAG genes, cytokine genes, and gene rearrangement allow us to put forward the following differentiation scheme, as shown in FIGURE 1.

Human Immunodeficiency Virus nef *Gene Expression Affects Generation and Function of Human T Cells*

We exploited the retroviral gene transfer and T-cell assay techniques both in FTOC and in SCID/hu to study the effect of expression of HIV genes on T-cell development. We have expressed *nef* as the only HIV gene in immature thymocytes and hematopoietic precursor cells, using φ-LZRS-*nef* NL4-3-IRES-EGFP virus.[25] Cells transduced with this virus produce the two different proteins Nef and GFP, from the same bicistronic mRNA. Thymopoiesis from these precursors was then assayed in FTOC and in SCID/hu. We could show that *nef* hampers T-cell development. CD4 and CD8β surface expression is down-modulated, leading to a reduced DP thymocyte population. In FTOC, the total thymocyte number generated from ISP4⁺ cells is greatly reduced. Mature thymocytes generated *in vivo* are functional and could be expanded *in vitro* to hyperresponsive T cells. These observations show that *nef* expression alone can reproduce the thymic alterations observed after infection of human thymus with HIV, supporting the idea that this gene is a major determinant of HIV pathogenesis and progression toward AIDS.

REFERENCES

1. PLUM, J., M. DE SMEDT, M.P. DEFRESNE, G. LECLERCQ & B. VANDEKERCKHOVE. 1994. Human CD34+ fetal liver stem cells differentiate to T cells in a mouse thymic microenvironment. Blood **84:** 1587.

2. FISHER, A., L. LARSON, L. GOFF, D. RESTALL, L. HAPPERFIELD & M. MERKENSCHLAGER. 1991. Human thymocytes development in organ culture. Int. Immunol. **3:** 1.

3. YEOMAN, H., R. GRESS, C. BARE, A. LEARY, E. BOYSE, J. BARD, L. SCHULZ, D. HARRIS & D. DELUCA. 1993. Human bone marrow and umbilical cord blood cells generate CD4+CD8+ single positive T cells in murine fetal organ cultures. Proc. Natl. Acad. Sci. USA **90:** 10778.

4. DE SMEDT, M., G. LECLERCQ, B. VANDEKERCKHOVE & J. PLUM. 1994. Human fetal liver cells differentiate into thymocytes in chimeric mouse fetal thymus organ culture. Adv. Exp. Med. Biol. **355:** 27.

5. GALY, A., S. VERMA, A. BARCENA & H. SPITS. 1993. Precursors of CD3+CD4+CD8+ cells in the human thymus are defined by expression of CD34. Delineation of early events in human thymic development. J. Exp. Med. **178:** 391.

6. BARCENA, A., M.O. MUENCH, M.G. RONCAROLO & H. SPITS. 1995. Tracing the expression of CD7 and other antigens during T- and myeloid-cell differentiation in the human fetal liver and thymus. Leuk. & Lymphoma **17:** 1.

7. PLUM, J., M. DE SMEDT, B. VERHASSELT, F. OFFNER, T. KERRE, D. VANHECKE, G. LECLERCQ & B. VANDEKERCKHOVE. 1999. In vitro intrathymic differentiation kinetics of human fetal liver CD34+CD38− progenitors reveals a phenotypically defined dendritic/T-NK precursor split. J. Immunol. **162:** 60.

8. PLUM, J., M. DE SMEDT, G. LECLERCQ, B. VERHASSELT & B. VANDEKERCKHOVE. 1996. Interleukin 7 is a critical growth factor in early human T cell development. Blood **88:** 4239.

9. VANHECKE, D., G. LECLERCQ, J. PLUM & B. VANDEKERCKHOVE. 1995. Characterization of distinct stages during the differentiation of human CD69+CD3+ thymocytes and identification of thymic emigrants. J. Immunol. **155:** 1862.

10. VANHECKE, D., B. VERHASSELT, M. DE SMEDT, B. DEPAEPE, G. LECLERCQ, J. PLUM & B. VANDEKERCKHOVE. 1997. MHC class II molecules are required for initiation of positive selection but not during terminal differentiation of human CD4 single positive thymocytes. J. Immunol. **158:** 3730.

11. VERHASSELT, B., M. DE SMEDT, R. VERHELST, E. NAESSENS & J. PLUM. 1998. Retrovirally transduced CD34(++) human cord blood cells generate T cells expressing high levels of the retroviral encoded green fluorescent protein marker in vitro. Blood **91:** 431.

12. MCCUNE, J.M., B. PEAULT, P.R. STREETER & L. RABIN. 1991. Preclinical evaluation of human hematolymphoid function in the scid-hu mouse. Immunol. Rev. **124:** 45.

13. MCCUNE, J., H. KANESHIMA, J. KROWKA, R. NAMIKAWA, H. OUTZEN, B. PEAULT, L. RABIN, C.C. SHIH, E. YEE, M. LIEBERMAN et al. 1991. The SCID-hu mouse: a small animal model for HIV infection and pathogenesis. Annu. Rev. Immunol. **9:** 399.

14. PEAULT, B., I.L. WEISSMAN, C. BAUM, J.M. MCCUNE & A. TSUKAMOTO. 1991. Lymphoid reconstitution of the human fetal thymus in SCID mice with CD34+ precursor cells. J. Exp. Med. **174:** 1283.

15. VERHASSELT, B., M. DE SMEDT, R. VERHELST, E. NAESSENS & J. PLUM. 1998. Retrovirally transduced CD34++ human cord blood cells generate T cells expressing high levels of the retroviral encoded Green Fluorescent Protein marker in vitro. Blood **91:** 431–440.

16. DEXTER, M. & T. ALLEN. 1992. Haematopoiesis. Multi-talented stem cells? Nature **360:** 709.

17. HUANG, S. & L.W. TERSTAPPEN. 1994. Lymphoid and myeloid differentiation of single human CD34+, HLA-DR+, CD38− hematopoietic stem cells. Blood **83:** 1515.

18. KELLER, G. 1992. Hematopoietic stem cells. Curr. Opin. Immunol. **4:** 133.

19. BENDER, J.G., K.L. UNVERZAGT, D.E. WALKER, W. LEE, D.E. VAN EPPS, D.H. SMITH, C.C. STEWART & T. BIK. 1991. Identification and comparison of CD34 positive cells and their subpopulations from normal peripheral blood and bone marrow using flow cytometry. Blood **77:** 2591.

20. GOODELL, M.A., M. ROSENZWEIG, H. KIM, D.F. MARKS, M. DEMARIA, G. PARADIS, S.A. GRUPP, C.A. SIEFF, R.C. MULLIGAN & R.P. JOHNSON. 1998. Dye efflux studies suggest that hematopoietic stem cells expressing low or undetectable levels of CD34 antigen exist in multiple species. Nat. Med. **3:** 1337.

21. GALY, A., M. TRAVIS, D. CEN & B. CHEN. 1995. Human T, B, Natural Killer, and dendritic cells arise from a common bone marrow progenitor cell subset. Immunity **3:** 459.
22. KONDO, M., I.L. WEISSMAN & K. AKASHI. 1997. Identification of clonogenic common lymphoid progenitors in mouse bone marrow. Cell **91:** 661.
23. VANHECKE, D., B. VERHASSELT, V. DEBACKER, G. LECLERCQ, J. PLUM & B. VANDEKERCKHOVE. 1995. Differentiation to T helper cells in the thymus. Gradual acquisition of T helper cell function by CD3+CD4+ cells. J. Immunol. **155:** 4711.
24. OFFNER, F., K. VANBENEDEN, V. DEBACKER, D. VANHECKE, B. VANDEKERCKHOVE, J. PLUM & G. LECLERCQ. 1997. Phenotypic and functional maturation of tcr gamma delta cells in the human thymus. J. Immunol. **158:** 4634.
25. B. VERHASSELT, E. NAESSENS, C. VERHOFSTEDE, M. DE SMEDT, S. SCHOLLEN, T. KERRE, D. VANHECKE & J. PLUM. 1999. Human immunodeficiency virus nef gene expression affects generation and function of human T cells, but not dendritic cells. Blood **94:** 2809–2818.

Role of Glucocorticoids in Early T-Cell Differentiation

ROSA SACEDÓN,[a] ANGELES VICENTE,[b] ALBERTO VARAS,[a] EVA JIMÉNEZ,[a] JUAN JOSÉ MUÑOZ,[a] AND AGUSTÍN G. ZAPATA[a,c]

[a]*Department of Cell Biology, Faculty of Biology, Complutense University, 28040 Madrid, Spain*

[b]*Department of Cell Biology, Faculty of Medicine, Complutense University, 28040 Madrid, Spain*

ABSTRACT: The results of the T-cell differentiation in the progeny of adrenalectomized pregnant rats (Adx fetuses), an experimental model that ensures the absence of glucocorticoids (GCs) during the first stages of development, are summarized. In Adx thymuses there is an accelerated maturation of thymocytes that is reversed by *in vivo* GC replacement. In addition, Adx thymuses show decreased cell content, which correlates with both the increased numbers of apoptotic cells and an early migration of DP (CD4$^+$CD8$^+$) and SP (both CD4$^+$CD8$^-$ and CD4$^-$CD8$^+$) thymocytes to the spleen. As shown by *in vitro* recolonization assays, accelerated T-cell differentiation is a consequence of changes in the biology of lymphoid precursors occurring in the fetal liver of Adx fetuses. They arrive at the thymic primordium earlier and mature faster than the fetal liver lymphoid progenitors from Sham control fetuses. After the establishment of a fetal hypothalamus–pituitary-gland–adrenal-gland (HPA) axis, there is a gradual normalization of the T-cell development Adx fetuses.

INTRODUCTION

For many years, glucocorticoids (GCs) have been extensively used as anti-inflammatory agents by their known effects on lymphocytes.[1] Although GCs are necessary for the normal development of mammalian embryos,[2] their effects on the development of the immune system have been examined only recently and the results obtained are remarkably contradictory. Mice with either targeted disruption of the GR gene[3] or expressing a GR unable to bind DNA[4] do not show apparent changes in the thymus. On the other hand, mice that express a targeted GR antisense transgene that results in an important impairment of the GR expression in thymocytes show blockage of the normal progression of DN thymocytes to the DP cell compartment.[5,6] However, in one study[5] but not in the other[6] there is additionally an important increase in the numbers of apoptotic cells.

We have used another experimental approach in which the adrenal glands in pregnant rats are removed to ensure the absence of circulating GCs in their progeny until

[c]Address for correspondence: Agustin G. Zapata, Department of Cell Biology, Faculty of Biology, Complutense University, 28040 Madrid, Spain. Voice: 34-91-394-49-79; fax: 34-91-394-49-81.

zapata@eucmax.sim.ucm.es

the establishment of the fetal HPA axis at day 18 of gestation. In the present report, we extend previous results[7] on thymocyte maturation in this experimental model in which the appearance and maturation of thymic cell precursors occur in the absence of circulating GCs. In other studies, we have demonstrated that not only T-cell differentiation but also thymic epithelium and DC maturation are profoundly altered in the progeny of adrenalectomized pregnant rats.[8,9]

MATERIAL AND METHODS

Protocols used in the current study are described in detail in Sacedón *et al.*[7] Briefly, Wistar rats were either bilaterally adrenalectomized or sham adrenalectomized using the dorsal approach under ether on the first day of pregnancy. To reconstitute the fetal circulating corticosterone levels, an osmotic minipump (Alza Corporation, CA), which continuously infuses 23 μg/h of corticosterone, was subcutaneously implanted in pregnant rats during the adrenalectomy. A commercial double antibody RIA kit (Gamma B- [125]I- corticosterone RIA, IDS, UK) was used for the determination of serum corticosterone levels.

Flow Cytometry

Cell suspensions were stained with specific monoclonal antibodies labeled with either PE, FITC, or Cychrome for 15 minutes in PBS/2%FCS at 4°C and analyzed in a FACScan (Becton Dickinson, San Jose, CA) from the "Servicio Común de Investigación" (UCM, Spain). The data were analyzed using PC-Lysis research software (Becton Dickinson). Cell cycle analysis was cytofluorometrically performed by staining with 7-AAD (Sigma Chemicals, St. Louis, MO), and the number of cycling cells was determined from individual gated populations on the basis of surface marker expression. *In vivo* thymic basal apoptosis was determined on freshly isolated thymocytes by using an annexin-V fluos kit (Boehringer, Mannheim, Germany) for detecting apoptotic cells by flow cytometry.

Recolonization Assays

Alymphoid lobes were prepared by culturing thymic lobes from 15-day-old fetal Swiss mice in fetal organ culture (FTOC) in the presence of 1.35-mM 2'deoxiguanosine (Sigma) for 5 days. Single depleted lobes were plated with 5×10^4 cells from either Adx or Sham 13-day-old fetal liver in a total volume of 30 μL Terasaki plates. The plates were then inverted to combine lobe and cells at the bottom of the hanging drop. After 48 hours, recolonized lobes were cultured in FTOC for 12 days before harvesting for analysis by flow cytometry.

RT-PCR

Total RNA from either adult adrenal gland and thymuses as well as Adx or Sham control 16-day-old thymuses was purified using TRI reagent (Molecular Research Centre, Inc., Cincinnati, OH). Total cDNA was synthesized with Superscript II RT polymerase (Life Technologies, Barcelona, Spain) according to the instructions of the commercial supplier and used as a target in the PCR amplifications performed with specific primers for either glucocorticoid receptor (GR) (5′ primer: CGAGAGTC-CCTGGAGATCAG and 3′ primer: CCATGAACAGAAATGGCAGA) or steroid 11 β-hydroxylase (Cyp11β-1) (5′ primer CGGGTGTGAAGAACACTT and 3′ primer: TTATGAATGTCCCCAGCA). PCR products obtained in Cyp11β-1 amplification were blotted to a nylon membrane and hybridized with a Dig-labeled PCR product of the expected size, obtained from the adrenal glands.

RESULTS AND DISCUSSION

In the absence of circulating GCs the progeny of adrenalectomized pregnant rats (Adx fetuses) show both decreased numbers and accelerated maturation of thymocytes. On day 15 of fetal life, the Adx thymuses already contain the intermediate CD4$^-$CD8$^+$TcRαβ$^{-/lo}$ cell population (40%) as well as DP (CD4$^+$CD8$^+$) thymocytes (20%) that appear for the first time in Sham thymuses on fetal day 18 (see FIGURE 1). One day later, most Adx thymocytes have reached the DP stage and there is an important proportion of mature SP (both CD4$^+$CD8$^-$ and CD4$^-$CD8$^+$) TcRαβ^{hi} cells, whereas in Sham thymuses they appear on days 20–21 of fetal life (FIG. 1). When the circulating GCs increase to the normal level in Adx fetuses by implantation of osmotic minipumps in the adrenalectomized pregnant rats, both thymic cellularity and the percentage of thymocyte populations recover normal values, demonstrating the relationship between the lack of circulating GCs and the altered thymocyte development (FIG. 1).

Because ultrastructural evidence supported the suggestion that thymic primordium was colonized by lymphoid progenitors earlier in Adx fetuses than in Sham ones,[7,9] we looked for presumptive phenotypical and/or functional differences between fetal liver cell precursors from 13-day-old Adx and Sham fetuses. Although

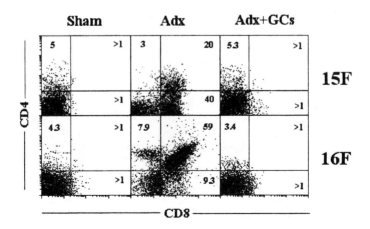

FIGURE 1. Flow cytometry analysis of thymic T-cell populations defined by CD4/CD8 expression in 15 (*up*) and 16 (*down*) -day-old Sham, *Adx,* and *Adx in vivo* supplied with corticosterone embryos.

both the numbers and phenotype of CD45+ (OX-1+) cells are similar in Adx and Sham 13-day-old fetal livers, d-Guo-pretreated thymic lobes from 15-day-old fetal mice *in vitro* reconstituted for 12 days with fetal liver Adx precursors contained a significantly higher proportion of TcRαβ^{hi} cells, which represented both mature SP (both CD4+CD8− and CD4−CD8+) cells and DP thymocytes, than those receiving Sham ones (see FIGURE 2). In addition, analysis of the percentage of cycling cells occurring in the cultures (Sham: 8.3 ± 1.3; Adx: 9.7 ± 2.4) demonstrated that the higher porportion of mature thymocytes was not generated by expansion of preexisting cells but by *in vitro* accelerated maturation of Adx fetal liver cell progenitors, which are therefore affected by the absence of GCs before their arrival at the thymic primordium.

On the other hand, the reduced thymic cell content found in Adx fetuses correlates with increased percentages of apoptotic cells (see FIGURE 3). Moreover, there are no significant differences in the proportion of cycling cells between Sham and Adx fetuses after 15 (Sham: 31 ± 3.1; Adx: 30 ± 4.5) and 16 days of gestation (Sham: 33 ± 5; Adx: 27 ± 3). The increased proportion of apoptotic cells in the thymus of 16–17-day-old fetuses, in agreement with the results obtained in mice that express a limited numbers of GR,[5] could be related to changes in the intrathymic production of GCs that was demonstrated by other authors.[10,11] There is considerable evidence

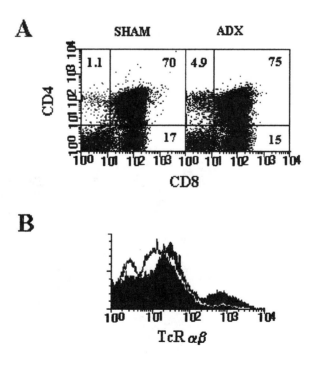

FIGURE 2. CD4/CD8 (**a**) and TcRαβ (**b**) expression in rat thymocytes recovered from dGuo-treated murine fetal thymic lobes after 12 days of in vitro reconstitution with fetal liver cells from either 13-day-old Sham or Adx fetuses.

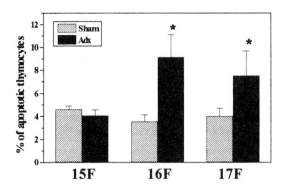

FIGURE 3. Percentage of apoptotic thymocytes in the thymus of either Sham or *Adx* fetuses on days 15 to 17 of gestation. Data are average values of three to four experiments ± SD. Statistical significance for differences between sham and Adx fetuses: * $p \leq 0.05$.

suggesting that GCs and TcR ligation are antagonistic in inducing programmed cell death.[12–15] It is therefore possible that altered endogenous production of GCs in the Adx fetal thymus could modify the balance between GR and TcR signals, resulting in increased apoptosis of DP thymocytes. Remarkably, a semiquantitative PCR analysis demonstrates a slight decrease (see FIGURE 4a) in the expression of GR mRNA

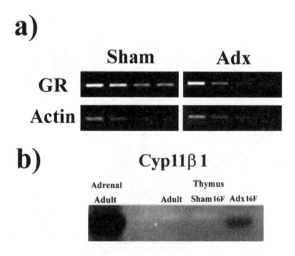

FIGURE 4. (a) Semiquantitative PCR analysis of the GR expression in 16-day-old fetal thymuses from either Sham or Adx fetal rats. 1:2 serial dilutions of total thymus cDNA were used as target for PCR amplification using either specific GR or actin primers. (b) RT-PCR analysis of the Cyp11β-1 expression in thymus from adult control rats, and 16-day-old Sham and *Adx* fetuses. Adrenal glands are used as a positive control. Amplification products were blotted to a nylon membrane and hybridized with a 460-pb Dig-labeled PCR product amplified from the adrenal gland.

in the 16-day-old Adx fetal thymuses as compared to Sham ones. In addition, mRNA for Cyp11β-1, a key enzyme in the GC synthesis pathway, could be amplified by RT-PCR from a 16- day-old fetal Adx thymus, whereas the expression of this enzyme in a Sham thymus was below detection levels for these PCR conditions, indirectly suggesting increased production of GCs in the Adx thymuses (FIG. 4b). However, DP and SP cells found in 16-day-old Adx thymuses were not present one day later and, on fetal day 18, both cell subsets were detected in the spleens of these animals but not in Sham fetuses, whose spleens did not contain any T lymphocyte until day 21 of gestation. Therefore, between days 16 and 17 of fetal life, an important population of thymocytes *in situ* dies or migrates to the spleen in Adx fetuses.

On the other hand, in this period, the absolute number of DN (CD4⁻CD8⁻) thymocytes increases, without significant changes in the percentage of cycling cells, in Adx, but not in Sham thymuses, suggesting that a new wave of lymphoid progenitors is beginning to differentiate in the Adx fetal thymus.

The recovery of circulating GC levels after the establishment of the fetal HPA axis (fetal day 18) gradually normalizes the T-cell differentiation, although this allows the maturation of new waves of cell progenitors. On day 18, the proportion of DP (CD4⁺CD8⁺) and DN (CD4⁻CD8⁻) cells in the Adx thymus was lower and higher, respectively, than that found in the control rats (see TABLE 1). Thus, the Adx thymuses contained only 10% of mature TcRαβ⁺ thymocytes compared to the 30% found in the Sham ones (TABLE 1). On day 19, the percentage of thymocytes defined by the surface expression of CD4/CD8 cell markers was similar in both groups of embryos, but approximately 50% of the thymic cells from Sham fetal rats were TcRαβ⁺, whereas in Adx thymuses less than 25% expressed this molecule (TABLE 1). This difference disappeared in the next stage studied (day 20). In contrast, in 17–19-day-old Adx embryos, the lower values of total cycling cells observed must be explained by the lower proportion of total CD8⁺ thymocytes that appeared in those embryos, because the percentages of both CD8⁺ and CD8⁻ cycling cells were similar in both groups of animals.

Both the percentage and the absolute numbers of DN thymocytes increased significantly between days 20 and 21 in the Adx fetuses and one day later in the Sham ones. As described earlier, this increase in the DN cell population was not correlated for 17-day-old Adx fetuses with increased numbers of cycling CD8⁻ cells. These results support the existence of a new wave of cell progenitors, the third one in the case of the Adx embryos and the second one in the Sham rats, which colonized the thymus around birth, just when mature T cells were leaving the organ to migrate to the peripheral lymphoid organs.

We can therefore conclude that GCs are necessary for the normal development of T lymphocytes during ontogeny. In the absence of circulating GCs, there is an accelerated maturation of T lymphocytes due to changes in the biology of fetal liver T-cell precursors that early colonize the thymic primordium and show altered proliferative capacity. In addition, a decreased thymic cellularity occurs that correlates well with increased programmed cell death and early migration of both DP (CD4⁺CD8⁺) and SP (both CD4⁺CD8⁻ and CD4⁻CD8⁺) thymocytes to the periphery.

TABLE 1. Flow cytometry analysis of thymic T-cell subsets In Either Sham or *Adx* rats from the establishment of fetal HPA axis (fetal day 18) to adult[a]

		18 F	19 F	20 F	21 F	Birth	1 PN	7 PN	14 PN	21 PN	Adult
CD4+CD8−	Sham	1.3 ± 0.12	0.4 ± 0.07	0.9 ± 0.2	6.7 ± 1.71	9.2 ± 0.3	7.1 ± 2.3	6.6 ± 1.9	8.7 ± 0.9	8 ± 2.3	8.8 ± 2.3
	Ads	1.6 ± 0.55	0.5 ± 0.4	1.5 ± 0.9	5.7 ± 0.7	**6.6 ± 0.7***	7.76 ± 1.8	6.47 ± 2.4	7.8 ± 1.2	9 ± 2.6	8.9 ± 1.8
CD4+CD8+	Sham	42.1 ± 2.16	67.5 ± 0.8	69.5 ± 2.7	74 ± 1.6	67.5 ± 1.1	81.3 ± 3.5	86 ± 1.9	82.56 ± 5	82.5 ± 2.3	84 ± 3.5
	Adx	**19.7 ± 3.5***	68.1 ± 2.4	77.1 ± 7	70.9 ± 3	68 ± 3.1	79.9 ± 1.2	85.8 ± 3	83.1 ± 4.1	79.5 ± 3.5	83.6 ± 4
CD4+CD8−	Sham	25.4 ± 0.9	12.9 ± 0.6	7.6 ± 1	8 ± 0.92	13.7 ± 0.7	4.9 ± 1.5	3.93 ± 1	3.84 ± 1.3	3.7 ± 0.6	2.47 ± 0.6
	Ads	**34.1 ± 4.5**	13.2 ± 2.5	6.4 ± 3.2	**12 ± 1.5***	11.1 ± 6	4.5 ± 0.5	3.31 ± 0.8	4.03 ± 1	5.93 ± 1.5	2.5 ± 0.7
CD4+CD8−	Sham	31.2 ± 1.6	19.2 ± 2.4	22 ± 2.4	22 ± 3.5	9.6 ± 2	6.7 ± 1.6	4.46 ± 0.4	4.9 ± 1	5.65 ± 0.3	4.8 ± 1
	Ads	**44.6 ± 2.3***	18.2 ± 4	15 ± 4.3	11.4 ± 5	14.3 ± 5.2	7.84 ± 2	4.38 ± 0.7	4.66 ± 2	6.52 ± 0.6	5 ± 1.2
TcRαβ^lo	Sham	31 ± 4	50 ± 4.5	54 ± 3	61 ± 5	50 ± 4	49.5 ± 7	53.8 ± 2.8	55.8 ± 2.3	57.1 ± 4	57.7 ± 5.3
	Ads	**10 ± 5***	**19 ± 4***	53 ± 6	48 ± 4	47 ± 2	52.5 ± 5	53.1 ± 1.9	52.8 ± 1.9	54.8 ± 5.3	55.3 ± 4.2
TcRαβ^hi	Sham	0 ± 0	1 ± 0.5	7.8 ± 0.6	13.7 ± 3	18 ± 3	13.25 ± 1.5	10.2 ± 1	14 ± 2	10.9 ± 0.6	15.6 ± 3
	Ads	0 ± 0	0 ± 0	8 ± 1	**20.5 ± 5***	19.6 ± 3	16.22 ± 2	10.1 ± 0.9	12.7 ± 1.7	11.7 ± 1.6	15.2 ± 2.1

[a]Data are average values of three to four experiments ± SD. Statistical significances for differences between sham and Adx rat: *p ≤ 0.05; **p ≤ 0.01.

ACKNOWLEDGMENTS

This work was supported by Grants PB97-0332 from the Spanish Ministry of Education and Culture, 98/0041 from the Fondo de Investigaciones Sanitarias (FIS), and 08.30014/1997 and 08.3/0027.1/1998 from the Comunidad de Madrid. The technical assistance of Alfonso Cortés and Catalina Escribano is greatly apreciated. We also thank the Centro Común de Investigación of the Faculty of Biology of UCM for the use of the facilities. Three of the authors (R.S., J.J.M., E.J.) are recipients of a fellowship from the Spanish Ministry of Education and Culture.

REFERENCES

1. BERCZI, I., Ed. 1986. Pituitary Function and Immunity. CRC Press. Boca Raton, FL.
2. MUGLIA, L., L. JACOBSON, P. DIKKES & J.A. MAJZOUB. 1995. Corticotropin-releasing hormone deficiency reveals major fetal but not adult glucocorticoid need. Nature **373:** 427–432.
3. COLE, T.J., J.A. BLENDY, A.P. MONAGHAN, K. KRIEGLSTEIN, W. SCHMID, A. AGUZZI, G. FANTUZZI, E. HUMMLER, K. UNSICKER & G. SCHUTZ. 1995. Targeted disruption of the glucocorticoid receptor gene blocks adrenergic chromaffin cell development and severely retards lung maturation. Genes & Dev. **9:** 1608–1621.
4. REICHARDT, H.M., K.H. KAESTNER, J. TUCKERMANN, O. KRETZ, O. WESSELY, R. BOCK, P. GASS, W. SCHMID, P. HERRLICH, P. ANGEL & G. SCHUTZ. 1998. DNA binding of the glucocorticoid receptor is not essential for survival. Cell **93:** 531–541.
5. KING, L.B., M.S. VACCHIO, K. DIXON, R. HUNZIKER, D.H. MARGULIES & J.D. ASHWELL. 1995. A targeted glucocorticoid receptor antisense transgene increases thymocyte apoptosis and alters thymocyte development. Immunity **3:** 647–656.
6. SACEDÓN, R., A. VICENTE, A. VARAS, M.C. MORALE, N. BARDEN, B. MARCHETTI & A.G. ZAPATA. 1999. Partial blockade of T-cell differentiation during ontogeny and marked alterations of the thymic microenvironment in transgenic mice with impaired glucocorticoid receptor function. J. Neuroimmunol. **98:** 157–167.
7. SACEDÓN, R., V. VICENTE, A. VARAS, E. JIMÉNEZ, J. MUÑOZ & A.G. ZAPATA. 1999. Early maturation of T-cell progenitors in the absence of glucocorticoids. Blood. In press.
8. SACEDÓN, R., A. VARAS, E. JIMÉNEZ, J. MUÑOZ, A. VICENTE & A.G. ZAPATA. 1999. Accelerated maturation of the thymic stroma in the progeny of adrenalectomized pregnant rats. Neuroimmunomodulation **6:** 23–30.
9. SACEDÓN, R., A. VICENTE, A. VARAS, E. JIMÉNEZ, J. MUÑOZ & A.G. ZAPATA. 1999. Early differentiation of thymic dendritic cells in the absence of glucocorticoids. J. Neuroimmunol. **94:** 103–108.
10. VACCHIO, M.S., V. PAPADOPOULOS & J.D. ASHWELL. 1994. Steroid production in the thymus: implications for thymocyte selection. J. Exp. Med. **179:** 1835–1846.
11. PAZIRANDEH, A., Y. XUE, I. RAFTER, J. SJOVALL, M. JONDAL & S. OKRET. 1999. Paracrine glucocorticoid activity produced by mouse thymic epithelial cells. FASEB J. **13:** 893–901.
12. IWATA, M., S. HANAOKA & K. SATO. 1991. Rescue of thymocytes and T cell hybridomas from glucocorticoid-induced apoptosis by stimulation via the T cell receptor/CD3 complex: a possible *in vitro* model for positive selection of the T cell repertoire. Eur. J. Immunol. **21:** 643–648.
13. ZACHARCHUK, C.M., M. MERCEP, P.K. CHAKRABORTI, S.S. SIMONS, JR. & J.D. ASHWELL. 1990. Programmed T lymphocyte death. Cell activation- and steroid-induced pathways are mutually antagonistic. J. Immunol. **145:** 4037–4045.
14. JONDAL, M., S. OKRET & D. MCCONKEY. 1993. Killing of immature CD4+ CD8+ thymocytes in vivo by anti-CD3 or 5'-(N- ethyl)-carboxamide adenosine is blocked by glucocorticoid receptor antagonist RU-486. Eur. J. Immunol. **23:** 1246–1250.

15. GRUBER, J., R. SGONC, Y.H. HU, H. BEUG & G. WICK. 1994. Thymocyte apoptosis induced by elevated endogenous corticosterone levels. Eur. J. Immunol. **24:** 1115–1121.

The Thymus at the Crossroad of Neuroimmune Interactions

MARELLA MARODER,[a] DIANA BELLAVIA,[b] ALESSANDRA VACCA,[b]
MARIA PIA FELLI,[c] AND ISABELLA SCREPANTI[b,d]

[a]Institute of General Pathology, University of Palermo, 90100 Palermo, Italy

[b]Department of Experimental Medicine and Pathology,
University "La Sapienza," 00161 Roma, Italy

[c]Department of Experimental Medicine, University of L'Aquila, 67100 L'Aquila, Italy

ABSTRACT: The numerous relationships existing between the nervous and the immune systems suggest that the neural networks present in the intrathymic microenvironment may influence T-cell development. We previously reported that thymic neural-crest-derived stromal cells are involved in a neural differentiation pathway and are able to produce neurotrophic factors and neurokines that are in turn able to increase and/or modulate thymic-stromal cell neuronal phenotype. We also showed that EGF promotes a neural phenotype in thymic epithelial cells by enhancing the expression of neuronal-specific markers, neurotransmitters, and neuropoietic cytokines, such as IL-6 and CNTF. More recently we showed that the effect of EGF in directing thymic epithelial cells toward a neural-oriented cell fate is mediated by modulating the expression of genes directly involved in neurotypic differentiation (i.e., thrombospondin-1). EGF-induced regulation of stromal cells may also affect T-cell differentiation, as we observed that an EGF-pretreatment reduces the ability of thymic epithelial cells to sustain thymocyte differentiation *in vitro*. Finally, we demonstrated that a complex network involving the neurotrophin BDNF and its specific receptors may have a role in sustaining thymocyte precursor survival and supporting the thymocyte differentiation process. All toghether, our results suggest that the thymus may be the site of integration of different neuroimmune networks that are potentially involved in the regulation of thymocyte survival and/or differentiation.

INTRODUCTION

Multiple cell interactions can control developmental cell fate and morphogenesis in many districts of the organism. The thymus represents one of the most striking examples in which the variety of phenotypes resulting from T-lymphoid cell developmental pathways and the acquisition of either the ability to react to external antigens or the tolerance against self-antigens arise through the action of instructive and/or selective differentiation signals generated by the different cell components of thymic

[d]Address for correspondence: Dr. Isabella Screpanti, Department of Experimental Medicine and Pathology, University "La Sapienza", Viale Regina Elena 324, 00161 Roma, Italy. Voice: 39-6-44700816; fax: 39-6-4454820.
screpant@caspur.it

stroma in close association with precursors and differentiating lymphoid cells (reviewed in Ref. 1).

Neural-crest-derived cells populate the thymus, and their coexistence with epithelial cells has been shown to be required for proper organ development and T-cell education and function.[2] Moreover the presence of neural-crest-derived cells in thymic stroma and the expression of a number of neuronal markers, neuropeptides, and neurotrophic factors in both thymic epithelium *in vivo* and thymic-stroma-derived cell cultures have been described by us and a number of research groups.[3–8]

The coexistence of epithelial and neural-crest-derived cells within the thymic stroma raises the question as to the nature of the regulatory signals that determine the development and survival of the neuronal cell component and as to the role of the neural cell microenvironment with respect to the T-cell survival, selection, and/or differentiation.

In the present paper we will briefly review recent evidence we obtained on the possible role of intrathymic neural networks, sustained by the neural-crest-derived stromal cell component, on thymocyte survival and/or differentiation.

NEURAL-CREST-DERIVED CELLS AS A COMPONENT OF THYMIC STROMA: ROLE OF THE INTRATHYMIC NEUROTROPHIC MICROENVIRONMENT

The heterogeneous ontogeny of thymic stromal cells has been shown to be necessary for the differentiation of T-cell progenitors into the complex spectrum of thymocyte subsets.[9] Moreover the dependence of thymus development on neural-crest derivatives has been suggested by experiments showing that ablation of the chicken embryo cephalic neural crest results in thymic aplasia/hypoplasia.[2] For this reason, an intrathymic neurotrophic microenvironment would be important for sustaining neural-crest derivatives in thymic stroma. We previously proved this prediction by identifying neural cells in several murine and human thymic-stromal-cell primary cultures[7] and by demonstrating a neuromodulatory loop, mediated by the expression of NGF and IL-6, that is able to enhance the neural phenotype of stromal cells in an autocrine/paracrine way.[7]

The coexistence of epithelial and neural cells within the thymic stroma raises the question as to the nature of the growth and/or differentiation factors that may regulate such a coexistence. The mechanisms involved in the regulation of this process are likely to require the local production of factors with multifunctional properties with regard to neural and other cell lineage trophisms. EGF was a likely candidate as a soluble regulatory signal. Indeed, in addition to being a potent growth factor for several epithelial cell types,[10] EGF promotes both neuron survival and mitogenesis of neuronal progenitors[11,12] and has been shown to be expressed in human thymic epithelial cell cultures.[13] Given these observations, we recently demonstrated that EGF plays a crucial role in directing thymic stromal cell lines toward a neural-oriented cell fate by modulating the expression of genes involved in neurotypic differentiation, such as the neurokines IL-6 and CNTF, that are able to increase the expression of several neuronal-specific markers, such as synapsin 1, tyrosine hydroxylase, and neurofilaments.[8] Moreover we demonstrated that the EGF-induced neurotypic response in thymic stromal cells included an increase in cells able to

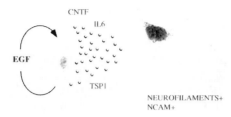

FIGURE 1. Autocrine/paracrine production of EGF promotes neurotypic differentiation in thymic stromal cells.

express the preprotachykinin A gene , encoding the substance P and neurokinin A neurotransmitters.[8] We also showed that EGF was able to promote a multivalent response, since it was able not only to promote the expression of a neuronal phenotype, but also to increase the proliferation of the neurodifferentiated cells, suggesting a possible modulation of different signaling pathways.[8] For this reason, in the attempt to identify different genes that are selectively expressed and/or modulated during the neurotypic differentiation process of thymic stromal cells induced by EGF, we recently applied a modification of RNA fingerprinting, a PCR-based differential screening technique, that allowed us to individuate a number of known and unknown genes, differentially expressed by EGF-treated with respect to untreated cells. Among them, the thrombospondin-1 (Tsp-1) encoding gene showed a significant increased expression at both RNA and protein levels, as revealed by Western blot and immunohistochemistry.[14] We also demonstrated that, similarly to what was observed in several types of neurons in CNS and PNS, Tsp-1 was able to enhance the outgrowth of neurite-like processes from thymic stromal cells. Moreover, thymic stromal cell cultured on Tsp-1-coated slides displayed an increased expression of neurofilaments and neural-cell adhesion molecule N-CAM.[14] All toghether, these results suggest that Tsp-1 contributes to the EGF-induced neurotypic differentiation of thymic stromal cells (see FIGURE 1).

THE NEUROTYPIC DIFFERENTIATION OF THYMIC STROMA MAY INFLUENCE THYMOCYTE DIFFERENTIATION

It is evident that the neurodifferentiative networks described, involving NGF, EGF, and the related neurokines and neurotransmitters, have an important effect in the reshaping of thymic stromal cells, and presumably affect their interactions with the lymphoid component of the thymus. We and others previously demonstrated that direct cell-to-cell lympho–stromal interaction play a crucial role in sustaining thymocyte survival and differentiation.[15] In particular, by using an *in vitro* thymocyte differentiation model, based on the coculture of thymocyte precursors on thymic-stromal-cell monolayers,[15] we have demonstrated the crucial role played by the fibronectin–integrin receptor interaction in the thymocyte differentiation process.[15] Tsp-1, which is significantly increased in thymic stromal cells during the EGF-induced neurotypic differentiation, is known to share with fibronectin the ability to interact with $\alpha4\beta1$ and $\alpha5\beta1$ integrin receptors. Therefore we can speculate that signals that modulate Tsp-1 and evoke an imbalance in the composition of ECM in lympho–stromal interactions could impair the *in vitro* differentiation process. Indeed, we observed that a pretreatment of thymic stromal cells with EGF, which evokes the morphological and biochemical changes described before[14] and increases the proliferation rate of neurodifferentiated cells,[8] is able to interfere with the generation of more mature thymocytes *in vitro* (our unpublished results).

These data show that the enhancement of a neurodifferentiative pathways in the thymus environment impairs the thymocyte differentiation process and suggest that the imbalance in the cell-type composition of the thymic stroma (i.e., the increased proportion of neurodifferentiated cells), together with the imbalance of extracellular matrix composition, could be, at least in part, responsible for this effect.

THE INTRATHYMIC NEUROTROPHIC MICROENVIRONMENT AS A REGULATOR OF THYMOCYTE FUNCTIONS

The intrathymic neural network involves several neuronal-related factors with different pleiotropic activities, as some of them are more active in inducing neurotypic differentiation and others in sustaining cell survival. Several components of the immune system previously have been regarded as potential targets of exogenous neurotrophins. The presence of high-affinity NGF trkA receptors has been reported in monocytes and activated CD4+ mature T lymphocyte;[16] moreover, both B and mature T-lymphocyte functions have been shown to be modulated by NGF.[17] In order to extend the study of the neurotrophin effects on intrathymic T-cell differentiation-related events, we investigated the expression of different neurotrophins and specific receptors in lymphoid and stromal components of the thymus, by using a previously established *in vitro* differentiation model.[15] We first demonstrated that the neurotrophic microenvironment of thymic stromal cells, besides NGF, also includes BDNF and NT4 neurotrophins. We also reported that the pattern of neurotrophin receptor expression depends on the developmental stage of T cells, as thymocytes only express trkB, the high-affinity receptors specific for BDNF and NT4 neurotrophins, in contrast to the expression of trkA described in mature Ag-activated CD4+ T cells. Moreover, we observed a differential expression of trkB receptors in different thymocyte subsets that inversely correlated with their maturation stage and their differentiation potential, being more expressed in immature thymocytes and progressively declining in more mature subsets.[18] Interestingly, we observed that BDNF, in analogy with its surviving effect on neuronal cells,[19] is able to sustain immature thymocyte survival.

It has been suggested that the thymic epithelium-assisted survival of thymocyte precursors is one of the crucial early phases of T-cell development.[20] Indeed our observations suggest that the thymic stroma-derived neurotrophin BDNF may be one of the factors that play a role in sustaining the intrathymic survival of thymocyte precursors, allowing their subsequent maturation.

CONCLUSIONS

The discovery of a functionally active neurotrophic microenvironment within the thymus and the link between epithelial and neural cells are intriguing, considering that relationships between the nervous and immune systems and their deregulation have been implicated in the pathogenesis of several autoimmune and/or neurodegenerative diseases. The neuromodulatory role of EGF in the thymus reveals a novel characteristic of this growth factor in the relationship between neural networks and the immune system. Indeed, the EGF-regulated bipotential neuro- and lymphopoietic cytokines (CNTF and IL-6) or the growth factor itself might either directly influence thymic lymphoid cells or sustain an appropriate intrathymic neuronal cell population and neurotransmitter production, which in turn may affect thymocyte development. Thus, the composite spectrum of EGF activity upon the thymus suggests that this organ may be the site at which a novel regulatory activity of the growth factor upon neural–immune interactions could occur.

Moreover, the presence of receptors for neurotrophins in developing T cells and the expression of neurotrophins in thymic stromal cells broaden the range of interactions between the nervous and immune systems. Indeed, the expression and the modulation of both trkB receptors and their specific ligand BDNF in thymocytes and thymic stromal cells, and the ability of BDNF to rescue thymocytes from cell death, suggest the presence of feedback mechanisms based on autocrine/paracrine neurotrophin–receptor interactions that may highlight novel mechanisms potentially involved in the thymocyte differentiation pathway. In conclusion, the data we summarized in this paper show that different lymphoid- and neural-related differentiation pathways and neurotrophic networks intercross in the thymus (see FIGURE 2),

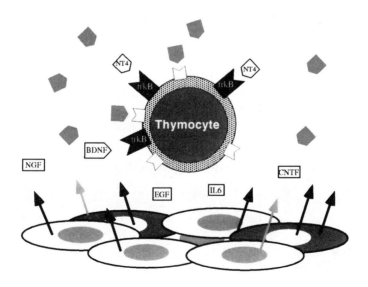

FIGURE 2. Different lymphoid- and neural-related differentiation pathways and neurotrophic networks intercross in the intrathymic microenvironment.

suggesting that a cross talk between the neural and immune systems may occur inside the thymus at the lympho–stromal interaction level.

AKNOWLEDGMENTS

This work was supported in part by the National Research Council (CNR Biotechnology Project), Associazione Italiana per la Ricerca sul Cancro (AIRC), and MURST 40%.

REFERENCES

1. SCREPANTI, I., A MODESTI & A. GULINO. 1993. Heterogeneity of thymic stromal cells and thymocyte differentiation: a cell culture approach. J. Cell Sci. **105:** 601–606.
2. BOCKMAN, D.E. & M.L. KIRBY. 1984. Dependence of thymus development on derivatives of the neural crest. Science **223:** 498–500.
3. ERICSSON, A., V. GEENEN, F. ROBERT, J.-J. LEGROS, Y. VRINDTS-GEVAERT, P. FRANCHIMONT, S. BRENE & H. PERSSON. 1990. Expression of preprotachykinin-A and neuropeptide-Y messenger RNA in the thymus. Mol. Endocrinol. **4:** 1211–1218.
4. FULLER, P.J. & K. VERITY. 1989. Somatostatin gene expression in the thymus gland. J. Immunol. **143:** 1015–1017.
5. GEENEN, V., F. ROBERT, M. FATEMI, H. MARTENS, M.-P. DEFRESNE, J. BONIVER, J.J. LEGROS & P. FRANCHIMONT. 1989. Neuroendocrine-immune interactions in T cell ontogeny. Thymus **13:** 131–140.
6. NAKAMURA, H. & C. AYER-LE LIÈVRE. 1986. Neural crest and thymic myoid cells. Curr. Top. Dev. Biol. **20:** 111–115.
7. SCREPANTI, I., D. MECO, S. SCARPA, S. MORRONE, L. FRATI, A. GULINO & A. MODESTI. 1992. Neuromodulatory loop mediated by nerve growth factor and interleukin 6 in the thymic stromal cell cultures. Proc. Natl. Acad. Sci. USA **89:** 3209–3212.
8. SCREPANTI, I., S. SCARPA, D. MECO, D. BELLAVIA, L. STUPPIA, L. FRATI, A. MODESTI & A. GULINO. 1995. Epidermal growth factor promotes a neural phenotype in thymic epithelial cells and enhances neuropoietic cytokine expression. J. Cell Biol. **130:** 183–192.
9. GUTIERREZ, J.C. & R. PALACIOS. 1991. Heterogeneity of thymic epithelial cells in promoting T-lymphocyte differentiation in vivo. Proc. Natl. Acad. Sci. USA. **88:** 642–646.
10. CARPENTER, G. & M.I. WAHL. 1990. *In* Peptide Growth Factors and Their Receptors. M.B. Sporn & A.B. Roberts, Eds.: 69–171. Springer-Verlag. Berlin.
11. ANCHAN, R.M., T.A. REH, J. ANGELLO, A. BALLIET & M. WALKER. 1991. EGF and TGF-a stimulate retinal neuroepithelial cell proliferation in vitro. Neuron **6:** 923–936.
12. REYNOLDS, B.A. & S. WEISS. 1992. Generation of neurons and astrocytes from isolated cells of the adult mammalian central nervous system. Science **255:** 1707–1710.
13. LE, P.T., S. LAZORICH, L.P. WHICHARD, B.F. HAYNES & K.H. SINGER. 1991. Regulation of cytokine production in the human thymus: epidermal growth factor and transforming growth factor a regulate mRNA levels of interleukin 1a (IL-1a), IL-1b, and IL-6 in human thymic epithelial cells at a post-transcriptional level. J. Exp. Med. **174:** 1147–1157.
14. VACCA, A., L. DI MARCOTULLIO, G. GIANNINI, M. FARINA, S. SCARPA, A. STOPPACCIARO, A. CALCE, M. MARODER, L. FRATI, I. SCREPANTI & A. GULINO. 1999. Thrombospondin-1 is a mediator of the neurotypic differentiation induced by EGF in thymic epithelial cells. Exp. Cell Res. **248:** 79–86.

15. MECO, D., S. SCARPA, M. NAPOLITANO, D. BELLAVIA, M. RAGANO-CARACCIOLO, A. MODESTI, L. FRATI, A. GULINO & I. SCREPANTI. 1994. Modulation of fibronectin and thymic stromal cell-dependent thymocyte maturation by retinoic acid. J. Immunol. **153:** 73–83.

16. EHRHARD, P.B., P. ERB, U. GRAUMANN & U. OTTEN. 1993. Expression of nerve growth factor and nerve growth factor receptor tyrosyn kinase trk in activated CD4− positive T-cell clones. Proc. Natl. Acad. Sci. USA **90:** 5423–5425.

17. OTTEN, U., P. EHRHARD & R. PECK. 1989. Nerve growth factor induces growth and differentiation of human B lymphocytes. Proc. Natl. Acad. Sci. USA **86:** 10059–10061.

18. MARODER, M., D. BELLAVIA, D. MECO, M. NAPOLITANO, A. STIGLIANO, E. ALESSE, A. VACCA, G. GIANNINI, L. FRATI, A. GULINO & I. SCREPANTI. 1996. Expression of trkB neurotrophin receptor during T cell development. Role of brain-derived neurotrophic factor in immature thymocyte survival. J. Immunol. **157:** 2864–2872.

19. BUCHMAN, V.L. & A.M. DAVIS. 1993. Different neurotrophins are expressed and act in a developmental sequence to promote the survival of embryonic sensory neurons. Development **118:** 989–993.

20. VON BOEHEMER, H., H.S. TEH & P. KISIELOW. 1989. The thymus selects the useful, neglects the useless and destroys the harmful. Immunol. Today **10:** 57–61.

Is There a Role for Growth Hormone upon Intrathymic T-Cell Migration?

WILSON SAVINO,[a,d] SALETE SMANIOTTO,[a,b] VALÉRIA DE MELLO-COELHO,[a] AND MIREILLE DARDENNE[c]

[a]Laboratory on Thymus Research, Department of Immunology, Institute Oswaldo Cruz, Foundation Oswaldo Cruz, Rio de Janeiro, Brazil

[b]Department of Morphology, Center for Biological Sciences, Federal University of Alagoas, Maceió, Brazil

[c]CNRS UMR-1083, Hôpital Necker, Paris, France

ABSTRACT: Intrathymic T-cell differentiation is essentially driven by the thymic microenvironment, a tridimensional network formed by thymic epithelial cells and to a lesser extent, dendritic cells, macrophages, fibroblasts, and extracellular matrix components. Thymocyte migration throughout the thymus is partially dependent on extracellular-matrix (ECM) -mediated interactions. Herein we investigated the putative role of growth hormone (GH) upon events related to intrathymic T-cell migration. We demonstrated that GH upregulates the expression of ECM ligands and receptors in distinct preparations of cultured thymic epithelial cells TECs). We also showed that adhesion of thymocytes to thymic epithelial cells was significantly increased by GH treatment, an effect that could be consistently abrogated when TECs were treated to antifibronectin, anti-VLA5, antilaminin, or anti-VLA6 antibodies before addition of thymocytes to the cultures. We also studied thymic nurse cells (TNCs), lymphoepithelial complexes that can be isolated *ex vivo* from the thymus. In this system, we had previously demonstrated that ECM ligands and receptors control both inward and outward thymocyte traffic. We then showed that GH enhances thymocyte release from TNCs, as well as the reconstitution of these lymphoepithelial complexes. Lastly, we evaluated the *in vivo* influence of GH on thymocyte exit. This was done by means of intrathymic injection of GH plus fluorescein isothiocyanate (FITC), and further analysis of recent thymic emigrants (FITC[+] cells) in peripheral lymphoid organs, as defined by CD4/CD8-based cytofluorometric phenotyping. The proportions of FITC[+] T cells appeared augmented in lymph nodes in GH-treated mice, as compared to controls. Taken together, these data indicate that GH stimulates intrathymic T-cell traffic, an effect that is at least partially mediated by extracellular matrix-mediated interactions.

[d]Address for correspondence: Wilson Savino, Laboratory on Thymus Research, Department of Immunology, Oswaldo Cruz Institute, Oswaldo Cruz Foundation, Avenue Brasil 4365—Manguinhos, 21045-000 Rio de Janeiro, RJ, Brazil. Voice: 55-21-280-1486/55-21-598-4326/55-21-598-4327; fax: 55-21-280-1589.

savino@gene.dbbm.fiocruz.br or savino@ioc.fiocruz.br

748

INTRODUCTION

The thymus is a primary lymphoid organ in which bone-marrow-derived T-cell precursors undergo a complex process of maturation, eventually leading to the migration of mature thymocytes to the T-dependent areas of peripheral lymphoid organs. This differentiation process involves sequential expression of a variety of membrane proteins and rearrangements in T-cell receptor genes. Most potentially self-reactive thymocytes are negatively selected by clonal deletion, whereas some cells are rescued from death through positive selection, eventually yielding the vast majority of the T-cell repertoire.[1] Key events of intrathymic T-cell differentiation are driven by the influence of the thymic microenvironment, a tridimensional network composed of distinct cell types such as epithelial cells, macrophages, and dendritic cells, as well as extracellular matrix (ECM) elements.[1-3]

The thymic epithelium is the major component of the thymic microenvironment and has an important and multifaceted influence on early events of T-cell differentiation, by secretion of various polypeptides, including thymic hormones and cytokines,[4-5] and cell–cell contacts, such as the interactions involving major histocompatibility complex gene products expressed by thymic epithelial cells (TECs) with the T-cell receptor,[1] and those occurring through classic adhesion molecules.[6] Lastly, TECs can bind to and interact with maturing thymocytes by means of ECM ligands and their respective receptors.[3,7] Interestingly, it is possible that supramolecular ECM arrangements function as a conveyor belt, allowing an ordered migration of thymocytes within the organ.[8]

It is currently well documented that the physiology of the thymus is under hormonal control.[9] In particular, growth hormone (GH) is able to upregulate the secretion of thymic hormone thymulin in humans, mice, and dogs.[10-12] Additionally, GH likely exerts a pleiotropic effect upon the thymic epithelium, since it also stimulates TEC proliferation.[10] Interestingly, both effects seem to be modulated by insulin-like growth factor 1 (IGF-1), since they could be prevented by treatment with anti-IGF-1 or anti-IGF-1 receptor monoclonal antibodies (mAb).[10] Moreover, the molecular basis for such a role of GH upon TECs was provided with the demonstration of specific GH receptors on TEC membrane.[13-14]

Taken together, these data prompted us to design experiments aimed at defining whether GH could also be involved in thymocyte migration events.

THYMOCYTE ADHESION TO THYMIC EPITHELIAL CELLS IS INCREASED BY GH

Cell adhesion is a necessary step for any cell migration. In this context, we searched whether GH could modulate thymocyte adhesion to TECs. In fact, when GH-treated cultured TEC lines were cocultured with freshly isolated thymocytes, thymocyte adhesion was consistently enhanced, an effect that could be abrogated with an anti-GH mAb. Again this effect likely occurs through IGF-1: this growth

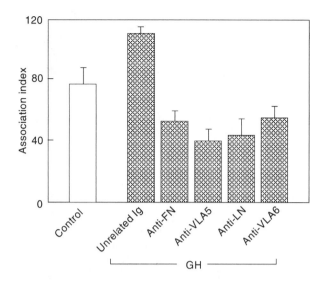

FIGURE 1. Involvement of extracellular matrix ligands and receptors in GH-stimulated TEC/thymocyte adhesion. TEC Cultures remained untreated □ or were treated with 10^{-8}-M GH alone, or in the presence of antifibronectin (anti-FN), anti-VLA-5, antilaminin (anti-LN), or anti-VLA6 ▨ antibodies. Data were expressed as the means ± SE of association indexes. The adhesion index was calculated using the following formula, which takes into account the numbers of thymocytes adhered to TEC as well as the numbers of TEC containing adhered thymocytes:

$$AI = \frac{\text{Numbers of TEC with thymocytes}}{\text{Total TEC number}} \times \frac{\text{Numbers of thymocytes per TEC}}{\text{Total TEC number}} \times 100.$$

Values of the GH-treated cultures were statistically different from the corresponding untreated control ($p < 0.01$). Blocking effects of GH with anti-extracellular matrix or anti-extracellular matrix receptor antibodies were also significant as compared to the hormonal treatment alone ($p < 0.05$). (Modified from Ref. 15.)

factor was able to increase thymocyte adhesion, and anti-IGF-1 or anti-IGF-1 receptor mAb could block the effects of GH.[15]

We had previously demonstrated that the heterocellular adhesion of thymocytes to TECs is mediated by various ECM proteins, including fibronectin and laminin, together with their corresponding receptors, VLA-5 and VLA-6, which are expressed on TEC membranes.[16–18] With respect to the effects of GH, this was also the case, since the enhancement of thymocyte/TEC adhesion was consistently prevented when TEC cultures were subjected to antifibronectin, anti-VLA-5, antilaminin, or anti-VLA-6 mAb,[15] as shown in FIGURE 1.

We also defined the molecular mechanism involved in such an effect, showing that GH actually yields an increase in the production of laminin and fibronectin by a murine TEC line, and also enhances the expression of VLA-5 and VLA-6 on TEC membranes, as ascertained by immunocytochemistry and cytofluorometry. Moreover, these changes could also be seen when TEC cultures were treated by IGF-1.[15]

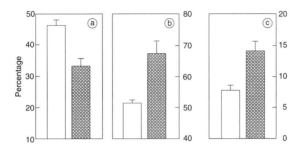

FIGURE 2. Growth hormone accelerates thymocyte traffic in thymic nurse cell complexes. (**a**) and (**b**) show, respectively, lymphocyte-containing and lymphocyte-free TNCs, which were cultured in the absence □ or in the presence ▨ of GH. Results are expressed in percentages of means ± SE, and the differences between control and hormone-treated TNCs were statistically significant ($p < 0.01$). (**c**) Shows the reconstitution of thymic nurse complexes from 5-day cultures of TNC-derived TEC cultures, which were treated or not with GH, as seen in the respective columns □ and ▨. Differences between control and GH-treated cultures were statistically different ($p < 0.05$). (Modified from Ref. 15.)

GH ENHANCES THYMOCYTE MIGRATION
IN THYMIC NURSE CELL COMPLEXES

In addition to the data described for a murine TEC line, we found that GH promotes an enhancement of ECM ligands and receptors in primary cultures of thymic nurse cells (TNCs). Considering that this lymphoepithelial complex can be used as an *in vitro* model for studying thymocyte migration,[19] we searched whether thymocyte exit from and entrance into TNCs could be under GH influence.

In the first series of experiments we showed that the thymocyte release from freshly isolated TNCs was enhanced in the presence of GH, as ascertained by lower values of lymphocyte-containing TNC complexes together with an increase in lymphocyte-free epithelial cells in hormone-treated cultures (see FIGURE 2). Furthermore, we found an increase in TNC reconstitution when TNC-derived lymphocyte-free five-day TEC primary cultures were treated with GH and then cocultured with freshly isolated fetal thymocytes.[15] Again, similar effects were observed when GH was replaced by IGF-1.

DOES GH INFLUENCE THE ENTRANCE AND
EXIT OF THYMOCYTES IN THE THYMUS?

In addition to its influence in thymocyte migration within the thymic parenchyma (mostly represented *in vivo* by the tridimensional TEC network), it is important to define whether GH modulates the entrance of bone-marrow-derived T-cell precursors, as well as the exit of mature thymocytes from the organ. Unfortunately, very few data concerning this issue are yet available. It was shown in one study that recombinant human GH did stimulate *in vitro* migration of peripheral blood-derived

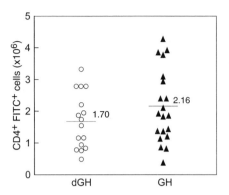

FIGURE 3. Growth hormone enhances the relative numbers of CD4$^+$CD8$^-$ recent thymic emigrants in lymph nodes. In this experiment, mice were injected intrathymically with GH (10^{-8} M in 10 μL) diluted in an FITC-containing PBS solution. Sixteen hours thereafter, lymph-node cells were recovered, labeled with the anti-CD4 and anti-CD8 mAb, and analyzed by three-color cytofluorometry. Data are expressed as relative cell numbers of CD4$^+$FITC$^+$ cells. This relative cell number was calculated out of the total number of FITC-labeled cells in the thymus + spleen + lymph nodes.

resting or activated human T cells, and favored *in vivo* T lymphocyte engraftment in the thymus of SCID mice. Interestingly, the authors showed that this GH effect was dependent on β1 and β2 integrin-mediated interactions.[20]

More recently, we initiated an *in vivo* study attempting to define whether the exit of thymocytes from the organ as well as their colonization in peripheral lymphoid organs could be under GH influence. This was done by means of intrathymic injection of GH in a PBS solution containing fluorescein isothiocyanate (FITC). This fluorochrome labels thymocyte membranes, thus allowing the tracing of recent thymic emigrants (FITC$^+$ cells) in peripheral lymphoid organs.[21] As compared to the values obtained when denatured (boiled) GH was used, we noticed that native GH apparently increases both the absolute and the relative numbers of CD4$^+$ recent thymic emigrants in both subcutaneous and mesenteric lymph nodes (see FIGURE 3). Interestingly, this effect was not seen in the spleen, thus suggesting that GH may affect the differential homing of recent thymic emigrants in the periphery of the immune system.

CONCLUDING REMARKS

The data just summarized strongly indicate that GH stimulates intrathymic T-cell traffic, a role that is exerted at least partially by modulating extracellular matrix-mediated interactions, likely after triggering an IGF-dependent circuitry.

Lastly, the data discussed herein should be placed in the context of the findings showing the intrathymic production of GH as well as IGF-1. The expression of GH by TECs was ascertained by immunocytochemistry, *in situ* hybridization, and

RT-PCR.[14,22,23] Additionally, the production of IGF-1 by the thymic epithelium was demonstrated.[24,25]

In a second vein, production of GH by thymocytes was also demonstrated both in murine and human thymuses.[14,26–28] Moreover, from a functional point of view, it was found that thymocyte-derived GH can enhance thymocyte proliferation through an IGF-1-mediated circuit.[28]

Taken together, these findings raise the hypothesis that, besides the endocrine influences of pituitary hormones on TEC/thymocyte interactions, an autocrine/paracrine circuitry mediated by the same hormones may be involved. Yet, the functional relevance of such thymus-derived GH-mediated interactions, which ultimately modify the pattern of intrathymic T-cell migration, is to be determined.

ACKNOWLEDGMENTS

This work was financially supported by FIOCRUZ, CNPq, PRONEX/CNPq PADCT/CNPq, and FAPERJ (Brazil), as well as CNRS (PICS grant) and INSERM (France). We thank Mrs. D. Broneer for the English review.

REFERENCES

1. ANDERSON, G., N.C. MOORE, J.T.T. OWEN & E.J. JENKINSON. 1996. Cellular interactions in thymocyte development. Annu. Rev. Immunol. **14:** 73–99.
2. BOYD, R.L., C.L. TUCEK, D.I. GODFREY, D.J. IZON, T.J. WILSON, N.J. DAVIDSON, A.G.B. BEAN, H.M. LADYMAN, M.A. RITTER & P. HUGO. 1993. The thymic microenvironment. Immunol. Today **14:** 445–459.
3. SAVINO, W., D.M.S. VILLA-VERDE & J. LANNES-VIEIRA. 1993. Extracellular matrix proteins in intrathymic T cell migration and differentiation? Immunol. Today **14:** 158–161.
4. SAVINO, W. & M. DARDENNE. 1984. Thymic hormone containing cells. VI. Immunohistologic evidence for the simultaneous presence of thymulin, thymopoietin and thymosin α-1 in normal and pathological human thymuses. Eur. J. Immunol. **14:** 987–991.
5. LE, P.T., D.T. TUCK, C.A. DINARELLO, B.F. HAYNES & K.H. SINGER. 1988. Human thymic epithelial cells produce IL-1. J. Immunol. **138:** 2520–2525.
6. PATEL, D.D. & B.F. HAYNES. 1993. Cell adhesion molecules involved in intrathymic T cell development. Semin. Immunol. **5:** 283–292.
7. SAVINO, W., S.R. DALMAU & V. COTTA-DE-ALMEIDA. 2000. Role of extracellular matrix-mediated interactions in thymocyte migration. Dev. Immunol. In press.
8. SAVINO, W., M. DARDENNE & C. CARNAUD. 1996. Conveyor belt hypothesis for intrathymic cell migration: possible relationship with extracellular matrix. Immunol. Today **27:** 97–98.
9. DARDENNE, M. & W. SAVINO. 1994. Neuroendocrine control of thymus physiology by peptidic hormones and neuropeptides. Immunol. Today **15:** 518–523.
10. TIMSIT, J., W. SAVINO, B. SAFIEH, P. CHANSON, M.C. GAGNERAULT, J.F. BACH & M. DARDENNE. 1992. Effects of growth hormone and insulin-like growth factor 1 in thymic hormonal function in man. J. Clin. Endocrinol. Metab. **75:** 183–188.
11. GOYA, R.G., M.C. GAGNERAULT, M.C. LEITE-DE-MORAES, W. SAVINO & M. DARDENNE. 1992. In vivo effects of growth hormone on thymus fuction in aging mice. Brain Behav. Immun. **6:** 341–350.
12. GOFF, B.L., J.A. ROTH, L.H. ARP & G.S. INCEFY. 1987. Growth hormone treatment stimulates thymulin production in aged dogs. Clin. Exp. Immunol **68:** 580–587.

13. BAN, E., M.C. GAGNERAULT, H. JAMMES, M.C. POSTEL-VINAY, F. HAOUR & M. DARDENNE. 1990. Specific binding sites for growth hormone in cultured mouse thymic epithelial cells. Life Sci. **48:** 2141–2148.

14. MELLO-COELHO, V., M.C. GAGNERAULT, J.C. SOUBERBIELLE, C.J. STRASBURGER, W. SAVINO, M. DARDENNE & M.C. POSTEL-VINAY. 1998. Growth hormone and its receptor are expressed in human thymic cells. Endocrinology **139:** 3837–3842.

15. MELLO-COELHO, V., D.M.S. VILLA-VERDE, M. DARDENNE & W. SAVINO. 1997. Pituitary hormones modulate by extracellular matrix-mediated interactions between thymocyte and thymic epithelial cell mediated ligands and receptors. J. Neuroimmunol. **76:** 39-49.

16. LANNES-VIEIRA, J., R. CHAMMAS, D.M.S. VILLA-VERDE, M.A. VANNIER-DOS-SANTOS, S.J. SOUZA, R.R. BRENTANI & W. SAVINO. 1993. Thymic epithelial cells express laminin receptors that may modulate interactions with thymocytes. Int. Immunol. **5:** 1421-1430.

17. VILLA-VERDE, D.M.S., R. CHAMMAS, J.M. LAGROTA-CÂNDIDO, R.R. BRENTANI & W. SAVINO. 1994. Exracellular matrix components of the mouse thymic microenvironment. IV. Thymic nurse cells express extracellular matrix ligands and receptors. Eur. J. Immunol. **24:** 659–664.

18. DALMAU, S.R., C.S. FREITAS & W. SAVINO. 1999. High expression of fibronectin receptors and L-selectin as a hallmark of early steps of thymocyte differentiation: lessons from sublethally irradiatad mice. Blood **93:** 974–990.

19. VILLA-VERDE, D.M.S., V. MELLO-COELHO, J.M. LAGROTA-CÂNDIDO & W. SAVINO. 1995. The thymic nurse cell complex: an in vitro model for extracellular matrix-mediated intrathymic T cell migration. Braz. J. Med. Biol. Res. **28:** 907–912.

20. TAUB, D.D., G. TSARFATY, A.R. LLOYD, S.K. DURUM & W.J. MURPHY. 1994. Growth hormone promotes human T cell adhesion and migration to both human and murine matrix proteins in vitro and directly promotes xenogeneic engraftment. J. Clin. Invest. **94:** 293–300.

21. SCOLLAY, R., E.C. BUTCHER & I. WEISSMAN. 1980. Thymus cell migration. Quantitative aspects of cellular traffic from the thymus to the periphery in mice. Eur. J. Immunol. **10:** 210–218.

22. MAGGIANO, N., M. PIANTELLI, R. RICCI, L. LAROCCA, A. CAPELLI & F.O. RANELLETTI. 1994. Detection of growth hormone-producing cells in human thymus by immunohistochemistry and non-radioactive in situ hybridization. J. Histochem. Cytochem. **42:** 1349–1354.

23. WU, H., R. DEVI & W.B. MAMARKEY. 1996. Localization of growth hormone messenger ribonucleic acid in the human immune system—a clinical research center study. J. Clin. Endocrinol. Metabol. **81:** 1278–1282.

24. GEENEN, V., I. ACHOUR, F. ROBERT, E. VANDERSMISSEN, J. SODOYEZ, M.P. DEFRESNE, J. BONIVER, P.J. LEFEBVRE & P. FRANCHIMONT. 1993. Evidence that insulin-like growth factor 2 (IGF-2) is the dominant thymic peptide of the insulin superfamily. Thymus **21:** 115–124.

25. MELLO-COELHO, V. 1997. Neuroencodrine Control of Thymic Epithelial Cells and T Lymphocytes: Effects of Prolactin and Gronth Hormone. Ph.D. Thesis, Federal Univ. of Rio de Janeiro, Rio de Janeiro.

26. WEIGENT, D.A & J.E. BLALOCK. 1991. The production of growth hormone by subpopulations of rat mononuclear leukocytes. Cell. Immunol. **135:** 55–65.

27. KOOIJMAN, R., A. MALUR, S.C. VAN BUUL-OFFERS & E.L. HOOGHE-PETERS. 1997. Growth hormone expression in murine bone marrow cells is independent of the pituitary transcription factor PIT-1. Endocrinology **138:** 3949–3955.

28. SABHARWAL, P. & S. VARMA. 1996. Growth hormone synthesized and secreted by human thymocytes acts via insulin-like growth factor I as an autocrine and paracrine growth factor. J. Clin. Endocrinol. Metab. **81:** 2663–2669.

The Opioid Antagonist Naloxone Induces a Shift from Type 2 to Type 1 Cytokine Pattern in Normal and Skin-Grafted Mice

PAOLA SACERDOTE,[a] LEDA GASPANI, AND ALBERTO E. PANERAI

Department of Pharmacology, School of Medicine,
University of Milano, 20129 Milano, Italy

ABSTRACT: Opioid peptides affect different immune functions. We present evidence that these effects could be mediated by the modulation of Th1/Th2 cytokine production. The acute and chronic treatment with the opioid receptor antagonist naloxone decreased the production of IL-4 by splenocytes of C57BL/6 and Balb/cJ mice, that present a Th1/ Th2 dominance, respectively, immunized with the protein antigen KLH. In contrast, IL-2 and IFN-γ levels were increased after naloxone treatment. These results indicate that naloxone increases Th1 and decreases Th2 cytokine production. Moreover in C57BL/6 mice, naloxone treatment was able to accelerate skin-graft rejection, a Th1-mediated phenomenon, by increasing Th1 cytokine production. The effect of naloxone could be ascribed to the removal of the regulatory effects exerted by endogenous opioid peptides, which could activate Th2 and suppress Th1 cytokines.

INTRODUCTION

The involvement of the endogenous opioid peptides β-endorphin (BE) and met-enkephalin in the regulation of immune function is well known.[1,2,3] We have shown that BE exerts a physiological inhibitory effect[4,5] on some cellular-mediated immune responses, while the administration in the rodent of the opiate receptor antagonist naloxone or of immunoglobulins that neutralize the activity of BE, induces an increase of Natural Killer activity and of mitogen-induced splenocyte proliferation within minutes.[5]

In this work, we explore the possibility that the target of the effect of BE in the immune system could be the activation of the two types of mature T-helper cells, Th1 and Th2. The Th1 and Th2 cells produce different patterns of cytokines: Th1 cells produce IL-2, IFN-γ, and lymphotoxins, whereas Th2 cells produce IL-4, IL-5, IL-6, IL-10, and IL-13. Th1 cells are mostly involved in cell-mediated reactions, while the Th2 cytokines are commonly found in association with strong antibody and allergic responses. Moreover, the characteristic cytokine products of Th1 and Th2 cells are inhibitory for the differentiation and effector function of the opposite subset.[6] Strains of mice in which one type dominates over the other have been described.

[a]Address for correspondence: Department of Pharmacology, via Vanvitelli 32, 20129 Milano, Italy. Fax: 39-02-730470.
paola.sacerdote@unimi.it

Balb/cJ mice are susceptible to infection by intracellular pathogens, have a weak cell-mediated immune response, and consistently present a Th2 dominance.[7] In contrast, the C57BL/6 mice, which are resistant to intracellular pathogens and have a highly effective cell-mediated response, present a Th1 dominance.[7]

In an attempt to define a possible physiological role for opioid peptides in the modulation of the balance between Th1 and Th2 cell types, we analyze the effect of the *in vivo* treatment with the opioid receptor antagonist naloxone on splenocyte production of the Th1 cytokines IFN-γ and IL-2 and of the Th2 cytokine IL-4 in Balb/cJ and C57BL/6 mice immunized with the protein antigen keyhole limpet hemocyanin (KLH).

The disruption of a correct Th1/Th2 balance is involved in the development of immune diseases.[8] As a consequence, the effects that opioid peptides and naloxone exert on Th cell types can be relevant in immunopathology. Recently, the Th1/Th2 paradigm also has been involved in immune responses to organ transplantation.[9] Under certain experimental conditions, in fact, graft rejection has been associated with the presence of Th1 cytokines, while Th2 cytokines have been linked to graft survival. Therefore we also investigate the effect of the opioid receptor antagonist naloxone on the onset of allograft skin rejection in mice, and on the production of IL-2, IFN-γ, and IL-4 during the development of the rejection.

MATERIALS AND METHODS

KLH Experiments

Balb/cJ and C57BL/6 male mice, 18–20-g body weight (Charles River, Calco, Italy) were used in the study. Animals were kept on a 12-h light–dark cycle with water and food *ad libitum.*

Mice were injected i.p. with 100 μg of the protein antigen KLH (Sigma, St. Louis, MO) in a volume of 0.2 mL of saline.

The opioid receptor antagonist naloxone HCl (S.A.L.A.R.S., Como, Italy) was injected s.c. at the dose of 5 mg/kg. One group of mice received only one acute injection of naloxone at the moment of immunization, while a second group of animals was chronically treated with s.c. naloxone once daily starting from the immunization day. The animals received the last naloxone injection 30 min before sacrifice. Control animals were immunized with KLH, and treated acutely or chronically with saline.

One week after immunization, animals were killed, splenocytes suspended in complete RPMI supplemented with 10% FCS, and plated at 7×10^6 cells, containing a final concentration of 80 μg/mL KLH in a total volume of 1 mL. Plates were incubated at 37°C in 5% CO_2 and 95% air. Supernatants were collected after 48 and 72 h in culture and stored frozen at −80°C for cytokine analysis.

The levels of IL-2, IL-4, and IFN-γ in 48 h and 72 h supernatants were determined by ELISA protocol as standardized by Pharmingen (San Diego, CA), as previously described.[10]

Graft Experiments

Female C57BL/6N and C3H/HeN mice aged 7–8 weeks and 20–24-g body weight were used as skin recipients and donors, respectively.

Skin grafting was carried out in accordance with the procedure described by Billingham and Nedawar, slightly modified as previously described.[10] Grafts were controlled daily. The rejection was evaluated considering, for each mouse, the days when 50% (50% graft rejection) of the graft surface was necrosed.

Animals were injected twice daily, from the day of transplantation until the day of rejection, with naloxone (5 mg/kg) or saline; a third group of animals was injected with naloxone starting from day 5 after grafting. As control, a group of untreated transplanted animals was killed before the onset of rejection, that is, 6 days after surgery, corresponding at the mean time of rejection in naloxone-treated animals. A group of control animals, without treatment and/or surgery was also included as naive controls. On the rejection day, or when indicated, animals were killed by cervical dislocation, and their spleens removed for cytokines analysis.

Splenocytes were plated at 4×10^6 cells in 24 well plates, with and without a final concentration of 2.5 μg Con-A in a total volume of 1 mL. Plates were incubated at 37°C in 5% CO_2 and 95% air. Supernatants were collected after 24 and 48 h in culture and stored frozen at -80°C for cytokine analysis by ELISA.

Statistical Analysis

Data were analyzed using one-way analysis of variance (ANOVA), followed by Bonferroni's *t*-test for multiple comparisons.

RESULTS

As expected, Balb/cJ mice produced significantly more KLH-stimulated IL-4 than C57BL/6 mice (48-h cultures: 12.1 ± 2.23 pg/mL versus 6.7 ± 0.99, respectively, $p = 0.043$; 72-h cultures 23.8 ± 2.6 pg/mL vs. 15.1 ± 3.9, $p = 0.0001$), while the two strains made similar amounts of IL-2 and IFN-γ.

FIGURE 1 reports the effect of the acute and chronic treatment with naloxone on IL-2, IFN-γ, and IL-4 production by splenocytes obtained from Balb/cJ mice. In the acute experiment these animals were treated with one injection of naloxone or saline at the moment of *in vivo* KLH immunization, and 6 days later splenocytes were cultured *in vitro* with or without KLH. After 48 h in the culture, both spontaneous and KLH-stimulated IL-2 production by splenocytes were significantly higher than in the control animals. After 72 h in the cultures, IL-2 levels were very low, and no effect of naloxone was present. Increased IFN-γ production after acute naloxone treatment was observed after 48 h in KLH-stimulated culture, and in both *in vitro* KLH-stimulated and -nonstimulated cultures after 72 h. On the other hand, the spontaneous and KLH-induced IL-4 production of mice splenocytes acutely treated with naloxone was significantly lower than control after 72-h in the culture, while the effect did not reach statistical significance in the 48-h cultures.

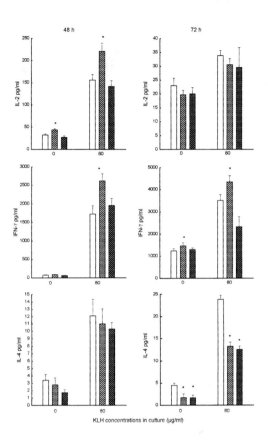

FIGURE 1. Effect of acute and chronic naloxone treatment on KLH-stimulated cytok-ine production *in vitro* by splenocytes from Balb/cJ mice. **Top panels**: IL-2; **middle panels**: IFN-γ; **lower panels**: IL-4. Animals were killed 6 days after immunization. Spleen cells were cultured with 0 or 80 µg/mL KLH for 48 h and 72 h. Results are expressed as mean ± SE of 10 animals per group. *, $p < 0.01$ vs. corresponding saline control; ☐, saline, ▨, acute naloxone, ▧, chronic naloxone.

When mice were treated with naloxone for six days, from immunization to the day of sacrifice, the effect on IL-2 and IFN-γ was lost, while the production of IL-4 was still significantly lower.

The effect of the acute and chronic naloxone treatment on cytokine production by splenocytes obtained from C57BL/6 mice is reported in FIGURE 2.

In this strain of animals, IL-2 and IFN-γ production were not affected by the acute naloxone treatment, while the production of IL-4 was significantly decreased in comparison to control animals both in unstimulated and in KLH-stimulated cultures. When animals were treated for one week with naloxone, the IL-2 levels were higher than controls, both in unstimulated and *in vitro* KLH-stimulated cultures in 48-h

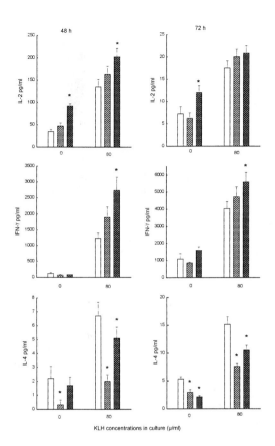

FIGURE 2. Effect of acute and chronic naloxone treatment on KLH-stimulated cytokine production *in vitro* by splenocytes from C57BL/6 mice. **Top panels**: IL-2; **middle panels**: IFN-γ; **lower panels**: IL-4. Animals were killed 6 days after immunization. Spleen cells were cultured with 0 or 80 μg/mL KLH for 48 and 72 h. Results are expressed as mean ± SE of 10 animals per group. *, $p < 0.01$ vs. corresponding saline control. ☐, saline; ▨, acute naloxone; ▦, chronic naloxone.

cultures and only in unstimulated 72-h supernatants. Also IFN-γ concentrations increased in the chronic naloxone group, but the rise reached a significant difference only in the cultures stimulated *in vitro* with KLH. Spontaneous and KLH-stimulated IL-4 production, which was already reduced after acute naloxone, is also lower than controls after chronic treatment with the drug.

FIGURE 3 shows the days at which 50% of the graft surface was rejected in the different treatment groups. Naloxone significantly accelerated the graft rejection when administered, starting at the time of grafting (control value, 9.05 ± 0.4 days, mean ± S.E.M.), while it was not effective when administered five days after surgery.

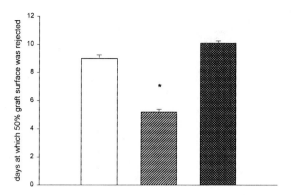

FIGURE 3. Effect of naloxone treatment on skin-graft rejection. Grafts were scored daily until 50% of the grafted surface was necrosed: this day was scored as rejection day. Results are the mean ± SEM of a group of eight animals. *, $p < 0.01$ vs. saline. ☐, saline; ▨, naloxone (day 0); ▦, naloxone (day 5).

TABLE 1 reports cytokine concentrations assayed in resting and Con-A-stimulated splenocytes cultures from different experimental groups: naive nontransplanted mice (control); saline-treated transplanted mice killed when 50% of the graft surface was rejected; saline-treated transplanted mice killed before the onset of rejection, that is, 6 days after transplantation; naloxone-treated animals killed the day when 50% of the graft surface was rejected. Neither transplantation nor naloxone treatment affected IL-2 concentrations in unstimulated cultures. In contrast, a significant effect of rejection was observed in Con-A-stimulated IL-2 production. IL-2 concentrations were lower in cultures of splenocytes obtained from mice at the moment of rejection, but not in mice killed before the rejection had began, although a not significant trend toward a decrease is present ($p = 0.055$). A significant effect of naloxone was present. In fact, in both acutely and chronically naloxone-treated animals killed at the moment of rejection, IL-2 levels did not differ from naive controls or from transplanted mice that had not yet started to reject the graft. IL-4 and IFN-γ were assayed in 48-h culture supernatant. IL-4 secretion was not affected by transplantation or naloxone treatment, but a trend toward the increase of spontaneous IFN-γ production was present in transplanted animals in comparison with controls. Naloxone treatments significantly enhanced both spontaneous and Con-A-stimulated IFN-γ production.

DISCUSSION

The administration of the opioid antagonist naloxone profoundly affects the pattern of cytokine production by splenocytes of Balb/cJ and C57BL/6 mice immunized with the protein antigen KLH. In both strains of mice, acute as well as chronic naloxone treatments decrease IL-4 production, both in unstimulated and *in vitro* KLH-stimulated splenocyte cultures. On the other hand, production of the Th1 cytokines, IL-2 and IFN-γ, is increased in both strains of mice by naloxone. Although no qualitative difference is observed in the two strains with the two treatment regimens used

TABLE 1. Splenocyte production of cytokines in transplanted animals

	IL-2 (pg/ml)		IFN-g (pg/ml)		IL-4 (pg/ml)	
	Medium	Con-A	Medium	Con-A	Medium	Con-A
Control	15.3 ± 2.9	3369 ± 692	21 ± 12.0	81260 ± 15319	6.9 ± 3.4	15.9 ± 5.5
Graft + saline at rejection[a]	12.6 ± 2.5	943 ± 89.7*	100 ± 15.6	84202 ± 21859	7.4 ± 1.3	19.5 ± 9.3
Graft + saline before rejection[b]	19.6 ± 4.1	1745 ± 288	170 ± 41.5	136190 ± 19042	12.7 ± 4.3	15.8 ± 1.7
Graft + naloxone at rejection[a]	22.1 ± 3.9	2965 ± 417	579 ± 116*,**	336186 ± 19420*	12.4 ± 4.5	20.1 ± 9.8

[a]Measurements were performed when 50% of graft surface was rejected.
[b]Measurements were performed before onset of rejection, at day six after grafting.
NOTE: Results are expressed as the mean (± SEM) of groups of eight animals; * $p < 0.05$ vs. control; ** $p < 0.01$ vs. graft + saline.

(acute vs. chronic) on Th1 cytokine production, which always increased, a temporal difference is present. While, in fact, the effect of naloxone on IL-2 and IFN-γ production by splenocytes obtained from Balb/cJ mice is already present after acute treatment with the drug, IL-2 and IFN-γ production increased in C57BL/6 mice only after chronic treatment. This difference in the sensitivity of the two strains could be explained by the fact that a strong Th1 dominance has been reported for the C57BL/6 mice[7]: it is therefore conceivable that this strain needs a longer drug regimen in order to further increase an already upregulated Th1 cytokine pattern. Although the IFN-γ concentrations are not different in Balb/cJ and C57BL/6 mice, the highest IL-4 production observed in Balb/cJ mice causes a reduction of the IFN-γ/IL-4 ratio, suggesting a Th2 dominance in this strain.

Given the fact that naloxone is an almost pure antagonist at the μ-opioid receptor, devoid of any intrinsic activity, the effects of the drug are likely to be due to the removal of a regulatory tone exerted by endogenous opioid peptides. We previously showed that, in rat and human, naloxone increased T lymphocyte proliferation, NK activity, and worsened the development of inflammatory responses.[11,12] Similar effects were achieved by our laboratory, also with a neutralizing antibody against the opioid peptide BE.[11] It can therefore be hypothesized that the modulation of Th1/Th2 cytokine pattern induced by naloxone could be due to the removal of BE effects, although the involvement of other opioid peptides, that is, met-enkephalin, also could be possible. Moreover, the observation that naloxone is able to also affect cytokine production after a single acute injection at the moment of immunization, suggests that BE is involved in the early events following immunization. Since we and others have demonstrated that BE is produced and released by the cells of the immune system,[2,3] and that it can bind specific opioid receptors present on immunocytes,[1–3] there is strong evidence for an autocrine/paracrine activity of the opioid.

The data reported in this paper offer a new insight into the role of opioid peptides in the modulation of the immune system. In fact, it becomes questionable to claim an absolute immunosuppressive or immunostimulatory role for opioid peptides and BE. Instead it can be suggested that the peptide might exert an inhibitory control on Th1 cell populations, probably throughout the stimulation of Th2 cell types. In line with this hypothesis, the literature on the effects of opioid peptides on the immune system is often contradictory.[1,2] Depending on the immune function evaluated, cellular vs. humoral, and on the preexisting Th1/Th2 balance due, for example, to the earlier exposure of animals to different pathogens or to genetic predisposition, inhibition or stimulation of classic laboratory immune parameters have been reported.

The disruption of the correct Th1/Th2 balance is involved in the development of immune diseases.[8] As a consequence, the effects that opioid peptides and naloxone exert on Th cell types can be relevant in immunopathology. Our data show that the opioid receptor antagonist naloxone accelerates the time of graft rejection, most probably through the blockade of an immunosuppressive tone exerted by endogenous opioids. In fact, we show that naloxone, without the BE tone, accelerates graft rejection, but also that this effect is present only when the administration of the opiate receptor antagonist starts at the time of grafting, but not at a later time. The latter observation is consistent with the finding of Kavelaars,[12] who demonstrated that opioid peptides modulate the phosphorylation of the CD3-gamma chain of T-cell antigen receptor function, that is, the early activation of transduction pathways to the biological effect.

The effects on graft rejection that we observe with naloxone could be due to the role of the opioid in the Th1/Th2 balance. Consistent with what we observed in normal healthy animals after the antigenic challenge with KLH, naloxone treatment further increased IFN-γ production, confirming a stimulation of Th1 cells by the opioid antagonist. A significant decrease of IL-2 production in the culture supernatants is indeed present when spleens are removed at the moment of rejection. These low IL-2 concentrations could indicate a very rapid and massive utilization of the cytokine by T lymphocytes. It is possible therefore that naloxone, by stimulating IL-2 production, leads to a reduction in the time necessary to reach the amount of IL-2 that is critical for the onset of rejection. On the whole, these data seem to confirm that the modulation of graft rejection by naloxone could be due to its effects on cytokine production.

In conclusion, our data suggest a role for opioid peptides in the modulation of the Th1/Th2 balance, in the complex network of immunoregulatory signals. We can hypothesize that the use of opioid peptides or their modulation, and/or opioid antagonists, in order to achieve immune deviation might be interesting.

REFERENCES

1. BESEDOWSKY, H.O. & A. DEL REY. 1996. Immune-neuro-endocrine interactions: facts and hypothesis. Endocrine Rev. **17:** 64–102.
2. HEIJNEN, C.J., A. KAVELAARS & R.E. BALLIEUX. 1991. β-Endorphin, cytokine and neuropeptide. Immunol. Rev. **119:** 41–63.
3. PANERAI, A.E. & P. SACERDOTE. 1997 Beta-endorphin in the immune system: a role at last? Immunol. Today **18:** 317–319.
4. MANFREDI, B., P. SACERDOTE, M. BIANCHI *et al.* 1993. Evidence for an opioid inhibitory effect on T cell proliferation. J. Neuroimmunol. **44:** 43–48.
5. PANERAI, A.E., B. MANFREDI, F. GRANUCCI *et al.* 1995. The beta-endorphin inhibition of mitogen-induced splenocytes proliferation is mediated by central and peripheral paracrine/autocrine effects of the opioid. J. Neuroimmunol. **58:** 71–76.
6. MOSMAN, T.R. & S. SAD. 1996. The expanding universe of T-cell subsets; Th1,Th2 and more. Immunol. Today **17:** 138–146.
7. KRUSZEWSKA, B., S.J. FELTEN & J.A. MOYNIHAN. 1995. Alterations in cytokine and antibody production following chemical sympathectomy in two strains of mice. J. Immunol. **155:** 4613–4620.
8. ROMAGNANI, S. 1994. Lymphokine production by human T cell in disease states. Annu. Rev. Immunol. **12:** 227–230.
9. STROM, T., P. ROY-CHAUNDHURY, R. MANFRO *et al.* 1996. The Th1/Th2 paradigm and the allograft response. Curr. Opin. Immunol. **8:** 688–693.
10. SACERDOTE, P., V.E.M. ROSSO DI SAN SECONDO, G. SIRCHIA *et al.* 1998. Endogenous opioids modulate allograft rejection time in mice: possible relation with Th1/Th2 cytokines. Clin. Exp. Immunol. **113:** 465–469.
11. SACERDOTE, P., M. BIANCHI & A.E. PANERAI. 1996. Involvement of Beta-endorphin in the modulation of paw inflammatory edema in the rat. Reg. Peptides **63:** 79–83.
12. PANERAI, A.E., J. RADULOVIC, G. MONASTRA *et al.* 1994. Beta-endorphin concentrations in brain areas and peritoneal macrophages in rats susceptible and resistant to experimental allergic encephalomyelitis: a possible relationship between tumor necrosis factor-α and opioids in the disease. J. Neuroimmunol. **51:** 169–176.
13. KAVELAARS, A., B.J. EGGEN, P.N. DE GRAAN *et al.* 1990. The phosphorylation of the CD3 gamma chain of T lymphocytes is modulated by beta-endorphin. Eur. J. Immunol. **20:** 943–945.

Expression of Delta Opioid Receptors and Transcripts by Splenic T Cells

BURT M. SHARP,[a] MING D. LI, SHANNON G. MATTA,
KATHY McALLEN, AND NAHID A. SHAHABI

Department of Pharmacology, University of Tennessee, Memphis, Tennessee 38163, USA

ABSTRACT: Delta opioid receptors (DORs) and preproenkephalin-A-derived opiate peptides are expressed by mononuclear cells in various lymphoid organs. DOR ligands modulate a variety of immune functions, such as T-cell proliferation, calcium mobilization, and cytokine production. Recently, quiescent T cells were found to express low levels of DOR transcripts, which increased due to the following: cell culture of unstimulated murine splenocytes (depending on cell density); cross-linking the T-cell receptor (TCR) with anti-CD$_3$-ε; and a single *in vivo* exposure to staphylococcal enterotoxin B (SEB). Enhanced expression of DOR mRNA was mediated transcriptionally. Moreover, PMA + ionomycin, which mimic the proliferative signal of anti-CD$_3$, inhibited the expression of DOR mRNA. Using semiquantitative immunofluorescence to detect DORs, SEB was found to increase the fraction of T cells that expressed DOR and to enhance the relative level of DOR expression per T cell. Previous studies have shown that DOR agonists inhibited the anti-CD$_3$-stimulated production of interleukin-2 and T-cell proliferation. Therefore, the enhanced expression of DORs by activated T cells may be capable of downregulating the T-cell activation program.

INTRODUCTION

The opioid peptides produced by lymphoid tissues appear to be capable of modulating diverse physiological responses of the immune system (reviewed in Ref. 1). Opioids such as β-endorphin and the enkephalins have been shown to modulate thymic and splenic T-cell proliferation, calcium mobilization, and interleukin-2 production.[2–5] Furthermore, delta opioid peptides modulate the mitogen-induced expression of preproenkephalin A mRNA by thymocytes.[6] Although some of the actions of β-endorphin are mediated by naloxone-resistant mechanisms, enkephalins appear to act through opioid receptors sensitive to selective antagonists, such as naltindole (NTI; effective on delta opioid receptors).

Several laboratories have reported that transcripts encoding the neuronal delta opioid receptor (DOR) are detectable in a variety of immune cell types. Following the original report of DOR mRNA in simian peripheral blood mononuclear cells,[7] another group showed that human peripheral blood lymphocytes and lymphoid cell

*a*Address for correspondence: Burt Sharp, Department of Pharmacology, University of Tennessee, Memphis, 874 Union Avenue, Crowe Bldg., Memphis, TN 38163. Voice: 901-448-6000; fax: 901-448-7206.

bsharp@utmem.edu
Supported by NIH DA-04196.

lines expressed DOR transcripts that were nearly identical to the known sequence found in the human brain.[8] DOR mRNA was also detected in murine splenic CD4[+] and CD8[+] T cells stimulated by concanavalin A *in vitro.*[9] Low levels of DOR mRNA have consistently been detected by our laboratory in freshly obtained murine splenocytes and enriched T-cell fractions;[10,11] the sequence of these PCR transcripts was 98% identical to the known murine brain DOR. These studies demonstrated that DOR mRNA is expressed by quiescent and activated T cells from several species. However, the factors regulating its expression are largely unknown.

Few laboratories have successfully detected DORs on leukocytes, using radioligand binding or immunological approaches. One group reported a single high-affinity site for [^{3}H]-deltorphin on membranes from human peripheral blood polymorphonuclear leukocytes.[12] Experiments that covalently cross-linked selective delta ligands provide supporting evidence for the existence of DORs on macrophages and lymphocytes. Specific binding was found on macrophage, T- and B-cell lines,[13] and on both B- and T-cell-enriched murine splenocytes.[14] Recently, Western immunoblotting was utilized in a brief report, suggesting that DORs are present on mitogen-stimulated murine splenic T cells.[15]

The present studies were performed to further characterize the regulated expression of DORs and their transcripts by murine splenocytes and T cells. Experiments determined the effects of cell density (in the absence of mitogen) on DOR mRNA expression. In other studies, the *in vitro* effects of cross-linking the T-cell receptor (TCR) and of activating T cells with phorbol myristate acetate and ionomycin were evaluated, using quantitative competitive RT-PCR amplification. Then, the effects of stimulation *in vivo* with staphylococcal enterotoxin B (SEB; Ref. 16) were studied. In addition, immunofluorescence was used to detect DORs on quiescent and stimulated T cells from mice treated with SEB.

METHODS

Cell isolation, enrichment, identification, culture, proliferation, RNA isolation, and RT-PCR (both semi- and quantitative) were performed using published protocols.[3,12]

For immunofluorescence studies, splenocytes were fixed with 4% paraformaldehyde for 10 min at 4°C, rinsed, incubated for 1 h at 22°C in a solution containing rabbit anti-DOR antiserum (Chemicon Int., Inc., Temecula, CA; 1:500 dilution), and goat anti-CD$_3$-ε, and then incubated for 30 min with biotinylated anti-rabbit-IgG and Cy3-conjugated anti-goat-IgG. Thereafter, cells were washed extensively, incubated for 10 min at 4°C with fluorescein-avidin-DCS (Vector Labs., Burlingame, CA), again washed, and then centrifuged onto glass slides.

RESULTS AND DISCUSSION

We have previously shown that freshly obtained, quiescent murine splenic T cells (from BALB/c) expressed DOR transcripts at low levels.[10,11] Using quantitative competitive RT-PCR amplification, we observed approximately one DOR transcript per T cell in extracts prepared from fresh T-cell-enriched populations (CD1) that

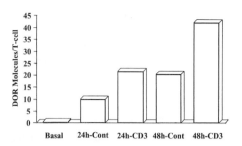

FIGURE 1. The effects of cell culture [control (Cont)] and anti-CD_3-ε on the number of DOR mRNA copies per T cell. T-cell enriched fractions were isolated from pooled splenocytes (from 12 spleens) that had been cultured (for 24 or 48 h) or from fresh, unstimulated cells (basal). The number of DOR molecules per T cell were estimated by quantitative competitive RT-PCR.[11] A representative experiment is shown. Reprinted with permission of J. Leukocyte Biol.

were 85% positive for Thy-1 (see FIGURE 1). Thus, the basal expression of DOR mRNA does not appear to be strain-dependent.

Cell culture, itself, in the absence of mitogens, was sufficient to increase transcript expression by 10- to 20-fold after 24 and 48 h, respectively (FIG. 1). Additional experiments were performed to further understand the effects of cell culture. FIGURE 2

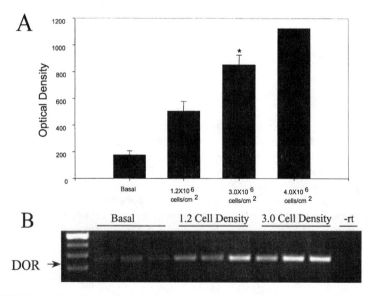

FIGURE 2. The effects of cell density on the level of DOR mRNA expressed by splenocytes. Pooled splenocytes were cultured ($N = 3$ flasks per group, except for the highest density) at increasing densities for 48 h in the absence of mitogens. DOR mRNA levels present in cultured cells were compared to the levels in freshly obtained cells (basal). DOR mRNA levels were assayed by RT-PCR; all reactions were performed with RNA extracted from the same number of cells. *$P = 0.002$ compared to basal.

shows the effect of increasing cell density on splenocyte DOR expression after 48 h of cell culture compared to levels in fresh cells (basal). RT-PCR reactions, performed with RNA extracted from a constant number of cells, showed that DOR transcript expression increased linearly with cell density. To determine whether these effects reflect the secretion of a soluble factor, supernatant transfer experiments were performed in which cells were cultured at low density (1.2×10^6 cells/cm^2) in a medium containing supernatant from cells that previously had been cultured at either low or high density (3.0×10^6 cells/cm^2). FIGURE 3 indicates that DOR expression was not enhanced by supernatants from cells cultured at high density. Therefore, direct cell–cell interactions, rather than a soluble factor(s), appear to mediate the enhanced expression of DOR mRNA by splenocytes cultured in the absence of mitogenic stimulation.

FIGURE 1 shows that cross-linking the TCR (with anti-CD$_3$-ε) further enhanced splenocyte DOR expression at 24 and 48 h; DOR levels increased by 20- and 40-fold, respectively, compared to basal. Additional experiments with actinomycin D showed that the apparent half-life of DOR mRNA was about six hours in the presence or absence of anti-CD$_3$-ε.[11] DOR mRNA stability was similar in basal and anti-CD$_3$-ε-treated cells, indicating that the TCR-enhanced expression of DOR mRNA is mediated transcriptionally.

FIGURE 4 shows that PMA inhibited both the culture-induced (control) and the anti-CD$_3$-ε-induced expression of DOR mRNA. The suppressive effects of PMA depended, to some extent, on when it was added relative to anti-CD$_3$-ε. Thus, pretreatment (PMA-CD3) and cotreatment (PMA/CD3) with PMA had the greatest effect, which diminished with delayed addition (CD3-PMA). Other studies have shown that PMA + ionomycin, which mimics the proliferative effects of cross-linking

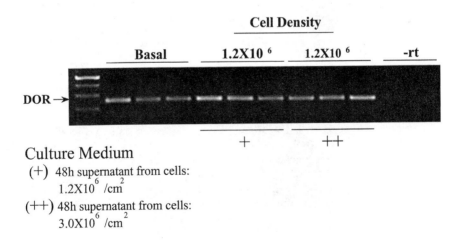

FIGURE 3. The effects of supernatant transfer on the expression of DOR mRNA by splenocytes. Pooled splenocytes were cultured ($N = 3$ flasks per group) at low density (1.2×10^6 splenocytes per cm^2) in medium containing supernatants from splenocytes that previously had been cultured (48 h) at either low or high density (3.0×10^6 splenocytes per cm^2). DOR mRNA levels present in cultured cells were compared to the levels in freshly obtained cells (basal). No effect of supernatants obtained from high-density cells was observed.

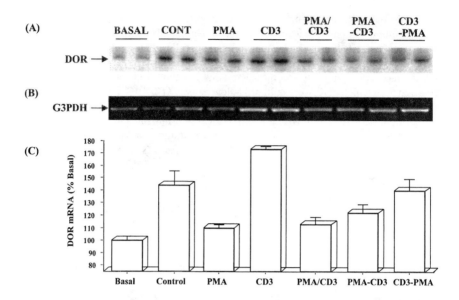

FIGURE 4. The effects of culture alone (control), PMA, anti-CD$_3$-ε, or combinations of PMA and anti-CD$_3$-ε on the expression of DOR mRNA in splenocytes. Splenocytes were pooled (12 spleens) and each treatment group ($N = 2$) was cultured for 24 h. For PMA/CD3, cells were incubated with PMA and anti-CD$_3$-ε simultaneously; for PMA-CD3, PMA treatment for 4 h preceded the addition of anti-CD$_3$-ε; and for CD3-PMA, the addition of anti-CD$_3$-ε preceded PMA by 4 h. DOR mRNA levels present in cultured cells were compared to the levels in freshly obtained cells (basal). PMA suppressed both the cell-culture-induced and the anti-CD$_3$-ε-induced expression of DOR mRNA. Similar results were observed in experiments in which DOR mRNA was measured using extracts obtained from splenic T cells, purified after cell culture.[11] Reprinted with permission of J. Leukocyte Biol.

the TCR by anti-CD$_3$-ε, also suppressed DOR mRNA expression by enriched splenic T cells at 24 and 48 h compared to unstimulated, cultured cells.[11] Both anti-CD$_3$-ε and PMA/ionomycin stimulated T-cell proliferation,[11] yet PMA/ionomycin suppressed DOR expression in the presence or absence of anti-CD$_3$-ε. Thus, the enhanced expression of DOR mRNA and T-cell proliferation appear to be independent events that may occur concurrently, depending on the specific T-cell stimuli that are present.

Inhibition of DOR mRNA expression by PMA was dominant over stimulation by anti-CD$_3$-ε. Since TCR signaling activates protein kinase C (PKC) and activation of PKC by PMA inhibits DOR gene expression, it is possible that other TCR-dependent intracellular effectors deliver a dominant positive signal(s), resulting in enhanced DOR transcription. The activation of PKC by PMA appears to shift this balance, perhaps due to the magnitude and duration of PKC activation by PMA.

We have recently observed that the expression of splenocyte DOR transcripts was dose-dependently enhanced by *in vivo* treatment with the superantigen, staphylococcal enterotoxin B (SEB 20 μg, i.p.), which is recognized by the TCR of virtually all T cells bearing the Vβ7, 8.1, 8.2, and 8.3 alleles;[16] DOR mRNA levels were significantly

TABLE 1. DOR+ and CD3+ immunofluorescent murine splenocytes

%Positive cells (Mean ± SEM)						
Saline			SEB			
CD3+	DOR+	CD3+ DOR+/CD3+	CD3+	DOR+	CD3+ DOR+/CD3+	
23.3 ± 3.8	4.2 ± 1.5	8.3 ± 4.6	21.5 ± 2.2	20.9 ± 3.4	51.1 ± 7.8*	

NOTE: Five random images per slide were visualized by epifluorescence on an Olympus BX60, and captured with a Spot CCD camera (Diagnostics Instruments, Sterlings Hts., MI). Images were analyzed with NIH Image 1.6.1 (zippy.nimh. nih.gov), and statiscal analyses were performed with Statview 1.03. Comparison by of the two double-positive groups as a percentage of total CD3$^+$ cells (CD3$^+$ + DOR$^+$/CD3$^+$) showed that saline was less than SEB (*$p < 0.001$; $n = 6$ experiments per group).

elevated by 24 h after a single injection (unpublished data). The effects of this treatment on DOR protein expression were studied by double-labeling cells with complexes containing FITC/anti-DOR and Cy3/anti-CD$_3$. TABLE 1 shows the results of studies in which the percent of positive splenocytes was determined by blind cell counts. In saline-treated mice, approximately one-third of splenocytes were T cells (CD3$^+$) compared to 25% after SEB treatment. The DOR-positive fraction of the total splenocyte population increased from approximately 28% to 43% with SEB treatment. Furthermore, the fraction of the T-cell population that expressed DOR increased significantly, from approximately 8% to 51% with SEB. In saline-treated animals, low levels of FITC-DOR fluorescence were typically observed in most cells. This increased substantially after SEB stimulation. Thus, SEB can significantly increase DOR expression *in vivo,* affecting both mRNA and protein levels. These effects occur largely within the T-cell population.

In summary, the expression of DORs by T cells can be stimulated by the following TCR-dependent mechanisms: (1) a superantigen (SEB) administered *in vivo,* and (2) cross-linking the TCR with anti-CD$_3$-ε *in vitro.* In addition, *in vitro* studies have shown that undefined cell–cell interactions can enhance DOR expression. T-Cell proliferation and the enhanced expression of DOR mRNA appear to be independent events that can occur concurrently, depending on the specific T-cell stimuli that are present (i.e., anti-CD$_3$-ε vs. PMA + ionomycin).

The DORs expressed by activated T cells may be involved in downregulating the T-cell activation program. This is supported by the antiproliferative effects of DOR agonists, which have been demonstrated with thymic and splenic T cells. Both T-cell DORs and locally produced DOR peptides appear to be involved in the downregulation of activated T cells.

REFERENCES

1. SHARP, B.M., S. ROY & J.M. BIDLACK. 1998. Evidence for opioid receptors in cells involved in host defense and the immune system. J. Neuroimmunol. **83:** 45–56.
2. LINNER, K.M., H.E. QUIST & B.M. SHARP. 1995. Met-eknephalin-containing peptides encoded by proenkephalin A mRNA expressed in activated murine thymocytes inhibit thymocyte proliferation. J. Immunol. **154:** 5049–5060.

3. SHAHABI, N.A. & B.M. SHARP. 1995. Antiproliferative effects of delta opioids on highly purified CD4⁻ and CD8⁻ murine T cells. J. Pharmacol. Exp. Therap. **273:** 1105–1113.

4. GILMORE, W. & L.P. WEINER. 1988. Beta-endorphin enhances interleukin-2 (IL-2) production in murine lymphocytes. J. Neuroimmunol. **18:** 125–138.

5. BESSLER, H., M.B. SZTEIN & S.A. SERRATE. 1990. Beta-endorphin modulation of IL-1-induced IL-2 production. Immunopharmacology **19:** 5–14.

6. LINNER, K.M., H.E. QUIST & B.M. SHARP. 1995. Met-enkephalin-containing peptides encoded by proenkephalin A mRNA expressed in activated murine thymocytes inhibit thymocyte proliferation. J. Immunol. **154:** 5049–5060.

7. CHUANG, L.J., T.K. CHUANG, K.F. KILLAM, JR., A.J. CHUANG, H.F. KUNG, L. YU & R.Y. CHUANG. 1994. Delta opioid receptor gene expression in lymphocytes. Biochem. Biophys. Res. Commun. **202:** 1291–1299.

8. WICK, M.J., S.R. MINNERATH, S. ROY, S. RAMAKRISHNAN & H.H. LOH. 1996. Differential expression of opioid receptor genes in human lymphoid cell lines and peripheral blood lymphocytes. J. Neuroimmunol. **64**(1): 29–36.

9. MILLER, B. 1996. Delta opioid receptor expression is induced by concanavalin A in CD4⁺ T cells. J. Immunol. **157:** 5324–5328.

10. SHARP, B.M., D.J. MCKEAN, M.D. LI & K. MCALLEN. 1997. Detection of basal levels and induction of delta opioid receptor mRNA in murine splenocytes. J. Neuroimmunol. **78:** 198–202.

11. LI, M.D., K. MCALLEN & B.M. SHARP. 1999. Regulation of delta opioid receptor expression by anti-CD₃-ε, PMA, and ionomycin in murine splenocytes and T cells. J. Leukocyte Biol. **65:** 707–714.

12. STEFANO, G.B., P. MELCHIORRI, L. NEGRI, T.K. HUGHES, JR. & B. SCHARRER. 1992. [D-Ala2]-deltorphin I binding and pharmacological evidence for a special subtype of delta opioid receptor on human and invertebrate immune cells. Proc. Natl. Acad. Sci. USA **89:** 9316–9320.

13. CARR, D.J.J., B.R. DeCOSTA, C.-H. KIM, A.E. JACOBSON, V. GUARECELLO, K.C. RICE & J.E. BLALOCK. 1989. Opioid receptors on cells of the immune system: evidence for δ and κ-classes. J. Endocrinol. **122:** 161–168.

14. CARR, D.J., C.H. KIM, B. DeCOSTA, A.E. JACOBSON, K.C. RICE & J.E. BLALOCK. 1988. Evidence for delta-class opioid receptor on cells of the immune system. Cell Immunol. **116**(1): 44–51.

15. MILLER, B.C. 1998. Western blot analysis of the delta-opioid receptor in activated murine T cells. Adv. Exp. Med. Biol. **437:** 159–167.

16. KAPPLER, J., B. KOTZIN, L. HERRON, E. GELFAND, R. BIGLER, A. BOYLSTON, S. CARREL, D. POSNETT, Y. CHOI & P. MARRACK. 1989. Vβ-specific stimulation of human T cells by staphylococcal toxins. Science **244:** 811–813.

Acute Effects of Morphine on Blood Lymphocyte Proliferation and Plasma IL-6 Levels

RICHARD A. HOUGHTLING,[a] R. DANIEL MELLON,[a]
RODERICK J. TAN,[b] AND BARBARA M. BAYER[c,d]

[a]Department of Pharmacology, Georgetown University Medical Center,
Washington, DC 20007, USA

[b]Department of Biology, Georgetown University Medical Center,
Washington, DC 20007, USA

[c]Department of Neuroscience, Georgetown University Medical Center,
Washington, DC 20007, USA

ABSTRACT: Administration of morphine (10 mg/kg) to rats was found to decrease the proliferative potential of blood lymphocytes by 60–80% and concurrently elevate circulating levels of the cytokine, interleukin-6 (IL-6), 2- to 4-fold. Both parameters were similarly altered upon the central administration of morphine and were blocked upon pretreatment of animals with the opioid receptor antagonist, naltrexone. These results suggest that the activation of central opioid receptors is involved in morphine-induced inhibition of lymphocyte proliferation as well as increases in circulating levels of IL-6. Studies addressing the potential peripheral mechanisms demonstrated that intact ganglionic transmission was required for both effects of morphine. Although the suppression by morphine of lymphocyte proliferation appeared to be largely independent of stimulation of the hypothalamic–pituitary–adrenal axis, the elevation of IL-6 was completely abolished in adrenalectomized animals. Collectively, these results suggest that central opioid receptor activation results in changes in different immune parameters that can be mediated through distinct peripheral mechanisms.

INTRODUCTION

The potential immunomodulatory role of opioid receptors within the central nervous system has been examined by several laboratories (for review, see Ref. 1). For example, our laboratory has demonstrated that acute morphine to the rat leads to a decreased blood lymphocyte proliferation response to the T-cell mitogen concanavalin A (ConA) mediated by central opioid receptors.[2,3] Recently, we have determined that this effect was mediated primarily by central μ-opioid receptors.[3] The autonomic nervous system has been implicated as the primary mediator in this response, since blockade of the peripheral ganglia with chlorisondamine prevented this effect,[4] and stimulation of the ganglia by nicotine or epibatidine led to a similar decreased

[d]Address for correspondence: Barbara M. Bayer, Ph.D., Department of Neuroscience, Georgetown University Medical Center, 3970 Reservoir Road, N.W., Washington, DC 20007. Voice: 202-687-1616; fax: 202-687-4226.
bayerb@gusun.georgetown.edu

blood lymphocyte proliferation response.[5] Although it is well known that opioids increase plasma corticosterone levels, the effect of morphine on blood lymphocyte proliferation appears to be largely independent of adrenal-derived factors.[6]

Recently, central opioid receptors have been indirectly implicated in interleukin-1-induced elevations of plasma interleukin-6 (IL-6).[7] In contrast to the well-characterized effects of morphine in the lymphocyte proliferation response, however, mechanisms involved in the effects of morphine on plasma IL-6 levels are relatively uncharacterized. Since both of these potential immunomodulatory effects appear to be mediated, at least in part, by central opioid receptors, the studies described here compare and contrast the effects of morphine on both blood lymphocyte proliferation and plasma IL-6.

MATERIALS AND METHODS

Animals

Sprague-Dawley rats (200–225 g) were purchased from Taconic Laboratories (Germantown, NY) and group housed three per cage in a light (12-h light:dark) and temperature (23 ± 1°C) controlled room for one week prior to surgery or experiments. Animals were provided free access to food (Purina Rat Chow) and water *ad libitum*. Sham-operated and adrenalectomized animals were purchased from Taconic Laboratories. For microinjection studies, one week prior to experimentation, animals were implanted with intraventricular guide cannula into the lateral ventricle corresponding to the following coordinates measured from bregma: AP $= -0.92$ mm, ML $= -1.6$ mm, and DV $= -3.4$ mm.[8] Standard surgical procedures for microinjection studies were similar to those previously described.[3]

Drugs

Morphine sulfate was generously provided by The National Institute on Drug Abuse (Research Triangle, NC). Chlorisondamine chloride was a kind gift from Ciba-Geigy. All other drugs were purchased from the Sigma Chemical Company (St. Louis, MO).

Blood Proliferation

Blood lymphocyte proliferation to the polyclonal T-cell mitogen ConA was measured as previously described.[3]

Plasma IL-6

Plasma IL-6 levels were determined using the 7TD1 cell line,[9] as recently described.[10] For these studies, half-maximal proliferation of the cell line determined by recombinant rat IL-6 corresponded to 1 U of activity.

RESULTS

Effects of Central Administration of Morphine

To determine if the effect of morphine on blood lymphocyte proliferation or plasma IL-6 levels could be elicited by central administration of morphine, animals were cannulated in the lateral ventricle one week prior to experiments. On the day of the experiment, animals were centrally microinjected with either saline (5 μL/rat) or morphine (10 μg/5 μL) and blood lymphocyte proliferation and plasma IL-6 levels were examined. Central morphine administration significantly decreased blood lymphocyte proliferation responses ($P < 0.01$) compared to saline-treated animals (see FIGURE 1A). In contrast to the suppression of blood lymphocyte proliferation, central morphine administration elevated plasma levels of the proinflammatory cytokine IL-6 by 54% (FIG. 1B).

Effects of Ganglionic Blockade

To determine if the effect of morphine on both blood lymphocyte proliferation and plasma IL-6 levels required stimulation of peripheral ganglia, the effect of pretreatment with a low dose of chlorisondamine (a bisquaternary, neuronal nicotinic

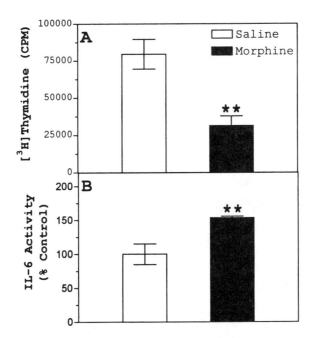

FIGURE 1. Effect of central morphine administration. Animals ($n = 6$–7 per group) were treated intraventricularly with either saline or morphine (10 μg/5 μL, lateral ventricle) and sacrificed 1 hour later. (**A**) Blood lymphocyte proliferation, and (**B**) plasma IL-6 levels. **$p < 0.01$ compared to saline-treated animals (unpaired *t*-test).

receptor antagonist) was examined. Previous studies from our laboratory demonstrated that a high dose of chlorisondamine (5 mg/kg, i.p.) prevented morphine-induced suppression of blood lymphocyte proliferation.[4] As depicted in FIGURE 2A, morphine administration (10 mg/kg, s.c.) significantly decreased blood lymphocyte proliferation (52%, $P < 0.01$) compared to saline-injected controls. Chlorisondamine pretreatment (0.5 mg/kg, i.p.) had no effect on blood lymphocyte proliferation alone, but it completely blocked the effect of morphine. Plasma IL-6 activity (FIG. 2B) was significantly increased following morphine administration ($P < 0.01$). Similar to blood lymphocyte proliferation, chlorisondamine pretreatment had no effect on its own, but completely blocked the effect of morphine on that of plasma IL-6.

Effects of Adrenalectomy

Since opioids lead to activation of the HPA axis, the role of the adrenal gland in the effect of morphine on blood lymphocyte proliferation and plasma IL-6 activity was evaluated. Due to the loss of both mineralocorticoids and glucocorticoids by adrenalectomy, and since glucocorticoids negatively regulate IL-6,[11] adrenalecto-mized (ADX-CORT) animals were provided drinking saline supplemented with

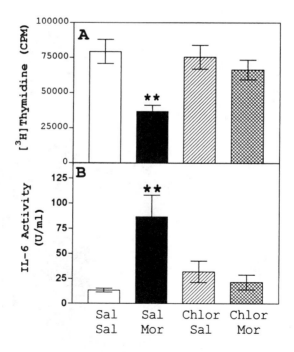

FIGURE 2. Effect of chlorisondamine pretreatment. Animals ($n = 10–11$ per group) were treated with either saline (Sal) or chlorisondamine (Chlor, 0.5 mg/kg, i.p.) 30 minutes prior to a systemic injection of either morphine (Mor, 10 mg/kg, s.c.) or saline (Sal) and sacrificed 1 hour later. (**A**) Blood lymphocyte proliferation, and (**B**) plasma IL-6 levels. **$p < 0.01$ compared to all other groups (ANOVA, Newman-Keuls).

corticosterone (25 µg/mL). This supplementation has been shown to minimize elevations of basal IL-6 levels.[12] Sham-operated and adrenalectomized animals were
treated with either saline (1 mL/kg, s.c.) or morphine (20 mg/kg, s.c.) and sacrificed
1 h following treatment. As shown in FIGURE 3A, sham-operated animals injected
with morphine had significantly decreased blood lymphocyte proliferation responses
($P < 0.05$) compared to saline-injected controls. Blood lymphocyte proliferation in
saline-treated ADX-CORT animals was significantly higher than that of saline-treated sham-operated animals ($P < 0.001$). Similar to the previous finding that adrenalectomy did not block the effect of morphine on blood lymphocyte proliferation,[6]
adrenalectomy with corticosterone replacement did not prevent morphine-induced
inhibition (45%) of blood lymphocyte proliferation in ADX-CORT animals. Morphine administration significantly increased plasma IL-6 levels in sham-operated
animals (FIG. 3B). In contrast to the effect of morphine on the blood proliferation
response in ADX-CORT animals, the effect of morphine on plasma IL-6 levels was
completely blocked in ADX-CORT animals (FIG. 3B).

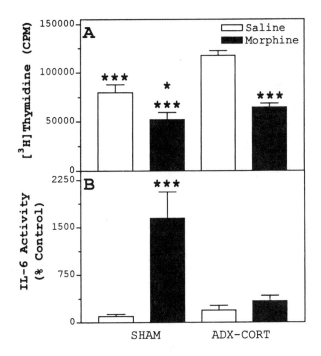

FIGURE 3. Effect of adrenalectomy with corticosterone replacement. Animals ($n =$
5–6 per group) were either sham-operated (SHAM) or adrenalectomized (ADX) 1 week pri-
or to experiments. ADX animals were provided drinking water supplemented with corticosterone (25 µg/mL). Animals were treated with either saline or morphine (20 mg/kg, s.c.)
and sacrificed 1 hour later. (**A**) Blood lymphocyte proliferation *$p < 0.05$ compared to
SHAM saline treatment and ***$p < 0.001$ compared to ADX-CORT, and (**B**) Plasma IL-6
levels, ***$p < 0.001$ compared to all groups (ANOVA, Newman-Keuls).

DISCUSSION

A comparison of the effects of morphine on blood lymphocyte proliferation and plasma IL-6 levels demonstrated several clear similarities. First, both effects of morphine appear to be mediated predominantly by central opioid receptors, since administration of morphine to the lateral ventricle led to a decreased proliferation response as well as increased plasma IL-6. Second, both effects appear to be mediated by classic opioid receptors, since both of these responses to morphine are blocked by naltrexone (data not shown). Third, both effects were prevented by blockade of peripheral nicotinic receptors, suggesting a role of the autonomic nervous system (ANS). A role of the ANS has been suggested previously for lymphocyte proliferation,[4,5] as well as for IL-1-induced plasma IL-6.[13] Thus, similar to the effects of acute morphine on lymphocyte proliferation, morphine-induced elevation of plasma IL-6 also appears to be mediated by activation of the autonomic ganglia.

Although the effect of morphine on blood lymphocyte proliferation and plasma IL-6 levels share several similarities, one distinct difference was evident in these studies. Previously, Flores *et al.*[6] demonstrated that the effect of morphine on lymphocyte proliferation was largely independent of adrenal activation. Consistent with this observation, morphine treatment of adrenalectomized animals that received basal corticosterone replacement had decreased blood lymphocyte proliferation compared to saline-injected controls (FIG. 3A). Although ADX-CORT alone significantly increased blood lymphocyte proliferation compared to sham controls, the effect of morphine in sham-operated and ADX-CORT animals were not significantly different. Taken together, these data suggested that blood lymphocyte proliferation responses to morphine were largely adrenal-independent. In contrast, the effect of morphine on plasma IL-6 levels appears to be largely dependent upon the adrenal gland (FIG. 3B). Thus, these data suggested that the mechanism of morphine-induced alterations of both blood lymphocyte proliferation and plasma IL-6 occur through either a common pathway that diverges or through two separate pathways leading to adrenal-independent and adrenal-dependent responses, respectively.

ACKNOWLEDGMENTS

This work was supported by NIH grants DA04358 (BMB), DA05849 (RAH), and DA05779 (RDM).

REFERENCES

1. MELLON, R.D. & B.M. BAYER. 1998. Evidence for central opioid receptors in the immunomodulatory effects of morphine: review of potential mechanism(s) of action. J. Neuroimmunol. **83:** 19–28.
2. HERNANDEZ, M.C., L.R. FLORES & B.M. BAYER. 1993. Immunosuppression by morphine is mediated by central pathways. J. Pharmacol. Exp. Ther. **267:** 1336–1341.
3. MELLON, R.D. & B.M. BAYER. 1998. Role of central opioid receptor subtypes in morphine-induced alterations in peripheral lymphocyte activity. Brain Res. **789:** 56–67.
4. FLORES, L.R., K.L. DRETCHEN & B.M. BAYER. 1996. Potential role of the autonomic nervous system in the immunosuppressive effects of acute morphine administration. Eur. J. Pharmacol. **318:** 437–446.

5. MELLON, R.D. & B.M. BAYER. 1999. The effects of morphine, nicotine and epibatidine on lymphocyte activity and hypothalamic-pituitary-adrenal axis responses. J. Pharmacol. Exp. Ther. **288:** 635–642.
6. FLORES, L.R., M.C. HERNANDEZ & B.M. BAYER. 1994. Acute immunosuppressive effects of morphine: lack of involvement of pituitary and adrenal factors. J. Pharmacol. Exp. Ther. **268:** 1129–1134.
7. DE SIMONI, M.G., A. DE LUIGI, L. GEMMA, M. SIRONI, A. MANFRIDI & P. GHEZZI. 1993. Modulation of systemic interleukin-6 induction by central interleukin-1. Am. J. Physiol. **265:** R739–R742.
8. PAXINOS, G. & C. WATSON. 1997. The Rat Brain in Stereotaxic Coordinates, 3rd edit. Academic Press. New York.
9. VAN SNICK, J., S. CAYPHAS, A. VINK, C. UYTTENHOVE, P.G. COULIE, M.R. RUBIRA & R.J. SIMPSON. 1986. Purification and NH_2-terminal amino acid sequence of a T-cell-derived lymphokine with growth factor activity for B-cell hybridomas. Proc. Natl. Acad. Sci. USA **83:** 9679–9683.
10. HOUGHTLING, R.A. & B.M. BAYER. 2000. Role of opioids in elevating plasma interleukin-6 (IL-6): pharmacological characterization and dependence on adrenal activation. J. Neuroimmunol. Submitted.
11. RAY, A., K.S. LAFORGE & P.B. SEHGAL. 1999. On the mechanism for efficient repression of the interleukin-6 promoter by glucocorticoids: enhancer, TATA box, and RNA start site (Inr motif) occlusion. Mol. Cell. Biol. **10:** 5736–5746.
12. ZHOU, D., A.W. KUSNECOV, M.R. SHURIN, M. DEPAOLI & B.S. RABIN. 1993. Exposure to physical and psychological stressors elevates plasma interleukin 6: relationship to the activation of hypothalamic-pituitary-adrenal axis. Endocrinology **133:** 2523–2530.
13. KITAMURA, H., S. OKAMOTO, Y. SHIMAMOTO, M. MORIMATSU, A. TERAO & M. SAITO. 1998. Central IL-1 differentially regulates peripheral IL-6 and TNF synthesis. Cell. Mol. Life Sci. **54:** 282–287.

Expression of Preproenkephalin mRNA and Production and Secretion of Enkephalins by Human Thymocytes

ANNEMIEKE KAVELAARS[a] AND COBI J. HEIJNEN

Department of Pediatric Immunology, Wilhelmina Children Hospital of the University Medical Center Utrecht, Utrecht, The Netherlands

ABSTRACT: Human thymocytes were tested for the capacity to express the preproenkephalin (PPE) gene and for production of the end product metenkephalin (MENK). It is shown here for the first time that the cytokines IL-2, IL-4, IL-6, and TGF-β are capable of inducing PPE mRNA expression. Moreover, a culture of thymocytes with the cytokines results in intracellular expression of MENK as determined by immunohistochemistry. Thymocytes do not secrete detectable amounts of MENK, however, but only the larger MENK-containing peptides or proteins. Cytokines IL-1β and IL-10 increase the expression of PPE mRNA in 50% of the thymuses tested, whereas IFN-γ does not induce changes in PPE mRNA expression.

INTRODUCTION

The immune system and the neuroendocrine system communicate via shared mediators and receptors.[1] One clear example of this phenomenon is that cytokines produced by the immune system can signal to the brain.[2] Conversely, neuroendocrine mediators, like neuroepeptides, can modulate immune functioning.[3] Interestingly, neuroepeptides are not only produced within the neuroendocrine system, but also within the immune system.[1,3]

One of the peptides that can be produced by both the neuroendocrine and immune system is the opioid peptide met-enkephalin (MENK).[4–7] This peptide is encoded by the preproenkephalin (PPE) gene, which is translated to the prohormone preproenkephalin A (PEA). PEA is processed into biologically active, MENK-containing peptides such as BAM-20P and -22P, amidorphin, peptide E, F, and B, and ultimately into the pentapeptides MENK and leu-enkephalin.[8]

Earlier studies by Linner *et al.*[9,10] showed that murine thymocytes express and produce enkephalins after stimulation with the mitogen concanavalin A. We are interested in the effect of cytokines on opioid peptide expression in the immune system. Cytokines, such as IL-2 and IL-4, promote proliferation and differentiation of immature thymocytes *in vitro*.[11] We have shown that human peripheral blood cells

[a]Address for correspondence: Dr. Annemieke Kavelaars, Department of Pediatric Immunology, Room KC 03.068.0, Wilhelmina Children Hospital of the University Medical Center Utrecht, PO BOX 85090, 3508 AB Utrecht, The Netherlands. Voice: 31-30-250-4360; fax: 31-30-250-5311.

a.kavelaars@wkz.azu.nl

respond to Th2 cytokines with increased expression of PPE mRNA and increased production of the gene product. In contrast, Th1 cytokines like IFN-γ do not induce detectable changes in PEA protein or in MENK, although small increases in PPE mRNA could be induced by Th1 cytokines in human peripheral blood cells.[5]

The aim of the present study was to investigate whether cytokines can induce the expression of the PPE gene and its gene products in human thymocytes.

MATERIALS AND METHODS

Thymocytes

Thymus tissue of children that had to be removed during cardiac surgery was used. Thymocytes were released by gently teasing through a mesh wire and further isolated by Ficoll-paque density centrifugation.

Thymocytes (5×10^6/mL) were cultured in RPMI-1640 supplemented with 5% FCS (Gibco, Grand Island, NY) and antibiotics.

Analysis of PPE Gene Expression

At the end of the culture period, RNA was isolated by RNAzol extraction. The expression of the PPE gene was determined by quantitative RT-PCR using a deletion mutated RNA as the internal standard, as described.[5]

Immunohistochemistry

Cells were spun onto glass slides, fixed in ethanol/acetic acid, and stained using a polyclonal rabbit-anti-MENK antibody (Campro Scientific) and a swine–anti-rabbit– peroxidase conjugate, as described.[5]

Radioimmunoassay

The concentration of MENK in culture supernatant was determined using a radio-immunoassay according to the manufacturers protocol (Incstar, Stillwater, MN). In part of the experiments, culture supernatants were treated with trypsin and carbox-ypeptidase B, as described.[5]

RESULTS

Human thymocytes were cultured with IL-1β, IL-2, IL-4, IL-6, IL-10, or IFN-γ for 24 h. The data depicted in FIGURE 1 demonstrate that unstimulated thymocytes do express very low levels of the PPE gene. Culture of the cells with IL-2, IL-4, IL-6, or TGF-β induces a marked increase in PPE mRNA levels. In contrast, addition of IFN-γ to cultures of thymocytes does not result in increased expression of the PPE gene. For IL-10 and IL-1β, mixed results were obtained. In 50% of the thymuses we did observe an increase in PPE mRNA expression after culture with either IL-1β or IL-10, whereas in the other half of the experiments we did not observe any change in PPE mRNA levels. β-Globin mRNA levels were similar in all samples.

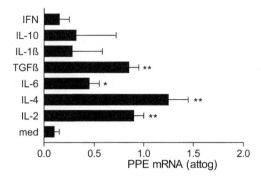

FIGURE 1. Effect of cytokines on PPE mRNA expression. Freshly isolated thymocytes were cultured in the presence of cytokines in the concentrations indicated in TABLE 1 for 24 h. RNA was isolated and PPE mRNA expression was determined by quantitative RT-PCR. Data represent mean and SEM of 8 independent experiments. * $p < 0.05$; ** $p < 0.01$ versus controls.

To investigate whether thymocytes can translate PPE mRNA and process PEA into the pentapeptide MENK, we determined the presence of MENK by immunohistochemistry. Thymocytes were cultured for 72 h in the presence of cytokines and stained with an anti-MENK antibody. The data in Table 1 demonstrate that IL-2, IL-4, IL-6, and TGF-β induce a significant increase in the percentage of MENK-positive cells. IL-1, IL-10, and IFN-γ do not induce significant changes in the percentage of MENK-positive cells.

To control for the specificity of the staining, we preincubated the anti-MENK antibody with a 100-fold excess of synthetic MENK. After this procedure, the antibody did not detect MENK-positive cells anymore (data not shown).

TABLE 1. Immunohistochemical detection of MENK-positive thymocytes after culture with cytokines

Stimulus	MENK positive cells (%)
Control	15 ± 4
IL-2 (40 U/mL)	65 ± 6*
IL-4 10 ng/mL	70 ± 4*
IL-6 100 U/mL	60 ± 3*
TGF-β 1.6 ng/mL	62 ± 5*
IL-1β 25 pg/mL	19 ± 5
IL-10 2 ng/mL	19 ± 5
IFN-γ 200 U/mL	15 ± 5

NOTE: Thymocytes were cultured for 72 h in the presence of the indicated cytokines and stained for MENK. Data represent mean and SEM of six independent experiments. *$P < 0.01$ versus control cultures.

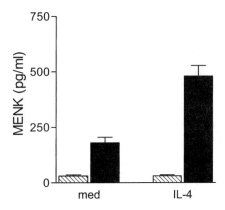

FIGURE 2. MENK secretion by thymocytes. Thymocytes were cultured with IL-4 (10 ng/mL) for 72 h. Culture supernatants were harvested and, directly (*open bars*) or after treatment with trypsin and carboxypeptidase A (*black bars*), tested for MENK by RIA. Data represent mean and SEM of three experiments.

The amount of MENK in culture supernatants of thymocytes was determined by radioimmunoassay. Since IL-4 is a potent inducer of gene expression and of intracellular MENK (FIG. 1 and TABLE 1), thymocytes were stimulated with IL-4 and supernatants assayed for MENK. Surprisingly, IL-4 did not induce an increase in the MENK level in the culture supernatant, suggesting that thymocytes do not secrete MENK.

In previous studies[6] it was shown that lymphocytes are capable of secreting larger MENK-containing peptides rather than the fully processed end product MENK. To examine this possibility, supernatants of thymocytes cultured with IL-4 and control cultures were treated with trypsin and carboxypeptidase B. The data in FIGURE 2 demonstrate that digestive treatment of the IL-4-stimulated culture supernatant results in a significant increase in the amount of MENK. Therefore, we conclude that thymocytes do not secrete detectable amounts of MENK, but are capable of secreting larger MENK-containing propeptides.

DISCUSSION

The present study demonstrated that human thymocytes express the PPE gene. The cytokines IL-2, IL4, IL-6, and TGF-β are potent inducers of PPE gene expression in freshly isolated human thymocytes. Although thymocytes do express IFN-γ receptors, the Th1 cytokine IFN-γ does not induce PPE gene expression in these cells. In this respect, thymocytes behave like peripheral blood T cells. In an earlier study, we showed that IFN-γ cannot induce PPE mRNA expression in human peripheral blood T cells. In contrast, Th2 cytokines, such as IL-4, are potent inducers of the PPE gene in T cells.[5]

IL-1β and IL-10 enhanced PPE gene expression in only 50% of the thymocyte samples. We do not know the reason for this inconsistent result. One possibility could be that there is a differential expression of receptors for these cytokines, depending on age or clinical condition of the thymus donors.

The cytokines that induce PPE gene expression in thymocytes also give rise to the translation of the mRNA into proenkephalin A and further processing into MENK. Immunohistochemical analysis of thymocytes revealed that MENK is not the only PEA product that can be detected intracellularly. IL-4 stimulation also results in 20–25% of peptide F postivie cells. Moreover, 15% of the cells are stained positively with an antibody-recognizing BAM-22p. Therefore, we conclude, that thymocytes can process PEA into MENK, but that larger processing intermediates are also retained in the cell.

With respect to secretion of PEA-derived peptides by thymocytes, we showed that cytokine stimulation does not results in detectable increases in MENK in the medium. There are two possible explanations for this phenomenon. Either MENK in the culture medium is very unstable or it is rapidly bound to receptors on thymocytes and therefore not recognized in the radioimmunoassay. Interestingly, thymocytes do appear to secrete larger processing intermediates after IL-4 stimulation. Treatment of the culture supernatant with processing enzymes results in significant amount of MENK. Kuis et al.[6] have shown that human peripheral blood T cells also secrete intermediary PEA products after mitogenic stimulation. These data are supported by our earlier results indicating that IL-4 can induce peripheral blood T cells to secrete MENK-containing peptides, but no MENK. In contrast, monocytes can secrete the fully processed end product MENK after proper activation.

Tissue-specific processing of MENK has also been observed when comparing adrenal medulla and neuronal cells. In the adrenal medulla the initial cleavage of PEA is thought to occur near the carboxy terminal of the molecule, giving rise to large products (8.6–18.2 kD). At the nerve terminals, only pentapeptides are detectable, suggesting a different, more complete processing.[12] Although most of the attention has been focused on the immunomodulatory effects of MENK, intermediate products like peptide F and peptide F also have been shown to have immunomodulatory effects, for example, on T-cell-dependent antibody responses.[13]

There is controversy in the literature with respect to expression of opioid receptors on immune cells. Although membrane receptors for MENK have been described on T cells, we propose that human T cells and thymocytes recognize and respond more to endogenous intermediate MENK-containing peptides than to MENK. The possibility remains, however, that the intracellular pentapeptide influences cellular metabolism via an intracellular pathway, without the necessity of being secreted.

Linner et al.[10] have demonstrated that murine thymocyte-derived enkephalins inhibit murine thymocyte division. In this respect it is of interest that endogenous opioids also inhibit cell proliferation and promote cell differentiation of astrocytes and cardiac muscle cells.[14] Moreover, PEA (and no other opioids) is also expressed abundantly in embryonic mesenchymal tissues during differentiation into cartilage, bone, dermis, kidney tubules, and choroid plexus of the eyes.[15] As soon as the differentiation process stops, the PEA mRNA is shut down. In addition, we have shown earlier that PEA or its processed intermediates produced by T cells can inhibit their own proliferation. Therefore, it is likely to assume that in the human thymus, thymocyte division and differentiation will be modulated by its own PEA products.

REFERENCES

1. BLALOCK, J.E., D.V. HARBOUR-MCMENAMIN & E.M. SMITH. 1985. Peptide hormones shared by the neuroendocrine and immunologic systems. J. Immunol. **135:** 858s–860s.
2. BESEDOVSKY, H.O. & A. DEL REY. 1996. Immune-neuro-endocrine interactions: facts and hypotheses. Endocr. Rev. **17:** 64–102.
3. HEIJNEN, C.J., A. KAVELAARS & R.E. BALLIEUX. 1991. β-Endorphin: cytokine and neuropeptide. Immunol. Rev. **119:** 41–63.
4. KAMPHUIS, S., F. ERIKSSON, A. KAVELAARS, J. ZIJLSTRA, M. VAN DE POL, W. KUIS & C.J. HEIJNEN. 1998. Role of endogenous pro-enkephalin A derived peptides in human T cell proliferation and monocyte IL-6 production. J. Neuroimmunol. **84:** 53–60.
5. KAMPHUIS, S., A. KAVELAARS, R. BROOIMANS, W. KUIS, B.J.M. ZEGERS & C.J. HEIJNEN. 1997. T Helper 2 cytokines induce preproenkephalin mRNA expression and proenkephalin A in human peripheral blood mononuclear cells. J. Neuroimmunol. **79:** 91–99.
6. KUIS, W., P.M. VILLIGER, H.G. LASER & M. LOTZ. 1991. Differential processing of proenkephalin-A by human perihperal blood moncytes and T lymphocytes. J. Clin. Invest. **88:** 817–824.
7. ZURAWSKI, G., M. BENEDIK, B.J. KAMB, J.S. ABRAMS, S.M. ZURAWSKI & F.D. LEE. 1986. Activation of mouse T-helper cells indues abundant preproenkephaline mRNA synthesis. Science **232:** 772–775.
8. UDENFRIEND, S. & D.L. KILPATRICK. 1984. Proenkephalin and the products of its processing: chemistry and biology. Peptides **7:** 339.
9. LINNER, K.M., H.S. BEYER & B.M. SHARP. 1991. Induction of the messenger ribonucleotidic acid for proenkephalin A in cultured murine CD4-positive thymocytes. Endocrinology **128:** 717–724.
10. LINNER, K.M., H.E. QUIST & B.M. SHARP. 1995. Met-enkephalin-containing peptides encoded by proenkephalin A mRNA expressed in activated murine thymocytes inhibit thymocyte proliferation. J. Immunol. **154:** 5049–5060.
11. VAN EWIJK, W. 1991. T cell differentiation is influenced by thymic microenvironments. Ann. Rev. Immunol. **9:** 591.
12. DILLEN, L., M. MISEREZ, A. YASSOURIDIS & A. HERZ. 1993. Posttranslational processing of proenkephalins and chromogranins/secretogranins. Neurochem. Int. **22:** 315.
13. HIDDINGA, H.J., D.D. ISAAK & R.V. LEWIS. 1994. Enkephalin-containing pepetides processed from proenkephalin significantly enhance the antibody forming cell responses to antigen. J. Immunol. **152:** 3748.
14. HAUSER, K.F., J.G. OSBORNE, A.S. MARTIN & M.H. MELNER. 1990. Cellular localization of proenkephalin mRNA and enkephalin peptide products in cultured astrocytes. Brain Res. **522:** 347.
15. SPRINGHORN, J.P. & W.C. CLAYCOMB. 1989. Preproenkephalin mRNA expression in developing rat heart and in cultured ventricular cardiac muscle cells. Biochem. J. **258:** 73.

Susceptibility to Autoimmune Disease and Drug Addiction in Inbred Rats

Are There Mechanistic Factors in Common Related to Abnormalities in Hypothalamic–Pituitary–Adrenal Axis and Stress Response Function?

RONALD L. WILDER,[a,d] MARIE M. GRIFFITHS,[b] GRANT W. CANNON,[b] RACHEL CASPI,[c] AND ELAINE F. REMMERS[a]

[a]*Inflammatory Joint Diseases Section, Arthritis and Rheumatism Branch, National Institute of Arthritis and Musculoskeletal and Skin Diseases, National Institutes of Health, Bethesda, Maryland 20892, USA*

[b]*Research Service, Veteran Affairs Medical Center, Department of Medicine, University of Utah School of Medicine, Salt Lake City, Utah 84132, USA*

[c]*Laboratory of Immunology, National Eye Institute, National Institutes of Health, Bethesda, Maryland 20892, USA*

ABSTRACT: DA and LEW inbred rats are extraordinarily susceptible to a wide range of experimental autoimmune diseases. These diseases include rheumatoid arthritis models such as collagen-induced arthritis (CIA) and adjuvant-induced arthritis (AIA), multiple sclerosis models such as myelin-basic-protein (MBP)–induced experimental autoimmune encephalomyelitis (MBP-EAE), and autoimmune uveitis models such as retinal S antigen (SAG) and interphotoreceptor-retinoid-binding-protein (IRBP) -induced experimental autoimmune uveitis (SAG-EAU and IRBP-EAU, respectively). DA and LEW rats are also addiction-prone to various drugs of abuse, such as cocaine. Moreover, they exhibit a variety of behavioral and biochemical characteristics that appear to be related to their susceptibility to addiction. By contrast, F344 and BN rats show quite different phenotypes. They are relatively resistant to CIA, AIA, MBP-EAE, SAG-EAU, and IRBP-EAU, and they are relatively resistant to addiction. Interestingly, both DA and LEW rats, in contrast to F344 and BN rats, have abnormalities in hypothalamic–pituitary–adrenal (HPA) axis function. For example, circadian production of corticosteroids is very abnormal in DA and LEW rats; that is, they exhibit minimal circadian variation in corticosterone levels. Since corticosteroids potentially have significant influences on immune function and autoimmune disease susceptibility and may also influence sensitivity to drugs of abuse, we have begun to dissect genetic control of these various phenotypic differences, focusing initially on the regulation of autoimmune disease expression. Using genomewide scanning techniques involving F2 crosses of DA × F344 (CIA and AIA), DA × BN (CIA), and LEW × F344 [IRBP-EAU and streptococcal-cell-wall arthritis (SCWA)], we have

[d]Address for correspondence: Ronald L. Wilder, M.D., Ph.D., Chief, Inflammatory Joint Diseases Section, ARB, NIAMS, NIH, Bldg. 10, Room 9N240, Bethesda, Maryland 20892. Voice: 301-496-6499; fax: 301-402-0012.

wilderr@exchange.nih.gov

identified, to date, 14 genomic regions [quantitative trait loci (QTL)] that regulate disease expression in these crosses. Development and analysis of QTL-
congenic rats involving these loci are in progress and should permit us to
address the relationships among autoimmune disease susceptibility, drug
addiction, and HPA axis and stress response function. These initial data, however, indicate that the genetic control of the autoimmune disease traits is highly
complex.

INTRODUCTION

Numerous lines of evidence, primarily clinical and epidemiological, now support
the view that neuroendocrine hormonal factors are involved in regulating the expression of autoimmune diseases in humans, such as rheumatoid arthritis (RA).[1–3] However, dissecting the molecular mechanisms underlying these observations in humans
is extraordinarily difficult because they are intermixed with variable contributions
of environmental, genetic, age, gender, and reproductive factors. Neuroendocrine
hormonal factors also appear to play a prominent role in regulating the expression
of experimental autoimmune diseases in animals,[1,4] and it appears that several of
these experimental models, particularly inbred rats, provide a powerful approach to
investigate relevant mechanisms in human autoimmune diseases. Of potential additional interest, studies of drug addiction in inbred rats also suggest that neuroendocrine hormonal factors may play a role in susceptibility and maintenance of the
addiction.[5–10] Review of the available inbred rat data stimulates one to ask if factors
influencing susceptibility to drug addiction may interrelate, in part, with those that
control autoimmune disease susceptibility. It is the purpose of the review presented
here to discuss these relationships and to describe some of our ongoing efforts to
address these hypotheses more incisively.

EXPERIMENTAL AUTOIMMUNE DISEASE
SUSCEPTIBILITY IN INBRED RATS

DA and LEW inbred rats are used widely for the study of experimental autoimmune and/or autoinflammatory diseases.[11] DA rats are extraordinarily susceptible to
collagen-induced arthritis (CIA) in response to immunization with either heterologous and homologous type II collagen in incomplete Freund's adjuvant (IFA).[12,13]
They also develop autoimmune arthritis when immunized with another cartilage
macromolecule, cartilage oligomeric matrix protein (COMP).[14] Moreover, they are
highly susceptible to various forms of adjuvant oil-induced arthritis (mycobacteria
[MTB-AIA], pristane-induced arthritis [PIA], avridine-induced arthritis, and IFA-
only induced arthritis [OIA]).[15–17] In addition, DA rats are highly susceptible to
experimental autoimmune encephalomyelitis (EAE) induced with whole spinal cord
homogenate, with myelin basic protein (MBP-EAE) or with myelin oligodendrocyte
glycoprotein (MOG-EAE),[18–22] and are susceptible to interphotoreceptor retinoid-
binding-protein (IRBP) -induced experimental autoimmune uveitis (EAU; R. Caspi,
unpublished data). Recent publications have provided evidence indicating that DA
rats are relatively unresponsive to antigen tolerization protocols and are uniquely

prone to develop pathogenic autoreactive T cells that produce proinflammatory cytokines, such as tumor necrosis factor alpha.[22]

LEW rats are also unusually susceptible to a wide variety of experimental models of autoimmune or autoinflammatory disease. For example, they are susceptible to arthritis in response to heterologous type II collagen in IFA, but they, interestingly, do not develop disease in response to homologous type II collagen in IFA, as do DA rats.[11] LEW rats are also extremely susceptible to MTB-AIA,[11] PIA,[23] avridine-induced arthritis, but again, unlike the DA rats, they are not susceptible to arthritis induction with the IFA alone (OIA).[15] In addition, LEW inbred rats are highly susceptible to various forms of bacterial-cell-wall-induced arthritis such as streptococcal-cell-wall arthritis (SCWA).[24] Moreover, they are highly susceptible to MBP-EAE[22,25] and to experimental autoimmune uveitis (EAU) induced with any one of several retinal antigens [e.g., retinal S antigen (SAG) or IRBP];[26] however, they develop only mild MOG-EAE.[20,27] In contrast to DA rats, LEW rats can be tolerized by vaccination with MBP, and rendered resistant to MBP-EAE.[22] Thus, although LEW rats are highly susceptible to a variety of experimentally induced autoimmune diseases, some aspects of the autoimmune disease susceptibility in LEW rats appear to be less marked than observed in DA rats.

In striking contrast to DA and LEW inbred rats, specific-pathogen-free F344 inbred rats are relatively resistant to most, but not all, forms of experimentally induced autoimmune disease. For example, specific-pathogen-free and conventionally housed F344 inbred rats are highly resistant to CIA, PIA, avridine-induced arthritis, OIA, SCWA, MBP-EAE, SAG-EAU, and IRBP-EAU.[11,12,17,24,26,28] They are also generally resistant or develop very mild MTB-AIA.[17] Interestingly, germ-free F344 rats are susceptible to MTB-AIA and SCWA, but disease resistance can be reestablished by recolonizing their GI tracts with a conventional microbial flora.[29–31] In contrast, the microbial flora does not suppress disease susceptibility in DA and LEW rats.[32] In other words, the gut flora appears to play a role in controlling autoimmune disease susceptibility in F344 rats, but DA and LEW rats are not similarly influenced.

BN rats have an unusual autoimmune disease susceptibility profile. They are highly resistant to CIA, avridine-induced arthritis, PIA, OIA, SAG-EAU, and MBP-EAE.[11,21,28] They are mildly susceptible to MTB-AIA and SCWA,[11] moderately susceptible to IRBP-EAU (R. Caspi, unpublished data), and, most interestingly, are highly susceptible to MOG-induced EAE.[27] The susceptibility to MOG-EAE but not MBP-EAE appears to reflect fundamental differences in pathogenetic mechanisms for these two EAE models. MBP-EAE in LEW and DA rats appears to be primarily a Th1-dependent disease in which antibodies are not involved. In contrast, MOG-EAE involves antibody-dependent effector pathways that are highly expressed in BN rats.[19,20,27] BN rats, in contrast to LEW rats, are also noted for their extreme susceptibility to mercury-chloride-induced autoimmune disease, which is characterized by arthritis, necrotizing vasculitis and glomerulonephritis, and high levels of the Th2 cytokine IL-4.[33] In other words, BN rats, in contrast to DA and LEW rats, appear to develop autoimmune disease pathology in the context of Th2 cytokines and pathogenic antibodies.[11]

SUSCEPTIBILITY TO DRUG ADDICTION
AND HPA AXIS ABNORMALITIES IN INBRED RATS

As in studies of autoimmune disease, inbred LEW and F344, and more recently, DA rats have been studied intensively in efforts to identify genetically determined traits related to addiction.[6,10,34,35] LEW rats have a higher preference, compared with F344 inbred rats, to self-administer or develop place preference for cocaine, morphine, ethanol, and nicotine.[36–40] In addition to these behavioral differences, drug-naive LEW and F344 rats exhibit many differences in brain biochemistry suspected to be relevant to addiction, particularly in mesolimbic dopamine pathways.[34,37,41–53] Similarly, in studies of morphine-induced-locomotor activation and sensitivity, DA, unlike F344, rats develop sensitization to a second morphine injection.[35] Drug-naive DA and F344 rats have also been compared for several brain proteins thought to be involved in susceptibility to addiction. DA rats show higher levels of tyrosine hydroxylase and glial fibrillary acidic protein, and lower levels of neurofilament proteins, in the ventral tegmental area.[35]

Corticosteroids clearly play an important role in regulating autoimmune disease expression,[1,3,4] and they also appear to be involved in regulating susceptibility to addiction.[54,55] For example, central administration of dexamethasone produces feedback inhibition of cocaine-induced corticosteroid production, and, notably, LEW rats are more sensitive to dexamethasone suppression of cocaine-induced corticosteroid production than are F344 rats.[54,55] In other words, corticosteroids appear to modulate sensitivity to drug addiction. Of relevance to these observations, both autoimmune-disease-prone and addiction-prone LEW and DA rats, in striking contrast to relatively resistant F344, BN, and most other inbred rat strains, show marked abnormalities in hypothalamic-pituitary-adrenal (HPA) axis function. For example, F344 and most other inbred rat strains, particularly females, display a marked rise in basal plasma corticosterone levels in the late light phase and early dark phase of the 24-h circadian cycle. In contrast, LEW and DA rats show minimal or no significant circadian variation in plasma corticosterone levels.[34,35,54,56–58] Moreover, most inbred rat strains, including F344 and BN, show marked increases in plasma corticosterone levels in response to a wide variety of stressful stimuli, but this response is profoundly blunted, depending on the intensity of the stimulus, in LEW rats; that is, dose-response relationships are shifted to the right.[57–68] Numerous biochemical studies of relevance to basal and stress-activated HPA axis function have been reported that compare autoimmune disease- and addiction-prone and -resistant rats, particularly LEW and F344. These studies further document multiple differences in these rat strains.[34,35,43,44,48,49,54,57,58,60,69] Thus, the available data support the notion that susceptibility to autoimmune diseases and drug addiction, as well as abnormalities in basal and stress-induced activation in HPA axis function, may share common mechanistic components. Since this hypothesis is based on studies in a limited number of inbred rat strains, it is certainly possible that the associations noted are coincidental. The possibility, however, clearly warrants additional investigation.

TABLE 1. Chromosomal locations of loci regulating autoimmune-disease-related phenotypes in crosses involving DA, LEW, F344, or BN inbred rats

Rat Chr. No.	Autoimmune regulatory locus	Phenotype regulated	Rat strains crossed, generation used for locus identification	Ref.
1	Cia2	Severity of CIA	DA × F344, F2	(12)
2	Cia7	Severity of CIA (homologous CII)	DA × ACI, F2	(13)
	Cia10	Suggestive locus for severity of CIA	DA × ACI, F2	(13)
	Pia	Suggestive locus for PIA-COMP day 35	DA × E3, F2	(72)
	Pia	Suggestive locus for PIA-COMP day 49	DA × E3, F2	(72)
	Eae	Suggestive locus of severity of EAE induced with spinal cord homogenate	DA × BN, F2	(21)
3	Cia11	Severity of CIA	DA × BN, F2	(71)
4	Cia3	Severity of CIA	DA × F344, F2	(12)
	Aia2	Severity of MTB-AIA	DA × F344, F2	(17)
	Aia3	Severity of MTB-AIA	DA × F344, F2	(17)
	Oia2	Incidence and severity of OIA	DA × LEW. 1Av1, F2	(78)
	Pia2	Onset of PIA	DA × E3, F2	(72)
	Pia5	Chronicity of PIA	DA × E3, F2	(72)
	Cia13	Severity of CIA	DA × BN, F2	(71)
	Scwia1	Suggestive locus for severity of SCW arthritis	LEW × F344, F2	(71)
	Eau2	Suggestive locus for susceptibility to IRBP-EAU	LEW × F344, F2	(26)
	Eae	IgG1, IgE antibody levels in MOG-EAE	DA × PVG.RT1a, F2	(21)
5	Pia	Suggestive locus for severity of PIA	DA × E3, F2	(72)
6	Pia3	Onset of PIA	DA × E3, F2	(72)
	Pia	Suggestive locus for number of affected paws on day 24 in PIA	DA × E3, F2	(72)

TABLE 1/continued.

Rat Chr. No.	Autoimmune regulatory locus	Phenotype regulated	Rat strains crossed, generation used for locus identification	Ref.
7	*Cia4*	Severity of CIA	DA × F344, F2	(12)
	Cia8	Severity of CIA	DA × F344, F2	(70)
	Eae	Suggestive locus of severity of EAE (spinal cord homogenate)	DA × BN, F2	(21)
8	*Cia6*	Suggestive locus for severity of CIA	DA × F344, F2	(12)
9	*Ciaa3*	Locus for antibody titer in CIA	DA × BN, F2	(71)
	Eae4	Incidence of EAE (spinal cord homogenate)	DA × BN, F2	(21)
10	*Cia5*	Severity of CIA	DA × F344, F2; DA x BN, F2	(12, 71)
	Ciaa2	Anti-type II collagen antibody titer	DA × F344, F2	(71)
	Oia3	Incidence and severity of OIA	DA × LEW.1Av1, F2	(78)
12	*Cia12*	Severity of CIA	DA × BN, F2	(71)
	Pia4	Severity and joint erosion in PIA	DA × E3, F2	(72)
	Eau3	Suggestive locus for susceptibility to IRBP-EAU	LEW × F344, F2	(26)
	Eae	Suggestive locus for EAE inflammation (spinal cord model)	DA × BN, F2	(21)
14	*Pia6*	Chronicity of PIA	DA × E3, F2	(72)
15	*Aia4*	Suggestive locus for severity of MTB-AIA	DA × F344, F2	(17)
19	*Cia14*	Suggestive locus for severity of CIA	DA × BN, F2	(71)
20	*Cia1/Ciaa1*	Severity of CIA/anti-type II collagen antibody titer	DA × F344, F2 DA × BN, F2	(12, 71)
	Aia1	Severity of MTB-AIA	DA × F344, F2	(17)
	Pia1	Chronicity of PIA		(72)
	Oia1	Susceptibility to OIA	DA × LEW.1Av1, F2	(78)
Y	*Cia9*	Severity of CIA (homologous rat CII)	DA × ACI, F2	(13)

GENETIC LINKAGE STUDIES INVOLVING
LEW, DA, F344, AND BN INBRED RATS

Genetic linkage studies provide a potentially incisive approach to investigate whether susceptibility to autoimmune diseases and drug addiction are mechanistically linked to abnormalities in basal and stress-activated HPA axis function. Identification of genomic loci containing regulatory genes in common to all of these traits would provide a strategy to delineate the underlying biochemical pathways that can causally link the traits. Our groups are conducting genetic linkage studies, focused on rat CIA, AIA, and EAU, in an effort to identify regulatory loci for these experimental autoimmune diseases. We have applied quantitative trait locus (QTL) analysis techniques to evaluate F2 intercrosses between autoimmune disease-prone (DA and LEW) and relatively resistant (F344 and BN) inbred rat strains (see TABLE 1). For CIA induced with heterologous bovine type II collagen, 11 quantitative trait loci (QTL), including the major MHC-related QTL (*Cia1*) and non-MHC QTL on chromosomes 1 (*Cia2*), 3 (*Cia11*), 4 (*Cia3* and *Cia13*), 7 (*Cia4* and *Cia8*), 8 (*Cia8**), 10 (*Cia5*), 12 (*Cia12*), and 19 (*Cia14**), control arthritis severity in the F2 progeny of DA × F344 rats and or DA × BN rats.[12,17,70,71] Only *Cia1* (Chr20) and *Cia5* (Chr10) are regulatory loci in both crosses. These studies indicate that the genetically determined regulation of CIA severity is polygenic and dependent upon the genetic background provided by the parental strains.

The genetic control of MTB-adjuvant-induced arthritis has also been evaluated in F2 progeny of DA × F344 rats (TABLE 1). At least four QTL regulate severity. The MHC-linked QTL, *Aia1*, is on chromosome 20, and two non-MHC QTL, *Aia2* and *Aia3*, are on chromosome 4.[17] *Aia1* overlaps with *Cia1*, and *Aia3* overlaps with *Cia3* supporting the view that AIA and CIA have pathogenetic mechanisms in common. Another locus, *Aia4**, is located on chromosome 15.

We have also evaluated crosses involving F2 progeny of LEW × F344 inbred rats in additional experimental autoimmune/inflammatory models (TABLE 1). Interestingly, a suggestive locus has been identified that regulates severity of streptococcal-cell-wall arthritis. This locus, *Scwa1**, maps to the same region of rat chromosome 4 that contains *Cia3* and *Aia3*.[71] Similarly, we identified a locus, which also maps to this region of chromosome 4, that regulates EAU. An additional regulatory locus for EAU was identified on Chr12.[26]

Of significant interest (TABLE 1), the genomic interval of rat chromosome 4 containing *Cia3, Aia3, Scwa1*, Eau2** also overlaps with susceptibility loci identified in other crosses: (1) a locus regulating chronicity in pristane-induced arthritis (PIA) in DA × E3 rats (*Pia5*),[72] (2) a QTL regulating severity in MOG-EAE in DA × PVG.RT1a rats,[18] (3) a locus regulating susceptibility to insulin-dependent diabetes (IDDM, *Iddm1*),[73,74] and /or thyroiditis[75] in BB-DP rats. The genomic interval containing *Aia2* also overlaps with loci regulating PIA (*Pia2*) in DA × E3 rats,[72] and IDDM (*Iddm4*) in BB × WF rats.[74]

An analysis of conserved chromosomal homology among rats, mice, and humans suggests that rat chromosome 4 segments that contain the regulatory loci for CIA, MTB-AIA, SCWA, IRBP-EAU, PIA, MOG-EAE, and IDDM in the rat contain candidate genes for several autoimmune/inflammatory diseases in mice and humans. These include CIA and IDDM in mice, and systemic lupus erythematosus, inflammatory bowel disease, asthma/atopy, multiple sclerosis, and RA in humans.[11,17,76] It remains to be determined if these homologous segments truly contain allelic variants regulating autoimmune/inflammatory disease susceptibility within and across species, but the observation that multiple regulatory loci appear to cluster is provocative.

It is unknown whether any of the regulatory loci that have been identified to date have regulatory effects on drug addiction or HPA axis function in rats. Interestingly, a QTL regulating alcoholism has also been identified, in a cross between Preferring (P) and Nonpreferring (NP) inbred rats, that colocalizes with the chromosome 4 loci that regulate autoimmune disease.[77] The investigators that identified the alcohol QTL locus have been particularly interested in the NPY gene that maps in the interval. To date, genomic variants of the NPY gene have not been identified (L. Carr, personal communication, and R. Wilder and E. Remmers, unpublished data). Almost certainly, the most incisive approach to address the hypothesis that common mechanisms underlie susceptibility to autoimmune disease and drug addiction, as well as HPA axis abnormalities, will require the development and analysis of congenic rats. A QTL-congenic strain has a relatively small region (10–25 centimorgans) of the genome from one strain (e.g., LEW or DA) introgressed onto the comparison strain (e.g., F344 or BN), or vice versa, through a successive series of backcrosses. For example, introgression of the genomic region of chromosome 4 containing *Cia3/ Aia3* from F344 rats onto the DA rats would result in a congenic, DA.F344(Chr4-*Cia3/Aia3*). The reverse procedure would result in a congenic, F344.DA(Chr4-*Cia3/ Aia3*). We currently are developing QTL-congenic strains of this type. Analysis of these strains for HPA axis function and addiction-related phenotypes, as well as autoimmune disease phenotypes, should generate data that either support or contradict a mechanistic link among these diverse phenotypes.

SUMMARY

The hypothesis addressed in this manuscript is intended to stimulate further discussion. Moreover, these concepts can be explored experimentally. There are clearly very interesting associations among inbred rats, particularly DA, LEW, F344, and BN, with regard to susceptibility to a variety of autoimmune diseases and addiction. Moreover, while the available data that the HPA axis and stress response play a role in regulating susceptibility are very compelling, they do not establish causal links. The genetic linkage data involving these inbred rat strains indicate that the underlying molecular regulatory mechanisms are very complex, and, thus, multiple strategies will be required to comprehensively investigate the interrelationships.

REFERENCES

1. WILDER, R.L. 1995. Neuroendocrine-immune system interactions and autoimmunity. Annu. Rev. Immunol. **13**: 307–338.

2. WILDER, R.L. 1996. Adrenal and gonadal steroid hormone deficiency in the pathogenesis of rheumatoid arthritis. J. Rheumatol. Suppl. **44**: 10–12.

3. WILDER, R.L. & I.J. ELENKOV. 1999. Hormonal regulation of tumor necrosis factor-alpha, interleukin-12 and interleukin-10 production by activated macrophages. A disease-modifying mechanism in rheumatoid arthritis and systemic lupus erythematosus? Ann. N.Y. Acad. Sci. **876:** 14–31.

4. WILDER, R.L. 1996. Hormones and autoimmunity: animal models of arthritis. Baillieres Clin. Rheumatol. **10:** 259–271.

5. NESTLER, E.J., M.T. BERHOW & E.S. BRODKIN. 1996. Molecular mechanisms of drug addiction: adaptations in signal transduction pathways. Mol. Psychiatry **1:** 190–199.

6. NESTLER, E.J. 1997. Molecular mechanisms of opiate and cocaine addiction. Curr. Opin. Neurobiol. **7:** 713–719.

7. NESTLER, E.J. & G.K. AGHAJANIAN. 1997. Molecular and cellular basis of addiction. Science **278:** 58–63.

8. KOOB, G.F. & M. LE MOAL. 1997. Drug abuse: hedonic homeostatic dysregulation. Science **278:** 52–58.

9. KOOB, G.F., P.P. SANNA & F.E. BLOOM. 1998. Neuroscience of addiction. Neuron **21:** 467–476.

10. KOOB, G.F. & E.J. NESTLER. 1997. The neurobiology of drug addiction. J. Neuropsychiatry Clin. Neurosci. **9:** 482–497.

11. WILDER, R.L., E.F. REMMERS, Y. KAWAHITO, P.S. GULKO, G.W. CANNON & M.M. GRIFFITHS. 1999. Genetic factors regulating experimental arthritis in mice and rats. *In* Genes and Genetics of Autoimmunity, Vol. 1, Current Directions in Autoimmunity, A.N. Theophilopoulos, Ed.: 121–165. Karger. Basel.

12. REMMERS, E.F., R.E. LONGMAN, Y. DU, A. O'HARE, G.W. CANNON, M.M. GRIFFITHS & R.L. WILDER. 1996. A genome scan localizes five non-MHC loci controlling collagen-induced arthritis in rats. Nat. Genet. **14:** 82–85.

13. GULKO, P.S., Y. KAWAHITO, E.F. REMMERS, V.R. REESE, J. WANG, S.V. DRACHEVA, L. GE, R.E. LONGMAN, J.S. SHEPARD, G.W. CANNON, A.D. SAWITZKE, R.L. WILDER & M.M. GRIFFITHS. 1998. Identification of a new non-major histocompatibility complex genetic locus on chromosome 2 that controls disease severity in collagen-induced arthritis in rats. Arthritis Rheum. **41:** 2122–2131.

14. CARLSEN, S., A. HANSSON, H. OLSSON, D. HEINEGARD & R. HOLMDAHL. 1998. Cartilage oligomeric matrix protein (COMP)-induced arthritis in rats. Clin. Exp. Immunol. **114:** 477–484.

15. KLEINAU, S., H. ERLANDSSON, R. HOLMDAHL & L. KLARESKOG. 1991. Adjuvant oils induce arthritis in the DA rat. Characterization of the disease and evidence for an immunological involvement. J. Autoimmun. **4:** 871–880.

16. VINGSBO, C., R. JONSSON & R. HOLMDAHL. 1995. Avridine-induced arthritis in rats; a T cell-dependent chronic disease influenced both by MHC genes and by non-MHC genes. Clin. Exp. Immunol. **99:** 359–363.

17. KAWAHITO, Y., G.W. CANNON, P.S. GULKO, E.F. REMMERS, R.E. LONGMAN, V.R. REESE, J. WANG, M.M. GRIFFITHS & R.L. WILDER. 1998. Localization of quantitative trait loci regulating adjuvant-induced arthritis in rats: evidence for genetic factors common to multiple autoimmune diseases. J. Immunol. **161:** 4411–4419.

18. DAHLMAN, I., J.C. LORENTZEN, K.L. DE GRAAF, A. STEFFERL, C. LININGTON, H. LUTHMAN & T. OLSSON. 1998. Quantitative trait loci disposing for both experimental arthritis and encephalomyelitis in the DA rat; impact on severity of myelin oligodendrocyte glycoprotein-induced experimental autoimmune encephalomyelitis and antibody isotype pattern. Eur. J. Immunol. **28:** 2188–2196.

19. STORCH, M.K., A. STEFFERL, U. BREHM, R. WEISSERT, E. WALLSTROM, M. KERSCHENSTEINER, T. OLSSON, C. LININGTON & H. LASSMANN. 1998. Autoimmunity to myelin oligodendrocyte glycoprotein in rats mimics the spectrum of multiple sclerosis pathology. Brain Pathol. **8:** 681–694.

20. WEISSERT, R., E. WALLSTROM, M.K. STORCH, A. STEFFERL, J. LORENTZEN, H. LASSMANN, C. LININGTON & T. OLSSON. 1998. MHC haplotype-dependent regulation of MOG-induced EAE in rats. J. Clin. Invest. **102:** 1265–1273.

21. DAHLMAN, I., L. JACOBSSON, A. GLASER, J.C. LORENTZEN, M. ANDERSSON, H. LUTHMAN & T. OLSSON. 1999. Genome-wide linkage analysis of chronic relapsing experimental autoimmune encephalomyelitis in the rat identifies a major susceptibility locus on chromosome 9. J. Immunol. **162:** 2581–2588.

22. LENZ, D.C., N.A. WOLF & R.H. SWANBORG. 1999. Strain variation in autoimmunity: attempted tolerization of DA rats results in the induction of experimental autoimmune encephalomyelitis. J. Immunol. **163:** 1763–1768.

23. VINGSBO, C., P. SAHLSTRAND, J.G. BRUN, R. JONSSON, T. SAXNE & R. HOLMDAHL. 1996. Pristane-induced arthritis in rats: a new model for rheumatoid arthritis with a chronic disease course influenced by both major histocompatibility complex and non-major histocompatibility complex genes. Am. J. Pathol. **149:** 1675–1683.

24. WILDER, R.L., G.B. CALANDRA, A.J. GARVIN , K.D. WRIGHT & C.T. HANSEN. 1982. Strain and sex variation in the susceptibility to streptococcal cell wall-induced polyarthritis in the rat. Arthritis Rheum. **25:** 1064–1072.

25. KIM, G., K. KOHYAMA, N. TANUMA, H. ARIMITO & Y. MATSUMOTO. 1998. Persistent expression of experimental autoimmune encephalomyelitis (EAE)-specific Vbeta8.2 TCR spectratype in the central nervous system of rats with chronic relapsing EAE. J. Immunol. **161:** 6993–6998.

26. SUN, S.H., P.B. SILVER, R.R. CASPI, Y. DU, C.C. CHAN, R.L. WILDER & E.F. REMMERS. 1999. Identification of genomic regions controlling experimental autoimmune uveoretinitis in rats. Int. Immunol. **11:** 529–534.

27. STEFFERL, A., U. BREHM, M. STORCH, D. LAMBRACHT-WASHINGTON, C. BOURQUIN, K. WONIGEIT, H. LASSMANN & C. LININGTON. 1999. Myelin oligodendrocyte glycoprotein induces experimental autoimmune encephalomyelitis in the "resistant" Brown Norway rat: disease susceptibility is determined by MHC and MHC-linked effects on the B cell response. J. Immunol. **163:** 40–49.

28. CASPI, R.R., C.C. CHAN, Y. FUJINO, S. ODDO, F. NAJAFIAN, S. BAHMANYAR, H. HEREMANS, R.L. WILDER & B. WIGGERT. 1992. Genetic factors in susceptibility and resistance to experimental autoimmune uveoretinitis. Curr. Eye Res. **11:** 81–86.

29. KOHASHI, O., Y. KOHASHI, T. TAKAHASHI, A. OZAWA & N. SHIGEMATSU. 1986. Suppressive effect of Escherichia coli on adjuvant-induced arthritis in germ-free rats. Arthritis Rheum. **29:** 547–553.

30. VAN DE LANGERIJT, A.G., P.L. VAN LENT, A.R. HERMUS, L.B. VAN DE PUTTE & W.B. VAN DEN BERG. 1993. Regulation of resistance against adjuvant arthritis in the Fisher rat. Clin. Exp. Immunol. **94:** 150–155.

31. VAN DEN BROEK, M.F., M.C. VAN BRUGGEN, J.P. KOOPMAN, M.P. HAZENBERG & W.B. VAN DEN BERG. 1992. Gut flora induces and maintains resistance against streptococcal cell wall-induced arthritis in F344 rats. Clin. Exp. Immunol. **88:** 313–317.

32. BJORK, J., S. KLEINAU, T. MIDVEDT, L. KLARESKOG & G. SMEDEGARD. 1994. Role of the bowel flora for development of immunity to hsp 65 and arthritis in three experimental models. Scand. J. Immunol. **406:** 548–652.

33. KIELY, P.D., S. THIRU & D.B. OLIVEIRA. 1995. Inflammatory polyarthritis induced by mercuric chloride in the Brown Norway rat. Lab. Invest. **73:** 284-293.

34. BRODKIN, E.S., W.A. CARLEZON, JR., C.N. HAILE, T.A. KOSTEN, G.R. HENINGER & E.J. NESTLER. 1998. Genetic analysis of behavioral, neuroendocrine, and biochemical parameters in inbred rodents: initial studies in Lewis and Fischer 344 rats and in A/J and C57BL/6J mice. Brain Res. **805:** 55–68.

35. BRODKIN, E.S., T.A. KOSTEN, C.N. HAILE, G.R. HENINGER, W.A. CARLEZON, JR., P. JATLOW, E.F. REMMERS, R.L. WILDER & E.J. NESTLER. 1999. Dark Agouti and Fischer 344 rats: differential behavioral responses to morphine and biochemical differences in the ventral tegmental area. Neuroscience **88:** 1307–1315.

36. SUZUKI, T., F.R. GEORGE & R.A. MEISCH. 1988. Differential establishment and maintenance of oral ethanol reinforced behavior in Lewis and Fischer 344 inbred rat strains. J. Pharmacol. Exp. Ther. **245:** 164–170.

37. KOSTEN, T.A., M.J. MISERENDINO, S. CHI & E.J. NESTLER. 1994. Fischer and Lewis rat strains show differential cocaine effects in conditioned place preference and behavioral sensitization but not in locomotor activity or conditioned taste aversion. J. Pharmacol. Exp. Ther. **269:** 137–144.

38. KOSTEN, T.A., M.J. MISERENDINO, C.N. HAILE, J.L. DECAPRIO, P.I. JATLOW & E.J. NESTLER. 1997. Acquisition and maintenance of intravenous cocaine self-administration in Lewis and Fischer inbred rat strains. Brain Res. **778:** 418–429.

39. HORAN, B., M. SMITH, E.L. GARDNER, M. LEPORE & C.R. ASHBY, JR. 1997. (–)-Nicotine produces conditioned place preference in Lewis, but not Fischer 344 rats. Synapse **26:** 93–94.

40. SUZUKI, T., Y. ISE, J. MAEDA & M. MISAWA. 1999. Mecamylamine-precipitated nicotine-withdrawal aversion in Lewis and Fischer 344 inbred rat strains. Eur. J. Pharmacol. **369:** 159-162.

41. BEITNER-JOHNSON, D., X. GUITART & E.J. NESTLER. 1991. Dopaminergic brain reward regions of Lewis and Fischer rats display different levels of tyrosine hydroxylase and other morphine- and cocaine-regulated phosphoproteins. Brain Res. **561:** 147-150.

42. GUITART, X., D. BEITNER-JOHNSON, D.W. MARBY, T.A. KOSTEN & E.J. NESTLER. 1992. Fischer and Lewis rat strains differ in basal levels of neurofilament proteins and their regulation by chronic morphine in the mesolimbic dopamine system. Synapse **12:** 242–253.

43. BURNET, P.W., I.N. MEFFORD, C.C. SMITH, P.W. GOLD & E.M. STERNBERG. 1992. Hippocampal 8-[3H]hydroxy-2-(di-n-propylamino) tetralin binding site densities, serotonin receptor (5-HT1A) messenger ribonucleic acid abundance, and serotonin levels parallel the activity of the hypothalamopituitary-adrenal axis in rat. J. Neurochem. **59:** 1062–1070.

44. GUITART, X., J.H. KOGAN, M. BERHOW, R.Z. TERWILLIGER, G.K. AGHAJANIAN & E.J. NESTLER. 1993. Lewis and Fischer rat strains display differences in biochemical, electrophysiological and behavioral parameters: studies in the nucleus accumbens and locus coeruleus of drug naive and morphine-treated animals. Brain Res. **611:** 7–17.

45. CAMP, D.M., K.E. BROWMAN & T.E. ROBINSON. 1994. The effects of methamphetamine and cocaine on motor behavior and extracellular dopamine in the ventral striatum of Lewis versus Fischer 344 rats. Brain Res. **668:** 180–193.

46. NYLANDER, I., M. VLASKOVSKA & L. TERENIUS. 1995. Brain dynorphin and enkephalin systems in Fischer and Lewis rats: effects of morphine tolerance and withdrawal. Brain Res. **683:** 25–35.

47. CHAOULOFF, F., A. KULIKOV, A. SARRIEAU, N. CASTANON & P. MORMEDE. 1995. Male Fischer 344 and Lewis rats display differences in locomotor reactivity, but not in anxiety-related behaviours: relationship with the hippocampal serotonergic system. Brain Res. **693:** 169–178.

48. BURNET, P.W., I.N. MEFFORD, C.C. SMITH, P.W. GOLD & E.M. STERNBERG. 1996. Hippocampal 5-HT1A receptor binding site densities, 5-HT1A receptor messenger ribonucleic acid abundance and serotonin levels parallel the activity of the hypothalamo-pituitary-adrenal axis in rats. Behav. Brain Res. **73:** 365–368.

49. FLORES, G., G.K. WOOD, D. BARBEAU, R. QUIRION & L.K. SRIVASTAVA. 1998. Lewis and Fischer rats: a comparison of dopamine transporter and receptors levels. Brain Res. **814:** 34–40.

50. MINABE, Y., E.L. GARDNER & C.R. ASHBY, JR. 1998. Differential effects of chronic haloperidol administration on midbrain dopamine neurons in Sprague-Dawley, Fischer 344, and Lewis rats: an in vivo electrophysiological study. Synapse **29:** 269–271.

51. WERME, M., P. THOREN, L. OLSON & S. BRENE. 1999. Addiction-prone Lewis but not Fischer rats develop compulsive running that coincides with downregulation of nerve growth factor inducible-B and neuron-derived orphan receptor 1. J. Neurosci. **19:** 6169–6174.

52. MARTIN, S., J. MANZANARES, J. CORCHERO, C. GARCIA-LECUMBERRI, J.A. CRESPO, J.A. FUENTES & E. AMBROSIO. 1999. Differential basal proenkephalin gene expression in dorsal striatum and nucleus accumbens, and vulnerability to morphine self-administration in Fischer 344 and Lewis rats. Brain Res. **821:** 350–355.

53. LINDLEY, S.E., T.G. BENGOECHEA, D.L. WONG & A.F. SCHATZBERG. 1999. Strain differences in mesotelencephalic dopaminergic neuronal regulation between Fischer 344 and Lewis rats. Brain Res. **832:** 152–158.

54. ORTIZ, J., J.L. DECAPRIO, T.A. KOSTEN & E.J. NESTLER. 1995. Strain-selective effects of corticosterone on locomotor sensitization to cocaine and on levels of tyrosine hydroxylase and glucocorticoid receptor in the ventral tegmental area. Neuroscience **67:** 383–397.

55. SIMAR, M.R., D. SAPHIER & N.E. GOEDERS. 1997. Dexamethasone suppression of the effects of cocaine on adrenocortical secretion in Lewis and Fischer rats. Psychoneuroendocrinology **22:** 141–153.

56. GRIFFIN, A.C. & C.C. WHITACRE. 1991. Sex and strain differences in the circadian rhythm fluctuation of endocrine and immune function in the rat: implications for rodent models of autoimmune disease. J. Neuroimmunol. **35:** 53–64.

57. DHABHAR, F.S., B.S. MCEWEN & R.L. SPENCER. 1993. Stress response, adrenal steroid receptor levels and corticosteroid-binding globulin levels—a comparison between Sprague-Dawley, Fischer 344 and Lewis rats. Brain Res. **616:** 89–98.

58. OITZL, M.S., A.D. VAN HAARST, W. SUTANTO & E.R. DE KLOET. 1995. Corticosterone, brain mineralocorticoid receptors (MRs) and the activity of the hypothalamic-pituitary-adrenal (HPA) axis: the Lewis rat as an example of increased central MR capacity and a hyporesponsive HPA axis. Psychoneuroendocrinology **20:** 655–675.

59. STERNBERG, E.M., J.M. HILL, G.P. CHROUSOS, T. KAMILARIS, S.J. LISTWAK, P.W. GOLD & R.L. WILDER. 1989. Inflammatory mediator-induced hypothalamic-pituitary-adrenal axis activation is defective in streptococcal cell wall arthritis-susceptible Lewis rats. Proc. Natl. Acad. Sci. USA **86:** 2374–2378.

60. STERNBERG, E.M., W.S.D. YOUNG, R. BERNARDINI, A.E. CALOGERO, G.P. CHROUSOS, P.W. GOLD & R.L. WILDER. 1989. A central nervous system defect in biosynthesis of corticotropin-releasing hormone is associated with susceptibility to streptococcal cell wall-induced arthritis in Lewis rats. Proc. Natl. Acad. Sci. USA **86:** 4771–4775.

61. GLOWA, J.R., M.A. GEYER, P.W. GOLD & E.M. STERNBERG. 1992. Differential startle amplitude and corticosterone response in rats. Neuroendocrinology. **56:** 719–723.

62. STERNBERG, E.M., J.R. GLOWA, M.A. SMITH, A.E. CALOGERO, S.J. LISTWAK, S. AKSENTIJEVICH, G.P. CHROUSOS, R.L. WILDER & P.W. GOLD. 1992. Corticotropin releasing hormone related behavioral and neuroendocrine responses to stress in Lewis and Fischer rats. Brain Res. **570:** 54–60.

63. GLOWA, J.R., E.M. STERNBERG & P.W. GOLD. 1992. Differential behavioral response in LEW/N and F344/N rats: effects of corticotropin releasing hormone. Prog. Neuropsychopharmacol. Biol. Psychiatry **16:** 549–560.

64. ARMARIO, A., A. GAVALDA & J. MARTI. 1995. Comparison of the behavioural and endocrine response to forced swimming stress in five inbred strains of rats. Psychoneuroendocrinology **20:** 879–890.

65. VACCARINO, A.L. & L.C. COURET, JR. 1995. Relationship between hypothalamic-pituitary-adrenal activity and blockade of tolerance to morphine analgesia by pain: a strain comparison. Pain. **63:** 385–389.

66. GOMEZ, F., A. LAHMAME, E.R. DE KLOET & A. ARMARIO. 1996. Hypothalamic-pituitary-adrenal response to chronic stress in five inbred rat strains: differential responses are mainly located at the adrenocortical level. Neuroendocrinology **63:** 327–337.

67. MARTI, J. & A. ARMARIO. 1996. Forced swimming behavior is not related to the corticosterone levels achieved in the test: a study with four inbred rat strains. Physiol. Behav. **59:** 369–373.

68. GROTA, L.J., T. BIENEN & D.L. FELTEN. 1997. Corticosterone responses of adult Lewis and Fischer rats. J. Neuroimmunol. **74:** 95–101.

69. OPP, M.R. 1997. Rat strain differences suggest a role for corticotropin-releasing hormone in modulating sleep. Physiol. Behav. **63:** 67–74.

70. DRACHEVA, S.V., E.F. REMMERS, P.S. GULKO, Y. KAWAHITO, R.E. LONGMAN, V.R. REESE, G.W. CANNON, M.M. GRIFFITHS & R.L. WILDER. 1999. Identification of a new quantitative trait locus on chromosome 7 controlling disease severity of collagen-induced arthritis in rats. Immunogenetics **49:** 787–791.

71. WILDER, R.L., M.M. GRIFFITHS, E.F. REMMERS, G.W. CANNON, R.R. CASPI, Y. KAWAHITO, P.S. GULKO, R.E. LONGMAN, S.V. DRACHEVA, Y. DU, S.H. SUN, J. WANG, J.S. SHEPARD, B. JOE, L. GE, S. CHEN, L. CHANG, J. HOFFMAN, P.B. SILVER & V.R. REESE. 1999. Localization in rats of genetic loci regulating susceptibility to experimental erosive arthritis and related autoimmune diseases. Transplant. Proc. **31:** 1585–1588.

72. VINGSBO-LUNDBERG, C., N. NORDQUIST, P. OLOFSSON, M. SUNDVALL, T. SAXNE, U. PETTERSSON & R. HOLMDAHL. 1998. Genetic control of arthritis onset, severity and chronicity in a model for rheumatoid arthritis in rats. **Nat. Genet. 20:** 401–404.

73. JACOB, H.J., A. PETTERSSON, D. WILSON, Y. MAO, A. LERNMARK & E.S. LANDER. 1992. Genetic dissection of autoimmune type I diabetes in the BB rat. Nat. Genet. **2:** 56–60.

74. MARTIN, A.M., E.P. BLANKENHORN, M.N. MAXSON, M. ZHAO, J. LEIF, J.P. MORDES & D.L. GREINER. 1999. Non-major histocompatibility complex-linked diabetes susceptibility loci on chromosomes 4 and 13 in a backcross of the DP-BB/Wor rat to the WF rat. Diabetes **48:** 50–58.

75. PETTERSSON, A., D. WILSON, T. DANIELS, S. TOBIN, H.J. JACOB, E.S. LANDER & A. LERNMARK. 1995. Thyroiditis in the BB rat is associated with lymphopenia but occurs independently of diabetes. J. Autoimmun. **8:** 493–505.

76. GRIFFITHS, M.M., J.A. ENCINAS, E.F. REMMERS, V.K. KUCHROO & R.L. WILDER. 1999. Mapping autoimmune genes. Curr. Opin. Immunol. **11:** 689–700.

77. CARR, L.G., T. FOROUD, P. BICE, T. GOBBETT, J. IVASHINA, H. EDENBERG, L. LUMENG & T.K. LI. 1998. A quantitative trait locus for alcohol consumption in selectively bred rat lines. Alcohol Clin. Exp. Res. **22:** 884–887.

78. LORENTZEN, J.C., A. GLASER, L. JACOBSSON, J. GALLI, H. FAKHRAI-RAD, L. KLARESKOG & L.H. 1998. Identification of rat susceptibility loci for adjuvant-oil-induced arthritis. Proc. Natl. Acad. Sci. USA **95:** 6383–6387.

Neuroendocrine Manifestations in Sjögren's Syndrome

Relation to the Neurobiology of Stress

ELIZABETH O. JOHNSON[a,c] AND HARALAMPOS M. MOUTSOPOULOS[b]

[a]*Department of Anatomy, School of Medicine,*
University of Ioannina, Ioannina, Greece

[b]*Department of Pathophysiology, Medical School,*
National University of Athens, Athens, Greece

ABSTRACT: Evidence suggests that autoimmune rheumatic diseases are associated with neuroendocrine dysfunction. Sjögren's syndrome (SS) is proposed as an ideal model to study perturbations in the neuroimmune axis, since patients tend to be medication free and studies are not confounded by the effects of chronic immunosuppressive therapy. The functional integrity of the adrenal, gonadal, and thyroid axes was assessed in SS. Pituitary function of the HPA axis was evaluated directly by determining the ACTH released during oCRH stimulation, while adrenal function was assessed indirectly by endogenous ACTH released during oCRH stimulation. Low basal activity of the HPA axis was associated with pituitary hyporesponsiveness to exogenous CRH, as well as hyporesponsiveness of the adrenal glands to endogenous ACTH. These findings are compatible with a central deficiency of the adrenal axis. An overall attenuated and delayed LH and FSH response to LHRH stimulation was also indicative of central dysfunction of the gonadal axis in SS. SS patients demonstrated elevated basal TSH levels and evidence of mild hypothyroidism. Basal prolactin concentrations were also elevated in SS, and both TSH and PRL showed relatively increased responses to TRH stimulation. The data suggest a central deficiency in all three neuroendocrine axes: adrenal, gonadal, and thyroid. It is not clear if any one system plays a primary role in the expression of the disease. Rather, it is likely that the net effect involves the synergistic and antagonistic effects of multiple hormones. Taken together, adrenal and gonadal steroid hormone deficiency, plus elevated PRL levels, probably greatly affect immune function in SS patients.

INTRODUCTION

Cellular and molecular biological techniques have demonstrated that immune and inflammatory processes bidirectionally communicate with the central nervous system (CNS). A body of evidence now suggests that disruptions of this communication may be associated with susceptibility to or severity of autoimmune/inflammatory disease.[1] One working hypothesis is that a relationship between autoimmunity and

[c]Address for correspondence: Elizabeth O. Johnson, Ph.D., Assistant Professor of Anatomy, Department of Anatomy, School of Medicine, University of Ioannina, Ioannina 45 110, Greece. Voice: +30-651-97 584; fax: +30-651-67 860.

stress-related brain disorders is rooted in common defects where neuroendocrine factors involved in the stress response may play a critical role.[2] In addition to the stress axis, there is considerable evidence indicating that sex and thyroid hormones play an important role in the neuroendocrine–immune regulatory network.

Sjögren's syndrome (SS) is a chronic autoimmune disorder characterized by diminished lacrimal and salivary gland secretion.[3] The glandular insufficiency is secondary to lymphocytic and plasma cell infiltration, and the disease may extend to a systemic process. Patients with SS often express a wide range of constitutional symptoms, such as fatigue, arthralgias, myalgias, or low-grade fever, as well as neuropsychiatric features, including anxiety, depressed mood, and personality structure disorders.[4] SS patients are proposed as an ideal model to study the immune-neuroendocrine feedback network, since they tend not to be treated with corticosteroids or other hormonal steroids that may confound findings.

HYPOTHALAMIC–PITUITARY–ADRENAL AXIS IN SS

Psychological stress has long been thought to be associated with the onset and exacerbations of autoimmune/inflammatory disease with recent developments indicating that a relationship between stress-related brain disorders and autoimmunity may be rooted in a common neuroendocrine defect.[1] Both behavioral and inflammatory stresses, through stimulation of the CRH neuron, activate a final common neuroendocrine pathway: the hypothalamic–pituitary–adrenal (HPA) axis.[2] This suggests that an association between stress and development of inflammatory disease may be related to alterations of this common pathway, or to defects in its intricate feedback loops.

The immunosuppressive effects of glucocorticoids represent a major effector end point of the immune-system–CNS counterregulatory loop.[2] The feedback effects of corticosteroids in regulating the immune system suggest several possible mechanisms by which clinical hyperimmune or autoimmune states can arise.[5] For example, inadequate corticosterone production during an invasive challenge could hypothetically induce self-injurious inflammation or immune disease. Alternatively, abnormally rapid or altered catabolism of corticosteroids, resulting in functionally deficient levels of anti-inflammatory glucocorticoids, or any form of glucocorticoid resistance at the cellular level could contribute to a predisposition to autoimmune disease.

We have assessed the functional integrity of the HPA axis in SS patients as assessed by ovine (o) CRH stimulation in the evening in medication-free, female patients with sequential SS during the prefollicular phase.[6] Adrenocorticotropin (ACTH) response to oCRH was used as a direct measure of corticotrophic function, and the plasma cortisol response to ACTH released during oCRH stimulation was an indirect measure of adrenal function. SS was associated with low basal activity of the HPA axis expressed by low basal concentrations of ACTH and cortisol in the early evening. Mean basal plasma ACTH levels in pSS (5.1 ± 0.5 pg/mL) were significantly lower than in normal controls (11.4 ± 1.5 pg/mL; $p \leq 0.05$). SS patients also demonstrated significantly lower basal cortisol concentrations compared to normal volunteers in the evening (2.4 ± 0.6 vs 5.9 ± 1.2 µ/mL, respectively; $p \leq 0.05$).

The evening is when the HPA axis is normally at its nadir, making the reduction in the mean evening basal ACTH and cortisol concentrations in patients with SS more notable. It is noteworthy that a subgroup of patients with SS and FM had basal ACTH and cortisol concentrations that were similar to controls, but intermediate to those measured in patients with either FM or SS alone (see TABLE 1).

The functional integrity and reactivity of the HPA axis was evaluated by the responses of ACTH and cortisol concentrations at various time points. Although patients with SS responded to the oCRH injection with an increase in ACTH and cortisol, the low basal activity was associated with both pituitary and adrenal hyporesponsiveness (see FIGURE 1). Compared to healthy controls, the basal hypocortisolism in patients with SS was associated with a significant attenuation of the ACTH response to the evening administration of oCRH, with peak ACTH responses of 61.5 ± 3.8 pg/mL versus 46.2 ± 5.4 pg/mL ($p \leq 0.05$), respectively. This reduction in pituitary corticotropin responsiveness, in turn, was associated with a blunted response in the cortisol time course; specifically, the peak cortisol response in patients vs. controls was of 15.7 ± 1.6 vs. 19.6 ± 0.7 μ/mL ($p \leq 0.05$). In a small number of patients tested, we have found that the tendency for basal hypercortisolism in FM is associated with an exaggerated ACTH response to intravenous oCRH. Patients with SS and FM, on the other hand, demonstrate HPA-axis activity intermediate to either SS or FM alone (unpublished findings).

These results indicate a relative hyporesponsiveness of the adrenal glands to the endogenous ACTH released during the course of stimulation by CRH. Such a hyporesponsivenss of the adrenal cortex could occur in the context of a primary adrenal insufficiency in which the adrenals are themselves intrinsically hypoactive, or in the context of insufficient stimulation of the adrenal cortex by ACTH, owing either to a pituitary or hypothalamic defect. Since we observed a blunted rather than exaggerated ACTH response to oCRH despite basal hypocortisolism, the data strongly suggest that either the pituitary or hypothalamus was hyporesponsive. In this regard, the blunted ACTH response to CRH in the presence of hypocortisolism probably resuls from insufficient priming of the pituitary corticotrophs by endogenous CRH.

IL-1 is a potent mediator of the stress response.[7] In addition to its effects on immune cells, IL-1 directly stimulates the HPA axis to release corticosteroids, which

TABLE 1. oCRH stimulation test in primary and secondary Sjögren's patients compared to normal controls and fibromyalgia patients

	pSS	SS + FM	FM	Control
Plasma ACTH (pg/mL)				
Basal	5.1 ± 0.5*	11.8 ± 6.3	16.2 ± 6.2	11.4 ± 1.5
Peak	46.2 ± 5.4*	56.9 ± 15.9	74.0 ± 14.3	61.5 ± 3.8
Delta	41.1 ± 5.7	45.1 ± 10.4	57.7 ± 11.8	50.1 ± 4.1
Plasma cortisol (mg/mL)				
Basal	2.4 ± 0.6*	6.8 ± 2.5	7.9 ± 1.7	5.9 ± 1.2
Peak	15.7 ± 1.6*	20.0 ± 4.4	22.0 ± 1.3	19.6 ± 0.7
Delta	13.3 ± 1.4	13.2 ± 3.0	14.0 ± 2.6	13.7 ± 1.3

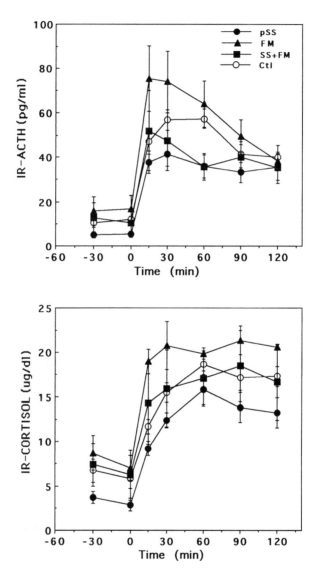

FIGURE 1. ACTH (**upper panel**) and cortisol (**lower panel**) responses to oCRH stimulation test in patients with pSS, SS + FM, and FM compared to normal controls. oCRH was injected at time zero, and the data are shown as mean ± SEM. Compared to normal controls, the basal hypocortisolism in patients with pSS was associated with a significant attenuation of the ACTH response to the evening administration of oCRH. On the other hand, the tendency for basal hypercortisolism in patients with FM was associated with an exaggerated ACTH and cortisol response. A subgroup of patients with SS and FM demonstrated an ACTH and cortisol response that tended to be similar to normal controls and intermediate to pSS and FM patients (*$p \leq 0.05$).

in turn feedback to inhibit macrophage release of IL-1,[29] thereby preventing the overproduction of proinflammatory mediators that otherwise could generate deleterious self-injury, including autoimmune disease. Additional evidence that the neuroimmune axis is impaired in SS patients is the significantly higher levels of plasma IL-1 (SS vs. control: 214.0 ± 59.5 vs. 17.4 ± 11.7 pg/mL; $p \leq 0.005$; unpublished findings) in the context of significant basal hypocorisolism and HPA-axis hyporesponsiveness. We have found that IL-6 is also significantly elevated in SS patients (SS vs. control: 3.4 ± 0.2 vs. 1.9 ± 0.5; $p \leq 0.05$; unpublished findings); other authors also have reported elevated IL-6 levels in serum and saliva of pSS.[8] In contrast, we have found that TNFα plasma levels tend to be only slightly elevated compared to normal controls.

HYPOTHALAMIC–PITUITARY–GONADAL AXIS IN SS

Although there are multiple observations that implicate the gonadal axis in the immunopathogenesis of autoimmune-inflammatory diseases, the most widely appreciated evidence is that these diseases affect females more than males.[5,9] Overall a profound female predilection exists for a variety of model autoimmune diseases in animals and several human autoimmune diseases. SS is characterized by striking age–sex disparities. The incidence in women increases steadily from the age of menarche to its maximal incidence around menopause. pSS in men is an uncommon condition, with variable clinical and serological differences from women.[10] Disease onset appears to occur more commonly at an older age in men than in women. In one study, 26% of the men compared to 12% of the women had an elderly onset of SS (after the age of 70 years).[11] These observations suggest that androgens may play an important immunosuppressive role in SS.

Estrogens, testosterone, and progesterone have varying immunologic effects, which partially explains the enhanced immune response in females and their predisposition to develop autoimmune disease. In animal models, castration of males or administration of estrogen has been shown to enhance development and severity of the disease, while administration of testosterone suppresses the disease. In humans, sex differences in the expression of autoimmune disease may also be related to the immunosuppresive effects of testosterone.[5,9,12] We have found that female patients with pSS tend to have low plasma testosterone levels (0.25 ± 0.04 ng/mL compared to the normal range 0.3–1.4 ng/mL; unpublished findings from a limited number of patients). Despite these apparently low circulating levels of testosterone in female SS patients, estradiol, testosterone, and dihydrotestosterone have been reported positive in the epithelial cells of the duct labial minor salivary glands using the peroxidase-antiperoxidase method, while only estradiol was positive in normal controls.[12] Moreover, androgens have been found to regulate both lacrimal and meibomian gland function, indicating that androgen deficiency may be a critical etiologic factor in the pathogenesis of dry eye syndromes.[14] These findings suggest that the epethilial cells in SS may serve as target cells for sex hormone modulation of cellular function. In turn, the role of corticosteroid regulation of this interaction is implicated by our findings that glucocorticoids regulate sex hormone receptors.[15]

Recent findings from our team identify the CRISP-3 gene in the minor salivary glands of female SS patients.[16] The human CRISP-3 gene is expressed in the testis, and the male salivary glands under the control of androgens and several androgen-responsive elements have been detected in the sequence. The identification of the CRISP-3 gene in female SS patients in addition to the characterization of this gene as a possible early activated gene, may reflect a molecular communication link between the immune and the neuroendocrine systems.

We have assessed the hypothalamic–pituitary–gonadal (HPG) axis in female patients with pSS using the GnRH Stimulation Test during the follicular phase. We found an overall attenuated and delayed LH responses to GnRH stimulation in SS patients compared to normal controls (unpublished findings). Similarly, FSH responses to GnRH were also delayed and often failed to demonstrate a peak at 30 minutes. Although the GnRH stimulation test is not considered a diagnostic test, delayed LH and FSH responsiveness has been associated with central dysfunction. This interpretation is compatible with the findings of central HPA-axis dysfunction. Despite this apparent central dysfunction of the HPG axis, fertility, parity, and sexual activity are apparently not affected. [17]

SS tends to present in women during the fourth and fifth decades of life, a period when sex hormone levels are in fluctuation at the onset of menarche. This peak incidence suggests that estrogen and/or progesterone deficiency may play a role in the disease, although investigations of the effects of estrogens in SS have produced contradictory results. Estrogens were reported to induce the development of autoantibodies and promote salivary gland lymphoid infiltrates in normal mice, suggesting that estrogens accelerate the development of autoimmune salivary gland lesions.[18] Mice prenatally exposed to estrogens had accelerated development of autoimmune salivary-gland lesions similar to those observed in SS patients, suggesting that estrogen may have an effect during prenatal development of immune function. In contrast, in a murine model for autoimmune exocrinopathy of SS, estrogen deficiency was associated with dysfunction of regulatory T cells, resulting in severe destructive autoimmune lesions in the salivary and lacrimal glands. These lesions recovered with estrogen administration, suggesting that dysfunction of regulatory T cells by the estrogen deficiency may play a crucial role in the acceleration of the organ-specific autoimmune lesions. In two autoimmune disease animal models, near-physiological doses of ethinylestradiol did not significantly affect disease symptoms.[19] On the other hand, supraphysiological doses produced indications of toxicity (wasting of organs and tissues), as well as autoimmunity (increased proteinuria and mononuclear cell infiltrations). Taken together, the findings suggest that mortality by estrogens may be due to toxic rather than accelerated autoimmunity, and that the sexual dichotomy in autoimmunity reflects the protective effects of androgens. In summary, however, the available evidence does not allow a definitive response to the question of a primary versus secondary role of sex hormone perturbations in SS.

HYPOTHALAMIC–PITUITARY–THYROID AXIS IN SS

Hypoactivity of the adrenal axis in SS was associated with elevated basal TSH concentrations and evidence of mild hypothyroidism. This is intriguing in light of our data showing that clinical and experimentally induced hypothyroidism is associated with a hypothalamic CRH deficiency, thus further supporting our view of a central adrenal deficiency in SS patients. [20]

The role of thyroid hormone in HPA axis dysfunction and in the pathogenesis of autoimmune/inflammatory disorders is not known, but there appears to be an epidemiological association between thyroid dysfunction and both neuropsychiatric and autoimmune/inflammatory diseases. Prolactin (PRL), a lactotropic polypeptide hormone, is now recognized as a growth factor for lymphocytes and accelerates T-cell-dependent immune responses.[21] A number of reports have shown that PRL is an immune-stimulating hormone that is capable of stimulating organ-specific inflammatory disease in humans.[22] In this regard, hyperprolactinemia has been associated with the active phase of SLE and autoimmune thyroiditis in humans. Similarly, in experimental animals, PRL has been implicated in stimulating a number of immune-mediated diseases that affect specific organs or joints.

Autoimmune thyroiditis (chronic thyroidistis) is the most frequent organ-specific autoimmune disease recognized in both pSS and sSS patients.[23] On the other hand, about one-third of the patients with autoimmune thyroid disease have been found to have SS features, perhaps indicating that the two diseases may be related pathogenetically.[24] About one-half of Sjögren's patients have subclinical thyroid disease,[25] with a greater incidence of serological and functional thyroid abnormalities in pSS compared to sSS. We have reported evidence of altered thyroid function as assessed by basal TSH levels and the thyrotropin-releasing hormone stimulation test in SS.[6] SS patients had significantly higher basal plasma TSH concentrations compared to controls (1.3 ± 0.2 vs. 0.9 ± 0.05 µIU/mL, respectively; $p \leq 0.05$) (see FIGURE 2). In addition, SS patients had a slightly higher TSH and PRL response to TRH stimulation compared to controls (see FIGURE 3). In this regard, it should be noted that patients with mild degrees of hypothyroidism, may show elevated serum TSH

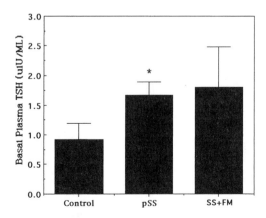

FIGURE 2. Basal plasma TSH concentrations in pSS patients and a subgroup of patients with SS + FM compared to normal controls. *Bars* represent group mean ± SEM. Basal plasma TSH levels were significantly elevated in pSS patients compared to normal controls.

concentrations with an exaggerated TSH response to TRH with normal levels of T3 and T4.

We searched for an autoimmune basis of thyroid insufficiency in our study by evaluating the sera for antithyroid antiboidies.[6] No patient was positive for antibodies to TSH receptor; however, about half of the patients were positive for antithyroid

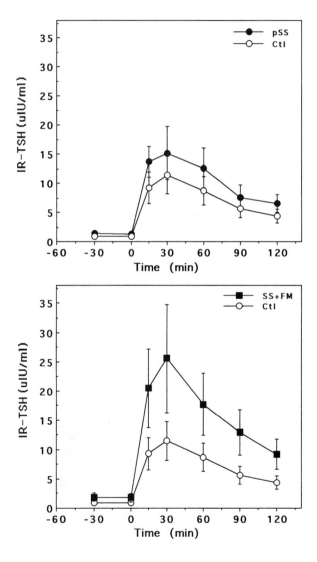

FIGURE 3. TSH response to TRH stimulation test in patients with pSS (**upper panel**) and patients with SS + FM (**lower panel**). TRH was injected at time 0 min, and the data are shown as mean ± SEM. Both patient groups demonstrated a somewhat exaggerated TSH response to TRH stimulation (*$p \leq 0.05$).

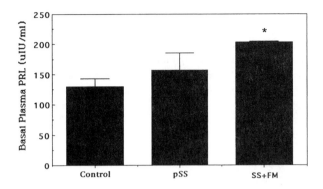

FIGURE 4. Basal plasma concentrations of prolactin in pSS patients and patients with SS + FM compared to normal controls. *Bars* represent group mean ± SEM.

antibodies, either to thyroid peroxidase or to thyroglobulin. Patients with autoimmune thyroid disease commonly develop antibodies to thyroid antigens. When interpreting thyroid hormone parameters, it should be noted that low titers of antithyroid antibodies may be found in patients with a wide variety of thyroid disorders and also in apparently asymptomatic patients who have no evidence of thyroid disease.

PRL is known to exert profound proinflammatory effects.[26] SS patients demonstrate PRL levels that were relatively elevated compared to controls (150 ± 25 vs. 140 ± 10, μIU/dL)[6] (see FIGURE 4). These patients also had a tendency for an exaggerated PRL response to TRH stimulation. In addition, patients with sSS (SS-FM) also had significantly increased basal PRL levels and a prolonged exaggerated response to TRH administration, while FM patients did not demonstrate an exaggerated PRL response (unpublished findings). Compatible with our own findings, others have reported that patients with pSS have moderately increased levels of serum PRL.[27] The authors report that this was particularly evident in patients diagnosed at a young age with active disease. It is interesting to note that in this study serum PRL was correlated to internal organ disease.[27] In association with a deficient HPA response, PRL may be a mechanism that contributes to the etiopathogenesis of human autoimmune disease. PRL secretion in SS appears excessive and dysregulated when the HPA-axis defect is taken into account. Thus, it can be hypothesized that there is a proinflammatory bias in patients with SS.

BEHAVIORAL AND PSYCHIATRIC PROFILE IN SS

A detailed study of psychiatric dysfunction in pSS showed that 25 out 40 patients exhibited various psychiatric abnormalities, the most common of which were affective disturbances.[4] The authors note that the symptoms expressed by their patient population closely fulfilled the criteria for "atypical depression" rather than those of a major depressive episode. In our study, we found that the majority of women with

SS experienced a stressful life event six months to two years before the onset of their symptoms.[6] These events, including death or major illness of a loved one, or the like, were considered by the patients to be highly significant. Patients expressed feelings of anxiety, fatigue, irritability, and impaired sleep quality.

Because perturbations of neurohormones and neurotransmitters that make up the central stress response are associated with behavioral disorders, perturbations of the normal immune-system–CNS interaction may also be associated with changes in behavior. Perturbations in the CRH system in humans have been clearly associated with depressive symptoms.[28,29] In contrast to the arousal seen in melancholic depression, atypical depression represents an excessive counterregulation of the generalized stress response, featuring lethargy, apathy, and passivity. This syndrome also occurs during various diseases including Cushing's disease, hypothyroidism, chronic fatigue syndrome, and RA.[7] Studies that examined the activity of the HPA axis in patients with seasonal affective disorder reported a delayed and significantly blunted ACTH response to exogenous CRH in the setting of low–normal cortisol levels suggest.[28–30] The attenuated ACTH response despite the hypocortisolism suggests that either the pituitary or hypothalamus was hyporesponsive.

Patients with SS demonstrate behavioral traits, including easy fatigability, lethargy, and mood disorders, which are similar in nature to those expressed in patients with atypical depression, chronic fatigue syndrome, among others. Furthermore, these disorders have also been associated with HPA-axis hypoactivity. Specifically, central adrenal insufficiency has been proposed in atypical depression,[31] seasonal affective disorder (SAD),[30] postoperative Cushing's syndrome,[31] and hypothyroidism.[20] Demetrac and colleagues[32] suggested that the lethargy and fatigue in patients with chronic fatigue syndrome also appeared to occur in the context of a hypofunctioning CRH system. The blunted ACTH response to CRH stimulation in the context of hypocortisolism observed, was hypothesized to reflect insufficiently primed pituitary corticotrophs. It is noteworthy that in one study, an unusually large cohort (16%) of chronic fatigue syndrome patients with complaints of severe, dominating, chronic fatigue, were detected to also have SS.[33]

Taken together, the clinical relevance of our data is not yet clear, although the data suggest that patients with SS often show signs of the atypical form of major depression. Whether the clinical picture of SS and possibly other forms of autoimmune disease in humans represents a confluence of immunological and behavioral deficits, both attributable to a relative deficiency in CRH responsiveness, remains to be determined.

In summary, female SS patients indicated a central deficiency in all three neuroendocrine axes: adrenal, gonadal, and thyroid. At present, it is not clear if any one system plays a primary role in the expression of the disease. Rather, it is likely that the net effect involves the synergistic and antagonistic effects of multiple hormones, making the specific effects of individual hormones difficult to discern. Taken together, adrenal and gonadal steroid hormone deficiency, plus elevated PRL levels, probably greatly facilitate cellular immunity in SS patients.

REFERENCES

1. JOHNSON, E.O. & H.M. MOUTSOPOULOS. 1992 Neuroimmunological axis and rheumatic diseases (editorial). Eur. J. Clin. Invest. **22:** 2–5.

2. JOHNSON, E.O., T.C. KAMILARIS, G.P. CHROUSOS & P.W. GOLD. 1992. Mechanisms of stress: a dynamic overview of hormonal and behavioral homeostasis. Neurosci. Biobehav. Rev. **16:** 115–130.
3. TALAL, N., H.M. MOUTSOPOULOS & S.S. KASSAN, Eds. 1987. Sjögren's Syndrome: Clinical and Immunological Aspects. Springer Verlag. Berlin.
4. MALINOW, K.L., R. MOLINA & B. GORDON *et al.* 1985. Neuropsychiatric dysfunction in primary Sjögren's syndrome. Ann. Intern. Med. **103:** 344–349.
5. WILDER, R.L. & E.M. STERNBERG. 1990. Neuroendocrine hormonal factors in rheumatoid arthritis and related conditions. Curr. Opin. Rheumatol. **2:** 436–440.
6. JOHNSON, E.O., P. VLACHOYIANNOPOULOS & F.N. SKOPOULI *et al.* 1998. Hypofunction of the stres axis in Sjögren's syndrome. J. Rheumatol. **25:** 1508–1514.
7. STERNBERG, E.M., G.P. CHROUSOS, R.L. WILDER & P.W. GOLD. 1992. The stress response and the regulation of inflammatory disease. Ann. Intern. Med. **177:** 854–866.
8. GRISIUS, M.M., D.K. BERMUDEZ & P.C. FOX. 1997. Salivary and serum Interleukin 6 in primary Sjögren's syndrome. J. Rheumatol. **24:** 1089–1091.
9. WILDER, R.L. 1996. Adrenal and gonadal steroid hormone deficiency in the pathogenesis of rheumatoid arthritis. J. Rheumatol. Suppl. **44:** 10–12.
10. ANAYA, J.M., G.T. LIU & E. D'SOUZA *et al.* 1995. Primary Sjögren's syndrome in men. Ann. Rheum. Dis. **54:** 748–751.
11. GARCIA-CARRASCO, M., R. CERVERA & J. ROSAS *et al.* 1999. Primary Sjögren's syndrome in the elderly: clinical and immunological characteristics. Lupus **8:** 20–23.
12. CARLSTEN, H., R. HOLMDALH & A. TARKOWSKI *et al.* 1989. Oestradiol- and testosterone-mediated effects on the immune system in normal and autoimmune mice are genetically linked and inherited as dominant traits. Immunology **68:** 209.
13. KUMAGAMI, H. & T. ONITSUKA. 1993. Estradiol and testosterone in minor salivary glands of Sjögren's syndrome. Auris Nasus Larynx **20:** 137–143.
14. SULLIVAN, D.A., L.A. WICKHAM & E.M. ROCHA *et al.* 1999. Androgens and dry eye in Sjögren's syndrome. Ann. N.Y. Acad. Sci. **876:** 312–324.
15. RABIN, D.S., E.O. JOHNSON & D.D. BRANDON *et al.* 1990. Glucocorticoids inhibit estradiol-mediated uterine growth: possible role of the uterine estradiol receptor. Biol. Reprod. **42:** 74–80.
16. TAPINOS, N.I., M. POLIHRONIS & H.M. MOUTSOPOULOS. 1999. Identification and characterization of CRISP-3 mRNA transcripts in minor salivary glands from patients with Sjögren's syndrome. *In* Programs and Abstracts of the VII International Symposijm on Sjögren's Syndrome, Venice, Italy.
17. SKOPOULI, F.N., S. PAPANIKOLAOU & K. MALAMOU-MITSI *et al.* 1994. Obstetric and gynaecological profile in patients with primary Sjögren's syndrome. Ann. Rheum. Dis. **53:** 569–573.
18. AHMED, S.A., T.B. AUFDEMORTE & J.R. CHEN, JR. *et al.* 1989. Estrogen induces the development of autoantibodies and promotes salivary gland lymphoid infiltrates in normal mice. J. Autoimmun. **2:** 543–552.
19. VERHEUL, H.A., M. VERVELD, S. HOEFAKKER & A.H. SCHUURS. 1995. Effects of ethinylestradiol on the course of spontaneous autoimmune disease in NZB/W and NOD mice. Immunopharmacol. Immunotoxicol. **17:** 163–180.
20. KAMILARIS, T.C., C.R. DEBOLD & E.O. JOHNSON *et al.* 1991. Effects of short and long duration hypothyroidsim and hyperthyroidism on the plasma adrenocorticotropin and corticosterone responses to ovine corticotropin-releasing hormone in rats. Endocrinology **128:** 2567–2576.
21. JARA, L.J., C. LAVALLE & A. FRAGA *et al.* 1991. Prolactin, immunoregulation and autoimmune diseases. Semin. Arthritis Rheum. **20:** 273–284.
22. WALKER, S.E., S.H. ALLEN & R.W. MCMURRAY. 1993. Prolactin and autoimmune disease. Trends Endocrinol. Metab. **4:** 147–151.
23. ICHIKAWA, Y. & R. FUKUDA. 1995. Clinical and pathological features of Sjögren's syndrome associated with autoimmune thyroid diseases. Nippon Rinsho. **53:** 2545–2550.

24. COLL, J., J. ANGLADA & S. TOMAS *et al.* 1997. High prevalence of subclinical Sjögren's syndrome features in patients with autoimmune thyroid disease. J. Rheumatol. **24:** 1719–1724.
25. KARSH, J., N. PAVLIDIS, B.D. WEINTRAUB & H.M. MOUTSOPOULOS. 1980. Thyroid disease in Sjögren's syndrome. Arthritis Rheum. **23:** 1326–1329.
26. CHIKANZA, I.C. & G.S. PANAYI. 1991. Hypothalamic-pituitary mediated modulation of immune function: prolactin as a neuroimmune peptide. Br. J. Rheumatol. **30:** 203–207.
27. HAGA, H.J. & T. RYGH. 1999. The prevalence of hyperprolactinemia in patients with primary Sjögren's syndrome. J. Rheumatol. **26:** 1291–1295.
28. GOLD, P.W., F.K. GOODWIN & G.P. CHROUSOS. 1988. Clinical and biochemical manifestations of depression: relation to the neurobiology of stress (1). N. Engl. J. Med. **319:** 384–393.
29. GOLD, P.W., F.K. GOODWIN & G.P. CHROUSOS. 1988. Clinical and biochemical manifestations of depression: relation to the neurobiology of stress (2). N. Engl. J. Med. **319:** 413–420.
30. VANDERPOOL, J., N. ROSENTHAL & G.P. CHROUSOS *et al.* 1991. Evidence for hypothalamic CRH deficiency in patients with seasonal affective disorder. J. Clin. Endocrinol. Metab. **72:** 1382–1387.
31. GOLD, P.W., D.L. LORIAUX & A. ROY *et al.* 1986. Responses to corticotropin-releasing hormone in the hypercortisolism of depression and Cushing's disease. N. Engl. J. Med. **314:** 1329–1335.
32. DEMITRACK, M.A., J.K. DALE & S.E. STRAUS *et al.* 1991. Evidence for impaired activation of the hypothalamic-pituitary-adrenal axis in patients with chronic fatigue syndrome. J. Clin. Endocrinol. Metab. **73:** 1224–1234.
33. CALABRESE, L.H., M.E. DAVIS & W.S. WILKE. 1994. Chronic fatigue syndrome and a disorder resembling Sjögren's syndrome: preliminary report. Clin. Infect. Dis. **18**(Suppl. 1): S28–S31.

Gonadotropin-Releasing Hormone and G Proteins: Potential Roles in Autoimmunity

J.D. JACOBSON

Section of Endocrinology, Children's Mercy Hospital, University of Missouri-Kansas City School of Medicine, Kansas City, Missouri 64108, USA

ABSTRACT: The hypothalamic homone gonadotropin-releasing hormone (GnRH) displays gender-specific actions. Pituitary responsiveness to GnRH is generally increased by estrogens and decreased by androgens. GnRH is now known to be produced by the immune system and to exert potent immunologic actions. Our central hypothesis is that gender differences in responsiveness to GnRH in the immune system play a pivotal role in the gender differences in immunity and autoimmunity. Studies in lupus-prone mice demonstrate that GnRH exacerbates murine lupus in a gender-specific fashion. Subsequent studies from our laboratory suggest that the gender differences in immunologic responsiveness to GnRH may relate to differences in the expression of the signal transducers through which GnRH acts, namely, the G proteins, Gs, and Gq/11. We have further demonstrated gender differences in second messengers for GnRH, IP3, and cAMF in immune cells. We have also demonstrated that GnRH agonist increases the quantities and/or activity of G proteins in immune cells in a gender-specific fashion. We speculate that gender differences in GnRH production and action, and in G protein expression play a role in a variety of autoimmune diseases that affect females predominantly.

INTRODUCTION

The gender differences in the immune system are well established. Perhaps the most clinically relevant difference between males and females is the markedly increased incidence of certain autoimmune diseases that occur in females. The gender differences have been attributed to differences between the sexes in androgens and estrogens.[1,2] However, the mechanisms by which gonadal steroids modulate the immune system remain elusive.

Investigators have long speculated that the immunomodulatory effects of androgens and estrogens may be mediated indirectly.[3] One of the best-characterized targets for feedback actions of gonadal steroids is the hypothalamic hormone gonadotropin-releasing hormone (GnRH). Rising estradiol levels are known to increase GnRH production at the level of the hypothalamus and GnRH action at the level of the pituitary.[4,5] Androgen exposure is known to decrease GnRH responsiveness at the level of the pituitary.[6,7] We speculate that gonadal steroids might exert similar effects on GnRH production and/or action at the level of the immune system (see FIGURE 1). GnRH itself has been shown to be immunostimulatory. Immune cells produce bioactive GnRH[8,9] and express receptors for GnRH.[10,11] Studies in rodents show that GnRH exerts stimulatory influences on expression of the interleukin-2 receptor, on B and T lymphocyte proliferation, and on serum IgG levels (see FIGURE 2).[12-16] Our

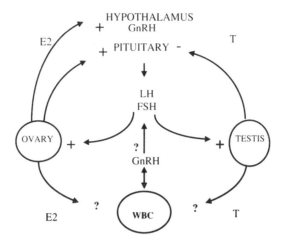

FIGURE 1. Rising estradiol, as seen in women during the reproductive years, leads to increased hypothalamic GnRH production and increased GnRH action at the level of the pituitary, evidenced by increased gonadotropin production. Androgens lead to a decrease in pituitary responsiveness to GnRH and a reduction in gonadotropin levels. Because immune cells produce GnRH and express GnRH receptor, we propose that androgens and estrogens affect production of and/or responsiveness to GnRH in the immune system in a similar manner.

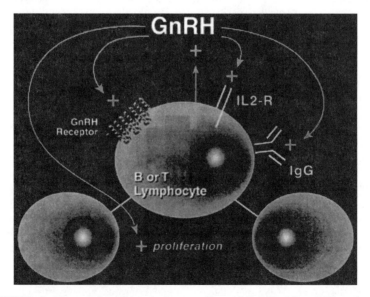

FIGURE 2. Diagram describing the known effects of GnRH on B and T lymphocytes. Immune cells from rats and humans produce immunoreactive and bioactive GnRH. Porcine and human immune cells express GnRH receptors. Acute treatment with GnRH increases expression of GnRH receptor mRNA in murine thymocytes.[29] Studies in mice and rats show that GnRH exerts stimulatory influences on expression of the interleukin-2 receptor, on B and T lymphocyte proliferation, and on serum IgG levels. (Modified from Jacobson et al.[36])

overall hypothesis is that gender differences in production and/or action of GnRH contribute to gender differences in immunity and/or autoimmunity.

We have previously demonstrated that administration of GnRH antagonists ameliorated murine lupus, as assessed by autoantibody levels, renal disease, and survival.[14] Effects of GnRH antagonists were similar in males and females and in intact and gonadectomized mice, demonstrating that the effects of GnRH antagonists were independent of gonadal steroids. We later demonstrated that, in contrast to the results observed with GnRH antagonists, GnRH agonists exerted sexually dimorphic actions. GnRH administration led to a worsening of disease, but this effect was restricted to females.[16]

We next hypothesized that the gender differences in immunological responsiveness to GnRH might relate to increased GnRH receptor expression in immune cells in females. We measured GnRH receptor mRNA and GnRH binding in lupus-prone mice after *in vivo* exposure to GnRH or vehicle. Vehicle-treated females expressed more GnRH receptor in immune cells than did vehicle-treated males. GnRH administration itself also yielded gender-specific results. Lymphoid cells from females demonstrated a marked reduction in expression of GnRH receptor mRNA and decreased GnRH binding after exposure to GnRH. GnRH administration exerted no effect on GnRH mRNA or binding in males.[16]

The above results led us to study postreceptor gender differences. Previous studies have shown that GnRH responsiveness in pituitary cells does not correlate with the expression of the GnRH receptor. Authors have suggested that postreceptor differences may explain these observations.[17–19] GnRH is known to exert its actions largely through two related G proteins, namely $G\alpha_q$ and $G\alpha_{11}$ (collectively termed $G\alpha_{q/11}$), at least at the pituitary level.[20] We hypothesized that the gender differences in responsiveness to GnRH might relate to gender differences in expression of these stimulatory G proteins in immune cells. We measured $G\alpha_{q/11}$ mRNA and protein in immune cells. Gender differences were confirmed, with females expressing more $G\alpha_{q/11}$ mRNA and protein than did males.[16]

MATERIALS AND METHODS

Mice. All experiments were carried out in accordance with the National Institutes of Health (NIH) Guide for the Care and Use of Laboratory Animals and with the University of Missouri-Kansas City Animal Care and Use Committee. Studies were done in male and female (SWR × NZB) F1 and (NZB × NZW) F1 hybrid mice and in DBA/2 mice, bred in our animal facilities or purchased from Jackson Labs (Bar Harbor, ME). Both lupus-prone models had been characterized to display gender differences in severity of disease, with females affected earlier and more severely than males. Anti-DNA antibody levels correlate directly with disease severity in both models of murine lupus.[21,22] In all experiments, gonadectomized mice were used in order to eliminate the variable of sex hormone production. Gonadectomized animals were randomized at 14 to 18 days of age to treatment with GnRH, GnRH antagonist, or vehicle.

Gonadectomy. Each male was castrated via a scrotal incision, and each female was ovariectomized via a dorsal incision between 14 and 18 days of age under pentobarbital anesthesia.

Injections. GnRH (native decapeptide) was purchased from Sigma Chemical Co. (St. Louis, MO). GnRH antagonist Antide (acetyl-β-[2-naphthyl]-D-Ala-D-*p*-chloro-phe-β-[3-pyridyl]-D-Ala-Ser-Nε-[nicotinoyl]-Lys-Nε-[nicotinoyl]-D-Lys-Leu-Nε-[Isopropyl]-Lys-Pro-D-Ala-NH2, was synthesized at the Salk Institute under contract numbers N01-HD-2-2824, N01-HD-0-2906, and N01-HD-2905 with NIH and were made available for these studies by the Contraceptive Development Branch, Center for Population Research, National Institute of Child Health and Human Development. Animals were injected subcutaneously in the nape of the neck six times weekly, with 100 μg of GnRH, Antide, or 100 μl of vehicle consisting of 0.9 N saline.

Sera. Sera were collected from blood obtained at six weeks by retroorbital puncture after isoflorane anesthesia.

Anti-DNA antibody levels. Anti-DNA antibody levels were measured by a previously described ELISA technique.[23] Sera for anti-DNA antibody measurements were stored at $-20°C$. All samples from each time point were run in the same assay in an effort to avoid interassay variability.

RNA purification. RNA was isolated by the technique of Chomczynski, using TRI Reagent (Molecular Research Center, Inc, Cincinnati, OH).[24]

Reverse transcription. RNA (5 μg) from each individual organ was transcribed into cDNA in a total volume of 50 μl using random hexamers to prime the reaction (Perkin Elmer-Cetus, Norwalk, CT), and mouse murine leukemia virus reverse transcriptase (BRL, Gaithersberg, MD). Control reaction tubes were identical except for the omission of reverse transcriptase in one set and RNA in another set.[25]

Primer design. We used the published sequences of the murine GnRH receptor mRNA[26] and the homologous genes $G\alpha_q$ and $G\alpha_{11}$ $(G\alpha_{q/11})$[27] to amplify GnRH receptor and $G\alpha_{q/11}$. We used commercially available primers for PCR of murine β-actin (Clontech, Palo Alto, CA). All primers also flank intron-exon boundaries.

Competitor construction. Because quantitation is important, we used a competitive PCR technique for all genes. We used mimic construction kits (Clontech, Palo Alto, CA) to construct nonhomologous DNA fragments flanked by the primer templates for all genes.[28]

Competitor titration. In order to optimize the working concentration of each competitor, a standard curve was produced by amplifying serial tenfold dilutions of competitor in the presence of a constant amount of cDNA from a positive sample. The log ratio of target:competitor was plotted against the log of femtomoles of competitor. We have previously demonstrated a linear relationship between the log ratio target:competitor versus log competitor using our primers for the GnRH receptor.[29] A linear relationship was observed between the log ratio of target to competitor for all genes. Competitor was added to the samples within these linear ranges.

Amplification efficiency. In order to establish that the target cDNA and competitor cDNA were amplified at similar efficiencies, the log density of target DNA and competitor cDNA were plotted against cycle number. For each gene, the linear portions of the two curves exhibited very similar slopes, indicating that the amplification efficiencies of the target DNA and competitor DNA were equal.

PCR. PCR was performed by mixing 5 μl of the cDNA with PCR buffer, 2 mM $MgCl_2$, 0.2 mM dNTP's, 2 ng/ml sense and antisense primers, five units of Taq polymerase, 2 μl of mimic and 27 μl of RNAase- and DNAase-free H_2O in a total volume of 50 μl. For radiolabeled PCR, 0.5 μl of ^{32}P-labeled dCTP was added to the reaction mixture. PCR cycles were programmed as follows: 95° for 2 min; 1 cycle: 95° for 1 min, 60° or 65° for 1 min; 35 cycles: 72° for 7 min; 1 cycle: 4° soak.[29]

Electrophoresis. Aliquots (5 μl) of PCR reactions were subjected to electrophoresis through 5% polyacrylamide gels or 1.8% agarose gels. Product and competitor bands were quantitated using densitometry (Molecular Dynamics, Sunnyvale, CA). Data are expressed as ratio of product:competitor, which correlates linearly with the amount of competitor added for each gene.

Statistics. Anti-DNA antibody measurements and densitometric data were analyzed using a one-way ANOVA and further analyzed by Student's *t* test. Graphic data are expressed as mean ± SEM of all experiments.

RESULTS

Anti-DNA antibody levels. Males and females responded to administration of GnRH antagonist with a reduction in anti-DNA antibody levels. Ovariectomized females responded to GnRH agonist with a significant increase in anti-DNA antibody levels compared to vehicle at 6 and 12 weeks of treatment ($p < 0.05$). In contrast to females, gonadectomized males did not display an increase in anti-DNA antibody levels with GnRH treatment at any point (see FIGURE 3).

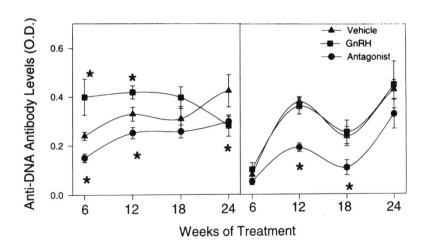

FIGURE 3. Anti-DNA antibody levels in gonadectomized (SWR X NZB) F1 hybrid female and male mice after various weeks of treatment with vehicle, GnRH, or GnRH antagonists. Serum anti-DNA antibody levels were measured by a standard ELISA technique as described in MATERIALS AND METHODS and expressed as optical density (O.D.). Results are mean ± SEM ($n = 14$–22). *Significantly different ($p < 0.05$) from vehicle. (Modified from Jacobson *et al.*[16])

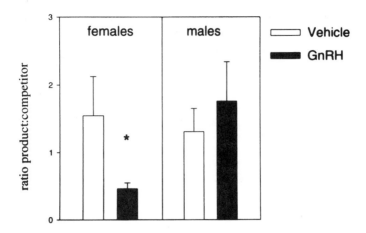

FIGURE 4. GnRH receptor mRNA expression in spleen in gonadectomized (NZB × NZW) F1 hybrid male and female mice treated with vehicle or GnRH for two weeks. Graphic representation of ratio target:competitor in spleen with various treatments from all experiments (n = 6–10/group). GnRH significantly decreases the splenic expression of the GnRH receptor mRNA compared to vehicle in the spleen in females (p = 0.004). Data were quantitated by densitometry and are expressed as mean ± SEM. (Modified from Jacobson *et al.*[16])

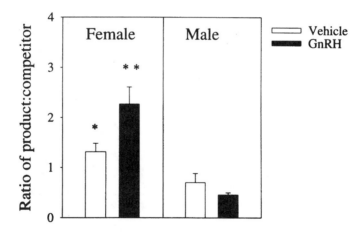

FIGURE 5. G$\alpha_{q/11}$mRNA expression in spleen in gonadectomized (NZB × NZW) F1 mice treated with vehicle or GnRH for two weeks. Graphic representation of ratio target:competitor for all experiments. *Vehicle-treated females express more G$\alpha_{q/11}$mRNA than do vehicle-treated males, in spite of prepubertal gonadectomy (p < 0.05). **GnRH administration further increases expression of G$\alpha_{q/11}$mRNA compared to vehicle in the spleen in females (p < 0.01), but not in males. Data were quantitated by densitometry and are expressed as mean ± SEM (n = 10–12/group). (Modified from Jacobson *et al.*[36])

Expression of GnRH receptor mRNA. The observation that GnRH exacerbated disease in females only led us to the initial speculation that females expressed more GnRH receptor than did males. We measured GnRH receptor mRNA by competitive RT-PCR after treatment with GnRH or vehicle. GnRH agonist treatment was associated with significantly decreased expression of the GnRH receptor compared to vehicle in spleen in females at the two-week time point ($p < 0.005$). GnRH agonist administration exerted no demonstrable effect on expression of the GnRH receptor in males (see FIGURE 4). Binding studies revealed similar results (data not shown).[16]

Expression of G protein mRNA. GnRH is known to work through G proteins, specifically through $G\alpha_{q/11}$. We measured $G\alpha_{q/11}$ mRNA by competitive RT-PCR after administration of GnRH or vehicle. Females expressed significantly more $G\alpha_{q/11}$ mRNA than did males ($p < 0.05$). GnRH agonist administration significantly increased expression of the $G\alpha_{q/11}$ compared to vehicle in spleen in females ($p < 0.01$). GnRH agonist administration exerted no demonstrable effect on expression of the $G\alpha_{q/11}$ mRNA in males (see FIGURE 5). Data were quantitated by densitometry and are expressed as mean $\pm$ SEM ($n = 6$ to 7 mice/group).

DISCUSSION

Much of the field of neuroimmunoendocrinology has focused on roles for CRH and prolactin in immunity and autoimmunity. The possibility that GnRH affects autoimmune disease represents an understudied area of immunoendocrine research. GnRH is immunostimulatory and has been demonstrated to exert effects on the expression of autoimmune disease.[14] We have recently demonstrated that some of the immune actions of GnRH appear to be gender-specific. GnRH exacerbates murine lupus *in vivo* in females only.[16] GnRH stimulates T lymphocyte proliferation *in vitro* in females only.[30] We speculate that GnRH plays a pivotal role in the gender differences in the immune system. We have investigated the mechanisms for the gender dimorphism in immune responsiveness to GnRH. We first examined the expression of the GnRH receptor on immune cells.[16] We found that females expressed more GnRH receptor than did males. Because GnRH is known to exert its actions through one or more guanine nucleotide binding signal transducing proteins,[31–33] we next sought gender differences in the expression of these G proteins. Previous studies in pituitary cultures in rats show that prior exposure to estradiol *in vivo* has a major stimulatory influence on gonadotropin production, a measure of GnRH responsiveness.[17] On the other hand, exposure to testosterone induces a long-lasting suppression in gonadotropin production and therefore GnRH responsiveness in pituitary cultures.[34] Our studies showed increased levels of the G protein in females compared to males, supporting the concept that gender differences in G proteins in immune cells may parallel gender differences in G proteins in pituitary cells. The literature contains few reports of gender differences in G protein expression. One study demonstrated increased cAMP generation in response to β–adrenergic stimulation in female compared to male rats. A stimulatory G protein related to $G\alpha_{q/11}$, namely, $G\alpha_s$, was increased with β–adrenergic exposure in female rats but not in male rats.[35] Beyond these studies, little is known about gender differences or hormonal control of G proteins. We have initiated studies to try to identify the factor or factors that lead to differential modulation of $G\alpha_{q/11}$ between males and females. Among the possibilities are GnRH itself, pulsatile GnRH, estrogen or cyclical estrogen, or androgens. We found that short-term administration of daily pulses of GnRH does in fact increase $G\alpha_{q/11}$ mRNA in thymus and spleen in females. It exerts no effects on G protein in mRNA in males. Immunoblot studies also suggest that daily pulses of GnRH increase $G\alpha_{q/11}$ protein expression in females but not in males.

Our observations are consistent with the possibility that gender differences in expression of certain G proteins contribute to gender differences in responsiveness to GnRH. We speculate that these gender differences contribute to the gender differences in the expression autoimmune disease.

On a broader scope, G proteins are the signal transducers for a variety of hormones, including CRH, LH, FSH, TSH, ADH, PTH, MSH, and melatonin. If gender differences in the ubiquitously expressed G proteins exist, they may play a role in a variety of other non–autoimmune diseases affecting females predominantly, including perhaps osteoporosis, precocious puberty, and McCune Albright syndrome.

ACKNOWLEDGMENTS

This study was supported by NIH grant 1R29AR43152 and by grants from the Philip S. Astrowe Trust, the Lupus Foundation of America, the Sarah Morrison Bequest, and Children's Mercy Research Vision.

REFERENCES

1. ANSAR AHMED, S., W. J. PENHALE & N. TALAL. 1985. Sex hormones, immune responses, and autoimmune diseases. Mechanisms of sex hormone action. Am. J. Pathol. **121:** 531–551.

2. NELSON, J.L. & A.D. STEINBERG. 1987. Sex steroids, autoimmunity, and autoimmune diseases. *In* Hormones and Immunity. I. Berczi & K. Kobazs, Eds.: 93–119. M.P. Press. Lancaster.

3. GRAFF, R.J., M.A. LAPPE & G.D. SNELL. 1969. The influence of the gonads and adrenal glands on the immune response to skin grafts. Transplantation **7:** 105–111.

4. QUINONES-JENAB, V., S. JENAB, S. OGAWA, T. FUNABASHI, G.D. WEESNER & D.W. PFAFF. 1996. Estrogen regulation of gonadotropin-releasing hormone receptor messenger RNA in female rat pituitary tissue. Brain Res. Mol. Brain Res. **38:** 243–250.

5. BAUER-DANTOIN, A.C., J. WEISS & J.L. JAMESON. 1995. Roles of estrogen, progesterone, and gonadotropin-releasing hormone (GnRH) in the control of pituitary GnRH receptor gene expression at the time of the preovulatory gonadotropin surges. Endocrinology **136:** 1014–1019.

6. MCARDLE, C.A., E. SCHOMERUS, I. GRONER & A. POCH. 1992. Estradiol regulates gonadotropin-releasing hormone receptor number, growth and inositol phosphate production in alpha T3-1 cells. Mol. Cell. Endocrinol. **87:** 95–103.

7. YASIN, M., A.C. DALKIN, D.J. HAISENLEDER, J.R. KERRIGAN & J.C. MARSHALL. 1995. Gonadotropin-releasing hormone (GnRH) pulse pattern regulates GnRH receptor gene expression: augmentation by estradiol. Endocrinology **136:** 1559–1564.

8. MAIER, C.C., B. MARCHETTI, R.D. LE BOEUF & J.E. BLALOCK. 1992. Thymocytes express a mRNA that is identical to hypothalamic luteinizing hormone-releasing hormone mRNA. Cell. Mol. Neurobiol. **12:** 447–454.

9. EMANUELE, N.V., M.A. EMANUELE, J. TENTLER, L. KIRSTEINS, N. AZAD & A.M. LAWRENCE. 1990. Rat spleen lymphocytes contain an immunoactive and bioactive luteinizing hormone-releasing hormone. Endocrinology **126**: 2482–2486.

10. WEESNER, G.D., B.A. BECKER & R.L. MATTERI. 1997. Expression of luteinizing hormone-releasing hormone and its receptor in porcine immune tissues. Life Sci. **61**: 1649–1649.

11. CHEN, H., E. JEUNG, M. STEPHENSON & P.C.K. LEUNG. 1999. Human peripheral blood mononuclear cells express gonadotropin-releasing hormone (GnRH),GnRH receptor, and interleukin-2 receptor γ-chain messenger ribonucleic acids that are regulated by GnRH *in vitro*. J. Clin. Endocrinol. Metab. **84**: 743–750.

12. MARCHETTI, B., V. GUARCELLO, M.C. MORALE, G. BARTOLONI, F. RAITI, G. PALUMBO, JR., Z. FARINELLA, S. CORDARO & U. SCAPAGNINI. 1989. Luteinizing hormone-releasing hormone (LHRH) agonist restoration of age-associated decline of thymus weight, thymic LHRH receptors, and thymocyte proliferative capacity. Endocrinology **125**: 1037–1045.

13. MORALE, M.C., N. BATTICANE, G. BARTOLONI, V. GUARCELLO, Z. FARINELLA, M.G. GALASSO & B. MARCHETTI. 1991. Blockade of central and peripheral luteinizing hormone-releasing hormone (LHRH) receptors in neonatal rats with a potent LHRH-antagonist inhibits the morphofunctional development of the thymus and maturation of the cell-mediated and humoral immune responses. Endocrinology **128**: 1073–1085.

14. JACOBSON, J.D., B.C. NISULA & A.D. STEINBERG. 1994. Modulation of the expression of murine lupus by gonadotropin-releasing hormone analogs. Endocrinology **134**: 2516–2523.

15. BATTICANE, N., M.C. MORALE, F. GALLO, Z. FARINELLA & B. MARCHETTI. 1991. Luteinizing hormone-releasing hormone signaling at the lymphocyte involves stimulation of interleukin-2 receptor expression. Endocrinology **129**: 277–286.

16. JACOBSON, J.D., M.A. ANSARI, M. KINEALY & V. MUTHUKRISHNAN. 1999. Gender-specific exacerbation of murine lupus by gonadotropin-releasing hormone: potential role of G alpha q/11. Endocrinology **140**: 3429–3437.

17. COLIN, I.M., A.C. BAUER-DANTOIN, S. SUNDARESAN, P. KOPP & J.L. JAMESON. 1996. Sexually dimorphic transcriptional responses to gonadotropin-releasing hormone require chronic *in vivo* exposure to estradiol. Endocrinology **137**: 2300-2307.

18. LAWS, S.C., J.C. WEBSTER & W.L. MILLER. 1990. Estradiol alters the effectiveness of gonadotropin-releasing hormone (GnRH) in ovine pituitary cultures: GnRH receptors versus responsiveness to GnRH. Endocrinology **127**: 381–386.

19. BALDWIN, D.M., G.A. BOURNE & J.C. MARSHALL. 1984. Pituitary LH responsiveness to GnRH *in vitro* as related to GnRH receptor number. Am. J. Physiol. **247**: E651–656.

20. STANISLAUS, D., J.H. PINTER, J.A. JANOVICK & P.M. CONN. 1998. Mechanisms mediating multiple physiological responses to gonadotropin-releasing hormone. Mol. Cell. Endocrinol. **144**: 1–10.

21. DATTA, S.K., N. MANNY, C. ANDRZEJEWSKI, J. ANDRE-SCHWARTZ & R.S. SCHWARTZ. 1978. Genetic studies of autoimmunity and retrovirus expression in crosses of New Zealand black mice I. Xenotropic virus. J. Exp. Med. **147**: 854–871.

22. MANNY, N., S.K. DATTA & R.S. SCHWARTZ. 1979. Synthesis of IgM by cells of NZB and SWR mice and their crosses. J. Immunol. **122**: 1220-1227.

23. KLINMAN, D.M. & A.D. STEINBERG. 1986. Proliferation of anti-DNA-producing NZB B cells in a non-autoimmune environment. J. Immunol. **137**: 69–75.

24. CHOMCZYNSKI, P. 1993. A reagent for the single-step simultaneous isolation of RNA, DNA and proteins from cell and tissue samples. Biotechniques **15**: 532–534, 536–537.

25. SAMBROOK, J., E.F. FRITSCH & T. MANIATIS, Eds. 1989. Molecular Cloning: A Laboratory Manual. Cold Spring Harbor Laboratory Press. New York.

26. TSUTSUMI, M., W. ZHOU, R.P. MILLAR, P.L. MELLON, J.L. ROBERTS, C.A. FLANAGAN, K. DONG, B. GILLO & S.C. SEALFON. 1992. Cloning and functional expression of a mouse gonadotropin-releasing hormone receptor. Mol. Endocrinol. **6**: 1163–1169.

27. STRATHMANN, M. & M.I. SIMON. 1990. G protein diversity: a distinct class of alpha subunits is present in vertebrates and invertebrates. Proc. Natl. Acad. Sci. USA **87:** 9113–9117.

28. LI, B., P.K. SEHAJPAL, A. KHANNA, H. VLASSARA, A. CERAMI, K.H. STENZEL & M. SUTHANTHIRAN. 1991. Differential regulation of transforming growth factor beta and interleukin 2 genes in human T cells: demonstration by usage of novel competitor DNA constructs in the quantitative polymerase chain reaction. J. Exp. Med. **174:** 1259-1262.

29. JACOBSON, J.D., L.J. CROFFORD, L. SUN & R.L. WILDER. 1998. Cyclical expression of GnRH and GnRH receptor mRNA in lymphoid organs. Neuroendocrinology **67:** 117–125.

30. JACOBSON, J.D., J.C. BAKER & L. SUN. 1996. Gender differences in immune responsiveness to gonadotropin-releasing hormone in mice. Pediatr. Res. **39:** 90A.

31. STANISLAUS, D., J.A. JANOVICK, T. JI, T.M. WILKIE, S. OFFERMANNS & P.M. CONN. 1998. Gonadotropin and gonadal steroid release in response to a gonadotropin-releasing hormone agonist in Gqalpha and G11alpha knockout mice. Endocrinology **139:** 2710–1717.

32. KUPHAL, D., J.A. JANOVICK, U.B. KAISER, W.W. CHIN & P.M. CONN. 1994. Stable transfection of GH3 cells with rat gonadotropin-releasing hormone receptor complementary deoxyribonucleic acid results in expression of a receptor coupled to cyclic adenosine $3',5'$-monophosphate-dependent prolactin release via a G-protein. Endocrinology **135:** 315–320.

33. JANOVICK, J. & P. CONN. 1994. Gonadotropin-releasing hormone (GnRH)-receptor coupling to inositol phosphate and prolactin production in GH3 cells stably transfected with rat GnRH receptor complementary deoxyribonucleic acid. Endocrinology **135:** 2214–2219.

34. FATTINGER, K.E., D. VEROTTA, H.C. PORCHET, A. MUNAFO, J.Y. LE COTONNEC & L.B. SHEINER. 1996. Modeling a bivariate control system: LH and testosterone response to the GnRH antagonist antide. Am. J. Physiol. **271:** E775–787.

35. YAGAMI, T., M. TOHKIN & T. MATSUBARA. 1994. The involvement of the stimulatory G protein in sexual dimorphism of beta-adrenergic receptor-mediated functions in rat liver. Biochim. Biophys. Acta **1222:** 257–264.

36. JACOBSON, J.D., M.A. ANSARI, M.E. MANSFIELD, C.P. MCARTHUR & L.T. CLEMENT. 1999. Gonadotropin-releasing hormone increases $CD4^+$ T-lymphocyte numbers in an animal model of immunodeficiency. J. Allergy Clin. Immunol. **104:** 653–658.

Neuroendocrine and Other Factors in the Regulation of Inflammation

Animal Models

MEHRNAZ JAFARIAN-TEHRANI AND ESTHER M. STERNBERG[a]

National Institute of Mental Health-CNE/NIH, 10 Center Drive,
Building 10-2D46, Bethesda, Maryland 20892-1284, USA

ABSTRACT: A variety of animal models have been used to study the role of neuroendocrine responses in various aspects of autoimmune/inflammatory disease. Complex models of autoimmune disease, such as inflammatory arthritis
in rats and thyroiditis in chickens, indicate a role for blunted HPA axis and
dysregulated sympathoneuronal responses in susceptibility to autoimmune
disease. A variety of approaches including pharmacological, surgical (ablation,
transplantation), genetic linkage and segregation studies have been used to
identify factors contributing to the phenotypes of susceptibility or resistance to
inflammatory/autoimmune disease. Innate inflammation, or the earliest nonspecific form of the inflammatory response, which is characterized by fluid
exudation and migration of immune cells to inflammatory sites, is a subtrait of
these forms of inflammatory disease. Genetic linkage and segregation studies
in inflammatory susceptible and resistant rat strains indicate that this subtrait
is multigenic and polygenic; that is, that multiple loci on multiple chromosomes, each with a weak effect, control this trait, and that there is a large environmental component to the variability of this trait. Such information derived
from animal studies can be used to target candidate genes for further study
and to inform the design of human studies.

A variety of approaches have been previously taken to define different aspects of
neural immune interactions. These include *in vitro* molecular and pharmacological
studies utilizing primary organ or cell cultures or cell lines, as well as *in vivo* studies.
In these studies, the particular immune molecule in question, such as a cytokine, is
added to cell culture or may be injected *in vivo* through various routes (e.g., intraperitoneal, intravenous), and a variety of neural or glial responses are measured. In *in
vivo* studies, response measures may include *in situ* expression of neuropeptides or
early genes, hormonal secretion, or behavioral responses. An added level of precision in analyzing these complex interactions in animal models is added by surgical
intervention, such as ablation, cutting or chemically deleting specific nerve pathways, or reconstituting specific brain regions through fetal tissue transplantation.
Such *in vivo* systems can also be manipulated further at the stimulus end if the question of interest involves the effects of stress on the system. Such studies now indicate
that exposures to stressful stimuli can variably affect immune responses and disease

[a]Address for correspondence: Esther M. Sternberg, M.D., Director, Integrative Neural-
Immune Program, NIMH/NIH, Bldg. 10 Rm. 2D-46, 10 Center Drive, MSC 1284,
Bethesda, MD 20892-1284.

outcome, depending on the timing, specific nature, duration of exposure of the stressor in relation to the immune outcome measured. In fundamental design, however, all these approaches constitute a blend between immunopharmacology and neuropharmacology—a sort of immunoneuropharmacological approach.

Taken together, this body of literature has shown that many molecular, hormonal, neuronal routes exist by which the immune system can activate the central nervous system and by which the central nervous system can affect immune responses and inflammatory or infectious disease outcome.[1] Such studies have indicated, for example, that cytokines can stimulate the hypothalamic-pituitary-adrenal axis and can activate the central nervous system via vagal nerve pathways[2,3]; that HPA axis responses, including corticosteroid responses, alter patterns of immune response; and that sympathetic nervous system responses affect inflammatory responses.[4,5] Such studies indicate that the HPA axis plays an important role in susceptibility and resistance to inflammatory and infectious disease,[6,7] with blunted HPA axis responses being associated with enhanced susceptibilty to inflammation[8–10] and excess HPA axis activity, such as in chronic stress conditions, associated with enhanced susceptibility to infection.[11,12] More precise control of various types of stressful stimuli has indicated that different neuroendocrine and neural pathways are activated in response to different stresses.[13,14] Furthermore, more precise analyses of outcome measures have shown that different patterns of immune responses are affected depending on the duration and type of stress involved.[15,16]

These types of studies have also shown that cytokines released by glial cells or by activated macrophages entering the central nervous system in the course of infection play an important role in neuronal cell death and survival.[17–20] They have shown that at different times after neuronal trauma immune cell activation and cytokines can play a role both in neural regeneration and in neurodegeneration.[21] These findings have important implications for potential new therapeutic agents, such as the endogenous interleukin-1 receptor antagonist (IL-1ra) for treatment of nerve trauma, neurodegeneration, and stroke. Conversely, such studies have shown that neural factors, such as noradrenergic innervation of the spleen, play a role in immunosuppression of aging,[22] opening up new avenues for therapeutic agents to enhance the immunosuppression of aging.

An additional level of analysis may be added by assessing genetic and developmental factors involved in pre-morbid animal susceptibility and resistance to inflammatory disease. Such studies[23–25] have shown that several regions of many chromosomes, containing many unknown genes, but also many known, potentially relevant, candidate genes, link to inflammatory/autoimmune disease expression. The number and chromosomal location of linkage regions that have been identified to be associated with inflammatory/autoimmune diseases are determined by the particular phenotype or trait under study, as well as by the parental inbred strains used to generate the crosses. The more complex the phenotype, the more linkage regions are associated with it. Thus, inflammatory arthritis is associated with linkage regions on more than 15 different chromosomes.[23] The number of linkage regions identified may be limited by using as an outcome measure a subtrait of the more complex disease in question.

Thus, in our linkage and segregation studies in inflammatory susceptible Lewis (LEW/N) and resistant Fischer (F344/N) rat strains, we used the quantitative trait of inflammatory response to carrageenan, a model for innate inflammatory response, as a subtrait.[25] Our previous studies had shown that this phenotype was modified by manipulations of the HPA axis, including intracerebroventricular transplantation of fetal hypothalamic tissue from inflammatory-resistant to inflammatory-susceptible rats.[26] Several findings emerged from the linkage studies that have relevance to the application of this approach to the study of neural-immune interactions. First, as in other such linkage and segregation studies, multiple chromosome regions linked to the inflammatory trait. Second, there was a large environmental component to the expression of this trait, with genotypic variance accounting for only approximately 35–40%. This is consistent with the literature indicating that susceptibility and resistance to inflammatory/autoimmune disease is multigenic and polygenic, that is, controlled by multiple genes each with weak effect, and has a large environmental component. Nonetheless, the main linkage region on rat chromosome 10 for the subtrait of innate inflammation was the same as one region that links with inflammatory arthritis in rats.[23,24] This region was also syntenic with a region on human chromosome 17 that links with these diseases in humans.[27] This is consistent with the findings of the literature that many molecular pathways contribute to overall susceptibility and resistance to inflammatory diseases, and that the overall likelihood of developing a given autoimmune disease is determined by the load of susceptibility and resistance genes that an individual inherits, and by the environmental factors to which that individual is exposed.

What do these sorts of studies tell us about neural-immune factors that might predispose the host to develop such illnesses? From a genetic point of view, such studies can point to new pathways that might play a role in pathogenesis of such illnesses. The presence of novel candidate genes within the linkage regions may suggest a role for molecules regulating neural-immune networks that might not have been previously considered. The caveat in such studies is that the presence of a likely candidate gene within a linkage region does not prove that it is the cause of disease. Many additional studies are necessary to determine whether mutations exist in such genes. If a mutation is found, it may or may not result in a functional alteration in activity of the protein it encodes. Even if a functional mutation is identified, the relevance of the mutated gene to the disease in question must be tested in vivo with pharmacologic or transgenic knock-out or knock-in animal models. If such animal models are not associated with development of disease expression, the mutated gene may still contribute to disease expression; however, more than one gene or environmental factor combined may be necessary for full disease expression.

Several candidate genes are present within the chromosome 10 inflammatory resistance linkage region in F344/N rats. Some of these play a role in HPA axis as well as immune regulation, including the corticotrophin-releasing hormone (CRH) receptor type 1, angiotensin-converting enzyme (ACE), and several transcription factors (STATs).[25] Our preliminary studies indicate that the CRH receptor coding region sequence does not differ in these strains. Current studies are ongoing to determine the functional relevance of a mutation in the *ACE* gene in F344/N rats.[28]

There is a debate among geneticists as to when it is appropriate to sequence and study potential candidate genes within large regions of chromosomes that are found to link to a given trait. Some feel that before such sequencing is tackled, it is more appropriate to narrow the linkage region by performing additional manipulations including fine mapping and production and evaluation of congenic animals.[24,29] On the other hand, if genes of obvious pathophysiological interest lie within a linkage region, such genes can be sequenced and studied simultaneously as further genetic studies are carried out.

The fact that multiple genes contribute to disease expression indicates that new approaches with the capacity to analyze expression of multiple genes simultaneously must be applied if we are to successfully identify interacting factors and pathways that contribute to complex disease. Such technologies exist and are currently being perfected. One powerful approach that can shed light on differences in expression of thousands simultaneously is expression microarrays.[30] In this technique, mRNA is extracted from selected sources and the corresponding labeled cDNA is probed to a glass slide or a filter microarray containing the PCR products of up to 8,000–10,000 ESTs or cDNA clones. The patterns of differences in expression of groups of genes may be analyzed using complex mathematics. This approach is a powerful method that will help define multiple genes and gene pathways which together contribute to disease expression.

The complexity of the results of such genetic studies reflects the complexity of factors which together contribute to disease expression. In addition to genes predisposing to disease, as well as the nature, load, and route of exposure to environmental triggers, other factors such as developmental factors, aging and social factors, such as crowding or isolation, may all contribute to variability in disease expression. The ability to control for genetic factors and identify regions of chromosomes, if not specific genes, which link to disease susceptibility, will make identification of these many environmental factors more feasible. As an example, in addition to differences in inflammatory susceptibility, HPA axis responsiveness and differences in behavioral responses to a variety of stressors, LEW/N and F344/N rats exhibit large differences in maternal behaviors. LEW/N dams retrieve all pups within 3 min after separation, while F344/N dams do not retrieve pups during the entire 15-min period of observation.[31] Such differences in maternal behavior could be related to stress responsiveness, and could contribute to later phenotypic differences in these strains.

Thus, in designing future studies to identify neural-immune factors in complex disease, a variety of approaches *in vivo* will be needed. These include immuno- and neuropharmacological approaches, surgical ablation and transplantation, genetic linkage and segregation studies, and microarray technology. Behavioral, developmental and social manipulations must be superimposed on such approaches, as well as manipulations of environmental triggers to which the host is exposed. It is only through studies carefully controlling for all these variables that the ways in which these many factors interact will begin to be elucidated.

REFERENCES

1. STERNBERG, E.M. 1997. Neural-immune interactions in health and disease. J. Clin. Invest. **100:** 2641–2647.
2. LAYE, S., R.M. BLUTHE, S. KENT, C. COMBE, C. MEDINA, P. PARNET, K. KELLEY & R. DANTZER. 1995. Subdiaphragmatic vagotomy blocks induction of IL-1 beta mRNA in mice brain in response to peripheral LPS. Am. J. Physiol. **268:** R1327–1331.

3. Maier, S.F., L.E. Goehler, M. Fleshner & L.R. Watkins. 1998. The role of the vagus nerve in cytokine-to-brain communication. Ann. N.Y. Acad. Sci. **840:** 289–300.

4. Green, P.G., J. Luo, P.H. Heller & J.D. Levine. 1993. Further substantiation of a significant role for the sympathetic nervous system in inflammation. Neuroscience **55:** 1037–1043.

5. Levine, J.D., S.J. Dardick, M.F. Roizen, C. Helms & A.I. Basbaum. 1986. Contribution of sensory afferents and sympathetic efferents to joint injury in experimental arthritis. J. Neurosci. **6:** 3423–3429.

6. Mason, D., I. MacPhee & F. Antoni. 1990. The role of the neuroendocrine system in determining genetic susceptibility to experimental allergic encephalomyelitis in the rat. Immunology **70:** 1–5.

7. Edwards, C.K.D., L.M. Yunger, R.M. Lorence, R. Dantzer & K.W. Kelley. 1991. The pituitary gland is required for protection against lethal effects of *Salmonella typhimurium.* Proc. Natl. Acad. Sci. USA **88:** 2274–2277.

8. Sternberg, E.M., J.M. Hill, G.P. Chrousos, T. Kamilaris, S.J. Listwak, P.W. Gold & R.L. Wilder. 1989. Inflammatory mediator-induced hypothalamic-pituitary-adrenal axis activation is defective in streptococcal cell wall arthritis-susceptible Lewis rats. Proc. Natl. Acad. Sci. USA **86:** 2374–2378.

9. Sternberg, E.M., W.S.D. Young, R. Bernardini, A.E. Calogero, G.P. Chrousos, P.W. Gold & R.L. Wilder. 1989. A central nervous system defect in biosynthesis of corticotropin- releasing hormone is associated with susceptibility to streptococcal cell wall-induced arthritis in Lewis rats. Proc. Natl. Acad. Sci. USA **86:** 4771–4775.

10. Wick, G., Y. Hu, S. Schwarz & G. Kroemer. 1993. Immunoendocrine communication via the hypothalamo-pituitary-adrenal axis in autoimmune diseases. Endocr. Rev. **14:** 539–563.

11. Kiecolt-Glaser, J.K., R. Glaser, S. Gravenstein, W.B. Malarkey & J. Sheridan. 1996. Chronic stress alters the immune response to influenza virus vaccine in older adults. Proc. Natl. Acad. Sci. USA **93:** 3043–3047.

12. Sheridan, J.F., C. Dobbs, J. Jung, X. Chu, A. Konstantinos, D. Padgett & R. Glaser. 1998. Stress-induced neuroendocrine modulation of viral pathogenesis and immunity. Ann. N. Y. Acad. Sci. **840:** 803–808.

13. Bluthe, R.M., B. Michaud, K.W. Kelley & R. Dantzer. 1996. Vagotomy blocks behavioural effects of interleukin-1 injected via the intraperitoneal route but not via other systemic routes. Neuroreport **7:** 2823–2827.

14. Licinio, J. & M.L. Wong. 1997. Pathways and mechanisms for cytokine signaling of the central nervous system. J. Clin. Invest. **100:** 2941–2947.

15. Dominguez-Gerpe, L. & I. Lefkovits. 1996. Lymphocyte protein synthesis: evidence that murine T cells are more affected by stress than B cells. Immunol. Lett. **52:** 109–123.

16. Millan, S., M.I. Gonzalez-Quijano, M. Giordano, L. Soto, A.I. Martin & A. Lopez-Calderon. 1996. Short and long restraint differentially affect humoral and cellular immune functions. Life Sci. **59:** 1431–1442.

17. Brenneman, D.E., M. Schultzberg, T. Bartfai & I. Gozes. 1992. Cytokine regulation of neuronal survival. J. Neurochem. **58:** 454–460.

18. Brenneman, D.E., S.W. Page, M. Schultzberg, F.S. Thomas, P. Zelazowski, P. Burnet, R. Avidor & E.M. Sternberg. 1993. A decomposition product of a contaminant implicated in L-tryptophan eosinophilia myalgia syndrome affects spinal cord neuronal cell death and survival through stereospecific, maturation and partly interleukin-1-dependent mechanisms. J. Pharmacol. Exp. Ther. **266:** 1029–1035.

19. Rothwell, N.J. & P.J. Strijbos. 1995. Cytokines in neurodegeneration and repair. Int. J. Dev. Neurosci. **13:** 179–185.

20. Pasinelli, P., D.R. Borchelt, M.K. Houseweart, D.W. Cleveland & R.H. Brown, Jr. 1998. Caspase-1 is activated in neural cells and tissue with amyotrophic lateral sclerosis-associated mutations in copper-zinc superoxide dismutase. Proc. Natl. Acad. Sci. USA **95:** 15763–15768. [Erratum appears in Proc. Natl. Acad. Sci. USA 1999 Mar 16; **96**(6): 3330].

21. LOTAN, M. & M. SCHWARTZ. 1994. Cross talk between the immune system and the nervous system in response to injury: implications for regeneration. FASEB J. **8:** 1026–1033.
22. FELTEN, S.Y., K.S. MADDEN, D.L. BELLINGER, B. KRUSZEWSKA, J.A. MOYNIHAN & D.L. FELTEN. 1998. The role of the sympathetic nervous system in the modulation of immune responses. Adv. Pharmacol. **42:** 583–587.
23. REMMERS, E.F., R.E. LONGMAN, Y. DU, A. O'HARE, G.W. CANNON, M.M. GRIFFITHS & R.L. WILDER. 1996. A genome scan localizes five non-MHC loci controlling collagen-induced arthritis in rats. Nat. Genet. **14:** 82–85.
24. LORENTZEN, J.C., A. GLASER, L. JACOBSSON, J. GALLI, H. FAKHRAI-RAD, L. KLARESKOG & H. LUTHMAN. 1998. Identification of rat susceptibility loci for adjuvant-oil-induced arthritis. Proc. Natl. Acad. Sci. USA **95:** 6383–6387.
25. LISTWAK, S., R.M. BARRIENTOS, G. KOIKE, S. GHOSH, M. GOMEZ, B. MISIEWICZ & E.M. STERNBERG. 1999. Identification of a novel inflammation-protective locus in the Fischer rat. Mamm. Genome **10:** 362–365.
26. MISIEWICZ, B., M. POLTORAK, R.B. RAYBOURNE, M. GOMEZ, S. LISTWAK & E.M. STERNBERG. 1997. Intracerebroventricular transplantation of embryonic neuronal tissue from inflammatory resistant into inflammatory susceptible rats suppresses specific components of inflammation. Exp. Neurol. **146:** 305–314.
27. BECKER, K.G., R.M. SIMON, J.E. BAILEY-WILSON, B. FREIDLIN, W.E. BIDDISON, H.F. MCFARLAND & J.M. TRENT. 1998. Clustering of non-major histocompatibility complex susceptibility candidate loci in human autoimmune diseases. Proc. Natl. Acad. Sci. USA **95:** 9979–9984.
28. JAFARIAN-TEHRANI, M., S. LISTWAK, R.M. BARRIENTOS, A. MICHAUD, P. CORVOL & E.M. STERNBERG. 2000. Characterization of a missense mutation in the angiotensin I-converting enzyme cDNA in exudative-inflammation resistant F344/N rats. **6**(4): 319–331
29. GROOT, P.C., C.J. MOEN, W. DIETRICH, J.P. STOYE, E.S. LANDER & P. DEMANT. 1992. The recombinant congenic strains for analysis of multigenic traits: genetic composition. FASEB J. **6:** 2826–2835.
30. DUGGAN, D.J., M. BITTNER, Y. CHEN, P. MELTZER & J.M. TRENT. 1999. Expression profiling using cDNA microarrays. Nat. Genet. **21:** 10–14.
31. GOMEZ, M.A., A.L. RILEY & E.M. STERNBERG. 1997. Maternal differences between Lewis and Fischer rat strains. 27th Annual Meeting of the Society for Neuroscience, New Orleans, LA. Abstr. 459.20.

Perturbations of Arginine Vasopressin Secretion during Inflammatory Stress

Pathophysiologic Implications

IAN C. CHIKANZA,[a,d] PETROS PETROU,[b] AND GEORGE CHROUSOS[c]

[a]*Bone & Joint Research Unit, St. Bartholomews & Royal London School of Medicine and Dentistry, New Science Building, Charterhouse Square, London EC1 6BQ, UK*

[b]*Rheumatology Clinic, Appolonion Hospital, Strovolos, Nicosia, Cyprus*

[c]*National Institute of Child Health & Human Development, Endocrinology Section, Bethesda, Maryland, USA*

ABSTRACT: Pro-inflammatory cytokines, such as interleukin-1β (IL-1β), interleukin-6 (IL-6), and tumor necrosis factor-α (TNFα), released from inflammatory foci, can activate the hypothalamus to produce corticotrophin-releasing hormone (CRH) and arginine vasopressin (AVP). These hypothalamic peptides in synergy increase ACTH production by the pituitary gland and hence corticosteroid (CS) secretion by the adrenal cortices. CS dampens inflammation. The pituitary also produces prolactin (PRL), which is pro-inflammatory, and macrophage inhibitory factor (MIF), which by counteracting the anti-inflammatory and immunosuppressive effects of CS, is pro-inflammatory. Lewis rats develop a variety of induced-autoimmune inflammatory conditions, such as streptococcal cell wall arthritis, whereas the histocompatible F344 Fisher rats are resistant to this condition. Lewis rats have a defective hypothalamic-pituitary adrenal (HPA) response to a variety of hypothalamic stimuli, but have augmented systemic secretion of AVP. Patients with rheumatoid arthritis (RA) have deficient CS with exaggerated PRL responses to inflammatory stimuli. Within inflammatory foci, CRH is pro-inflammatory. AVP, which augments autologous mixed lymphocyte reactions, can replace the IL-2 requirement for γIFN production by T cells via V_{1a} receptors, and potentiates primary antibody responses, is also pro-inflammatory. Lewis rats have significantly high plasma levels, hypothalamic content, and *in vitro* release of AVP in comparison to the inflammatory disease-resistant Fischer rats. Immunoneutralization of AVP attenuates inflammatory responses. In Sprague-Dawley rats, AVP potentiates PRL secretion. Preliminary studies in patients with RA have shown that the circulating levels of AVP are significantly increased, which might be a compensatory response to low CS levels or a result of elevated levels of IL-6 in these patients but could nevertheless contribute to rheumatoid inflammation. A similar observation has been made in patients with ankylosing spondylitis.

[d]Address for correspondence: Dr. I.C. Chikanza, M.B., Ch.B., M.R.C.P. F.R.C.P.C.H., M.D., Consultant/Senior Lecturer in Rheumatology, Bone & Joint Research Unit, St. Bartholomews & Royal London Hosp. School of Medicine & Dentistry, New Science Bldg., Charterhouse Square, London EC1M 6BQ, UK. Voice: +44-020-7882 6127; Fax: +44-020-7882 6121.

i.c.chikanza@mds.qmw.ac.uk

INTRODUCTION

The neuroendocrine and immune systems interact with each other during inflammatory stress. Cytokines and chemokines released in inflammatory sites, such as the joints of patients with rheumatoid arthritis (RA), stimulate leukocytes such as monocytes, macrophages, and T cells and activate the endothelium to express adhesion molecules that facilitate the local accumulation of inflammatory cells.[1,2] These cytokines also initiate the hepatic and systemic acute-phase response and trigger a cascade of neuroendocrine changes that help with the control and eventual termination of inflammation.[3,4] These mechanisms include the activation of the HPA axis and the sympathetic nervous system,[4,5] the generation of fever, somnolence, and slow wave sleep,[6,7] and the release of a variety of neuropeptides involved in the stress response including CRH, AVP, ACTH, αMSH, and prolactin.[8]

HYPOTHALAMIC-PITUITARY RESPONSES TO INFLAMMATION

The stress of inflammation in the course of an infectious disease, active autoimmune inflammatory process, and accidental or operative trauma is associated by a coordinated complex series of adaptive responses involving the immune, nervous, and endocrine systems. Inflammatory signals reach the brain via the blood stream or more rapidly via the vagus nerve and stimulate the hypothalamus to increase the release of CRH and AVP, which synergistically enhance ACTH secretion by the pituitary gland; ACTH in turn increases the production of corticosteroid (CS) by the adrenal cortices.[9] CS dampens the inflammatory response by inhibiting pro-inflammatory cytokine production, while upregulating anti-inflammatory cytokine secretion.[4] The pituitary gland also releases prolactin, β-endorphin, macrophage inhibitory factor (MIF), and other neuropeptides.[4,10] Prolactin exerts pro-inflammatory effects, while αMSH and β-endorphin are anti-inflammatory and αMSH exerts anti-pyretic effects.[11,12] MIF counteracts the immunosuppressive effects of CS on T cells and macrophages.[13]

In addition to the changes in the production of pro-inflammatory and anti-inflammatory cytokines, there is also local release in inflammatory lesions of pro-inflammatory neuropeptides, such as CRH, prolactin, and substance P.[14–18] CRH potentiates pro-inflammatory cytokine production, while substance P potentiates pain, T-cell activation, and proliferation.[16,19] In the baseline, immune tone is modulated by the diurnal rhythm of corticosteroids, catecholamines, pro-inflammatory cytokines, and prolactin, all regulated by the hypothalamic circadian pacemaker.[20] The variation in circulating T cell numbers and subsets, as well as their immune reactivity and several markers, follow such a pattern.[21,22] Transgenic mice lacking an effective CS receptor have marked immunological abnormalities, including hyperresponsive T helper-1 cells.[23]

Studies in a number of animal models of human autoimmune inflammatory disorders have shown that abnormalities in the interactions between the neuroendocrine and immune systems can contribute to the pathogenesis of chronic autoimmune inflammatory diseases.[24,25] For instance, female Lewis (LEW/N) rats develop streptococcal cell wall peptidoglycan (SCW)-induced chronic arthritis and basic myelin-induced experimental allergic encephalomyelitis unlike the histocompatible Fischer

(F344/N) rats that are resistant to these conditions.[26,27] Similarly, the obese strain of chicken develops spontaneous autoimmune thyroiditis.[28] The susceptibility to developing chronic inflammatory diseases in Lewis rats, and to developing autoimmune thyroiditis in the obese strain of chicken, is directly linked to an inability to mount an adequate ACTH and CS response to inflammation.[28,30] Lewis rats also fail to respond adequately to injections of inflammatory cytokines such as IL-1, and hypothalamic catecholaminergic, serotonergic, and cholinergic stimulants. Fischer rats (F344/N) only develop acute transient polyarthritis, and mount a normal or mildly exaggerated ACTH and corticosterone response.[26,29]

End-organ unresponsiveness to CS may also contribute to inflammation. This may be the case in the NOD mice and, to a lesser extent, BB rats, which develop spontaneous autoimmune diabetes mellitus as a consequence of autoimmune-mediated β-cell insulitis.[31,32] Immune cells from NOD mice are resistant to the effects of CS, and the T and B cells from this animal model exhibit an extended life span.[32] Interestingly, in the BB rat, the transportation of CS is altered. This strain has a mutation in the corticosteroid binding globulin gene, which reduces the affinity of this protein for corticosterone; it is doubtful, however, that this explains immune cell resistance to CS.[33]

The observations in the Lewis rats and obese strain of chicken are of direct relevance to a number of human inflammatory conditions. Patients with Addison's disease face dire consequences if not given appropriate high-dose cortisol replacement during infectious and inflammatory stress. Low basal or defective cortisol responses to ACTH have been associated with high mortality in septicemic patients.[34] Neuroendocrine immune studies in patients with rheumatoid arthritis (RA) show defective HPA axis responses to inflammation characterized by inappropriately low levels of circulating ACTH and cortisol for the degree of ongoing joint inflammation,[24,25,35–37] as well as excessive and dysregulated prolactin production.[25,38]

AVP production, like that of corticosteroids and prolactin, has a diurnal rhythm of secretion with a peak in the morning[39] and like these hormones is also involved in the exercise-induced stress response.[40] Since it synergizes with CRH to induce ACTH secretion by the pituitary, it indirectly suppresses inflammation. Like its functional companion CRH, which has direct pro-inflammatory effects, AVP also exerts direct pro-inflammatory actions at the inflammatory site.

REGULATION OF ARGININE VASOPRESSIN SECRETION

Although AVP production is widely distributed in the central nervous system, the main sources of AVP in the brain are the magnocellular and parvicellular neurons of the paraventricular nucleus (PVN) of the hypothalamus, as well as the magnocellular neurons of the supraoptic nucleus (SON).[41–43] The parvicellular neurons that may co-express both AVP and CRH secrete both peptides into the median eminence from where they are transported via the hypophyseal portal vessels to the pituitary.[9] Parvicellular neuron AVP is suppressed by direct action of glucocorticosteroids, while the regulation of magnocellular AVP by CS in not clear.[44,45] Magnocellular AVP reaches the hypophyseal portal system via collateral nerve terminals.[46]

The osmoreceptor cells situated in the anterior hypothalamus and the organum vasculosum of the lamina terminalis regulate the release of AVP from the posterior pituitary.[10] Other stimuli include hypotension, decreased blood volume, morphine, nicotine, carbamazepine, chlorpromazine, hypoglycemia, and angiotensin II, whereas alcohol inhibits its secretion.[10] Atrial natriuretic peptide reduces magnocellular AVP secretion in man.[47,48] The gene which codes for AVP in man is on chromosome 20p13, while in mice it is on chromosome 2, which also carries the IL-1 gene.[49,50] Like CRH, AVP gene expression and synthesis are positively regulated by catecholamines, acetylcholine, and serotonin;[51] γ-aminobutyric acid and corticosteroids are inhibitory.[52]

PHYSIOLOGIC ROLE OF ARGININE VASOPRESSIN

AVP has many biological effects which include antidiuresis, synergy with CRH to stimulate ACTH secretion, vasoconstriction, enhancement of memory and arousal.[9,10,53,54] These biologic effects are mediated by V_1, V_2, and V_3 (V_{1b}) receptors that show specific tissue distribution, allowing design of selective targeting approaches.[55–58] V_1 receptors mediate the vascular effects of AVP.[55,58] V_2 receptors mediate renal effects, while V_3 (V_{1b}) receptors are involved in the regulation of ACTH secretion.[58]

IMMUNOMODULATORY EFFECTS OF ARGININE VASOPRESSIN

Many studies have shown that AVP has immunomodulatory properties.[59] This neuropeptide, acting via V_1 receptors, enhances autologous mixed lymphocyte reactions in a dose-dependent manner and can replace the IL-2 requirement for interferon-γ (IFN-γ) production.[60–61] Furthermore, high-affinity V_1 receptors are found on human peripheral blood mononuclear cells and splenic lymphocytes.[62,63] In experimental animals, AVP potentiates primary antibody responses *in vivo*.[54] As reviewed above, Lewis (LEW/N) rats are highly susceptible to developing severe chronic inflammatory disease, whereas the near histocompatible Fischer rats (F344/N) are resistant.[26] Lewis rats also have significantly high plasma levels, hypothalamic content, and *in vitro* release of AVP in comparison with the F344/N rats.[64,65] It is possible that these findings represent a compensatory adaptation to deficient CRH and corticosterone secretion. Since systemic immunoneutralization of AVP in Lewis rats attenuates inflammatory responses, the high levels of circulating AVP may be an additional neuroendocrine factor contributing to the susceptibility to developing chronic inflammatory disease.[66,67] Given the T helper-1 suppressive and stimulatory effects of CS and AVP, respectively, the low corticosterone and high levels of AVP would favor the development of predominantly T helper-1 cellular responses in these animals.[68]

Although the effects of IL-1β, TNFα, and IL-6 on the magnocellular AVP system are not fully characterized, most studies in rats suggest a stimulatory effect of the cytokines on AVP secretion.[4,69,73] IL-6 infusions increase AVP secretion in a dose-dependent manner in man.[74] AVP, on the other hand, attenuates endotoxin-induced fever via V_1 receptors in rats.[75] Of further interest is the observation that in Sprague-

Dawley rats, AVP potentiates the secretion of prolactin, while infusions of substance P increase scrum levels of AVP in a dose-dependent manner.[76–78] Whether enhanced AVP secretion is the mechanism responsible for the excessive and dysregulated secretion of prolactin seen in patients with RA remains to be determined. Such a link could be of relevance to disease pathophysiology because both hormones are pro-inflammatory.

EVIDENCE FOR A PRO-INFLAMMATORY ROLE FOR AVP IN HUMAN CHRONIC INFLAMMATORY DISEASE

Patients with RA have inappropriately low levels of cortisol for the degree of joint inflammation, a situation reminiscent of the Lewis rat.[8,24,26,29,35–37] CRH is produced in the joints of RA patients, where it might potentiate inflammation.[79] In addition, patients with RA also have excessive and rather dysregulated prolactin responses.[34] The lack of a corticosterone response, increased local CRH in inflammatory sites, and high circulating levels of AVP in Lewis rats, contribute to their susceptibility to developing inflammatory disease.[26,29,64,67] Thus, like Lewis rats, RA patients have a pro-inflammatory hormonal milieu, which may contribute to the chronicity of their disease.

Preliminary studies of AVP in RA patients have demonstrated significantly higher circulating levels of the neuropeptide, than in normal and chronic osteomyelitis control subjects, and higher AVP responses to surgery than in patients with osteoarthritis and those with chronic osteomyelitis, who had similar levels of inflammation in terms of ESR and chronicity.[80] This observation suggests that the high levels of AVP in RA are not simply a reflection of inflammation or amount of stress. IL-6 can increase AVP secretion, but the levels of IL-6 in RA patients were not significantly different from those seen in subjects with chronic osteomyelitis, suggesting that the levels of IL-6 cannot explain the pronounced dysregulation of AVP in RA patients.

Excessive prolactin production appears to play a role in the pathophysiology of experimental SLE, autoimmune uveitis, and experimental allergic encephalomyelitis.[81–83] Patients with systemic lupus erythematosus (SLE), RA, scleroderma, Reiter's and Sjogren's syndromes have significantly elevated levels of prolactin.[34,84–88] Because AVP can enhance prolactin secretion, it can be hypothesized that the enhanced prolactin secretion might be a consequence of dysregulated AVP production in these chronic autoimmune inflammatory diseases. This possibility is worthy of further investigation because it may lead to a better understanding of the neuroendocrine immune mechanisms in these disorders and to the development of novel therapeutic options.

We have recently shown that patients with ankylosing spondylitis (AS) have appropriate CS responses for the degree of their inflammatory disease, but with low ACTH and high AVP circulating levels.[89] The underlying mechanisms of these changes remain to be determined.

SUMMARY AND CONCLUSIONS

AVP is involved in the regulation of ACTH secretion by the pituitary gland and, therefore, of corticosteroids by the adrenal glands. It is also involved in the inflammatory stress response and has anti-pyretic and behavioral effects. Infusions of IL-6 increase levels of AVP in a dose-dependent manner. AVP has direct immune effects on inflammatory cells via V_{1A} receptors. Immunoneutralization of AVP attenuates carragheenin-induced inflammation in rats. It can thus be hypothesized that perturbations of AVP physiology may contribute to susceptibility to develop chronic inflammatory disease. Lewis rats, which have a defective HPA axis and excessive AVP secretion, can be induced to develop a variety of chronic autoimmune inflammatory disorders. Similar neurohormonal observations have been made in patients with RA.

REFERENCES

1. AKIRA, S., T. HIRANO, T. TAGA & L. KISHIMOTO. 1990. Biology of multi-functional cytokines: IL-6 and related molecules (IL-1 and TNF). FASEB J. **4:** 2860–2867.
2. ALBELDA, S.M. & C.A. BUCK. 1990. Integrins and other cell adhesion molecules. FASEB J. **4:** 2868–2880.
3. RAMADORI, G., J. VAN DARNINE, R. RIEDER & K.H. MEYER. 1988. IL-6, the third mediator of acute phase reaction modulates hepatic protein synthesis in humans and mouse. Comparison with IL-Iβ and TNF-α. Eur. J. Immunol. **18:** 1259–1264.
4. CHIKANZA, I.C. & A. GROSSMAN. 1996. Neuroendocrine immune responses to inflammation: the concept of the neuroendocrine immune loop. Bailliere's Clin. Rheumatol. **10:**199–226.
5. TSAGARAKIS, S., J.M.P. HOLLY, L.H. REES, G.M. BESSER & A. GROSSMAN. 1988. Acetylcholine and norepinephrin stimulate CRF-41 release from the rat hypothalamus *in vitro*. Endocrinology **123:** 1962–1969.
6. FONTANO, A., E. WEBER & J-M. DAYER. 1984. Synthesis of interleukin-l/endogenous pyrogen in the brain of endotoxin-treated mice: a step in fever induction. J. Immunol. **133:** 1696–1701.
7. KRUEGER, J.M., J. WALTER, C.A. DINARELLO, S.M. WOLFF & L. CHEDID. 1984. Sleep-promoting effects of endogenous pyrogen (interleukin-1). Am. J. Physiol. **264:** R994–1009.
8. CHIKANZA, I.C., G. CHROUSOS & G.S. PANAYI. 1992. Abnormal neuroendocrine immune communications in rheumatoid arthritis. Eur. J. Clin. Invest. **22:** 635–637.
9. ANTONI, F.A. 1993. Vasopressinergic control of pituitary adrenocorticotropin secretion comes of age. Front. Neuroendocrinol. **14:** 72–122.
10. GANONG, W.E. 1985. Review of Medical Physiology, 12th edit. Lange Medical Publications.: 190–203. Los Altos, CA.
11. CHIKANZA, I.C. & G.S. PANAYI. 1991. Hypothalamic-pituitary mediated modulation of immune function: prolactin as a neuroimmune peptide. Br. J. Rheumatol. **30:** 203–207.
12. CANONG, J.G., J.B. TATRO, S. REICHLIN & C.A. DINARELLO. 1986. αMSH inhibits immunostimulatory and inflammatory actions of IL-1. J. Immunol. **137:** 2232–2236.
13. CALANDRA, T. & R. BUCALA. 1997. Macrophage inhibitory factor: a glucocorticoid counter-regulator within the immune system. Crit. Rev. Immunol. **17:** 77–88.
14. AREND, W.P., M. MALYAK, M.F. SMITH, T.D. WHISENAND, X. SLACK, J.E. SIMS *et al.* 1994. Binding of IL-1α and IL-1β and IL-lRa by soluble receptors and levels of soluble IL-1 receptors in synovial fluid. J. Immunol. **153:** 4766–4774.
15. DAYER, J.M. 1991. Chronic inflammatory joint disease: natural inhibitors of IL-1 and TNFα. J. Rheumatol. **18:** 71–75.

16. KARALIS, K., H. SANO, J. REDWINE, S. LISTWAK, R. WILDER & G. CHROUSOS. 1991. Autocrine or paracrine inflammatory actions of corticotropin-releasing hormone *in vivo*. Science **254:** 421–423.

17. MARSHALL, K.W., B. CHIU & R.D. INMAN. 1990. Substance P and arthritis; analysis of plasma and synovial fluid levels. Arthritis Rheum.**33:** 87–90.

18. AKAHOSHI, T., J.J. OPPENHEIM & K. MATSUSHIMA. 1988. Induction of high affinity interleukin-1 receptor on human peripheral blood lymphocytes by glucocorticosteroid hormones. J. Exp. Med. **167:** 924–936.

19. MATUCCI-CERINIC, M. & G. PARTSCH. 1992. The contribution of the perpherial nervous system and the neuropeptide network to the development of synovial inflammation. Clin. Exp. Rheumatol. **10:** 211–215.

20. TAKAHASHI, J.S. 1992. Circadian clock genes are ticking. Science **258:** 238–239.

21. FAUCI, A.S. & D.C. DALE. 1974. The effects of *in vivo* hydrocortisone on subpopulations of human lymphocytes. J. Clin. Invest. **53:** 240–245.

22. POWNALL, R. & M.S. KNAPP. 1980. A circadian study of cortico-steroid suppression of delayed hypersensitivity. Int. J. Pharmacol. **1:** 293–298.

23. MORALE, M.C., N. BATTICANE, F. GALLO, N. BARDEN & B. MARCHETTI. 1995. Disruption of hypothalamic pituitary adrenocortical system in transgenic mice expressing type 2 glucocorticoid receptor antisense ribonucleic acid permanently impairs T cell function: effects on trafficking and T cell responsiveness during postnatal development. Endocrinology **136:** 3949–3960.

24. CHIKANZA, I.C. 1996. The neuroendocrine immunology of rheumatoid arthritis. Bailliere's Clin. Rheumatol. **10:** 273–294.

25. JORGENSEN, C., N. BRESSOT, C. BOLOGNA & J. SANY. 1995. Dysregulation of hypothalamo-pituitary axis in rheumatoid arthritis. J. Rheumatol. **22:** 1825–1833.

26. STERNBERG, E.M., J.M. HILL, G. CHROUSOS, T. KAMLARIS, S.J. LISTWAK, P.W. GOLD *et al.* 1989. Inflammatory mediator induced arthritis is defective in streptococcal cell arthritis susceptible Lewis rats. Proc. Natl. Acad. Sci. USA **86:** 2374–2378.

27. MASON, D. 1991. Genetic variation in the stress response: susceptibility to experimental allergic encephalomyelitis and implications for human inflammatory disease. Immunol. Today **12:** 57–61.

28. SCHAUENSTEIN, K., R. FESSLER, H. DIETRICH, S. SCHWARZ, G. KREMER & G. WICK. 1987. Disturbed immune endocrine communication in autoimmune disease. Lack of corticosterone response to immune signals in obese strain chickens with spontaneous autoimmune thyroiditis. J. Immunol. **139:** 1830–1837.

29. STERNBERG, E.M., W.S. YOUNG, R. BERNADINI, A.E. CALGERO, G.P. CHROUSOS, P.W. GOLD *et al.* 1989. A central nervous system defect in the biosynthesis of CRH is associated with susceptibility to streptococcal cell wall induced arthritis in Lewis rats. Proc. Natl. Acad. Sci. USA **86:** 4771–4775.

30. FESSLER, R., K. SCHAUENSTEIN, G. KREMER, S. SCHWARZ & G. WICK. 1986. Elevation of corticosteroid binding globulin in obese strain (OS) chickens: possible implications for the disturbed immunoregulation and the development of spontaneous autoimmune thyroiditis. J. Immunol. **136:** 3657–3663.

31. FITZPATRICK, F., N. CHRISTEFF, S. DURANT *et al.* 1992. Glucocorticoids in the non-obese (NOD) mouse: basal serum levels, effect of endocrine manipulation and immobilization stress. Life Sci. **150:** 1063–1069.

32. LEIJON, K., B. HAMMARSTROM & D. HOLMBERG. 1994. Non-obese diabetic (NOD) mice display enhanced immune responses and prolonged survival of lymphoid cells. Int. Immunol. **6:** 339–345.

33. HAMMOND, G.L. & C.L. SMITH. 1991. An amino acid substitution in BioBreeding rat corticosteroid binding globulin results in reduced steroid binding affinity. J. Biol. Chem. **266:** 18555–18559.

34. ROTHWELL, P.M., Z.F. UDWADIA & P.G. LAWLER. 1991. Cortisol response to corticotropin and survival in septic shock. Lancet **337:** 582–583.

35. CHIKANZA, I.C., P. PETROU, G. KINGSLEY, G. CHROUSOS & G.S. PANAYI. 1992. Defective hypothalamic response to immune and inflammatory stimuli in patients with rheumatoid arthritis. Arthritis Rheum. **35:** 1281–1288.

36. NEECK, G., K. FEDERLIN, V. GRAEF, D. RUSCH & K.I. SCHMIDT. 1990. Adrenal secretion of cortisol in patients with rheumatoid arthritis. J. Rheumatol. **17:** 24–29.

37. HALL, J., E.F. MORAND, S. MEDBAK, M. ZAMAN, L. PERRY, N.J. GOULDING et al. 1994. Abnormal hypothalamic pituitary adrenal function in rheumatoid arthritis. Arthritis Rheum. **37:** 1132–1137.

38. CHIKANZA, I.C., P. PETROU, G. KINGSLEY, G. CHROUSOS & G.S. PANAYI. 1993. Excessive and dysregulated secretion of prolactin in rheumatoid arthritis: immunopathogenctic and therapeutic implications. Br. J. Rheumatol. **32:** 445–448.

39. BURBACK, J.P., B. LITI, T.A. VOORHIUS & F.I.H. VAN TOT. 1988. Diurnal variation in vasopressin and oxytocin mRNA in hypothalamic nuclei of the rat. Brain Res. **464:** 157–160.

40. WITTERT, G.A., D.E. STEWART, M.P. GRAVES, M.J. ELLIS, M.J. EVANS, J.E. WELLS et al. 1991. Plasma CRF and vasopressin responses to exercise in normal man. Clin. Endocrinol. **35:** 311–317.

41. DU VIGNEAUD, V., C. RESSLER, J.M. SWAN, P.G. KATSOYANNIS & C.W. ROBERTS. 1954. Synthesis of oxytocin. J. Am. Chem. Soc. **76:** 3115–3121.

42. MOURI, T., K. ITOI, K. TAKAHUSHI, T. SUDA, O. MURAKAMI, N. ANDOH et al. 1993. Localisation of corticotropin-release factor and vasopressin in the paraventricular nucleus of the human hypothalamus. Neuroendocrinology **57:** 34–39.

43. HOLMES, M.C., L.A. ANTONI, G. AGUILERA & K.I. CATT. 1986. Magnocellular axons in passage through the median eminence release vasopressin. Nature **319:** 326–329.

44. KISS, J., J.A.M. EEKELEN, J.M.H.M. REUL, H.M. WESTPHAL & E.R. DE KLOET. 1988. Glucocorticoid receptors in magnocellular neurosecretory cells. Endocrinology **122:** 444–449.

45. RAFF, H., J. SHINSAKO, L. KEIL & M.F. DALLMAN. 1984. Feedback inhibition of ACTH and AVP responses to hypoxia by physiological increases in endogenous corticosteroids in dogs. Endocrinology **114:** 1245–1259.

46. PAGE, R.B. 1982. Pituitary blood flow. Am. J. Physiol. **241:** E427–442.

47. RUSSI, W.F. 1993. Effect of endothelin-3 on vasopressin release *in vitro* and water excretion *in vivo* in Long-Evans rats. J. Physiol. **461:** 501–511.

48. ESPINER, E.A., A.M. RICHARDS, R.A. DONALD, J.H. LIVESEY & T.G. YANDLE. 1993. Atrial natriuretic factor reduces vasopressin and angiotensin 11 but not ACTH response to acute hypoglycaemic stress in normal man. Clin. Endocrinol. **38:** 183–189.

49. RAO, V.V., C. LOFFIER, J. BATTEY & L. HANSMANN. 1992. The human gene for oxytocin-neurophysin-1 is physiologically mapped to chromosome 20pl 3 by *in situ* hybridisation. Cytogenet. Cell Genet. **61:** 271–273.

50. MARINI, J.C., K.K. NELSON, J. BATTEY & L.D. SIRACUSA. 1993. The pituitary hormones arginine vasopressin-neurophysin 11 and oxytoein-neurophysin 1 show close linkage with IL-1 on mouse chromosome 2. Genomics **15:** 200–202.

51. PLOTSKY, P.M. 1987. Regulation of hypophysiotropic factors mediating ACTH secretion. Ann. N.Y. Acad. Sci. **512:** 205–217.

52. OTAKE, K., K. KONDO & Y. OSIO. 1991. Possible involvement of endogenous opiod peptides in the inhibition of arginine vasopressin release by γ-aminobutyric acid in conscious rats. Neuroendocrinology **54:** 170–174.

53. DODT, C., R. PICTROWSK, A. SEWING, A. ZABEL, H.L. FELM & J. BORN. 1994. Effects of vasopressin on event-related potential indicators of cognitive processing in young and old humans. J. Gerontol. **49:** M183–188.

54. CROISET, G., C.J. HEIJNEN & D. DEWIED. 1990. Passive avoidance behaviour, vasopressin and the immune system. A link between avoidance latency and immune response. Neuroendocrinology **51:** 156–161.

55. MITCHELL, R.H., C.J. KIRK & M.M. BILLAH. 1979. Hormonal stimulation of phosphatidylinositol breakdown with particular reference to hepatic effects of vasopressin. Biochem. Soc. Trans. **7:** 861–865.

56. JARD, S., C. BARBERIS, S. AUDIGIER & E. TRIBOLLET. 1997. Neurohypophyseal hormone receptor systems in brain and periphery. Prog. Brain Res. **72:** 173–187.

57. JARD, S. 1988. Mechanisms of action of vasopressin antagonists. Kidney Int. **34:** 538–542.

58. NORSZCZYK, B., S. LON & E. SZCZEPANSKA-SADOWSK. 1993. Central cardiovascular effects of AVP and AVP analogues V1, V2 & V3 agonistic or antagonistic properties in conscious dog. Brain Res. **610:** 115–126.

59. CHIKANZA, I.C. & A.G. GROSSMAN. 1998. Hypothalamic-mediated immunomodulation: arginine vasopressin is a neuroendocrine immune mediator. Br. J. Rheumatol. **37:** 131–136.

60. JOHNSON, H.M., W.L. FARRAR & B. TORRES. 1982. Vasopressin replacement of IL-2 requirement in gamma interferon production: lymphokine activity of a neuroendocrine hormone. J. Immunol. **129:** 983–986.

61. TORRES, B.A. & H.M. JOHNSON. 1988. AVP replacement of helper cell requirement in IFN production. Evidence for a novel AVP receptor on mouse lymphocytes. J. Immunol. **140:** 2179–2182.

62. BELL, J., M.W. ADLER, J.I. GREENSTEIN & L.Y. LITI-CELM. 1993. Identification and characterisation of [125] arginine vasopressin binding sites on human peripheral blood mononuclear cells. Life Sci. **52:** 95–105.

63. ELANDS, J., A. RESINK & E. R. DE KLOET. 1990. Neurohypophyseal hormone receptors in the rat thymus, spleen and lymphocytes. Endocrinology **126:** 2703–2710.

64. PATCHEV, V.K., K.T. KALOGERAS, P. ZELAZOWSKI, R.L. WILDER & G.P. CHROUSOS. 1992. Increased plasma concentrations, hypothalamic content and *in vitro* release of AVP in inflammatory disease-prone, hypothalamic CRH deficient Lewis rats. Endocrinology **131:** 1453–1457.

65. MILLAN, M.J., M.H. MILLAN, F.C. COLPAERT & A. HERZ. 1985. Chronic arthritis in the rat: differential changes in discrete brain pools of vasopressin as compared to oxytocin. Neurosci. Lett. **54:** 33–37.

66. PATCHEV, V.K., G. MASTORAKOS, L.S. BRADY, J. REDIVINE, R.L. WILDER & G.P. CHROUSOS. 1993. Increased AVP secretion may participate in the enhanced susceptibility of Lewis rats to inflammatory disease. Neuroendocrinology **58:** 106–110.

67. CROFFORD, U., H. SANO, K. KARALIS, E.L. WEBSTER, E.A. GOLDMURIZ, G.P. CHROUSOS *et al.* 1992. Local secretion of CRH in the joints of Lewis rats with inflammatory arthritis. J. Clin. Invest. **90:** 2555–2564.

68. LIBLAU, R.S., S.M. SINGER & H.O. MCDEVITT. 1995. TH1 and TH2 CD4 T cells in the pathogenesis of organ-specific autoimmune disease. Immunol. Today **16:** 34–38.

69. HERMUS, A.R.M.M. & M. SWEEP. 1990. Cytokines and the hypothalamic pituitary adrenal axis. J. Steroid Biochem. **37:** 867–871.

70. SAPOLSKY, R., C. RIVIER, G. YAMAMOTO, P. PLOTSKY & W. VALE. 1987. Interleukin-1 stimulates the secretion of hypothalamic corticotropin-releasing factor. Science **238:** 522–524.

71. CHRISTENSEN, J.D., E.W. HANSEN & B. FJALLAND. 1989. IL-1B stimulates the release of vasopressin from rat neurohypophysis. J. Pharmacol. **171:** 233–235.

72. NAKATSURA, K., S. OHGO, Y. OKI & S. MATSUKURA. 1991. IL-1 stimulates AVP release from superfused rat hypothalamo-neurohypophyseal complexes independently of cholinergic mechanism. Brain Res. **554:** 38–45.

73. YASIN, S.A., A. COSTA & A. GROSSMAN. 1994. IL-1β and IL-6 stimulate neurohypophyseal hormone release *in vitro*. J. Neuroendocrinol. **6:** 179–184.

74. MASTORAKOS, G., J.S. WEBER, M.A. MAGIAKOU, H. GUNN & G.P. CHROUSOS. 1994. Hypothalamic-pituitary-adrenal axis activation and stimulation of systemic vasopressin secretion by recombinant interleukin 6 in humans: potential implications for the syndrome of inappropriate vasopressin secretion. J. Clin. Endocrinol. Metab. **79:** 934–939.

75. JANSKY, L. 1992. A discrete mode of the anti-pyretic action of AVP, MSH and ACTH. Physiol. Res. **41:** 57–61.

76. KJAER, A., U. KNIGGE, L.L. VILHARDT & J. WARBERG. 1993. Involvement of vasopressin in histamine and stress induced prolactin release: permissive, mediating or potentiating role? Neuroendocrinology **57:** 314–321.

77. CHOWDREY, H.S., D.S. LESSOP & S.L. LIGHTMAN. 1990. Substance P stimulates arginine vasopressin and inhibits ACTH release *in vivo* in the rat. Neuroendocrinology **52:** 90–93.

78. CHIODERA, P. & V. COIRO. 1992. Effects of intravenous infusion of substance P on arginine vasopressin and oxytocin secretion in normal man. Brain Res. **569:** 173–176.
79. CROFFORD, U., H. SANO, K. KARALIS, H.R. EPPS, P. MANTHERN, G.P. CHROUSOS *et al.* 1993. Corticotropin–releasing hormone in synovial fluids and tissues of patients with rheumatoid arthritis and osteoarthritis. J. Immunol. **151:** 1587–1596.
80. CHIKANZA, I.C., P. PETROU & G. CHROUSOS. 1998. Dysregulation of AVP secretion in rheumatoid arthritis: pathophysiological implications. Clin. Exp. Rheum. **16:** 640.
81. MCMURRAY, R., D. KEISLER, K. KANUCKEL, S. IZIII & S.E. WALKER. 1991. Prolactin influences autoimmune disease activity in the female B/W mouse. J. Immunol. **147:** 3780–3787.
82. PALESTINE, A.G., C.G. MUELLENBURG-COULOMBRE, M.K. KIM, M. GELATO & R.B. NUSSENBLATT. 1987. Bromocriptine and low dose cyclosporine in the treatment of experimental uveitis in the rat. J. Clin. Invest. **79:** 1078–1081.
83. CANONICO, P.L., M.A. SORTINO, A. FAVIT, G. ALEPPO & U. SCAPAGNINI. 1993. Dihydroergocryptine protects from acute experimental allergic encephalomyelitis in the rat. Funct. Neurol. **8:** 183–188.
84. JARA, I.J., C. GOMEZ-SANCHEZ, P. MARTINEZ-OSUNA, F.B. VSEY & L.R. ESPINOZA. 1992. Hyperprolactinaemia in systemic lupus erythematosus. Association with disease activity. Am. J. Med. Sci. **303:** 222-226.
85. GUTIERREZ, M.A., J.M. ANAYA, E. SCOPELITIS, G. CITERA, L.H. SILVEIRA & L.R. ESPINOZA. 1994. Hyperprolactinaemia in primary Sjogren's syndrome. Ann. Rheum. Dis. **53:** 425-428.
86. JARA, I.J., C. GOMEZ-SANCHEZ & C. PINNEDA. 1991. Hyperprolactinaemia in reactive arthritis. Arthritis Rheum. **34**(1)**:** 187.
87. CHIKANZA, I.C., P. PETROU, G. CHROUSOS & G. PANAYI. 1995. Arginine vasopressin secretion in rheumatoid arthritis: pathophysiological implications. Arthritis Rheum. **38:** S216.
88. KUCHARZ, E.J., R. JARCZYK, G. JONDERKO, J. RUBISZ-BRZEZISNKA & L. BREZEZISNKA-WASLO. 1996. High serum levels of prolactin in patients with systemic sclerosis. Clin. Rheumatol. **15**(3)**:** 314.
89. CHIKANZA, I.C., P. PETROU & G. CHROUSOS. 1996. The circadian hypothalamic-pituitary-adrenal axis responses in patients with active ankylosing spondylitis. Br. J. Rheumatol. **36**(Suppl. 1)**:** 126.

The Hypothalamic-Pituitary-Adrenal and Gonadal Axes in Rheumatoid Arthritis

MAURIZIO CUTOLO,[a,b] BARBARA VILLAGGIO,[b] LUCA FOPPIANI,[c] MELANIA BRIATA,[b] ALBERTO SULLI,[b] CARMEN PIZZORNI,[b] FRANCESCA FAELLI,[b] CAMILLA PRETE,[b] LAMBERTO FELLI,[d] BRUNO SERIOLO,[b] AND MASSIMO GIUSTI[d]

[b]Division of Rheumatology, Department of Internal Medicine, University of Genova, Italy

[c]Division of Endocrinology, Department of Metabolic and Endocrinologic Sciences, University of Genova, Italy

[d]Division of Orthopedics, Department of Motor Sciences, University of Genova, Italy

ABSTRACT: The hypothalamic-pituitary-adrenal (HPA) and the hypothalamic-pituitary-gonadal (HPG) axes involvement or response to immune activation seems crucial for the control of excessive inflammatory and immune conditions such as autoimmune rheumatic diseases, including rheumatoid arthritis (RA). However, female patients seem to depend more on the HPA axis, whereas male patients seem to depend more on the HPG axis. In particular, hypoandrogenism may play a pathogenetic role in male RA patients because adrenal and gonadal androgens, both products of the HPA and HPG axes, are considered natural immunosuppressors. A significantly altered steroidogenesis of adrenal androgens (i.e., dehydroepiandrosterone sulfate, DHEAS and DHEA) in nonglucocorticoid-treated premenopausal RA patients has been described. The menopausal peak of RA suggests that estrogens and/or progesterone deficiency also play a role in the disease, and many data indicate that estrogens suppress cellular immunity, but stimulate humoral immunity (i.e., deficiency promotes cellular Th1-type immunity). A range of physical and psychosocial stressors are also implicated in the activation of the HPA axis and related HPG changes. Chronic and acute stressors appear to have different actions on immune mechanisms with experimental and human studies indicating that acute severe stressors may be even immunosuppressive, while chronic stress may enhance immune responses. The interactions between the immunological and neuroendocrine circuits is the subject of active and extensive ongoing research and might in the near future offer highly promising strategies for hormone-replacement therapies in RA.

[a]Address for correspondence: Maurizio Cutolo, MD, Division of Rheumatology, Department of Internal Medicine, Via D. Chiodo 25 c/7, 16136 Genova, Italy. Voice and fax: +39 010 353 7994.

Address for reprint requests: Maurizio Cutolo, MD, Division of Rheumatology, Department of Internal Medicine, Viale Benedetto XV,6, 16132 Genova, Italy.

mcutolo@unige.it

INTRODUCTION

Rheumatoid arthritis is considered as a multifactorial autoimmune rheumatic disease that originates from the patient's excessive immune and inflammatory response to a pathogenic antigen (i.e., an infective agent) which, in "normal" people, is handled without complications.[1]

The abnormal response results from the combination of several predisposing factors, that include the relationships between epitopes of the agent and histocompatibility epitopes, the status of the stress response system (i.e., HPA) and the gonadal hormones (i.e., HPG), with estrogens implicated as enhancers of the immune response and androgens and progesterone as natural suppressors.[2–5] Other mechanisms besides HPA/HPG dysfunction might chronically alter microvascular function and contribute to increased susceptibility to RA, such as aging effects, being female, and chronic, heavy cigarette smoking.[6]

THE HYPOTHALAMUS-PITUITARY-ADRENOCORTICAL AXIS FUNCTION IN RA

An intricate balance between soluble mediators released by activated cells of the immune/inflammatory system and products of the neuroendocrine system mantains the homeostasis in the presence of an inflammatory stress. Inflammatory cytokines (i.e., IL-6, IL-1, TNFα), as soluble products of the activated immune system, stimulate the production of corticotropin-releasing hormone (CRH) in the hypothalamus: CRH release leads to pituitary production of adrenocorticotropic hormone (ACTH), followed by glucocorticoid secretion by adrenal cortex and indirect perturbations of gonadal function (see FIGURE 1). Vascular endothelial system (VES) interactions with hormones and immunologic mediators are also involved.[8]

Young females, affected by recent intensive stressful conditions (interpersonal stressors, surgical or infectious events) activating the HPA, with associated low plasma adrenal androgens (i.e., DHEAS) and recent use of contraceptive pills, are the best candidates for the onset of autoimmune disorders, including RA.[8–10]

The existence of a sort of afferent pathway to the central nervous system (CNS) from the immune system implies that the latter should be regarded as a diffuse, receptor-sensorial organ.[11] The physiologic balance between the stress and the immune system may be disrupted as a consequence of various pathological insults, including sustained exposure to stress, abnormal immune reactions to infections or both.[12] Recently, intact ACTH secretion but impaired cortisol response in patients with active RA has been described, and this observation was consistent with a relative adrenal glucocorticoid insufficiency, the latter already suggested 40 years earlier.[13,14]

Increased HPA axis function is a normal response to the stress of inflammation and might be mediated by central and peripheral actions of circulating cytokines. Besides IL-1 and tumor necrosis factor-α (TNFα), IL-6 appears a major factor mediating interactions between the activated immune system and both the anterior pituitary cells and the adrenal steroidogenesis.[15] However, recent studies in patients with RA have shown that the overall activity of the HPA axis remains inappropriately

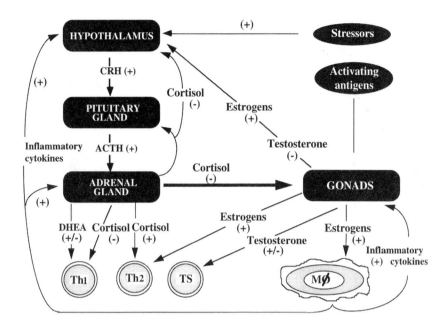

FIGURE 1. Relationships between the hypothalamus-pituitary-adrenocortical (HPA) and gonadal (HPG) axes activation and the immune response in rheumatoid arthritis. Stressors and inflammatory cytokines stimulate the production of corticotropin-releasing hormone (CRH) in the hypothalamus: the release of CRH leads to pituitary production of adrenocorticotropic hormone (ACTH), followed by glucocorticoid secretion by adrenal cortex (cortisol), affecting the immune cells and, indirectly, gonadal functioning. Testosterone and estrogens also modulate the immune response affecting both lymphocytes and macrophages/monocytes. Inflammatory cytokines (i.e., IL-6, IL-1, TNFα), as soluble products of the activated immune system, stimulate both the anterior pituitary cells and the adrenal steroidogenesis. Mφ, macrophages; DHEAS, dehydroepiandrosterone sulfate; Th1-Th2, T helper lymphocytes; Ts, T suppressor lymphocytes.

normal and apparently is insufficient to inhibit ongoing inflammation at least in early untreated arthritic patients.[16]

In general, in patients with RA, the relative deficiency of adrenal glucocorticoid production with compensatory ACTH hypersecretion is frequently observed, and chronically elevated cytokines might directly cause the decrease of the adrenal production.[17]

Recently, DHEA and DHEAS basal concentrations were found to be significantly lower ($p < 0.05$) in premenopausal RA patients than in controls. As expected, significantly higher basal levels of IL-6 and IL-12 ($p < 0.05$) were found in RA patients.[18] After the low-dose ACTH testing, the DHEA AUC was found to be significantly lower ($p < 0.01$) in RA patients than controls. Similar results, but without statistical significance, were observed after the oCRH stimulation. DHEA levels showed, at basal time, a significant negative correlation with the ESR and platelet count, as well as with the Steinbrocker class of the disease ($p < 0.05$). Normal plasma cortisol levels during oCRH and ACTH testing were found in RA patients in spite of their inflammatory condition.[18]

THE HYPOTHALAMUS-PITUITARY-ADRENOCORTICAL AND GONADAL AXES PRODUCT INTERACTIONS

Androgens seem implicated in the pathophysiology of autoimmune disorders, including RA as natural immunosuppressors. The disease is uncommon in men under age 45, but its incidence increases rapidly in older men and approaches the incidence in women. Low plasma and synovial fluid testosterone concentrations are observed in male RA patients; low plasma DHEAS is mainly observed in female RA patients.[5]

Direct exposure of T cells, T cell clones or T cell hybridomas to low concentrations of DHEA was found to increase the secretion of type 1 cytokines (Th1), at least IL-2 (see FIG. 1). Similar results have been observed in cultured T cells from patients with systemic lupus erythematosus (SLE) that are characterized by low DHEA serum levels.[19] Therefore, a causative role for reduced levels of gonadal (testosterone) and adrenal androgens (DHEA and DHEAS) has been suggested in the pathogenesis of RA, as well as in other immune/inflammatory arthritis (i.e., SLE).[10,20]

Recently, a significantly altered steroidogenesis of adrenal androgens (DHEA and DHEAS) in non-glucocorticoid-treated premenopausal RA patients has been confirmed.[21] Similar results were observed after desmopressin testing in RA patients.[22] Testosterone replacement therapy in RA patients is characterized by concomitant changes of DHEAS concentrations.[23] The reduced basal concentration of adrenal androgens in RA might be due both to a decreased pooling and a reduced sensitivity of the adrenal gland to exogenous corticotropin or, alternatively, to a partial enzymatic defect (i.e., 17,20-lyase).

Low levels of plasma DHEA and DHEAS in RA patients have been found significantly correlated with early morning low cortisol concentrations and high basal levels of IL-6.[21] Recently, higher IL-6 early morning peak values have been found in RA patients than in controls and significantly correlated to morning C-reactive protein (CRP) levels and Ritchie's index.[24]

The observation of reduced DHEA production combined with unexpected normal cortisol levels during oCRH and ACTH testing further support the concept of the presence of an adrenal hypofunction in patients with active RA in the setting of a sustained inflammatory process as shown by high IL-6 and IL-12 concentrations. In addition, adrenal and gonadal androgens, in particular DHEAS and both testosterone and dihydrotestosterone (DHT), have been found to repress the expression and activity of the human IL-6 gene promoter, thus supporting the concept of anti-inflammatory/immunosuppressive effects of androgens.[25,26] Therefore, the well-assessed deficiency of gonadal and adrenal androgens in RA patients seems to represent a relevant factor involved in the pathophysiology of the disease.[27–29]

The menopausal peak of RA suggests that estrogens and/or progesterone deficiency also play a role in the disease, and many data indicate that estrogens suppress cellular immunity, but stimulate humoral immunity (i.e., deficiency promotes cellular

Th1-type immunity).[30] On the other hand, recent observations suggest that progesterone, as well as pregnancy (elevated estrogens, progesterone, corticosteroids and testosterone), stimulates switch from Th1- to Th2-type immune responses.[30]

These data, taken together, indicate that gonadal and adrenal steroid deficiency (altered HPA/HPG axis), plus prolactin increase (i.e., breastfeeding), probably facilitates the expression of Th1-type immunity, which is now considered to be critical in the pathogenesis of RA.[30] In contrast, normal levels of adrenal and gonadal steroids seem to suppress the development of RA. In addition, recent studies suggest that testosterone may directly suppress anti-DNA antibody production in peripheral blood mononuclear cells from SLE patients by inhibiting B cell hyperactivity and, indirectly, by downregulating IL-6 production in monocytes.[31] Furthermore, in an *in vivo* investigation of testosterone therapy ameliorated experimental autoimmune encephalomyelitis and induced a T helper-2 bias in the autoantigen-specific T lymphocyte response.[32]

ASPECTS OF THE ACTIVATION OF THE STRESS SYSTEM

The immune system is directly linked to the stress system, and is profoundly influenced by the effectors of the stress response[33,34] (see FIG. 1). The stress response is associated with the activation of several neuroendocrine systems including the HPA and hypothalamic-pituitary-gonadal (HPG) axes, and the sympathetic nervous system.[35] For example, activation of the HPA axis may occur when confronted by a psychosocial stressor, which, if appraised as threatening, can result in associated affective and behavioral (i.e., coping) responses, as well as elevated serum levels of cortisol.[29,30] Hence, the HPA axis provides an essential interface between the internal and external environments and enables the individual to adapt to diverse noxious stimuli, whether they be psychological, physical or otherwise.[36,37]

The role of the increased cortisol release is adaptational and attempts to counteract the effects of stressors in order to reestablish homeostasis.[38] However, failure to mount an appropriate HPA axis response to a stress trigger may be detrimental, and may represent a significant contributory factor in the etiology of a variety of disease processes, including autoimmune and inflammatory disorders such as RA.[39] Some research indicates that psychosocial stressors, and a range of other psychosocial variables (e.g., coping, personality), may influence disease onset and/or exacerbations.[40] In fact, stress is the cause most given by patients for flare-ups in their RA.[41]

Psychosocial stressors may influence disease activity by disturbing the homeostasis of the neuroendocrine and immune systems in RA. However, recent research indicates that different psychosocial stressors may have differing effects on the neuroendocrine and immune systems in individuals with RA, as well as those with other rheumatic conditions. Acute stressors and interpersonal conflicts are associated with increases in cortisol, catecholamines, and prolactin.[42] In addition, chronic stressors may generally alter baseline neuroendocrine levels. Furthermore, chronic and acute stressors appear to have different actions on immune mechanisms with experimental and human studies indicating that acute severe stressors may even be immunosuppressive, while chronic stress may enhance immune responses.[43]

It is possible that major as well as small life events may in fact operate via different neuroendocrine pathways, in turn leading to different alterations in immune mechanisms, and subsequent disease outcomes.[44]

ANDROGEN MODULATION OF CYTOKINES IN RA

Adrenal and gonadal androgens, both products of the HPA and HPG axes, are considered natural immunosuppressors.[45] DHEA has been found to have immunomodulatory activities. *In vitro* studies showed that DHEA increases secretion of IL-2 by activated T lymphocytes (even in SLE patients) and decreases production of IL-4, IL-5, and IL-6, thus stimulating Th1-type cytokines.[46,47] In particular, DHEAS has been found to repress the expression and activity of the human IL-6 gene promoter, thus supporting the concept of anti-inflammatory/immunosuppressive effects exerted by androgenic steroids.[48] Specific receptors for the free active adrenal androgen DHEA have been found in T cells and particularly in activated Th1 subtype of T cells; however, further studies are needed to elucidate their significance.[49]

Testosterone administration in cultures of RA synovial macrophages showed that testosterone was metabolized and was found to inhibit at least IL-1 production.[50,51] Similar inhibition of IL-1 and IL-6 was found on PBMC of RA patients in the presence of testosterone.[52] In contrast, estradiol was found to increase IL-1 secretion in rat peritoneal macrophages and IL-1 and IL-6 production in human PBMC.[53] DHT, the active metabolite of testosterone, has been found to repress the expression and activity of the human IL-6 gene promoter via inhibition of NFkB activity through maintenance of IkBa levels.[54]

Human and murine macrophages exhibit functional cytoplasma and nuclear testosterone receptors, and both site I (high-affinity, low-binding) and site II (low- affinity, high-binding) androgen receptors were found in HLA-DR positive human synovial macrophages.[55] Therefore, in RA, synovial macrophages appear to be the "link" at least between the sex hormone environment (HPG) and the immune response effectors (i.e., cytokine modulation)[30,56,57] (see FIG. 1).

These functional and molecular interactions between the immunological and neuroendocrine circuits are the subject of active and extensive ongoing research and might in the near future offer highly promising strategies for hormone-replacement terapies in RA.[58–60]

REFERENCES

1. FORD, D.K. 1997. Understanding rheumatoid arthritis. J. Rheumatol. **24:** 1464–1466.
2. CUTOLO, M. & S. ACCARDO. 1991. Sex hormones, HLA and rheumatoid arthritis. Clin. Exp. Rheumatol. **9:** 641–646.
3. WILDER, R.L. 1995. Neuroendocrine-immune system interactions and autoimmunity. Annu. Rev. Immunol. **13:** 307–338.
4. CUTOLO, M., A. SULLI, B. SERIOLO *et al.* 1995. Estrogens, the immune response and autoimmunity. Clin. Exp. Rheumatol. **13:** 217–226 .
5. CUTOLO, M. & L. CASTAGNETTA. 1996. Immunomodulatory mechanisms mediated by sex hormones in rheumatoid arthritis. Ann. N.Y. Acad. Sci . **784:** 534–541.

6. MASI, A.T., S.L. FEIGENBAUM & M. CUTOLO. 1995. Integrated hormonal-immunological-vascular ("H-I-V" triad) system interactions in rheumatic diseases. Clin. Exp. Rheumatol. **13:** 203–216.

7. CHROUSOS, G.P. 1995. The hypothalamic-pituitary-adrenal axis and immune-mediated inflammation. N. Engl. J. Med. **332:** 1351–1362.

8. MASI, A.T., J.W.J. BIJLSMA, M. CUTOLO *et al.* 1999. Neuroendocrine, immunologic and microvascular systems interactions in rheumatoid arthritis: physiopathogenic and therapeutic perspectives. Semin. Arthritis Rheum. **29:** 65–81.

9. HALLER, C., B. HOLZNER, E. MUR *et al.* 1997. The impact of life events on patients with rheumatoid arthritis: a psychological myth? Clin. Exp. Rheumatol. **15:** 175–179.

10. MASI, A.T., J.A.P. DA SILVA & M. CUTOLO. 1996. Perturbations of the hypothalamic pituitary gonadal axis in rheumatoid arthritis. *In* Neuroendocrine Immune Mechanisms of Rheumatic Diseases. I.C. Chikanza, Ed. Ballière's Clin. Rheumatol. **10:** 295–331.

11. BESEDOVSKY, H.O. & A. DEL REY. 1996. Immune-neuro-endocrine interactions: facts and hypothesis. Endocr. Rev. **17:** 64–102.

12. PIETRINI, P. & M. GUAZZELLI. 1997. Life events in the course of chronic diseases: a psychological or a psycho-neuro-biochemical loop? Clin. Exp. Rheumatol. **15:** 125–128.

13. GUDBJÖRNSSON, B., B. SKOGSEID, B. ÖBERG *et al.* 1996. Intact adrenocorticotropic hormone secretion but impaired cortisol response in patients with active rheumatoid arthritis. Effect of glucocorticoids. J. Rheumatol. **23:** 596–602.

14. WEST, H.F. 1957. Corticosteroid metabolism and rheumatoid arthritis. Ann. Rheum. Dis. **16:** 173–181.

15. TEMPL, E., M. KOELLER, M. RIEDEL *et al.* 1996. Anterior pituitary function in patients with newly diagnosed rheumatoid arthritis. Br. J . Rheumatol. **35:** 350–356.

16. CROFFORD, L.J., K. KALOGERAS, G. MASTORAKOS *et al.* 1997. Circadian relationship between interleukin (IL)-6 and hypothalamus-pituitary-adrenocortical axis hormones: failure of IL-6 to cause hypercortisolism in patients with early, untreated rheumatoid arthritis. J. Clin. Endocr. Metab. **82:** 1279–1283.

17. MASI, A.T. & G. P. CHROUSOS. 1996. Hypothalamic-pituitary-adrenal-glucocorticoid axis function in rheumatoid arthritis. J. Rheumatol. **23:** 577–581.

18. CUTOLO, M., L. FOPPIANI, C. PRETE *et al.* 1999. Hypothalamic-pituitary-adrenocortical axis function in premenopausal rheumatoid arthritis patients: not treated with glucocorticoids. J. Rheumatol. **26:** 282–288.

19. SUKUKI, N., T. SUZUKI & T. SAKANE. 1996. Hormones and lupus: defective DHEA activity induces impaired interleukin-2 activity of T lymphocytes in patients with systemic lupus erythematosus. Ann. Med. Interne **147:** 248–252.

20. HENNEBOLD, J.D., M.E. POYNTER & R.A. DAYNES. 1995. DHEA and immune function: activities and mechanism of action. Semin. Reprod. Endocrinol. **13:** 257–269.

21. CUTOLO, M., L. FOPPIANI, M. GIUSTI *et al.* 1997. The adrenal response to oCRH and low dose ACTH in premenopausal rheumatoid arthritis patients. Arthritis Rheum. **40:** S253–1331.

22. FOPPIANI, L., A. SULLI, M. CUTOLO *et al.* 1999. Desmopressin, ovine CRH, and low-dose ACTH tests: tools for the study of the hypothalamic-pituitary-adrenal axis in premenopausal rheumatoid arthritis patients. Ann. N.Y. Acad. Sci. **876:** 83-87.

23. CUTOLO, M. 1996. Effects of gonadal androgens on adrenal androgens. Clin. Endocrinol. **44:** 490-491.

24. ARVIDSON, G.N., G. GUDBJØRSSON, L. ELFMAN *et al.* 1994. Circadian rhythm of serum interleukin-6 in rheumatoid arthritis. Ann. Rheum. Dis. **53:** 521–524.

25. BELLIDO, T., R. JILKA, B. BOYCE *et al.* 1995. Regulation of interleukin-6, osteoclastogenesis and bone mass by androgens. J. Clin. Invest. **95:** 2886–2895.

26. KELLER, T., C. CHANG & W.B. ERSHLER. 1996. Inhibition of NFkB activity through maintenence of IkBa levels contributes to dihydrotestosterone-mediated repression of IL-6 promoter. J. Biol. Chem. **271:** 26267–26275.

27. CUTOLO, M., S. ACCARDO, B. VILLAGGIO *et al.* 1996. Androgen and estrogen receptors are present in primary cultures of human synovial macrophages. J. Clin. Endocrinol. Metab. **81:** 820–827.

28. JAMES, W.H. 1997. Further evidence that low androgen values are a cause of rheumatoid arthritis: the response of rheumatoid arthritis to seriously stressful life events. Ann. Rheum. Dis. **56:** 566.

29. CUTOLO, M. 1997. Do sex hormones modulate synovial macrophages in rheumatoid arthritis? Ann. Rheum. Dis. **56:** 281–284.

30. WILDER, R.L. & I.J. ELENKOV. 1999. Hormonal regulation of tumor necrosis factor-α, interleukin-12 and interleukin-10 production by activated macrophages. Ann. N.Y. Acad. Sci. **876:** 14–31.

31. KANDA, N., T. TSICHIDA & K. TAMAKI. 1997. Testosterone suppress anti-DNA antibody production in peripheral blood mononuclear cells from patients with systemic lupus erythematosus. Arthritis Rheum. **40:** 1703–1711.

32. MIRA, D., K. SOOKHYUN & R.R. RHONDA. 1997. Testosterone therapy ameliorates experimental autoimmune encephalomyelitis and induces a T helper 2 bias in the autoantigen-specific T lymphocyte response. J. Immunol. **159:** 3–6.

33. CUTOLO, M. 1998. The role of the hypothalamus-pituitary-adrenocortical and -gonadal axis in rheumatoid arthritis. Clin. Exp. Rheumatol. **16:** 3–6.

34. CUTOLO, M., A. SULLI, B. VILLAGGIO *et al.* 1998. Relations between steroid hormones and cytokines in rheumatoid arthritis and systemic lupus erythematosis. Ann. Rheum. Dis. **57:** 573–577.

35. CHROUSOS, G.P. & P.W. GOLD. 1992. The concepts of stress and stress system disorders: overview of physical and behavioral homeostasis. JAMA **267:** 1244–1252.

36. BRANTLEY, P.J., L.S. DIETZ, G.T. MCKNIGHT *et al.* 1988. Convergence between the daily stress inventory and endocrine measures of stress. J. Consult. Clin. Psychol. **56:** 459–461.

37. CUTOLO, M. 1998. The roles of steroid hormones in arthritis. Br. J. Rheumatol. **37:** 597–601.

38. BESEDOVSKY, H.O. & A. DEL REY. 1996. Immune-neuro-endocrine interactions: facts and hypothesis. Endocr. Rev. **17:** 64–71.

39. WALKER, J.G., G. LITTLEJOHN & M. CUTOLO. 1999. Stress system activation in rheumatoid arthritis: a multilevel approach. Rheumatology. **38:** 1050–1057.

40. MERCENARO, M., C. PRETE, A. SULLI *et al.* 1999. Rheumatoid arthritis, personality, stress response style and copying with illness: a preliminary survey. Ann. N.Y. Acad. Sci. **876:** 419–426.

41. CUTOLO, M., C. PRETE & J. WALKER. 1999. Is stress a factor in the pathogenesis in autoimmune rheumatic diseases? Clin. Exp. Rheum. **17:** 515–518 .

42. BESEDOVSKY, H.O., A.E. DEL REY & E. SORKIN. 1985. Immune-neuroendocrine interactions. J. Immunol. **135:** 750s–754s.

43. MONJAN, A.A. & M.I. COLLECTOR. 1977. Stress-induced modulation of the immune response. Science **196:** 307–308.

44. ZAUTRA, A.J., N.A. HAMILTON, P. POTTER *et al.* 1999. Field research on the relationships between stress and disease activity in rheumatoid arthritis. Ann. N.Y. Acad. Sci. **876:** 397–412.

45. BIJLSMA, J.W.J., M. CUTOLO, A.T. MASI *et al.* 1999. Neuroendocrine immune basis of the rheumatic diseases. Immunol. Today **20:** 298–301.

46. DAYNES, R.A., D.J. DUDLEY & B.A. ARANEO. 1990. Regulation of murine lymphokine production *in vivo*. Dehydroepyandrosterone is a natural enhancer of interleukin 2 synthesis by helper T cells. Eur. J. Immunol. **20:** 793–80I.

47. SUZUKI, T., N. SUZUKI, E.G. ENGLEMAN *et al.* 1995. Low serum levels of dehydroepiandrosterone therapy may cause deficient IL-2 production by lymphocytes in patients with SLE. Clin. Exp. Immunol. **99:** 251–255.

48. BELLIDO, T., R. JILKA, B. BOYCE *et al.* 1995. Regulation of interleukin-6, osteoclastogenesis and bone mass by androgens. J. Clin. Invest. **95:** 2886–2895.

49. ROOK, G.A.W., R. HERNANDEZ-PANDO & S.L. LIGHTMAN. 1994. Hormones, peripherally activated prohormones and regulation of Th1/Th2 balance. Immunol. Today **135:** 301–303.

50. CUTOLO, M., B. VILLAGGIO, A. BARONE *et al.* 1996. Primary cultures of human synovial macrophages metabolize androgens. Ann. N.Y. Acad. Sci. **784:** 237–251.
51. CUTOLO, M., S. ACCARDO, B. VILLAGGIO *et al.* 1993. Cultured synovial macrophages from rheumatoid arthritis synovium metabolize testosterone and exhibit inhibition of IL-1β production. Arthritis Rheum. **36:** S158.
52. LI, Z.G., V.A. DANIS & P.M. BROOKS. 1993. Effect of gonadal steroids on the production of IL-1 and IL-6 by blood mononuclear cells *in vitro.* Clin. Exp. Rheumatol. **11:** 157–162.
53. HU, S.K., Y.L. MITCHO & N.C. RATH. 1987. Effect of estradiol on interleukin-1 synthesis by macrophages. Int. J. Immunopharmacol. **10:** 247–252.
54. KELLER, T., C. CHANG & W.B. ERSHLER. 1996. Inhibition of NFkB activity through maintenance of IkBa levels contributes to dihydrotestosterone-mediated repression of IL-6 promoter. J. Biol. Chem. **271:** 26267–26275.
55. CUTOLO, M., S. ACCARDO, B. VILLAGGIO *et al.* 1992. Evidence for androgen receptors in the synovial tissue of rheumatoid arthritis patients and healthy controls. Arthritis Rheum. **35:** 1007–1015.
56. DA SILVA, J.A.P., A. PINTO, M. CUTOLO *et al.* 1999. Gender differences in adrenal and gonadal responses in inflammatory aggression. Ann. N.Y. Acad. Sci. **876:** 148–151.
57. CUTOLO, M. 1999. Macrophages as effectors of the immunoendocrinologic interactions in autoimmune rheumatic diseases. Ann. N.Y. Acad. Sci. **876:** 32–43.
58. MASI, A.T. & M. CUTOLO. 1995. Perspectives on sex hormones and the systemic rheumatic diseases. Clin. Exp. Rheumatol. **13:** 201–202.
59. HARBUZ, M.S. & D.S. JESSOP. 1999. Is there a defect in cortisol production in rheumatoid arthritis? Rheumatology **38:** 298–302.
60. ROBINZON, B. & M. CUTOLO. 1999. Viewpoint: Should dehydroepiandrosterone (DHEA) replacement therapy be provided with glucocorticoids? Rheumatology **38:** 488–495.

Environmental Factors Favoring the Allergen-specific Th2 Response in Allergic Subjects

MARIE-PIERRE PICCINNI,[a] ENRICO MAGGI, AND SERGIO ROMAGNANI

Department of Internal Medicine, Immunoallergology Unit, University of Florence, 85 viale Morgagni, 50134 Florence, Italy

ABSTRACT: Allergen-reactive type 2 helper T cells (Th2) play a triggering role in the activation and/or recruitment of IgE antibody-producing B cells, mast cells, and eosinophils, i.e., the cellular triad involved in the allergic inflammation. Interleukin (IL)-4 production at the time of antigen presentation to the Th cell is critical for the development of Th2 cells. Other cytokines, such as IL-1 and IL-10, and hormones, such as calcitriol and progesterone, also play a positive role. In contrast, cytokines such as interferon (IFN)-α, IFN-γ, IL-12, and transforming growth factor (TGF)-β, and relaxin play a negative regulatory role on the development of Th2 cells. However, the mechanisms underlying the preferential activation by environmental allergens of Th2 cells in atopic individuals still remain obscure. Some gene products selectively expressed in Th2 cells or selectively controlling the expression of IL-4 have recently been described. Moreover, cytokines and other gene products that dampen the production of IL-4, as well as the development and/or the function of Th2 cells, have been identified. These findings allow us to suggest that the upregulation of genes controlling IL-4 expression and/or abnormalities of regulatory mechanisms of Th2 development and/or function may be responsible for Th2 responses against common environmental allergens in atopic subjects.

INTRODUCTION

Atopy is a genetically determined group of disorders characterized by an increased ability of B lymphocytes to synthesize IgE antibodies against ubiquitous antigens (allergens) able to activate the immune system after inhalation or ingestion, and perhaps after penetration through the skin. IgE antibodies are able to bind to high-affinity Fcϵ receptors (FcϵRI) present on the surface of mast cells/basophils, and allergen-induced FcϵRI cross-linking triggers the release of vasoactive mediators, chemotactic factors, and cytokines that are responsible for the allergic events. In addition, eosinophils also appear to be involved in the pathogenesis of allergic reactions because they usually accumulate at the site of allergic inflammation, and their toxic products significantly contribute to tissue damage.

The mechanisms linking IgE-producing B cells, mast cells/basophils, and eosinophils in the pathogenesis of allergic reactions have remained unclear until distinct subsets of CD4+ T helper (Th) cells, based on their profile of cytokine secretion, were

[a]Address for correspondence: Dr. Marie-Pierre Piccinni, Dipartimento di Medicina Interna- sezione: Immunoallergologia, Viale Morgagni, 85, Firenze 50134, Italy. Voice: +39-055-4271353; fax: +39-055-412867.

mppiccinni@hotmail.com

discovered. At least three different subsets of Th cells have been described in both mouse and man: Th1 cells that produce interleukin (IL)-2, interferon-γ (IFN-γ), and tumor necrosis factor (TNF)-β; Th2 cells that produce IL-4, IL-5, and IL-10; Th0 cells that produce both Th1- and Th2-type cytokines.[1,2] IL-3, GM-CSF, and TNF-α are variably produced by all Th subsets. It is of note that IL-3, IL-4, and IL-10 are growth factors for mast cells, and IL-5 is a selective activating and differentiating factor for eosinophils.[1,2] It has been clearly shown that IgE synthesis results from the collaboration between Th2 cells and B cells.[3] Recently, a less restrictive definition has been introduced for Th1/Th2 cell subsets: Th2 are generally defined as cells able to actively produce IL-4, whereas Th1 cells are cells that have lost this function. The knowledge of Th cell properties has allowed clarification of the mechanisms linking IgE-producing B cells, mast cells/basophils, and eosinophils; this is known as the "Th2 hypothesis" for the pathogenesis of allergic reactions.

REGULATION OF IgE SYNTHESIS

In 1986 it was reported that IL-4 was able to induce the production of IgE and IgG1 by murine B cells stimulated *in vitro* with lipopolysaccharide (LPS), and that its activity was strongly inhibited by IFN-γ.[4] This has been confirmed *in vivo* by injection of a monoclonal anti-IL-4 antibody that abolishes IgE production and, more importantly, also has this effect in IL-4 K.O. mice, which exhibited no IgE synthesis.[5] The role of IL-4 in the induction of human IgE synthesis was shown by the use of T-cell clones.[6,7] Recently, IL-13, a cytokine showing poor homology with IL-4 (30%) but having similar IgE-switching activity, was discovered.[8] It has recently been shown that receptors for IL-4 and IL-13 are distinct, but share a common subunit (γ chain).[9] Even though both IL-4 and IL-13 are sufficient to begin germline transcription through the ε locus, a physical interaction between T and B cells is needed for the expression of mature ε mRNA transcripts and for production of IgE protein (designed "two-signal model" for the induction of human IgE synthesis). Molecule(s) involved in the contact-mediated noncognate signaling required for IgE production has recently been clarified. The most critical signaling is provided by the interaction of CD40 present on the B cell with its ligand (CD40L) expressed by the activated T cell.[10] In addition, the 26-kDa membrane form of TNF-α (m-TNF-α), expressed on activated CD4+ cells, is a molecule associated with productive T-cell/B-cell interactions.[11] Recently, another member of the TNF superfamily, the CD30 ligand (CD30L) was found to be very active in inducing CD40L-independent IgE secretion.[12]

The T-cell/IL-4-dependent IgE synthesis can be modulated by cytokines other than IL-4. IL-2, IL-5, IL-6, TNF-α, and IL-9 enhance IL-4-induced IgE synthesis.[13,14] IL-6 is known to act at a late stage in B cell differentiation with no isotype preference. The mechanisms responsible for the enhancing effect of IL-2 and TNF-α on IgE synthesis are not completely clear. Both cytokines are indeed active in the proliferation of both T and B lymphocytes, as well as in the differentiation of B cells into antibody-producing cells.[15] Factors, such as IFN-α, IFN-γ, TGF-β, IL-8, IL-10, IL-12, PAF-acether, and prostaglandin E_2 have been shown to downregulate IgE synthesis.[6,7,16–20] IFN-γ profoundly suppressed the expression of ε germline transcripts in murine B cells stimulated with LPS plus IL-4, whereas no inhibition was observed when IFN-γ was added to highly purified human B cells stimulated with IL-4, suggesting that activation of ε germline transcription and switch recombination may not be associated. The ability of IL-8 to block spontaneous IgE synthesis appeared to be mediated by its ability to decrease the production of IL-6 and TNF-α.[17] On the other hand, IL-10 blocks IgE synthesis by peripheral mononuclear cells by inhibiting some monocyte functions, but, conversely, it also directly stimulates B cells cultured in the presence of IL-4 and anti-CD40 mAbs cross-linked to CD32 (FcγRII) on murine L cells.[8,21] The mechanism responsible for the inhibitory activity of IL-12 on IgE synthesis is probably mediated by IFN-γ, because IL-12 is a powerful inducer of IFN-γ by T and NK cells.[22]

ROLE OF TH2 CELLS IN ATOPY

Evidence exists that Th2-like cells accumulate at the level of target organs in different allergic disorders by using either cloning techniques or *in situ* hybridization. The majority of T-cell clones generated from the conjunctival infiltrates of patients with vernal conjunctivitis were found to develop into Th2 clones.[23] Using *in situ* hybridization, cells showing mRNA for Th2 cytokines, but not for Th1, were detected at the site of late-phase skin reactions in skin biopsies from atopic patients, in mucosal bronchial biopsies or bronchoalveolar lavage (BAL) from patients with asthma,[24,25] and after local allergen challenge in nasal mucosa of patients with allergen-induced rhinitis.[26] Likewise, increased levels of IL-4 and IL-5 were measured in the BAL of allergic asthmatics, whereas in nonallergic asthmatics IL-2 and IL-5 predominated.[27]

Inhaled allergens induce activation and recruitment of allergen-specific Th2 cells in the airway mucosa of patients with respiratory allergy and in the skin of patients with atopic dermatitis (AD) taken after contact challenge with dermatophagoides pteronyssinus (DP), suggesting that transcutaneous sensitization to aeroallergens may be essential in the induction of skin lesions in patients with AD.

Recently, we have shown that CD30, a member of the TNF-R superfamily, is preferentially expressed by T-cell clones able to produce Th2-type cytokines.[28,29] No CD4+CD30+ cells were detected in any nonatopic or atopic donors examined before the grass pollination season, whereas the majority of grass-sensitive donors assessed during the season showed small proportions of circulating CD4+CD30+ cells (from 0.08 to 0.3%). When sorted into CD30+ and CD30– cells, only CD30+ cells proliferated in response to Lolium perenne (Lol p 1) and exhibited the ability to produce IL-4 and IL-5, whereas production of Th1-cytokines were prevalent in the CD30– cell fractions.[29] These findings demonstrate that grass allergen-reactive CD4+CD30+ Th2 cells can circulate in the peripheral blood of grass-sensitive patients during the *in vivo* natural exposure to grass pollen allergens.

MECHANISMS INVOLVED IN THE
REGULATION OF TH2 DEVELOPMENT

The mechanisms responsible for the preferential development of allergen-reactive Th2 cells in atopic subjects have not yet been completely clarified. Attention has been focused on the possible role of antigen-presenting cells (APC), the T cell repertoire, and soluble factors present in the microenvironment at the time of allergen presentation. It has been suggested that atopic patients with asthma have higher numbers of intraepithelial dendritic cells than nonasthmatic subjects and that these cells (in the presence of allergen) can trigger T cells to release IL-4 and IL-5.[30] However, the actual role of APC in driving the development of allergen-reactive Th2-like cells remains obscure.

The role of hormones in promoting the differentiation of Th cells or in favoring the shifting of differentiated Th cells from one to another cytokine profile has also been suggested. Glucocorticoids enhance Th2 activity and synergize with IL-4, whereas dehydroepiandrostenone sulfate enhances Th1 activity.[31] Another major prohormone, 25-hydroxy cholecalciferol [25 (OH) vitamin D3] may have a reverse effect on the Th1/Th2 balance. The intense conversion of 25 (OH) vitamin D3 to 1,25 (OH)2 vitamin D3 (calcitriol) decreases secretion of IL-2 and IFN-γ and increases a Th2 pattern of response.[31] Lastly, progesterone favors the *in vitro* development of human T cells producing Th2-type cytokines and promotes both IL-4/IL-5 production and membrane CD30 expression in established human Th1 clones.[32] It represents one of the mechanisms involved in the Th1/Th2 switch occurring at the maternal-fetal interface in order to promote successful pregnancy.[33] The mechanisms by which the maternal immune system does not reject the fetus during pregnancy despite the presence of paternal histocompatibility antigens, are still unclear. Because Th1-type cytokines (IFN-γ, TNF-β) promote allograft rejection and may compromise pregnancy, the production of Th2-type cytokines (i.e., IL-4 and IL-10) which inhibit Th1 responses has been suggested to account for allograft tolerance and fetus survival. We demonstrated that progesterone, a hormone that is locally produced at high levels during pregnancy, favors the development of both IL-4- and LIF-producing cells.[33,34] LIF is a cytokine involved in the successful implantation of blastocyst. Interestingly, we recently found that relaxin, another hormone produced by corpus luteum during pregnancy, also influences the cytokine profile of CD4+ effector T cells by upregulating the production of IFN-γ.[35] Based on these findings, we suggest that a hormonal-cytokine network at the level of maternal-fetal interface plays an important role in both blastocyst implantation and maintenance of successful pregnancy.[34] Therefore, during fetal life, a maternal environment could favor a Th2-skewed priming at the moment that aeroallergen sensitization occurs.[37]

IL-10 and IL-1[36] favor the development of Th2-like clones. IL-6 produced by APC has been found to be one of the Th2-skewing factors in the primary response.[38] In both murine and human systems, IL-4 appears to be the most dominant factor in determining the likelihood for Th2 polarization in cultured cells.[39,40] Accordingly, IL-4–gene-targeted mice fail to generate mature Th2 cells *in vivo* and to produce IgE antibodies,[41] suggesting that early IL-4 production by other cell types is involved.

One of the most intriguing points is the source of IL-4 in the primary response capable of modulating Th2 differentiation. Possible candidates include mast cells and basophils, CD4+NK1.1+, T-cell subset or the T helper cells themselves.[42]

GENETIC ALTERATIONS FAVORING THE ALLERGEN-SPECIFIC TH2-RESPONSES IN ATOPIC PATIENTS

The new insights on the pathogenesis of allergic disorders allows to hypothesize that the preferential development of allergen-specific Th2-like responses in atopic subjects is determined by the genetic dysregulation of atopic subjects at the level of Th-cell-derived IL-4. It is supported by several observations: (1) CD4+ T-cell clones from atopic individuals are able to produce noticeable amounts of IL-4 and IL-5 in response to bacterial antigens, usually evoking Th1-like responses in nonatopic individuals;[43] (2) atopic donors have a higher frequency of IL-4-producing T cells when compared to normal subjects;[44] (3) T-cell clones generated from cord blood lymphocytes of newborns with atopic parents produce higher IL-4 concentrations than these from newborns with nonatopic parents;[45] and (4) peptide-specific T-cell clones generated from donors with high IgE serum levels produced high amounts of IL-4 and low IFN-γ, whereas T-cell clones generated from "low IgE" donors showed a Th1-like profile.

Genetic mechanisms underlying heightened IgE responsiveness seen in the atopic diseases may be divided into two types, antigen-specific and non-antigen-specific.[46] In the past the possible role of MHC class II molecules has been extensively investigated by both genetic and molecular approaches. Significant associations between some HLA haplotypes and specific immune responses to different allergens (such as Amb a V, Amb a VI, and Lol p I, II and III) have been observed.[46] However, weaker associations for other allergens have been reported, thus suggesting that class II molecules on APC can play a permissive role in the binding of allergen peptides, but other non-MHC-associated genes are more important in the overall IgE immune responsiveness to allergens (prevalent Th2-type response). A recent finding has shown a linkage of overall IgE to markers in chromosome 5q31.1, expecially to the IL-4 gene.[46]

The entire IL-4 gene has been scanned for possible atopy-associated polymorphisms based on the hypothesis that they may reside in transcriptional regulatory elements.[46] Analysis of the IL-4 promoter has revealed functionally important binding sites for several transcription factors (including NF-AT, CCAAT box binding protein NF-Y, Oct 1, HMGI(Y), AP-1 members, NF-kB, and an as yet unpurified factor termed PCC) and silencer elements (that bind factors termed NRE).[48] Moreover, the nuclear extracts from individuals with atopic dermatitis exhibited a higher affinity for a consensus P-element, suggesting that polymorphic residues in NF-AT family members themselves or in their posttranslationally modified versions may be involved.[44] More recently, it has been shown that the proto-oncogene c-*Maf*, a transcription factor, controls tissue-specific expression of IL-4. c-*Maf* is expressed in Th2 but not Th1 clones and is induced during normal precursor cell differentiation along a Th2 but not Th1 lineage.[49] These data indicate that *c-Maf* is a factor responsible for dictating Th2-selective IL-4 gene transcription and make c-*Maf* as an obvious candidate for an atopy gene. Another good candidate for an atopy gene is STAT6, a protein that binds to DNA sequences found in the promoters of IL-4–responsive genes.[50] The experiments on K.O. mice have shown that this member of the STAT family of proteins is required for the development of Th2 cells.[51,52] Moreover, it has been shown that the transcription factor GATA-3 is necessary for Th2 cytokine gene expression in CD4 T cells.

Downregulation of the mechanisms dampening IL-4 production can also be involved in the development of prevalent Th2 responses in atopy. IL-12 induces tyrosine phosphorylation and DNA-binding of STAT3 and STAT4.[53] STAT-deficient mice have impaired Th1 development and show enhanced ability to develop Th2 cells.[54] A locus that controls the maintenance of IL-12 responsiveness, and therefore favors the preferential development of Th1 cells, has recently been described in B10.D2 mice.[55] This locus maps on a region of chromosome 11, which is syntenic with the locus on human chromosome 5q31.1, shown to be associated with elevated serum IgE levels.[46] Several other genes map within 5q31.1, including possible candidates which might influence IgE production. One of them is IRF1, whose gene product upregulates IFN-α, which downregulates IgE production and inhibits Th2 cell development, and IL12B, which encodes the β chain of IL-12, another downregulator of Th2 cells.

Either alterations of molecular mechanisms directly involved in the regulation of IL-4 gene expression, or deficient regulatory activity of cytokines responsible for inhibition of Th2-cell development, or both, may account for the the preferential Th2-type response in atopic people and for the production by Th2 cells of the cytokines involved in the allergic inflammation, and therefore may explain the persistent histological, pathophysiological, and clinical aspects of allergic disorders.

CONCLUDING REMARKS

Evidence exists that suggests allergen-reactive Th2 cells play a essential role in the activation and/or recruitment of IgE antibody-producing B cells, mast cells and eosinophils, the cellular triad involved in allergic inflammation. Th2 cells provide B cell help for IgE isotype with at least two signals: soluble IL-4 and a T-B cell-to-cell physical interaction, occurring between the CD40L expressed on the activated Th cell and the CD40 molecule on the B cell. The Th2-cell-derived IL-4 induces germline e expression on the B cell, whereas the CD40L/CD40 interaction is required for the expression of productive mRNA and for the synthesis of IgE protein. Other soluble factors produced by both T cells and non-T cells have also been shown to have negative or positive regulatory effects on the human IgE synthesis. Th2 cells are generated from precursor naive Th cells when they encounter the specific antigen in an IL-4-containing microenvironment. Several gene products expressed in Th2 cells selectively or controlling selectively the expression of IL-4 have recently been described. This suggests that the upregulation of genes controlling IL-4 expression and/or abnormalities in the regulatory mechanisms of Th2 development and function may be responsible for Th2 responses against common environmental allergens in atopic people. These findings provide opportunities for the development of novel immunotherapeutic strategies for atopic diseases.

REFERENCES

1. MOSMANN, T.R. *et al.* 1989. TH1 and TH2 cells: different patterns of lymphokine secretion lead to different functional properties. Annu. Rev. Immunol. **7:** 145–173.
2. ROMAGNANI, S. 1994. Lymphokine production by human T cells in disease states. Annu. Rev. Immunol. **12:** 227–257.
3. VERCELLI, D. *et al.* 1991. Regulation of IgE synthesis in humans: a tale of two signals. J. Allergy Clin. Immunol. **8:** 285–295.
4. COFFMAN, R.L. *et al.* 1986. A T cell activity that enhances polyclonal IgE production and its inhibition by interferon. J. Immunol. **136:** 949–954.
5. KUHN, R. *et al.* 1991. Generation and analysis of IL-4-deficient mice. Science **254:** 707–710.
6. DEL PRETE, G.F. *et al.* 1988. IL-4 is an essential factor for the IgE synthesis induced *in vitro* by human T cell clones and their supernatants. J. Immunol. **140:** 4193–4198.
7. PENE, J. *et al.* 1988. IgE production by normal human B cells is induced by interleukin 4 and suppressed by interferon γ and α and prostaglandin E2. Proc. Natl. Acad. Sci. USA **85:** 6880–6884.
8. PUNNONEN, J. *et al.* 1993. Interleukin 13 induces interleukin 4-independent IgG4 and IgE synthesis and CD23 expression by human B cells. Proc. Natl. Acad. Sci. USA **90:** 3730–3734.
9. ZURAWSKI, G. *et al.* 1994. Interleukin 13, an interleukin 4-like cytokine that acts on monocytes and B cells, but not on T cells. Immunol. Today **15:** 19–26.
10. ARMITAGE, R. *et al.* 1992. Molecular and biological characterization of a murine ligand for CD40. Nature **357:** 80–82.
11. AVERSA, G. *et al.* 1993. The 26-kD transmembrane from tumor necrosis factor α on activated CD4+ T cell clones provides a co-stimulatory signal for human B-cell activation. J. Exp. Med. **177:** 1575–1585.
12. SHANEBECK, K.D. *et al.* 1995. Regulation of murine B cell growth and differentiation by CD30 ligand. Eur. J. Immunol. **25:** 2147–2153.
13. PUNNONEN, J. *et al.* 1994. Role of interleukin-4 and interleukin-13 in synthesis of IgE and expression of CD23 by human B cells. Allergy **49:** 576–586.
14. DUGAS, B. *et al.* 1993. Interleukin-9 potentiates the interleukin-4-induced immunoglobulin (IgG, IgM and IgE) production by normal human B lymphocytes. Eur. J. Immunol. **23:** 1687–1692.
15. VAN KOOTEN, C. *et al.* 1992. Both naive and memory T cells can provide help for human IgE production, but with different cytokine requirements. Eur. Cytokine Netw. **3:** 289–297.
16. GAUCHAT, J.-F. *et al.* 1992. Modulation of IL-4-induced germline e RNA synthesis in human B cells by tumor necrosis factor-α, anti-CD40 monoclonal antibodies or transforming growth factor-β correlates with levels of IgE production. Int. Immunol. **4:** 397–406.
17. KIMATA, H. *et al.* 1992. Interleukin 8 (IL-8) selectively inhibits immunoglobulin E production induced by IL-4 in human B cells. J. Exp. Med. **176:** 1227–1231.
18. PUNNONEN, J. *et al.* 1993. IL-10 and viral IL-10 prevent IL-4-induced IgE synthesis by inhibiting the accessory cell function of monocytes. J. Immunol. **151:** 1280–1289.
19. KINIWA, M. *et al.* 1992. Recombinant interleukin-12 suppresses the synthesis of immunoglobulin E by interleukin-4 stimulated human lymphocytes. J. Clin. Invest. **90:** 262–266.
20. DERYCKX, S. *et al.* 1992. Immunoregulatory functions of paf-acether. VIII. Inhibition of IL-4-induced human IgE synthesis. J. Immunol. **148:** 1465–1470.
21. ROUSSET, F. *et al.* 1992. Interleukin-10 is a potent growth and differentiation factor for activated human B lymphocytes. Proc. Natl. Acad. Sci. USA **89:** 1890–1894.
22. CHEHIMI, J. *et al.* 1995. Interleukin-12: a bridge between innate resistance and adaptive immunity with a role in infection and acquired immunodeficiency. J. Clin. Immunol. **14:** 149–161.
23. MAGGI, E. *et al.* 1991. Accumulation of Th2-like helper T cells in the conjunctiva of patients with vernal conjunctivitis. J. Immunol. **146:** 1169–1174.

24. KAY, A.B. *et al.* 1991. Messenger RNA expression of the cytokine gene cluster, interleukin 3 (IL-3), IL-4, IL-5, and granulocyte/macrophage colony-stimulating factor, in allergen-induced late-phase cutaneous reactions in atopic subjects. J. Exp. Med. **173:** 775–778.
25. ROBINSON, D.S. *et al.* 1992. Predominant Th2-like bronchoalveolar T-lymphocyte population in atopic asthma. N. Engl. J. Med. **326:** 295–304.
26. BRADDING, P. *et al.* 1993. Immunolocalization of cytokines in the nasal mucosa of normal and perennial rhinitic subjects: the mast cells as a source of IL-4, IL-5, and IL-6 in human allergic mucosal inflammation. J. Immunol. **151:** 3853–3860.
27. WALKER, C. *et al.* 1992. Allergic and nonallergic asthmatic have distinct patterns of T-cell activation and cytokine production in peripheral blood and bronchoalveolar lavage. Am. Rev. Respir. Dis. **146:** 109–115.
28. SMITH, C.A. *et al.* 1993. CD30 Antigen, a marker for Hodgkin's lymphoma, is a receptor whose ligand defines an emerging family of cytokines with homology to TNF. Cell **73:** 1349–1360.
29. DEL PRETE, G.-F. *et al.* 1995. Preferential expression of CD30 by human CD4+ T cells producing Th2-type cytokines. FASEB J. **9:** 81-86.
30. SCHON-HEGRAD, M.A. *et al.* 1991. Studies on the density, distribution and surface phenotype of intraepithelial class II MHC (Ia) antigen-bearing dendritic cells in the conductive airways. J. Exp. Med. **173:** 1345–1356.
31. ROOK, G.A.W. *et al.* 1994. Hormones, peripherally activated prohormones and regulation of the Th1/Th2 balance. Immunol. Today **15:** 301–303.
32. PICCINNI, M.-P. *et al.* 1995. Progesterone favors the development of human T helper (Th) cells producing Th2-type cytokines and promotes both IL-4 production and membrane CD30 expression in established Th1 clones. J. Immunol. **155:** 128–133.
33. PICCINNI, M.-P. *et al.* 1998. Defective production of both leukemia inhibitory factor and type 2 T-helper cytokines by decidual T cells in unexplained recurrent abortions. Nature Med. **9:** 1020-1024.
34. PICCINNI, M.-P. *et al.* 1996. Regulation of fetal allograft survival by hormone-controlled Th1 and Th2-type cytokines. Immunol. Res. **15:** 141–150.
35. PICCINNI, M.-P. *et al.* 1999. Relaxin favors the development of activated human T cells into Th1-like effectors. Eur. J. Immunol. **29:** 2241–2247.
36. MANETTI, R. *et al.* 1994. Interleukin-1 favors the *in vitro* development of type 2 T helper (Th2) human T-cell clones. Res. Immunol. **145:** 93–100.
37. PICCINNI, M.-P. *et al.* 1993. Aeroallergen sensitization can occur during fetal life. Int. Arch. Allergy Immunol. **102:** 301–303.
38. RINCON, M. *et al.* 1997. Interleukin-(IL)-6 directs the differentiation of IL-4-producing CD4+ T cells. J. Exp. Med. **185:** 461–469.
39. MAGGI, E. *et al.* 1992. Reciprocal regulatory role of IFN-γ and IL-4 on the *in vitro* development of human Th1 and Th2 cells. J. Immunol. **148:** 2142–2147.
40. SWAIN, S.L. *et al.* 1990. IL-4 directs the development of Th2-like helper effectors. J. Immunol. **145:** 3796–3806.
41. KOPF, M. *et al.* 1993. Disruption of the murine IL-4 gene blocks Th2 cytokine responses. Nature **362:** 245–248.
42. PICCINNI, M.P. *et al.* 1991. Human bone marrow non-B, non-T cells produce interleukin-4 in response to cross-linkage of Fcε and Fcγ receptors. Proc. Natl. Acad. Sci. USA **88:** 8656–8660.
43. PARRONCHI, P. *et al.* 1992. Aberrant interleukin (IL)-4 and IL-5 production *in vitro* by CD4+ helper T cells from atopic subjects. Eur. J. Immunol. **22:** 1615–1620.
44. CHAN, S.C. *et al.* 1996. Abnormal IL-4 gene expression by atopic dermatitis T lymphocytes is reflected in altered nuclear protein interactions with IL-4 transcriptional regulatory element. J. Dermatol. Invest. **106:** 1131–1136.
45. PICCINNI, M.P. *et al.* 1996. Abnormal production of Th2-type cytokines (IL-4 and IL-5) by T cells from newborns with atopic parents. Eur. J. Immunol. **26:** 2293–2298.
46. MARSH, D.G. *et al.* 1994. Linkage analysis of IL-4 and other chromosome 5q31.1 markers and total serum immunoglobulin E concentrations. Science **264:** 1152–1156.

47. ROSENWASSER, L.J. *et al.* 1995. Promoter polymorphisms in the chromosome 5 gene cluster in asthma and atopy. Clin. Exp. Allergy **25:** 74–78.
48. LI-WEBER, M. *et al.* 1992. T cell-specific negative regulation of transcription of the human cytokine IL-4. J. Immunol. **148:** 1913–1918.
49. HO, C.I. *et al.* 1996. The proto-oncogene c-maf is responsible for tissue-specific expression of interleukin-4. Cell **85:** 973–983.
50. LEDERER, J.A. *et al.* 1996. Regulation of NF-kB activation in T helper 1 and T helper 2 cells. J. Immunol. 156: 56–63.
51. TAKEDA, K. *et al.* 1996. Essential role of Stat6 in IL-4 signalling. Nature **380:** 627–630.
52. SHIMODA, K. *et al.* 1996. Lack of IL-4-induced Th2 response and IgE class switching in mice with disrupted Stat6 gene. Nature **380:** 630–632.
53. BACON, C.M. *et al.* 1995. Interleukin 12 (IL-12) induces tyrosine phosphorylation of JAK2 and TYK2: differential use of Janus family tyrosine kinases by IL-2 and IL-12. J. Exp. Med. **181:** 399–404.
54. KAPLAN, M.H. *et al.* 1996. STAT 6 is required for mediating responses to IL-4 and for development of Th2 cells. Immunity **4:** 313–319.
55. GORHAM, J.D. *et al.* 1996. Genetic mapping of a locus controlling development of Th1/Th2 type responses. Proc. Natl. Acad. Sci. USA **93:** 12467–12472.

Conditioning Rhinitis in Allergic Humans

JUDITH E. BARRETT,[a,d] MAURICE G. KING,[b] AND GERALD PANG[c]

[a]Department of Psychology, University of Newcastle, NSW, 2308, Australia

[b]Institute for Behavioural Research in Health, Curtin University of Technology, WA, 6845, Australia

[c]Faculty of Medicine, University of Newcastle, NSW, 2308, Australia

ABSTRACT: A classical Pavlovian paradigm pairing an olfactory cue with allergen challenge for a single training trial was used to produce conditioned histamine release and conditioned nasal airflow decrease in seasonal allergic rhinitis sufferers. There was no conditioned increase in subjective symptoms. Histamine release and airflow decrease showed evidence of extinction by a second test trial. A second study comparing the effects of the number of training trials showed that three training trials produced greater histamine release and airflow decrease than a single training trial, suggesting stronger effects with additional training.

INTRODUCTION

Pavlovian conditioning of the immediate hypersensitivity response was first demonstrated in animal studies.[1,2,3] Gauci et al.[4] used human sufferers of perennial rhinitis to study conditioned release of the mast cell mediator, tryptase, by pairing a distinctive drink with nasal allergen challenge for a single training trial. Reexposure to the drink with placebo challenge resulted in an increase in mast cell tryptase, but no increase in subjectively rated symptoms.

The present studies used nasal challenge with seasonal grass allergens to investigate conditioning of the immediate hypersensitivity reaction in hay fever (seasonal allergic rhinitis) sufferers. An olfactory cue was used as the conditioned stimulus (CS) to simulate the environmental occurrence of allergens and facilitate conditioning through belongingness of stimuli or preparedness of associations.[5,6] Salience of the odor CS was further enhanced by requiring subjects to report on the odor qualities. Responses assessed were release of histamine, the predominant preformed mediator present in mast cells, as well as the physiological response of peak nasal inspiratory airflow, and subjective symptoms.

The first study used an independent groups design and a classical Pavlovian paradigm with a single training trial followed by two test (extinction) trials. Control groups were limited to three in consideration not only of volunteer availability and processing time required but also of the ethical considerations of exposing humans to unpleasant procedures carrying some risk of severe reactions. When the first study

[d]Address for correspondence: J.E. Barrett, Information Technology Division, Defence Science and Technology Organisation, PO Box 1500, Salisbury, SA, 5108, Australia. Voice: +61 8 8259 5445; fax: +61 8 8259 5589.

judy.barrett@dsto.defence.gov.au

had shown that a conditioned response could be learned with a single training trial, a second study used the same conditioning procedures to compare the effects of one, two, or three training trials on the response measures. The training trials were again followed by two extinction trials.

METHODS

Subjects for both experiments were otherwise healthy volunteers who suffered from seasonal allergic rhinitis, and whose allergic status was confirmed by a positive result to skin prick test with seasonal Grass Mix #7 test allergen (Miles Inc., Elkhart, USA).

For Experiment 1, subjects were randomly allocated to one of four groups: placebo control, CS control, conditioning (experimental), and UCS control groups. These groups allowed controls for effects of the procedure, the olfactory CS, and any environmental cues. Subjects were tested individually in sessions approximately one week apart, with timing of session controlling for possible circadian effects. The experimental protocol is summarized in TABLE 1.

For Experiment 2, subjects were randomly allocated to groups that were to receive either one, two, or three training trials, with each group then receiving two test (extinction) trials. The experimental protocol is summarized in TABLE 2.

Testing session procedures were the same for both experiments. Peak nasal inspiratory flow (PNIF) was recorded with a Youlten Meter (Clement Clarke International, London), nasal washing carried out in the manner first described by Naclerio et al.,[7] and subjective symptom scores (SSS) assessed using a Visual Analogue Scale for each of 10 symptoms. Subjects who were administered the olfactory CS were given standardized instructions before the odor (provided by 10 mL benzaldehyde in a brown glass bottle) was presented, and after the allergen or placebo drops were placed in their nostrils they completed a form rating the odor qualities. For each session, recordings of SSS and PNIF, and a nasal washing were carried out prechallenge and again at 5- and 15-min postchallenge, after which the postchallenge PNIF was recorded.

The histamine assay used was adapted from the enzymatic–isotopic microassay described by Taylor et al.,[8] with modifications made for the low levels of histamine in nasal washing samples. For the present studies samples were first concentrated by freeze-drying and resuspension in distilled water. Other assay modifications included use of a higher specific activity methyl donor, S-adenosyl-L-[methyl-^{3}H] methionine (^{3}H-SAME, 15 Ci/mmol, from Amersham Australia).

TABLE 1. Experimental protocol for single-trial conditioning study

Group	Conditioning	Test 1	Test 2
Placebo control	No CS, Plac	No CS, Plac	No CS, Plac
CS control	CS, Plac	CS, Plac	CS, Plac
Experimental	CS, All	CS, Plac	CS, Plac
UCS control	No CS, All	No CS, Plac	No CS, Plac

NOTE: $n = 15$ for each group. All, allergen; plac, placebo.

TABLE 2. **Experimental protocol for study of additional training trials**

	Conditioning Trials			Test Trials	
Group	1	2	3	1	2
One trial	CS, All	—	—	CS, Plac	CS, Plac
Two trial	CS, All	CS, All	—	CS, Plac	CS, Plac
Three trial	CS, All	CS, All	CS, All	CS, Plac	CS, Plac

NOTE: $n = 5$ for each group. All, allergen; plac, placebo.

RESULTS

Experiment 1

As with previous research,[4] histamine levels and symptoms were measured as peak increases from prechallenge. PNIF was measured as decrease from prechallenge. Each dependent measure was analyzed as a 4×3 (Group $\times$ Trial) mixed two-factor analysis of variance, and within-subject degrees of freedom adjusted using the Greenhouse-Geisser ε factor.[9] Significant interactions were examined by simple effects analyses, and followed up with planned linear comparisons.

FIGURE 1 illustrates the significant differences in histamine release between groups and across trials. On the conditioning trial, contrasts showed the only significant effect to be that of allergen challenge ($F(1,164) = 77.28, p < 0.001$). On the first test trial, the experimental group released more histamine than the placebo and CS

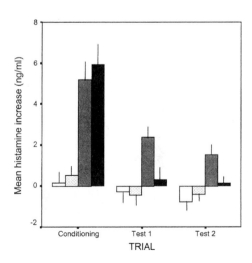

FIGURE 1. Mean increase in histamine relese measured from nasal washings in response to allergen or placebo challenge for each group on the conditioning trial and each of the two test trials. Group: ☐, placebo control; ▨, CS control; ▨, conditioned; ■, UCS control. Error bars show SEM.

controls ($F(1,164) = 14.19$, $p < 0.001$) or the UCS control ($F(1,164) = 6.15$, $p < 0.02$), confirming conditioned histamine release. The UCS control did not differ from other controls. On the second test trial, the experimental group differed from placebo and CS controls ($F(1,164) = 8.23$, $p < 0.01$), but not from the UCS control, and control groups did not differ from each other.

FIGURE 2 shows the similar significant differences in PNIF. The planned contrasts again showed the significant effect of allergen challenge ($F(1,147) = 124.67$, $p < 0.001$) on the conditioning trial. On the first test trial, the experimental group had a significantly greater decrease in PNIF than did the placebo and CS controls ($F(1,147) = 12.95$, $p < 0.001$) or the UCS control ($F(1,147) = 5.37$, $p < 0.05$), while the control groups did not differ from each other. On the second test trial the experimental group and controls did not differ.

SSS were summed for the 10 individual symptoms. While the overall analysis showed a significant difference between groups, trials, and a significant interaction, the simple effects analysis showed that the groups differed only for the conditioning trial ($F(3,150) = 20.77$, $p < 0.001$), indicating that there was no conditioned increase in subjective symptoms.

On the conditioning trial, histamine increase was correlated with PNIF decrease ($r = 0.68$, $df = 58$, $p < 0.001$) and with SSS increase ($r = 0.52$, $df = 58$, $p < 0.001$). However, on the first test trial only histamine and PNIF were correlated ($r = 0.27$, $df = 58$, $p < 0.05$), since neither was correlated with SSS.

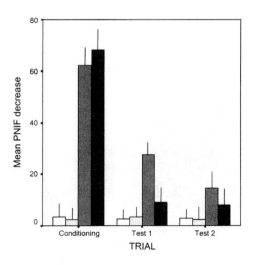

FIGURE 2. Mean decrease in peak nasal inspiratory flow in response to allergen or placebo challenge for each group on the conditioning trial and each of the two test trials. Units of PNIF approximate to liters/min, but cannot be considered absolute due to meter design. Group: □, placebo control; ▨, CS control; ▓, conditioned; ■, UCS control. Error bars show SEM.

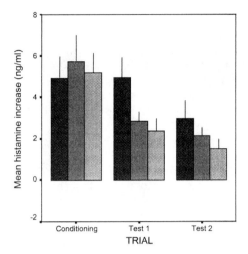

FIGURE 3. Mean increase in histamine release measured from nasal washings in response to allergen or placebo challenge for each group on the first conditioning trial and each of the two test trials. Group: ■, three trial conditioned; ▨, two trial conditioned; ▨, one trial conditioned. Error bars show SEM.

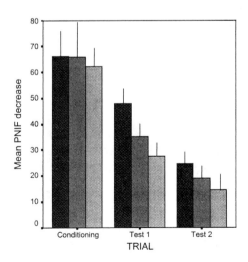

FIGURE 4. Mean decrease in peak nasal inspiratory flow in response to allergen or placebo challenge for each group on the first conditioning trial and each of the two test trials. Units of PNIF approximate to liters/min, but cannot be considered absolute due to meter design. Group: ■, three trial conditioned; ▨, two trial conditioned; ▨, one trial conditioned. Error bars show SEM.

Experiment 2

Peak increase in histamine, PNIF, and SSS were each analyzed by one-way analysis of variance for the first conditioning trial, and for the first and second test trials. FIGURE 3 presents the results for histamine release, which showed no difference between groups on the conditioning trial. On the first test trial the groups differed significantly $(F(2,42) = 3.73, p < 0.05)$, with Fisher's least significant difference (LSD) showing the three-training-trial group to have a greater increase in histamine than either the two- $(p < 0.05)$ or single-training-trial group $(p < 0.05)$. The groups receiving one and two training trials did not differ. On the second test trial there was no difference between the groups.

FIGURE 4 shows the pre- to postchallenge decrease in PNIF for the compared trials. Again the groups did not differ for the conditioning trial, while there was a significant difference for the first test trial $(F(2,42) = 3.79, p < 0.05)$. Fisher's LSD indicated that the three-training-trial group had a greater PNIF decrease than the single-training-trial group $(p < 0.05)$, while the two-training-trial group did not differ significantly from the others. The apparently similar trend on the second test trial was not significant.

The analyses of peak increase in SSS for the first conditioning, and first and second test trials, showed that the groups did not differ for any of the compared trials.

DISCUSSION

The results of the first experiment gave evidence of conditioning of an immediate hypersensitivity response in hay fever sufferers. Following a single conditioning trial, in which an olfactory cue was paired with nasal allergen challenge, reexposure to the cue alone resulted in an increase in histamine release accompanied by a decrease in peak nasal inspiratory flow, but no increase in subjective symptoms. Both conditioned responses were a little less than half the magnitude of the unconditioned responses to allergen. A similar result for both the physiological and the biochemical measure, and the correlation between the two, support the validity of the conditioning.

These results are in agreement with those of Gauci et al.,[4] who found a conditioned increase in mast cell tryptase after a single training trial, an increase of approximately one-third the magnitude of the unconditioned response. The Gauci study also found no conditioned increase in subjective symptoms. The results are also consistent with animal studies of conditioned release of histamine[1,2] and rat mast cell protease II,[3] although following the several training trials given in these studies, the conditioned release was of a magnitude comparable to the response to allergen.

The larger conditioned effects found in the animal studies after several cue pairings are consistent with the findings of the second experiment. This study showed that, compared to a single cue pairing, three pairings of the olfactory cue with grass allergen challenge resulted in stronger histamine release and airflow decrease on first reexposure to the cue. For histamine release this stronger effect was comparable in size to the response to allergen, while for airflow decrease, it was approximately three-quarters the unconditioned effect. By the second reexposure, the groups receiving different training no longer differed. However, to confirm that these stronger effects were true conditioned responses requires further experimentation with appropriate controls.

The first experiment also demonstrated the effectiveness of the olfactory CS in eliciting a conditioned response, as the UCS control group that differed from the experimental group only by the absence of the olfactory cue showed no conditioned responses. This suggests that there was no learned response to environmental cues alone and is consistent with predictions of preparedness or belongingness theory.

As can be seen in FIGURES 1 and 2, the histamine and airways responses conditioned with a single training trial were considerably reduced by the second test trial, and no longer differed significantly from controls. This indicates that they were undergoing rapid extinction, and suggests that responses learned with a single training trial are not robust. Further studies could show whether stronger responses learned with additional training were more resistant to extinction.

In conclusion, by concurrently conditioning both histamine release and airflow decrease, the first experiment provided evidence of Pavlovian conditioning in humans of an IgE-mediated immediate hypersensitivity response. It also showed the responses to be undergoing extinction by a second test trial. The second experiment provided suggestive evidence that learned responses can be strengthened by additional training.

REFERENCES

1. RUSSELL, M., K.A. DARK, R.W. CUMMINS, G. ELLMAN, E. CALLAWAY & H.V.S. PEEKE. 1984. Learned histamine release. Science **225:** 733–734.
2. PEEKE, H.V.S., K. DARK, G. ELLMAN, C. McCURRY & M. SALFI. 1987. Prior stress and behaviorally conditioned histamine release. Physiol. Behav. **39:** 89–93.
3. MACQUEEN, G., J. MARSHALL, M. PERDUE, S. SIEGEL & J. BIENENSTOCK. 1989. Pavlovian conditioning of rat mucosal mast cells to secrete rat mast cell protease II. Science **243:** 83–85.
4. GAUCI, M., A.J. HUSBAND, H. SAXARRA & M.G. KING. 1994. Pavlovian conditioning of nasal tryptase release in human subjects with allergic rhinitis. Physiol. Behav. **55:** 823–825.
5. SELIGMAN, M.E.P. 1970. On the generality of the laws of learning. Psychol. Rev. **77:** 406–418.
6. SELIGMAN, M.E.P. 1971. Phobias and preparedness. Behav. Ther. **2:** 307–320.
7. NACLERIO, R.M., H.L. MEIER, A. KAGEY-SOBOTKA, N. ADKINSON, D.A. MEYERS, P.S. NORMAN & L.M. LICHTENSTEIN. 1983. Mediator release after nasal airway challenge with allergen. Am. Rev. Respir. Dis. **128:** 597–602.
8. TAYLOR, K.M., S. KRILIS & B.A. BALDO. 1980. An enzymatic-isotopic microassay for measuring allergic release of histamine from blood and mast cells *in vitro*. Int. Arch. Allergy Appl. Immunol. **60:** 19–27.
9. HOWELL, D.C. 1992. Statistical methods for psychology, 3rd edit. Duxbury Press. Belmont, California.

Androstenetriol and Androstenediol

Protection Against Lethal Radiation and Restoration of Immunity After Radiation Injury

R.M. LORIA,[a,c] D.H. CONRAD,[a] T. HUFF,[a] H. CARTER,[b] AND D. BEN-NATHAN[b]

[a]Virginia Commonwealth University, Medical College of Virginia, Richmond, Virginia 23298-0678, USA

[b]The Institute of Biological Research, Ness-Ziona, Israel

ABSTRACT: Androstenetriol (AET) and Androstenediol (AED) upregulate host immunity, leading to increased resistance against infections. AET augments IL-2, IL-3, IFNγ levels, and counteracts hydrocortisone immune suppression. AET and AED at a dose of 0.75 mg/- and 8.0 mg/25-g mouse, protected 60 and 70%, respectively, of C57/BL/6J mice irradiated with a lethal dose. These hormones also protected mice irradiated with 6 Gy and infected with a coxsackievirus B4 LD50. AET significantly increased spleen lymphocyte numbers at 7, 14, and 21 days after a 6-Gy exposure. Fluorescent activated cell-sorter analysis of irradiated mice, spleen, and bone marrow showed that AET significantly augmented the myeloid precursor markers, CD11b/Mac-1, and B220 (pan B), as well as the absolute numbers of CD4+/CD8+ cells over the 21 days of testing. Overall, the data are consistent with AET/AED inducing a more rapid recovery of all hematopoietic precursors from the small number of surviving stem cells.

INTRODUCTION

Previously we reported that several native steroid hormones upregulate the immune response. The downstream metabolites of dehydroepiandrostrone (5-androstene-3β-ol-17-one, DHEA)—particularly androstenediol (5-androstene-3β,17β-diol, AED) and Androstenetriol (5-androstene-3β,7β,17β-triol, AET)—markedly prevent morbidity and mortality from infections by several diverse pathogens.[1–12] Indeed, a single subcutaneous (s.c.) injection of DHEA or AED to mice resulted in protection from coxsackievirus B4 (CB4), herpesvirus type-2 encephalitis, and *Enterococcus faecalis* lethality. Subsequent tests of AED showed that this hormone is 10,000 times more efficacious than DHEA, when tested for protection against lethal virus infections.[3] Experiments with AET, the second downstream metabolite of DHEA, that is, DHEA→AED→AET, have shown that *in vitro*, AET increases the production of both IL-2 and IL-3. AET also counteracts the suppressive effects of glucocorticosteroids on cell proliferation and on cytokine production. These hormones upregulate host

[c]Address for correspondence: Roger M. Loria, Professor, Department of Microbiology, Immunology and Pathology, Commonwealth University of Virginia, Medical College of Virginia, Richmond, VA 23298-0678. Voice: 804-828-9717; fax: 804-828-5862.

Loria@hsc.vcu.edu

resistance against a wide range of lethal infections by bacterial and viral agents; they also counteract stress-mediated immune suppression.

There are many similarities between corticosteroid and radiation-mediated immune injury. Whole-body or localized irradiation will result in the destruction of lymphoid cells and is toxic to proliferating cells. Similarly, hydrocortisone has a direct destructive effect on lymphoid cells, alters RNA synthesis, inhibits inflammation, and sequesters lymphocytes. This laboratory had previously shown that AED had significant radioprotecting effects. These findings were recently confirmed in a collaborative study by Witnall *et al.*[13]

The present study's aim was to determine whether the ability of AET to counteract corticoids immune suppression could be extended to protection against radiation-mediated immune injury. The findings demonstrate that administration of AET/AED to animals exposed to whole-body irradiation of 6 to 8 Gy results in a more rapid recovery of hematopoietic precursors from the small number of surviving stem cells and upregulates the host resistance against a lethal infection.

MATERIAL AND METHODS

Six-week-old C57BL/6J male mice were obtained from Jackson Bar Harbor Laboratory. Animals were weighed three consecutive times to ascertain that they were gaining weight prior to experimentation. Animals were exposed to whole-body irradiation of 6 to 8 Gy, depending on the experiments, in a CS-137 gamma unit (Mark 68, JL Sheperd & Associates). A single s.c. injection of either AET 0.75 mg/25-g mouse or AED 8.0 mg/25-g mouse, suspended in 0.1 mL of dimethyl sulfoxide:ethanol 1:1 was used as the vehicle. Animals in survival experiments were monitored for 21 days. The sublethal dose of a human coxsackievirus B4 was determined previously and found to be 2×10^2 pfu/mouse. This virus dose was injected intraperitoneally (i.p.) after whole-body radiation exposure. Spleen and bone marrow preparation were stained for either one- or two-color FACS analysis, as previously described.[14]

RESULTS

Protection Against Whole-body Lethal Irradiation

The results of the protective effects against lethal radiation are presented in FIGURE 1. Either AED at a concentration of 8.0 mg/25-g mouse (320 mg/kg) or AET at 0.75 mg/25-g mouse (30 mg/kg) as a single s.c. injection significantly protected animals from a lethal radiation exposure of 8 Gy; $p < 0.01$. The dose of AED required to achieve a protective effect was more than ten times greater than the dose of AET; nevertheless, both agents caused a significant protective effect from lethal radiation.

Restoring Resistance of Irradiated Animals Against Infection

In the following experiments, we tested whether AET or AED would restore resistance to irradiated animals infected with a human coxsackievirus B4. The virus

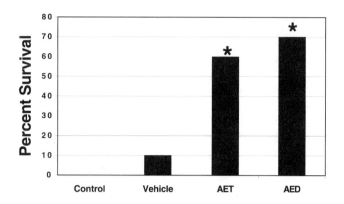

FIGURE 1. AET and AED protect against an 8-Gy lethal whole-body irradiation. Nine-week-old C57BL/6J male mice were exposed to whole-body irradiation of 8 Gy. A single s.c. injection of 0.75 mg AET or 8.0 mg AED or vehicle (DMSO:ethanol 1:1) were administered. AET or AED effects were statistically different from control $p < 0.001$. The difference between AET and AED is not significant.

challenge dose did not cause mortality in normal control mice; however, the mortality of animals exposed to 6-Gy whole-body radiation and infected with coxsackievirus B4 reached 50%. Treatment with either AED or AET restored host resistance against virus challenge to irradiated mice, resulting in 88% and 75% survival, respectively; $p < 0.01$ (see FIGURE 2).

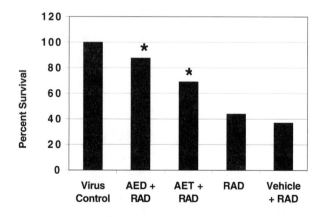

FIGURE 2. AET and AED protect irradiated mice from virus-mediated mortality. C57BL/6J mice were exposed to whole-body irradiation of 6 Gy and challenge with 100 plaque-forming units of coxsackievirus B4. Control animals not exposed to irradiation survived this infectious challenge; however, only 44% of irradiated mice survived. A single s.c. injection of 0.75 mg AET or 8.0 mg AED protected the irradiated mice from mortality resulting from coxsackievirus B4 challenge. The vehicle (DMSO:ethanol 1 : 1) did not have any protective effect against virus infection.

AET Restores Spleen-Cell Counts in Irradiated Mice

The protective effects of AETs are clearly associated with its ability to enhance the recovery of a small number of lymphocytes surviving the radiation-mediated destruction. The results presented in FIGURE 3 illustrate this point. Spleen-cell counts of animals exposed to 6-Gy whole-body irradiation and treated with AET were performed and compared with untreated or vehicle-injected irradiated control mice over a 14-day period. Irradiation resulted in about 90% or more spleen-cell destruction. Treatment with AET was associated with an increased spleen-cell count at day three, by about 104% over irradiated control. At day seven the increase was 151%, while at 14 days, AET-treated animals' spleen-cell counts were 738% above the nontreated irradiated controls; $p < 0.001$.

Effects of AET on Spleen CD4 and CD8 Cell Numbers

FACS analysis was subsequently performed over a period of 21 days on spleen- and bone marrow cells of mice exposed to 6-Gy whole-body irradiation and treated with AET and compared with untreated irradiated animals. Spleen cells were stained for $CD4^+$ and $CD8^+$, while bone marrow cells were stained for CD11b/Mac-1 and B220. All FACS analysis utilized acquisition of 10,000 events. The FACS analysis results of spleen- and bone marrow cells were multiplied by the actual number of cells in the particular organ of the given group. The results for spleen CD4 and CD8 counts in irradiated, untreated, and AET-treated irradiated animal at 7, 14, and 21 days are presented in FIGURE 4. Irradiated animals treated with AET had remarkable increases in the numbers of CD4 and CD8 cells, as compared to irradiated controls.

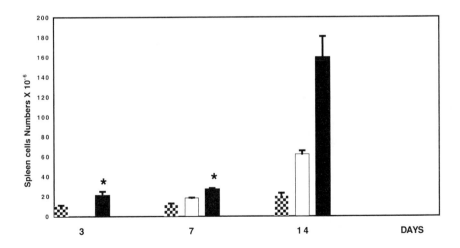

FIGURE 3. AET restores spleen-cell counts after whole-body irradiation. Spleen-cell counts of animals exposed to whole-body irradiation of 6 Gy and treated with a single s.c. injection of 0.75 mg AET or vehicle (DMSO:ethanol 1 : 1). Spleen-cell counts were done at 3, 7, and 14 days after irradiation. KEY: ▨, radiation only; ☐, radiation + vehicle; ■, radiation + AET.

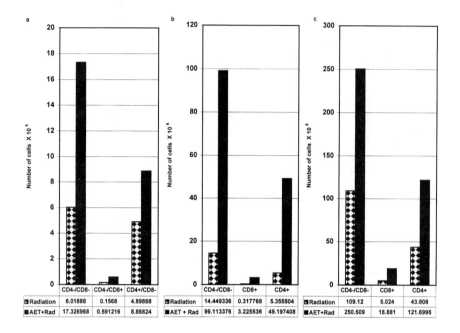

FIGURE 4. Effects of AET on CD4 and CD8 spleen-cell numbers after 6-Gy irradiation. (**a**) Results at seven days; (**b**) 14 days; (**c**) 21 days. Result are expressed as the number of CD4+ and CD8+ cells in irradiated and AET-treated irradiated animals. FACS analysis was used to obtain the particular percent of CD4/CD8 distribution and multiplied by the total spleen-cell count of either irradiated or AET + irradiation group.

AET treatment of irradiated mice resulted in an increase of 287% of CD4−/CD8−, 377% of CD8+, 181% of CD4+ cells, respectively, as compared to untreated irradiated mice. Fourteen days after whole-body irradiation and AET treatment, these numbers are considerably higher, with a 685% increase of CD4−/CD8−, 1,015% increase of CD8+, 918% increase of CD4+ cells, as compared to irradiated control, respectively (FIG. 4b). By 21 days after radiation exposures, these numbers were still 230% for CD4−/CD8−, 376% for CD8+, 278 for CD4+ and cells, as compared to irradiated control (FIG. 4c).

Effects of AET on Bone Marrow CD11b/Mac-1 and B220 Cell Numbers

The results of AET treatment on the number of bone marrow cells at seven days are presented in FIGURE 5a. AET increased the numbers of CD11b/Mac-1−/− cells by 146%, CD11b/Mac-1+ by 200%, and B220+ cells by 219%, respectively, as compared to the irradiated untreated group. At 14 days after irradiation, AET treatment augmented the counts CD11b/Mac-1+ by 1,194%. However, the levels of B220+ were lower in AET treated than the irradiated control by 30% (FIG. 5b). By 21 days after whole-body irradiation, the remarkable effects of AET were evident, since the

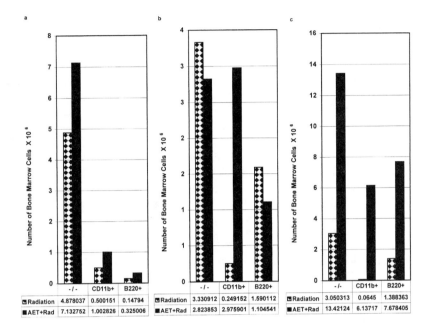

FIGURE 5. Effects of AET on CD11b/Mac-1 and B220 bone marrow cells numbers after 6-Gy irradiation. (**a**) Results at seven days; (**b**)14 days; (**c**) 21 days. Results are expressed as the number of CD11b/Mac-1 and B220 cells in irradiated and AET-treated irradiated animals. FACS analysis was used to obtain the particular percent of CD11b/Mac-1 and B220 distribution and multiplied by the total bone marrow cell count of either irradiated or AET + irradiation group.

number of CD11b/Mac-1$^{-/-}$ cells was increased by 439%, CD11b/Mac-1^{+} by 9,514%, and B220^{+} cells by 553%, respectively (FIG. 4c).

DISCUSSION

The results show that AET is effective in protecting animals from a lethal radiation exposure of 8 Gy. AED also was protective, albeit at a higher concentration. Both hormones also protected the irradiated host from a viral infection that was lethal only in the irradiated immune-suppressed host, but was not lethal for the normal host. This paradigm is particularly relevant to the increased susceptibility to infections observed in individuals due to radiation or chemotherapy treatment as well as stress-mediated immune suppression. Recently, Whitnall *et al.*[13] reported that a single injection of AED was effective in protecting B6D2F1/J female mice irradiated with three Gy from *Kaufman's pneumonia* infection.

The results of the FACS analysis demonstrate the ability of AET to restore cells with the precursor markers, CD11b/Mac-1, and B220 (pan B) in bone marrow, as well as the absolute numbers of CD4^{+}/CD8^{+} cells over the 21 days of testing. In addition, the results show a significant and consistent elevation of both bone marrow and spleen double-negative cells, suggesting numerous effects in restoring other cellular elements. Based on previous observations, it is evident that AED,[13] and most likely AET, restore platelet counts as well as peripheral neutrophils counts.

The findings reported are consistent with the overall observation that AET/AED induce a more rapid recovery of all hematopoietic precursors from the small number of surviving stem cells.

ACKNOWLEDGMENT

In memory of: Dr. Sidney Kibrick, M.D. Ph.D., who unexpectedly passed away on August 3, 2000. Sid was one of the fathers of the field of human virology. As part of Dr. John Enders' team, he participated in the development of tissue culture procedures for the isolation and production of human viruses, which led to the development of viral vaccines. He served as assistant director in poliovirus vaccine field trials. Sid was also a pioneer on herpes virus research and, above and beyond, a true healer. Dr. Kibrick was my teacher and mentor. Leter he became my colleague and dear friend. He will be missed profoundly.

This work was supported in part by a gift from the SCDR Cancer Research Fund.

REFERENCES

1. LORIA, R.M. et al. 1988. Protection against acute lethal viral infections with the native steroid dehydroepiandrosterone (DHEA). J. Med. Virol. **26:** 301–314.
2. LORIA, R.M., W. REGELSON & D.A. PADGETT. 1990. Immune Response facilitation and resistance to virus and bacterial infections with dehydroepiandrosterone (DHEA). In The Biologic Role of Dehydroepiandrosterone (DHEA), M. Kalimi and W. Regelson, Eds.: 107–130. Walter De Gruyter. New York.
3. LORIA, R.M. & D.A. PADGETT. 1992. Androstenediol regulates systemic resistance against lethal infections in mice. Arch. Virol. **127:** 103–115.
4. LORIA, R.M. & D.A. PADGETT. 1992. Mobilization of cutaneous immunity for systemic protection against infections. Ann. N.Y. Acad. Sci. **650:** 363–366.
5. PADGETT, D.A. & R.M. LORIA. 1994. In-vitro potentiation of lymphocyte activation by dehydroepiandrosterone, androstenediol, and androstenetriol. J. Immunol. **153:** 1544–1552.
6. LORIA, R.M., D.A. PADGETT & N.H. PHUONG. 1996. Regulation of the immune response by DHEA and its metabolites. J. Endocrinol. **150:** S209–S219.
7. PADGETT, D.A., R.M. LORIA & J.F. SHERIDAN. 1997. Endocrine regulation of the immune response to influenza virus infection with a metabolite of DHEA—Androstenediol. J. Neuroimmunol. **78:** 203–211.
8. PADGETT, D.A. & R.M. LORIA. 1998. Endocrine regulation of murine macrophage function: effects of dehydroepiandrosterone, androstenediol, and androstenetriol. J. Neuroimmunol. **84:** 61–68.
9. LORIA, R.M. & D. BEN-NATHAN. 1998. Steroids, stress and the neuroimmune axis. In New Frontiers in Stress Research, Modulation of Brain Function, A. Levy, E. Grauer, D. Ben-Nathan, and E.R. de Kloet, Eds.: 163–173. Hardwood. Amsterdam.
10. LORIA, R.M. 1997. Anti-glucocorticoid function of androstenetriol. Psychoneuroendocrinology **22**(S1): S103–S108.

11. BEN NATHAN, D. *et al.* 1998. Stress induced central nervous system penetration by non-invasive attenuated encephalitis viruses. *In* New Frontiers in Stress Research, Modulation of Brain Function, De Kloet, Grauer, Levy, and D. Ben Nathan, Eds.: 227–283. Hardwood. Amsterdam.

12. BEN-NATHAN, D., D.A. PADGETT & R.M. LORIA. 1999. Androstenediol and dehydroepiandrosterone protect mice against lethal bacterial infections and LPS toxicity. J. Med. Microbiol. **48:** 1–7.

13. WHITNALL, W.M. *et al.* 2000. Androstenediol stimulates myelopoiesis and enhances resistance to infection in gamma-irradiated mice. Int. J. Immunopharmacol. **22:** 1–14.

14. PAYET, M.E., E.C. WOODWARD & D.H. CONRAD. 1999. Humoral response suppression observed with CD23 transgenics. J. Immunol. **163:** 217–223.

Altered Glucocorticoid Regulation of the Immune Response in the Chronic Fatigue Syndrome

JEROEN T.J. VISSER,[a,b,d] E. RONALD DE KLOET,[b] AND LEX NAGELKERKEN[a,c]

[a]TNO Prevention and Health, Division of Immunological and Infectious Diseases, Leiden, The Netherlands

[b]Division of Medical Pharmacology, Leiden Amsterdam Center of Drug Research, Leiden, The Netherlands

ABSTRACT: It is increasingly recognized that glucocortiocoids (GCs) can have subtle modulatory effects in immunoregulation rather than having generalized immunosuppressive effects. GCs suppress Th1 cells and cellular immunity, but may favor Th2 responses and humoral immunity. The chronic fatigue syndrome (CFS) appears to be associated with a disturbed HPA-axis. Moreover, CFS patients show several immunological changes suggestive of decreased cellular immunity. It is postulated herein that in CFS patients a decreased Th1/Th2 balance may be the result of selective effects of GC on the IL-10/IL-12 regulatory circuit.

ROLE OF THE HPA-AXIS IN IMMUNE DYSFUNCTION AND AUTOIMMUNITY

The hypothalamus–pituitary–adrenal gland (HPA)-axis plays a major role in the crosstalk between the immune system and the neuroendocrine system. The immune system can influence the functionality of the HPA-axis through cytokines, like tumor-necrosis-factor-α (TNF-α), interleukin(IL)-1, IL-6, and interferons.[1,2] These cytokines, for instance, induce the release of corticotropin-releasing hormone (CRH) in the hypothalamus, which in turn activates the HPA-axis. Furthermore, these cytokines cause fever and a general feeling of malaise. On the other hand, hormones associated with the HPA-axis have potent immunomodulatory properties. For instance, adrenocorticotropic hormone (ACTH) and CRH have been shown to activate macrophages and to recruit monocytes to the site of inflammation.[1,2] However, the most potent immunomodulatory hormones are glucocorticoids (GCs), which are widely applied because of their immunosuppressive characteristics. GCs can influence the functionality of the cells of the immune system by inducing apoptosis,

[c]Address for correspondence: Dr. Lex Nagelkerken, TNO Prevention and Health, Division of Immunological and Infectious Diseases, P.O. Box 2215, 2301 CE Leiden, The Netherlands. Voice: + 31 71 5181398; fax : + 31 71 5181901.

am.nagelkerken@pg.tno.nl

[d]Current address: Department of Histology and Cell Biology, Immunology Section, University of Groningen, Groningen, The Netherlands.

inhibition of proliferation, interfering with cytokine production, and specific modulation of the capacity of antigen-presenting cells (APCs) to activate T cells.[1-3]

The integrity of the HPA-axis plays an important role in the development of experimental autoimmune encephalomyelitis (EAE) in Lewis rats. These rats show an impaired release of GCs upon stressful events, and this feature is suggested to be a determinant of susceptibility for EAE.[4,5] On the other hand, the relatively resistant PVG rat becomes sensitive to EAE induction after adrenalectomy, and this can be reversed by corticosterone treatment.[4] The impaired capacity of animals to increase GC levels has also been demonstrated to contribute to their sensitivity for streptococcal cell-wall-induced arthritis.[6]

The idea that the integrity of the HPA-axis is a major determinant in the development of autoimmunity is further supported by observations in humans. Patients with rheumatoid arthritis (RA) display decreased levels of GCs, as a result of an impaired functioning of the HPA-axis.[7] These patients show a decreased induction of CRH and ACTH after a challenge with IL-1. On the other hand, increased activity of the HPA-axis has been reported in multiple sclerosis (MS) patients.[8] Because these diseases are widely thought to be due to the activity of Th1 cells, which may promote inflammatory responses by the secretion of interferon-γ (IFN-γ) and lymphotoxin, it has been postulated that the integrity of the HPA-axis, that is, the capacity to produce GCs, may determine the development of autoimmunity via selective effects on Th1 and Th2 responses.[2,3]

SELECTIVE EFFECTS OF GLUCOCORTICOIDS ON TH1 AND TH2 RESPONSES

The balance between Th1 and Th2 cells—two important subsets of $CD4^+$ T cells—is important for the nature of the immune response to pathogens. Th1 cells, which produce high levels of IFN-γ, promote cellular immunity by stimulating the activity of NK cells, macrophages, and cytotoxic T cells. Th2 cells, on the other hand, produce high levels of IL-4, IL-5, and IL-13, and are supportive for humoral immunity, by providing help for B cells in the production of antibodies.[9,10] The differentiation of naive $CD4^+$ T cells into either Th1 or Th2 cells is regulated by several factors. In particular, the type of APC, cytokines, and hormones present in the microenvironment of the differentiating T cell play a major role.[9-12] The presence of IL-4 during a developing immune response has been shown to favor Th2 responses.[10] On the other hand, IL-12 has been shown to be crucial in the development of Th1 responses.[11] In addition, the activation state of APC might be of importance: it was demonstrated that APCs, which secrete prostaglandin E_2, inhibit Th1 development.[12]

In 1994 it was hypothesized by Rook *et al.*[3] that GCs selectively suppress Th1 responses while promoting Th2 responses. Several observations have substantiated this hypothesis and indicate that GC may use several mechanisms for this Th2 skewing effect. First of all, GCs have selective effects on the cytokines that contribute to the polarization of Th1 or Th2 cells: proinflammatory and Th1-inducing cytokines are strongly suppressed by GCs, while the anti-inflammatory and Th2-inducing cytokines are much less affected (see FIGURE 1). In the mouse this was demonstrated

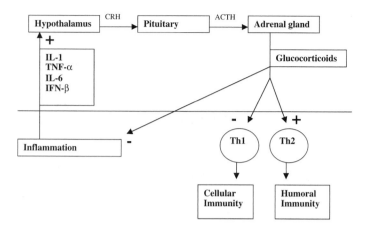

FIGURE 1. Effects of glucocorticoids on Th1 and Th2 responses. Cytokines produced upon an inflammatory reaction are capable of activating the HPA-axis, leading to the production of GCs by the adrenal gland. These GCs suppress the production of these proinflammatory cytokines and are favorable for Th2 responses. (Figure adapted from Rook *et al.*[3])

by showing that dexamethasone suppressed IL-2 and IFN-γ production by Th1 cells, but not the IL-4 production by Th2 cells.[13] Also in humans GCs have selective effects on CD4[+] T-cell subsets, which appear to depend on the activation pathway.[14] Addition of GCs during restimulation of primed human naive CD4[+] T cells stimulated the IL-4 and IL-10 production and suppressed IL-5 and IFN-γ production.[14] Moreover, GCs increase the production of IgE by IL-4-stimulated B cells.[15]

In addition to direct effects on the developing T cell, GCs inhibit the expression of the costimulatory molecules CD80 and CD86 on macrophages and dendritic

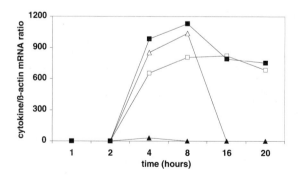

FIGURE 2. Selective suppression of IL-12p40 mRNA by dexamethasone. Whole blood was stimulated with 0.25 μg/mL LPS in the absence (*open symbols*) or presence (*closed symbols*) of 1 μM dexamethasone. RNA was isolated at different time points and used for the detection of IL-12p40 mRNA (*triangles*) and IL-10 mRNA (*squares*) by PCR, as described previously.[18] Results are expressed as a ratio of cytokine mRNA over β-actin mRNA.

cells.[16] This downregulation of costimulatory molecules by GCs might render the APC to become tolerogenic, because loss of this costimulatory signal causes anergy in T cells. In fully activated monocytes or fully matured dendritic cells, GCs only slightly affect the antigen presentation potential and instead enhance their Th2 skewing potential via the downregulation of IL-12.[17] Recently, we have demonstrated that dexamethasone inhibits IL-12 production in whole blood cultures, whereas effects on IL-10 range from a slight inhibition to stimulation.[18]

As shown in FIGURE 2, dexamethasone is potent in inhibiting LPS-induced IL-12p40 mRNA expression, whereas IL-10 mRNA is rather increased. We postulate that GCs can suppress Th1 responses in favor of Th2 responses by increasing the IL-10/IL-12 ratio. Also, treatment of MS patients with GCs can affect the IL-10/IL-12 ratio. A relapsing–remitting MS-patient who received a high-dose methylprednisolone treatment showed a one-million-fold increase of the IL-10/IL-12 mRNA ratio (van Boxel-Dezaire *et al.*, unpublished observation). A recent study by Gayo *et al.*[19] showed that methylprednisolone treatment increases IL-10 in MS patients. Moreover, healthy controls treated with hydrocortisone showed increased plasma levels of IL-10, and an increase of LPS induced IL-10 in whole blood cultures.[20]

Besides selective effects on cytokines, GCs also have selective effects on the expression of cytokine receptors. Wu and coworkers[21] demonstrated that the expression of the IL-12 receptor on T cells is downregulated by GCs and that the cells remain unresponsive for at least 24 h. Interestingly, Michel *et al.*[22] demonstrated that GCs can enhance the expression of the IL-10 receptors on keratinocytes.

Our observations that the glucocorticoid receptor antagonist RU486 synergized with anti-IL-10 in the enhancement of IL-12,[18] suggests that GCs and IL-10 can also act in synergy in suppressing IL-12 and inflammatory responses. Accordingly, Herfarth *et al.* have recently demonstrated that dexamethasone enhances the anti-inflammatory actions of IL-10 in inflammatory bowel disease.[23]

MOLECULAR MECHANISMS IN CYTOKINE MODULATION BY GLUCOCORTICOIDS

GCs exert their immunomodulatory effect via binding of the activated glucocorticoid receptors (GRs) to specific glucocorticoid-responsive elements (GREs) in the promoter regions of regulatory genes, which in turn leads to activation or silencing of the gene.[24] Another mechanism is the selective effect on transcription factors that are involved in the regulation of cytokine genes. The activated GR complex is inhibitory for the activity of activator protein 1 (AP-1) via protein–protein interaction with its two subunits c-jun and c-fos.[25] Also other transcription factors that are important for the induction of immune responses, that is, NFκB and CREB, are downregulated by GCs via protein–protein interaction.[26] Importantly, GCs were demonstrated to upregulate IκB, a protein that maintains NFκB in its inactive state in the cytosol[27,28] by an as yet unidentified mechanism involving transactivation.

GCs are only capable of exerting their effects by binding to the GRs. Alterations in the functionality of these receptors will interfere with the responsiveness of cells to GCs. Changes in the affinity and density of the GRs have been shown to interfere with the responses to GCs *in vitro* and *in vivo*.[29] However, other studies suggest that

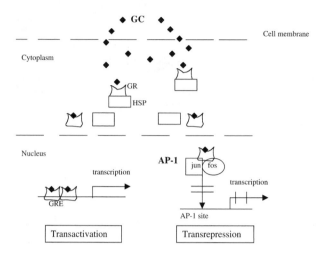

FIGURE 3. Regulation of gene transcription by glucocorticoids. GCs passively diffuse through the membrane and bind to their receptors in the cytosol. After formation of a GR–GC complex, this complex can act as a transcription factor by binding to a GRE in a promoter region of genes and can enhance or silence transcription, a mechanism known as transactivation. On the other hand, the activated GR can bind to transcription factors via protein–protein interaction, preventing the binding of this transcription factor to its responsive elements. This phenomenon is termed transrepression.

an altered sensitivity may be observed despite a normal density and affinity of the GRs. Possibly, an altered sensitivity in these studies is due to an impaired interaction between transcription factors and the occupied GRs.

Taken together, GCs exploit several mechanisms in controlling immune responses (see FIGURE 3), and the responsiveness to GCs depends on the affinity and density of the GRs, their interaction with transcription factors, and the presence of GRE in promoter regions of regulatory genes. It remains to be established to what extent these mechanisms result in selective effects of GCs on IL-10 and IL-12 gene expression.

THE CHRONIC FATIGUE SYNDROME

The chronic fatigue syndrome (CFS) is a disease of unknown origin characterized by severe disabling fatigue with a duration of more than six months and a reduction in normal activity of at least 50%.[30] Several causes have been held responsible for the onset and maintenance of the syndrome, including viral infections, a disturbed HPA-axis, and an altered immune function.[31–33] Infectious agents can cause fatigue complaints known as the postviral fatigue syndrome, and several groups therefore suggested an infectious etiology for the disease.[32,33] The idea that CFS might be caused by an infectious trigger or another event, leading to a chronic activation and imbalance of the immune system, became a major hypothesis in the etiology of CFS.[32,33]

Several authors have demonstrated alterations in immunological parameters in CFS patients. Cytokines, like IL-1, IL-6, and TNF-α, that are strongly augmented by viral or bacterial infections were shown to be normal or increased in CFS patients.[32,33] The observed immunological disturbances in CFS patients suggest a slight reduction in the cellular immunity because of reduced NK cell activity.[34] Furthermore, a reduced IFN-γ production[35] and one report regarding a reduced delayed-type hypersensitivity (DTH) response[36] were also found. The observed differences in the immunological parameters, however, are not consistent and show diversity. An explanation for this inconsistency could be variations in the group of patients under investigation. In fact, a study with a well-defined patient group and a well-matched control group showed that when the patients were subgrouped according to disease onset or severity, more pronounced differences were found.[37]

Certain immunological alterations may be unique to certain lymphocyte subsets. We recently demonstrated that a reduced production of IFN-γ in CFS became particularly evident when purified CD4$^+$ T cells were used. Simultaneously, these cells showed a normal proliferation and a normal IL-4 production, which indeed points to a selective decrease in (the activity of) CD4$^+$ T cells.[38] Taken together differences in immune parameters in CFS patients shown so far are subtle, and this appears to be dependent on the parameter under investigation, the composition of the patient population, and the nature of the control group.

NEUROENDOCRINOLOGY IN RELATION TO IMMUNE FUNCTION IN CFS

Endrocrinological studies have demonstrated an impaired functioning of the HPA-axis in CFS patients.[39] CFS patients show significantly reduced levels of urinary-free cortisol and a reduced production of ACTH upon stimulation with CRH. Furthermore, a blunted response in cortisol production to ACTH challenge has been demonstrated.[39] These alterations are quite different from those found in depression, because patients with depression are characterized by hyperfunctioning of the HPA-axis, resulting in high levels of cortisol.[40] Accordingly, most of the people suffering from depression show a reduced dexamethasone suppression, probably because of a reduced functioning of the glucocorticoid receptors.[40]

The alterations of the HPA-axis found in CFS patients might be due to an increased negative feedback as a consequence of an increased responsiveness to GCs. In view of the importance of GCs in the regulation of immune responses, the reduced Th1 activity in CFS-patients also might be due to an increased sensitivity for GCs. We have indeed demonstrated recently that CD4$^+$ T cells from CFS patients have an increased sensitivity to dexamethasone.[38]

In lipopolysaccharide-stimulated whole blood cultures of CFS patients, increased levels of IL-10 and decreased levels of IL-12 are found (submitted for publication). Although the differences are subtle and represent group effects, they might explain the decreased Th1 activity. Interestingly, IL-10 in particular appeared useful in identifying patients with an increased sensitivity to GC.

The increased responsiveness to GCs by lymphocytes of CFS patients might be due to several mechanisms. As indicated earlier, the density and affinity of the GRs are important factors for GC sensitivity. Preliminary data indicate that the increased sensitivity of lymphocytes from CFS patients cannot be explained by the number or affinity of the GRs, but should rather be attributed to the molecular processes beyond the actual binding of the ligand to the GRs. Taken together, HPA-axis abnormalities may not only increase the vulnerability to affective disorders and fatigue syndromes but also modify immune function via selective effects on the IL-10/IL-12 regulatory circuit.

ACKNOWLEDGMENT

This work was supported by Zorg Onderzoek Nederland, Grant 28-2908.

REFERENCES

1. BLALOCK, J.E. 1994. The syntax of immune-neuroendocrine communication. Immunol. Today **15**(11): 504–511.
2. WILDER, R.L. 1995. Neuroendocrine-immune system interactions and autoimmunity. Annu. Rev. Immunol. **13**: 307–338.
3. ROOK, G.A.W. et al. 1994. Hormones, peripherally activated prohormones and regulation of the Th1/Th2 balance. Immunol. Today **15**: 301–303.
4. MACPHEE, I.A. et al. 1989. Spontaneous recovery of rats from experimental allergic encephalomyelitis is dependent on regulation of the immune system by endogenous adrenal corticosteroids. J. Exp. Med. **169**: 431–435.
5. MASON, D. 1991. Genetic variation in the stress response: susceptibility to experimental allergic encephalomyelitis and implications for human inflammatory disease. Immunol. Today **12**: 57–60.
6. STERNBERG, E.M. et al. 1989. A central nervous system defect in biosynthesis of corticotropin-releasing hormone is associated with susceptibility to streptococcal cell wall-induced arthritis in Lewis rats. Proc. Natl. Acad. Sci. USA **86**(12): 4771–4775.
7. CHIKANZA, I.C. et al. 1992. Defective hypothalamic response to immune and inflammatory stimuli in patients with rheumatoid arthritis. Arthritis Rheum. **35**: 1281–1288.
8. MICHELSON, D. et al. 1994. Multiple sclerosis is associated with alterations in hypothalamic-pituitary-adrenal axis function. J. Clin. Endocrinol. & Metab. **79**(3): 848–853.
9. MOSMANN, T.R. & R.L. COFFMAN. 1989. Th1 and Th2 cells: different patterns of lymphokine secretion lead to different functional properties. Annu. Rev. Immunol. **7**: 145–173.
10. PAUL, W.E. & R.A. SEDER. 1994. Lymphocyte responses and cytokines. Cell **76**: 241–251.
11. TRINCHIERI, G. 1995. Interleukin-12: a proinflammatory cytokine with immunoregulatory functions that bridge innate resistance and antigen specific adaptive immunity. Annu. Rev. Immunol. **13**: 251–276.
12. HILKENS, C.M. et al. 1996. Accessory cell derived IL-12 and prostaglandin-E2 determine the IFN-γ level of activated human CD4+ T cells. J. Immunol. **156**: 1722–1727.
13. DAYNES, R.A. & B.A. ARANEO. 1989. Contrasting effects of glucocorticoids on the capacity of T cells to produce growth factors Interleukin-2 and Interleukin-4. Eur. J. Immunol. **19**: 2319–2325.
14. BRINKMANN, V. et al. 1995. Regulation by corticosteroids of Th1 and Th2 cytokine production in human CD4+ effector T cells generated from CD45RO− and CD45RO+ subsets. J. Immunol. **155**: 3322–3328.
15. WU, C.Y. et al. 1991. Glucocorticoids increase the synthesis of immunoglobulin E by interleukin-4 stimulated human lymphocytes. J. Clin. Invest. **87**: 870–877.

16. MOSER, M. et al. 1995. Glucocorticoids down-regulate dendritic cell function in vitro and in vivo. Eur. J. Immunol. **25:** 2818–2824.
17. DEKRUYFF, R. et al. 1998. Corticosteroids enhance the capacity of macrophages to induce Th2 cytokine synthesis in CD4$^+$ lymphocytes by inhibiting IL-12 production. J. Immunol. **160:** 2231–2237.
18. VISSER, J. et al. 1998. Differential regulation of IL-10 and IL-12 by glucocorticoids in vitro. Blood **91**(11): 4255–4264.
19. GAYO, A. et al. 1998. Glucocorticoids increase IL-10 expression in multiple sclerosis patients with acute relapse. J. Neuroimmunol. **85**(2): 122–130.
20. VAN DER POLL, T. et al. 1996. Hypercortisolemia increases plasma Interleukin-10 concentration during human endotoxemia—a clinical research center study. J. Clin. Endocrinol. Metab. **81:** 3604–3606.
21. WU, C.Y. et al. 1998. Prostaglandin E2 and dexamethasone inhibit IL-12 receptor expression and IL-12 responsiveness. J. Immunol. **161**(6): 2723–2730.
22. MICHEL, G. et al. 1997. Demonstration and functional analysis of IL-10 receptors in human epidermal cells. J. Immunol. **159:** 6291–6297.
23. HERFARTH, H.H. et al. 1998. Subtherapeutic corticosteroids potentiate the ability of Interleukin-10 to prevent chronic inflammation in rats. Gastroenterology **115:** 856–865.
24. BAMBERGER, C.M. et al. 1996. Molecular determinants of glucocorticoid receptor function and tissue sensitivity to glucocorticoids. Endocrine Rev. **17**(3): 245–261.
25. YANG-YEN, H.F. et al. 1990. Transcriptional interference between c-Jun and the glucocorticoid receptor: mutual inhibition of DNA-binding due to direct protein-protein interaction. Cell **62:** 1205–1215.
26. ADCOCK, I.M. et al. 1995. Effects of glucocorticoids on transcription factor activation in human peripheral blood mononuclear cells. Am. J. Physiol. **268:** 331–338.
27. SCHEINMAN, R.I. et al. 1995. Role of transcriptional activation of IkBα in mediation of immunosuppression by glucocorticoids. Science **270:** 283–286.
28. AUPHAN, N. et al. 1995. Immunosuppression by glucocorticoids: inhibition of NF-kB activity through induction of IkB synthesis. Science **270:** 286–290.
29. BARNES, P.J. et al. 1995. Glucocorticoid resistance in asthma. Am. J. Respir. Crit. Care Med. **152:** 125–142.
30. FUKUDA, K. et al. 1994. The chronic fatigue syndrome: a comprehensive approach to its definition and study. Ann. Intern. Med. **121:** 953–959.
31. BEARN, J. & S. WESSELY. 1994. Neurobiological aspects of the chronic fatigue syndrome. Eur. J. Clin. Invest. **24:** 79–90.
32. STRAUSS, S.E. et al. 1994. Chronic fatigue syndrome: point and counterpoint. J. Infect. Dis. **170:** 1–6.
33. KOMAROFF, A.L. et al. 1998. Chronic fatigue syndrome: an update. Ann. Rev. Med. **49:** 1–13.
34. CALIGUIRI, M. et al. 1987. Phenotypic and functional deficiency of natural killer cells in patients with chronic fatigue syndrome. J. Immunol. **139:** 3306–3313.
35. KLIMAS, N.G. et al. 1990. Immunologic abnormalities in chronic fatigue syndrome. J. Clin. Microbiol. **28:** 1404–1410.
36. LLOYD, A. et al. 1992. Cell mediated immunity in patients with chronic fatigue syndrome, healthy control subjects and patients with major depression. Clin. Exp. Immunol. **87:** 76–79.
37. MAWLE, A.C. et al. 1997. Immune responses associated with chronic fatigue syndrome: a case-control study. J. Infect. Dis. **175:** 136–141.
38. VISSER, J.T.J. et al. 1998. CD4 T lymphocytes from patients with chronic fatigue syndrome have decreased interferon-γ production and increased sensitivity to dexamethasone. J. Infect. Dis. **177:** 451–454.
39. DEMITRACK, M.A. et al. 1991. Evidence for impaired activation of the hypothalamic-pituitary-adrenal axis in patients with chronic fatigue syndrome. J. Clin. Endocrinol. Metab. **73:** 1224–1234.
40. MODELL, S. et al. 1997. Corticosteroid receptor function is decreased in depressed patients. J. Neuroendocrinol. **65**(3): 216–222.

Acute Stress Enhances While Chronic Stress Suppresses Skin Immunity

The Role of Stress Hormones and Leukocyte Trafficking

FIRDAUS S. DHABHAR[a]

College of Dentistry and College of Medicine, Ohio State University, 4179 Postle Hall, Columbus Ohio 43210-1241, USA

ABSTRACT: Delayed-type hypersensitivity (DTH) reactions are antigen-specific, cell-mediated immune responses that, depending on the antigen, mediate beneficial (resistance to viruses, bacteria, fungi) or harmful (allergic dermatitis, autoimmunity) aspects of immunity. Contrary to the widely held notion that stress is immunosuppressive, we have shown that under certain conditions, stress can enhance immune function. DTH reactions can be studied in rats or mice by challenging the pinnae of previously sensitized animals with antigen. Studies have shown that acute stress administered immediately before antigen exposure significantly enhances skin DTH. In contrast, chronic stress significantly suppresses skin DTH. Stress-induced changes in leukocyte distribution may contribute to these bidirectional effects of stress, since acute stress induces a significant mobilization of leukocytes from the blood to the skin, whereas chronic stress suppresses leukocyte mobilization. In order to identify the hormonal mediators of the observed effects of stress, we first showed that adrenalectomy (ADX) eliminates the stress-induced enhancement of DTH. Acute administration (to ADX animals) of low doses of corticosterone and/or epinephrine significantly enhances skin DTH. In contrast, acute administration of high doses of corticosterone, low doses of dexamethasone, or chronic administration of moderate doses of corticosterone suppress skin DTH. Thus, the timing and duration of stress may significantly affect the nature (enhancing versus suppressive) of the effects of stress on skin immune function. These results suggest that during acute stress, stress hormones may help enhance immune function by informing the immune system about impending challenges (e.g., wounding or infection) that may be imposed by a stressor (e.g., an aggressor). Thus, during acute stress, the brain may send a warning signal to the immune system, just as it does to other fight/flight systems in the body.

INTRODUCTION

Stress is a term that means different things to different people, but generally has a negative connotation. Yet, stress is a familiar aspect of modern life, being a stimu-

[a]Address for correspondence: College of Dentistry, Ohio State University, 4179 Postle Hall, 305 W. 12th. Ave., #192, Columbus OH 43210-1241. Voice: 614-688-8562; fax: 614-292-6087.

dhabhar.1@osu.edu

lant for some individuals, but a problem for many others. We have defined *stress* as a constellation of events, which begins with a stimulus (*stressor*) that precipitates a reaction in the brain (*stress perception*), which subsequently activates physiologic systems in the body (*stress response*).[1,2] The physiologic stress response results in the release of neurotransmitters and hormones that serve as the brain's messengers to the rest of the body. The consequences of this physiologic response are generally adaptive in the short run,[1,3] but can be damaging when stress is chronic and long lasting.[1,4]

Important distinguishing characteristics of stress include its duration and intensity. We define *acute stress* as stress that lasts for a period of minutes to hours, and *chronic stress* as stress that persists for days to months. The magnitude of stress can be gauged by the peak levels of stress hormones, neurotransmitters, and other physiological changes, such as increases in heart rate and blood pressure, and by the amount of time for which these changes persist during and following stressor exposure. Thus, the magnitude of stress can be regarded as a combination of its intensity and duration. An important marker for deleterious effects of chronic stress is a breakdown in the regularity of the circadian corticosterone rhythm in rodents[1] and cortisol rhythm in humans.[5]

Stress has long been suspected of playing a role in the etiology of many diseases. Numerous studies have shown that stress can be immunosuppressive, and hence that it can be detrimental to health.[6–18] Moreover, glucocorticoid stress hormones are regarded widely as being immunosuppressive,[7] and are used clinically as anti-inflammatory agents.[19] In contrast to the generally accepted idea that stress and stress mediators are harmful, this chapter examines the beneficial effects of stress and stress hormones in preparing the immune system for dealing with potential immunologic challenges (e.g., wounding or infection) that may be imposed by the actions of a stressor (e.g., a predator).

AN EVOLUTIONARY PERSPECTIVE

An evolutionary perspective has guided our approach to the study of stress and immune function. When viewed from this perspective, suppression of immune function under all stress conditions does not appear to be evolutionarily adaptive because stress is an intrinsic part of life for most organisms. Dealing successfully with stressors is what enables survival. Environmental challenges and most evolutionary selection pressures are stressors that might be psychological (fear, anxiety), physical (wounding, infection), or physiological (food or water deprivation). One of the primary functions of the brain is to perceive stress, warn of danger, and enable an organism to deal with the consequences. This function is accomplished through the release of stress-responsive neurotransmitters and hormones. For example, when a gazelle sees a charging lion, the gazelle's brain detects a threat and orchestrates a physiologic response to first prepare, and then enable, the gazelle to flee. We have suggested that under such conditions, just as the stress response prepares the nervous, cardiovascular, musculoskeletal, and neuroendocrine systems for fight or flight, it may also prepare the immune system for challenges (e.g., wounding or infection) that may be imposed by the stressor.[1,3,20–22] A focus of our research has been to elucidate the cellular and molecular mechanisms mediating the beneficial versus harmful effects of stress on the overall health of an organism.

PARADOXICAL OBSERVATIONS ON
THE EFFECTS OF STRESS ON IMMUNE FUNCTION

Three paradoxes present themselves when one reviews the extensive literature examining the relationship between stress, immune function, and health: First, as the preceding discussion suggests, it is paradoxical that organisms should have evolved to suppress immune function at a time when an active immune response may be critical for survival—for example, under conditions of stress when an organism may be injured or infected by the actions of the stress-inducing agent (e.g., an attacking predator). Second, on the one hand stress is thought to suppress immunity and increase susceptibility to infections and cancer,[13,15,23-25] but on the other hand it is thought to exacerbate inflammatory diseases[26-31] such as psoriasis, asthma, arthritis, and lupus erythematosus (which should be ameliorated by a suppression of immune function). Third, stress is known to exacerbate autoimmune and inflammatory diseases,[26-28] however, stress hormones (glucocorticoids) are used clinically to treat these diseases.[19]

Keeping these paradoxical observations in mind, and based on our initial studies on the effects of stress on blood leukocyte distribution, we hypothesized that under certain conditions, stress may enhance rather than suppress immune function. The studies described here were designed to test this hypothesis.

STRESS-INDUCED CHANGES IN
LEUKOCYTE NUMBERS IN THE BLOOD

Immune cells or leukocytes circulate continuously from the blood, into various organs, and back into the blood. This circulation is essential for the maintenance of an effective immune defense network,[32] The numbers and proportions of leukocytes in the blood provide an important representation of the state of distribution of leukocytes in the body and of the state of activation of the immune system. Numerous studies have shown that stress and stress hormones induce significant changes in absolute numbers and relative proportions of leukocytes in the blood. In fact, decreases in blood leukocyte numbers were used as an indirect measure for increases in plasma corticosterone before methods were available to directly assay the hormone.[33] Stress-induced decreases in blood leukocyte numbers have been reported in fish,[34] mice,[35] rats,[20,21,36-38] rabbits,[39] horses,[40] non-human primates,[41] and humans.[12,42] This suggests that the phenomenon of stress-induced leukocyte distribution has been conserved through evolution, and that perhaps this redistribution has an important adaptive and functional significance.

Studies have shown that stress-induced increases in plasma corticosterone are accompanied by a significant decrease in numbers and percentages of lymphocytes, and by an increase in numbers and percentages of neutrophils. Dhabhar et al. have shown that stress-induced changes in blood leukocyte distribution are apparent within

30 min of applying the stressor.[21] These authors reported a large decrease (45–60% lower than baseline) in total blood leukocyte numbers. FACS analyses revealed that absolute numbers of peripheral blood helper T cell (Th), cytolytic T cell (CTL), B cells, natural killer (NK) cells, and monocytes all show a rapid and significant decrease (40–70% lower than baseline) during stress.[21] Further experiments revealed that stress-induced decreases in blood leukocyte numbers are rapidly reversed with leukocyte numbers returning to prestress baseline levels within three hours after the cessation of stress.[21]

Dhabhar et al. have also shown that the stress-induced changes in leukocyte distribution are mediated by hormones released by the adrenal gland.[22,43] Thus, the magnitude of the stress-induced changes in blood leukocyte numbers is significantly reduced in adrenalectomized animals.[21,22] Cyanoketone treatment, which virtually eliminates the corticosterone stress response, also virtually eliminates the stress-induced decrease in blood lymphocyte numbers, and significantly enhances the stress-induced increase in blood neutrophil numbers.[22] Several studies have shown that glucocorticoid treatment induces changes in leukocyte distribution in mice,[44–47] guinea pigs,[48] rats,[22,49,50] rabbits,[51] and humans.[52–54] It has been shown in rats that both adrenalectomy (which eliminates the corticosterone and epinephrine stress response)[21,22,35,55] or cyanoketone treatment (which eliminates only the corticosterone stress response), virtually eliminate the stress-induced redistribution of blood leukocytes.[22]

Since adrenal steroids act at two distinct receptor subtypes, both of which show a heterogeneity of expression in immune cells and tissues,[56–59] Dhabhar et al. investigated the role played by each receptor subtype in mediating changes in leukocyte distribution.[22] Acute administration of aldosterone (a specific Type I adrenal steroid receptor agonist) to adrenalectomized animals did not have a significant effect on blood leukocyte numbers. In contrast, acute administration of corticosterone (the endogenous Type I and Type II receptor agonist) or RU28362 (a specific Type II receptor agonist) to adrenalectomized animals induced changes in leukocyte distribution that were similar to those observed in intact animals during stress. These results suggest that corticosterone, acting at the Type II adrenal steroid receptor, is a major mediator of the stress-induced decreases in blood lymphocyte and monocyte distribution. Taken together, these studies show that stress and glucocorticoid hormones induce a significant decrease in blood lymphocyte numbers when administered under acute or chronic conditions.

In apparent contrast to glucocorticoid hormones, catecholamine hormones have been shown to increase blood leukocyte numbers in rats[60] and humans.[61] On closer examination it is observed that, following adrenaline or noradrenaline administration, neutrophil and NK cell numbers increase rapidly and dramatically whereas T and B cell numbers decrease.[62–65] Carslon et al. have shown that catecholamine pretreatment results in increased accumulation of lymphocytes in the spleen and lymph nodes,[66] an observation that is in agreement with a catecholamine-induced decrease in lymphocytes in the blood. By acutely administering epinephrine, norepinephrine, selective α and β adrenergic receptor agonists, or corticosterone to adrenalectomized animals, Dhabhar and McEwen have shown that increases in blood granulocyte numbers may be mediated by the α_1 and β adrenergic receptors, and are counteracted by corticosterone acting at the Type II adrenal steroid receptor.[43] Increases in lymphocytes may be mediated by the α_2 receptor while decreases in lymphocytes may be mediated by β adrenergic and Type II adrenal steroid receptors.[43]

Therefore, the absolute number of specific blood leukocyte subpopulations may be significantly affected by the ambient concentrations of epinephrine, norepinephrine, and corticosterone. Differences in concentrations and combinations of these hormones may explain reported differences in blood leukocyte numbers during different stress conditions (e.g., short- versus long-duration acute stress, acute versus chronic stress) and during exercise.

A STRESS-INDUCED DECREASE IN BLOOD LEUKOCYTE NUMBERS REPRESENTS A REDISTRIBUTION RATHER THAN A DESTRUCTION OR NET LOSS OF BLOOD LEUKOCYTES

From the above discussion it is clear that stress and glucocorticoid hormones induce rapid and significant decreases in blood lymphocyte, monocyte, and NK cell numbers. The decrease in blood leukocyte numbers may be interpreted in two possible ways. The decrease in cell numbers could reflect a large-scale destruction of circulating leukocytes. Alternatively, it could reflect a redistribution of leukocytes from the blood to other organs in the body. Several studies have shown that glucocorticoid-induced decrease in blood leukocytes reflects a redistribution rather than a destruction of immune cells.[44–47,67,68]

Dhabhar *et al.* conducted experiments to test the hypothesis that acute stress induces a redistribution of leukocytes from the blood to other compartments in the body.[21,69] The first series of experiments examined the kinetics of recovery of the stress-induced reduction in blood leukocyte numbers. It was hypothesized that if the observed effects of stress represented a redistribution rather than a destruction of leukocytes, one would see a relatively rapid return of leukocyte numbers back to baseline upon the cessation of stress. Results showed that all leukocyte subpopulations that showed a decrease in absolute numbers during stress, showed a complete recovery with numbers reaching prestress baseline levels within three hours after the cessation of stress.[21] Plasma levels of lactate dehydrogenase (LDH), a marker for cellular damage, were also monitored in the same experiment. If the stress-induced decrease in leukocyte numbers were the result of a destruction of leukocytes, one would expect to observe an increase in plasma levels of LDH during or following stress. No significant changes in plasma LDH were observed, further suggesting that a redistribution rather than a destruction of leukocytes was primarily responsible for the stress-induced decrease in blood leukocyte numbers.[21]

It is important to recognize that glucocorticoids induce changes in various immune parameters,[7,70] and in immune cell distribution,[20,21,46–48,52,67,71] in the absence of cell death even though these hormones are also known to induce leukocyte apoptosis.[72] It has been suggested that some species may be *steroid-resistant* and others may be *steroid-sensitive*, and that glucocorticoid-induced changes in blood leukocyte numbers represent changes in leukocyte redistribution in steroid-resistant species (humans and guinea pig), and leukocyte lysis in steroid-sensitive species (mouse and rat).[73] However, a large body of evidence now indicates that even in species previously thought to be steroid-sensitive, adrenal steroids induce leukocyte redistribution rather than leukocyte destruction.[46,74–76]

Based on the above discussion, the obvious question one might ask is: Where do blood leukocytes go during stress? Numerous studies using stress or stress hormone treatments, have investigated this issue. Using gamma imaging to follow the distribution of adoptively transferred radio-labelled leukocytes in rabbits, Toft *et al.* have shown that stress induces a redistribution of leukocytes from the blood to lymphatic tissues.[39] It has been reported that anesthesia stress, as well as the infusion of adrenocorticotropic hormone (ACTH) and prednisolone in rats results in decreased numbers of labelled lymphocytes in the thoracic duct, while the cessation of drug infusion results in normal circulation of labelled lymphocytes.[71] This suggests that hormonal changes similar to those observed during stress induce the retention of circulating lymphocytes in different body compartments, thus resulting in a decrease in lymphocyte numbers in the thoracic duct and a concomitant decrease in numbers in the peripheral blood.[71] Fleshner *et al.* have shown that acute stress results in an increase in the percentage of CD4 and a decrease in the percentage of CD8 in the mesenteric lymph nodes and have suggested that these changes in lymphocyte composition may mediate changes in antibody production by the affected lymph nodes.[77] It has also been reported that a single injection of hydrocortisone, prednisolone, or ACTH results in increased numbers of lymphocytes in the bone marrow of mice,[46] guinea pigs,[48] and rats.[68] Fauci *et al.* have suggested that glucocorticoid-induced decreases in blood leukocyte numbers in humans may also reflect a redistribution of immune cells to other organs in the body.[52,78,79] Finally, corticosteroids have been shown to induce the accumulation of lymphocytes in mucosal sites,[80] and the skin has been identified as a target organ to which leukocytes traffic during stress.[3]

It is important to note that in these studies, a return to basal glucocorticoid levels is almost always followed by a rapid return to baseline numbers of blood lymphocytes, further supporting the hypothesis that the decrease in blood leukocyte numbers is the result of a glucocorticoid-induced redistribution rather than a glucocorticoid-induced destruction of blood leukocytes.

STRESS-INDUCED REDISTRIBUTION OF BLOOD LEUKOCYTES—FUNCTIONAL CONSEQUENCES

Dhabhar *et al.* were the first to propose that a stress-induced decrease in blood leukocyte numbers represents an adaptive response.[1–3,20–22] These authors have suggested that this decrease in blood leukocyte numbers represents a redistribution of leukocytes from the blood to other organs, such as the skin, mucosal lining of gastrointestinal and urinary-genital tracts, lung, liver, and lymph nodes that may serve as "battle stations" should the body defenses be breached. They have also suggested that such a leukocyte redistribution may enhance immune function in compartments into which leukocytes traffic during stress.[1–3,20–22]

Thus, an acute stress response may direct the body's "soldiers" (leukocytes), to exit their "barracks" (spleen and bone marrow), travel the "boulevards" (blood vessels), and take position at potential "battle stations" (skin, lining of gastro-intestinal and urinary-genital tracts, lung, liver, and lymph nodes) in preparation for immune challenge.[1,3,20–22] In addition to "redeploying" leukocytes to potential "battle stations" stress hormones may also better equip them for "battle" by enhancing processes like antigen presentation, phagocytosis, and antibody production. Thus, a hormonal alarm signal released by the brain upon detecting a stressor, may "prepare" the immune system for potential challenges (wounding or infection) that may arise due to the actions of the stress-inducing agent (e.g., a predator or attacker).

An important, but under appreciated function of endocrine mediators released during of acute stress may be to ensure that appropriate leukocytes are present in the right place and at the right time to respond to an immune challenge that might be initiated by the stress-inducing agent (e.g., attack by a predator or invasion by a pathogen). The modulation of immune cell distribution by acute stress, may be an adaptive response designed to enhance immune surveillance and increase the capacity of the immune system to respond to challenge in immune compartments (such as the skin, epithelia of lung, and gastro-intestinal and urinary-genital tracts) that serve as major defense barriers for the body. Thus, endocrine mediators released during stress may serve to enhance immune preparedness for potential (or ongoing) immune challenge.

STRESS-INDUCED ENHANCEMENT OF IMMUNE FUNCTION

Although a majority of studies in the field of psychoneuroimmunology have focussed on the immunosuppressive effects of stress, several studies have also revealed that, under certain conditions, stress can be immunoenhancing. In general, acute stress is found to be immunoenhancing whereas chronic stress is found to be immunosuppressive (in some cases the effects of stress on leukocyte numbers and proportions in the compartment being assayed need to be taken into consideration for this statement to hold). Dhabhar *et al.* have suggested that a stress-induced enhancement of immune function may be an adaptive response to prepare an organism for potential immunologic challenges (e.g., a wound or infection inflicted by an attacker) for which stress perception by the brain, and subsequent stress hormone and neurotransmitter release, may serve as an early warning.[1–3,21]

As discussed above, acute stress induces a significant redistribution of leukocytes from the blood to other organs (e.g., skin and lymph nodes) in the body,[21,69] and adrenal stress hormones are major mediators of this leukocyte redistribution.[22] Since the skin is one of the targets to which leukocytes traffic during stress, Dhabhar and McEwen hypothesized that a stress-induced leukocyte redistribution may increase immune surveillance in the skin and consequently enhance immune function should the skin be exposed to antigen following acute stress.[3]

To test this hypothesis, they examined the effects of acute stress on skin immunity, using a rodent model for a skin delayed type hypersensitivity (DTH) response.[3] In order to induce DTH, animals were initially sensitized to 2,4-dinitro-1-fluorobenzene (DNFB) by administering the chemical antigen to the skin of the dorsum. The *sensitization* phase of a DTH reaction is one in which the organism develops an immunologic memory (through the generation of memory T cells) for the antigen with which it is immunized. Following sensitization, the ability of the animals to mount a DTH response against DNFB was examined by administering DNFB to the dorsal aspect of the pinna. The DTH response was subsequently measured as an increase in pinna thickness proportional to the intensity of the ongoing immune reaction.[81,82] This phase, also known as the elicitation or *challenge* phase, involves recruitment of memory T cells and effector cells (such as, neutrophils, macrophages, CTLs, and NK cells) that mount an immune response against the antigen to which the animal was previously sensitized. Acute restraint stress administered immediately before the challenge with antigen resulted in a large and long-lasting enhancement of skin DTH.[3] Histological analysis revealed significantly larger numbers of leukocytes in the skin of stressed animals both before and after exposure to antigen, and suggested that a stress-induced redistribution of leukocytes was one of the factors mediating the stress-induced enhancement of skin immunity.[3] Acute stress has similarly been shown to enhance skin DTH in mice.[83]

Dhabhar and McEwen subsequently showed that acute stress administered at the time of sensitization also significantly enhances a skin DTH response following challenge.[84] In these studies animals were stressed acutely (2-h restraint) before the administration of the sensitizing antigen. Compared to control animals, stressed animals showed a significantly larger DTH response following challenge although no stress was applied at the time of challenge. These results showed that acute stress administered either during sensitization or challenge, can significantly enhance a skin DTH response.[84]

STRESS-INDUCED SUPPRESSION OF IMMUNE FUNCTION

Numerous studies have shown that stress can be immunosuppressive and hence may be detrimental to health. Since these studies have been reviewed and discussed extensively,[8–10,85–88] the reader is referred to these papers and to other papers in this volume for a more detailed account of the subject. It may be worth noting here that most stress conditions that are found to be immunoenhancing involve acute stress, and those that are found to be immunosuppressive involve chronic stress (with the effects of stress on leukocyte distribution being an important factor to be taken into account).

It has been shown that in contrast to acute stress, chronic stress suppresses the skin DTH response.[1,89] A chronic stress-induced decrease in leukocyte mobilization from the blood to other body compartments is thought to be one of the mediators of this stress-induced suppression of skin DTH.[1] Similarly, in human and animal studies, chronic stress has also been shown to suppress different immune parameters examples of which include: delayed type hypersensitivity,[89,90] antibody production,[91,92] NK activity,[18,93–95] leukocyte proliferation,[93,94,96] skin homograft rejection,[97] virus-specific T cell and NK cell activity [98], and antimycobacterial activity of macrophages from susceptible mouse strains.[99]

ADRENAL HORMONES MEDIATE THE BIDIRECTIONAL
EFFECTS OF STRESS ON SKIN IMMUNE FUNCTION

It was the immunosuppressive effects of glucocorticoid hormones that led Philip Hench and Edward Kendall to the Nobel Prize in 1950, awarded for their discovery of the use of corticosteroids in the treatment of autoimmune disease.[100,101] Hench observed that patients suffering from autoimmune diseases showed recovery from these diseases during periods of other illnesses such as hepatitis. He postulated that the inflammatory response accompanying the other disease was stimulating the production of an endogenous immunosuppressive mediator that was responsible for inhibiting the autoimmune disease. Together with Kendall he determined that cortisol was that endogenous mediator, and their finding revolutionized the treatment of autoimmune disease and a host of other inflammatory disorders. Since that time, glucocorticoid hormones have been widely used as immunosuppressive agents in various clinical and experimental situations (for reviews see References 19 and 102–104).

In contrast to the well-known immunosuppressive effects of glucocorticoids, several studies have revealed that glucocorticoid hormones also exert immunomodulating (for reviews see References 105 and 106) and immunoenhancing effects (see References 107 and 108). In general, pharmacological concentrations of glucocorticoids exert immunosuppressive effects, whereas under different conditions, physiologic concentrations may exert immunomodulatory, immunoenhancing, or immunosuppressive effects. It is important to recognize that the source (natural versus synthetic) and concentration (physiologic versus pharmacologic) of glucocorticoid hormones, the effects of other physiologic factors (hormones, cytokines, and neurotransmitters), and the state of activation of an immune parameter (naïve versus activated leukocyte, early versus late activation, *etc.*), are all important factors that ultimately determine the nature of the effects of glucocorticoids on a given immune response.

Dhabhar and McEwen have demonstrated that the acute stress-induced enhancement of skin DTH is mediated by adrenal stress hormones.[2] Adrenalectomy, which eliminates the glucocorticoid and epinephrine stress response, eliminated the stress-induced enhancement of skin DTH.[2] Low dose corticosterone or epinephrine administration significantly enhanced skin DTH and caused a significant increase in T cell numbers in lymph nodes draining the site of the DTH reaction.[2] Moreover, simultaneous administration of these two stress hormones, produced an additive increase in the skin DTH response. These results showed that hormones released during an acute stress response may help prepare the immune system for potential challenges (e.g., wounding or infection) for which stress perception by the brain may serve as an early warning signal.[2] In contrast to the effects of physiologic doses of natural hormones, high dose corticosterone, chronic corticosterone, or low dose dexamethasone administration, all significantly suppressed skin DTH.[2]

Thus, adrenal stress hormones mediate the bidirectional effects of stress on skin immunity. Low doses of acutely administered corticosterone and epinephrine have immunoenhancing effects, whereas high doses of corticosterone, chronic corticosterone, or low doses of the synthetic steroid, dexamethasone, all exert immunosuppressive effects.[2] Moreover, dexamethasone shows a significantly greater immunosuppressive potency than corticosterone.[2] The cellular and molecular mechanisms mediating these bidirectional effects of stress hormones on skin immune function need to be investigated further.

STRESS-INDUCED ENHANCEMENT OF IMMUNE FUNCTION: IMPLICATIONS FOR DISEASE

In view of the above discussion, we hypothesize that a stress-induced enhancement of immune function may be beneficial in case of wound healing, infection or cancer, but could also be harmful in case of autoimmune or inflammatory disorders. The hypothesis that acute stress may increase in resistance to infections or cancer needs to be rigorously investigated. However, numerous studies have reported stress-induced exacerbation of autoimmune and inflammatory diseases. Over thirty years ago, Solomon and Moos described an association between stress and autoimmune disorders.[26] Rimon and Laakso have classified two categories of rheumatoid arthritis, a disease form more associated with genetic factors, and another more associated with psychodynamic factors such as stress.[109] Thomason et al. found that minor stress events such as day to day irritants were associated with exacerbations of rheumatoid arthritis.[28] Similarly, stress has been shown be related with the onset and exacerbation of psoriasis.[31] Stress has also been reported to precede the onset and exacerbation of multiple sclerosis,[27] in some cases however, it was chronic but not acute stress that was reported to precipitate disease.[110] It must be mentioned here that many studies have also failed to discover consistent relationships between life stress and autoimmune disease.[111,112]

We suggest that certain stress conditions, may enhance immune function and increase resistance to infections and cancer, but may also exacerbate autoimmune or inflammatory disorders. In contrast, chronic stress may suppress immune function and increase susceptibility to infections and cancer, but ameliorate autoimmune and inflammatory disorders.

STRESS-INDUCED SUPPRESSION OF IMMUNE FUNCTION: IMPLICATIONS FOR DISEASE

In addition to suppressing different immune parameters, human as well as animal studies have shown that chronic stress increases susceptibility to the common cold,[24] and to infection with viruses such as influenza,[15] and bacteria such as Toxoplasma,[113] and Salmonella.[91] Stress has also been shown to increase susceptibility to cancer.[23,114,115] Similarly, chronic stress has been shown to delay wound healing in mice[16] and humans,[14] and to impair the immune response to vaccination in human subjects.[13,116]

If chronic stress suppresses immune function and increases susceptibility to infectious disease and cancer, it may also be hypothesized that under these conditions, stress should ameliorate autoimmune or inflammatory diseases. Numerous studies have investigated the effects of environmental or psychological stress on autoimmune reactions. Levine et al. in 1962, demonstrated that the administration of prolonged restraint stress to rats before the induction of experimental allergic encephalomyelitis (EAE) resulted in a suppression of the incidence and severity of disease.[117] Rogers *et al.* in 1980, showed that exposure of rats to a variety of stressors results in a marked suppression of the clinical and histological manifestations of type II collagen-induced arthritis. Similarly, Griffin *et al.* demonstrated suppression of EAE by chronic stress.[118]

Thus, it is evident that under certain conditions, stress suppresses different immune parameters. Although this increases susceptibility to infectious disease and cancer, it may also confer protection against autoimmune and proinflammatory diseases. It is clear that further studies are needed to rigorously examine the mechanisms mediating both, stress-induced enhancement in resistance to infections and cancer, and stress-induced exacerbation of autoimmune and inflammatory disorders.

THE STRESS SPECTRUM HYPOTHESIS

Dhabhar and McEwen have proposed that a stress response and its consequent effects on immune function may be viewed in the context of a *stress spectrum* (see FIGURE 1).[1] One region of the stress spectrum is characterized by *eustress*; that is, conditions of acute or short-duration stress that may result in immunopreparatory, or immunoenhancing physiological conditions. An important characteristic of eustress is a rapid physiologic stress response mounted in the presence of the stressor, followed by a rapid shut-off of the response once the stress has subsided. The other end

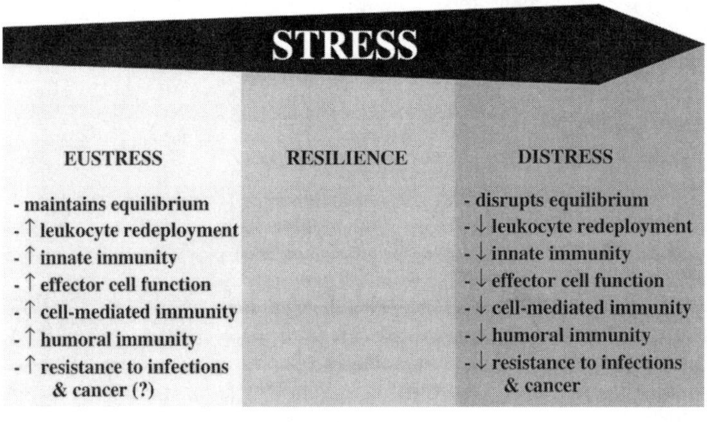

FIGURE 1. Hypothetical model representing the *stress spectrum* and its relationship to immune function.[1] One region of the stress spectrum is characterized by *eustress,* that is, conditions of acute or circumscribed amounts of stress, which may result in immunopreparatory, or immunoenhancing conditions. The other end of the stress spectrum is characterized by *distress,* that is, chronic, repeated, or physiologically exhausting stress, that may result in immunosuppressive conditions. Between eustress and distress is an area that represents *resilience,* that is, the ability of physiologic systems to enable survival for extended periods of time under increasingly demanding conditions. (From Dhabhar and McEwen.[1] Reproduced by permission.)

of the stress spectrum is characterized by *distress*; that is, chronic, repeated, or physiologically exhausting stress that may result in immunosuppression. An important characteristic of distress is that the physiologic stress response either persists long after the stress has subsided, or is activated repeatedly to result in an overall integrated increase in exposure of the organism to stress hormones. Recently, the concept of *allostatic load* has been proposed to define the constant wear and tear that takes place while different physiologic systems respond to the exhausting demands placed by internal and external stressors under conditions of distress (see Reference 4 for a review). We suggest that conditions of high allostatic load results in deleterious immunosuppression. Importantly, a disruption of the circadian corticosterone rhythm may be an indicator and/or mediator of distress or high allostatic load.[1,5] The stress spectrum model also proposes that between eustress and distress is an area that represents *resilience*, which we define as the ability of physiologic systems to enable survival for extended periods of time under increasingly demanding conditions.

CONCLUSIONS

Stress has long been suspected to play a role in the etiology of many diseases, and numerous studies have shown that stress can be immunosuppressive and, hence, may be detrimental to health. Moreover, glucocorticoid stress hormones are widely regarded as being immunosuppressive, and are used clinically as anti-inflammatory agents. However, this paper shows that under certain conditions, stress and glucocorticoid hormones exert immunoenhancing effects. Dhabhar *et al.* have suggested that the physiologic stress response may play a critical evolutionarily adaptive role, with stress hormones and neurotransmitters serving as messengers to prepare the immune system for potential immunologic challenges (e.g., wounding or infection) that are perceived in advance by the brain (e.g., the detection of predator or attacker).[1–3,20,21] However, it is important to recognize that, although a stress-induced enhancement of immune function may increase resistance to infections or cancer, it may also exacerbate autoimmune and inflammatory disease. In contrast, a stress- or glucocorticoid-induced suppression of immune function may increase susceptibility to infections or cancer, but may ameliorate autoimmune and inflammatory disorders. Therefore, there exists a Yin-Yang principle with respect to the effects of stress on immune function, and perhaps on most physiological parameters. Since these effects may potently influence the overall health of an organism, one might hypothesize that a physiologic equilibrium among these different systems would be most favorable for the maintenance of health.

It is also important to recognize that humans as well as animals experience stress as an intrinsic part of life, and in conjunction with many standard diagnostic, clinical, and experimental manipulations. Unintended stressors may significantly affect these diagnostic and clinical measures and overall health outcomes. Thus, when conducting clinical, diagnostic, or experimental manipulations, it may be important to account for the effects of stress on the specific physiologic parameter or health outcome being measured.

A determination of the physiologic mechanisms through which stress and stress hormones enhance or suppress immune responses may help our understanding and treatment of diseases thought to be affected by stress. The cellular and molecular mechanisms by which stress and stress hormones up- or downregulate an immune response merit further investigation. A greater understanding of these mechanisms would help in the development of biomedical treatments which could harness an individual's physiology to selectively enhance (during vaccination, wounding, infections, or cancer) or suppress (during autoimmune or inflammatory disorders) the immune response depending on what would be most beneficial for the patient.

ACKNOWLEDGMENT

This work was supported by The John D. & Catherine T. MacArthur Foundation, and by a DeWitt Wallace Foundation Fellowship.

REFERENCES

1. DHABHAR, F.S. & B.S. MCEWEN. 1997. Acute stress enhances while chronic stress suppresses immune function *in vivo*: a potential role for leukocyte trafficking. Brain Behav. Immun. **11**: 286–306.
2. DHABHAR, F.S. & B.S. MCEWEN. 1999. Enhancing versus suppressive effects of stress hormones on skin immune function. PNAS **96**: 1059–1064.
3. DHABHAR, F.S. & B.S. MCEWEN. 1996. Stress-induced enhancement of antigen-specific cell-mediated immunity. J. Immunol. **156**: 2608–2615.
4. MCEWEN, B.S. 1998. Protective and damaging effects of stress mediators: allostasis and allostatic load. N. Engl. J. Med. **338**: 171–179.
5. SEPHTON, S.E., R.M. SAPOLSKY, H.C. KRAEMER & D. SPIEGEL. 2000. Early mortality in metastatic breast cancer patients with absent or abnormal diurnal cortisol rhythms. J. Nat. Cancer Inst. In press.
6. ADER, R., D.L. FELTEN & N. COHEN. 1991. Psychoneuroimmunology, 2nd edit.: 1217. Academic Press, San Diego.
7. MUNCK, A., P.M. GUYRE & N.J. HOLBROOK. 1984. Physiological functions of glucocorticoids in stress and their relation to pharmacological actions. Endocr. Rev. **5**: 25–44.
8. BORYSENKO, M. & J. BORYSENKO. 1982. Stress, behavior, and immunity: animal models and mediating mechanisms. Gen. Hosp. Psychiatry **4**: 59–67.
9. KHANSARI, D.N., A.J. MURGO & R.E. FAITH. 1990. Effects of stress on the immune system. Immunol. Today **11**: 170–175.
10. KORT, W.J. 1994. The effect of chronic stress on the immune system. Adv. Neuroimmunol. **4**: 1–11.
11. MAIER, S.F., L.R. WATKINS & M. FLESHNER. 1994. Psychoneuroimmunology—The interface between behavior, brain, and immunity. Am. Psychol. **49**: 1004–1017.
12. HERBERT, T.B. & S. COHEN. 1993. Stress and immunity in humans: a meta-analytic review. Psychosom. Med. **55**: 364–379.
13. KIECOLT-GLASER, J.K., R. GLASER, S. GRAVENSTEIN, W.B. MALARKEY & J. SHERIDAN. 1996. Chronic stress alters the immune response to influenza virus vaccine in older adults. Proc. Natl. Acad. Sci. USA **93**: 3043–3047.
14. MARUCHA, P.T., J.K. KIECOLT-GLASER & M. FAVAGEHI. 1998. Mucosal wound healing is impaired by examination stress. Psychosom. Med. **60**: 362–365.
15. SHERIDAN, J.F. 1998. Stress-induced modulation of anti-viral immunity—Normal Cousins Memorial Lecture 1997. Brain Behav. Immun. **12**: 1–6.
16. PADGETT, D.A., P.T. MARUCHA & J.F. SHERIDAN. 1998. Restraint stress slows cutaneous wound healing in mice. Brain Behav. Immun. **12**: 64–73.

17. COHEN, S. & R.B. HERBERT. 1996. Health psychology: psychological factors and physical disease from the perspective of human psychoneuroimmunology. Annu. Rev. Psychol. **47:**

18. IRWIN, M., T. PATTERSON, T.L. SMITH, C. CALDWELL, S.A. BROWN, C. J. GILLIN & I. GRANT. 1990. Reduction of immune function in life stress and depression. Biol. Psychiatry **27:** 22–30.

19. SCHLEIMER, R.P., H.N. CLAMAN & A. ORONSKY, Eds. 1989. Anti-inflammatory Steroid Action: Basic and Clinical Aspects. 564. Academic Press, San Diego.

20. DHABHAR, F.S., A.H. MILLER, M. STEIN, B.S. MCEWEN & R.L. SPENCER. 1994. Diurnal and stress-induced changes in distribution of peripheral blood leukocyte subpopulations. Brain Behav. Immun. **8:** 66–79.

21. DHABHAR, F.S., A.H. MILLER, B.S. MCEWEN & R.L. SPENCER. 1995. Effects of stress on immune cell distribution—Dynamics and hormonal mechanisms. J. Immunol. **154:** 5511–5527.

22. DHABHAR, F.S., A.H. MILLER, B.S. MCEWEN & R.L. SPENCER. 1996. Stress-induced changes in blood leukocyte distribution—Role of adrenal steroid hormones. J. Immunol. **157:** 1638–1644.

23. BEN-ELIYAHU, S., R. YIRMIYA, J.C. LIEBESKIND, A.N. TAYLOR & R.P. GALE. 1991. Stress increases metastatic spread of a mammary tumor in rats: evidence for mediation by the immune system. Brain Behav. Immun. **5:** 193–205.

24. COHEN, S., D. A.J. TYRRELL & A.P. SMITH. 1991. Psychological stress and susceptibility to the common cold. New Engl. J. Med. **325:** 606–612.

25. GLASER, R., D.K. PEARL, J.K. KIECOLT-GLASER & W.B. MALARKEY. 1994. Plasma cortisol levels and reactivation of latent Epstein-Barr virus in response to examination stress. Psychoneuroendocrinology **19:** 765–772.

26. SOLOMON, G.F. & R.H. MOOS. 1964. Emotions, immunity and disease. Arch. Gen. Psychiatry **11:** 657–669.

27. MEI-TAL, V., S. MEYEROWITZ & G. ENGEL. 1970. Role of psychological process in a somatic disorder: multiple sclerosis. Psychosom. Med. **32:** 67–86.

28. THOMASON, B.T., P.J. BRANTLEY, G.N. JONES, H.R. DYER & J.L. MORRIS. 1992. The relations between stress and disease activity in rheumatoid arthritis. J. Behav. Med. **15:** 215–220.

29. AMKRAUT, A.A., C.F. SOLOMON & H.C. KRAEMER. 1971. Stress, early experience and adjuvant-induced arthritis in the rat. Psychosom. Med. **33:** 203–214.

30. PAWLAK, C., H. HEIKER, T. WITTE, B. WIESE, C.J. HEIJNEN, R.E. SCHMIDT & M. SCHEDLOWSKI. 1999. A prospective study of daily stress and disease activity in patients with systemic lupus erythematosus. Neuroimmunomodulation **6:** 241.

31. AL'ABADIE, M.S., G.G. KENT & D.J. GAWKRODGER. 1994. The relationship between stress and the onset and exacerbation of psoriasis and other skin conditions. Brit. J. Dermatol. **130:** 199–203.

32. SPRENT, J. & D.F. TOUGH. 1994. Lymphocyte life-span and memory. Science **265:** 1395–1400.

33. HOAGLAND, H., F. ELMADJIAN & G. PINCUS. 1946. Stressful psychomotor performance and adrenal cortical function as indicated by the lymphocyte reponse. J. Clin. Endocrinol. **6:** 301–311.

34. PICKFORD, G.E., A.K. SRIVASTAVA, A.M. SLICHER & P.T. PANG. 1971. The stress response in the abundance of circulating leukocytes in the Killifish, Fundulus heteroclitus. I. The cold-shock sequence and the effects of hypophysectomy. J. Exp. Zool. **177:** 89–96.

35. JENSEN, M.M. 1969. Changes in leukocyte counts associated with various stressors. J. Reticuloendothel. Soc. **8:** 457–465.

36. JOHNS, M.W. 1967. Leukocyte response to sound stress in rats: role of the adrenal gland. J. Pathol. Bacteriol. **93:** 681–685.

37. RINNER, I., K. SCHAUENSTEIN, H. MANGGE, S. PORTA & R. KVETNANSKY. 1992. Opposite effects of mild and severe stress on *in vitro* activation of rat peripheral blood lymphocytes. Brain Behav. Immun. **6:** 130–140.

38. STEFANSKI, V., G.F. SOLOMON, A.S. KLING, J. THOMAS & S. PLAEGER. 1996. Impact of social confrontation on rat CD4 T cells bearing different CD45R isoforms. Brain Behav. Immun. **10:** 364–379.

39. TOFT, P., P. SVENDSEN, E. TONNESEN, J.W. RASMUSSEN & N.J. CHRISTENSEN. 1993. Redistribution of lymphocytes after major surgical stress. Acta Anesthesiol. Scand. **37:** 245–249.

40. SNOW, D.H., S.W. RICKETTS & D.K. MASON. 1983. Hematological responses to racing and training exercise in Thoroughbred horses, with particular reference to the leukocyte response. Equine Vet. J. **15:** 149–154.

41. MORROW-TESCH, J.L., J.J. MCGLONE & R.L. NORMAN. 1993. Consequences of restraint stress on natural killer cell activity, behavior, and hormone levels in Rhesus Macaques (*Macaca mulatta*). Psychoneuroendocrinology **18:** 383–395.

42. SCHEDLOWSKI, M., R. JACOBS, G. STRATMAN, S. RICHTER, A. HÄDIKE, U. TEWES, T.O.F. WAGNER & R.E. SCHMIDT. 1993. Changes of natural killer cells during acute psychological stress. J. Clin. Immunol. **13:** 119–126.

43. DHABHAR, F.S. & B.S. MCEWEN. 1999. Changes in blood leukocyte distribution: interactions between catecholamine and glucocorticoid hormones. Neuroimmunomodulation **6:** 213.

44. DOUGHERTY, R.F. & A. WHITE. 1945. Functional alterations in lymphoid tissue induced by adrenal cortical secretion. Am. J. Anat. **77:** 81–116.

45. SPAIN, D.M. & W. THALHIMER. 1951. Temporary accumulation of eosinophilic leucocytes in spleen on mice following administration of cortisone. Proc. Soc. Exp. Biol. Med. **76:** 320–322.

46. COHEN, J.J. 1972. Thymus-derived lymphocytes sequestered in the bone marrow of hydrocortisone-treated mice. J. Immunol. **108:** 841–844.

47. ZATZ, M.M. 1975. Effects of cortisone on lymphocyte homing. Isr. J. Med. Sci. **11:** 1368–1372.

48. FAUCI, A.S. 1975. Mechanisms of corticosteroid action on lymphocyte subpopulations. I. Redistribution of circulating T and B lymphocytes to the bone marrow. Immunology **28:** 669–680.

49. ULICH, T.R., M. KEYS, R.X. NI, J. DEL CASTILLO & E.B. DAKAY. 1988. The contributions of adrenal hormones, hemodynamic factors, and the endotoxin-related stress reaction to stable prostaglandin analog-induced peripheral lymphopenia and neutrophilia. J. Leukocyte Biol. **43:** 5–10.

50. MILLER, A.H., R.L. SPENCER, J. HASSET, C. KIM, R. RHEE, D. CIRA, F.S. DHABHAR, B.S. MCEWEN & M. STEIN. 1994. Effects of selective Type I and Type II adrenal steroid receptor agonists on immune cell distribution. Endocrinology **135:** 1934–1944.

51. VAN DEN BROEK, A.A., F.J. KEUNING, R. SOEHARTO & N. PROP. 1983. Immune suppression and histophysiology of the immune response I. Cortisone acetate and lymphoid cell migration. Virchows Arch. B Cell Pathol. **43:** 43–54.

52. FAUCI, A.S. & D.C. DALE. 1974. The effect of in vivo hydrocortisone on subpopulations of human lymphocytes. J. Clin. Invest. **53:** 240–246.

53. FAUCI, A.S. 1976. Mechanisms of corticosteroid action on lymphocyte subpopulations. II. Differential effects of in vivo hydrocortisone, prednisone, and dexamethasone on in vitro expression of lymphocyte function. Clin. Exp. Immunol. **24:** 54–62.

54. ONSRUD, M. & E. THORSBY. 1981. Influence of in vivo hydrocortisone on some human blood lymphocyte subpopulations. Scand. J. Immunol. **13:** 573–579.

55. KELLER, S.E., J.M. WEISS, S.J. SCHLEIFER, N.E. MILLER & M. STEIN. 1983. Stress-induced suppression of immunity in adrenalectomized rats. Science **221:** 1301–1304.

56. DHABHAR, F.S., B.S. MCEWEN & R.L. SPENCER. 1993. Stress response, adrenal steroid receptor levels, and corticosteroid-binding globulin levels—A comparison between Sprague Dawley, Fischer 344, and Lewis rats. Brain Res. **616:** 89–98.

57. DHABHAR, F.S., A.H. MILLER, B.S. MCEWEN & R.L. SPENCER. 1995. Differential activation of adrenal steroid receptors in neural and immune tissues of Sprague Dawley, Fischer 344, and Lewis rats. J. Neuroimmunol. **56:** 77–90.

58. MILLER, A.H., R.L. SPENCER, B.D. PEARCE, T.L. PISELL, Y. AZRIELI, P. TANAPAT, H. MODAY, R. RHEE & B.S. MCEWEN. 1998. Glucocorticoid receptors are differentially expressed in the cells and tissues of the immune system. Cell. Immunol. **186:** 45–54.

59. SPENCER, R.L., B.A. KALMAN & F.S. DHABHAR. 2000. Role of endogenous glucocorticoids in immune system function: Regulation and counterregulation. *In* Handbook of Physiology, B.S. McEwen, Ed. In press.

60. HARRIS, T.J., T.J. WALTMAN, S.M. CARTER & A.S. MAISEL. 1995. Effect of prolonged catecholamine infusion on immunoregulatory function: implications in congestive heart failure. J. Am. Coll. Cardiol. **26:** 102–109.

61. LANDMANN, R., F.B. MULLER, C.H. PERINI, M. WESP, P. ERNE & F.R. BUHLER. 1984. Changes of immunoregulatory cells induced by psychological and physical stress: relationship to plasma catecholamines. Clin. Exp. Immunol. **58:** 127–135.

62. LANDMANN, R. 1992. Beta-adrenergic receptors in human leukocyte subpopulations. Eur. J. Clin. Invest. **22**(Suppl. 1): 30–36.

63. TONNESEN, E., N.J. CHRISTENSEN & M.M. BRINKLOV. 1987. Natural killer cell activity during cortisol and adrenaline infusion in healthy volunteers. Eur. J. Clin. Invest. **17:** 497–503.

64. SCHEDLOWSKI, M., A. FALK, A. ROHNE, T.O.F. WAGNER, R. JACOBS, U. TEWES & R.E. SCHMIDT. 1993. Catecholamines induce alterations of distribution and activity of human natural killer (NK) cells. J. Clin. Immunol. **13:** 344–351.

65. BENSCHOP, R.J., M. RODRIGUEZ-FEUERHAHN & M. SCHEDLOWSKI. 1996. Catecholamine-induced leukocytosis: early observations, current research, and future directions. Brain, Behav. Immun. **10:** 77–91.

66. CARLSON, S.L., S. FOX & K.M. ABELL. 1997. Catecholamine modulation of lymphocyte homing to lymphoid tissues. Brain Behav. Immun. **11:** 307–20.

67. LUNDIN, P.M. & L.A. HEDMAN. 1978. Influence of corticosterone on lymphocyte recirculation. Lymphology **11:** 216–221.

68. COX, J.H. & W.L. FORD. 1982. The migration of lymphocytes across specialized vascular endothelium. IV. Prednisolone acts at several points on the recirculation pathway of lymphocytes. Cell. Immunol. **66:** 407–422.

69. DHABHAR, F.S. 1998. Stress-induced enhancement of cell-mediated immunity. *In* Neuroimmunomodulation: Molecular, Integrative Systems, and Clinical Advances, S.M. McCann, et al., Eds.: 359–372. New York Academic Scientific, New York.

70. CALLEWAERT, D.M., V.K. MOUDGIL, G. RADCLIFF & R. WAITE. 1991. Hormone specific regulation of natural killer cells by cortisol—direct inactivation of the cytotoxic function of cloned human NK cells without an effect on cellular proliferation. FEBS **285:** 108–110.

71. SPRY, C.J.F. 1972. Inhibition of lymphocyte recirculation by stress and corticotropin. Cell. Immunol. **4:** 86–92.

72. COHEN, J.J. 1992. Glucocorticoid-induced apoptosis in the thymus. Semin. Immunol. **4:** 363–369.

73. CLAMAN, H.N. 1972. Corticosteroids and lymphoid cells. N. Engl. J. Med. **287:** 388–397.

74. MOORHEAD, J.W. & H.N. CLAMAN. 1972. Thymus-derived lymphocytes and hydrocortisone: identification of subsets of theta-bearing cells and redistribution to bone marrow. Cell. Immunol. **5:** 74–86.

75. THOMPSON, J. & R. VAN FURTH. 1973. The effect of glucocorticoids on the kinetics of promonocytes and monocytes of the bone marrow. J. Exp. Med. **137:** 10–21.

76. HEDMAN, L.A. & P.M. LUNDIN. 1977. The effect of steroids on the circulating lymphocyte population. II. Studies of the thoracic duct lymphocyte population of the guinea pig after neonatal thymectomy and prednisolone treatment. Lymphology **10:** 192–198.

77. FLESHNER, M., L.R. WATKINS, L.L. LOCKWOOD, M.L. LAUDENSLAGER & S.F. MAIER. 1992. Specific changes in lymphocyte subpopulations: a potential mechanism for stress-induced immunomodulation. J. Neuroimmunol. **41:** 131–142.

78. FAUCI, A.S. & D.C. DALE. 1975. Alternate-day prednisone therapy and human lymphocyte subpopulations. J. Clin. Invest. **55:** 22–32.

79. YU, D.T.Y., P.J. CLEMENTS, H.E. PAULUS, J.B. PETER, J. LEVY & E.V. BARNETT. 1974. Human lymphocyte subpopulations. Effects of corticosteroids. J. Clin. Invest. **53:** 565–571.

80. WALZER, P.D., M. LABINE, T.J. REDINGTON & M.T. CUSHION. 1984. Lymphocyte changes during chronic administration of and withdrawal from corticosteroids: relation to *Pneumocystis carinii* pneumonia. J. Immunol. **133:** 2502–2508.

81. PHANUPHAK, P., J.W. MOORHEAD & H.N. CLAMAN. 1974. Tolerance and contact sensitivity to DNFB in mice. I. In vivo detection by ear swelling and correlation with in vitro cell stimulation. J. Immunol. **112:** 115–123.

82. KIMBER, I. & R. DEARMAN. 1993. Approaches to the identification and classification of chemical allergens in mice. J. Pharmacol. Toxicol. Methods **29:** 11–16.

83. BLECHA, F., R.A. BARRY & K.W. KELLEY. 1982. Stress-induced alterations in delayed-type hypersensitivity to SRBC and contact sensitivity to DNFB in mice. Proc. Soc. Exp. Biol. Med. **169:** 239–246.

84. DHABHAR, F.S. & B.S. MCEWEN. 1999. Enhancement of the immunization/sensitization phase of cell-mediated immunity: the role of acute stress & adrenal stress hormones. Neuroimmunomodulation **6:** 213.

85. SKLAR, L.S. & H. ANISMAN. 1981. Stress and cancer. Psychol. Bull. **89:** 369–406.

86. ZWILLING, B. 1992. Stress affects disease outcomes. Confronted with infectious disease agents, the nervous and immune systems interact in complex ways. ASM News. **58:** 23–25.

87. IRWIN, M. 1994. Stress-induced immune suppression: role of brain corticotropin releasing hormone and autonomic nervous system mechanisms. Adv. Neuroimmunol. **4:** 29–47.

88. BLACK, P.H. 1994. Immune system-central nervous system interactions: effect and immunomodulatory consequences of immune system mediators on the brain. Antimicrob. Agents Chemother. **38:** 7–12.

89. BASSO, A.M., M. DEPIANTE-DEPAOLI, L. CANCELA & V. MOLINA. 1993. Seven-day variable-stress regime alters cortical β-adrenoreceptor binding and immunologic responses: reversal by imipramine. Pharmacol. Biochem. Behav. **45:** 665–672.

90. KELLEY, K.W., R.E. GREENFIELD, J.F. EVERMANN, S.M. PARISH & L.E. PERRYMAN. 1982. Delayed-type hypersensitivity, contact sensitivity, and PHA skin-test responses of heat- and cold-stressed calves. Am. J. Vet. Res. **43:** 775–779.

91. EDWARDS, E.A. & L.M. DEAN. 1977. Effects of crowding of mice on humoral antibody formation and protection to lethal antigenic challenge. Psychosom. Med. **39:** 19–24.

92. FLESHNER, M., M.L. LAUDENSLAGER, L. SIMONS & S.F. MAIER. 1989. Reduced serum antibodies associated with social defeat in rats. Physiol. & Behav. **45:** 1183–1187.

93. BARTROP, R., L. LAZARUS, E. LUCKHURST, L.G. KILOH & R. PENNY. 1977. Depressed lymphocyte function after bereavement. Lancet **8016:** 834–836.

94. CHENG, G.J., J.L. MORROW-TESCH, D.I. BELLER, E.M. LEVY & P.H. BLACK. 1990. Immunosuppression in mice induced by cold water stress. Brain Behav. Immun. **4:** 278–291.

95. KIECOLT-GLASER, J.K., W. GARNER, C. SPEICHER, G.M. PENN, J. HOLLIDAY & R. GLASER. 1984. Psychosocial modifiers of immunocompetence in medical students. Psychosom. Med. **46:** 7–14.

96. REGNIER, J.A. & K.W. KELLEY. 1981. Heat- and cold-stress suppresses in vivo and in vitro cellular immune response of chickens. Am. J. Vet. Res. **42:** 294–299.

97. WISTAR, R. & W.H. HILDEMANN. 1960. Effect of stress on skin transplantation immunity in mice. Science **131:** 159–160.

98. BONNEAU, R.H., J.F. SHERIDAN, N. FENG & R. GLASER. 1991. Stress-induced effects on cell-mediated innate and adaptive memory components of the murine immune response to herpes simplex virus infection. Brain Behav. Immun. **5:** 274–295.

99. BROWN, D.H. & B.S. ZWILLING. 1994. Activation of the hypothalamic-pituitary-adrenal axis differentially affects the anti-mycobacterial activity of macrophages from BCG-resistant and susceptible mice. J. Neuroimmunol. **53:** 181–187.

100. HENCH, P.S., E.C. KENDALL, C.H. SLOCUMB & H. POLLEY. 1949. The effect of a hormone of the adrenal cortex (17-hydroxy-11-dehydrocorticosterone: compound E) and of pituitary adrenocorticotropic hormone on rheumatoid arthritis. Proc. Staff Meet. Mayo Clin. **24:** 181–197.

101. HENCH, P.S. 1952. The reversibility of certain rheumatic and nonrheumatic conditions by the use of cortisone or of the pituitary adrenocorticotropic hormone. Ann. Intern. Med. **36:** 1–25.

102. FAUCI, A.S. 1979. Immunosuppressive and anti-inflammatory effects of glucocorticoids. *In* Glucocorticoid Hormone Action, J.D. Baxter and G.G. Rousseau, Eds.: 449–465. Springer-Verlag, Berlin.

103. GOLDSTEIN, R.A., D.L. BOWEN & A.S. FAUCI. 1992. Adrenal corticosteroids. *In* Inflammation: Basic Principles and Clinical Correlates, J.I. Gallin, I.M. Goldstein, and R. Snyderman, Eds.: 1061–1081. Raven Press, New York.

104. MARX, J. 1995. How the glucocorticoids suppress immunity. Science **270:** 232–233.

105. WILCKENS, T. 1995. Glucocorticoids and immune function: physiological relevance and pathogenic potential of hormonal dysfunction. TIPS **16:** 193–197.

106. WILCKENS, T. & R. DERIJK. 1997. Glucocorticoids and immune function: unknown dimensions and new frontiers. Immunol. Today **18:** 418–424.

107. JEFFERIES, W.M. 1991. Cortisol and immunity. Med. Hypotheses **34:** 198–208.

108. SPENCER, R.L., B.A. KALMAN & F.S. DHABHAR. 2000. Role of endogenous glucocorticoids in immune system function: regulation and counterregulation. *In* Handbook of Physiology: Coping with the Environment, B.S. McEwen, Ed. Oxford University Press, Oxford. In press.

109. RIMON, R. & R.-L. LAAKSO. 1985. Life stress and rheumatoid arthritis. Psychother. Psychosom. **43:** 38–43.

110. PHILIPPOPOULOS, G.S., E.D. WITTKOWER & A. COUSINEAU. 1958. The etiologic significance of emotional factors in onset and exacerbation of multiple sclerosis. Psychosom. Med. **20:** 458–474.

111. HENDRIE, H.C., R. PARASEKVAS, F.D. BARAGAR & J.D. ADAMSON. 1971. Stress, immunoglobulin levels, and early polyarthritis. J. Psychosom. Res. **15:** 337–342.

112. ZAUTRA, A.J., M.A. OKUN, S.E. ROBINSON, D. LEE, S.H. ROTH & J. EMMANUAL. 1989. Life stress and lymphocyte alterations among patients with rheumatoid arthritis. Health Psychol. **8:** 1–14.

113. CHAO, C.C., P.K. PETERSON, G.A. FILICE, C. POMEROY & B.M. SHARP. 1990. Effects of immobilization stress on the pathogenesis of acute murine toxoplasmosis. Brain Behav. Immun. **4:** 162–169.

114. BRENNER, G.J., N. COHEN, R. ADER & J.A. MOYNIHAN. 1990. Increased pulmonary metastases and natural killer cell activity in mice following handling. Life Sci. **47:** 1813–1819.

115. ANDERSEN, B.L., W.B. FARRAR, D. GOLDEN-KREUTZ, L.A. KUTZ, R. MACCALLUM, M.E. COURTNEY & R. GLASER. 1998. Stress and immune responses after surgical treatment for regional breast cancer. J. Natl. Cancer Inst. **90:** 30–36.

116. GLASER, R., J.K. KIECOLT-GLASER, R.H. BONNEAU, W. MALARKEY, S. KENNEDY & J. HUGHES. 1991. Stress-induced modulation of the immune response to recombinant hepatitis B vaccine. Psychosom. Med. **54:** 22–29.

117. LEVINE, S. & A. SALTZMAN. 1987. Nonspecific stress prevents relapses of experimental allergic encephalomyelitis in rats. Brain Behav. Immun. **1:** 336–341.

118. GRIFFIN, A.C., D.L. WARREN, A.C. WOLNY & C.C. WHITACRE. 1993. Suppression of experimental autoimmune encephalomyelitis by restraint stress. J. Neuroimmunol. **44:** 103–116.

Social Disruption, Immunity, and Susceptibility to Viral Infection

Role of Glucocorticoid Insensitivity and NGF

J.F. SHERIDAN,[a] J.L. STARK, R. AVITSUR, AND D.A. PADGETT

Laboratory of Neuroendocrine Immunology, Section of Oral Biology,
College of Dentistry, and the Institute for Behavioral Medicine Research,
The Ohio State University Health Sciences Center, Columbus, Ohio 43210, USA

ABSTRACT: Glucocorticoid (cort) responses have been shown to suppress inflammatory reactions by inhibiting the trafficking of immune cells. Recently, it was demonstrated that restraint stress (RST) and psychosocial stress (social reorganization; SRO) differentially affected the pathophysiology and survival in the mouse influenza viral infection model. While both stressors activated the HPA axis, only SRO affected survival. In RST, elevated cort diminished recruitment of inflammatory cells following intranasal challenge of C57BL/6 mice with A/PR8 virus. However, infected SRO mice developed hypercellularity in the lungs and were more likely to die from lung consolidation than controls. Since elevated cort failed to be anti-inflammatory in SRO mice, the hypothesis that psychosocial stress induced steroid insensitivity was tested. An *in vitro* cort suppression test was performed by stimulating splenocytes from SRO and control mice with mitogen in the presence or absence of cort. Proliferation of ConA-stimulated cells was inhibited by cort in a dose-dependent fashion in controls, but splenocytes from SRO mice stimulated with ConA were resistant to cort-induced suppression. Thus, psychosocial stress induced a state of steroid insensitivity. SRO also induced the release of nerve growth factor (NGF) from the salivary glands into circulation; plasma NGF correlated with development of steroid insensitivity. NGF has been reported to negatively regulate the expression of type II glucocorticoid receptors, and thus may be a key factor in the induction of steroid insensitivity.

INTRODUCTION

Stress is generally defined as a state of altered homeostasis resulting from either an external or internal stimulus. The stress response involves a variety of adaptive neuroendocrine mechanisms designed to restore homeostasis.[1] Although the response to stress may be directed toward physiological adaptation and restoration of health, there is evidence to indicate that stress increases the susceptibility to and severity of inflammatory and infectious diseases.[2–4] The response to stress is initiated within the

[a]Address for correspondence: John F. Sheridan or David A. Padgett, Section of Oral Biology, Box 192 Postle Hall, The Ohio State University, 305 W.12th Ave., Columbus, OH 43210, USA.
padgett.11@osu.edu or sheridan.1@osu.edu

central nervous system and translated into action by the hypothalamic–pituitary–adrenal (HPA) axis and the autonomic nervous system. These neuroendocrine pathways have been shown to modulate inflammatory and immune responses.[3,5–9]

The nature of the stressor is a significant variable in determining the host's response. For example, in a model of social conflict utilizing male mice (social reorganization; SRO), aggressive behavioral interactions activate the HPA-axis and cause the release of nerve growth factor (NGF) from the salivary glands into the blood.[10,11] On the other hand, physical restraint stress (RST), which has been shown to suppress antiviral immunity,[3] activates the HPA axis, but does not stimulate the release of NGF. RST prevents the lung and lymph-node inflammation that normally occurs in response to an influenza viral infection; glucocorticoids (cort) mediate this effect, as cellular accumulation in these organs is normalized by treating with RU486, a glucocorticoid receptor antagonist.[12] In contrast, there is increased lymphadenopathy and tissue cellularity in SRO mice, despite the fact that circulating cort levels are similar to those seen in RST mice (unpublished observation). One explanation for this observation might be that the leukocytes of the SRO mice are cort resistant, and therefore unable to respond to the circulating corticosterone.

Previous studies have established that NGF and cort have opposing actions at both the cellular and molecular levels. For example, the synthetic glucocorticoid (GC), dexamethasone, has been found to decrease production of NGF receptor mRNA *in vitro* and *in vivo*.[13] Similarly, NGF suppresses the type II GC receptor in hippocampal cell cultures without affecting the expression of the type I mineralocorticoid receptor.[14] This finding raises the possibility that the type II receptors on leukocytes could be modulated by NGF *in vivo*, thus making these cells resistant to GC.

In the present study, social reorganization of established murine cohorts was examined as a stressor in the setting of a viral infection. This naturalistic social stressor elevated plasma cort and NGF, induced cort resistance in splenocytes, and increased mortality in influenza-virus-infected mice. In light of these observations, it is hypothesized that the stress of social reorganization causes a state of functional glucocorticoid resistance that results in hyperinflammatory responses; challenge of hosts that are cort resistant results in increased immunopathology during viral infection.

MATERIALS AND METHODS

Animals

Male and female C57BL/6 mice (Charles River, Inc., Wilmington, MA) were 6–16 weeks old and housed five per cage. Mice were allowed free access to water and standard laboratory chow (except during restraint stress) and were kept on a 12-h light/dark cycle. Before use, animals were given one to two weeks to recover from shipping stress. Aggressive male mice used for paired fighting studies were housed individually for at least two weeks prior to the experiment.

Blood Collection/ Processing

Whole blood (100–200 μL) was obtained from the retro-orbital plexus or tail vein, and serum was isolated and stored frozen until assayed.

Fighting Pairs Study

Baseline blood samples were obtained from 12 aggressive male mice that had been individually housed for at least two weeks. Subsequently, the animals were paired for a 20-min morning fighting session. The latency to the first attack was seconds to minutes, and timing began at the initiation of the first attack. The number of attacks occurring in each cage and the mouse initiating the attacks were noted. Mice were bled from the retro-orbital plexus immediately after the 20-min fighting session, and again at 1, 3, and 24 h after the fighting session.

Social Reorganization Paradigm

Upon arrival, mice were identified by ear tag and randomly distributed at five mice per cage. All mice were allowed to acclimate to the new surroundings for two weeks. During this time, definable social hierarchies formed. At this point "dominant" mice were identified in each cage using behavioral observations.[15] During observation, the number of social investigatory (sniffing), aggressive (chase, bite, tail-rattle, allogroom, aggressive upright, and aggressive sideways postures), and defensive (flee and submissive upright or sideways postures) behaviors were assessed for each individual animal. In addition, fur score was assessed ranging from 1 (no bald, damaged, or disheveled patches, fur well groomed) to 5 reflecting increasing incidence of damage to, or deterioration in the apparent condition, of the fur. Individuals within groups were ranked according to the ratio of the number of investigatory/aggressive interactions initiated and the number of defensive interactions.[16] Top- ranked "dominant" males had the highest attack ratio. Subsequently, for SRO, mice initially labeled as dominant were switched between cages at the beginning of the 12-h dark cycle (6:00 P.M.). SRO was performed every second day for a total of four times.

Restraint Stress

Mice were restrained in 50-mL conical tubes for four consecutive nights (16 h per night), as previously described.[2]

Virus Stock

Influenza A/Puerto Rico/8/34 (PR8) virus was obtained from the American Type Culture collection (Rockville, MD) and propagated in the allantoic cavity of 10-day-old embryonated chicken eggs as previously described.[2] Infectious allantoic fluid was collected, clarified by low-speed centrifugation, and stored at −70°C. The virus titer was determined to be 1280 hemagglutinating units (HAU) per mL, using human type-"O" erythrocytes.

Infection of Mice

Mice were infected with 0.05 mL containing influenza A/PR8 virus diluted in PBS and instilled intranasally. For challenge studies, mice were infected with 24 HAU A/PR8. Prior to infection, all mice were anesthetized with an intramuscular injection (0.05 mL) of 10% Rompun (Haver-Lockhart, Shawnee, KS) plus 10% Ketaset (Bristol Labs, Syracuse, NY). Infection was verified by seroconversion using an influenza-specific IgG ELISA. Preinfection serum samples were routinely screened for antibody to influenza virus to assure that all mice were seronegative prior to experimentation.

Nerve Growth Factor ELISA

This procedure was modified from a protocol provided by the manufacturer (Boehringer Mannheim, Indianapolis, IN). First, 96-well ELISA plates (Corning, Corning, NY) were coated with 50 μL of 0.5 μg/mL antimouse NGF monoclonal antibody and incubated overnight at 4°C. Excess antibody solution was removed and nonspecific binding sites were blocked by adding 100 μL of 0.5% BSA for one hour at 37°C, then plates were washed three times. Serial dilutions of mouse NGF standards (Harlan Bioproducts, Madison, WI) and serum samples (beginning at a 1:5 or 1:10 dilution) were added to the wells (final volume, 50 μL/well) and incubated overnight at 4°C. After three washes, 100 μL of 0.1U/mL antimouse NGF antibody conjugated to β-galactosidase was added to the wells and incubated overnight at 4°C. Unbound secondary antibody was removed by washing three times, and the plates were developed with 2 mg/mL substrate (chlorophenol red-β-D-galactopyranoside; Boehringer Mannheim) at 37°C for 10–12 h. Plates were read on an ELISA microplate reader at 570 nm. Sample concentrations were determined from the lowest dilution that fell within the standard curve. The lower range of detection for mouse NGF was approximately 0.015–0.032 ng/mL, and the high range was 0.5–1.0 ng/mL. If no detectable NGF was present in a sample, the low detection limit of the assay was multiplied by the dilution factor of the serum (5 or 10) to obtain a value for calculation.

Corticosterone Radioimmunoassay

Serum levels of corticosterone were quantified using the DA Rat Corticosterone kit (ICN Biomedicals, Costa Mesa, CA) according to the manufacturer's instructions. The detection range of the kit was 25–1000 ng/mL.

Testosterone Radioimmunoassay

Serum testosterone was assessed with a kit purchased from ICN Biomedicals according to the manufacturer's instructions. The sensitivity limit of the assay was 0.09 ng/mL.

Corticosterone Sensitivity Assay

Spleens were removed aseptically and mashed between glass slides to obtain single-cell suspensions. Red blood cells were lysed with 0.17 M ammonium chloride buffer, and the remaining pellet was washed once with HBSS/10% FBS and twice more with HBSS. Cells were resuspended in RPMI/10% FBS alone or with 2.5 μg/mL ConA at a concentration of 2.5×10^6 cells/mL, and were treated with various doses of cort (Sigma, St. Louis, MO). Cell suspensions were added in triplicate to flat-bottom 96-well plates at a volume of 100 μL/well and incubated at 37°C and 5% CO_2 for 48 h. The CellTiter 96 AQueous nonradioactive proliferation assay kit (Cat. #G5430) was purchased from Promega (Madison, WI). The substrate solution was prepared according to the instructions, and 20 μL were added to each well of the 96-well plate. Living cells convert this substrate to formazan, producing a brown precipitate. The plates were incubated at 37°C and 5% CO_2 for 2–3 h, and the color changes were quantified by obtaining optical density readings on an ELISA plate reader at 490 nm.

RESULTS

Kinetics of Serum NGF, Corticosterone, and Testosterone Following Paired Fighting Sessions

It has been reported in the literature that a fighting bout of 20 min causes a long-term increase in serum NGF in CD-1 male mice.[10] To determine the kinetics of serum NGF in C57BL/6 mice, 12 isolated aggressive males were paired for a 20-min fighting session and were bled immediately after and again at 1, 3, and 24 h. Serum samples were also assayed for cort as a general measure of stress, and for testosterone, which is involved in male-specific aggressive behaviors. In each of the six pairs, there was a clear aggressor (dominant) and a clear submissive mouse. The mean number of attacks during the fighting session was 21, with a low of 12 and a high of 36.

Hormonal data were analyzed using ANOVA with repeated measures. There was a significant effect of both social status ($F(1,54) = 7.517$, $p < 0.05$) and of bleeding time ($F(4,54) = 8.51$, $p < 0.05$) on NGF levels (see FIGURE 1A). In addition, there

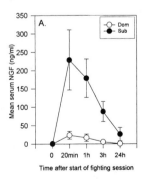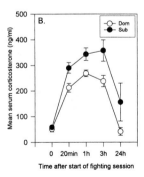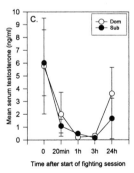

FIGURE 1. Effect of fighting on serum hormone kinetics: isolated aggressive male mice ($n = 12$) were paired for a 20-min fighting session in the morning when baseline cort is low. Blood was collected the morning before (*baseline*) and at the represented times after the fighting session. Each serum sample was analyzed by (**A**) ELISA for NGF, (**B**) by RIA for corticosterone, and (**C**) for testosterone. *Open circles* represent dominant mice, while *solid circles* represent subordinates. Values represent the mean ± standard error.

was an interaction between these two factors ($F(4,54) = 5.604, p < 0.005$). *Post hoc* analysis revealed that NGF was significantly increased after the fighting session in both dominant and submissive mice. However, submissive mice (in the range 20–563 ng/mL) had nearly a 10-fold greater peak response compared to dominant mice (in the range 0.57–57 ng/mL). Corticosterone levels were significantly affected by both social status ($F(1,54) = 14.774, p < 0.05$) and bleeding time ($F(4,54) = 64.521, p < 0.05$) (FIG. 1B). There was a rise in serum cort immediately, with peak concentrations occurring between 1 and 3 h after the 20-min session. As with NGF, the cort elevation was higher and more prolonged in the submissive mice. Serum testosterone levels did not differ between dominant and submissive mice (FIG. 1C). However, there was a significant effect of bleeding time ($F(4,53) = 3.422, p < 0.05$). In contrast to NGF and cort, serum testosterone declined as a result of the fighting. At 1–3 h following the session, all animals had low to undetectable levels of the hormone in serum. By 24 h, testosterone levels were rebounding, but remained below baseline levels.

Serum NGF Response Following a Single Social Reorganization Event

In contrast to pairing isolated males for a limited fighting session, the social context encountered during SRO is more complex. To induce social conflict through social reorganization, the existing social hierarchy (in a cage of five mice) was disrupted by replacing the resident dominant mouse with a dominant mouse from another cage. This caused increased investigative, offensive, and defensive behaviors. The purpose of this study was to determine the NGF responses of individual mice 3 h after a single SRO event (when the NGF concentrations remained elevated

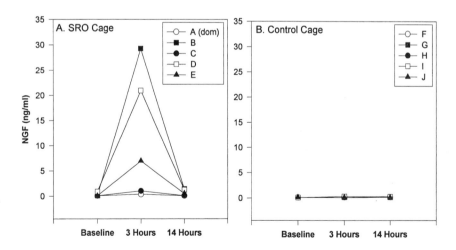

FIGURE 2. (A) Serum NGF in individual SRO or nonstressed mice: cages of mice were socially reorganized at 5 P.M. Blood samples were collected at 8 P.M. and at 10 A.M. the following morning. (B) A cage of nonreorganized controls was also bled at the same time points. Serum NGF was measured by ELISA for individual mice in the SRO (A–E) and the control (E–J) cages.

in the paired fighting paradigm described earlier) and again the following morning (14 h after SRO). FIGURE 2 shows the NGF concentrations for mice in control and SRO cages in which a substantial number of attacks occurred in the first hour after reorganization (one 7-min-long bout followed by four shorter ones). All five mice (labeled A through E) in the SRO cage (FIG. 2A) had elevated serum NGF levels following SRO. The individual NGF levels were variable (0.4–29.3 ng/mL). Serum samples from the nonfighting control mice (labeled F through J) (FIG. 2B) had low (less than 0.3 ng/mL) to undetectable levels of NGF. The dominant mouse (mouse A in the SRO cage) showed an attenuated NGF response to social disruption. The fact that a second mouse (mouse C) was a low responder suggests a codominant was present in the cage. The other mice had detectable NGF (0.53–1.4 ng/mL) the morning following SRO. In contrast to the SRO cage, serum NGF in the home-cage control group remained low to undetectable throughout the assay period.

Effect of Multiple Cycles of Social Reorganization or Restraint on Serum NGF Levels

To confirm that NGF was specifically induced by social reorganization of male mice, serum levels were compared in males stressed by SRO and RST, as well as in control and SRO female mice. Chi-square analysis showed that the percentages of animals testing positive for NGF in these groups were significantly different ($\chi^2(5) = 42.084$, $p < 0.001$). Aggressive behavior was observed in every SRO cage following the first reorganization, and variable levels of fighting were seen following the other three SRO cycles. All the observed attacks (in the 1-h observation period) were initiated by the dominant animals. SRO, but not RST, induced NGF secretion in male mice (see TABLE 1). In addition, the status of the SRO animals affected the likelihood of NGF secretion. Only SRO subordinates were more likely to have elevated NGF than control mice. NGF was not detected in any serum samples from control or stressed females.

Effects of SRO on Serum Cort and Survival from an Influenza Viral Infection

After a single cycle of SRO, serum cort levels were measured at 10:00 A.M. by radioimmunoassay. Similar to restraint stress,[17] SRO significantly increased plasma cort levels in all mice. The levels in the SRO groups increased almost threefold

TABLE 1. Effect of SRO and RST on serum nerve growth factor

	Percent mice positive	Number positive/Total
Control	20	2/10
Restraint	10	1/10
SRO dominant	40	2/5
SRO subordinate	95	18/19
Female control	0	0/10
Female SRO	0	0/8

TABLE 2. Serum cortisone levels in uninfected dominant dominant and subordinate mice subjected to social reorganization

	Base line	Peak	Δ^a
Dominants ($n = 8$)	78.4 ± 6.4^b	348.7 ± 18.7^b	270.3
Subordinates ($n = 32$)	64.4 ± 3.1	432.5 ± 32.2	368.1

NOTE: Serum corticosterone levels are expressed in ng/ml. Peak levels were determined after four rounds of social reorganization.
[a] Δ represents the difference between mean baseline and peak levels.
[b] Comparative difference between dominants and subordinates, $p \le 0.05$ by Mann-Whitney U-test.

(181.4 ± 75.2 ng/mL) compared to control animals (68.5 ± 5.3 ng/mL; $t = 6.71$; $p < 0.005$). Subsequent social reorganization events resulted in further elevation of serum cort. Compared to baseline levels, the change in cort was less pronounced in animals initially identified as dominant. Although the dominant mice had baseline cort levels higher than subordinate animals, their peak levels after seven days of social stress were 20% lower ($z = 3.12$; $p < 0.05$) (see TABLE 2).

Social disruption led to increased mortality (see TABLE 3). Compared to virus-infected control animals (infected with influenza A/PR8 virus, intranasally), in which a total of 32 of 36 mice survived infection, only 31 of 70 SRO mice survived to 10 days postinfection. Thus, the stress of SRO was associated with significantly increased mortality ($\chi^2 = 6.92$; $p < 0.001$). In addition, social rank was also important; animals identified as dominant at the beginning of the experiment were more likely than subordinates to die from the influenza infection ($\chi^2 = 3.59$; $p < 0.001$) (TABLE 3). Histopathologic analysis of the lungs from infected animals suggested that mice died of an excessive accumulation of mononuclear cells in the lungs (data not shown). Hypercellularity has been observed to disrupt the structure of the alveoli, and the resulting decrease in lung function has been identified as an important factor contributing to mortality.[12]

SRO and the Development of Functional Steroid Resistance in Splenocytes

The hypercellularity observed in the lungs of SRO stressed and infected mice suggested that despite high levels of plasma cort (which should have suppressed cell

TABLE 3. Effect of social reorganization on mortality in dominant and subordinate mice infected intranasally with influenza A/PR8 virus

	Dominants	Subordinates	Controls
Exp 1	3/4	5/16	0/10
Exp 2	5/6	14/24	1/11
Exp 3	4/4	8/16	3/15
Totals	12/14 (85.7%)	27/56 (48.2%)	4/36 (11.1%)

NOTE: Data presented as (number dead/total number of animals infected).

accumulation at the inflammatory site), mononuclear cells were trafficking to the lungs unabated. To determine if SRO induced a state of steroid resistance in these cells, an *in vitro* steroid-suppression test was performed. Normally, splenic T lymphocytes proliferate in response to a ConA mitogen challenge, and proliferation can be inhibited by the addition of cort. If SRO induced a state of steroid resistance, then splenocyte proliferation would be resistant to suppression by exogenously added cort. The data (see FIGURE 3) support the development of functional steroid resistance in the spleen of mice subjected to SRO. ConA-induced proliferation of splenocytes from home-cage controls (or mice subjected to RST) were suppressed by addition of cort in a dose-dependent fashion, while proliferation of splenocytes from SRO mice was unaffected.

DISCUSSION

The results of the present studies show that social reorganization (SRO) stress decreased resistance to infection with influenza A/PR8 virus. Higher infection-associated mortality was observed in the SRO group (56%) compared to home-cage controls (11%). In addition, SRO mice initially identified as the dominants in their

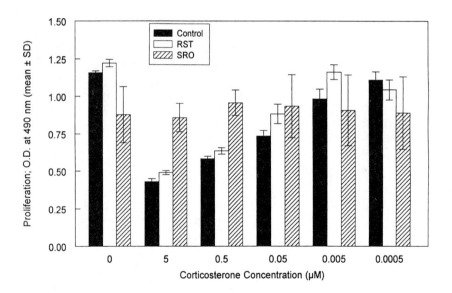

FIGURE 3. SRO induces glucocorticoid resistance in splenocytes: spleens were removed from home-cage control mice and from mice that had undergone four cycles of nightly restraint (RST) or four social reorganization (SRO) events occurring every other night. Splenocyte suspensions were prepared and treated with 2.5 μg/mL ConA and various doses of corticosterone in culture. Following 48 h of incubation, proliferation was assessed using a nonradioactive assay (CellTiter96 AQueous, Promega). *Solid bars* represent control mice; *open bars* represent restraint-stressed mice; and *crosshatched bars* represent socially reorganized mice. Data are presented as mean ± standard deviation of triplicate cultures.

cages were more likely to die than the subordinates (TABLE 3). The poor outcome of the infection during SRO appears to be due to hyperinflammatory responses to the virus, resulting in lung damage and consolidation.

In contrast to SRO, we have found that a nonsocial stressor, restraint (RST), suppressed inflammation and did not increase mortality from influenza infection.[2] RST significantly elevated plasma cort levels,[12] and by blocking the actions of cort with administration of the GC receptor antagonist, RU486, the accumulation of lymphocytes was restored to the lung.[17] Similar to RST, SRO significantly increased plasma corticosterone levels (TABLE 2). Therefore, it was surprising that the elevated cort levels seen during SRO did not have anti-inflammatory actions on cell trafficking as they did during RST.

One factor that has the potential to modulate the biological activity of cort during SRO is nerve growth factor (NGF). It has been reported that high levels of NGF are released from the salivary glands into the bloodstream during aggressive behavior in male mice.[10,11] NGF has been shown to negatively regulate the expression of type II corticosteroid receptors,[14] which mediate lymphocyte responses to cort.[18] These findings suggest that increased circulating levels of NGF may desensitize target cells to the actions of corticosterone.

To examine the relationship between NGF and cort, a paired fighting paradigm was used to establish the kinetics of the hormonal responses following a brief aggressive interaction between previously isolated male mice. A single 20-min episode of fighting resulted in the release of NGF into the blood, elevation of circulating cort, and diminished levels of plasma testosterone. In each fighting pair, a clear dominant and submissive mouse was observed. Dominant mice had lower NGF and cort responses than submissives, while no differences were observed in testosterone (FIG. 1).

Dominant animals subjected to SRO had higher baseline levels (prior to SRO) of cort than subordinate animals, but in response to SRO, subordinate animals had a higher peak response (TABLE 2). Subordinate animals were also more likely to have detectable NGF in circulation than dominant animals following social stress (FIG. 2 and TABLE 1).

The nature of the stressor was an important variable associated with the release of NGF. While the majority of mice exposed to SRO had elevated NGF in circulation, only a low percentage of restraint-stressed mice, home-cage controls, or female mice had detectable levels (TABLE 1). NGF release appeared to be specific to social stress in mice, since stressors such as inescapable footshock, cold water swimming, and forced immobilization do not alter serum NGF levels.[10]

The increased mortality observed in influenza-infected SRO mice, despite high circulating levels of cort, suggested that the immune cells of these animals may be less responsive to the inhibitory effects of cort. *In vitro* assessment of cort sensitivity in ConA-stimulated splenocytes revealed that cells from SRO mice were less sensitive to cort-induced suppression of proliferation than control cells (FIG. 3). Thus, the anti-inflammatory actions of cort, which are important in maintaining the balance between antiviral immune responses and immunopathology, were inoperative. Suppression of cort responses surgically or pharmacologically results in enhanced viral pathogenesis and severe tissue pathology.[17] The host must be able to limit the inflammatory cell trafficking, particularly to tissues whose function is architecturally dependent (e.g., lungs, heart, brain, kidneys, etc.), in order that organ damage and loss of function can be avoided. Thus, a state of cort resistance induced by social conflict was associated with enhanced inflammatory responses and diminished resistance to a viral infection. Studies are currently underway to elucidate the role of NGF in the development of steroid resistance in this psychosocial stress model.

ACKNOWLEDGMENT

This research was supported in part by grants from the John D. and Catherine T. MacArthur Foundation Mind-Body Network, the National Institute of Mental Health (RO1 MH46801, R29 MH56899, and F31 MH11792), and the National Institute on Aging (PO1 AG11585).

REFERENCES

1. RAMSEY, J.M. 1982. Basic Pathophysiology: Modern Stress and the Disease Process: 30–73. Addison-Wesley. Menlo Park, Calif.
2. HERMANN, G., C.A. TOVAR, F.M. BECK, C. ALLEN & J.F. SHERIDAN. 1993. Restraint differentially affects the pathogenesis of an experimental influenza viral infection in three inbred strains of mice. J. Neuroimmunol. 47: 83–94.
3. DOBBS, C.M., M. VASQUEZ, R. GLASER & J.F. SHERIDAN. 1993. Mechanisms of stress-induced modulation of viral pathogenesis and immunity. J. Neuroimmunol. 48: 151–160.
4. COHEN, S., D.A.J. TYRRELL & A.P. SMITH. 1991. Psychological stress and susceptibility to the common cold. N. Engl. J. Med. 325: 607–612.
5. KELLER, S.E., J.M. WEISS, S.J. SCHLEIFFER, N.E. MILLER & M. STEIN. 1983. Stress-induced suppression of immunity in adrenalectomized rats. Science 221: 1301–1304.
6. CUNNICK, J.E., D.T. LYSLE, A. ARMFIELD & B.S. RABIN. 1988. Shock-induced modulation of lymphocyte responsiveness and natural killer activity: differential mechanisms of induction. Brain Behav. Immun. 2: 102–113.
7. IRWIN, M.R., W. VALE & K.T. BRITTON. 1987. Central corticotropin-releasing factor suppresses natural killer cytotoxicity. Brain Behav. Immun. 1: 81–87.
8. SPRY, C.J. 1972. Inhibition of lymphocyte recirculation by stress and corticotropin. Cell. Immunol. 4: 86–92.
9. SUNDAR, S.K., M.A. CIERPIAL, C. KILTS, J.C. RITCHIE & J.M. WEISS. 1990. Brain IL-1 induced immunosuppression occurs through activation of both pituitary-adrenal axis and sympathetic nervous system by corticotropin-releasing factor. J. Neurosci. 10: 3701–3706.
10. ALOE, L., E. ALLEVA, A. BOHM & R. LEVI-MONTALCINI. 1986. Aggressive behavior induces release of nerve growth factor from mouse salivary gland into the bloodstream. Proc. Natl. Acad. Sci. USA 83: 6184–6187.
11. LAKSHMANAN, J. 1986. Aggressive behavior in adult male mice elevates serum nerve growth factor levels. Am. J. Phys. 250: E386–E392.
12. HERMANN, G., M.F. BECK & J.F. SHERIDAN. 1995. Stress-induced glucocorticoid response modulates mononuclear cell trafficking during an experimental influenza viral infection. J. Neuroimmunol. 56: 179–186.
13. YAKOVLEV, A.G., M.A. DE BERNARDI, M. FABRAZZO, G. BROOKER, E. COSTA & I. MOCCHETTI. 1990. Regulation of nerve growth factor receptor mRNA content by dexamethasone. Neurosci. Lett. 116: 216–220.
14. SARRIEAU, A., D. O'DONNELL, R. ALONSO & M.J. MEANEY. 1996. Regulation of glucocorticosteroid receptor expression in rat hippocampal cell cultures by nerve growth factor. Neurosci. Lett. 206: 207–211.
15. ADAMS, H.E. 1986. Handbook of Behavioral Assessment, 2nd edit. Wiley-Interscience. New York.

16. BARNARD, C.J., J.M. BEHNKE & J. SEWELL. 1993. Social behavior, stress and susceptibility to infection in house mice (*Mus musculus*): effects of duration of grouping and
aggressive behaviour prior to infection on susceptibility to *Babesia microti.* Parasi-
tology **107:** 183–192.
17. HERMANN, G., C.A. TOVAR, F.M. BECK & J.F. SHERIDAN. 1994. Kinetics of glucocorticoid response to restraint stress and/or experimental influenza viral infection in two
inbred strains of mice. J. Neuroimmunol. **49:** 25–33.
18. SPENCER, R.L., A.H. MILLER, M. STEIN & B.S. MCEWEN. 1991. Corticosterone regulation of type I and type II adrenal steroid receptors in brain, pituitary, and immune
tissue. Brain Res. **549:** 236–246.

The Role of Oxidative Stress in Viral Infections

M.A. BECK,[a,b] J. HANDY,[c] AND O.A. LEVANDER[d]

Departments of Pediatrics[a] and Nutrition,[b] University of North Carolina at Chapel Hill, Chapel Hill, North Carolina 27599-7220, USA

[c]Departments of Microbiology and Immunology and Pathology and Laboratory Medicine, University of North Carolina at Chapel Hill, Chapel Hill, North Carolina 27599-7220, USA

[d]Nutrient Requirements and Functions Laboratory, USDA, Beltsville Human Nutrition Research Center, Beltsville, Maryland, USA

ABSTRACT: Oxidative stress is implicated as a pathogenic factor in a number of viral infections. Our work has shown that nutritionally induced oxidative stress exacerbates the pathogenesis of coxsackievirus B3 (CVB3) infection in mice. Of particular note, mice fed on a diet deficient in antioxidants developed myocarditis when infected with a normally benign strain of CVB3. This change in virulence was found to be due to changes in the viral genome. Immune functions of the oxidatively stressed mice were also altered. Another example of the effect of oxidative stress on a viral pathogen took place in Cuba in the 1990s. An epidemic of optic and peripheral neuropathy in the population occurred that was associated with a lack of dietary antioxidants and with smoking (a pro-oxidant). A coxsackie-like virus was isolated from the cerebrospinal fluid from 84% of patients cultured. Thus, oxidative stress can have profound effects, not only on the host, but on the pathogen as well.

INTRODUCTION

Malnutrition is known to increase the susceptibility of the human host to a variety of disease agents. Most studies have focused on how poor diets affect the immune system, and impairment has been demonstrated in a number of functions, including antibody titers, complement function, and activity of T-cells, natural killer cells, and macrophages. However, little is known about the effect that impaired host nutrition may have on the virus and its overall interaction with the host. This report discusses two human disease outbreaks that provide models for study of the virus and its interaction with the nutritionally compromised host. Both involve human diseases associated with demonstrated nutritional deficiency and coxsackievirus infection.

[a]Address for correspondence: Melinda A. Beck, Ph.D., Department of Pediatrics, 535 Burnett-Womack, CB #7220, University of NC at Chapel Hill, Chapel Hill, NC 27599-7220, USA. Voice: 919-966-6809; fax: 919-966-0135.
melinda_beck@unc.edu

KESHAN DISEASE

Keshan disease is a cardiomyopathy that occurred among people living in areas of China where the soil, and hence the diet, was deficient in selenium.[1] Although dietary selenium supplementation prevented the disease, virologists in China noted that the illness also showed an annual peak incidence that coincided with the peak season for transmission of enteroviruses. This observation was of interest because coxsackieviruses, which are members of the enterovirus family of picornaviruses, are well recognized in association with myocarditis and dilated cardiomyopathy throughout the world. Indeed, coxsackieviruses were isolated from blood and tissues of some Keshan disease patients, and coxsackievirus genome fragments could be demonstrated in heart tissue by reverse-transcriptase PCR.[2,3]

These observations prompted laboratory experiments using a mouse model, which indeed showed that selenium-deficient mice were more susceptible to myocarditis when infected with a myocarditic strain of coxsackievirus B3 (CVB3/20) than were control mice fed a diet adequate in selenium.[4] Pathology was more severe, as measured by microscopic examination of the myocardium, and virus titers were higher in the hearts of selenium-deficient mice. The experiments were carried a step further, to investigate whether replication in a selenium-deficient host affected the virus itself. Coxsackievirus B3 was re-isolated from the hearts of infected mice and was used to

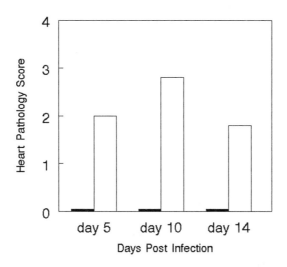

FIGURE 1. CVB3/0-induced inflammation: mice were injected intraperitoneally with 10^5 tissue culture infectious dose-50 ($TCID_{50}$) of CVB3/0. Histologic sections of hearts were stained with hematoxylin and eosin from CVB3/0-infected Se-adequate (*solid bars*) and Se-deficient (*open bars*) mice. Inflammation was graded on a scale of 0 to 4+. Pathologic scores: 0, no lesions; 1+, foci of mononuclear cell inflammation associated with myocardial cell reactive changes without myocardial cell necrosis; 2+, inflammatory foci clearly associated with myocardial cell reactive changes; 3+, inflammatory foci clearly associated with myocardial cell necrosis and dystrophic calcification; and 4+, extensive inflammatory infiltration, necrosis and dystrophic calcification.

infect a second group of mice fed a selenium-adequate diet. Myocarditis appeared earlier, developed to greater severity as measured by heart muscle pathology, and virus titers were three orders of magnitude higher in these secondary, selenium-adequate, mice when the infecting virus was obtained from selenium-deficient primary mice than when it was obtained from primary mice fed a selenium-adequate diet. These observations suggested that the dietary deficiency not only lowered the resistance of the host, but also increased the virulence of the virus replicating in that host.

The next experiments addressed the effect of diet on a CVB3 strain of lesser virulence, which does not produce myocarditis in normal mice. This strain, known as CVB3/0, was benign in mice fed a selenium-adequate diet, but produced myocarditis and replicated to higher titers in selenium-deficient mice (see FIGURES 1 and 2).[5] Again the result of passage into secondary mice was investigated (see FIGURE 3). Virus re-isolated from the hearts of selenium-adequate mice and passed into a second group of selenium-adequate mice remained benign, causing no heart damage. However, virus of the normally amyocarditic strain, when isolated from the inflamed hearts of mice fed a selenium-deficient diet, then produced significant heart pathology in secondary selenium-adequate mice as well. An avirulent virus had acquired virulence as a result of passage through a selenium-deficient host.

In this model, it was also possible to investigate the genotype of those viruses that were phenotypically altered with respect to virulence. Coxsackieviruses have a single-stranded RNA genome of approximately 7,400 nucleotides, and the entire genomic sequences of both virus strains are known. There are only seven nucleotide differences between the virulent strain, CVB3/20, and the amyocarditic strain, CVB3/0. After this latter strain had been re-isolated from the hearts of selenium-deficient mice, which developed myocarditis, it was renamed CVB3/0Se⁻. Sequence analysis revealed that this virus had mutated to the virulent genotype at six of these

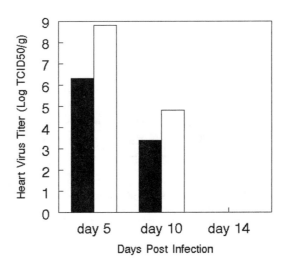

FIGURE 2. Virus titers of heart tissue from Se-adequate (*solid bars*) and Se-deficient (*open bars*) mice at various times post inoculation with CVB3/0.

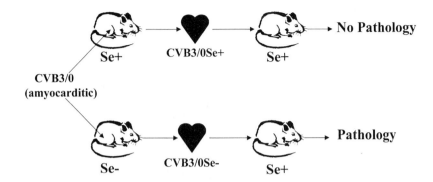

FIGURE 3. Viral passage experiment demonstrating virulence of CVB3/0 after passage through a Se-deficient mouse.

seven nucleotide positions.[6] This was the first report of a specific nutritional deficiency driving changes in a viral genome, permitting an avirulent virus to acquire virulence due to genetic mutation.

What are the possible mechanisms of these effects of selenium deficiency on the host-virus interaction? Selenium is an essential cofactor for glutathione peroxidase, an antioxidant enzyme that decomposes H_2O_2 and organic peroxides. Therefore, similar experiments were performed using mice fed on a diet adequate in selenium, but deficient in another antioxidant nutrient, vitamin E, a fat-soluble, free-radical scavenger that appears to partially spare the need for glutathione peroxidase. Vitamin E deficiency had the same potentiating effects on the infection of mice with CVB3 as were seen with selenium deficiency.[7] Fish oil, long known to be a tocopherol antagonist, further increased the pathology. The myocarditic CVB3/20 strain caused greater heart damage in vitamin E-deficient compared with vitamin E-adequate mice, and vitamin E deficiency allowed the amyocarditic CVB3/0 virus to become myocarditic. Moreover, the same six nucleotide changes, in every case changing to the nucleotide present in myocarditic CVB3, were observed in CVB3/0 after passage through vitamin E-deficient mice. With both strains of virus, higher virus titers were seen in the hearts of vitamin E-deficient animals.

Because nutritional deficiencies often lead to impaired host immunity, the immune response was studied in relation to nutritional status in the mouse myocarditis model.[4,5,7] Neutralizing antibody titers to CVB3 were not affected by deficiency of selenium or vitamin E. Spleen cell proliferation to both antigen (CVB3) and the mitogen concanavalin A was significantly decreased in mice deficient in either selenium or vitamin E. Natural killer cell activity was decreased only in the fish oil treated groups, with or without vitamin E.

Inflammation is the hallmark of myocarditis. For this reason, the role of the specific proinflammatory chemokine MIP-1α was investigated in coxsackievirus-induced myocarditis. MIP-1α is chemotactic for activated, but not resting, CD8[+] cells. It induces integrin expression and enhances binding of CD8[+] cells to endothelium. It induces expression of TNF-α, IL-1, and IL-6; and it is expressed in monocytes on binding to the endothelium. In order to study the role of MIP-1α, knockout mice, which do not produce this chemokine, were used. In the first experiment, all mice were fed a normal, adequate diet. As expected, the myocarditic strain CVB3/20 produced myocardial pathology in about 50% of the wildtype mice, but pathology was not seen in any of the MIP-1α knockout mice.[8] However, when the MIP-1α knockout mice were fed a diet deficient in both selenium and vitamin E, more than half of these animals then developed myocarditis when infected with the myocarditic strain of CVB3. Thus, a combined nutritional deficiency of selenium and vitamin E was able to override the protective effect of the absence of MIP-1α.

The fact that both selenium deficiency and vitamin E deficiency produced similar exacerbation of CVB3 infection in mice supports the hypothesis that increased oxidative stress may be the mechanism for the increased pathology and changes in viral virulence. This hypothesis was investigated using another strain of knockout mice that do not produce glutathione peroxidase 1 (GPx1). These mice develop normally and show no compensatory increase in other antioxidant enzymes.[9] However, when infected with the amyocarditic virus CVB3/0, more than 50% of these mice developed cardiac pathology, but wildtype mice did not.[10] The virus replicated to similar titers in both groups of mice. The GPx1 knockout mice produced decreased levels of neutralizing antibody to CVB3 compared to wildtype mice, although their spleen cell proliferative responses were similar. Following infection, both selenium-deficient and GPX1-knockout mice, compared to adequately nourished wildtype mice, had increased lymph node mRNA expression of the proinflammatory chemokines MIP-1α and MCP-1. This observation again suggests that these chemokines may play a critical role in the development of the inflammation.

The genomic sequence of CVB3/0 virus was studied after passage through the GPx1-knockout mice. Seven nucleotide changes were observed, and six of these were identical to the changes previously observed in this virus when passed through selenium-deficient mice; that is, each of the six nucleotides mutated to that seen in the myocarditic virus CVB3/20.[10] Importantly, these genomic changes were found only in those GPx1-knockout mice that developed pathology. This evidence again points to the importance of adequate host defenses against oxidative stress to protect from viral challenge.

EPIDEMIC NEUROPATHY

An epidemic of optic and peripheral neuropathy occurred in Cuba from late 1991 until 1994, affecting more than 50,000 people in a national population of about 11 million.[11] The symptoms of optic neuropathy included severe decreases in visual acuity, often progressing to near blindness over the course of several months. Some patients had defects in color vision or narrowing of the visual field. Centrocecal scotomata and visible changes in the nerve fiber layer accompanied these changes. A sensory peripheral neuropathy, with burning and tingling of the hands and feet, occurred in some patients, alone or in combination with the optic form of the illness.

This illness occurred at a time of severe economic difficulty in Cuba and was clearly associated with impaired nutrition. After patients were shown to respond to therapy with parenteral vitamins, oral vitamin supplementation was instituted for the entire Cuban population in May, 1993. This measure coincided with the peak of the epidemic, which subsequently declined rapidly until only sporadic cases were occurring by the end of that year.

Population-based and case-control epidemiologic studies showed that this disease was strongly associated with a diet low in animal proteins, fats, B-group vitamins, and several antioxidant nutrients, including vitamin E, selenium, alpha- and beta-carotenes, and especially lycopene—the strongest antioxidant among the carotenoids.[12] Smoking, especially of cigars, was implicated as an associated risk factor, but was not independently implicated in the multivariate analysis. Extensive search did not implicate other toxic cofactors.

In an effort to rule out the possibility of an infectious agent, virus cultures were performed on cerebrospinal fluid (CSF) of 125 patients with optic and/or peripheral neuropathy. Coxsackievirus A9 (CVA9) and closely related viruses were isolated from 105 (84%) of these specimens.[13] Five of the isolates were typical coxsackieviruses and could be identified as CVA9 by the standard technique of neutralization with pooled antisera. The other 100 isolates were antigenically related to CVA9, but were not identical with it; these viruses grew slowly in cell culture, requiring blind passage for initial detection, and produced a very mild cytopathic effect and pinpoint plaques that were much smaller than those of typical coxsackieviruses. Analysis by immunoblotting showed that the capsid proteins, which form the surface of coxsackieviruses and contain the major epitopes for neutralization by antibody, were not present in their native form in the variant viruses. Instead, a higher molecular weight protein was present that may represent a precursor of the capsid proteins. The variant viruses also persisted in the CSF of patients whose symptoms persisted; virus was reisolated from CSF of these patients up to one year after the first isolation. The CSF of one patient yielded CA9 when first cultured, and a virus of the variant type when recultured one month later.

CVA9 was the major picornavirus that circulated in Cuba in the year before onset of the neuropathy epidemic, as shown by virus isolations from patients with acute viral meningitis and also by seroprevalence studies.[14] The evidence suggests the development of a variant coxsackievirus concurrent with a nutritional deficiency in the host population. The resulting epidemic disease was not identical with any of the previously described vitamin deficiency diseases, nor with any syndrome previously attributed to coxsackievirus infection. Ongoing laboratory studies of these viruses, in collaboration with Dr. Pedro Más, are being undertaken in an effort to elucidate the nature of this virus-host interaction.

In summary, both Keshan disease and epidemic neuropathy in Cuba represent diseases that may have arisen due to the interaction between nutritionally-induced oxidative stress and a viral pathogen. Our work points to the importance of examining the impact of oxidative stress not only on the host, but on the infecting pathogen as well.

REFERENCES

1. GU, B.Q. 1983. Pathology of Keshan disease. A comprehensive review. Chin. Med. J. **96:** 251–261.
2. SU, C., C. GONG, J. LI *et al.* 1979. Preliminary results of viral etiology of Keshan disease. Chin. J. Med. **59:** 466–472.

3. LI, Y., H. ZHANG, Y. YANG et al. 1995. High prevalence of enteroviral genomic sequences in an endemic cardiomyopathy (Keshan disease) detected by nested polymerase chain reaction [abstract]. Prog. Clin. Virol. 1995 Joint Meeting. 172.
4. BECK, M.A., P.C. KOLBECK, Q. SHI et al. 1994. Increased virulence of a human enterovirus (coxsackievirus B3) in selenium-deficient mice. J. Infect. Dis. **170:** 351–357.
5. BECK, M.A., P.C. KOLBECK, L.H. ROHR et al. 1994. Benign human enterovirus becomes virulent in selenium-deficient mice. J. Med. Virol. **43:** 166–170.
6. BECK, M.A., Q. SHI, V.C. MORRIS et al. 1995. Rapid genomic evolution of a nonvirulent coxsackievirus B3 in selenium-deficient mice results in selection of identical virulent isolates. Nature Med. **1:** 433–436.
7. BECK, M.A., P.C. KOLBECK, L.H. ROHR et al. 1994. Vitamin E deficiency intensifies the myocardial injury of coxsackievirus B3 infection in mice. J. Nutr. **124:** 345–358.
8. COOK, D.N., M.A. BECK, T. COFFMAN et al. 1995. Requirement of MIP-1α (for inflammatory response to viral infection. Science **269:** 1583–1585.
9. HO, Y.-S., J.L. MAGNENAT, R.T. BRONSON et al. 1997. Mice deficient in cellular glutathione peroxidase develop normally and show no increased sensitivity to hypoxia. J. Biol. Chem. **272:** 16644–16651.
10. BECK, M.A., R.S. ESWORTHY, Y.-S. HO et al. 1998. Glutathione peroxidase protects mice from viral-induced myocarditis. FASEB J. **12:** 1143–1149.
11. ROMÁN, G.C. 1994. An epidemic in Cuba of optic neuropathy, sensorineural deafness, peripheral sensory neuropathy and dorsolateral myeloneuropathy. J. Neurol. Sci. **127:** 11–28.
12. CUBA NEUROPATHY FIELD INVESTIGATION TEAM. 1995. Epidemic optic neuropathy in Cuba–Clinical characterization and risk factors. New Engl. J. Med. **333:** 1176–1182.
13. MAS, P., J.L. PELEGRINO, M.G. GUZMAN et al. 1997. Viral isolation from cases of epidemic neuropathy in Cuba. Arch. Pathol. Lab. Med. **121:** 825–833.
14. BELLO, M., P. MAS, R. PALOMERA et al. 1997. Meningoencefalitis virales por enterovirus en Cuba en el periodo 1990–1995. Revista Argentina de Microbiologia **29:** 176–183.

Local Regulation of Glucocorticoid Activity in Sites of Inflammation

Insights from the Study of Tuberculosis

G. ROOK,[a,b] R. BAKER,[b] B. WALKER,[c] J. HONOUR,[b] D. JESSOP,[d]
R. HERNANDEZ-PANDO,[e] K. ARRIAGA,[e] R. SHAW,[f] A. ZUMLA,[b] AND S. LIGHTMAN[d]

[b]*Royal Free and University College Medical School, London, United Kingdom*

[c]*University Department of Medicine, Western General Hospital, Edinburgh, Scotland*

[d]*Department of Medicine, Bristol Royal Infirmary, Bristol, United Kingdom*

[e]*Instituto Nacional de Ciencias Medicas y Nutricion, "Salvador Zubiran," Mexico*

[f]*Hammersmith Hospital, London, United Kingdom*

ABSTRACT: In sites of inflammation there is a change in the equilibrium between the enzymes that inactivate cortisol by conversion to cortisone and those that reactivate cortisone by conversion to cortisol. Current evidence suggests that during an immune response with a Type 1 cytokine profile such as tuberculosis, there is locally enhanced reductase activity with locally increased cortisol concentrations due to recruitment of cortisone. This results in enhanced cortisol mediated feedback on the inflammatory process, and deviation of the response towards Type 2. Preliminary data suggest that eventually, in the presence of Type 2 cytokine polarization, the enzyme equilibrium may reverse again and cortisol is then locally inactivated to cortisone. Together with changes in glucocorticoid receptor expression and function this may result in local cortisol resistance and susceptibility to tissue damage mediated by proinflammatory cytokines. These observations help to explain the sequence of events in several infectious, inflammatory and autoimmune diseases.

INTRODUCTION

Recent discoveries have totally altered the way in which we perceive the interaction between sites of inflammation and the hypothalamo–pituitary–adrenal axis. For some years it had been assumed that the presence of inflammation was signalled by cytokines released into the circulation that crossed the blood–brain barrier. With hindsight this was an improbable notion, since the brain would not know where the inflammation was situated. Moreover the brain uses nerves to detect other changes in the periphery, so why would this principle not apply to the detection of inflammation? Recent work has proved that, although the fever response may be mediated by cytokines crossing the blood–brain barrier under some circumstances,[1] the activation of

---

[a]Address for correspondence: Graham A.W. Rook, Dept. Bacteriology, UCL Medical School, Windeyer Institute of Medical Sciences, 46 Cleveland Street, London W1P 6DB, U.K. Voice: +44 171 504 9489; fax: +44 171 636 8175.

g.rook@ucl.ac.uk

the HPA axis and the induction of behavioral changes are not. The release of proin-flammatory cytokines from the gut and peritoneal cavity is detected locally, within the inflamed site, and the signal is conveyed to the central nervous system by vagal afferents.[2] We now know that the same is true for inflammation within the lung (Lowry *et al.*, in preparation). It is still not clear how proinflammatory cytokines are detected by the vagal afferents in the lesion, but structures such as neuroepithelial bodies and paraganglia are likely candidates.[3,4] Indeed the latter are rich in receptors that will bind IL-1ra, implying that they are rich in IL-1 receptors, and they are also richly innervated with vagal afferent terminals.

The efferent loop of the interaction between inflammation and the HPA axis also needs to be restated. Most current literature suggests that activation of the HPA axis results in a nonspecific outpouring of cortisol from the adrenal, which then circulates indiscriminately to all tissues. It would clearly make more sense if the cortisol were in some way targeted to the site of inflammation. The only mechanism for doing this that is commonly described is an increased release of cortisol from cortisol-binding globulin (CBG) in the site of inflammation. This release is attributable to enzymes such as elastase associated with activated neutrophils and monocytes.[5] However, common sense suggests that there are other mechanisms, so that the inflammation can be terminated by enhancing local cortisol activity, or perpetuated by blocking it, because this feed-back role of cortisol is crucial in models of autoimmunity in which it can terminate the inflammation,[6,7] and in infection where it can prematurely curtail the protective response and contribute to disease progression.[8,9]

REGULATION OF THE LOCAL EFFECTS OF CORTISOL IN SITES OF INFLAMMATION

It is not difficult to conceive of mechanisms that could have evolved to control the function of cortisol at the level of the target tissue. This could be achieved by: (1) modulating access of cortisol to the site,[5] (2) modulating the concentration of cortisol in the site,[10] (3) modulating the numbers of glucocorticoid receptors, (4) modulating the affinity of the receptors for cortisol,[11,12] or (5) changing the local efficacy of other compounds or receptors with antiglucocorticoid activity.[8,9] Indeed all of these mechanisms exist, thus the questions are: (a) to what extent do they act as physiological regulators of inflammation, and (b) what are the pathways that control them?

Such regulatory mechanisms could theoretically be controlled by the innervation of the inflamed site (since, as discussed above, the brain "knows" where the inflam-mation is), or by signals derived from the inflammation itself, such as cytokines. The possibility that neural connections to the site of inflammation regulate the local effects of cortisol appears not to have been investigated. This is surprising because we know that neuropeptide release from sensory afferents can either attenuate or exacerbate various models of inflammation and wound healing,[13,14] and there is evi-dence that sympathetic efferents can also play a role.[14,15] We know so little of the detailed effects of neuropeptides and catecholamines that it remains entirely possible that neural influences can operate via any of mechanisms (1) to (5) above. It seems likely that such pathways will be found if they are sought.

Although the possibility of neural pathways remains unexplored, there is already evidence that the inflammatory process itself can modulate the local activity of cortisol by changing the function or expression of the enzymes that interconvert cortisol and cortisone.

REGULATING THE CORTISOL-CORTISONE EQUILIBRIUM: 11 β-HYDROXYSTEROID DEHYDROGENASE ENZYMES

A major mechanism for the regulation of local cortisol levels is the interconversion of active cortisol (11-hydroxy) and inactive cortisone (11-keto). Most interconversion was thought to occur in two sites, the kidney and the liver. In the kidney the enzyme 11β-hydroxysteroid dehydrogenase type 2 (11βHSD-2) converts cortisol into inactive cortisone, and hence stops cortisol from binding to the mineralocorticoid receptors.[16] In the liver, on the other hand a reversible oxidoreductase, 11β-hydroxysteroid dehydrogenase type 1 (11βHSD-1), converts cortisone back to active cortisol. Thus, effective cortisol concentrations in the liver and kidney are totally different from each other, and both are different from the values found in the serum. The importance of this concept is illustrated by considering other tissues. For instance, 11-hydroxy and 11-keto compounds are equally effective on vascular smooth muscle cells, either because in these cells 11βHSD acts as an efficient reductase[17] or because 11βHSD-2 is also present in the vessel wall.[18] Either way the 11-keto forms are reactivated. In contrast, a tissue in which dehydrogenase rather than reductase activity is dominant, will show no response to cortisone. Granulosa cells express 11βHSD-1 at some stages of the ovulatory cycle (luteinising) and consequently at that time may be sensitive both to cortisone (after conversion) and to cortisol, whereas at other times in the cycle (non-luteinised) the cells express only 11βHSD-2 and so will not be sensitive to either steroid.[19]

THE CORTISOL-CORTISONE EQUILIBRIUM IN HUMAN TUBERCULOSIS

The first clue that tuberculosis patients have a change in the balance of the cortisol to cortisone emerged from studies of steroid metabolites in 24-hour urine collections (see FIGURE 1). Gas chromatography and mass spectrometry revealed a striking excess of metabolites of cortisol relative to metabolites of cortisone.[20] This imbalance returned to normal during treatment. This investigation was subsequently repeated using urine taken before initiation of treatment in order to eliminate any possibility that the effect was due to the drugs. The results were identical and were further supported by the observation that tuberculosis patients more rapidly converted an oral load of cortisone into cortisol (measured in plasma) than did control individuals or cured tuberculosis patients.[21]

This observation raised a further question. Where was the extra conversion of cortisone to cortisol happening? We could deduce that the shift to metabolites of cortisol could not be due to a failure of 11βHSD-2 in the kidney, since this would result in hypertension and salt retention.[22] In fact, tuberculosis patients do not show these

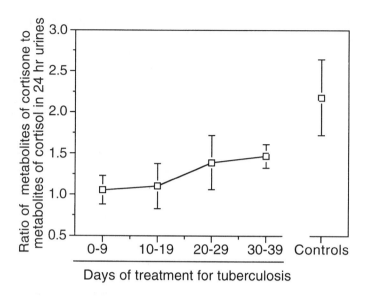

FIGURE 1. The ratio of metabolites of cortisone to metabolites of cortisol in 24-hour urine collections from 23 patients with tuberculosis sampled during the first five weeks of treatment, and nine controls. Note the tendency for the ratio to correct itself during treatment. Subsequent studies have proved that the effect is not caused by the chemotherapy itself, and that the ratio is normal in cured patients more than six months after completion of chemotherapy.

symptoms, and if anything show the opposite. Another alternative was an increased activity of 11βHSD-1 in the liver. However, our hypothesis was that the change in the cortisol-cortisone equilibrium must be a part of the *local* regulation of cortisol activity within the site of inflammation itself. This hypothesis was investigated in murine models and in human tuberculosis.

INTERCONVERSION OF CORTISOL AND CORTISONE IN MICE INFECTED WITH THE BACILLE CALMETTE GUÉRIN

Preliminary experiments were performed in a model of intravenous infection of Balb/c mice with BCG. An i.p. injection of 10 μCi of H3-cortisol reached an equilibrium of cortisol/cortisone in each organ in 30 min. Thus, 30 min after administration of the H3-cortisol, organs were snap-frozen in liquid nitrogen, steroids were extracted from the still frozen powdered tissues, and after addition of unlabeled cortisol and cortisone the steroids were separated by thin layer chromatography. The tritium in the cortisol and cortisone spots was assayed by liquid scintillation counting. Full details will be published elsewhere (Baker *et al.*, in preparation). Three days after an intravenous injection of BCG there is significantly less conversion of cortisol to cortisone in the lungs, implying a relative increase in reductase activity (see

FIGURE 2). Interestingly, there was a significant change in the reverse direction by day 10 (FIG. 2), implying a relative increase in dehydrogenase activity (i.e., *inactivation* of cortisol). No such changes were seen in the liver, where the ratio of H3-cortisol to H3-cortisone remained constant throughout the experiment (data not shown).

In order to confirm this finding and to look for any relationship with cytokine profiles, the experiment was repeated in a model where the precise sequence of cytokine expression is already known. Following intratracheal infection with virulent *M. tuberculosis* in Balb/c mice, there is an early phase of response dominated by Type 1 cytokine production (IFNγ and IL-2) together with the proinflammatory cytokines IL-1 and TNFα. Subsequently a Type 2 response develops (IL-4),[23] and TNFα and IL-1 expression decrease.[24] In this model the same biphasic sequence of events was seen, with a shift in the equilibrium towards reductase activity during the early phase of Type 1 cytokine production, followed by a switch to increased dehydrogenase activity during the phase of Type 2 cytokine production (Baker *et al.*, in preparation).

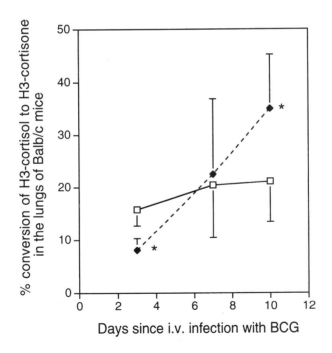

FIGURE 2. The percent conversion of H3-cortisol to H3-cortisone in the lungs of Balb/c mice at intervals after an intravenous injection of 5×10^7 live BCG organisms (◆) or saline (□). At three days there is reduced dehydrogenase activity, but by 10 days this increased relative to controls. See text for methods. *Asterisks* indicate results that differ significantly from the controls ($p < 0.01$).

THE CORTISOL-CORTISONE EQUILIBRIUM
IN THE LUNGS IN HUMAN TUBERCULOSIS

To provide evidence for the relevance of these findings to human tuberculosis, we examined the ratio of cortisol to cortisone in alveolar lavage samples from controls and from patients with tuberculosis. The results indicate that alveolar lavage fluid from tuberculosis patients, but not from normal subjects, has a higher cortisol/cortisone ratio than is found in the corresponding plasma sample.[21]

PROINFLAMMATORY CYTOKINES AND THE ENZYMES
OF THE CORTISOL-CORTISONE EQUILIBRIUM

The mouse and human data, therefore, imply that during the phase of Type 1 and proinflammatory cytokine production there is an increase in reductase activity at the site of infection, relative to dehydrogenase activity. This may be explained by the observation that TNFα and IL-1β both increased the expression levels and reductase

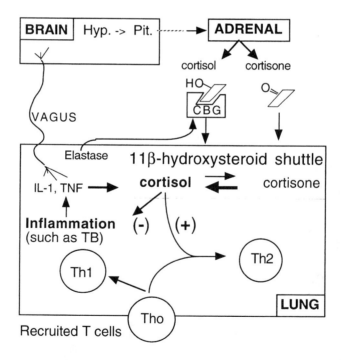

FIGURE 3. The hypothetical sequence of events in the local enzymatic control of cortisol levels in sites of inflammation. The initial Type 1 response with accompanying proinflammatory cytokine release increases the reductase activity of 11β-HSD-1 (or decreases activity of 11βHSD-2), hence local cortisol concentrations rise. Eventually this may cause development of lymphocytes with a Type 2 cytokine profile and decreased inflammation.[26,27]

activity of 11β-HSD-1 in a cell line *in vitro*.[25] However, the relative increase in reductase activity could also be due to a decrease in the activity of 11βHSD-2, since it has recently become apparent that this enzyme is present in lung.[26] Further enzymological and quantitative RT-PCR studies will be required to answer this question. Perhaps both enzymes are involved.

Whatever the mechanism, a shift in the equilibrium toward reductase activity will increase local cortisol concentrations (see FIGURE 3). This in turn can inhibit lymphocyte and macrophage function, and also cause newly recruited T cells to express a Type 2 cytokine profile (IL-4, IL-13, IL-5, etc.) (FIG. 3). Thus glucocorticoids (GC) stop IL-12 production by macrophages, but enhance IL-10.[27] The same is true for dendritic cells. After GC exposure they make less IL-12 and more IL-10, but still take up antigen, express CD40, CD80, and HLA-DR, and present antigen to T cells. Therefore, GC-treated dendritic cells cause the T cells to make IL-5 rather than IFNγ and deviate the response towards a Type 2 profile.[28] These are the changes seen in HPA-axis dependent termination of inflammation in models of autoimmunity,[6,7] and in infections where there is premature downregulation of the protective response.[8,9]

TYPE 2 CYTOKINES AND THE ENZYMES CONTROLLING THE LOCAL CORTISOL–CORTISONE EQUILIBRIUM

As described above, after the initial increase in relative reductase activity, in both mouse models the enzyme equilibrium eventually switches toward increased dehydrogenase activity. This coincides with the appearance of a Type 2 (IL-4) cytokine profile and implies increased local *inactivation* of corticosterone (the most important glucocorticoid in mice) by conversion to the 11-keto derivative, dehydrocorticosterone, during a Type 2 response. Clearly this observation needs to be confirmed and explained. However, it is interesting that in a human community, where allergies (Type 2 cytokine-mediated) are common, the ratio of metabolites of cortisone in urine increases relative to the metabolites of cortisol during the summer,[29] and we have observed an even greater seasonal shift in this ratio in urine samples from patients with hayfever (unpublished observations). Such shifts may be explained by mechanisms unrelated to cytokine profiles, but we hypothesize that cytokines associated with the Type 2 response may push the equilibrium towards dehydrogenase activity, and hence, towards inactivation of cortisol in the site of inflammation (see FIGURE 4). This activity would, if correct, aggravate a state of local cortisol resistance, because in the presence of IL-4 and/or IL-13 both T cells and macrophages can become inherently cortisol-resistant.[11,12] Thus dehydrogenase activity would exacerbate the situation by depleting cortisol and could contribute to glucocorticoid-resistant allergic inflammation,[11] and also to the Th2 or IL-4-dependent susceptibility to TNFα-mediated tissue damage seen in some infections such as tuberculosis[30] and *Trichinella spiralis* infection.[31]

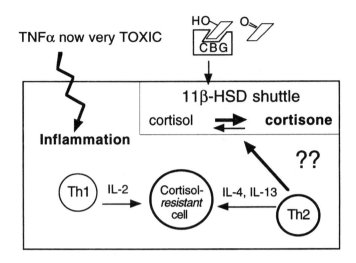

FIGURE 4. A hypothetical diagram. Preliminary data suggest that at a later stage than is depicted in FIGURE 3, when Type 2 cytokines are abundant, the enzyme equilibrium may reverse so that cortisol is depleted. Meanwhile, simultaneous exposure to IL-4, IL-2, and IL-13 increases cortisol resistance of the local cells.[11,12] As a consequence of these two effects working together, the site may become cortisol resistant and susceptible to damage mediated by TNFα.[29,30]

CONCLUSIONS

It is important to ascertain how the effects of cortisol are targeted to sites of inflammation, and how this is locally regulated. We provide evidence that the enzymes that interconvert active cortisol and inactive cortisone are involved, and are themselves regulated. by components of the inflammatory response. Moreover, treatment of mice with glycyrrhetinic acid to inhibit these enzymes increases susceptibility to *Listeria monocytogenes*,[32] and coadministration of such inhibitors can increase the effect of glucocorticoids on the skin of mice[33] or humans.[34] Therefore, in these situations *inactivation* of cortisol in the relevant sites was dominant and could be opposed by the inhibitors. In contrast we show that in human tuberculosis the equilibrium is changed and these enzymes may increase local cortisol concentrations by reduction of cortisone. These concepts are likely to be generally applicable to inflammatory disorders and the enzymes that mediate these interconversions provide interesting targets for therapeutic intervention.[35]

REFERENCES

1. CALDWELL, F.J., D.B. GRAVES & B.H. WALLACE. 1999. Humoral versus neural pathways for fever production in rats after administration of lipopolysaccharide. J. Trauma **47:** 120–129.

2. DANTZER, R., S. LAYE, E. GOUJAN *et al.* 1997. Mechanisms of action of cytokines on the central nervous system. Interaction with glucocorticoids. *In* Steroid Hormones and the T Cell Cytokine Profile. G.A.W. Rook & S. Lightman, Eds.: 1–13. Springer. London.
3. VAN LOMMEL, A., T. BOLLE, W. FANNES *et al.* 1999. The pulmonary neuroendocrine system: the past decade. Arch. Histol. Cytol. **62:** 1–16.
4. GOEHLER, L.E., J.K. RELTON, D. DRIPPS *et al.* 1997. Vagal paraganglia bind biotinylated interleukin-1 receptor antagonist: a possible mechanism for immune-to-brain communication. Brain Res. Bull. **43:** 357–364.
5. HAMMOND, G.L., C.L. SMITH, C.M. UNDERHILL *et al.* 1990. Interaction between corticosteroid binding globulin and activated leukocytes in vitro. Biochem. Biophys. Res. Commun. **172:** 172–177.
6. CALOGERO, A.E., E.M. STERNBERG, G. BAGDY *et al.* 1992. Neurotransmitter-induced hypothalamic–pituitary–adrenal axis responsiveness is defective in inflammatory disease-susceptible Lewis rats. Neuroendocrinology **55:** 600–608.
7. MACPHEE, I.A.M., F.A. ANTONI & D.W. MASON. 1989. Spontaneous recovery of rats from experimental allergic encephalomyelitis is dependent on regulation of the immune system by endogenous adrenal corticosteroids. J. Exp. Med. **169:** 431–445.
8. HERNANDEZ-PANDO, R., M. DE LA LUZ STREBER, H. OROZCO *et al.* 1998. Emergent therapeutic properties of a combination of glucocorticoid and anti-glucocorticoid steroids in tuberculous Balb/c mice. Q. J. Med. **91:** 755–766.
9. HERNANDEZ-PANDO, R., M. DE LA LUZ STREBER, H. OROZCO *et al.* 1998. The effects of androstenediol and dehydroepiandrosterone on the course and cytokine profile of tuberculosis in Balb/c mice. Immunology **95:** 234–241.
10. ESKAY, R.L. & L.E. EIDEN. 1992. Interleukin-1 alpha and tumor necrosis factor-alpha differentially regulate enkephalin, vasoactive intestinal polypeptide, neurotensin, and substance P biosynthesis in chromaffin cells. Endocrinology **130:** 2252–2258.
11. KAM, J.C., S.J. SZEFLER, W. SURS *et al.* 1993. Combination IL-2 and IL-4 reduces glucocorticoid receptor-binding affinity and T cell response to glucocorticoids. J. Immunol. **151:** 3460–3466.
12. SPAHN, J.D., S.J. SZEFLER, W. SURS *et al.* 1996. A novel action of IL-13: induction of diminished glucocorticoid receptor-binding affinity. J. Immunol. **157:** 2654–2659.
13. REINSHAGEN, M., G. FLAMIG, S. ERNST *et al.* 1998. Calcitonin gene-related peptide mediates the protective effect of sensory nerves in a model of colonic injury. J. Pharmacol. Exp. Ther. **286:** 657–661.
14. LEVINE, J.D., E.J. GOETZL & A.I. BASBAUM. 1987. Contribution of the nervous system to the pathophysiology of rheumatoid arthritis and other polyarthritides. Rheum. Dis. Clin. North Am. **13:** 369–383.
15. JASMIN, L., G. JANNI, H.J. MANZ *et al.* 1998. Activation of CNS circuits producing a neurogenic cystitis: evidence for centrally induced peripheral inflammation. J. Neurosci. **18:** 10016–10029.
16. WALKER, B.R. 1994. Organ-specific actions of 11 beta-hydroxysteroid dehydrogenase in humans: implications for the pathophysiology of hypertension. Steroids. **59:** 84–89.
17. MUTO, S., J. NEMOTO, S. EBATA *et al.* 1998. Corticosterone and 11-dehydrocorticosterone stimulate Na,K-ATPase gene expression in vascular smooth muscle cells. Kidney Int. **54:** 492–508.
18. BRAY, P.J., B. DU, V.M. MEJIA *et al.* 1999. Glucocorticoid resistance caused by reduced expression of the glucocorticoid receptor in cells from human vascular lesions. Arterioscler. Thromb. Vasc. Biol. **19:** 1180–1189.
19. TETSUKA, M., F.J. THOMAS, M.J. THOMAS *et al.* 1997. Differential expression of messenger ribonucleic acids encoding 11beta-hydroxysteroid dehydrogenase types 1 and 2 in human granulosa cells. J. Clin. Endocrinol. Metab. **82:** 2006–2009.
20. ROOK, G.A.W., J. HONOUR, O.M. KON *et al.* 1996. Urinary steroid metabolites in tuberculosis; a new clue to pathogenesis. Q. J. Med. **89:** 333–341.
21. BAKER, R.W., B.R. WALKER, J. HONOUR, D. JESSOP, R.J. SHAW, S.L. LIGHTMAN, A. ZUMLA & G.A.W. ROOK. 2000. Increased cortisol:cortisone ratio in acute pulmonary tuberculosis. Am. J. Resp. Crit. Care Med. In press.

22. WALKER, B.R., P.M. STEWART, C.H.L. SHACKLETON *et al.* 1993. Deficient inactivation of cortisol by 11β-hydroxysteroid dehydrogenase in essential hypertension. Clin. Endocrinol. **39:** 221–227.
23. HERNANDEZ-PANDO, R., H. OROZCO, A. SAMPIERI *et al.* 1996. Correlation between the kinetics of Th1/Th2 cells and pathology in a murine model of experimental pulmonary tuberculosis. Immunology **89:** 26–33.
24. HERNANDEZ-PANDO, R., H. OROZCO, K. ARRIAGA *et al.* 1997. Analysis of the local kinetics and localisation of interleukin 1a, tumour necrosis factor α and transforming growth factor β during the course of experimental pulmonary tuberculosis. Immunology **90:** 507–516.
25. ESCHER, G., E. GALLI, B.S. VISHWANATH *et al.* 1997. Tumour necrosis factor α and interleukin 1β enhance the cortisone/cortisol shuttle. J. Exp. Med. **186:** 189–198.
26. SUZUKI, T., H. SASANO, S. SUZUKI *et al.* 1998. 11β-hydroxysteroid dehydrogenase type 2 in human lung: possible regulator of mineralocorticoid action. J. Clin. Endocrinol. Metab. **83:** 4022–4025.
27. VISSER, J., A. VAN BOXEL-DEZAIRE, D. METHORST *et al.* 1998. Differential regulation of interleukin-10 (IL-10) and IL-12 by glucocorticoids in vitro. Blood **91:** 4255–4264.
28. VIEIRA, P.L., P. KALINSKI, E.A. WIERENGA *et al.* 1998. Glucocorticoids inhibit bioactive IL-12p70 production by in vitro generated human dendritic cells without affecting their T cell stimulatory potential. J. Immunol. **161:** 5245–5251.
29. WALKER, B.R., R. BEST, J.P. NOON *et al.* 1997. Seasonal variation in glucocorticoid activity in healthy men. J. Clin. Endocrinol. Metab. **82:** 4015–4019.
30. HERNANDEZ-PANDO, R. & G. ROOK. 1994. The role of TNFα in T cell-mediated inflammation depends on the Th1/Th2 cytokine balance. Immunology **82:** 591–595.
31. LAWRENCE, C.E., J.C. PATERSON, L.M. HIGGINS *et al.* 1998. IL-4-regulated enteropathy in an intestinal nematode infection. Eur. J. Immunol. **28:** 2672–2684.
32. HENNEBOLD, J.D., H.-H. MU, M.E. POYNTER *et al.* 1997. Active catabolism of glucocorticoids by 11β-hydroxytseroid dehydrogenase *in vivo* is a necessary requirement for natural resistance to infection with *Listeria monocytogenes*. Int. Immunol. **9:** 105–115.
33. HENNEBOLD, J.D. & R.A. DAYNES. 1998. Inhibition of skin 11beta-hydroxysteroid dehydrogenase activity in vivo potentiates the anti-inflammatory actions of glucocorticoids. Arch. Dermatol. Res. **290:** 413–419.
34. TEELUCKSINGH, S., A.D. MACKIE, D. BURT *et al.* 1990. Potentiation of hydrocortisone activity in skin by glycyrrhetinic acid. Lancet **335:** 1060–1063.
35. ROOK, G.A.W., R. BAKER & A. ZUMLA. 1997. Steroid metabolism and immunity: therapeutic implications. BioDrugs **8:** 157–163.

Chemical Sympathectomy Alters Cytotoxic T Lymphocyte Responses to Herpes Simplex Virus Infection

NICOLE A. LEO AND ROBERT H. BONNEAU[a]

Department of Microbiology and Immunology and Program in Neuroscience,
The Pennsylvania State University College of Medicine,
Milton S. Hershey Medical Center, Hershey, Pennsylvania, USA

ABSTRACT: Numerous studies have sought to delineate the impact of neuroendocrine function on overall immune responsiveness. Using various murine models, we and others have previously shown that both adrenal-dependent and adrenal-independent mechanisms regulate components of the primary and memory cellular immune responses to herpes simplex virus type 1 (HSV-1) infection. We have extended these studies by determining the impact of 6-hydroxydopamine (6-OHDA)–induced peripheral sympathetic denervation on these responses. C57BL/6 mice treated with 6-OHDA (200 mg/kg) were inhibited in their ability to generate primary, HSV-specific cytotoxic T lymphocytes (CTL) in response to HSV infection. Sympathectomy also suppressed the activation and function of HSV-specific memory CTL (CTLm). In addition, administration of 6-OHDA resulted in a transient but substantial increase in levels of circulating corticosterone and hypothalamic Fos expression. Together, these findings suggest that peripheral sympathetic denervation may modulate immune function via activation of the hypothalamic–pituitary–adrenal (HPA) axis.

INTRODUCTION

The immune, nervous, and endocrine systems are functionally integrated such that each of these systems can receive and respond to signals originating from one another. Both the hypothalamic–pituitary–adrenal (HPA) axis and the sympathetic component of the autonomic nervous system (SNS) play roles in mediating the communication among these systems via the release of glucocorticoids and catecholamines, respectively. Numerous experimental models have provided evidence that glucocorticoids regulate a variety of immune parameters.[1] However, recent studies have indicated the important contribution of adrenal-independent mechanisms to the modulation of immunity.[2–7] Norepinephrine is a potential candidate for this adrenal-independent contributor for the following reasons: (1) lymphoid tissues are extensively innervated by noradrenergic fibers of the SNS,[2–7] (2) various types of immune cells express functional adrenergic receptors on their cell surfaces,[10] and

[a]Address for correspondence: Dr. Robert H. Bonneau, Department of Microbiology and Immunology, H107 The Pennsylvania State University College of Medicine 500 University Drive Hershey, PA 17033, USA. Voice: 717-531-4078; fax: 717-531-6522.
rbonneau@psu.edu

(3) norepinephrine has been shown to alter immune function.[11] Chemical sympathectomy by way of 6-hydroxydopamine (6-OHDA) administration is a widely practiced method to deplete tissue catecholamines[12] and has been used to study the role of norepinephrine in regulating a variety of immune responses. The norepinephrine content of the lymph nodes and spleen is substantially reduced as early as one day following 6-OHDA administration.[13-15] This neurotoxin selectively enters noradrenergic fibers of the SNS and then destroys the nerve terminal via oxidative damage. Because 6-OHDA does not cross the blood–brain barrier, when administered systemically only peripheral efferents are damaged and pools of norepinephrine in the central nervous system remain intact.[16] Treatment with 6-OHDA has been shown to alter numerous immune parameters including cytotoxic T lymphocyte (CTL) generation and proliferation,[17] antibody responses,[18] cytokine production,[19] and lymphocyte trafficking.[13] However, none of these have examined the effect of peripheral sympathectomy on the cellular immune response to a viral infection.

The studies described here were designed to investigate the effects of 6-OHDA–induced peripheral sympathetic denervation on both the primary and memory cellular immune responses to HSV-1 infection. We have demonstrated that administration of 6-OHDA inhibits the generation of functional herpes simplex virus (HSV)-specific primary CTL and suppresses HSV-specific memory CTL (CTLm) activation and function. These observations may be mediated, at least in part, by sympathectomy induced elevations in circulating levels of corticosterone. Overall, these studies contribute to the understanding of the mechanisms underlying neuroendocrine mediated modulation of antiviral immunity.

MATERIALS AND METHODS

Mice

Male C57BL/6 mice, 4–6 weeks of age, were obtained from Jackson Laboratories (Bar Harbor, ME), housed in metal cages at 3–5 mice per cage, and maintained on a 12:12-h light:dark cycle. Mice were allowed to adapt to such conditions for at least one week prior to any experimental manipulation. Food and water were provided *ad libitum.*

Cell Lines and Media

The B6/WT-3 cell line[20] was maintained in Dulbecco's modified Eagle's minimal essential medium supplemented with 5% (v/v) heat-inactivated fetal bovine serum (FBS), 20 mM Hepes buffer, and 0.075% (w/v) $NaHCO_3$. Lymphocyte cultures were maintained in Iscove's modified Dulbecco's medium (IMDM) supplemented with 10% FBS, 0.225% NaHCO3 (w/v), 25 mM Hepes buffer, and 50 µM 2-mercaptoethanol. All media contained 2 mM glutamine, 100 U/ml penicillin, and 100 µg/ml streptomycin sulfate.

Virus

HSV-1 strain Patton virus stocks were prepared in Vero cells at a multiplicity of infection of 0.01 and virus titers were determined by plaque assay. Virus stocks were stored at $-70°C$.

Chemical Sympathectomy

6-Hydroxydopamine (6-OHDA; Sigma, St. Louis) was dissolved in sterile saline containing 0.01% (w/v) ascorbic acid (vehicle) and was injected intraperitoneally (i.p.) at a concentration of 200 mg/kg. Control mice received i.p. injections of an equal volume of vehicle alone.

Assay for Serum Corticosterone

Mice were rapidly (less than 10 sec) anesthetized with Halothane (Halocarbon Laboratories, River Edge, NJ, USA) and serum was obtained from samples of trunk blood. Levels of corticosterone were determined by ^{125}I-radioimmunoassay (RIA; ICN, Costa Mesa, CA, USA).

Generation of Primary HSV-Specific CTL in the Spleen

Mice were infected i.p. with 1×10^7 PFU of HSV-1 Patton and five days later spleens were removed. Lymphocytes were collected and then assayed for HSV-specific activity by ^{51}Cr release assay.

In Vivo *Generation and* In Vitro *Activation of HSV-Specific CTLm*

Mice were immunized i.p. with 1×10^7 PFU of HSV-1 strain Patton. No less than four weeks later, splenic-derived lymphocytes were collected and cultured with syngeneic stimulator cells as described elsewhere.[21] Briefly, 1×10^7 lymphocytes were cultured in 12-well, flat-bottomed tissue culture plates with 5×10^5 mitomycin C-treated, HSV-infected B6/WT-3 cells (stimulator cells used to activate HSV-specific CTLm) for four days in supplemented IMDM.

Assay for Cell-Mediated Cytotoxicity by [51]*Cr Release*

The ^{51}Cr release assay for quantification of HSV-specific CTL was based on previously published methods.[22] Briefly, B6/WT-3 cells were infected with HSV-1 Patton. HSV- and mock-infected cells were then incubated at 37°C in the presence of ^{51}Cr for 12–14 h. These target cells were added at a concentration of either 1×10^4 or 2.5×10^3 cells in 0.1 ml to wells of a 96-well microtiter plate. An equal volume of effector cells was added at a concentration necessary to give the desired effector-to-target (E:T) cell ratio. The plates were centrifuged at $60g$ for five minutes and incubated at 37°C for 4–5 h. The percentage of specific ^{51}Cr released from the target cells was determined as previously described.[22]

Statistical Analysis

Statistical significance was assessed by analysis of variance (ANOVA). A p value no greater than 0.05 represents findings that are statistically different.

RESULTS

Effect of Chemical Sympathectomy on Splenic Norepinephrine Content

To verify that the route (i.p.) and dose (200 mg/kg) of 6-OHDA administration we were using significantly depleted levels of norepinephrine in the spleen, we examined the norepinephrine content of spleens from sympathectomized mice. Mice ($n = 4$ per group) were injected with either 6-OHDA or an equal volume of vehicle. Three days later, spleens were removed and splenic norepinephrine content was determined by a previously described method of high performance liquid chromatography (HPLC).[23] Spleens from 6-OHDA-treated mice displayed substantially reduced levels of norepinephrine in comparison with controls ($p = 0.003$) (see FIGURE 1).

Effect of Chemical Sympathectomy on the Generation of Splenic-Derived, HSV-Specific, Primary CTL Following Systemic Infection

To examine the effect of peripheral sympathetic denervation on the generation of a primary cellular immune response to HSV infection, we determined the levels of HSV-specific cytolytic activity of lymphocytes derived from the spleens of mice treated with either 6-OHDA or vehicle. Mice ($n = 7$ or 9 per group from two

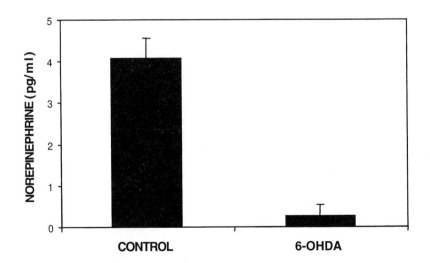

FIGURE 1. The effect of peripheral sympathetic denervation on splenic norepinephrine content. Mice were injected with either 6-OHDA (200 mg/kg) or an equal volume of vehicle three days prior to spleen removal. Levels of splenic norepinephrine were determined by HPLC analysis. Values represent mean ± SEM.

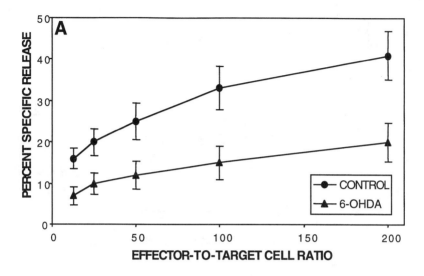

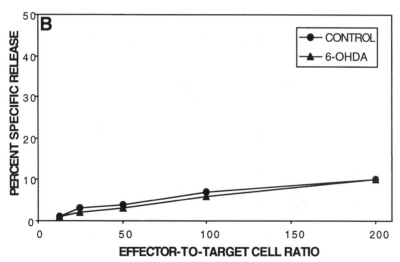

FIGURE 2. The effect of peripheral sympathetic denervation on the generation of primary, HSV-specific CTL in response to infection. Mice were infected with 1×10^7 PFU of HSV-1 and then injected with 6-OHDA (200 mg/kg) or an equal volume of vehicle 24 hours later ($n = 7$ or 9 per group from two independent experiments). Five days after infection, lytic activity of splenic-derived lymphocytes against HSV-infected (**A**) or mock-infected (**B**) target cells was assessed by ^{51}Cr release assay. Values represent mean ± SEM.

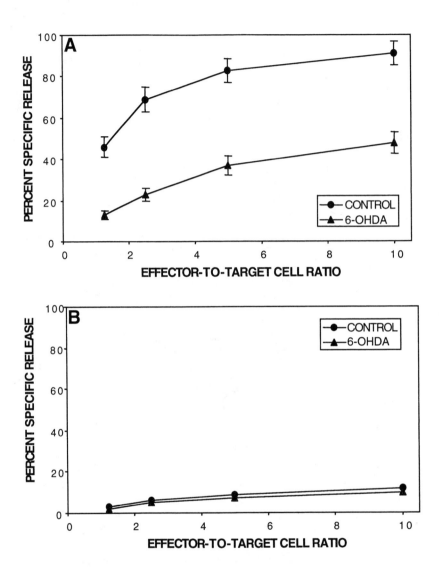

FIGURE 3. The effect of peripheral sympathetic denervation on the activation and function of HSV-specific CTLm. Mice were immunized with 1×10^7 PFU of HSV-1. No less than four weeks later, mice received injections of 6-OHDA (200 mg/kg) or an equal volume of vehicle three days prior to spleen removal ($n = 12$ per group from two independent experiments). Splenic-derived lymphocytes were cultured with mitomycin C-treated, HSV-infected B6/WT-3 cells (stimulator cells) for four days. Lytic activity of cells from these cultures against HSV-infected (**A**) or mock-infected (**B**) target cells was determined by ^{51}Cr release assay. Values represent mean ± SEM.

independent experiments) were infected i.p. with 1×10^7 PFU of HSV-1 and, 24 hours later, were injected with either 6-OHDA or vehicle. Five days after infection, splenic-derived lymphocytes from individual mice were examined for HSV-specific lytic activity by ^{51}Cr release assay. No significant differences between groups in splenic lymphoid yield were found (control, $4.61 \times 10^7 \pm 0.51 \times 10^7$; 6-OHDA, $5.21 \times 10^7 \pm 0.77 \times 10^7$; $p = 0.563$). However, lymphocytes from 6-OHDA–treated mice displayed a decreased level of HSV-specific lytic activity as compared to controls ($p = 0.0001$) (see FIGURE 2A). Lysis of mock-infected target cells was at background levels (FIG. 2B). These results indicate that peripheral sympathetic denervation inhibits the ability to generate HSV-specific, primary CTL in response to infection.

The Effect of Chemical Sympathectomy on the Activation and Function of HSV-Specific CTLm

To examine the effect of peripheral sympathetic denervation on the memory cellular immune response to HSV infection, we determined the ability of splenic-derived, HSV-specific CTLm from mice treated with either 6-OHDA or vehicle to be activated to a lytic phenotype. Mice were immunized i.p. with 1×10^7 PFU of HSV-1. At least four weeks later, mice were injected with either 6-OHDA or vehicle three days prior to spleen removal ($n = 12$ per group from two independent experiments). Sympathectomized mice demonstrated a significant decrease in splenic lymphoid cell yield in comparison with controls (control, $4.69 \times 10^7 \pm 0.40 \times 10^7$; 6-OHDA, $2.83 \times 10^7 \pm 0.37 \times 10^7$; $p = 0.011$). Lymphocytes from individual mice

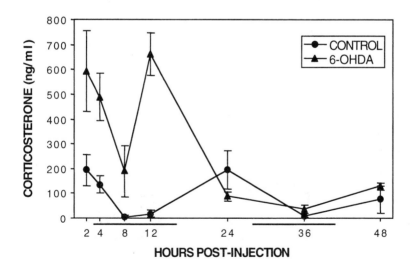

FIGURE 4. The effect of peripheral sympathetic denervation on levels of serum corticosterone. Mice were injected with either 6-OHDA (200 mg/kg) or an equal volume of vehicle and samples of trunk blood were obtained at various times following injection. Serum corticosterone levels were determined by RIA. The *solid bars* indicate the dark phase of the light/dark cycle. Values represent mean ± SEM.

were cultured with HSV-infected, B6/WT-3 cells (stimulator cells) and HSV-specific lytic activity was determined by ^{51}Cr release assay. Cells from cultures derived from 6-OHDA–treated mice demonstrated reduced HSV-specific lytic activity compared to controls ($p = 0.0001$), indicating a reduction in HSV-specific CTLm activation and function (see FIGURE 3A). Lysis of mock-infected target cells was at background levels (FIG. 3B).

The Effect of 6-OHDA Administration on Levels of Serum Corticosterone

To investigate the possibility that peripheral sympathetic denervation mediated its effects on HSV-specific CTL function via activation of the HPA axis, levels of serum corticosterone were examined in mice treated with either 6-OHDA or vehicle. At times ranging from 2 to 48 hours postinjection of 6-OHDA ($n = 3$ per group) or vehicle ($n = 2$ per group), mice were sacrificed and blood samples were obtained. Sympathectomized mice demonstrated a transient, but substantial increase in levels of corticosterone in comparison with controls ($p = 0.0001$), suggesting that 6-OHDA administration increases HPA axis activity (see FIGURE 4). Changes in corticosterone associated with circadian rhythm were observed in both control and 6-OHDA-treated mice.

DISCUSSION

Both adrenal-dependent and adrenal-independent mechanisms play a role in modulating the primary and memory CTL responses to infections such as herpes simplex virus and influenza virus.[3,4,6,7] To determine whether noradrenergic innervation of lymphoid tissues provided the adrenal-independent factor that played a role in the regulation of the cellular immune response to HSV infection, we employed 6-OHDA-induced chemical sympathectomy. In the studies described here, we have demonstrated that peripheral sympathetic denervation inhibits both the generation of primary and the activation of memory HSV-specific CTL.

To examine the possibility that corticosterone may have been responsible for the observed alterations in HSV-specific activity following sympathectomy in our model, we examined serum obtained from 6-OHDA-treated mice. Interestingly, sympathectomized mice displayed a substantial increase in circulating levels of corticosterone, suggesting that 6-OHDA administration increases the activity of the HPA axis. However, this response was not long lived, since baseline levels of corticosterone returned as early as 20 hours postinjection. As another indicator of HPA axis activation, we and others[24] determined the levels of Fos expression in the paraventricular nucleus (PVN) of the hypothalamus in 6-OHDA-treated mice. Expression of the immediate early gene c-fos is commonly used as marker for neural activation.[25] Compared to vehicle-injected controls, mice that were administered 6-OHDA exhibited substantially elevated levels of Fos as early as two hours postinjection. These levels were still strong at 12 hours postinjection and returned to baseline by 24 hours postinjection (data not shown). As expected, the changes in Fos expression paralleled the kinetic changes that we observed in levels of circulating corticosterone. Although the mechanisms by which peripheral sympathetic denervation elevates levels of corticosterone have yet to be addressed, it is possible that the destruction of the nerve terminal by 6-OHDA leads to the recruitment of phagocytic cells.[26] These cells could, in turn, release cytokines that mediate the increase in HPA axis activity.[27] It is also possible that the destruction of peripheral noradrenergic fibers stimulates feedback or "stress response" signals that ultimately activate the HPA axis.

Corticosterone is known to inhibit a variety of elements that are crucial to CTL activation and function such as IL-2 production[28,29] and effectiveness of antigen presentation.[30] Thus, it is likely that elevations in levels of circulating corticosterone play a role in the suppression of both the primary and memory HSV-specific CTL function that we have demonstrated. Corticosterone also regulates immune cell distribution,[31–33] trafficking, and retention.[34] These parameters contribute to the magnitude of an immune response in secondary lymphoid tissues. In the present studies, 6-OHDA administration induced a loss of splenic cellularity in mice that were in an immunologically quiescent state. Other studies have also associated 6-OHDA treatment with alterations in lymphocyte migration.[13] It is possible that the sympathectomy induced increase in levels of circulating corticosterone is responsible for the changes in lymphoid tissue cellularity that we and others have observed. However, the loss of functional sympathetic fibers from the spleen or the "bolus" of norepinephrine released upon denervation[16] may also play a role. We did not detect a loss in spleen cellularity in sympathectomized mice undergoing active HSV infection. This suggests that the influences of corticosterone and/or norepinephrine on lymphoid tissue cellularity may not be as great during an active viral infection. This is likely due to the significant increase in cellularity incited by the infection itself.

When examining the role of sympathetic innervation of lymphoid tissues in modulating immune responses, it is important to consider not only the loss of norepinephrine in these tissues associated with sympathectomy and the elevation in levels of corticosterone, as we have shown here, but also the large quantity of norepinephrine released into the tissue on destruction of the nerve terminal. Norepinephrine has been shown to suppress IL-2 production and receptor expression, via β-adrenergic receptor-induced elevation of cAMP,[35,36] as well as other components involved in CTL activation and function, such as IFN-γ production.[37] Furthermore, other molecules colocalized with norepinephrine in sympathetic nerve endings,[38] such as substance P, must also be considered when investigating the mechanisms underlying sympathectomy-induced modulation of immune function.

Recent studies from our laboratory using both glucocorticoid and β-adrenergic receptor antagonists have helped to delineate the roles of corticosterone and norepinephrine in sympathectomy-induced alterations of the cellular immune response to HSV infection. We have found that the suppression of HSV-specific primary CTL generation and CTLm activation observed following treatment with 6-OHDA is mediated via both glucocorticoid and β-adrenergic receptors. This is indicated by the restoration of both of these measures of CTL function in mice treated with either of two glucocorticoid receptor antagonists, RU486 or spironolactone, or with the β-adrenergic receptor antagonist nadolol prior to 6-OHDA administration (data not shown).

It is clear that the interconnections between the immune, nervous, and endocrine systems are complex. These studies reveal how intricate the communication among these systems can be and provide possible mechanisms underlying peripheral sympathectomy-induced alterations in immune function.

REFERENCES

1. McEwen, B.S., C.A. Biron, K.W. Brunson, K. Bulloch, W.H. Chambers, F.S. Dhabhar, R.H. Goldfarb, R.P. Kitson, A.H. Miller, R.L. Spencer & J.M. Weiss. 1997. The role of adrenocorticoids as modulators of immune function in health and disease: Neural, endocrine and immune interactions. Brain Res. Rev. **23:** 79–133.
2. Keller, S.E., J.M. Weiss, S.J. Schleifer, N.E. Miller & M. Stein. 1983. Stress-induced suppression of immunity in adrenalectomized rats. Science. **221:** 1301–1304.
3. Bonneau, R.H., J.F. Sheridan, N. Feng & R. Glaser. 1993. Stress-induced modulation of the primary cellular immune response to herpes simplex virus infection is mediated by both adrenal-dependent and independent mechanisms. J. Neuroimmunol. **42:** 167–176.
4. Bonneau, R.H., K.M. Zimmerman, S.C. Ikeda & B.C. Jones. 1998. Differential effects of stress-induced adrenal function on components of the herpes simplex virus-specific memory cytotoxic T lymphocyte response. J. Neuroimmunol. **82:** 191–199.
5. Esterling, B. & B.S. Rabin. 1987. Stress-induced alteration of T-lymphocyte subsets and humoral immunity in adrenalectomized rats. Behav. Neurosci. **101:** 115–119.
6. Dobbs, C.M., M. Vasquez, R. Glaser & J.F. Sheridan. 1993. Mechanisms of stress-induced modulation of viral pathogenesis and immunity. J. Neuroimmunol. **48:** 151–160.
7. Dobbs, C.M., N. Feng, M. Beck & J.F. Sheridan. 1996. Neuroendocrine regulation of cytokine production during experimental influenza viral infection: effects of restraint stress-induced elevation in endogenous corticosterone. J. Immunol. **157:** 1870–1877.
8. Felten, D.L., K.D. Ackerman, S.J. Wiegand & S.Y. Felten. 1987. Noradrenergic sympathetic innervation of the spleen: I. Nerve fibers associate with lymphocytes and macrophages in specific compartments of the splenic white pulp. J. Neurosci. Res. **18:** 28–36.
9. Felten, S.Y. & J.A. Olschowka. 1987. Noradrenergic sympathetic innervation of the spleen: II. Tyrosine hydroxylase (TH)-positive nerve terminals form synaptic-like contacts on lymphocytes in the splenic white pulp. J. Neurosci. Res. **18:** 37–48.
10. Livnat, S., S.Y. Felten, S.L. Carlson, D.L. Bellinger & D.L. Felten. 1985. Involvement of peripheral and central catecholamine systems in neural-immune interactions. J. Neuroimmunol. **10:** 5–30.
11. Madden, K.S., V.M. Sanders & D.L. Felten. 1995. Catecholamine influences and sympathetic neural modulation of immune responsiveness. Annu. Rev. Pharmacol. Toxicol. **35:** 417–448.
12. Picklo, M.J. 1997. Methods of sympathetic degeneration and alteration. J. Auton. Nerv. Syst. **62:** 111–125.
13. Madden, K.S., S.Y. Felten, D.L. Felten, C.A. Hardy & S. Livnat. 1994. Sympathetic nervous system modulation of the immune system: II. Induction of lymphocyte proliferation and migration in vivo by chemical sympathectomy. J. Neuroimmunol. **49:** 67–75.
14. Lyte, M., S. Ernst, J. Driemeyer & B. Baissa. 1991. Strain-specific enhancement of splenic T cell mitogenesis and macrophage phagocytosis following peripheral axotomy. J. Neuroimmunol. **31:** 1–8.
15. Felten, D.L., S. Livnat, S.Y. Felten, S.L. Carlson, D.L. Bellinger & P. Yeh. 1984. Sympathetic innervation of lymph nodes in mice. Brain Res. Bull. **13:** 693–699.

16. KOSTRZEWA, R.M. & D.M. JABOBWITZ. 1974. Pharmacological actions of 6-hydroxy-dopamine. Pharmacol. Rev. **26:** 199–288.

17. MADDEN, K.S., S.Y. FELTEN, D.L. FELTEN, P.R. SUNDARESAN & S. LIVNAT. 1989. Sympathetic neural modulation of the immune system: I. Depression of T cell immunity in vivo and in vitro following chemical sympathectomy. Brain Behav. and Immun. **3:** 72–89.

18. KASAHARA, K., S. TANAKA & Y. HAMASHIMA. 1977. Suppressed immune response to T-cell dependent antigen in chemically sympathectomized mice. Res. Commun. Chem. Pathol. Pharmacol. **18:** 533–542.

19. KRUSZEWSKA, B., S.Y. FELTEN & J.A. MOYNIHAN. 1995. Alterations in cytokine and antibody production following chemical sympathectomy in two strains of mice. J. Immunol. **155:** 4613–4620.

20. PRETELL, J., R.S. GREENFIELD & S.S. TEVETHIA. 1979. Biology of simian virus 40 (SV40) transplantation rejection antigen (TrAg): V. In vitro demonstration of SV40 TrAg in SV40-infected permissive mouse cells by the lymphocyte mediated cytotoxicity assay. Virology **97:** 32–41.

21. BONNEAU, R.H., J.F. SHERIDAN, N. FENG & R. GLASER. 1991. Stress-induced effects on cell-mediated innate and adaptive memory components of the murine immune response to herpes simplex virus infection. Brain Behav. Immun. **5:** 274–295.

22. CARTER, V.C., P.A. SCHAEFFER & S.S. TEVETHIA. 1981. The involvement of herpes simplex virus type I glycoproteins in cell-mediated immunity. J. Immunol. **126:** 1665–1661.

23. JONES, B.C., X. HOU & M.N. COOK. 1996. Effect of exposure to novelty on brain monoamines in C57BL/6 and DBA/2 mice. Physiol. Behav. **59:** 361–367.

24. CALLAHAN, T.A., J.A. MOYNIHAN & D.T. PIEKUT. 1998. Central nervous system activation following peripheral chemical sympathectomy: Implications for neural-immune interactions. Brain Behav. Immun. **12:** 230–241.

25. ERICSSON, A., K.J. KOVACS & P.E. SAWCHENKO. 1994. A functional anatomical analysis of central pathways subserving the effects of interleukin-1 on stress-related neuroendocrine neurons. J. Neurosci. **14:** 897–913.

26. PERRY, V.H., M.C. BROWN & S. GORDON. 1987. The macrophage response to central and peripheral nerve injury: A possible role for macrophages in regeneration. J. Exp. Med. **165:** 1218–1223.

27. WATKINS, L.R., S.F. MAIER & L.E. GOEHLER. 1995. Cytokine-to-brain communication: A review and analysis of alternative mechanisms. Life Sci. **57:** 1011–1026.

28. MOYNIHAN, J.A., T.A. CALLAHAN, S.P. KELLEY & L.M. CAMPBELL. 1998. Adrenal hormone modulation of type 1 and type 2 cytokine production by spleen cells: Dexamethasone and dehydroepiandrosterone suppress interleukin-2, interleukin-4, and interferon-gamma production in vitro. Cell. Immunol. **184:** 58–64.

29. NORTHROP, J.P., G.R. CRABTREE & P.A. MATTILA. 1992. Negative regulation of interleukin-2 transcription by the glucocorticoid receptor. J. Exp. Med. **175:** 1235–1245.

30. HIRSCHBERG, H., T. HIRSCHBERG, H. NAUSIANINEN, L.R. BRAATHEN & E. JOFFE. 1982. The effects of corticosteroid on the antigen presenting properties of human monocytes and endothelial cells. Clin. Immunol. Immunopathol. **23:** 577–585.

31. DHABHAR, F.S., A.H. MILLER, B.S. MCEWEN & R.L. SPENCER. 1996. Stress-induced changes in blood leukocyte distribution: Role of adrenal steroid hormones. J. Immunol. **157:** 1638–1644.

32. DHABHAR, F.S., A.H. MILLER, M. STEIN, B.S. MCEWEN & R.L. SPENCER. 1994. Diurnal and stress-induced changes in distribution of peripheral blood leukocyte subpopulations. Brain Behav. Immun. **8:** 66–79.

33. DHABHAR, F.S., A.H. MILLER, B.S. MCEWEN & R.L. SPENCER. 1995. Effects of stress on immune cell distribution: Dynamics and hormonal mechanisms. J. Immunol. **154:** 5511–5527.

34. OLSZEWSKI, W.L. 1987. Regulation of lymphocyte circulation by adrenal hormones. In In Vivo Migration of Immune Cells. W.L. Olszewski, Ed.: 135–140. CRC Press, Boca Raton.

35. CHEN, D. & E.V. ROTHENBERG. 1994. Interleukin 2 transcription factors as molecular targets of cAMP inhibition: Delayed inhibition kinetics and combinatorial transcription roles. J. Exp. Med. **179:** 931–942.
36. TAMIR, A. & N. ISAKOV. 1994. Cyclic AMP inhibits phophatidylinositol-coupled and uncoupled mitogenic signals in T lymphocytes: Evidence that cAMP alters PKC-induced transcription regulation of members of the jun and fos family of genes. J. Immunol. **152:** 3391–3399.
37. COLE, S.W., Y.D. KORIN, J.L. FAHEY & J.A. ZACK. 1998. Norepinephrine accelerates HIV replication via protein kinase A-dependent effects on cytokine production. J. Immunol. **161:** 610–616.
38. FELTEN, D.L., S.Y. FELTEN, D.L. BELLINGER & K.S. MADDEN. 1993. Fundamental aspects of neural-immune signaling. Psychother. Psychosom. **60:** 46–56.

Steroid Hormone Regulation of Antiviral Immunity

D.A. PADGETT,[a] R.M. LORIA, AND J.F. SHERIDAN[a]

Laboratory of Neuroendocrine Immunology, Section of Oral Biology,
College of Dentistry, and the Institute for Behavioral Medicine Research,
The Ohio State University Health Sciences Center, Columbus, Ohio 43210, USA

ABSTRACT: Recent observations in both humans and animals have demonstrated that stress is immunomodulatory and can alter the pathogenesis of microbial infections to the extent that it may be adverse to health. Stress disrupts homeostasis, and the body responds through endocrine and nervous system interactions in an effort to re-establish the health of the host. However, the resulting physiologic changes associated with stress, such as the rise in serum glucocorticoids (GCs), are implicated in suppression of antiviral immunity. Therefore, it would be of significance to counterregulate stress-mediated immunosuppression during viral infection to improve immune responses and limit virus-mediated damage. The data in this study focus upon the antiglucocorticoid influence of a native steroid hormone that has been shown to augment immune function and protect animals against lethal viral infections. Androstenediol (5-androstene-3β,17β-diol, AED), a metabolite of dehydroepiandrosterone (DHEA), confers protection against lethal infection with influenza A virus. The protective activity appears to counterbalance the function of the regulatory GCs because AED prevents GC-mediated suppression of IL-1, TNF-α, and IL-2 secretion. Furthermore, AED inhibits GC-induced transcription of a GC-sensitive reporter gene.

INTRODUCTION

Inflammatory cytokines such as IL-1 and IL-6 not only activate immune functions but also stimulate production of corticotrophin-releasing hormone (CRH) from the hypothalamus.[1] CRH production eventually leads to transient elevations of adrenal hormones such as cortisol/corticosterone.[2–3] The antiinflammatory role of these adrenal glucocorticoids (GCs) subsequently downregulates cytokine production and thus ensures that inflammatory responses are moderated. Therefore, GCs have an important role as messengers within a complex communication loop among the immune, endocrine, and nervous systems that controls homeostasis. Unfortunately, pathophysiologic perturbation of this feedback loop by exogenous stressors can have significant health-aversive consequences.[4–5] Although the response to stress may be directed toward restoration of health, there is evidence to indicate that stress increases the susceptibility to, and severity of, infectious diseases.[6–8]

[a]Address for correspondence: David A. Padgett or John F. Sheridan, Section of Oral Biology, Box 192 Postle Hall, The Ohio State University, 305 W. 12th Avenue, Columbus, Ohio 43210.Voice: 614-292-1176; fax: 614-292-6087.
padgett.11@osu.edu or sheridan.1@osu.edu.

Alternatively, a metabolite of another adrenal-derived hormone, dehydroepiandrosterone (5-androstene-3β-ol, 17-one, DHEA), has been shown to augment immune responses to viral infection. Androstenediol (5-androstene-3β, 17β-diol, AED) protected mice from lethal infection with either coxsackievirus B4,[9] influenza A virus,[10] or herpes simplex virus type 1.[11] Each of those studies showed that AED upregulated specific antiviral immune responses to control viral pathogenesis. The reported immunologic effects attributed to AED differed considerably from the well-established immunosuppressive influence of the glucocorticosteroid hormones[5,12–14] —so much, in fact, that it was hypothesized that AED may exert its immunologic influence in opposition to the glucocorticoids.

Therefore, these studies were designed to assess the ability of AED to counteract stress and prevent stress-mediated suppression of immune responses. In a mouse model for influenza virus infection, resolution of the acute respiratory infection is dependent on the recruitment of natural killer cells and lymphocytes to the site of infection as well as activation of their innate and virus-specific effector functions.[15–16] Repeated cycles of restraint stress, which elevates serum corticosterone levels, suppress many aspects of the immune response to influenza viral infection. To test AED's impact on the health-aversive influences of stress, the effects of AED treatment on survival associated with infection was tested. The ability of AED to counterbalance stress-mediated suppression of trafficking of inflammatory cells during infection, activation of innate and adaptive immune responses, NK cell cytotoxicity, and antigen-induced IFN-γ and IL-10 production were previously reported.[17] In an attempt to decipher the mechanism of action for AED, the ability of AED to block corticosterone-mediated suppression of IL-1, TNF-α, and IL-2 production was determined. And finally, the ability of AED to block glucocorticoid-induced gene expression was tested in a reporter gene system.

MATERIALS AND METHODS

Animals

Virus-antibody-free C57BL/6 male mice at four to eight weeks of age were obtained from Charles River, Inc. (Wilmington, MA) and allowed to acclimate to their surroundings for 7–10 days before initiation of any experimental procedures. All mice were housed five per cage and provided free access to food and water. The American Association for the Accreditation of Laboratory Animal Care (AAALAC) accredited facility is maintained on a 12-h light/dark cycle (lights on at 6:00 A.M.).

Virus Stock

Influenza A/Puerto Rico/8/34 (PR8) virus was obtained from the American Type Culture Collection (Rockville, MD) and propagated in the allantoic cavity of 10-day-old embryonated chicken eggs. Infectious allantoic fluid was collected, clarified by low-speed centrifugation, and stored at −70°C. The virus titer was determined to be 1280 hemagglutinating units (HAU) per ml, using human type O erythrocytes.

Route of Steroid Administration, Vehicle, and Dose

For injections, AED (Sigma, St. Louis, MO) was suspended in a 1:1 mixture of sterile dimethyl sulfoxide (DMSO) and 100% ethanol. Mice were injected subcutaneously in the dorsal area with 0.2 ml of AED (320 mg/kg) or the control vehicle four hours prior to infection with influenza A/PR8 virus. Previous experience with the time and dose of delivery has shown that while lower doses of AED protected mice from viral infection, the dose of 320 mg/kg injected four hours prior to infection was optimal for immunoregulation.[9–10,17]

Restraint Stress Paradigm

Mice were placed in well-ventilated 50-ml centrifuge tubes for one cycle of restraint prior to infection and six subsequent cycles. Individual mice were placed in tubes at 9:00 P.M. (lights out at 6:00 P.M.) and removed at 9:00 A.M. (lights on at 6:00 A.M.). Control mice were food and water deprived (FWD) during the same time period. However, these FWD animals were free to roam in their cages.

Infection of Mice

Mice were infected with 0.05 ml containing influenza A/PR8 virus diluted in PBS and instilled intranasally. For survival studies mice were infected with 24 HAU A/PR8. Prior to infection, all mice were anesthetized with an intramuscular injection (0.05 ml) of 10% Rompun (Haver-Lockhart, Shawnee, KS) plus 10% Ketaset (Bristol Labs, Syracuse, NY). Infection was verified by seroconversion using an influenza virus-specific IgG ELISA. Pre-infection serum samples were routinely screened for antibody to influenza virus to assure that all mice were seronegative prior to experimentation.

Preparation of Mononuclear Cell Cultures

Spleens were removed and pressed through wire screens (30 mesh). Cells were isolated by density gradient centrifugation on a Ficoll/metrizoate gradient. After centrifugation, the cells were resuspended in complete D-modified essential medium (DMEM) supplemented with 10% FCS, 200 μM L-glutamine, 20 mM Hepes, 2.5 U/ml penicillin, and 2.5 μg/ml streptomycin. Adherent cultures of 2×10^5 cells/well were stimulated with 1.0 μg/ml LPS to induce IL-1 production. Cultures were incubated at 37°C in an atmosphere containing 10% CO_2 for 24 hours. Unfractionated lymphocytes were maintained in RPMI 1640 containing the same supplements and an additional 5.0×10^{-5} M 2-mercaptoethanol. For IL-2 bioassays, 1.0 ml aliquots of 5.0×10^6 cells/ml were stimulated with 2.5 μg/ml concanavalin A (ConA) in 24-well tissue culture plates at 37°C in a 5% CO_2 incubator. Culture supernatants were collected after 48 h of stimulation, clarified by centrifugation and stored at −70°C.

Cytokine ELISAs

Each cytokine was assayed using a sandwich antigen ELISA. Primary, monoclonal cytokine-specific antibody was bound to enhanced protein binding 96-well plates (Corning 25805-96) at a concentration of 1 μg/ml. After overnight incubation at 4°C, excess antibody was removed and nonspecific binding was blocked with 10% FBS/PBS at room temperature for 2 h. Standards or samples were added and plates were incubated overnight at 4°C. Biotinylated anti-cytokine monoclonal antibody diluted to 1 μg/ml was added, and plates were incubated at room temperature for 45 min. After washing, avidin-horseradish peroxidase (Vector Laboratories A-2004) diluted 1:500 was added and plates incubated 30 min. Plates were washed and an ABTS substrate was added. Color was allowed to develop at room temperature. After the color reaction was stopped with SDS/DMF, optical density was read at 405 nm on a Bio-Tek Model EL310.

RESULTS

Effect of Androstenediol on Survival of Influenza-infected, Restraint-stressed Mice

AED's potential to protect male mice against infection with a lethal influenza A virus was tested. Mice were treated subcutaneously with 320 mg/kg AED four hours prior to the first and fourth cycles of restraint which began one day prior to infection. Mice were infected with 24 HAU influenza A/PR8 virus. As shown in TABLE 1, treatment of C57BL/6 mice with AED protected unstressed, control mice against infection with a lethal dose of influenza A virus. Data from three individual experiments were combined, and 28 of 40 infected control animals died (30% survival) within 10 days of infection. Pretreatment of unstressed mice with AED prevented mortality in all but 9 of 45 animals (80% survival) ($\chi^2 = 19.55$, $df = 1$, $p < 0.001$). Not only did AED reduce mortality associated with influenza in unstressed animals, but AED improved survival in restraint-stressed animals as well. Pretreatment with AED increased survival in RST mice from 33 to 67% ($\chi^2 = 8.71$, $df = 1$, $p = 0.003$).

Effects of AED on Macrophage Production of Proinflammatory Cytokines

The data from our previous published *in vivo* experiments[17] made it essential to determine the mode of action of AED. In contrast to glucocorticoids, AED upregulated the host's cellular immune response to limit virus-mediated pathology. This

TABLE 1. Effect of AED treatment on survival from influenza a virus infection

Treatment group	Survivors/Total	Percent survival
Infected control	12/40	30
AED 320 mg/kg	36/45	80
Restraint	15/45	30
Restraint + AED 320 mg/kg	30/45	67

NOTE: AED treatment improved survival of influenza-infected mice. Male C57BL/6 mice were infected intranasally with 24 HAU influenza A/PR8 virus, and RST was initiated one day prior to infection. AED (320 mg/kg) was injected subcutaneously four hours prior to the first and fourth cycles of RST.

observation provided a rationale to compare and contrast the function of AED in *in vitro* models where the effects of GCs are established.

Macrophages play an important role in the initiation of inflammatory responses and recruitment of cells into the lungs and lymph nodes of influenza-infected animals. Many proinflammatory cytokines such as IL-1α and TNF-α are downregulated by GCs.[14,18,19] This experiment was designed to determine whether AED could counterregulate the function of GCs *in vitro*. TABLE 2 shows that macrophages from C57BL/6 mice treated with 320 mg/kg AED produced higher levels of each proinflammatory cytokine when stimulated with LPS. Furthermore, when added *in vitro*, corticosterone failed to suppress the production of the proinflammatory cytokines from macrophages from those mice treated with AED. These data show that AED counterbalances the suppressive effects of GCs on macrophage proinflammatory cytokine production.

Effects of AED on IL-2 Production

Similar to macrophage activation, as described above, when administered to cultured lymphocytes, AED blocked the suppressive effect of GCs on IL-2 secretion. TABLE 3 shows that lymphocytes from C57BL/6 mice treated with 320 mg/kg AED produced significantly higher levels of IL-2 when stimulated with ConA. Furthermore, when added *in vitro*, corticosterone failed to suppress the production of the CD4+ T-cell cytokines from mice treated with AED as compared to cells from control animals. These data show direct evidence that AED possesses antiglucocorticoid activity.

TABLE 2. **Influence of AED on the production of proinflammatory cytokines**

In vivo treatment	*In vitro* treatment	TNF-α (ng/ml)	IL-1α (pg/ml)
Placebo	Vehicle	585 ± 45	856 ± 57
Placebo	Corticosterone	**256 ± 24**	**476 ± 30**
Placebo	AED	613 ± 67	826 ± 61
Corticosterone	Vehicle	312 ± 13	799 ± 23
Corticosterone	Corticosterone	187 ± 28	322 ± 24
Corticosterone	AED	**428 ± 56**	**638 ± 49**
AED	Vehicle	676 ± 75	1224 ± 84
AED	Corticosterone	**645 ± 72**	**1034 ± 91**
AED	AED	714 ± 84	1256 ± 123

NOTE: AED prevents corticosterone-mediated suppression of proinflammatory cytokines. Male C57BL/6 mice were implanted *in vivo* with 10 mg time-release pellets of corticosterone (25 mg/kg), AED (320 mg/kg) or placebo. After seven days, splenocytes were isolated, cultured at 5.0×10^6 cells/ml, and treated *in vitro* with corticosterone (1.0×10^{-7} M), AED (5.0×10^{-7} M) or control vehicle. Cultures were stimulated with 1.0 µg/ml LPS for 24 h, and supernatants were collected, and analyzed for TNF-α and IL-1α content by ELISA.

TABLE 3. Influence of AED on the production of IL-2

In vivo treatment	In vitro treatment	IL-2 (U/ml)
Placebo	Vehicle	92.5 ± 4.2
Placebo	Corticosterone	**77.0 ± 6.2**
Placebo	AED	90.1 ± 4.4
Corticosterone	Vehicle	74.3 ± 13.1
Corticosterone	Corticosterone	57.5 ± 7.5
Corticosterone	AED	**85.2 ± 9.0**
AED	Vehicle	115.8 ± 7.6
AED	Corticosterone	**97.7 ± 6.6**
AED	AED	133.0 ± 12.3

NOTE: AED prevents corticosterone mediated suppression of IL-2 production. Male C57BL/6 mice were implanted *in vivo* with 10 mg time-release pellets of corticosterone (25 mg/kg), AED (320 mg/kg) or placebo. After seven days, splenocytes were isolated, cultured at 5.0×10^6 cells/ml, and treated *in vitro* with corticosterone (1.0×10^{-7} M), AED (5.0×10^{-7} M) or control vehicle. Cultures were stimulated with 2.5 µg/ml concanavalin A for 48 h, and supernatants were collected and analyzed for IL-2 content by ELISA.

Effect of AED on Corticosterone-regulated Gene Expression

Based on the observations that AED counterbalanced the influence of GCs on cytokine production and because cytokine production is typically controlled at the transcriptional level, the control of gene expression by corticosterone and AED was examined. Mouse mammary tumor virus (MMTV) gene expression has been shown to be regulated by GCs.[20,21] In the MMTV long terminal repeat (LTR), a complex array of binding sites exists for the hormone receptors located between −202 and −59 upstream of the start of transcription that mediates hormonal induction of the provirus.[22–23] These HREs, when separated from the MMTV LTR promoter and cloned in front of an otherwise hormone-insensitive gene such as bacterial chloramphenicol acetyltransferase (CAT), confer hormone inducibility upon this gene.[24–26]

TABLE 4. Effects of AED on MMTV-driven cat activity by corticosterone

	Percent CAT conversion[a]	
Steroid concentration	Corticosterone	AED
1.0×10^{-7} M	**30.0 ± 2.2**	28.3 ± 4.1
5.0×10^{-7} M	—	28.7 ± 3.2
1.0×10^{-6} M	—	**22.8 ± 3.8**[b]
5.0×10^{-6} M	—	**20.1 ± 3.1**[b]

[a]The data show the influence of each of the respective concentrations of AED on CAT activity when simultaneously cocultured with 1.0×10^{-7} M corticosterone.
[b]Difference from control with $p < 0.05$ as determined by Student's t-test; $n = 6$.

Clone 1471.1 cells containing a stable MMTV-CAT construct were cultured in the presence of increasing concentrations of corticosterone for 48 h. AED did not induce independent transcription of the CAT gene (data not presented). However, when co-cultured with corticosterone, AED at doses at or above 1.0×10^{-6} M partially suppressed CAT expression by about one-third from the levels induced by corticosterone alone (TABLE 4). This shows that AED possesses antiglucocorticoid activity through the MMTV LTR, at least in the presence of corticosterone.

DISCUSSION

The results of these experiments described herein show that treatment of male mice with the steroid hormone androstenediol will ameliorate the physiologic effects of restraint stress. First, AED treatment increased the survival of influenza-infected animals and also augmented survival of stressed and infected mice. Second, mono-nuclear cells from animals treated with AED *in vivo* produced more IL-1 and IL-2 than did cells from control or corticosterone-treated mice. Additionally, AED treatment prevented GC-mediated suppression of cytokine production *in vitro*. Finally, AED suppressed GC-enhanced transcription in a GC-sensitive reporter gene construct. Taken together, these data provide support to the hypothesis that AED functions to counterbalance the physiologic influences of stress hormones such as corticosterone.

Riley[27] first promoted an antiglucocorticoid hypothesis to an adrenal-derived hormone when he showed that the involutional effects of stress on the spleen and thymus were antagonized by the subcutaneous injection of dehydroepiandrosterone (DHEA). Subsequent reports have shown that AED (a metabolite of DHEA) similarly prevented thymic and splenic involution associated with "restraint stress".[28] The enzyme 17β-hydroxysteroid dehydrogenase converts DHEA/DHEA-sulfate into AED/AED-sulfate.[29] From constant infusion experiments, it is known that about 75% of circulating AED is produced from DHEA peripherally,[30] and because it is a metabolite of DHEA, serum concentrations of AED closely follow those of DHEA. In healthy men and premenopausal women (mean age 34.5 years), circulating serum AED levels approximate 3.5 nmol/l.[31] However, during serious illness there is a shift in pregnenolone metabolism away from DHEA and AED production to that of the GCs.[32–33] The resulting increase in the cortisol to DHEA ratio in the blood may be partly responsible for the catabolic state that develops during stress and just the opposite of what occurs during fetal development and puberty when DHEA/AED levels are very high. Thus, it is reasonable to speculate that DHEA and AED may act to protect the host by counteracting GC-mediated immune suppression.

Stress and the resulting body-wide set of physiologic adaptations, mediated through the activation of neuroendocrine pathways, intersect and modulate inflammatory and immune response pathways, thus altering physiological processes such as the immune response to viral infection. Although the response to stress may be directed toward restoration of health, evidence indicates that stress increases the susceptibility to, and severity of, infectious diseases.[6–8] In contrast, these studies illustrated that AED counterregulated the suppressive function of GCs and preferentially augmented production of the cytokines necessary for inflammation and activation of cell-mediated immunity. Ultimately, AED improved the chances of survival of virus-infected animals subjected to a physiologic stressor.

ACKNOWLEDGMENTS

This research was supported in part by grants from the National Institute of Mental Health (RO1 MH46801, R29 MH56899) and the National Institute on Aging (PO1 AG11585).

REFERENCES

1. WEBSTER, E.L., D.J. TORPY, I.J. ELENKOV & G.P. CHROUSOS. 1998. Corticotropin-releasing hormone and inflammation. Ann. N.Y. Acad. Sci. **840:** 21–32.
2. SUNDAR, S.K., M.A. CIERPIAL, C. KILTS, J.C. RITCHIE & J.M. WEISS. 1990. Brain IL-1 induced immunosuppression occurs through activation of both pituitary-adrenal axis and sympathetic nervous system by corticotropin-releasing factor. J. Neurosci. **10:** 3701–3706.
3. KARALIS, K., L.J. MUGLIA, D. BAE, H. HILDERBRAND & J.A. MAJZOUB. 1997. CRH and the immune system. J. Neuroimmunol. **72:** 131–136.
4. CHROUSOS, G.P. & P.W. GOLD. 1992. The concepts of stress and stress system disorders. Overview of physical and behavioral homeostasis. JAMA **267:** 1244–1252.
5. MUNCK, A. & P.M. GUYRE. 1991. Glucocorticoids and immune function. *In* Psychoneuroimmunology, Vol. 2. R. Ader, D.L. Felton & N. Cohen, Eds.: 447–474. Academic Press. San Diego, CA.
6. HERMANN, G., C.A. TOVAR, F.M. BECK, C. ALLEN & J.F. SHERIDAN. 1993. Restraint differentially affects the pathogenesis of an experimental influenza viral infection in three inbred strains of mice. J. Neuroimmunol. **47:** 83–94.
7. DOBBS, C.M., M. VASQUEZ, R. GLASER & J.F. SHERIDAN. 1993. Mechanisms of stress-induced modulation of viral pathogenesis and immunity. J. Neuroimmunol. **48:** 151–160.
8. COHEN, S., D.A.J. TYRRELL & A.P. SMITH. 1991. Psychological stress and susceptibility to the common cold. N. Engl. J. Med. **325:** 606–612.
9. LORIA, R.M. & D.A. PADGETT. 1992. Androstenediol regulates systemic resistance against lethal infections in mice. Arch. Virol. **127:** 103–115.
10. PADGETT, D.A., R.M. LORIA & J.F. SHERIDAN. 1997. Endocrine regulation of the immune response to influenza A virus infection with a metabolite of deydroepiandrosterone—androstenediol. J. Neuroimmunol. **78:** 203–211.
11. DAIGLE, J. & D.J.J. CARR. 1998. Androstenediol antagonizes herpes simplex virus type 1-induced encephalitis through the augmentation of type I IFN production. J. Immunol. **160:** 3060–3066.
12. CRABTREE, G.R., A. MUNCK & K.A. SMITH. 1980. Glucocorticoids and lymphocytes. I. Increased glucocorticoid receptor levels in antigen stimulated lymphocytes. J. Immunol. **124:** 2430–2435.
13. KELLEY, K.W. 1988. Cross-talk between the immune and endocrine systems. J. Anim. Sci. **66:** 2095–2108.
14. RUSSO-MARIE, F. 1992. Macrophages and the glucocorticoids. J. Neuroimmunol. **40:** 281–286.
15. LEUNG, K.N. & G.L. ADA. 1980. Cells mediating delayed-type hypersensitivity in the lungs of mice infected with an influenza A virus. Scan. J. Immunol. **12:** 393–400.
16. LYNCH, F., P.C. DOHERTY & R. CEREDIG. 1989. Phenotypic and functional analysis of the cellular response in regional lymphoid tissue during an acute virus infection. J. Immunol. **142:** 3592–3598.

17. PADGETT, D.A. & J.F. SHERIDAN. 1999. Androstenediol (AED) prevents neuroendocrine-mediated suppression of the immune response to an influenza viral infection. J. Neuroimmunol. **98:** 121–129.

18. SNYDER, D.S. & E.R. UNANUE. 1992. Corticosteroids inhibit murine macrophage Ia expression and interleukin-1 production. J. Immunol. **129:** 1803–1805.

19. BENDRUPS, A., A. HILTON, A. MEAGER & J.A. HAMILTON. 1993. Reduction of tumor necrosis factor alpha and interleukin-1 beta levels in human synovial tissue by interleukin-4 and glucocorticoids. Rheumatol. Int. **12:** 217–220.

20. HYNES, H.E., B. GRONER & R. MICHALIDES. 1984. Mouse mammary tumor virus: transcriptional control and involvement in tumorigenesis. Adv. Cancer Res. **41:** 155–184.

21. MORRIS, D.W. & R.D. CARDIFF. 1987. Multistep model of mouse mammary tumor development. Adv. Viral Oncol. **7:** 123–140.

22. MINK, S., H. PONTA & A.C. CATO. 1990. The long terminal repeat region of the mouse mammary tumour virus contains multiple regulatory elements. Nucleic Acids Res. **18:** 2017–2024.

23. HARTIG, E., B. NIERLICH, S. MINK, G. NEBL & A.C. CATO. 1993. Regulation of expression of mouse mammary tumor virus through sequences located in the hormone response element: involvement of cell-cell contact and a negative regulatory factor. J. Virol. **67:** 813–821.

24. CATO, A.C., H. PONTA & P. HERRLICH. 1992. Regulation of gene expression by steroid hormones. Prog. Nucleic Acid Res. Mol. Biol. **43:** 1–36.

25. FUHRMANN, U., C. BENGTSON, G. REPENTHIN & E. SCHILLINGER. 1992. Stable transfection of androgen receptor and MMTV-CAT into mammalian cells: inhibition of cat expression by anti-androgens. J. Steroid Biochem. Mol. Biol. **42:** 787–793.

26. SOKOL-MISIAK, W., W.T. MARKIEWICZ, B. SZYDLOWSKA & A. PETRENKO. 1991. Introduction of the glucocorticoid binding sequences into the expression vector p delta SVE-CAT and its effect on the CAT gene expression in mammalian cells. Acta Biochim. Pol. **38:** 17–24.

27. RILEY, V. 1983. Psychoneuroendocrine influence on immune competence and neoplasia. Science **212:** 1100–1109.

28. MAY, M., E. HOLMES, W. ROGERS & M. POTH. 1990. Protection from glucocorticoid-induced thymic involution by dehydroepiandrosterone. Life Sci. **46:** 1627–1631.

29. ADAMS, J.B. 1985. Control of secrtion and function of C19-delta-5-steroids of the human adrenal gland. Ann. Clin. Biochem. **41:** 1–17.

30. POORTMAN, J., R. ANDRIESSE, A. AGEMA, G.H. DONKER, F. SCHWARZ & J.H.H. THIJSSEN. 1980. *In* Adrenal Androgens. A.R. Genazzani, J.H.H. Thijssen & P.K. Siiteri, Eds.: 219–240. Raven Press. New York.

31. DIKKESCHEI, L.D., P.H.B. WILLEMSE, B.G. WOLTHERS, A.W. DE RUYTER-BUITENHUIS & G.T. NAGEL. 1993. Delta-5-androstenediol and its sulphate in serum and urine of normal adults and patients with endocrine diseases. Clin. Endocrinol. **39:** 475–482.

32. PARKER, L.N., E.R. LEVIN & E.T. LIFRAK. 1985. Evidence for adrenocortical adaptation to severe illness. J. Clin. Endocrinol. Metab. **60:** 947–952.

33. PARKER, L.N., J. EUGENE, D. FARBER, E. LIFRAK, M. LAI & G. JULER. 1985. Dissociation of adrenal androgen and cortisol levels in acute stress. Horm. Metab. Res. **17:** 209–212.

34. STAHL, F., D. SCHNORR, C. PILZ & G. DORNER. 1992. Dehydroepiandrosterone (DHEA) levels in patients with prostatic cancer, heart diseases and under surgery stress. Exp. Clin. Endocrinol. **99:** 68–70.

CNS Penetration by Noninvasive Viruses Following Inhalational Anesthetics

D. BEN-NATHAN,[a,b] D. KOBILER,[b] S. RZOTKIEWICZ,[b]
S. LUSTIG,[b] AND Y. KATZ[c]

[b]Department of Infectious Diseases, Israel Institute for Biological Research,
Ness-Ziona, Israel

[c]Department of Anesthesiology, HaEmek Medical Center, Afula, and
Bruce Rappaport Faculty of Medicine Technion, Haifa, Israel

ABSTRACT: The effects of inhalational anesthetics on brain penetration by the neurovirulent noninvasive West Nile virus (WN-25) were studied in mice. WN-25 injected intracerebrally causes encephalitis and kills adult mice, but when injected intraperitoneally (i.p.) it is unable to invade the brain and kill. Under stress conditions, this strain causes encephalitis and death even after i.p. inoculation. In the study described in this paper, we used two inhalational anesthetics, a single short-term exposure to 2% halothane for 10 min in oxygen, or 70% nitrous oxide (N_2O) for 30 min in air. Both inhalational anesthetics induced WN-25 encephalitis and death in 33% and 20% of the tested mice, respectively. Exposure of inoculated mice to halothane for prolonged periods or for repeated exposures (two or three times) markedly increased the mortality rate (up to 75%). Exposure to 30% CO_2, a known modulator of blood–brain barrier (BBB) activity, was used as a positive control (80% mortality). No death was observed in the control non-exposed injected mice. Virus levels were found to be more than 10^7 plaque-forming units (PFU)/brain in all moribund mice. Additional parameter demonstrating the "stressor-like" nature of inhalation anesthetics was the induction of a significant decrease in weight of the lymphoid organs of inoculated mice. We suggest that inhalational anesthetics induces BBB breaching with subsequent entrance of the noninvasive WN-25 virus into the brain, causing encephalitis and death.

INTRODUCTION

Inhalation anesthetics used in operating rooms is considered to be a form of stress that might be responsible for the increased susceptibility to infectious diseases in patients subjected to anesthetics.[1,2] There are contradicting reports concerning the effect of inhalation anesthetics on the immune system.[3–5] Halothane attenuates the response of human lymphocytes to phytohemaglutinin and interferes with lymphocytic response to allogenic tumor cells as well as recruitment of alveolar immune cells in response to viral infection.[6–8] However, it does not influence the rejection of allogenic skin graft, neutrophil migration, chemotaxis, phagocytosis, degranulation,

[a]Address for correspondence: David Ben-Nathan, Dept. of Infectious Diseases, Israel Institute for Biological Research, Ness-Ziona, Israel. Voice: 972-8-9381632; fax: 972-8-9381639.

ben@iibr.gov.il

or nonmitochondrial oxidative metabolism.[9,10] Nitrous oxide (N_2O) reduces migration of human neutrophils, on the one hand, but enhances chemotaxis of polymorphonuclear leukocytes, on the other hand.[11,12] Most of the above observations were made on the *in vitro* measurable effects of inhalation anesthetics exposure on the immune response; however, little is known on the modulation of the response *in vivo* in the intact organism. Tait *et al.*[13] tested the effect of halothane anesthesia in mice and found that it inhibited the intra-alveolar recruitment of immune cells in response to influenza viral infection.

We have previously shown that several experimental stress paradigms were able to exacerbate the outcome of viral infections with attenuated encephalitic viruses.[14] Using the noninvasive neurovirulent viruses, WN-25 (a mutant of West Nile virus), and SVN (a variant of Sindbis virus), we developed a model capable of estimating the effect of environmental stressors on the defense mechanisms of the mouse.[15–17]

Three independent parameters can be used to estimate the immunosuppressive effect of stress: involution of lymphoid organs, viremia levels of attenuated viruses, and rate of mortality following brain neuroinvasion and encephalitis.[17,18] This model was validated by evaluation of the effects of known stressors, such as isolation and cold treatment.[18] We used this assay to demonstrate the effect of inhalational anesthetics on the outcome of the asymptomatic viral infection caused by the noninvasive WN-25. Furthermore, these studies demonstrated the hazardous consequences of the single and repeated use of inhalational anesthetics. The results reported herein demonstrate that inhalational anesthetics disrupt the blood–brain barrier (BBB) function, promoting viral neuroinvasion to cause encephalitis and death.

MATERIALS AND METHODS

Mice. OF-1 mice (IFFA-Credo, France), age 24 days, 10–12 g body weight, were used. In all studies, female mice of the same age and batch were compared.

Attenuated West Nile Virus (WN-25). The isolation of WN-25 is described elsewhere.[15]

Sindbis Virus. The process for neuroadaptation and isolation of neuroadapted strain – SVN has been described elsewhere.[16]

Virus inoculation. Immediately before exposure to inhalational anesthetics, WN-25 was inoculated intravenously (i.v. 0.2 ml) at a dose of 2×10^5 PFU/mouse.

Exposure Chambers. The exposure chamber was constructed from transparent glass and was perfectly sealed. At the roof of the chamber there were inlets to enable the introduction of various gases and sampling. Each gas was supplied via a flow meter, connected to a precalibrated agent-specific vaporizer. The actual concentrations of the gases inside the chamber were continuously measured by means of an anesthetic gas monitor (Ultima, Datex, Helsinki, Finland). In each experiment, 10–12 mice were introduced to the same chamber.

Titration of Virus in Tissue Culture. To determine WN-25 virus in the brain of infected mice, a dilution of brain suspension was added to Vero cell monolayers in Petri dishes and incubated (37°C, 5% CO_2) for 72 h. Plaques were counted after staining the monolayer with neutral red (0.05%).

RESULTS

An Experimental Model to Assess BBB Breaching by Different Modulators

Two attenuated encephalitic viruses, WN-25 and SVN, both of which are neu-rovirulent when injected i.c., but cause no overt symptoms when inoculated periph-erally, were used to estimate the effect of BBB modulators.

High dose CO_2, known to increase the BBB permeability, was used to demon-strate the efficacy of this assay.[15,19] The attenuated viruses, WN-25 (a noninvasive variant of WNV) and SVN (a neurovirulent noninvasive Sindbis virus) were inocu-lated intravenously (i.v.) at dose of 2×10^5 PFU/mouse. The inoculated mice were exposed to increasing concentrations of CO_2 (see FIGURE 1). A clear correlation was seen between the concentration of CO_2 to which the mice were exposed and the rate of mortality.

Exposure of inoculated mice to 30% CO_2 for two minutes resulted in a mortality rate of 83% for WN-25 and 67% for SVN, compared to no death in control inoculat-ed mice. These conditions were used as a positive control for all the experiments. The effects of environmental stressors, isolation, and cold treatment were used to validate this assay. Exposure to various stress paradigms, measured by this assay, resulted in mortality rate of 60–80% using both viruses.[17–18] Based on the above results, we used WN-25 to evaluate the stressor-like nature of inhalational anesthet-ics on the course of viral infection.

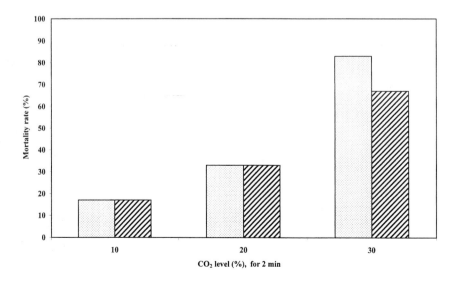

FIGURE 1. Effect of exposure to CO_2 on mortality of mice inoculated with attenuated encephalitic viruses. □, WN-25; ▨, SVN.

Effects of Exposure to Halothane or N_2O on the Mortality of Mice Inoculated with WN-25 Virus

Exposure of WN-25 infected mice to halothane 2% for 10 minutes induced a mortality rate of 37% (see TABLE 1). This effect markedly increased with prolongation of the exposure time.

As is shown in FIGURE 2, exposure to halothane for 30 and 45 min resulted in mortalities of 50% and 70%, respectively, as compared with no death in control inoculated mice. The effect of halothane is not unique to this anesthetic, as can be demonstrated by another commonly used gas, N_2O. Exposure to 70% N_2O for 30 min. induced a mortality rate of 20% (see TABLE 2) and prolonged exposure increased the mortality rate (60 min resulted in mortality of 40%, data not shown). These effects, on the background of no morbidity and no mortality in non-exposed inoculated mice, disclose the potential danger of the use of inhalational anesthetics in virus infected patients.

TABLE 1. The effects of repeated exposures to halothane on mortality of mice inoculated with WN-25 virus

Treatment group	Exposure time (min)	Mortality	
		D/T	%
Halothane 2%	10	3/8	37
Halothane 2%	10×2^a	4/8	50
Halothane 2%	10×3^b	6/8	75
CO_2 30%	2	5/6	83
Control (air)	20	0/6	0

[a]Exposure to halothane for 10 min on the day of inoculation and one day after.
[b]Mice were exposed to halothane for 10 min on the day of inoculation and on days 1 and 2 thereafter.

TABLE 2. Mortality rate of mice inoculated with WN-25 and treated with halothane plus N_2O

Treatment group	Exposure time (min)	Mortality	
		D/T	%
Halothane 2%	10	4/12	33
N_2O 70%	30	2/10	20
H (2%) + N_2O 70%	10/30	5/12	42
CO_2 30%	2	8/12	67
Control air	30	0/6	0

NOTE: Mice were injected i.v. with WN-25 virus and then exposed to halothane, N_2O, halothane plus N_2O, or to CO_2. D/T, death/total; H, halothane.

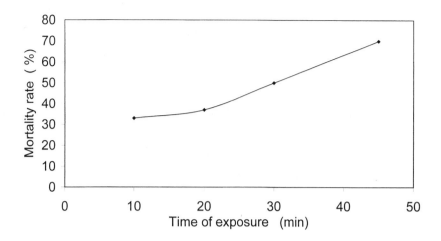

FIGURE 2. Effect of exposure time to halothane on mortality of WN-25 inoculated mice.

An additional parameter indicating the stressor-like nature of inhalational anesthetics was demonstrated. The exposure of the inoculated mice to the gaseous anesthetics resulted in the involution of the lymphoid organs (data not shown).

Effects of Repeated Exposures to Halothane

To simulate the situation of an operation room staff, we tested the effect of repeated exposures to inhalational anesthetics. In this experiment, mice were exposed to halothane 2% for 10 minutes for two or three consecutive days. The results presented in TABLE 1, demonstrate the accumulative effect of repeated exposures to inhalational anesthetics. As can be seen, a single exposure to halothane led to 40% mortality (TABLE 1), whereas two and three exposures led to 50% and 75% mortality, respectively. The high mortality rate due to repeated exposures to halothane is emphasized by the fact that no death was observed in inoculated non-exposed mice.

Effects of Exposure to a Mixture of Halothane and N_2O

Mixture of inhalation anesthetics is a common situation in the operation room. Therefore, we assessed the effect of exposure to the two gases halothane and N_2O. In this experiment, inoculated mice were exposed to 2% halothane for 10 min, 70% N_2O for 30 min, or a mixture of both gases (2% halothane for 10 min + 70% N_2O for 30 min). As can be seen from TABLE 2, there was no synergistic effect between the two gases; a moderate additive effect was noted. Exposure of mice for 10 min to halothane or 30 min to N_2O resulted in mortalities of 33% and 20%, respectively, for the inoculated mice. Exposure of inoculated mice to a mixture of both gases (halothane, 2% for 10 min, and N_2O, 70% for 30 min) increased the mortality rate to 42%.

In all moribund mice the brain virus levels were found to be more than 10^7 PFU/brain. No differences were detected between mice exposed to the various gases (CO_2

halothane or N_2O). This finding indicates that once the virus penetrates into the brain, it proliferates to a maximal titer.

DISCUSSION

The observations reported in this work disclose the *stressor-like* effect of inhalation anesthetics. Mice inoculated peripherally with WN-25 showed no overt symptoms, but exposure to the gaseous anesthetics induced encephalitis and death in those mice. The exacerbating effects of several environmental stressors on viral infections have been demonstrated previously. A similar effect was shown by the exposure to inhalation anesthetics, however, additional parameters are needed to define inhalation anesthetics as a classical stressor. In any case, this study demonstrated the hazardous consequences of exposure to inhalation anesthetics. The exacerbating effect of prolonged or repeated exposure emphasizes the problem. Patients or staff, bearing a symptomatic or asymptomatic viral infection can be prone to dangerous complications when submitted to inhalation anesthetics. Several reports alluded to the possibility that halothane induced an increase in BBB permeability by increasing membrane fluidity and breaching the tight junction.[20–21] However, no study has demonstrated the possibility of virus penetration to the brain due to inhalation anesthetics.

ACKNOWLEDGMENTS

This study was supported by the Research Center for Work Safety and Human Engineering, The Technion, Israel Institute of Technology, Haifa, and the Committee for Research and Prevention in Occupational Safety and Health, Israel Ministry of Labor and Social Affairs.

REFERENCES

1. SESSLER, D.I. 1997. Risks of occupational exposure to waste-anaesthetic gases. Acta Anaesthesiol. Scand. Suppl. **111:** 237–239.

2. ROWLAND, A.S., D.D. BAIRD, C.R. WEINBERG, D.L. SHORE, C.M. SHY & A.J. WILCOX. 1992. Reduced fertility among women employed as dental assistants exposed to high levels of nitrous oxide. N. Engl. J. Med. **327**(14): 993–997.

3. PERIC, M., M. PETROVECKI & M. MARUSIC. 1994. Age-dependent haematological disturbances in anaesthetic personnel chronically exposed to high occupational concentrations of halothane and nitrous oxide. Anaesthesia **49:** 1022–1027.

4. PERIC, M., Z. VRANES & M. MARUSIC. 1991. Immunological disturbances in anaesthetic personnel chronically exposed to high occupational concentrations of nitrous oxide and halothane. Anaesthesia **46:** 531–537.

5. ZIV, Y., B. SHOHAT, J. BANIEL, E. VENTURA, E. LEVY & M. DINTSMAN. 1988. The immunologic profile of anesthetists. Anesth. Analg. **67:** 849–851.

6. KOENIG, A., U.D. KOENIG, B. BINHOLD & H. STOECKEL. 1987. Differences in lymphocyte mitogenic stimulation pattern depending on anaesthesia and operative trauma. II. Combined neuroleptanaesthesia. Eur. J. Anaesthesiol. **4:** 25–33.

7. STEVENSON, G.W., S. HALL, P.J. MILLER, G. ALVORD, J.B. LEVENTHAL, F. SELENY & H.C. STEVENSON. 1986. The effect of anesthetic agents on human immune system function. I. Design of a system to deliver inhalational anesthetic agents to leukocyte cultures in vitro. J. Immunol. Meth. **88:** 277–283.

8. TAIT, A.R., B.A. DAVIDSON, K.J. JOHNSON, D.G. REMICK & P.R. KNIGHT. 1993. Halothane inhibits the intraalveolar recruitment of neutrophils, lymphocytes, and macrophages in response to influenza virus infection in mice. Anesth. Analg. **76:** 1106–1113.

9. BRUCE, D.L. 1975. Halothane inhibition of RNA and protein synthesis of PHA-treated human lymphocytes. Anesthesiol. **42:** 11–14.

10. NUNN, J.F., J.E. STURROCK, A.J. JONES, C. O'MORAIN, A.W. SEGAL, S.B. COADE, J. DORLING & D. WALKER. 1979. Halothane does not inhibit human neutrophil function in vitro. Br. J. Anaesth. **51:** 1101–1108.

11. NUNN, J.F. & C. O'MORAIN. 1982. Nitrous oxide decreases motility of human neutrophils in vitro. Anesthesiol. **56:** 45–48.

12. HILL, G.E., J.B. ENGLISH, T.H. STANLEY, R. KAWAMURA, E.A. LOESER & H.R. HILL. 1978. Nitrous oxide and neutrophil chemotaxis in man. Br. J. Anaesth. **50:** 555–558.

13. TAIT, A.R., P.M. DU-BOULAY & P.R. KNIGHT. 1988. Alterations in the course of histopathologic response to influenza virus infections produced by enflurane, halothane, and diethyl ether anesthesia in ferrets. Anesth. Analg. **67:** 671–676.

14. BEN-NATHAN, D., S. LUSTIG & G. FEUERSTEIN. 1989. The influence of cold or isolation stress on neuroinvasiveness and virulence of an attenuated variant of West Nile virus. Arch. Virol. **109:** 1–10.

15. KOBILER, D., L. LUSTIG, Y. GOZES, D. BEN-NATHAN & Y. AKOV. 1989. Sodium dodecylsulphate induces a breach in the blood-brain barrier and enables a West Nile virus variant to penetrate into mouse brain. Brain Res. **496:** 314–316.

16. LUSTIG, S., H.D. DANENBERG, Y. KAFRI, D. KOBILER & D. BEN-NATHAN. 1992. Viral neuroinvasion and encephalitis induced by lipopolysaccharide and its mediators. J. Exp. Med. **176:** 707–712.

17. BEN-NATHAN, D., S. LUSTIG & D. KOBILER. 1996. Cold stress-induced neuroinvasiveness of attenuated arboviruses is not solely mediated by corticosterone. Arch. Virol. **141:** 1221–1229.

18. BEN-NATHAN, D., S. LUSTIG & H. DANENBERG. 1991. Stress-induced neuroinvasiveness of a neurovirulent non invasive Sindbis virus in cold or isolation subjected mice. Life Sci. **48:** 1493–1500.

19. RAPOPORT, R.R. 1976. Blood-Brain Barrier in Physiology and Medicine. Raven Press, New York.

20. NEMOTO, E.M., S.W. STEZOSKI & D. MACMURDO. 1978. Glucose transport across the rat blood-brain-barrier during anesthesia. Anesthesiol. **49:** 170–176.

21. KARON, B.S. & D.D. THOMAS. 1993. Molecular mechanism of Ca-ATPase activation by halothane in sarcoplasmic reticulum. Biochem. **32:** 7503–7511.

Fat Redistribution in HIV-Infected Patients

A New Hormonal-Immune Disorder?

GUIDO NORBIATO,[a,b] GIULIANA TRIFIRÒ,[b] MASSIMO GALLI,[c]
CRISTINA GERVASONI,[c] AND MARIO CLERICI[d]

[b]Department of Endocrinology, University Hospital L. Sacco Milan, Italy

[c]Institute of Infectious Diseases, University Hospital L. Sacco Milan, Italy

[d]Institute of Immunology, University Hospital L. Sacco Milan, Italy

ABSTRACT: Multidrug antiretroviral regimes in HIV-infected patients may
have side effects. The most frequent side effects are changes in fat metabolism
and distribution. We describe a particular pattern of fat redistribution (FR),
characterized by a progressive enlargement of breast and abdominal girth and
fat loss in the lower limbs, which occurs in approximately 10% of HIV-infected
women treated with combined antiretroviral therapy. To elucidate the metabolic, endocrine, and immunologic consequences of the observed disturbance,
we measured serum lipids, glucose, C-peptide, ACTH, plasma, urinary cortisol, and cytokines IL-2, IFNγ, Il-4, IL-10, Il-12, and TNFα in 36 patients with
FR and in a control group without FR. There were no significant differences
in hormonal and metabolic laboratory testing between the two groups. Immunology studies showed that in vitro production of TNFα and IL-10 was lower
and IL-12 production higher in SR patients. Whether or not such immune
alterations may be reponsible or be caused by fat redistribution remains to be
explained. One year after the follow up, 50% of the patients treated with triple
therapy developed lipodystrophy, characterized by weight loss, face-wasting,
and hyperglycemia; the remaining 50% remained unchanged. In 13 patients
the 3TC withdrawal was followed by improvements of the syndrome in 50%
and of lipodystrophy in about 25%. These data suggest that the FR syndrome
is frequent in patients treated with 3TC and that it is associated with characteristic changes in the cytokine production.

INTRODUCTION

Since the development of antiretroviral therapies, a series of untoward effects
have been reported. Of particular interest are the fat tissue abnormalities[1–5] that frequently occur in these patients: accumulation of adipose tissue, in the dorso-cervical
region, visceral fat accumulation, fat-wasting of the face and limbs, central adiposity, and benign symetric lipomatosis.[4,5]

Among HIV-infected women treated with antiretroviral therapy at the L. Sacco
University Hospital, a complete change in bodily appearance, characterized by

[a]Address for correspondence: Guido Norbiato, Chief of Endocrinology L. Sacco
University Hospital, via G.B. Grassi 74, 20157 Milano Italy. Voice: 02 35799484;
fax: 02 38201160.

ircea@rdn.it

greater breast size and abdominal girth and wasting of the glutei and lower limbs was found in about 10% of patients. The study reported here was performed to describe the syndrome and to evaluate possible risk factors and pathogenetic mechanisms.

PATIENTS AND METHODS

Women seen as outpatients in the Institute of Infectious Diseases at the L. Sacco University Hospital, between December 1997 and February 1998, were evaluated and those receiving combined retroviral treatment for at least one year were included in the study. Clinical data for patients, including age, risk factors of HIV infection, stage of infection (CDC classification), type and duration of treatment, CD4 counts, and HIV-RNA levels were recorded.

The occurrence of a fat redistribution syndrome was diagnosed by means of physical examination and dual-energy X-ray absorptiometry (DEXA) to establish the percentage of body fat and lean body mass. The examination was carried out using a Hologic GDR –2000 X-ray bone densitometer (Waltham, MA, USA) and body composition was established by using BCA 7.20 software. Body composition was estimated in the trunk region and legs.

Endocrinological and metabolic characteristics were evaluated in patients with fat redistribution and compared with those of a group of patients who did not develop fat redistribution, matched for age, body mass index (BMI), CD4 cell counts, HIV-RNA levels, and type and duration of antiretroviral therapy. Serum was collected to determine cortisol, ACTH, GH, C-peptide, F testosterone, and prolactin and 24-hour urine collections were made to measure free cortisol.

Statistical Analyses

Statistical significance was determined by using χ^2 as the likelihood ratio, and the 95% confidence intervals of the odds ratio.

A final stepwise logistic regression was carried out to identify the significant and independently associated variables.

RESULTS

The cohort of study patients consisted of 306 HIV-infected women with an average age of 34 years (range 23–61). Fat redistribution was observed in 36 patients; the body changes were reported as having gradually emerged over a period of 3–8 months. Controls were 36 patients in whom body fat redistribution was not observed.

DEXA examinations revealed a similar fat percentage in the two groups of patients: median values were 27% (range 21–39%) in patients with fat redistribution and 31% (range 11–43%) in the control group. The FR group had significantly more fat on the trunk ($p < 0.01$) and significantly less leg fat ($p < 0.001$). Lean body mass was similar in the two groups (see TABLE 1). The two groups were also similar in their levels of C-peptide, prolactin, GH, F testosterone, ACTH, cortisol, glucose, cholesterol, and triglycerides. Twenty-four-hour free cortisol excretion was also normal in all cases (see TABLE 2). The glucose tolerance test analyzed in 16 patients (8

TABLE 1. DEXA data in patients with fat redistribution (median values)

	Patients with FR	HIV-control	p
Total fat (%)	27 (21–39)	31 (11–43)	0.6504
Trunk fat (%)	28 (19–43)	22 (3.1–4.0)	0.0135
Leg fat (%)	27 (18–45)	40 (19–56)	0.0012
Total LBM[a] (Kg)	38 (29–46)	34 (28–43)	0.0495
Trunk LBM[a] (Kg)	21 (16–25)	18 (16–22)	0.0147
Leg LBM[a] (Kg)	5.5 (3.9–7.1)	5.2 (3.9–7.1)	0.2505

[a]LBM: lean body mass.

patients and 8 controls) was normal and did not differ between the two groups. All women (18 out of 36) treated with Laminodine(3TC) developed fat redistribution. The FR was significantly correlated with the 3TC-including regimen ($p < 0.01$). Also, the use of Stavudine (d-4T) correlated with FR ($p < 0.001$). The risk was significantly lower in patients taking a combination including Zidovudine.

FR correlated with the duration of the therapy. The risk of FR for women who had received antiretroviral therapy for more than 1,000 days was ten times greater than in those who had received a shorter period of treatment. Production of cytokines IL-2, IFNα, and IL-4 was not different between the groups. IL-10 and TFNα were higher in the patients who did not present FR ($p = 0.0001$ and 0.01, respectively), but IL-12 was significantly higher in FR patients ($p = 0.001$) (see TABLE 3).

After a 12-month follow-up, 8 out of 16 patients under triple therapy presented a dystrophic-like syndrome characterized by weight loss, face-wasting, and/or

TABLE 2. Laboratory findings in patients with fat redistribution and controls: median (range)

	Patients	Controls	Normal values
C-Peptide (ng/ml)	2.7 (1.9–4.1)	2.3 (1.3–3.9)	0.4–4.0
Prolactin (ng/ml)	13.9 (7.6–27.8)	15.0 (8.5–25.9)	2.8–27
GH (ng/ml)	0.5 (0.1–5.8)	1.1 (0.5–4.3)	0–5.5
Testosterone (pg/ml)	0.8 (0.1–1.4)	1.1 (0.2–1.8)	< 3.2
ACTH (ng/ml)	20 (3–89)	26 (10–65)	3–52
Cortisol (ng/ml)	144.5 (13–237)	127.6 (41–354)	50–250
Urinary Free Cortisol (nmol/24h)	44 (21–58)	ND	10–90
Glucose (mg/dl)	87 (72–118)	89 (65–111)	70–110
Triglycerides (mg/dl)	167 (125–241)	194 (89–721)	< 170
Cholesterol (mg/dl)	180 (125–241)	164 (101–222)	< 200

* Normal glucose tolerance afterload in FR

TABLE 3. Cytokine *in vitro* production (pg/mL) in women with fat redistribution associated with ARV therapy

	Normal range	FR + median (range)	FR − median (range)	*p* value
IL-2	500–2000	112 (5–545)	75 (12–36)	0.2583
IFNγ	700–2000	98 (4–315)	141 (22–695)	0.1310
IL-4	0–25	2 (1–15)	2.5 (1–6)	0.5891
IL-10	50–200	50 (3–175)	245 (24–728)	0.0001
IL-12	800–2000	822 (169–2076)	163 (22–472)	0.0001
TNFα	5–80	9 (1–69)	30 (5–155)	0.0093

hyperglycemia. The withdrawal of 3TC was followed by an improvement of the syndrome in approximately 50% of the cases.

DISCUSSION

Reports of unexpected side effects involving lipid metabolism have appeared in the literature, usually represented by benign lipomatosis,[1] accumulation of adipose tissue in the dorso-cervical region,[3] accumulation of the visceral abdominal fat,[9] and an increase in the breast size and abdominal girth of female patients.[2,6,7] The majority of authors emphasize that these phenomena are not accompanied by changes in body weight, suggesting that they are secondary to fat redistribution.

Carr and coworkers[5] have recently described a syndrome characterized by fat loss in the face and limbs associated with central adiposity, hyperlipidemia, and insulin resistance.

We describe here a group of HIV-infected women treated with combined antiretroviral therapy to result in a progressive enlargement of breast and abdominal girth associated with wasting of the lower limbs. Fat redistribution was associated more frequently with 3TC treatment and with the duration of the therapy. DEXA data showed that the percentage of total body fat and the percentage of lean body mass were within normal levels, but leg fat was very much reduced ($p > 0.001$) and trunk fat increased ($p > 0.01$) in comparison with a control group without fat redistribution.

We were unable to find differences between the two groups concerning carbohydrates, lipid metabolism, and hormonal patterns. C-peptides, plasma and urinary cortisol, ACTH, and GH were within normal levels and had similar values in patients with or without fat redistribution.

Yanovski and coworkers[8] have described in immunodeficiency virus-infected patients with evidence of protease inhibitor–associated lipodystrophy, that urinary free cortisol excretion was lower and hydroxycorticoid excretion was greater than that of normal subjects. They also found that ACTH was higher in basal conditions than after CRH stimulation. Despite these findings, they concluded that changes in the pituitary–adrenal axis cannot explain the observed lipodystrophy.

We examined the possibility that the immune system may be involved in fat redistribution. Mitogen-stimulated interleukin IL-12 products was augmented and L-10 and TNFα production was reduced in FR patients. A peculiar cytokine pattern, mainly involving monocyte/macrophage, produced cytokines seems to be associated with this condition. Previous studies have suggested that TNFα is involved in fat metabolism. TNFα, also known as cachectin, has mediated weight loss in experimental animals by several mechanisms including suppression of food intake, suppression of lipoprotein and lipase, and catabolic effects on energy storage tissue.

However, the effects of TNFα in mediating fat loss in humans with cancer or chronic infectious disease has not yet been unequivocably demonstrated.[10] IL-12 therapy has been reported to increase estradiol production, which might influence fat distribution.

CONCLUSIONS

Fat redistribution, characterized by breast and abdominal girth enlargement and lower limb wasting is frequently observed in women treated with combined antiretroviral therapy. A preliminary survey does not reveal significant metabolic or hormonal alteration in FR patients. Immunological studies show that TNFα and Il-10 production is less efficient whereas IL-12 is more efficient in these patients. How such a peculiar immune profile may influence fat redistribution in HIV-infected patients remains to be explained. Interestingly, after a one-year follow up, 50% of the patients treated with triple therapy developed a lipodystrophy characterized by weight loss, face-wasting, and/or hyperglycemia. Another group of patients developed the same syndrome after 3TC withdrawal, which suggests that fat redistribution might be a condition that precedes lipodystrophy.

REFERENCES

1. HENGEL, R.L., N.B. WATTS & J.L. LENNOX. 1997. Benign symmetric lipomatosis associated with protease inhibitors. Lancet **350:** 1596.
2. HERRY, I., L. BERNARD, P. DE TRUCHIS & C. PERRONNE. 1997. Hypertrophy of the breasts in a patient treated with indinavir. Clin. Infect. Dis. **25:** 937–938.
3. LO, J.C., K. MULLIGAN, V.W. TAI, H. ALGREN & M. SCHAMBELAN. 1998. "Buffalo hump" in men with HIV-1 infection. Lancet **351:** 867–870.
4. VIRABEN, R. & C. AQUILINA. 1998. Indinavir-associated lipodystrophy. AIDS **12:** F37-39.
5. CARR, A., K. SAMARAS, S. BURTON *et al.* 1998. A syndrome of peripheral lipodystrophy, hyperlipidaemia and insulin resistance in patients receiving HIV protease inhibitors.AIDS **12:** F51–58.
6. LUI, A., D. KARTER & G. TURETT. 1998. Another case of breast hypertrophyin a patient treated with indinavir. Clin. Infect. Dis. **26:** 1482.
7. DONG, K., M.M. FLYNN, B.P. DICKINSON *et al.* 1998. Changes in body habitus in HIV(+) women after initiation of protease inhibitor therapy. 12th World AIDS Conference. Geneva. June 1998 (Abstract 12373).
8. YANOVSKI, J.A., K.D. MILLER, T. KINO, T.C. FRIEDMAN, G.P. CHROUSOS, C. TSIGOSIS & J. FALLOON. 1999. Endocrine and metabolic evaluation of human immunodeficiency virus infected patients with evidence of protease inhibitor-associated lipodystrophy. J. Off. Clin. End **84:** 1925–1931
9. MILLER, K.D., E. JONES, J.A. YANOVSKI, R. SHANKAR, I. FEUERSTEIN & J. FALLOON. 1998. Visceral abdominal-fat accumulation associated with use of indinavir. Lancet **351:** 870–975
10. OLIFF, A. 1988. The role of tumor necrosis factor (cachetin) in cachexia. Cell **54:** 141–142

Immunoendocrinologic Abnormalities in Human Immunodeficiency Virus Infection

MARIO CLERICI,[a,d] MASSIMO GALLI,[b] SIMONA BOSIS,[a]
CRISTINA GERVASONI,[b] MAURO MORONI,[b] AND GUIDO NORBIATO[c]

[a]Cattedra di Immunologia, Università di Milano, DISP LITA Vialba, Milano, Italy

[b]Divisione di Malattie Infettive, Università di Milano, Milano, Italy

[c]Reparto di Endocrinologia, Ospedale L. Sacco, Milano, Italy

ABSTRACT: Alterations in the production of adrenal steroids and a complex pattern of dysregulation in cytokine profiles accompany the progression of HIV infection. Cortisol levels increase in HIV infection, while those of dehydroepiandrosterone (DHEA), a physiologic antagonist of the immunoregulatory activities of cortisol, decrease. A shift from type-1 to type-2 cytokine production is also detected in most patients during disease progression. This shift is summarized as a defective production of interferon gamma (IFNγ), interleukin-2 (IL), and IL-12 accompanied by increased production of IL-4, IL-5, IL-6, and IL-10. IFNγ and IL-2 are suppressed, while the generation of IL-4 is stimulated by cortisol and pharmacological doses of glucocorticoids (GC). GC and IL-4 stimulate the differentiation of B lymphocytes into IgE-producing plasma cells, the concentration of which augments in HIV infection. Finally, GC induces programmed cell death (PCD) in a variety of different cells, including mature T lymphocytes. Because (1) TH1 but not TH2 undergo rapid Fas-mediated PCD upon antigen-stimulation, and (2) TH2 clones preferentially survive *in vitro* cell cultures, the progressive shift from type-1 to type-2 cytokine production observed in HIV infection could be at least partially provoked by the increase in the production of cortisol and the reduction of DHEA. Progression of HIV infection to AIDS can be controlled by highly active antiretroviral therapy (HAART); HAART drastically reduces HIV plasma viremia, but is less effective in immune reconstitution. Additionally HAART is associated in a sizable portion of patients by complex lypodistropyc phenomena that often involve the endocrine system.

CYTOKINE ALTERATIONS IN HIV INFECTION

Progression of HIV infection is associated with impairment of cell-mediated immunity (CMI) and the abnormal stimulation of humoral immunity (HI), which have both *in vivo* and *in vitro* correlates.[1] Thus, the inability to develop delayed-type hypersensitivity reactions (DTH) to ubiquitous antigens precedes and heralds the development of opportunistic infections and tumors. *In vivo* correlates of the abnormal activation of HI include hypergammaglobulinemia, hypereosinophylia,

[d]Address for correspondence: Mario Clerici, MD, Cattedra di Immunologia, Università di Milano, Via GB Grass, 74 20157 Milano, Italy. Voice: 39-02-3821-0354; fax: 39-02-3821-0350.

mago@mailserver.unimi.it

and augmented concentration of IgE. Defective production of the type-1 CMI-inducing cytokines interleukin IL-2, IL-12, and gamma interferon (IFN-γ), and augmented production of type-2 HI-inducing cytokines IL-4, IL-5, IL-6, and IL-10 are thus observed in HIV infection and are thought to be an *in vitro* immunologic marker of progression in HIV+ individuals.[1] The clinical relevance of these imbalances in cytokine profiles is reinforced by the observation that a strong type-1/weak type-2 cytokine production profile and a powerful CMI are present in HIV+ pediatric and adult patients with delayed or absent disease progression, whereas progression of HIV infection is correlated with a weak type-1/strong type-2 cytokine production profile.[2,3]

Type-1 and type-2 cytokines influence susceptibility of peripheral blood lymphocytes (PBL) in a strikingly opposing way.[4–6] Thus, type-1 cytokines reduce in vitro susceptibility of PBL to PCD, while type-2 cytokines increase cell death.

Changes in cytokine production could therefore lead to CD4 destruction via augmented PCD. On the other hand, the reduction in type-1 cytokine and the increase in type-2 cytokine production could be secondary to a different susceptibility of TH1 and TH2 cells to PCD. Thus, recent data showed that TH1 but not TH2 cells undergo rapid Fas-mediated PCD upon being stimulated by antigens;[7,8] TH2 clones were also seen to preferentially survive in *in vitro* cell cultures.[7,8] These findings were justified by the observation that, whereas both types of clone express Fas, only TH2 clones express high levels of a Fas-associated phosphates that inhibit Fas signaling.[8]

ALTERATIONS IN GLUCOCORTICOIDS ASSOCIATED WITH HIV INFECTION

The progression of HIV infection is also associated with increases in the levels of glucocorticoid hormones (GC) and by reduced concentration of the anticortisol hormones dehydroepiandrotestosterone sulfate (DHEAS) and DHEA.[9,10] In particular, a recent publication examined blood cortisol and DHEAS concentrations as well as CD4 T-cell counts in 44 HIV-infected patients. The results showed that (1) a significantly higher mean level of blood cortisol and greatly reduced mean DHEAS concentrations are present in HIV patients compared to controls, and (2) a significant correlation exists between low DHEAS levels and low CD4 T-cell counts in HIV-infected patients.[11] In recently infected asymptomatic patients, augmented concentration of GC could still be within physiologic values, but a string of data has shown that even circadian physiological variations in the endogen production of cortisol will regulate IgE-dependent cutaneous reactions.[12,13] The immunomodulatory role of DHEAS was further examined in a murine model of AIDS (MAIDS). Thus, the authors could demonstrate that the immune dysfunction provoked by LP-BM5 infection in susceptible mice strains, and characterized by reduction in IL-2 production and increases in the generation of IL-4 and IL-6, were prevented by DHEAS. DHEAS was also able to partially restore T- and B-cell proliferation, further suggesting a pathogenetic role for hormone imbalances in HIV infection.[14]

Based on these observations, reduction of cortisolemia could be beneficial in HIV infection. In particular, the correction of the cortisol/anticortisolic ratio might have a stimulating effect on type-1 cytokine production and CMI. The reduction of cortisolemia and the increased production of type-1 cytokines could in turn synergize in reducing PCD and, possibly, in containing viral replication in HIV-infected cells.

To summarize, in HIV infection (1) the concentration of GC is higher compared to HIV-seronegative controls; (2) cortisol response to ACTH stimulation is reduced, probably as a consequence of the chronically elevated concentration of GC; and (3) the concentration of DHEA and DHEAS is reduced.

ALTERATIONS OF THE IMMUNOENDOCRINOLOGIC AXIS ARE OBSERVED IN HIV INFECTION

Two different groups have independently proposed that endocrinological factors could be important in destroying the normal homeostasis of the immune response in the progression of HIV infection.[15,16] This would favor a type-1-to-type-2 switch in cytokine production. Most evidences indicate that GC suppress cell-mediated immunity and may stimulate humoral immunity. To summarize: (1) GC inhibit production of interleukin-1, which acts as a costimulator on T-cell activation; (2) GC suppress the production of IL-2 and IFN-γ by inhibiting the transcription of IL-2 and IFN-γ genes;[17] (3) GC favor the production of type-2 cytokines by directly stimulating the production of IL-4;[13,18] (4) GC synergize with IL-4 in the triggering and differentiation of B lymphocytes into IgE-producing plasmacells,[13,18] the concentration of which increases in HIV infection. Thus, the progressive shift from type-1 to type-2 cytokine production observed in HIV infection could be at least partially provoked by an imbalance in the cortisol/anticortisols ratio.

The alteration of the cortisol/anticortisol ratio could influence disease progression in more than one way, as GC are known to induce the transcription of murine retroviruses.[19–20] In particular, the *vpr* gene of HIV, involved in the regulation of HIV, directly interacts with a cellular protein that associates with the GC transcriptional complex. Additionally, the permissive action of *vpr* on HIV replication is suppressed by anti-GC agents, suggesting a possible role for such agents in the therapy of HIV infection.

GC also induce PCD in a variety of cells, including mature T lymphocytes.[21] This is particularly important, as an imbalance in type-1/type-2 cytokine production is a factor in the modulation of susceptibility of CD4+ T lymphocytes of HIV-seropositive individuals to PCD. To sumamrize, type-1 cytokines (IFN-γ, IL-2, and IL-12) block PCD, whereas IL-4 and IL-10 have either no effect or enhance *in vitro* T-cell PCD. GC and type-2 cytokines could therefore have a synergistic effect in the PCD-mediated reduction in CD4 counts characteristic of HIV infection. In short, the negative effects of cortisol in HIV infection could be the following: (1) suppression of CMI, at least in part secondarily to a suppression of the transcription of IL-2 and IFNγ, but not of IL-4; (2) stimulation of retroviruses transcription; and (3) induction of PCD.

A clinical picture of acquired glucocorticoids resistance (elevated cortisol concentration; reduction in the affinity of glucocorticoid receptors and lymphocyte resistance to cortisol) is described in a subgroup of AIDS patients.[22] Plasma cytokine concentrations were measured in AIDS patients with or without acquired glucocorticoids resistance (AGR), and results indicated that different cytokine profiles are present in these two subsets of HIV-seropositive individuals. Thus, a higher concentration of IL-2/lower concentration of IL-4 was observed in the serum of AGR-HIV-seropositive individuals. These data are consistent with the hypothesis that cortisol can directly modify cytokine profile in HIV infection.

FAT REDISTRIBUTION SYNDROMES IN HAART-TREATED PATIENTS

The development of the combined antiretroviral therapy, known as HAART, offered a significant advancement in the treatment of HIV infection. Although new antiretroviral drugs are generally well tolerated, a curious array of unique metabolic side effects characterized by abnormal fat distribution have been reported in a sizable portion of patients undergoing HAART.[23] One of the most frequent and unexpected side effects of combined antiretroviral therapy involves changes in normal body habits due to abnormal fat distribution. Two groups of conditions characterized by fat tissue abnormalities have been reported. One includes abnormal accumulation of fat tissue in particular body regions ("buffalo hump," benign symmetric lipomatosis, hypertrophy of breasts in women, visceral abdominal fat accumulation) without modifications of body weight and total fat mass. The other includes lipodystrophic syndromes involving the face, the lower limbs, and the upper trunk.[23] Although in the first group of conditions no abnormalities in methabolic or endocrinologic parameteres are generally reported, lypodystrophy is frequently associated with glucose metabolism disorders, mainly insulin resistence and diabetes mellitus type 2, hyperlipidemia, weight loss, and reduction of total fat mass.[23]

In a recent study we have described a particular pattern of fat distribution characterized by enlargement of breast and abdominal girth associated with wasting of glutei and lower limbs, observed in more than 10% of HIV-infected women treated with

TABLE 1. Clinical and endocrine parameters in HIV-infected and HAART-treated women with or without fat redistribution syndrome (mean values)

	With fat redistribution (N = 21)	Without fat redistribution (N = 14)
C-peptide (ng/ml)	2.9	2.3
Prolactin (ng/ml)	15.0	17.9
GH (ng/ml)	1.1	1
Testosteron (pg/ml)	0.8	1.1
ACTH (pg/ml)	22.2	26.3
Cortisol (ng/ml)	149	127
Urinary free cortisol (nmol/24)	41.7	—
Glucose (mg/dl)	83	94
Tryglycerides (mg/dl)	168	174
Cholesterol (mg/dl)	180	165

TABLE 2. SAC-stimulated IL-10 and IL-12 production (mean ± S.E.) in HIV-infected and HAART-treated women with or without fat redistribution syndrome

HIV-infected patients	SAC-stimulated cytokine production (pg/ml)	
	Interleukin-10	Interleukin-12
With fat redistribution ($N = 21$)	47 ± 11	560 ± 22
W/o fat redistribution ($N = 14$)	192 ± 51	142 ± 38

two or more antiretroviral drugs.[24] None of the women with this syndrome had variations of body weight and metabolic abnormalities, even if cortisol levels were slightly augmented in those women in whom fat redistribution was observed (149 vs. 122 ng/mL) (see TABLE 1). Interestingly, we observed that IL-12 production was significantly higher, while IL-10 was significantly lower in PBMC cultures from patients with fat redistribution compared to controls (see TABLE 2), suggesting an effect of these drugs on monocyte-produced cytokines. Moreover, women with the syndrome showed a more effective T-helper function, as evaluated by proliferation of PBMC upon stimulation with soluble antigens.

Interestingly, it was recently shown that in HIV-infected patients undergoing HAART, and in whom fat redistribution is observed, urinary-free cortisol is significanly reduced, but the excretion of 17-hydroxycorticosteroid is increased as compared to normal individuals. The authors also demonstrated that glucocorticoid receptors are quantitatively normal and that their affinity is comparable to the one of control individuals, suggesting that an indeed curious and atypical form of hypercortisolism might be associated with lipodystrophy.[25]

The correlation between immune and endocrine abnormality detected in the progression of HIV infection, and here briefly summarized, seem to be epitomized in HAART-treated patients in whom fat redistribution is observed. We therefore believe that the endocrinology of this condition should be explored in depth. We also believe that studies on the correlations between the endocrine and immunologic systems should be encouraged, as endocrine modulations could be extremely beneficial in this infection.

ACKNOWLEDGMENT

This work was supported by grants from Istituto Superiore di Sanità "II Programma Nazionale di Ricerca sull' AIDS 1998."

REFERENCES

1. CLERICI, M. & G.M. SHEARER. 1994. The TH1/TH2 hypothesis of HIV infection: new insights. Immunol. Today 15: 575–581.
2. CLERICI, M. et al. 1996. Type 1 cytokine production and low prevalence of viral isolation correlate with long term non progression in HIV infection. AIDS Res. Hum. Retroviruses 12: 1053–1061.

3. VIGANÓ, A. *et al.* 1995. Immunologic characterization of children vertically infected with human immunodeficiency virus, with slow or rapid disease progression. J. Pediatr. **126:** 368–374.

4. CLERICI, M. *et al.* 1994. Type1/type2 cytokine modulation of T cell programmed cell death as a model for HIV pathogenesis. Proc. Natl. Acad. Sci. USA **91:** 11811–11815.

5. ESTAQUIER, J. *et al.* 1995. T helper 1/T helper 2 cytokines and T cell death: preventive effect of IL-12 on activation-induced and CD95 (Fas/Apo-1)-mediated apoptosis of CD4+ T cells from human immunodeficiency virus-infected person. J. Exp. Med. **182:** 1759–1767.

6. RADDRIZZANI, M. *et al.* 1995. IL-12 inhibits apoptosis induced in a human Th1 clone by gp120/CD4 cross-linking and CD3/TcR activation or by IL-2 deprivation. Cell. Immunol. **161:** 14–21.

7. ZHANG, X. *et al.* 1997. Unequal death in T helper cell (Th)1 and Th2 effectors: Th1, but not Th2, effectors undergo rapid Fas/FasL-mediated apoptosis. J. Exp. Med. **185:** 1837–1849.

8. VARADHACHARY, A.S. *et al.* 1997. Differential ability of T cell subsets to undergo activation-induced cell death. Proc. Natl. Acad. Sci. USA **94:** 5778–5783.

9. CHRISTEFF, N. *et al.* 1992. Evidence of changes in adrenal and testicular steroids during HIV infection. J. AIDS **5:** 841–846.

10. GRINSPOON, S.K. & J.P. BILEZIKIAN. 1992. HIV disease and the endocrine system. N. Engl. J. Med. **327:** 1360–1365.

11. DE LA TORRE, B. *et al.* 1997. Blood cortisol and dehydroepiandrosterone sulphate (DHEAS) levels and CD4 T cell counts in HIV infection. Clin. Exp. Rheumatol. **15:** 87–90.

12. HERRSCHER, R.F. *et al.* 1992. Endogenous cortisol regulates immunoglobulin E dependent late phase reaction. J. Clin. Invest. **90:** 596–603.

13. WU, C.Y. *et al.* 1991. Glucocorticoids increase the synthesis of immunoglobulin E by interleukin-4 stimulated human lymphocytes. J. Clin. Invest. **87:** 870–877.

14. LEE, J. *et al.* 1999. Immune dysfunction during alcohol consumption and murine AIDS: the protective role of dehydroepiandrosterone sulfate. Alcohol. Clin. Exp. Res. **23:** 856–862.

15. ROOK, G.A.W. *et al.* 1993. TH1/TH2 switching and loss of CD4 T cells: an immunoendocrinological hypothesis not exclusive to HIV. Immunol. Today **14:** 568–569.

16. CLERICI, M. *et al.* 1994. An immunoendocrinologic hypothesis for HIV infection. Lancet **343:** 1552–1554.

17. VACCA, A. *et al.* 1992. Glucorticoid receptor mediated suppression of the interleukin-2 gene expression through impairment of the cooperativity between nuclear factors of activiated T cells and AP 1 enhancer elements. J. Exp. Med. **175:** 637–646.

18. DAYNES, R.A. & B.A. ARANEO. 1989. Contrasting effects of glucocorticoids on the capacity of T cells to produce the growth factors interleukin-2 and interleukin-4. Eur. J. Immunol. **19:** 2319–2325.

19. HELMBERG, A. *et al.* 1990. Glucocorticoid-regulated gene expression in the immune system. J. Immunol. **145:** 4332–4337.

20. REFAELI, Y. *et al.* 1995. The glucocorticoid receptor type II complex is a target for the HIV-1 vpr gene product. Proc. Natl. Acad. Sci. USA **92:** 3621–3625.

21. COHEN, I.J. *et al.* 1992. Apoptosis and programmed cell death in immunity Annu. Rev. Immunol. **10:** 267–293.

22. NORBIATO, G. *et al.* 1997. Cortisol resistance in acquired immunodeficiency syndrome. J. Clin. Endocrin. Metab. **74:** 608–613.

23. WANKE, C.A. 1999. Epidemiological and clinical aspects of the metabolic complications of HIV infection and the fat redistribution syndrome. AIDS **13:** 1287–1294.

24. GERVASONI, C. *et al.* 1999. Redistribution of body fat in HIV-infected women undergoing combined antiretroviral therapy. AIDS **13:** 473–479.

25. YANOVSKI, J.A. *et al.* 1999. Endocrine and metabolic evaluation of human immunodeficiency virus-infected patients with evidence of protease inhibitor-associated lipodystrophy. J. Clin. Endocrinol. Metabol. **84:** 1925–1931.

Changes in Cortisol/DHEA Ratio in HIV-Infected Men Are Related to Immunological and Metabolic Perturbations Leading to Malnutrition and Lipodystrophy

NÉVÉNA CHRISTEFF,[a,b] EMMANUEL A. NUNEZ,[b]
AND MARIE-LISE GOUGEON[a,c]

[a]*Viral Oncology Unit and CNRS URA 1930, AIDS and Retroviruses Department, Institut Pasteur, Paris, France*

[b]*Laboratoire d'Endocrinologie, Biochimie B, Hôpital X. Bichat, Paris, France*

ABSTRACT: HIV-1 infection is associated with immune deficiency and metabolic perturbations leading to malnutrition and lipodystrophy. Because immune response and metabolic perturbations (protein and lipid metabolism) are partly regulated by glucocorticoids and DHEA, we determined serum cortisol and DHEA concentrations, and the cortisol/DHEA ratio in HIV-positive men, either untreated or receiving various antiretroviral treatments (ART), including highly active antiretroviral therapy (HAART). Cortisol levels were found increased in all patients, whatever the stage of the disease and independently of the ART treatment. In contrast, serum DHEA was elevated in the asymptomatic stage, and it was below normal values in AIDS patients, either untreated or mono-ART-treated. The DHEA level was low in HAART-treated patients with lipodystrophy (LD+) and highly increased in HAART-treated patients without lipodystrophy (LD−). Consequently, the cortisol/DHEA ratio was similar to controls in asymptomatic untreated or mono-ART-treated patients, but increased in AIDS patients. Interestingly, this ratio was increased in LD+ HAART-treated men, but normalized in LD− HAART-treated patients. Changes in the cortisol/DHEA ratio were negatively correlated with the *in vivo* CD4 T-cell counts, with the malnutrition markers, such as body-cell mass and fat mass, and with the increased circulating lipids (cholesterol, triglycerides, and apolipoprotein B) associated to the lipodystrophy syndrome. Our observations show that the cortisol/DHEA ratio is dramatically altered in HIV-infected men, particularly during the syndromes of malnutrition and lipodystrophy, and this ratio remains elevated whatever the antiretroviral treatment, including HAART. These findings have practical clinical implications, since manipulation of this ratio could prevent metabolic (protein and lipid) perturbations.

[c]Address for correspondence: Marie-Lise Gougeon, Viral Oncology Unit and CNRS URA 1930, AIDS and Retroviruses Department, Institut Pasteur, Paris, France. Voice: 33-1 45-68-89-07; fax: 33-1 45-68-89-09.
mlgougeo@pasteur.fr

INTRODUCTION

The natural history of HIV-1 infection is characterized by severe immune deficiency and malnutrition (see FIGURE 1). Immune deficiency is mainly due to the selective depletion of CD4 T lymphocytes.[1] Malnutrition in HIV-infected men results in loss of both body-cell mass (protoplasmic mass that contains much of the body protein) and fat mass.[2] New highly active antiretroviral therapy (HAART), including HIV-1 protease inhibitors (PI), have a profound impact on both immune deficiency and malnutrition. A rise in the number of CD4 T lymphocytes[3] and an increase in body weight[4] have been observed in most of the treated patients. However, HAART can lead to new metabolic disorders. A syndrome of lipodystrophy, characterized by an increase in circulating lipids, particularly cholesterol and triglycerides, and abnormal fat distribution, including peripheral loss of fatty tissue and visceral abdominal fat accumulation, was recently reported.[5,6]

The immune response and metabolic perturbations (protein and lipid metabolism) are partly regulated by steroid hormones, such as glucocorticoids and androgens, particularly the adrenal androgen DHEA. Indeed, glucocorticoids decrease *in vitro* T-cell proliferation by inhibiting the production of cytokines.[7] DHEA stimulates helper T-cell function by enhancing the capacity of activated T cells to produce interleukin (IL)-2, and it also neutralizes the inhibitory effect of glucocorticoids on IL-2 synthesis.[8] Cortisol and DHEA also regulate the metabolism of muscle amino acids, which is altered in HIV infection, leading to the loss of body-cell mass.[9] Glucocorticoids stimulate amino-acid catabolism, but androgens increase amino-acid anabolism. Finally, lipid metabolism and fat mass distribution are notably regulated by glucocorticoids and androgens, particularly by their action on several lipases.[10] Indeed, glucocorticoids stimulate hormone-sensitive lipoprotein lipase (HSL)

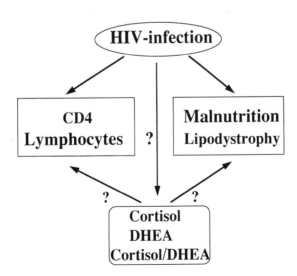

FIGURE 1. Are serum cortisol, DHEA, and the cortisol/DHEA ratio related to immunological and metabolic perturbations in HIV-1–infected men?

activity, and consequently increase peripheral lipolysis. DHEA is known to be a potent noncompetitive inhibitor of glucose-6-phosphate dehydrogenase (G6PD), an important enzyme in *de novo* lipogenesis, particularly in fatty-acid synthesis.[11] The decrease in DHEA is also associated with increases in pancreatic insulin secretion and insulin resistance.[12]

It is now accepted that glucocorticoids and DHEA profiles of HIV-1-infected men change during the course of the viral infection.[13-17] Indeed, the serum cortisol concentrations are elevated at all stages of the disease. In contrast, DHEA is elevated at early stages of infection and dramatically decreased in AIDS patients. These adrenal steroid modifications lead to an important rise in the cortisol/DHEA ratio at the AIDS stages, whereas this ratio is not altered in the asymptomatic phase of the infection.

Because antiretroviral treatments (ART) have an impact on the absolute number of CD4 lymphocytes, as well as on malnutrition and lipid metabolism, we asked (1) whether different antiretroviral therapies are associated with changes in serum cortisol and DHEA concentrations, and (2) whether CD4 cell counts, malnutrition, and lipod metabolism are related to serum glucocorticoids and DHEA modifications (FIG. 1). The present report is the first one to focus on the relationship between the cortisol/DHEA ratio and immunologic and metabolic perturbations observed in the course of HIV-1 infection. The mechanisms potentially involved in these perturbations are discussed.

METHODS

The data were obtained from patients included in six retrospective and prospective studies between 1987 and 1998 carried out on men with Western-blot-confirmed HIV-1 infection. Patients were followed in France at Claude Bernard Hospital, Paris,[13,18] Rothschild Hospital, Paris,[14] Avicenne University Hospital, Bobigny,[15,16] Compiègne Hospital,[15,16] and R. Poincaré Hospital, Garches.[18] Blood samples were collected between 8 A.M. and 10 A.M. and allowed to coagulate before separation of serum by centrifugation. Serum cortisol was measured by radioimmunoassay after extraction and chromatographic fractionation or by fluorescence polarization immunoassay (TDX System Cortisol, Abbott Diagnostics Division, USA). DHEA levels were determined by radioimmunoassay after extraction, or by commercial ELISA kits (DRG Diagnostics, Germany). The data were analyzed using different statistical tests appropriate to the individual studies.[18,19]

RESULTS

Effect of ART on Serum Cortisol, DHEA, and Cortisol/DHEA Ratio in HIV-Positive Men

The serum cortisol and DHEA concentrations and cortisol/DHEA ratio were determined in HIV$^+$ men either untreated ($n = 60$), or mono-ART-treated ($n = 119$), or bi-ART–treated ($n = 30$), or HAART-treated with lipodystrophy (LD$^+$) ($n = 23$), or HAART-treated without lipodystrophy (LD$^-$) ($n = 14$). All groups of HIV$^+$ men were compared to healthy donors ($n = 70$).

The serum cortisol concentrations were significantly higher in HIV-1-positive men than in seronegative controls, whatever the stage of the infection and independently of the treatment (see FIGURE 2). Cortisol levels were +50–80% ($p < 0.01$) in untreated asymptomatic and AIDS patients, +70–77% ($p < 0.001$) in mono-ART–treated men, +70% ($p < 0.001$) in bi-ART–treated men, and +45% ($p < 0.01$) in LD^+ or LD^- HAART–treated men. In contrast, modifications in serum DHEA levels were dependent on the regimens of ART and the stage of infection. In untreated or mono-ART-treated asymptomatic men, DHEA was increased compared to healthy donors (+25%, $p < 0.05$ and +85%, $p < 0.001$, respectively), and it was below normal values in untreated, in mono-ART–treated, or bi-ART–treated AIDS patients (−40%, $p < 0.01$; −25%, $p < 0.05$; and −35%, $p < 0.01$, respectively) (FIG. 2). Importantly, the serum DHEA level was quite elevated in LD^- HAART–treated men (+100% vs. controls, $p < 0.01$), but it was significantly decreased in LD^+ HAART–treated men (−125% vs. LD^-, $p < 0.0001$). Consequently, changes in the cortisol/DHEA ratio were observed in patients compared to seronegative controls. Indeed, this ratio was markedly elevated at the AIDS stage, both in untreated (+200%, $p < 0.001$) or mono-ART–treated (+125%, $p < 0.001$) or bi-ART–treated patients (+135%, $p < 0.001$). In contrast, this ratio remained similar to seronegative controls in untreated and mono-ART–treated asymptomatic men (FIG. 2). In HAART–treated men, the cortisol/DHEA ratio was dramatically elevated in LD^+ men (+100%, $p < 0.0001$) compared to LD^- patients or healthy donors (FIG. 2).

Correlations Between *In Vivo CD4 T-cell Counts and Serum Cortisol, DHEA, and Cortisol/DHEA Ratio*

Linear correlations between serum cortisol, DHEA, cortisol/DHEA ratio, and CD4 cell counts were assessed in HIV-positive men ($n = 179$) who had been either treated by mono-ART ($n = 119$) or untreated ($n = 60$) (see FIGURE 3). In these patients we found a significant positive correlation between the absolute number of CD4 T lymphocytes and the serum DHEA levels ($r = 0.51$, $p < 0.0003$). In contrast, the serum cortisol and the cortisol/DHEA ratio were negatively correlated with the absolute number of CD4 T cells ($r = −0.49$, $p < 0.0003$ and $r = −0.53$, $p < 0.0002$, respectively).

Correlations Between *Malnutrition Markers and Serum Cortisol, DHEA, and Cortisol/DHEA Ratio*

Correlation analyses between markers of malnutrition, such as body-weight loss, body-mass index, body-cell mass and free fat mass, and adrenal steroids were assessed in HIV-1–positive men ($n = 38$) submitted to mono ART.[18] Interestingly, the loss of body-cell mass, which is the more relevant marker of malnutrition during evolution of HIV-1 infection, was positively correlated with DHEA level ($r = +0.36$, $p < 0.03$) and negatively correlated with the cortisol/DHEA ratio ($r = −0.58$, $p < 0.0001$). In contrast, the body-weight loss was negatively correlated with serum DHEA ($r = −0.69$, $p < 0.0001$) and positively correlated with the cortisol/DHEA ratio ($r = 0.61$, $p < 0.0001$). In addition, fat-mass values were found negatively correlated with the cortisol/DHEA ratio ($r = −0.39$, $p < 0.02$). It is noteworthy that the serum cortisol level was not correlated to any of these malnutrition markers.

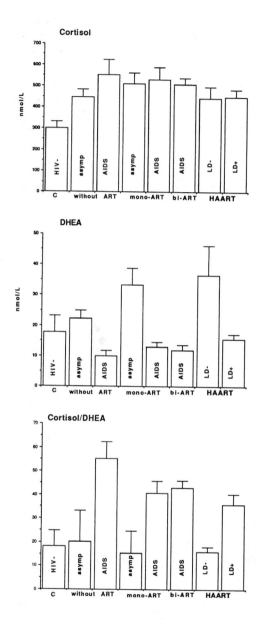

FIGURE 2. Serum cortisol, DHEA, and cortisol/DHEA ratio in HIV-1–positive men. HIV–infected men were either nontreated ($n = 60$), or mono-ART–treated ($n = 119$), or bi-ART–treated ($n = 30$), or HAART–treated patients with lipodystrophy (LD$^+$) ($n = 23$) and without lipodystrophy (LD$^-$). These patients were tested for cortisol and DHEA, and compared to healthy men ($n = 70$). The data are means ±SEM. Statistical analyses were performed with the Mann-Whitney test; $p < 0.05$ was considered significant. Statistical significances are mentioned in the RESULTS section.

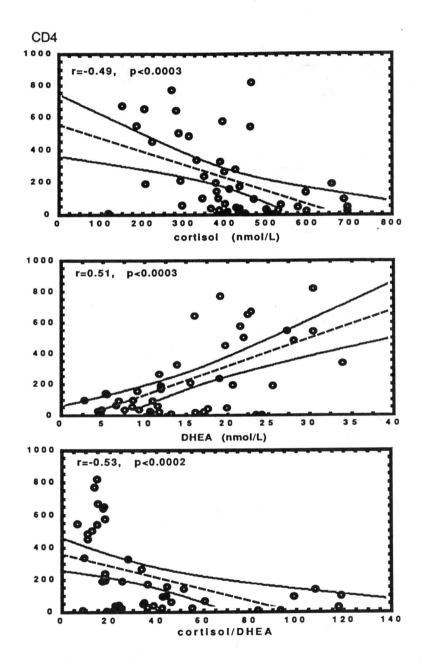

FIGURE 3. Correlations of the *in vivo* CD4 T-lymphocyte count and serum cortisol, DHEA, and cortisol/DHEA ratio in HIV-1–infected men (*n* = 179).

Correlations Between Lipid Alterations Associated With the Lipodystrophy Syndrome and Serum Cortisol, DHEA, and Cortisol/DHEA Ratio

We recently reported that in addition to dramatic lipid alterations (high levels of triglycerides, cholesterol, and apolipoprotein B), modifications in adrenal steroid hormone concentrations (increased cortisol levels, decreased DHEA concentration, and markedly elevated cortisol/DHEA ratio) occurred in LD⁺ HAART–treated patients compared to similarly treated LD⁻ patients.[19] In order to determine whether alterations in lipid metabolism were related to modifications in adrenal steroids, we looked for correlations between these parameters. Negative correlations were found between concentrations of DHEA and all lipids found increased in LD⁺ patients, such as cholesterol, triglycerides, and apolipoprotein B ($r = -0.39$, $p < 0.02$; $r = -0.35$, $p < 0.03$; and $r = -0.45$, $p < 0.006$, respectively). No correlations were found between lipid concentrations and cortisol levels. In contrast, the cortisol/DHEA ratio was positively correlated to cholesterol level ($r = 0.41$, $p < 0.01$), triglycerides ($r = 0.38$, $p < 0.02$), and apolipoprotein B ($r = 0.46$, $p < 0.005$).[19]

DISCUSSION AND CONCLUSION

The data of this report show that the cortisol/DHEA ratio, which reflects serum adrenal steroids profile, is progressively increased throughout HIV infection, reaching at the AIDS stage values corresponding to two to four times the control values. Following antiretroviral therapies, no modifications in the cortisol/DHEA ratio were observed when patients received either monotherapy (AZT) or bitherapy, including two reverse transcriptase inhibitors. In contrast, the cortisol/DHEA ratio was normalized following HAART. But this normalization was not observed in all HAART–treated men (FIG. 2). It is noteworthy that modifications in the cortisol/DHEA ratio were mainly due to alterations in DHEA concentrations, because cortisol levels remained elevated whatever the stage of HIV infection and independently of the antiretroviral treatment.

Changes in cortisol/DHEA ratio appear to be a crucial link between adrenal hormones and immunological and metabolic alterations (see FIGURE 4). Indeed, the increase of this ratio is correlated with the decreased number of CD4 lymphocytes, the loss of body-cell mass and fat mass, and the increase in circulating lipids. The drop in DHEA and concomitant elevated cortisol may contribute to (1) CD4 T-cell depletion by inhibiting IL-2 synthesis;[8] (2) the decrease in muscle protein anabolism consecutive to an imbalance between amino-acid anabolism and catabolism;[9] (3) the increase in the activity of HSL and G6PD,[10,11] which are probably responsible for the imbalance between lipolysis and lipogenesis in peripheral adipose tissue, leading to the lipodystrophy syndrome.

In conclusion, our observations suggest that the cortisol/DHEA ratio undoubtedly has a profound impact on the homeostasis and pathophysiological response of the organism. In particular, this ratio is dramatically altered during lipodystrophy. Because the cortisol/DHEA ratio is correlated with lipid alterations characteristic of this syndrome, we suggest that maintenance of increased cortisol/DHEA under HAART favors lipid perturbations already present in mono-ART-treated patients,[18] and leads to the abnormal fat-mass distribution, characteristic of lipodystrophy.[5]

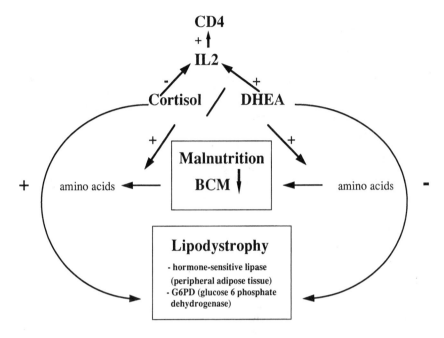

FIGURE 4. Relationship between the cortisol/DHEA ratio and both immunological and metabolic perturbations in malnutrition and lipodystrophy. This scheme is discussed in the DISCUSSION section.

These findings have practical clinical implications. Since lipodystrophy is observed whatever the antiretroviral treatment (bi-ART or HAART) currently given,[20] additional treatments by specific drugs, including steroid supplements, should be considered to manipulate the cortisol/DHEA ratio in order to prevent metabolic perturbations.

ACKNOWLEDGMENTS

This work was supported by grants from the Agence Nationale de Recherche sur le SIDA (ANRS), the Centre National de Recherche Scientifique (CNRS), and the Pasteur Institute. The authors are indebted to Drs. S. Gharakhanian, O. Lortholory, J.-C. Melchior, C. Michon, B. Trogoff, and P. de Truchis for their contribution to the clinical aspect of this work.

REFERENCES

1. GOUGEON, M.-L. & K.-M. DEBATIN. 1999. Molecular control of programmed cell death in HIV infection: contribution to the dysregulation of T cell homeostasis and to CD4 T cell depletion. *In* HIV and the New Viruses, 2nd edit. A.G. Dalgleish and R.A. Weiss, Eds.: 99–114. Academic Press, New York.

2. GRUNFELD, C. & D.P. KOTLER. 1992. Pathology of AIDS wasting syndrome. *In* AIDS Clinical Review, P. Volberding and M.A. Jacobson, Eds.: 191–199. Dekker, New York.

3. HO, D.D., A.U. NEUMANN, A.S. PERELSON *et al.* 1995. Rapid turnover of plasma virions and CD4 lymphocytes in HIV-1 infection. Nature **373:** 123–127.

4. CORCORAN, N.P. & S. GRINSPOON. 1999. Treatments for wasting in patients with the acquired immunodeficiency syndrome. N. Engl. J. Med. **340:** 1740–1750.

5. MILLER, K.K., P.A. DALY, J.D. SENTOCHINK *et al.* 1998. Pseudo-Cushing's syndrome in human immunodeficiency virus-infected patients. Clin. Infect. Dis. **27:** 68–72.

6. CARR, A., K. SAMARAS, S. BURTON *et al.* 1998. A syndrome of peripheral lipodystrophy, hyperlipidaemia and insulin resistance in patients receiving HIV-1-protease inhibitors. AIDS **12:** F51–F58.

7. HOMO-DELARCHE, F. 1988. Glucocorticoids, lymphokines and the cell response. *In* Progress in Endocrinology, H. Imura, K. Shizume, and S. Yoshida, Eds.: 349–354. Elsevier, Amsterdam.

8. DAYNES, R.A., D.J. DUBLEY & B.A. ARANEO. 1990. Regulation of murine lymphokine production in vivo II. Deydroepiandrosterone is a natural enhancer of interleukin 2 synthesis by helper T-cells. Exp. Clin. Endocrinol. Diabetes **20:** 793–802.

9. CAHILL, G.F. & O.E. OWEN. 1973. Metabolic effect of exogenous glucocorticoids in fasted man. J. Clin. Invest. **52:** 2596–2602.

10. NUNEZ, E.A. & N. CHRISTEFF. 1994. Steroid hormones, cytokines, lipids and metabolic disturbances in HIV infection. *In* The Endocrinology and Metabolism of HIV Infection, Vol. 8, G. Norbiato, Ed.: 803–821. Baillière Tindall, London.

11. OERTEL, G.W. & P. BENES. 1972. The effect of steroids on glucose-6-phosphate dehydrogenase. J. Steroid Biochem. **3:** 493–496.

12. CLORE, J.N. 1995. Deydroepiandrosterone and body fat. Obesity Res. **3:** 613S–616S.

13. CHRISTEFF, N., C. MICHON, G. GOEURTZ *et al.* 1988. Abnormal free fatty acids and cortisol concentrations in the serum of AIDS patients. Eur. J. Cancer Clin. Oncol. **24:** 1179–1183.

14. CHRISTEFF, N., S. GHARAKHANIAN, N. THOBIE *et al.* 1992. Evidence for changes in adrenal and testicular steroids during human imunodeficiency virus infection. J. AIDS **5:** 841–846.

15. CHRISTEFF, N., O. LORTHOLARY, P. CASASSUS *et al.* 1996. Relationship between sex steroid hormone levels and CD4 lymphocytes in HIV infected men. Exp. Clin. Endocrinol. **104:** 130–136.

16. LORTHOLARY, O., N. CHRISTEFF, P. CASASSUS *et al.* 1996. Hypothalamo-pituitary-adrenal function in HIV infected men. J. Clin. Endorcinol. Metab. **81:** 791–796.

17. SELLMEYER, D.E. & C. GRUNFELD. 1996. Endocrine and metabolic disturbances in human immunodeficiency virus infection and the acquired immune deficiency syndrome. Endocr. Rev. **17:** 518–532.

18. CHRISTEFF, N., J.C. MELCHIOR, O. MAMMES *et al.* 1999. Correlation between increased cortisol/DHEA ratio and malnutrition in HIV positive men. Nutrition **15:** 534–539.

19. CHRISTEFF, N., J.C. MELCHIOR, P. DE TRUCHIS *et al.* 1999. Lipodystrophy defined by a clinical score in HIV-infected men on HAART: correlation between dyslipidaemia and steroid hormone alterations. AIDS **13:** 2251–2260.

20. MERCIÉ, P., S. TCHAMGOUÉ, F. DABIS & J.L. PELLEGRIN. 1999. Lipodystrophy in HIV-1–infected patients. Lancet **354:** 867–68

7α-Hydroxy-Dehydroepiandrosterone and Immune Response

R. MORFIN,[a,b] P. LAFAYE,[c] A.C. COTILLON,[b] F. NATO,[c]
V. CHMIELEWSKI,[b] AND D. POMPON[d]

[b]Laboratoire de Biotechnologie, Conservatoire National des Arts et Métiers,
2 rue Conté, 75003 Paris, France

[c]Laboratoire d'Ingéniérie des Anticorps, Département des Biotechnologies,
Institut Pasteur, 25 rue du Docteur Roux, 75015 Paris, France

[d]Laboratoire d'Ingéniérie des Protéines Membranaires, Centre de Génétique
Moléculaire, Centre National de la Recherche Scientifique, 91190 Gif-sur
Yvette, France

ABSTRACT: In human and murine lymphoid organs, circulating 3β-hydroxys-
teroids, including pregnenolone (PREG), dehydroepiandrosterone (DHEA),
and epiandrosterone (EPIA), are 7α-hydroxylated by a cytochrome P450 identified in the hippocampus as P4507B1. Mouse and human lymphoid organs
produced different patterns of 3β-hydroxysteroid 7α-hydroxylation with the
absence of pregnenolone and epiandrosterone hydroxylation in human and
mouse, respectively. Both 7α-hydroxy-DHEA and 7α-hydroxy-EPIA triggered
a significant increase of antitetanus toxoid and anti-*Bordetella pertussis* toxins
IgGs production in cultures of activated B + T cells derived from human tonsils, whereas both 7α-hydroxy-PREG and 7α-hydroxy-DHEA increased the
immune response in mouse. Paracrine action of 7α-hydroxysteroids resulted
from their production in cells of the lymphoid organs. Comparison of P4507B1
sequences in rat, human, and two mouse species showed that one amino acid
change might explain important differences in K_M for 7α-hydroxylation, and
suggested that such differences might contribute to the extent of immune
response.

INTRODUCTION

Both human and murine species carry out the 7α-hydroxylation of dehydroepiandrosterone (DHEA) and produce 7α-hydroxy-DHEA, mainly in the liver and
brain,[1–3] and to a lesser extent in other tissues and organs.[4–8] Production in lymphoid
organs and immunoactivating potencies of the 7α-hydroxy-DHEA produced were
demonstrated in mouse[3,8] and led to the concept of a native steroid counteracting the
glucocorticoid-mediated immunosuppressive effects.[9,10] Whether this held true for
immunity in human lymphoid organs remained to be ascertained.

Furthermore, and due to the immunity-triggering action of 7α-hydroxy-DHEA in
mouse, activity of the cytochrome P450 responsible for 7α-hydroxylation of DHEA

[a]Address for correspondence: Prof. R. Morfin, Biotechnologie, CNAM, 2 rue Conté,
75003 Paris, France. Voice: 33-1 40272572; fax: 33-1 40272380.
morfin@cnam.fr

appeared to offer a key to this process.[3,8] The recent discovery of this $P450$ from rat and mouse, identified as CYP7B1 from its cDNA sequence,[11,12] and demonstration of its DHEA 7α-hydroxylating potencies when expressed in HeLa cells[13] provided valuable tools for studies of the relationships between cDNA sequences and activity of the resulting CYP7B1.

Data resulting from these studies could bring support for the implication of DHEA 7α-hydroxylation in the triggering of immune processes in human, and thus lead to new concepts for investigations of the known age-dependent and HIV-dependent decrease in both DHEA and immunity.

METHODS AND RESULTS

7α-Hydroxylation in Human and Murine Lymphoid Organs

Tonsillar tissues were obtained after routine surgery from four-year-old to 21-year-old patients, and thymus were collected from four-week-old C57BL/6 mice. Identical weights of both tissues were either processed for separation of lymphocytes (B+T cells or T cells) from stroma or were cut into small pieces.[14] Homogenization of intact tissues, of lymphocytes, and of stroma fractions was then performed in 67-mM phosphate buffer (pH 7.4) containing 1 mM EDTA. Incubation of homogenates with 0.5 μM [4-^{14}C]-DHEA in the 0.5-mM NADPH-fortified buffer was at 37°C for 30 min. Ethyl acetate extraction followed by thin-layer chromatography on silica gel plates developed once in the same solvent allowed separation of the [4-^{14}C]-DHEA substrate from its 7α-hydroxylated metabolite and quantification. Identification of the 7α-hydroxylated metabolites produced was ascertained by crystallization to constant specific activity after isotopic dilution with authentic carrier.[14] Results with human tonsils indicated that 7α-hydroxy-DHEA and 3β,7α-dihydroxy-5α-androstan-17-one (7α-hydroxy-EPIA) were produced only in homogenates of whole tonsil and of stroma fraction. No significant production was obtained in homogenates of isolated lymphocytes (see FIGURE 1A). Cultivation of the B+T tonsillar cells in supplemented (2 mM glutamine, 100 U/mL penicillin, 100 μg/mL streptomycin, 0.5 μM β-mercaptoethanol, 5 μg/mL insulin, 5 μg/mL transferin, 5 ng/mL Na$_2$SeSO$_3$, 10% heat-inactivated fetal calf serum) DMEM medium containing 0.1 μM [4-^{14}C]-DHEA, as well as the use of human PBMC, further confirmed the absence of 7α-hydroxylation in human lymphoid cells. Incubations with 0.5 μM [20-^{14}C]-pregnenolone (PREG) substrate led to no measurable production of 7α-hydroxy-PREG (FIG. 1A). In contrast, PREG was the preferred substrate in mouse thymus, and homogenates of thymocytes and thymus hydroxylated PREG in larger yields than DHEA and 3β-hydroxy-5α-androstan-17-one (EPIA) (FIG. 1B).

Triggering of Specific Immune Response in Human Tonsils

All tonsil glands were obtained from patients vaccinated against tetanus toxoid (TT) and *Bordetella pertussis* (*BP*) antigens. Cultivation of 10^6 isolated tonsillar B+T cells in supplemented DMEM medium under activation conditions (100 ng/mL anti-CD40 mAb, 5 ng/mL IL-2, 10 ng/mL IL-10) for eight days, led to secretion in the medium of anti-TT and anti-*BP* specific IgGs that were measured by ELISA.[14]

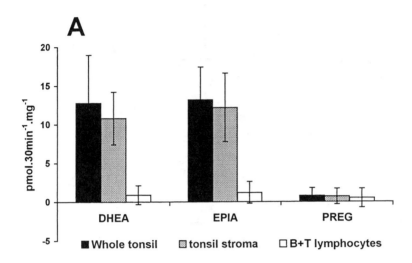

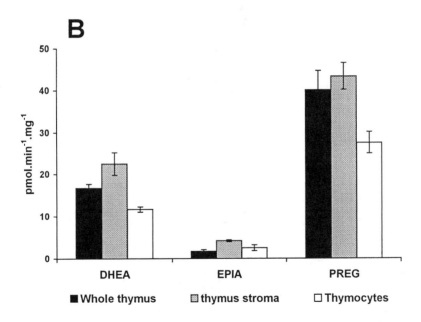

FIGURE 1. 7α-Hydroxylation of (**A**) 0.5-μM DHEA, 0.5-μM EPIA, and 0.5-μM PREG by NADPH-supplemented homogenate preparations of human tonsils, and (**B**) C57BL/6 mouse thymus. Data are means (±SEM) of triplicate measurements in four experiments.

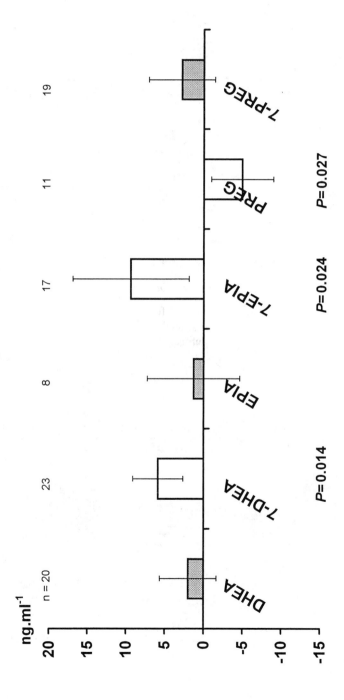

FIGURE 2. Differences ($\pm\Delta$ limit values)[15] in production of anti-TT IgGs by tonsillar B+T lymphocytes cultured under activation conditions for eight days. TT-Specific IgG amounts (ng/mL) produced by steroid-supplemented cultures were subtracted from those produced by steroid free control cutures. (*n* denotes the number of experiments.)

Changes in specific IgG production were tested after addition of 1 μM steroid to the culture medium. Supplementation with DHEA or EPIA or 7α-hydroxy-PREG resulted into no significant difference in anti-TT and anti-*BP* IgG production (see FIGURES 2 and 3). In marked contrast, and after examining the data of Gardner and Altman,[15] both 7α-hydroxy-DHEA and 7α-hydroxy-EPIA significantly increased specific IgG production, whereas PREG led to significantly decreased yields (FIGS. 2 and 3). Steroid effects were neither obtained when isolated B cells were cultured under stimulation conditions, nor when B+T cells were cultured without stimulation.

Under activation conditions, cultured tonsillar B+T lymphocytes produced three orders or magnitude more total IgGs than those of specific IgGs. Total IgG production was not changed by any of the 1-μM steroids tested, except for 1-μM PREG, which led to a significant decrease in total IgG production ($p = 0.008$). This effect was obtained with neither isolated B cells nor with B+T cells cultured without stimulation. Trypan blue exclusion test and proliferation experiments indicated that cell viability was not affected when PREG was added to the medium. These results imply that, through an effect on T lymphocytes, PREG likely led to decreased IgG production by B lymphocytes.

Sequence and Expression of Cytochrome P450 7B1

Total RNAs were isolated from hippocampal formations of C57BL/6 mice, then poly(A)$^+$ RNAs were selected and single- strand cDNAs were synthesized by RT-PCR. Primer sequences were based on the published sequence,[11] and the open reading frame in Cyp7b1 cDNA was amplified and reformatted by PCR, so as to be flanked by *Sal*I and *Eco*RI restriction sites. PCR-amplified fragments were then cloned into an *E. coli* intermediate vector (pCR-Script™ Amp SK$^{(+)}$ cloning kit, Stratagene) and sequenced. The open reading frame containing fragments was transferred to a multi-copy yeast expression vector, pYeDP63, belonging to the pYeDP60 series.[16] The W(hR) engineered yeast strain that over express human NADPH-cytochrome *P*450 reductase when grown in a galactose-containing medium was used as host.[17] Reductase and *P*450 expression were induced in the transformed yeast strain, as previously described,[18] except that the duration of derepression and of induction was 24 h and 4.5 h, respectively. Yeast and mouse brain microsomes were prepared as previously reported,[18,19] and were stored at −80°C before use. Incubation of microsomes with [4-^{14}C]-DHEA and [20-^{14}C]-PREG substrates in NADPH-fortified phosphate buffer and further processing of digests were as described elsewhere.[19,20]

After incubation of C57BL/6 mouse brain microsomes and of microsomes from the transformed yeast strain with either [4-^{14}C]-DHEA or [20-^{14}C]-PREG substrates, the K_M values obtained for 7α-hydroxylation of each substrate did not differ significantly (see TABLE 1), and V_{max} could not be compared with K_{cat} because of the impossibility of measuring the CYP7B1 content of brain microsomes. Nevertheless, when these kinetic parameters were compared with those obtained under identical conditions, either with brain microsomes from rat[7] or from HeLa cells expressing mouse CYP7B1,[13] the K_M values were found to be one order of magnitude larger than in C57BL/6 mouse (TABLE 1).

Whether differences in K_M could be due to sequence-specific differences in *P*450 7B1 was investigated. Alignment of Cyp *P*450 7b1 DNA sequence from C57BL/6

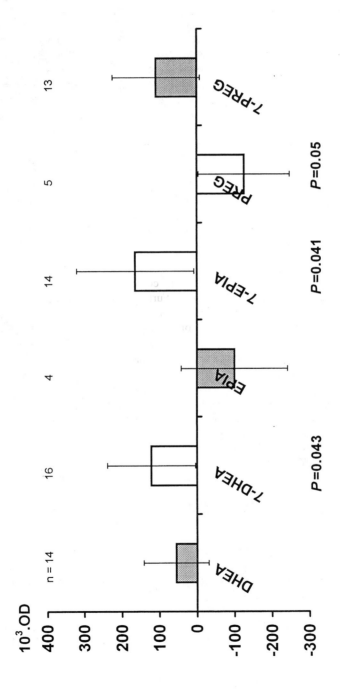

FIGURE 3. Differences (±Δ limit values)[15] in production of IgGs directed against *BP* antigens by tonsillar B+T lymphocytes cultured under activation conditions for eight days. *BP*-specific IgG amounts (O.D. units) produced by steroid-supplemented cultures were substracted from those produced by steroid free control cultures. (*n* denotes the number of experiments.)

TABLE 1. Kinetic parameters for DHEA and PREG 7α-hydroxylation resulting from incubations in phosphate buffer of murine brain microsomes and of microsomes of CYP7B1-transformed cells

7α-hydroxylating source	Ref	DHEA substrate			PREG substrate		
	#	$K_M{}^a$	$K_{cat}{}^b$	$V_{max}{}^c$	$K_M{}^a$	$K_{cat}{}^b$	$V_{max}{}^c$
Mus musculus P450 7B1 in HeLa cells	13	13.6	—	303	4.0	—	35.9
Rat brain microsomes	7	13.8	—	322	4.4	—	38.8
C57BL/6 mouse brain microsomes	3	1.3	—	4.2	0.5	—	4.2
C57BL/6 mouse P450 7B1 in yeast	—	1.9	42	—	0.3	11	—

^{a}μM.
^{b}min^{-1}.
^{c}pmol·min^{-1}·mg^{-1}.

mouse with that from *Mus musculus*[11] indicated the identical presence of the steroid and heme binding domains, and differences in nine bases out of the 1,524 analyzed. This resulted in eight codon changes with five mutations being silent at the amino-acid level and four mutations leading to amino-acid changes at positions 265, 278, 432, and 463 (see TABLE 2). These changes may constitute a natural polymorphism between C57BL/6 mouse and *Mus musculus*. Further alignment of C57BL/6 with rat[11] and recently available human[21] sequences showed conservation with minor changes in the steroid and heme binding domains, identity of amino acids 265 and 432, and the conservative M-463-I substitution (TABLE 2). Therefore, changes in amino acids 265, 432, and 463 were not likely to be responsible for the decreased K_M value measured in C57BL/6 mouse. In marked contrast, the change at position 278 was not conservative, and S-278-P as well as F-278-P, and L-278-P changes that take place within helix G, may lead to structural changes within the α-helix, resulting in modifications of P450-steroid affinities. This may contribute to the decreased K_M value in C57BL/6 mouse. This paradigm is being tested now with site-directed mutagenesis approaches.

TABLE 2. Differences (bold letters) in amino acids of CYP7B1 resulting from alignments of *Mus musculus* and C57BL/6 mouse sequences

cDNA P450 7B1	Ref	Amino acid number					
Species	#	265	278	348–362	432	440–453	463
		Helix G	Helix G	Steroid binding domain		Heme binding domain	Helix L
Mus musculus	11	**S**	**S**	LESTILEVLRLCSYS	**R**	FGLGTSKCPGRYFA	**E**
C57BL/6 mouse	—	**R**	**P**	LESTILEVLRLCSYS	K	FGLGTSKCPGRYFA	**M**
Rat	11	**R**	**F**	LESAILEVLRLCSYS	K	FGLGTSKCPGRYFA	I
Human	20	**R**	**L**	LESSIFEALRLSSYS	K	FGTGTSKCPGRFFA	I

NOTE: Further alignments with rat and human amino acid sequences are given for comparisons.

DISCUSSION

Because evidence for 7α-hydroxylation of DHEA in human adult and fetal liver, skin, mammary tissue, prostate, and adipose stromal cells were available,[2,5,6,22–25] and because previous work in mouse showed 7α-hydroxy-DHEA involvement in the triggering of immune response,[8] we investigated DHEA metabolism and its effects in a human lymphoid organ such as tonsil. Our findings demonstrate that 7α-hydroxylation of DHEA and EPIA is restricted to tonsillar cells other than B and T lymphocytes, and that specific IgGs produced by a mixture of T and B lymphocytes were significantly increased by 7α-hydroxy-DHEA and 7α-hydroxy-EPIA.[14] Moreover, this effect was triggered by neither DHEA nor EPIA, and this difference supports the key action of the 7α-hydroxylating enzyme for a putative paracrine action of the 7α-hydroxysteroid produced (see FIGURE 4). Another lymphoid organ (thymus) was used for comparison with mouse, and the results caused us to note the extensive differences between C57BL/6 mouse and humans. PREG was the preferred 7α-hydroxylated substrate in all mouse thymus fractions, and thymocytes as well as whole thymus provided 7α-hydroxylation of PREG, DHEA, and EPIA. These findings may explain why PREG and 7α-hydroxy-PREG were found to

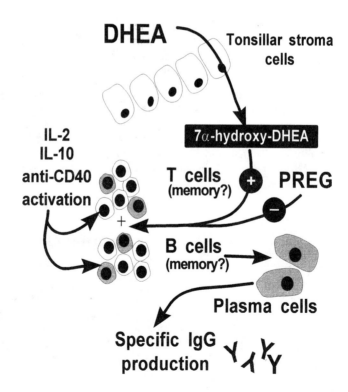

FIGURE 4. Production and paracrine action of 7α-hydroxy-DHEA leading to the control of specific IgG production in human tonsils.

trigger an immune response to a larger extent than DHEA and 7α-hydroxy-DHEA.[8] Because of such differences between human and mouse lymphoid organs, one may question the use of mouse as an animal model for DHEA-mediated immunoactivation studies in humans. One may also question antiglucocorticoid effects described *in vivo* for DHEA in mouse and other rodents and for which no *in vitro* mechanism of action could be obtained.[27] If 7α-hydroxylation is the key to DHEA effects, investigations in rodents should use 7α-hydroxy-DHEA, DHEA, and specific inhibitors of the 7α-hydroxylating enzyme system.[19,20] It is known that PREG is a precursor to glucocorticoids in mouse thymus where they participate in the regulation of antigen specific positive selection in a paracrine manner.[27–29] The 7α-hydroxylation of PREG and DHEA in mouse thymus may also provide the native 7α-hydroxylated antiglucocorticoids[3,8,10] necessary for the fine physiological control of this process.

In any case, the cytochrome P450 responsible for 7α-hydroxylation of DHEA and other 3β-hydroxysteroids is worth extensive investigation. At present, its identity (CYP7B1) and the cDNA sequence are known in the mouse and rat brain,[11] and in the human liver and hippocampus.[21] Mouse CYP7B1 carries out 7α-hydroxylation of DHEA, PREG, 5α-androstane-3β,17β-diol, 17β-estradiol, and 25-hydroxycholesterol,[13] and was shown to be responsible for an alternate pathway of bile acid synthesis in mouse liver,[30] as well as in that of humans.[31] Whether CYP7B1 is present in human and murine lymphoid organs remains to be proved, but evidence for 7α-hydroxylation in these organs[3,8] supports this proposition. Comparative examination of cDNA and amino-acid sequences and available K_M values for DHEA 7α-hydroxylation within different species may lead to an explanation of the variations in immune response according to species polymorphism. Here we report K_M values for 7α-hydroxylation of DHEA by recombinant CYP7B1 that are similar to those measured from C57BL/6 mouse brain microsomal enzyme under identical conditions.[3] It is interesting that the apparent K_M values for DHEA reported with HeLa-expressed CYP7B1 of *Mus musculus*[13] were very similar to the values recorded for the rat brain microsomal enzyme,[7] but ranged one order of magnitude lower than those obtained under identical conditions in C57BL/6 brain microsomes[3] and recombinant C57BL/6 CYP7B1. These differences between our K_M values and those reported by Rose et al.[13] cannot be explained by the nature of the NADPH-P450 reductase, because the same human reductase was present in microsomes of the W(hR) strain and in HeLa microsomes. An explanation may be found in the S-265-R, S-278-P, and E-463-M changes that are nonconservative and could affect the structure within the G helix, between the G and H helixes, and within the L helix, respectively, according to sequence alignment with $P450_{BM-3}$. These amino acid changes may explain the lower K_M in C57BL/6 CYP7B1 than in *Mus musculus* P450 7B1. The low K_M and the involvement of 7α-hydroxy-DHEA in the increase of cellular immunity[8] could be responsible for the good immune responsiveness of the C57BL/6 inbred strain. Other support for this hypothesis can be found in the facts that C57BL/6 mice are defective in melatonin synthesis[32] and that melatonin administration to C57BL/6 mice increased levels of circulating 7α-hydroxy-DHEA.[33] Even though this immune-promoting pineal hormone[34] is not produced in C57BL/6 mice, the notoriously good immune-responsiveness of this strain may result from the low K_M of DHEA 7α-hydroxylation. In order to clarify this issue and to provide new insight into the active CYP7B1 site, site-directed mutagenesis studies using the transformed yeasts are currently being carried out.

At present, the known cDNA sequence of the human CYP7B1[21] has not been expressed in transformed cells and tested for its ability to 7α-hydroxylate DHEA with K_M value measurements. Putative 7α-hydroxylation is inferred from sequence homologies between human, rat, and mouse CYP7B1 and the presence of both steroid-binding and heme-binding sites. If low K_M values are directly related to immune responsiveness through antiglucocorticoid action of the 7α-hydroxy-DHEA produced,[10] natural polymorphism of the CYP7B1 gene may be a key to the onset or to the avoidance of glucocorticoid-dependent diseases. Expression of the human cDNA in transformed yeasts and site-directed mutagenesis studies should provide answers to this hypothesis.

In any case, and given that glucocorticoids activate the 7α-hydroxylating enzyme,[35] a decrease in circulating DHEA in HIV-infected patients[36] should result in a dramatic decrease in 7α-hydroxy-DHEA production and lead to an immune process impairment. To our knowledge, AIDS-related variations in circulating and tissular PREG levels are not available, but normal concentrations in brain and nerves (0.1 μM)[37,38] are nearly two orders of magnitude larger than in plasma. Thus, PREG could aggravate the immune process impairment in AIDS through a decreased production of IgGs as reported here for a human lymphoid organ.

REFERENCES

1. STÁRKA, L. & J. KUTOVA. 1962. 7-Hydroxylation of dehydroepiandrosterone by rat liver homogenate. Biochim. Biophys. Acta **56:** 76–82.
2. ŠULCOVÁ, J., A. CAPKOVA, J.E.V. JIRASEK & L. STÁRKA. 1968. 7-Hydroxylation of dehydroepiandrosterone in human fetal liver, adrenals and chorion *in vitro*. Acta Endocrinol. **59:** 1–9.
3. DOOSTZADEH, J. & R. MORFIN. 1996. Studies of the enzyme complex responsible for pregnenolone and dehydroepiandrosterone 7α-hydroxylation in mouse tissues. Steroids **61:** 613–620.
4. ŠULCOVÁ, J. & L. STÁRKA. 1963. Extrahepatic 7α-hydroxylation of dehydroepiandrosterone. Experimentia **19:** 632–633.
5. FAREDIN, I., A.G. FAZEKAS, I. TÓTH, K. KOKAI & M. JULESZ. 1969. Transformation *in vitro* of [4-^{14}C]-dehydroepiandrosterone into 7-oxygenated derivatives by normal human male and female skin tissue. J. Invest. Dermatol. **52:** 357–361.
6. COUCH, R.A.F., S.J.M. SKINNER, C.J.P. TOBLER & T.W. DOOUSS. 1977. The *in vitro* synthesis of 7-hydroxy-dehydroepiandrosterone by human mammary tissue. Steroids **26:** 1–15.
7. AKWA, Y., R. MORFIN, P. ROBEL & E.E. BAULIEU. 1992. Neurosteroid metabolism. 7α-Hydroxylation of dehydroepiandrosterone and pregnenolone by rat brain microsomes. Biochem. J. **288:** 959–964.
8. MORFIN, R. & G. COURCHAY. 1994. Pregnenolone and dehydroepiandrosterone as precursors of native 7-hydroxylated metabolites which increase the immune response in mice. J. Steroid Biochem. Mol. Biol. **50:** 91–100.
9. MORFIN, R., D. CALVEZ & M.I. MALEWIAK. 1994. Native immunoactivating steroids interfere with the nuclear binding of glucocorticoids. IX Int. Congr. on Hormonal Steroids, Dallas, Sept. 24–29.
10. STÁRKA, L., M. HILL, R. HAMPL, M.I. MALEWIAK, A. BENALYCHERIF, R. MORFIN, J. KOLENA & S. SCSUKOVA. 1998. Studies on the mechanism of antiglucocorticoid action of 7α-hydroxy-dehydroepiandrosterone. Collect. Czech. Chem. Commun. **63:** 1683–1698.

11. STAPLETON, G., M. STEEL, M. RICHARDSON, J.O. MASON, K.A. ROSE, R.G.M. MORRIS & R. LATHE. 1995. A novel cytochrome P450 expressed primarily in brain. J. Biol. Chem. **270:** 29739–29745.

12. NELSON, D.R., L. KOYMANS, T. KAMATAKI, J.J. STEGEMAN, R. FEYEREISEN, D.J. WAXMAN, M.R. WATERMAN, O. GOTOH, M.J. COON, R.W. ESTABROOK, I.C. GUNSALUS & D.W. NEBERT. 1996. The P450 superfamily: update on new sequences, gene mapping, accession numbers, and nomenclature. Pharmacogenetics **6:** 1–42.

13. ROSE, K.A., G. STAPLETON, K. DOTT, M.P. KIENY, R. BEST, M. SCHWARZ, D.W. RUSSELL, I. BJÖRKHEM, J. SECKL & R. LATHE. 1997. Cyp 7b, a novel brain cytochrome P450, catalyzes the synthesis of neurosteroids 7α-hydroxy-dehydroepiandrosterrone and 7α-hydroxy-pregnenolone. Proc. Natl. Acad. Sci. USA **94:** 4925–4930.

14. LAFAYE, P., V. CHMIELEWSKI, F. NATO, J.C. MAZIÉ & R. MORFIN. 1999. The 7α-hydroxysteroids produced in human tonsils enhance the immune response to tetanus toxoid and *Bordetella pertussis* antigens. Biochim. Biophys. Acta. **1472:** 222–231.

15. GARDNER, M.J. & D.G. ALTMAN. 1986. Confidence intervals rather than *p* values: estimation rather than hypothesis testing. Brit. Med. J. **292:** 746–750.

16. URBAN, P., C. CULLIN & D. POMPON. 1990. Maximizing the expression of mammalian cytochrome P-450 monooxygenase activities in yeast cells. Biochimie **72:** 463–472.

17. URBAN, P., G. TRUAN, J.C. GAUTIER & D. POMPON. 1993. Xenobiotic metabolism in humanized yeast: engineered yeast cells producing human NADPH-cytochrome P450 reductase, cytochrome b_5, epoxide hydrolase and P-450s. Biochem. Soc. Trans. **21:** 1028–1034.

18. POMPON, D., B. LOUERAT, A. BRONINE & P. URBAN. 1996. Yeast expression of animal and plant P450s in optimized redox environments. Methods Enzymol. **272:** 51–64.

19. DOOSTZADEH, J., A.C. COTILLON & R. MORFIN. 1997. Dehydroepiandrosterone 7α- and 7β-hydroxylation in mouse brain microsomes. Effects of cytochrome P450 inhibitors and structure-specific inhibition by steroid hormones. J. Neuroendocrinol. **9:** 923–928.

20. DOOSTZADEH, J. & R. MORFIN. 1997. Effects of cytochrome P450 inhibitors and of steroid hormones on the formation of 7-hydroxylated metabolites of pregnenolone in mouse brain microsomes. J. Endocrinol. **155:** 343–350.

21. GENEBANK. Entrez, AF029403; NM_004820.

22. INGELMAN-SUNDBERG, M., A. RANE & J.Å. GUSTAFSSON. 1975. Properties of hydroxylase systems in the human fetal liver active on free and sulfoconjugated steroids. Biochem. **14:** 429–437.

23. KHALIL, M.W., B. STRUTT, D. VACHON & D.W. KILLINGER. 1993. Metabolism of dehydroepiandrosterone by human adipose stromal cells. Identification of 7α-hydroxy-dehydroepiandrosterone as a major metabolite using high performance liquid chromatography and mass spectrometry. J. Steroid Biochem. Molec. Biol. **46:** 585–595.

24. MORFIN, R., S. DISTÉFANO, J.F. CHARLES & H.H. FLOCH. 1980. 5α-Androstane-3β,17β-diol and 5α-androstane-3β,7α,17β-triol in the human hyperplastic prostate. J. Steroid Biochem. **12:** 529–532.

25. JACOLOT, F., F. BERTHOU, Y. DREANO, J.P. BERCOVICI & H.H. FLOCH. 1981. *In vivo* metabolism of ^{14}C-labelled 5α-androstane-3β,17β-diol. J. Steroid Biochem. **14:** 663–669.

26. KALIMI, M., Y. SHAFAGOJ, R. LORIA, D. PADGETT & W. REGELSON. 1994. Antiglucocorticoid effects of dehydroepiandrosterone [DHEA]. Molec. Cell. Biochem. **131:** 99–104.

27. VACCHIO, M., V. PAPADOPOULOS & J.D. ASHWELL. 1994. Steroid production in the thymus: implications for thymocyte selection. J. Exp. Med. **179:** 1835–1846.

28. VACCHIO, M. & J.D. ASHWELL. 1997. Thymus-derived glucocorticoids regulate antigen-specific positive selection. J. Exp. Med. **185:** 2033–2038.

29. PAZIRANDEH, A., Y. XUE, I. RAFTER, M.J. SJÖVALL & S. OKRET. 1999. Paracrine glucocorticoid activity produced by mouse thymic epithelial cells. FASEB J. **13:** 893–901.

30. SCHWARZ, M., E.G. LUND, R. LATHE, I. BJÖRKHEM & D.W. RUSSELL. 1997. Identification and characterization of a mouse oxysterol 7α-hydroxylase cDNA. J. Biol. Chem. **272:** 23995–24001.

31. SETCHELL, K.D.R., M. SCHWARZ, N.C. O'CONNELL, E.G. LUND, D.L. DAVIS, R. LATHE, H.R. THOMPSON, R.W. TYSON, R.J. SOKOL & D.W. RUSSELL. 1998. Identification of a new inborn error in bile acid synthesis: Mutation of the oxysterol 7α-hydroxylase gene causes severe neonatal liver disease. J. Clin. Invest. **102:** 1690–1703.

32. ROSEBOOM, P.H., A.M.A. NAMBOODIRI, D.B. ZIMOJIC, N.C. POPESCU, I.R. RODRIGUEZ, J.A. GASTEL & D.C. KLEIN. 1998. Natural melatonin 'knockdown' in C57BL/6J mice: rare mechanism truncates serotonin N-acetyltransferase. Molec. Brain Res. **63:** 189–197.

33. ATTAL-KHÉMIS, S., V. DALMEYDA & R. MORFIN. 1998. Change of 7α-hydroxy-dehydroepiandrosterone levels in serum of mice treated by cytochrome P450-modifying agents. Life Sci. **63:** 1543–1553.

34. GUERRERO, J.M., M. RAFII-EL-IDRISSI, A. GARCIA-PERGAÑEDA, S. GARCIA-MAURIÑO, M. GIL-HABA, D. POZO & J.R. CALVO. 1997. Mechanisms of action of melatonin on the human immune system. *In* Therapeutic Potential of Melatonin, Vol. 23, G.J.M. Maestroni, A. Conti & R.J. Reiter, Eds.: 43–51. Frontiers of Hormonal Research. Karger. Basel.

35. KHALIL, M.W., B. STRUTT, D. VACHON & D.W. KILLINGER. 1994. Effect of dexamethasone and cytochrome P450 inhibitors on the formation of 7α-hydroxy-dehydroepiandrosterone by human adipose stromal cells. J. Steroid Biochem. Molec. Biol. **48:** 545–552.

36. JACOBSON, M.A., R.E. FUSARO, M. GALMARINI & W. LANG. 1991. Decreased serum dehydroepiandrosterone is associated with an increased progression of human immunodeficiency virus infection in men with CD4 cell counts of 200-499. J. Infect. Dis. **164:** 864–868.

37. LACROIX, C., J. FIET, J.P. BENAIS, B. GUEUX, R. BONETE, J.M. VILLETTE, B. GOURMEL & C. DREUX. 1987. Simultaneous radioimmunoassay of progesterone, androst-4-enedione, pregnenolone, dehydroepiandrosterone and 17-hydroxy-progesterone in specific regions of human brain. J. Steroid Biochem. **28:** 317–325.

38. MORFIN, R., J. YOUNG, C. CORPÉCHOT, B. EGESTAD, J. SJÖVALL & E.E. BAULIEU. 1992. Neurosteroids: pregnenolone in human sciatic nerves. Proc. Natl. Acad. Sci. USA **89:** 6790–6793.

Index of Contributors